NSCA'S ESSENTIALS OF PERSONAL TRAINING

THIRD EDITION

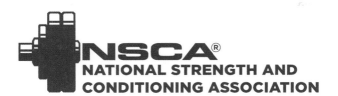

NSCA®
NATIONAL STRENGTH AND
CONDITIONING ASSOCIATION

Brad J. Schoenfeld, PhD, CSCS,*D, CSPS,*D, NSCA-CPT,*D, FNSCA

CUNY Lehman College

Ronald L. Snarr, PhD, CSCS,*D, NSCA-CPT,*D, TSAC-F,*D

Missouri State University

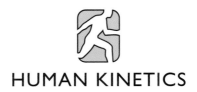

HUMAN KINETICS

Library of Congress Cataloging-in-Publication Data

Names: Schoenfeld, Brad J., 1962- editor. | Snarr, Ronald L., 1982- editor. |
National Strength & Conditioning Association (U.S.)
Title: NSCA's essentials of personal training / Brad J. Schoenfeld, Ronald
L. Snarr, editors.
Description: Third edition. | Champaign, IL : Human Kinetics, 2021. |
"National Strength & Conditioning Association." | Includes
bibliographical references and index.
Identifiers: LCCN 2020057946 (print) | LCCN 2020057947 (ebook) | ISBN
9781492596721 (hardback) | ISBN 9781492596738 (epub) | ISBN
9781492596745 (pdf)
Subjects: LCSH: Personal trainers. | Physical education and training. |
Muscle strength. | Physical fitness--Physiological aspects.
Classification: LCC GV428.7 .N73 2021 (print) | LCC GV428.7 (ebook) | DDC
796.071--dc23
LC record available at https://lccn.loc.gov/2020057946
LC ebook record available at https://lccn.loc.gov/2020057947

ISBN: 978-1-4925-9672-1 (print)

The web addresses cited in this text were current as of March 2021, unless otherwise noted.

Senior Acquisitions Editor: Roger W. Earle; **Developmental Editor:** Laura Pulliam; **Managing Editor:** Miranda K. Baur; **Copyeditor:** Patricia MacDonald; **Indexer:** Michael Ferreira; **Permissions Manager:** Martha Gullo; **Senior Graphic Designer:** Joe Buck; **Cover Designer:** Keri Evans; **Cover Design Specialist:** Susan Rothermel Allen; **Photographs (interior):** © Human Kinetics, unless otherwise noted; **Photo Asset Manager:** Laura Fitch; **Photo Production Specialist:** Amy M. Rose; **Photo Production Manager:** Jason Allen; **Senior Art Manager:** Kelly Hendren; **Illustrations**: © Human Kinetics, unless otherwise noted; **Printer:** Walsworth

We thank Matthew Sandstead, NSCA-CPT,*D and Mel Herl, MS, CSCS,*D, RSCC at the National Strength and Conditioning Association in Colorado Springs, Colorado, for overseeing the photo and video shoot for this book. We also thank Crunch Fitness in Champaign, Illinois, for providing a location for the photo and video shoot.

Printed in the United States of America

10 9 8 7 6 5 4 3 2 1

The paper in this book was manufactured using responsible forestry methods.

Human Kinetics
1607 N. Market Street
Champaign, IL 61820
USA

United States and International
Website: US.HumanKinetics.com
Email: info@hkusa.com
Phone: 1-800-747-4457

Canada
W*ebsite*: Canada.HumanKinetics.com
Email: info@hkcanada.com

E8021

Tell us what you think!
Human Kinetics would love to hear what we
can do to improve the customer experience.
Use this QR code to take our brief survey.

CONTENTS

Preface   vii   •   Acknowledgments   x   •   Credits   xi

Developed by the National Strength and Conditioning Association (NSCA), *NSCA's Essentials of Personal Training, Third Edition,* is the definitive reference for current and aspiring personal trainers. This comprehensive book continues its legacy to provide the most accurate and reliable information with clear explanations of supporting scientific evidence and practical applications related to personal training. Its 51 contributors include commercial-, corporate-, and community-integrated personal trainers and fitness instructors; fitness facility and wellness center owners, operators, and managers; community college, college, and professional school instructors; researchers; athletic trainers; physical therapists; lawyers; counselors; behavioral health professionals; registered dieticians; and nutritionists.

CONNECTION BETWEEN THIS BOOK AND THE NSCA-CPT CERTIFICATION EXAM

Readers will gain the knowledge, skills, and abilities (KSAs) required of personal trainers and the third edition's new content addresses the latest objectives found on the National Strength and Conditioning Association's Certified Personal Trainer (NSCA-CPT) exam, thereby maintaining this book's position as the single best exam preparation resource. The exam's objectives and associated KSAs are spread across four primary content domains and reflected in the 25 chapters of the *NSCA's Essentials of Personal Training* book. The domains and their associated chapters are as follows:

- Domain I: *Client consultation and assessment*—assessing a client, selecting and administering fitness tests, interpreting the results based on descriptive and normative data, understanding general nutrition, and determining proper scope of practice for providing nutritional information (chapters 7 and chapters 9-11)
- Domain II: *Program planning*—setting goals; determining effective motivational strategies; understanding how the body responds and adapts to exercise; designing safe, effective, and goal-specific warm-ups, flexibility, resistance (including body weight and stability ball exercises), aerobic, plyometric, and speed training programs; and recognizing the capacities and limitations of a client with a specialized need or condition (and modifying an exercise program accordingly or referring the client as needed) (chapters 5, 6, 8, 12, and 15-23)

- Domain III: *Techniques of exercise*—providing technique instruction for flexibility exercises; body weight, free weight, machine, and alternative resistance exercises; plyometric exercises; sprinting; and cardiovascular activities (chapters 12-14 and 17)
- Domain IV: *Safety, emergency procedures, and legal issues*—maintaining safe exercise environments and equipment; designing and organizing an exercise facility; effectively responding to emergencies; and practicing professional, legal, and ethical responsibilities (chapters 24 and 25)

The first four chapters of the book contain exercise science-related information about anatomy, physiology, bioenergetics, and biomechanics that are foundational to a personal trainer's understanding of the practical and applied content of the rest of the book. Lastly, the appendix, new for the third edition, covers the primary business concepts of personal training. Although business topics are not tested in the NSCA-CPT certification exam, their inclusion in the new edition more fully rounds out the book as a professional resource.

HIGHLIGHTS OF THIS BOOK

NSCA's Essentials of Personal Training, Third Edition, provides guidelines for the complex process of designing safe, effective, and goal-specific resistance, aerobic, plyometric, and speed training programs for clients of all ages and fitness levels. With comprehensive coverage of various categories of unique client needs, readers will learn how to make specific modifications and adjust exercise programs for each individual client. Multiple fitness testing protocols and norms for each component of fitness are all presented with detailed, yet easy-to-follow instructions, equipping personal trainers with modern, research-backed applications of client assessment and exercise prescription.

Over 300 full-color photos and accompanying instructions clearly describe and visually show proper technique for exercises and drills, including flexibility, stability ball, resistance, plyometric, and speed, as well as new sections on suspension training, manual resistance training, and common types of resistance training equipment. Plus, online videos demonstrate exercise technique in live action, preparing readers to instruct clients through safe exercise performance. Adopting instructors can use the chapter-specific summaries and resources that provide ideas for in-class activities, discussion topics, recommended readings, and tips for teaching complex concepts.

Study questions at the end of each chapter are written in a similar style and format as those found on the NSCA-CPT exam to facilitate learning of chapter content and fully prepare candidates for exam day. Further, practicing and aspiring professionals alike will benefit from a new appendix with advice on building a successful career as a personal trainer.

Unmatched in scope, *NSCA's Essentials of Personal Training, Third Edition,* is the most comprehensive reference for current and future personal trainers, exercise instructors, fitness facility and wellness center mangers, and other fitness professionals.

UPDATES TO THE THIRD EDITION

The third edition of *NSCA's Essentials of Personal Training* updates and expands on the information presented in the second edition with the goal to provide the latest scientific and practical information for personal trainers. Changes for this edition include the following:

- Updated research and references throughout
- New and revised end-of-chapter study questions to help readers test their knowledge of chapter content or prepare for the NSCA-CPT exam
- "Activities of daily living" examples for the planes of movement relative to the body in the anatomical position (chapter 4)
- Explanations about the role of the personal trainer regarding nutrition, who can provide nutrition counseling and education, and dietary supplement regulation in light of current practices and guidelines (chapter 7)
- Revised parameters of the USDA *MyPlate* program and the *2015-2020 Dietary Guidelines for Americans* (chapter 7)
- A new physical activity readiness questionnaire to reflect the *PAR-Q+* form, rather than the *PAR-Q* form (chapter 9)
- Updated information regarding coronary artery disease risk factors, identification of medical conditions and diagnosed disease, interpretation of results, referral process, and associated case studies based on the latest guidelines from prominent exercise science organizations (chapter 9)
- Revised normative and descriptive data associated with testing protocols and more tests for speed, agility, power, postural alignment, and movement assessment (chapter 11)
- New sections and guidelines about suspension training and manual resistance training and descriptions and photos for additional static flexibility, dynamic flexibility, body weight, suspension, manual resistance, and stability ball exercises (chapter 12)
- New section and guidelines about common types of resistance training equipment and descriptions and photos for additional anatomical core, back, arms, chest, hip and thigh, shoulders, and whole body exercises (chapter 13)
- Updated numerical guidelines for the program design variables and all sample programs for resistance training to reflect current research and to be specifically applicable to working with traditional clients, rather than athletes (chapter 15)
- Descriptions and photos for additional lower and upper body plyometric exercises (chapter 17)
- Revised guidelines for training pregnant women (chapter 18)
- Updated statistics and references related to overweight and obesity (chapter 19)
- Updated numerical guidelines for the program design variables and all sample programs to be specifically applicable to working with athletes (chapter 23)
- New section about the emergency response plan (chapter 24)
- Updated guidelines to reflect the benchmarks found in the NSCA's *Strength and Conditioning Professional Standards and Guidelines* and its *Code of Ethics* (chapter 25)
- Information and recommendations regarding the business of personal training (appendix)

INSTRUCTOR RESOURCES IN HK*PROPEL*

A variety of instructor resources (free to adopting instructors) are available online within the instructor pack in HK*Propel*:

- *Instructor guide.* Provides chapter-specific summaries and resources for in-class activities, discussion topics, recommended readings, and tips for teaching complex concepts.
- *Instructor video clips.* Includes 44 online video clips that teach proper exercise technique for instructors who may have insufficient demonstration expertise or lack facility equipment, space, access, or a combination of these reasons. Of these clips, 17 are unique for instructors to use to supplement their lectures (the remaining 27 clips are also available to students through their HK*Propel* Access).

- *Test package.* Includes 20 multiple-choice format questions per chapter. The files may be downloaded for integration with a learning management system or printed as paper-based tests. Instructors may also create their own customized quizzes or tests from the test bank questions to assign to students directly through HK*Propel.* Those questions are automatically graded, and students' scores can be reviewed by instructors in the platform.

- *Chapter quizzes.* Contains ready-made LMS-compatible quizzes (10 questions each) to assess student comprehension of the most important concepts in each chapter. Each quiz may be downloaded or assigned to students directly through HK*Propel.* The chapter quizzes are automatically graded, and students' scores can be reviewed by instructors in the platform.

- *Presentation package.* Features more than 750 PowerPoint slides of text, artwork, and tables from

the book that can be used for class discussion and presentation. Instructors can easily add, modify, and rearrange the order of the slides.

- *Image bank.* Includes most of the figures, content photos, and tables from the book, sorted by chapter. These can be used in developing a customized presentation based on specific course requirements.

Whether used for learning the fundamentals of personal training, preparing for a certification exam, or consulting it as a professional reference, *NSCA's Essentials of Personal Training, Third Edition,* will help individuals better understand how to develop and administer safe and effective personal training programs.

Instructor ancillaries are free to adopting instructors, including an ebook version of the text that allows instructors to add highlights, annotations, and bookmarks. Please contact your Sales Manager for details about how to access instructor resources in HK*Propel.*

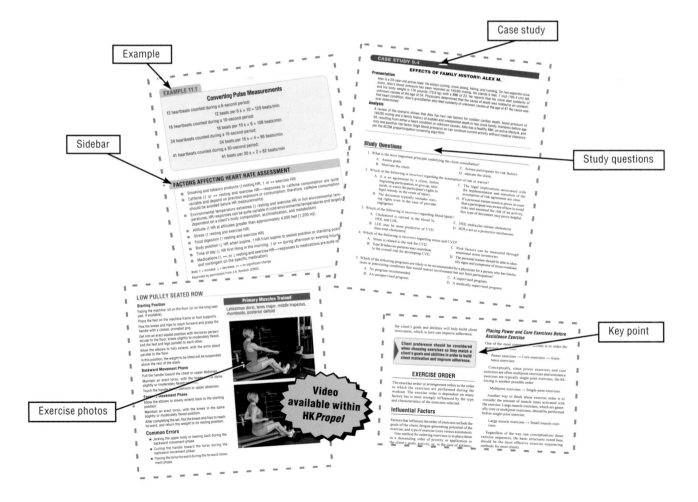

ACKNOWLEDGMENTS

From Brad J. Schoenfeld: It has been an honor to co-edit this edition of the Essentials of Personal Training. This was a true team effort that involved the coordinated actions of many people; the end result has set what I believe to be the new standard for evidence-based personal training education. Accordingly, I would like to acknowledge the following people for their work in facilitating the publication of this text:

First and foremost, I would like to thank the authors who contributed their expertise to each of the respective chapters. They displayed professionalism throughout the process, and were diligent in meeting the imposed deadlines for revisions so that the text was produced in a timely fashion. It was a pleasure to work with such a terrific group of fitness professionals.

Second, I would like to thank the Human Kinetics staff in guiding the publication process. In particular, I would like to acknowledge the efforts of Roger Earle, who went above and beyond the call in ensuring that the editing process progressed smoothly and efficiently.

Third, I would like to thank the NSCA for entrusting me with the task of co-editing this text. As a long-time member of the organization, I am truly honored to have served in this editorial role and to play a part in furthering their mission of bridging the gap between science and practice.

Finally, and most of all, I would like to thank my parents who instilled the importance of the scientific method from the time I was a child. These principles have guided my career path and continue to be instrumental in my development as an educator and researcher; I would not be where I am today without their guidance. R.I.P.

From Ronald L. Snarr: First, I would like to thank Human Kinetics and the National Strength and Conditioning Association for the amazing opportunity to co-edit and contribute to the third edition of the *NSCA's Essentials of Personal Training* textbook. It was an honor to work alongside of you all and to be a part of such an amazing project that I believe sets a new standard for evidence-based practice in the realm of personal training.

Undertaking this project would have not been possible without the consistent time and effort of the contributors and my co-editor, Dr. Brad Schoenfeld. Additionally, the key knowledge and insight provided by Roger Earle was crucial to the entire process, and I would like to thank him for assisting me through every step of the way.

My final, and most important, thanks go to my friends and family for supporting me throughout this entire process. Special thanks to my mother, Nancy, and sister, Michelle, for being the greatest support system that anyone could ask for. I would also like to thank my mentor and friend, Dr. Mike Esco, for teaching me how to become a better researcher, writer, and person. Lastly, thank you Michelle. You stood by my side through everything, and I cannot thank you enough.

Figures 2.1, 2.2, 6.1, 6.2, 6.3; tables 6.2, 6.4: Reprinted by permission from W.E. Kenney, J.H. Wilmore, and D.L. Costill, *Physiology of Sport and Exercise,* 7th ed. (Champaign, IL: Human Kinetics, 2020), 126, 189, 273, 275, 276, 287.

Figures 2.5, 2.11, 3.2, 3.3, 3.5-3.9, 4.3-4.6, 4.8, 4.9 (right), 4.11, 5.1, 13.3: Reprinted by permission from National Strength and Conditioning Association, *Essentials of Strength Training and Conditioning,* 4th ed., edited by G.G. Haff and N.T. Triplett (Champaign, IL: Human Kinetics, 2016), 14, 21, 22, 24, 31, 32, 47, 48, 52, 54, 57, 58, 91, 119, 352.

Figure 2.7: Reprinted by permission from P.O. Åstrand et al., *Textbook of Work Physiology: Physiological Bases of Exercise,* 4th ed. (Champaign, IL: Human Kinetics, 2003), 143.

Figures 3.4, 4.14; table 24.1: Reprinted by permission from National Strength and Conditioning Association, *Essentials of Strength Training and Conditioning,* 3rd ed., edited by T.R. Baechle and R.W. Earle (Champaign, IL: Human Kinetics, 2008), 28, 81, 551.

Figure 4.2: Adapted by permission from E.A. Harman, M. Johnson, and P.N. Frykman, "A Movement-Oriented Approach to Exercise Prescription," *NSCA Journal* 14, no. 1 (1992): 47-54.

Figure 4.9: Adapted by permission from W.C. Whiting and S. Rugg, *Dynatomy: Dynamic Human Anatomy* (Champaign, IL: Human Kinetics, 2006), 76.

Figures 4.13, 5.2: Reprinted by permission from National Strength and Conditioning Association, *Essentials of Strength Training and Conditioning*, 2nd ed., edited by T.R. Baechle and R.W. Earle (Champaign, IL: Human Kinetics, 2000).

Figure 6.4: Reprinted by permission from W.E. Kenney, J.H. Wilmore, and D.L. Costill, *Physiology of Sport and Exercise*, 6th ed. (Champaign, IL: Human Kinetics, 2015), 471.

Figure 9.1; table 9.1; Preparticipation Physical Examination Components text on p. 153; Contraindications for Exercising During Pregnancy text on p. 513: Reprinted by permission from American College of Sports Medicine, *ACSM's Guidelines for Exercise Testing and Prescription*, 11th ed., edited by G. Liguori et al. (Philadelphia: Wolters Kluwer, 2022), 35-36, 47, 54, 187.

PAR-Q+ on pp. 162-165: Reprinted with permission from the PAR-Q+ Collaboration and the authors of the PAR-Q+ (Dr. Darren Warburton, Dr. Norman Gledhill, Dr. Veronica Jamnik, and Dr. Shannon Bredin).

Health Risk Analysis Form on pp. 169-173: Adapted by permission from B.J. Sharkey and S.E. Gaskill, *Fitness & Health*, 7th ed. (Champaign, IL: Human Kinetics, 2013), 397-401.

Factors Affecting Heart Rate Assessment text on 199; Factors Affecting Blood Pressure Assessment text on p. 200: Reprinted by permission from J.A. Kordich, *Evaluating Your Client: Fitness Assessment and Protocol Norms* (Lincoln, NE: NSCA Certification Commission, 2002).

Figures 11.5, 11.11, 11.12, 11.14, 11.15, 11.17, 11.19, 11.20, 11.23, 11.24, 11.26, 11.27, 11.29, 11.35-11.38: Reprinted by permission from D.H. Fukuda, *Assessments for Sport and Athletic Performance* (Champaign, IL: Human Kinetics, 2019), 83, 84, 109, 112, 123, 132, 139, 142, 143, 148, 179, 267.

Tables 11.8, 11.11, 11.23, 11.24: Reprinted by permission from A.L. Gibson, D.R. Wagner, and V.H. Heyward, *Advanced Fitness Assessment and Exercise Prescription*, 8th ed. (Champaign, IL: Human Kinetics, 2019), 249, 274, 81, 168.

Table 11.9: Reprinted by permission from V.H. Heyward and D.R. Wagner, *Applied Body Composition Assessment*, 2nd ed. (Champaign, IL: Human Kinetics, 2004), 9.

Tables 11.13, 11.14: Adapted by permission from L.A. Kaminsky, R. Arena, and J. Myers, "Reference Standards for Cardiorespiratory Fitness Measured With Cardiopulmonary Exercise Testing: Data From the Fitness Registry and the Importance of Exercise National Database," *Mayo Clinic Proceedings* 90, no. 11 (2015): 1515-1523.

Tables 11.15-11.17: Adapted by permission from P.O. Åstrand, "Aerobic Work Capacity in Men and Women With Special References to Age," *Acta Physiologica Scandinavia* 49, suppl. 169 (1960): 45-60.

Table 11.18: Reprinted by permission from W.C. Beam and G.M. Adams, *Exercise Physiology Laboratory Manual*, 7th ed. (New York: McGraw-Hill, 2014).

Tables 11.19, 11.20: Reprinted by permission from J.R. Morrow, A.W. Jackson, J.G. Disch, and D.P. Mood, *Measurement and Evaluation in Human Performance*, 4th ed. (Champaign, IL: Human Kinetics, 2011), 200, 201.

Table 11.29: Source: CSEP Physical Activity Training for Health (CSEP-PATH®), 2nd Edition, 2019. Reprinted with permission of the Canadian Society for Exercise Physiology.

Table 11.33: Adapted by permission from L. Herrington and A. Munro, "A Preliminary Investigation to Establish the Criterion Validity of a Qualitative Scoring System of Limb Alignment During Single-Leg Squat and Landing," *Journal of Exercise Sport and Orthopedics* 1, no. 2 (2014): 1-6.

Table 13.1: Adapted by permission from D.T. McMaster, J. Cronin, and M. McGuigan, "Forms of Variable Resistance Training," *Strength and Conditioning Journal* 31, no. 1 (2009): 50-64.

Figure 14.6: © BikeFit

Figure 14.11: Adapted by permission from E.W. Maglischo, *Swimming Fastest* (Champaign, IL: Human Kinetics, 2003), 181.

Figure 15.1: Reprinted by permission from R.J. Robertson, *Perceived Exertion for Practitioners: Rating Effort With the OMNI Picture System* (Champaign, IL: Human Kinetics, 2004), 49.

Figure 15.2: Reprinted by permission from M.C. Zourdos, A. Klemp, C. Dolan, et al., "Novel Resistance Training-Specific RPE Scale Measuring Repetitions in Reserve," *Journal of Strength and Conditioning Research* 30, no. 1 (2016): 267-275.

Figure 17.1: Reprinted from *Eccentric Muscle Training in Sports and Orthopaedics*, 2nd ed., M. Albert, Copyright 1995, with permission from Elsevier.

Figure 18.1: Reprinted by permission from W. Westcott, *Building Strength and Stamina*, 2nd ed. (Champaign, IL: Human Kinetics, 2003), 9.

Figure 18.2: Reprinted by permission from W. Westcott and T. Baechle, *Fitness Professional's Guide to Strength Training Older Adults*, 2nd ed. (Champaign, IL: Human Kinetics, 2010), 22.

Figure 19.1: Reprinted by permission from C.W. Baker and K.D. Brownwell, "Physical Activity and Maintenance of Weight Loss: Physiological and Psychological Mechanisms," in *Physical Activity and Obesity*, edited by C. Bouchard (Champaign, IL: Human Kinetics, 2000), 311-328.

Figures 20.2, 20.3: Reprinted by permission from A.S. Fauci, E. Braunwald, K.J. Isselbacher, et al., *Harrison's Principles of Internal Medicine*, 14th ed. (New York: McGraw-Hill Companies, 1998), 1345-1352.

Tables 22.1, 22.2: Reprinted by permission from S.M. Tweedy, E.M. Beckman, T.J. Geraghty, et al, "Exercise and Sports Science Australia (ESSA) Position Statement on Exercise and Spinal Cord Injury," *Journal of Medicine and Science in Sport* 20, no. 2 (2017): 108-115.

Table 22.5: Adapted by permission from P.L. Jacobs, S.M. Svoboda, and A. Lepeley, "Neuromuscular Conditions and Disorders," in *NSCA's Essentials of Training Special Populations*, edited by P.L. Jacobs for the National Strength and Conditioning Association (Champaign, IL: Human Kinetics, 2018), 271.

Table 22.8: Adapted by permission from K. Kendall, G. Colquitt, and P. Hyde, "Therapeutic Physical Activities for Individuals With Cerebral Palsy," in *Therapeutic Physical Activities for People With Disability*," edited by L. Li and S. Zhang (Hauppauge, NY: Nova Science, 2015).

Table 22.9: Reprinted by permission from P. Rosenbaum, N. Paneth, A, Leviton, et al. "A Report: The Definition and Classification of Cerebral Palsy April 2006, *Developmental Medicine and Child Neurology* 49, suppl. 109 (2007): 8-14.

Table 22.11: Reprinted by permission from O. Verschuren, M.D. Peterson, A.C.J. Balemans, and E.A. Hurvitz. "Exercise and Physical Activity Recommendations for People With Cerebral Palsy," *Developmental Medicine & Child Neurology* 58, no. 8 (2016): 798-808.

CHAPTER 1

Structure and Function of the Muscular, Nervous, and Skeletal Systems

Jared W. Coburn, PhD, and Moh H. Malek, PhD

After completing this chapter, you will be able to

- describe the structure and function of skeletal muscle,

- list and explain the steps in the sliding filament theory of muscle action,

- explain the concept of muscle fiber types and how it applies to exercise performance,

- describe the structure and function of the nervous system as it applies to the control of skeletal muscle, and

- explain the role of exercise in bone health, as well as the function of tendons and ligaments in physical activity.

Physical activity occurs through the combined and coordinated efforts of the muscular, nervous, and skeletal systems. Nerves are responsible for initiating and modifying the activation of muscles. Muscles produce movement by generating forces to rotate bones around joints. This chapter explores the basic structure and function of these systems as they apply to the practice of personal training.

THE MUSCULAR SYSTEM

Muscles generate force when they are activated. This is referred to as a **muscle contraction** or **muscle action**. Of the three types of muscle—smooth, car-diac, and skeletal—it is the third type that attaches to bones, causing them to rotate around joints. It is this function of skeletal muscles that allows us to run, jump, and lift and throw things. The function of muscle is dictated by its structure.

Gross Anatomy (Macrostructure) of Skeletal Muscle

The system of skeletal muscles is illustrated in figure 1.1 (15). Each skeletal muscle (e.g., deltoid, pectoralis major, gastrocnemius) is surrounded by a layer of connective tissue referred to as **epimysium**. A muscle

The authors would like to acknowledge the significant contributions of Len Kravitz to this chapter.

is further divided into bundles of **muscle fibers**. A bundle of muscle fibers is called a **fasciculus** or **fascicle**. Each fasciculus is surrounded by connective tissue called **perimysium**. Within a fasciculus, each muscle fiber is surrounded and separated from adjacent fibers by a layer of connective tissue referred to as **endomysium**. Together, these connective tissues help transmit the force of muscle action to the bone via another connective tissue structure, the tendon. Figure 1.2 illustrates these connective tissue structures and their relationship to the muscle (15).

Microscopic Anatomy of Skeletal Muscle

Each muscle fiber is a cell, with many of the same structural components as other cells (figure 1.3; 15). For example, each muscle fiber is surrounded by a plasma membrane, referred to as the **sarcolemma**. The sarcolemma encloses the contents of the cell, regulates the passage of materials such as glucose into and out of the cell, and receives and conducts stimuli

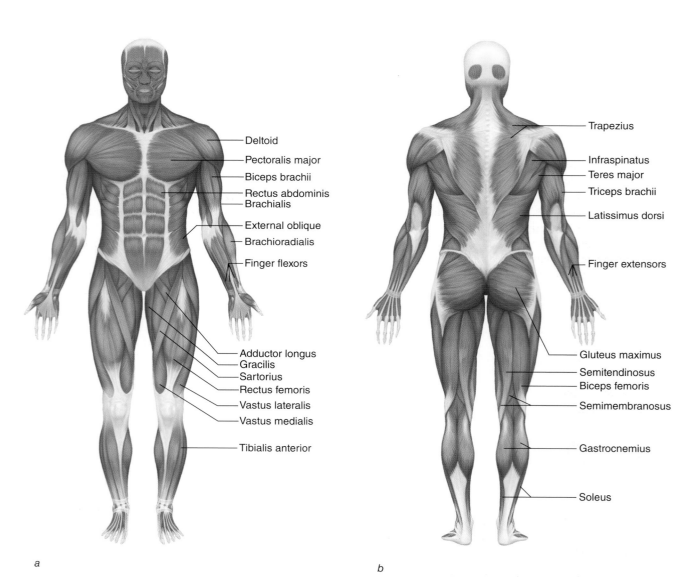

a

b

FIGURE 1.1   *(a)* Front view and *(b)* rear view of adult male human skeletal musculature.

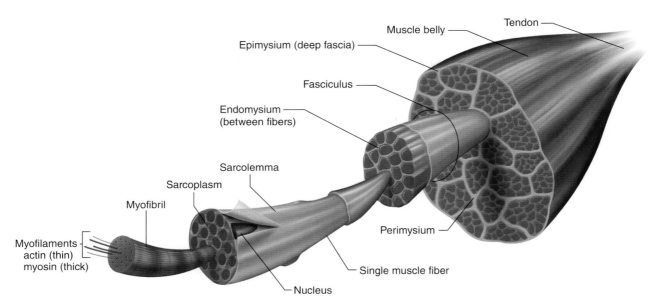

Muscle belly

Tendon

Epimysium (deep fascia)

Fasciculus

Endomysium
(between fibers)

Sarcolemma

Sarcoplasm

Myofibril

Myofilaments
actin (thin)
myosin (thick)

Perimysium

Single muscle fiber

Nucleus

FIGURE 1.2 The gross structure of skeletal muscle. The whole muscle, the fasciculus, and individual muscle fibers are surrounded by the connective tissues epimysium, perimysium, and endomysium, respectively.

in the form of electrical impulses or **action potentials**. Skeletal muscle cells are multinucleated, meaning they possess more than one nucleus. The nuclei contain the genetic material, or DNA, of the cell, and are largely responsible for initiating the processes associated with adaptations to exercise. Adaptations to resistance training and aerobic endurance training are discussed in chapters 5 and 6, respectively.

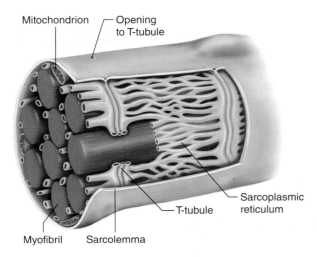

Mitochondrion

Opening
to T-tubule

Myofibril

Sarcolemma

T-tubule

Sarcoplasmic
reticulum

FIGURE 1.3 Single muscle fiber anatomy.

Within the boundary of the sarcolemma, but outside the nuclei, is the **cytoplasm**, referred to as **sarcoplasm** in muscle. This watery solution contains the cell's energy sources, such as **adenosine triphosphate (ATP)** (the only direct source of energy for muscle actions), phosphocreatine, glycogen, and fat droplets. Also suspended within the sarcoplasm are organelles. These include **mitochondria** (singular is *mitochondrion*), which are the sites of aerobic ATP production within the cell and thus of great importance for aerobic exercise performance. Another important organelle is the **sarcoplasmic reticulum**. This organelle stores calcium and regulates the muscle action process by altering the intracellular calcium concentration. Specifically, the sarcoplasmic reticulum releases calcium into the sarcoplasm of the cell when an action potential passes to the interior of the cell via structures called **transverse tubules**, or **T-tubules**. The T-tubules are channels that form from openings in the sarcolemma of the muscle cell.

> **Skeletal muscle fibers (cells) produce the force that allows for the movements common in sport, recreation, and daily activities.**

Myofibril

Each muscle cell contains columnar protein structures that run parallel to the length of the muscle fiber. These structures are known as **myofibrils** (figure 1.4; 15). Each myofibril is a bundle of **myofilaments**, which primarily consist of **myosin** (thick) and **actin** (thin) filaments. The myosin and actin filaments are arranged in a regular pattern along the length of the myofibril, giving it a striated, or striped, appearance.

Myosin filaments are formed from the aggregation of myosin molecules. Each myosin molecule consists of a head, neck, and tail. The head is capable of attaching to and pulling on the actin filament. Energy from the splitting, or hydrolysis, of ATP is used to perform the power stroke, an important step in the process of muscle activation. The neck structure connects the head to the tail. The middle of the myosin filament is oriented in a tail-to-tail fashion, such that the head portions project outward from the ends of the filament (figure 1.4). The protein **titin** maintains the position of the myosin filament relative to actin.

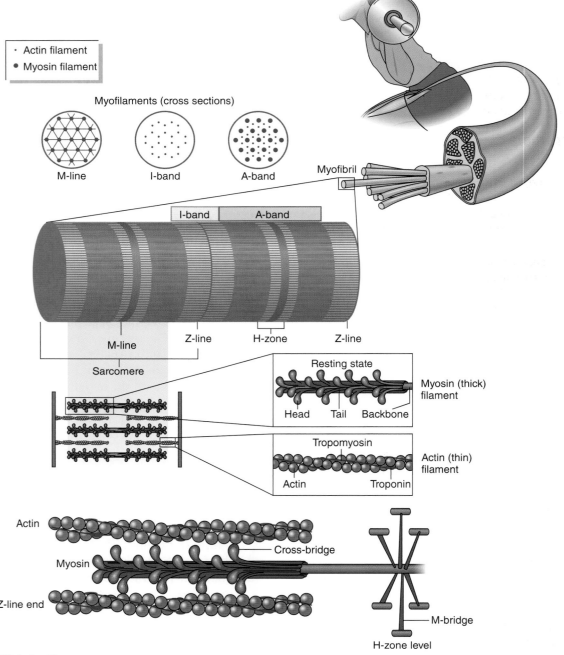

FIGURE 1.4 The structural arrangement of the myofilaments actin and myosin within the sarcomere, the basic functional unit of skeletal muscle.

Each actin filament is formed from individual globular, or G-actin, proteins (figure 1.4). Each G-actin has a binding site for a myosin head. The G-actin proteins assemble into strands of filamentous, or F-actin. Associated with the actin filament are two other protein structures: **tropomyosin** and **troponin**. Collectively, tropomyosin and troponin are considered regulatory proteins because they regulate the interaction of myosin and actin, the contractile proteins. Tropomyosin is a rod-like protein that spans the length of seven G-actin proteins along the length of the actin filament. When the muscle cell is at rest, tropomyosin lies over the myosin binding sites on actin. Each end of a tropomyosin filament is attached to troponin. When bound to calcium, troponin causes the movement of tropomyosin away from the myosin binding sites on actin. This allows the myosin head to attach and pull on actin, a critical step in the muscle activation process. The protein **nebulin** acts to ensure the actin filaments are the correct length.

Sarcomere

The **sarcomere** is the basic contractile unit of muscle (figure 1.4). It extends from one Z-line to an adjacent **Z-line**. The **A-band** is determined by the width of a myosin filament. It is the A-band that provides the dark striation of skeletal muscle. Actin filaments are anchored at one end to the Z-line. They extend inward to the center of the sarcomere. The area of the A-band that contains myosin but not actin is the **H-zone**. In the middle of the H-zone is a dark line called the **M-line**. The M-line helps align adjacent myosin filaments. The **I-band** spans the distance between the ends of adjacent myosin filaments. As such, each I-band lies partly in each of two sarcomeres. The I-bands are less dense than the A-bands, and thus they are responsible for giving skeletal muscle its light striation.

> **The basic functional and contractile unit of skeletal muscle is the sarcomere.**

Neuromuscular Junction

In order to contract, muscle fibers must normally receive a stimulus from the nervous system. This communication between the nervous and muscle systems occurs at a specialized region referred to as the **neuromuscular junction** (figure 1.5a; 9a). Each muscle fiber has a single neuromuscular junction, located at the approximate center of the length of the cell. Structures at the neuromuscular junction include the axon terminal of the neuron; a specialized region of the muscle cell membrane called the **motor endplate**; and the space between the axon terminal and motor endplate, referred to as the **synaptic cleft** or **neuromuscular cleft**.

Sliding Filament Theory

Although the exact details are still being determined, the **sliding filament theory** is still the most widely accepted theory of muscle action (9). This theory states that a muscle shortens or lengthens when the filaments (actin and myosin) slide past each other, without the filaments themselves changing in length. The following steps detail the series of events that occur during muscle action:

1. An action potential passes along the length of a neuron, leading to the release of the excitatory neurotransmitter **acetylcholine (ACh)** at the neuromuscular junction. When the neuron is at rest, ACh is stored in the axon terminal of the neuron within structures called **synaptic vesicles**. It is the action potential that leads to the release of stored ACh into the synaptic cleft between the axon terminal of the neuron and the muscle fiber.

2. The ACh migrates across the synaptic cleft and binds with ACh receptors on the motor endplate of the muscle fiber (figure 1.5a).

3. This leads to the generation of an action potential along the sarcolemma of the muscle fiber. In addition, this action potential will travel to the interior of the muscle fiber via T-tubules. The movement of the action potential down the T-tubule triggers the release of stored calcium from the sarcoplasmic reticulum (figure 1.5b; 9a).

4. Once released into the sarcoplasm, the calcium migrates to, and binds with, troponin molecules located along the length of the actin filaments (figure 1.5c; 9a).

5. The binding of calcium to troponin causes a conformational change in the shape of troponin. Because tropomyosin is attached to troponin, this moves tropomyosin such that binding sites on actin are exposed to the myosin head.

6. When a muscle is in a rested state, the myosin head is energized; that is, it is storing the energy released from the breakdown of ATP to adenosine diphosphate (ADP) and inorganic phosphate (P_i). When the binding sites on actin are exposed to the myosin head, it is able to attach, forming a **crossbridge**, and attempt to pull the actin filament toward the center of the sarcomere. Whether it is successful at pulling, and thus shortening the

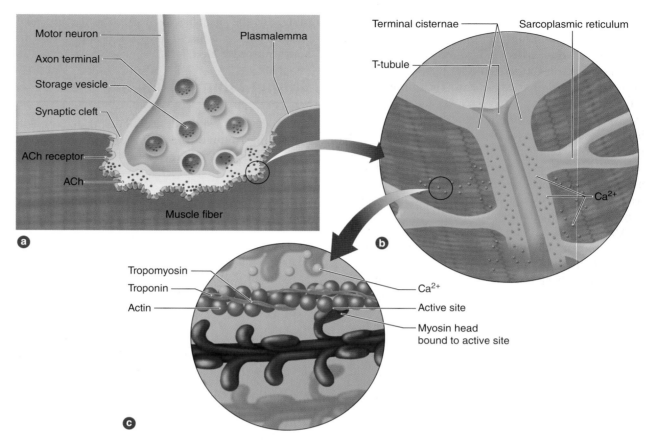

FIGURE 1.5 The sequence of events leading to muscle activation. *(a)* Acetylcholine (ACh) is released at the neuromuscular junction. *(b)* Calcium (Ca²⁺) is released from the sarcoplasmic reticulum, triggered by the propagation of an action potential down the T-tubules. *(c)* The binding of Ca²⁺ to troponin causes the movement of tropomyosin off the binding sites along actin. This allows for crossbridge formation between myosin and actin, and the process of force generation begins.

muscle, depends on the amount of force generated by the crossbridges that are pulling and the external force that opposes the crossbridges.

7. After pulling on the actin filament, the myosin head is now in a lower energy state. In order to cause detachment from the actin filament, as well as to energize the head, a fresh ATP molecule must be bound. Once it is bound, the myosin head detaches from actin, and the enzyme myosin **adenosine triphosphatase (ATPase)** causes the splitting of the ATP molecule. This once again energizes the myosin head. If the binding sites on actin are still exposed, the myosin head may once again form a crossbridge with actin, again attempting to pull toward the center of the sarcomere. This process will continue provided that the muscle fiber is being stimulated to contract by its motor neuron.

> **According to the sliding filament theory, a muscle shortens or lengthens because the actin and myosin filaments slide past each other, without the filaments themselves changing length.**

Types of Muscle Actions

It is important to recognize that when stimulated, muscle fibers always attempt to shorten. That is, the crossbridges always attempt to pull actin toward the center of the sarcomere, which would cause shortening of the sarcomere and thus the muscle. However, muscles are typically contracting against some type of external resistance, such as a barbell or dumbbell, which may be acting in opposition to the muscle force.

If the amount of force produced by a muscle is greater than the external resistance acting in the opposite direction, a **concentric muscle action** will result. During a concentric muscle action, the resistance is overcome and the muscle shortens. If the amount of force produced by a muscle is less than an opposing external resistance, the muscle will lengthen even as it attempts to shorten. This lengthening muscle action is known as an **eccentric muscle action**. Lastly, if the muscle force is equal and opposite to that of an external resistance, an **isometric (static) muscle action** results. In this case, the muscle neither shortens nor lengthens but remains the same length.

All three types of muscle actions are important during exercise, and all are used during a typical resistance exercise session. For example, in the starting position of the back squat exercise, the person will use isometric muscle actions to stabilize the barbell before the downward movement phase. During the downward movement phase, the knee and hip extensor muscles (quadriceps femoris and gluteus maximus) will produce force eccentrically, allowing the weight of the barbell to overcome the torque being produced around the knee and hip joints by the muscles, causing the barbell to be lowered. Meanwhile, the erector spinae and muscles of the abdomen will contract isometrically to stabilize the spine. Once the lowest position of the back squat has been reached, the erector spinae and abdominal muscles will continue their isometric muscle actions, while the person will increase force production and perform concentric muscle actions of the knee and hip extensors in order to overcome the weight of the barbell. These coordinated concentric and isometric muscle actions allow the person to stand upright and return to the starting position while protecting the low back.

During the performance of resistance training exercises, individuals perceive the concentric phase as more difficult than the eccentric phase. For example, during the bench press, lifting the barbell upward off the chest (concentric actions of the pectoralis major, anterior deltoid, and triceps brachii muscles) is more difficult than lowering the barbell to the chest (eccentric actions of the same muscles). This sometimes leads to the erroneous perception that the eccentric phase is less important than the concentric phase. However, there is evidence (3, 8) that an emphasis on both the concentric and eccentric action phases is important in order to maximize the benefits of resistance training.

Delayed-Onset Muscle Soreness (DOMS) and Eccentric Muscle Actions

It is not uncommon to experience muscular pain and discomfort 24 to 48 hours after beginning an exercise program or performing novel exercises. This **delayed-onset muscle soreness (DOMS)** was originally believed to be the result of lactic acid accumulation. However, it likely results from some combination of connective and muscle tissue damage followed by an inflammatory reaction that activates pain receptors (2). This damage is primarily caused by eccentric muscle actions and resulting micro-tears in connective and muscle tissues. The pain that results may last for days, reducing range of motion, strength, and the ability to produce force quickly (2, 13). Strategies to combat the pain and performance decrements resulting from DOMS have included nutritional supplements, massage, ice, and ultrasound (1, 2). It appears, however, that exercise itself may be the best means of decreasing pain associated with DOMS, although its analgesic effects are temporary (2).

Muscle Fiber Types

All muscle fibers are designed to contract and produce force, but not all fibers are alike when it comes to contractile performance and basic physiological characteristics. For example, muscle fibers from the same muscle may differ in the force they produce, the time they take to reach peak force, their preference for aerobic versus anaerobic metabolism, and fatigability. This has led to the concept of muscle fiber typing. That is, muscle fibers may be classified into types based on different characteristics of interest. To determine muscle fiber type, a muscle biopsy must be performed. This technique involves the removal of a small amount of muscle via insertion of a muscle biopsy needle through an incision in the muscle. After removal of the muscle tissue, it may be quickly frozen and then processed. Although many types of analyses may be performed, determination of the biochemical and contractile properties of the muscle fibers is likely of greatest practical significance to the personal trainer.

One biochemical property of muscle fibers is the ability to produce ATP aerobically, a characteristic called **oxidative capacity** since oxygen is necessary for aerobic metabolism. Fibers that have large and numerous mitochondria, and that are surrounded by an ample supply of capillaries to deliver blood and oxygen, are considered oxidative fibers. In addition, these fibers possess a large amount of **myoglobin**, which delivers oxygen from the muscle cell membrane to the mitochondria, enhancing aerobic capacity and lessening the reliance on anaerobic ATP production.

As explained previously, the enzyme myosin ATPase is responsible for splitting ATP, thus making energy available for muscle action. Several forms of myosin ATPase exist, and these differ in the rate at which they split ATP. Fibers with a myosin ATPase form that have high ATPase activity will have a high rate of shortening because of the rapid availability of energy from ATP to support the muscle action process. The opposite is true with fibers demonstrating low ATPase activity. This concept that the type of myosin ATPase affects maximal shortening velocity of a muscle fiber provides us with a link between the biochemical (type of myosin ATPase) and contractile (shortening velocity) characteristics of muscle.

In addition to maximal shortening velocity, two other contractile characteristics of muscle are maximal force production and fiber efficiency. For example, fibers may differ in the amount of force they produce relative to their size (cross-sectional area). This is referred to as **specific tension**. Fibers may also be described based on efficiency. An efficient fiber is able to produce more work with a given expenditure of ATP.

Differences in the biochemical and contractile properties of muscle fibers have led physiologists to classify muscle fibers into types. It is generally agreed that one type of slow fiber and two types of fast fibers exist. Slow fibers have alternatively been referred to as **type I**, slow oxidative (SO), or slow-twitch fibers. As can be inferred from the name, these fibers have high oxidative capacity and are fatigue resistant, but they contract and relax slowly. The two types of fast fibers are known as **type IIa**, fast oxidative glycolytic (FOG), and **type IIx**, fast glycolytic (FG), fibers. Both fast fiber types are large and powerful, with moderate to high anaerobic metabolic capability. The primary distinction between the two is that FOG fibers have moderate oxidative and anaerobic capacity, providing them with some fatigue resistance in comparison with the purely anaerobic and highly fatigable FG fibers (table 1.1).

It should be acknowledged, however, that the characteristics by which fibers are categorized into types lie on a continuum rather than being discrete categories. For example, at what point does a fiber have enough mitochondria to be classified as an oxida-

TABLE 1.1 Muscle Fiber Types and Their Use During Physical Activities

Activity	Type I	Type II	
Walking	High	Low	
Gardening or yard work	High	Low	
Moving heavy furniture	Low	High	
Firefighting	High	High	
Distance running or cycling	High	Low	
Sprinting	Low	High	
Olympic weightlifting	Low	High	
Baseball or softball	Low	High	
Football	Low	High	
Tennis	High	High	
Wrestling	High	High	
Volleyball	Low	High	
Throwing events	Low	High	
Resistance training for strength	Low	High	
Circuit weight or resistance training for muscular endurance	High	Low	

tive fiber? From a practical standpoint, muscle fibers will adapt based on the physiological stress placed on them. For example, both type I and type II fibers will increase in size in response to regular resistance training. More will be said about adaptations to resistance and aerobic endurance training in chapters 5 and 6, respectively.

THE NERVOUS SYSTEM

Although skeletal muscles produce the force that allows us to move and exercise, it is the nervous system that directs and controls the voluntary movement.

Organization of the Nervous System

Anatomically, the entire nervous system can be divided into the central nervous system and peripheral nervous system. The **central nervous system** consists of the brain and spinal cord. As its name implies, the **peripheral nervous system** lies outside the central nervous system and may be further divided into motor (efferent) and sensory (afferent) divisions. The motor branch of the peripheral nervous system relays nerve impulses from the central nervous system to the periphery (e.g., to skeletal muscles), while the sensory branch relays nerve impulses from the periphery back to the central nervous system.

The nervous system has **somatic** (voluntary) and **autonomic** (involuntary) functions. The somatic nervous system is responsible for activating skeletal muscles (e.g., the rhythmic actions of the quadriceps femoris muscles during cycling). The autonomic nervous system controls involuntary functions such as contraction of the heart and smooth muscle in blood vessels as well as glands. It is the flight-or-fight response of the sympathetic branch of the autonomic nervous system that causes increased blood flow from the heart, greater ventilation of the lungs, a redistribution of blood flow to the working skeletal muscles, and increased sweating, which is necessary for proper body temperature regulation. In this sense, the sympathetic branch of the autonomic nervous system supports the muscle actions initiated by the somatic nervous system. The parasympathetic division of the autonomic nervous system is primarily active during rest. It is responsible for processes such as digestion, urination, and gland secretion. The autonomic nervous system is discussed in more detail in later chapters. It is the

motor and sensory functions of the somatic nervous system that will be the focus of the rest of this chapter.

Neurons

The most basic unit of the nervous system is the nerve cell, or **neuron**. The neurons that conduct impulses from the central nervous system to the muscles are known as **motor neurons** or **efferent neurons**. It is these motor signals that cause skeletal muscles to contract. The neurons responsible for carrying impulses from the periphery toward the central nervous system are called the **sensory** or **afferent neurons**. Sensory neurons relay impulses from the periphery to the central nervous system regarding such information as tension, stretch, movement, and pain. The site of communication between two neurons or a neuron and a gland or muscle cell is known as a **synapse**. For example, the synapse between a motor neuron and a skeletal muscle fiber is called the neuromuscular junction, as discussed earlier in this chapter.

The structure of a typical motor neuron is presented in figure 1.6 (9a). **Dendrites** are projections from the neuron cell body. The dendrites receive excitatory or inhibitory signals (or both) from other neurons. Both the dendrites and the cell body of a motor neuron are located in the anterior gray horn of the spinal cord. If sufficiently excited, a neuron will transmit an action potential down its axon, away from the cell body. The axon extends outward from the spinal cord and may innervate a muscle that is a relatively great distance away from the spine. In the case of a motor neuron that activates skeletal muscle, the action potential causes the release of ACh at the neuromuscular junction. This leads to the process of muscle action discussed earlier (see "Sliding Filament Theory").

Sensory neurons convey information from the periphery, such as from the muscles and joints, back to the central nervous system. Two sensory structures with particular significance to exercise training are the muscle spindle and the Golgi tendon organ (GTO).

Muscle Spindle

As its name implies, the **muscle spindle** is a spindle-shaped sensory organ, meaning it is thicker in the middle and tapered at either end. It is a stretch receptor that is widely dispersed throughout most skeletal muscles. Muscle spindles are specialized to sense changes in muscle length, particularly when the muscle changes length rapidly. Each muscle

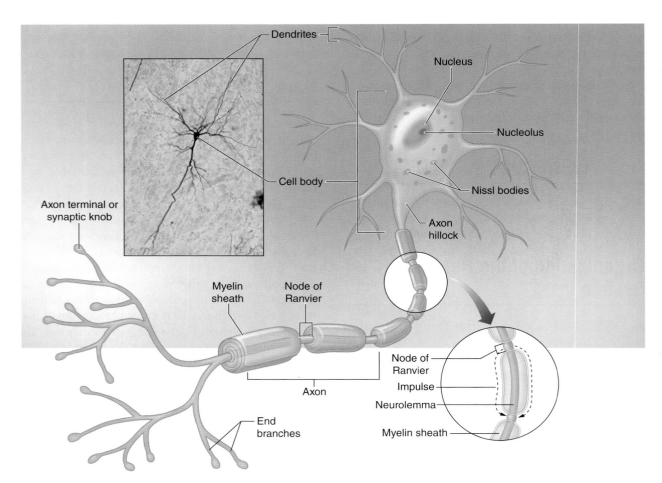

FIGURE 1.6   A schematic representation of a neuron, including its dendrites, cell body, and axon.

spindle is enclosed within a capsule (figure 1.7; 9a) and lies parallel to **extrafusal fibers** (ordinary skeletal muscle fibers). The muscle spindle contains specialized muscle fibers called **intrafusal fibers**. These intrafusal fibers have contractile proteins at each end (actin and myosin) and a central region that is wrapped by sensory nerve endings. Because the intrafusal fibers of the muscle spindle lie parallel to the extrafusal muscle fibers, a stretching force applied to the muscle will stretch both intrafusal and extrafusal muscle fibers. This will cause a sensory discharge from the muscle spindle that is carried toward the spinal cord. This leads to a motor response, activation of the muscle that was initially stretched. This reflex is known as the **myotatic** or **stretch reflex**. From a practical standpoint, static stretching exercises are typically done in such a way as to avoid activation of the muscle spindles. Moving slowly into a stretched position prevents activation of the muscle spindle.

This is important because muscles are most easily stretched when they are relaxed. There are other times, however, when activation of the muscle spindle is desired during training. For example, plyometric and weightlifting exercises (snatch, clean and jerk, and other derivatives), jumping, swinging a bat or tennis racket, and kicking and punching are commonly performed by rapidly stretching the muscles involved, followed immediately by a concentric action of the same muscles. This rapid stretch of the muscles will activate the stretch reflex, leading to a more powerful concentric action.

Golgi Tendon Organ

The **Golgi tendon organ** is located at the junction of the muscle and the tendon that attaches the muscle to the bone (figure 1.7). It appears to play a role in protecting the muscle from injury. The Golgi tendon

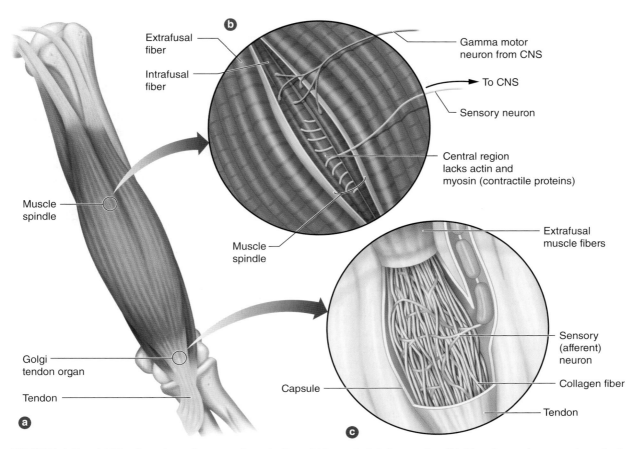

FIGURE 1.7   *(a)* The location of a muscle spindle within a skeletal muscle. *(b)* Structure of a muscle spindle. *(c)* Structure of a Golgi tendon organ.

organ is deformed when the muscle is activated. If the force of the muscle action is great enough, it will cause the Golgi tendon organ to convey sensory information to the spinal cord, which will lead to relaxation of the acting muscle and stimulation of the antagonist muscle. This protective reflex presumably prevents injury to the muscle and joint due to a potentially excessive force of muscle action. For example, during a **1-repetition maximum** (the heaviest weight that can be lifted one time) of a deadlift exercise, activation of the Golgi tendon organ may prevent a person from exerting themselves to the extent that muscles and associated connective tissues are damaged. Regular resistance training will strengthen the muscles and other tissues, while the Golgi tendon organ may have its sensitivity altered such that greater forces may be produced without initiating an inhibitory response.

The Motor Unit

A motor neuron and the muscle fibers it innervates is known as a **motor unit**. All fibers in a given motor unit are of the same fiber type. Indeed, it is the motor neuron that gives the fibers their metabolic and contractile characteristics. Motor units may vary in the number of fibers innervated. For example, motor units in small muscles, such as those in the hand, have relatively few fibers. Larger muscles, such as those in the thigh, contain a large number of fibers per motor unit.

> All fibers of a single motor unit are of the same muscle fiber type. The different muscle fiber types have distinct anatomical and physiological characteristics, which determine their functional capacities.

Gradation of Force

It is possible for the nervous system to vary the force produced by a muscle over a wide range of intensities. For example, individuals may be able to curl a 10-pound (5 kg) dumbbell but can also work their way up the dumbbell rack to curl a 60-pound (30 kg) dumbbell with maximal effort. In the simplest sense, there are two mechanisms the nervous system may use to vary, or grade, force production to accomplish these tasks. One method is to vary the number of motor units, and thus muscle fibers, that are activated. This is known as **motor unit recruitment**. The second method is to increase the firing rate of motor units already activated, a process known as **rate coding**.

When a light weight is lifted, a relatively small number of motor units are activated. As the resistance increases (i.e., as a heavier dumbbell is lifted), more motor units can be added, or recruited, to the active pool of motor units, and thus force is increased because more muscle fibers are contracting. Recruitment of all motor units would thus require the lifting of maximal or near-maximal weights at maximal intensity. Motor units are recruited in a specific order, known as the **size principle of motor unit recruitment** (7). The first motor units recruited are the smaller type I motor units, which have a lower threshold for being activated and thus are recruited even during low-force muscle actions. The next motor units recruited are the type IIa motor units, followed by the type IIx motor units. These type II motor units are larger than the type I motor units, and they have a higher threshold that must be reached before they are activated. It appears that most people are unable to activate all of their motor units but are able to recruit more motor units with training (10).

It is also possible to increase muscle force production by increasing the firing rate of already activated motor units (12). If a muscle is stimulated to contract before it has a chance to relax from a previous stimulus, it will produce greater force. Evidence suggests that well-trained weightlifters, even among older adults, have higher maximal motor unit discharge rates than untrained individuals (11).

THE SKELETAL SYSTEM

Movement and exercise are possible because skeletal muscles attach to bones, which are in turn connected at joints. The pulling of muscles on bones causes the bones to rotate. It is this combined functioning of muscles, bones, and joints that allows us to lift weights, run on a treadmill, and participate in a cycling class. Figure 1.8 shows the structure of a long bone (1a). In addition to providing a system of bony levers, the skeleton performs a number of other important anatomical and physiological functions. For example, bones are the primary storage site for minerals, such as calcium and phosphorus. They are also the location for blood cell formation, and they protect internal organs and the spinal cord.

Organization of the Skeletal System

The typical person has 206 bones that make up the skeletal system (figure 1.9; 15). The bones can be divided into two anatomical divisions: the axial skeleton and the appendicular skeleton. The **axial skeleton** consists primarily of the skull, vertebral column, sternum, and ribs. These bones protect important

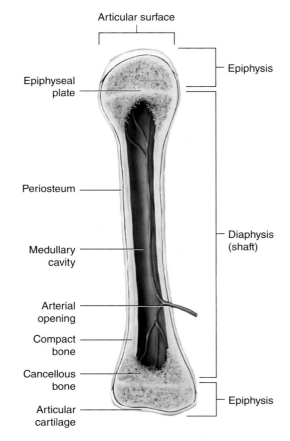

Articular surface

Epiphysis

Epiphyseal plate

Periosteum

Diaphysis (shaft)

Medullary cavity

Arterial opening

Compact bone

Cancellous bone

Articular cartilage

Epiphysis

FIGURE 1.8   The anatomy of a long bone.

internal organs, such as the brain, heart, and lungs, but also offer sites for skeletal muscle attachments. The **appendicular skeleton** includes the bones of the upper and lower limbs. The rotations of these bones around joints are responsible for most of the movements associated with exercise, such as lifting, running, throwing, kicking, and striking.

Osteoporosis and Exercise

Bone is a complex, living, and dynamic tissue. It is constantly undergoing a process called **remodeling**, in which bone-destroying cells called **osteoclasts** break down bone while other cells, called **osteoblasts**, stimulate bone synthesis. The two types, or categories, of bone are cortical (compact) bone and cancellous (trabecular) bone. **Cortical bone** is hard and dense and is found primarily in the outer layers of the shafts of long bones, such as the arms and legs. **Cancellous bone**, also called **spongy bone**, is much less dense than cortical bone and is found in the interior of long bones, the vertebrae, and the head of the femur. It is the site of **hematopoiesis**, the synthesis of blood cells. Calcium and phosphorus are two important minerals that help form the body's bones.

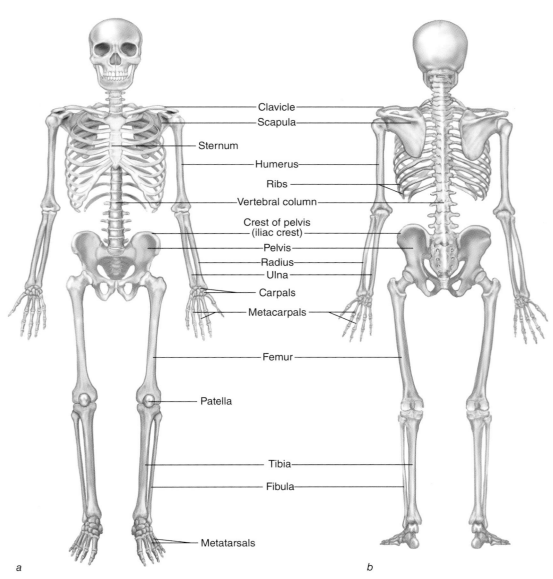

Clavicle
Scapula
Sternum
Humerus
Ribs
Vertebral column
Crest of pelvis (iliac crest)
Pelvis
Radius
Ulna
Carpals
Metacarpals
Femur
Patella
Tibia
Fibula
Metatarsals

a   *b*

FIGURE 1.9   *(a)* Front view and *(b)* rear view of an adult male human skeleton.

Osteoporosis, literally meaning "porous bones," is a condition in which the bones become weak and brittle. In this weakened condition, they are more susceptible to breaking, particularly in the spine and hip. Along with proper nutrition, including adequate calcium intake, exercise is an important component of bone health. According to Wolff's law, bone will adapt in response to stresses placed on it. For example, weight-bearing exercises, such as running, lead to increases in bone mineral density (5). Resistance training is also effective at increasing bone mineral density (4), with eccentric loading being an especially potent stimulus for bone growth (6, 14). This information has obvious implications for personal trainers, who should incorporate weight-bearing exercises like walking or running (or both) into a comprehensive resistance training program, along with an emphasis on eccentric loading, when training their clients.

> **Resistance training increases bone mass and strength and may decrease the likelihood of developing osteoporosis.**

Tendons and Ligaments

Associated with the skeletal system are two other connective tissues, tendons and ligaments. Tendons attach muscle to bone. They are primarily formed from the inelastic protein collagen and thus are well suited for withstanding the tensile forces produced when muscles pull on bones. **Ligaments** connect bones to other bones. Ligaments are formed from collagen as well, but they also contain an elastic protein called elastin. This affords ligaments some ability to stretch, thus allowing for a balance between stabilizing a joint and permitting some mobility.

CONCLUSION

In the simplest sense, exercise involves nervous system activation of muscles, which in turn pull on bones and their associated connective tissues. Personal trainers should have an intimate understanding of the structure and function of these tissues to appreciate how they work during exercise. This knowledge will help the personal trainer conduct safe and effective exercise programs and will provide a foundation for understanding the specific adaptations that occur with repeated bouts of varied types of physical activity.

Study Questions

1. What is the name of the connective tissue that surrounds skeletal muscle?
   A. epimysium
   B. endomysium
   C. perimysium
   D. fascicle

2. How many neuromuscular junctions does each muscle fiber have?
   A. 1
   B. 2
   C. 3
   D. 4

3. Which of the following branches of the nervous system is responsible for activating skeletal muscles?
   A. sensory
   B. autonomic
   C. afferent
   D. somatic

4. Which division of the skeleton contains the skull and vertebral column?
   A. axial skeleton
   B. appendicular skeleton
   C. central skeleton
   D. peripheral skeleton

5. Which of the following connective tissues connects muscle to bone?
   A. ligament
   B. tendon
   C. cartilage
   D. collagen

CHAPTER 2

Structure and Function of the Cardiorespiratory System

Michael R. Esco, PhD, and Moh H. Malek, PhD

After completing this chapter, you will be able to

- describe the anatomical and physiological characteristics of the cardiovascular system,
- describe the electrical conduction system of the heart and the basic electrocardiogram,
- describe the mechanisms that control the circulation of blood throughout the body,
- describe the anatomical and physiological characteristics of the respiratory system,
- explain the exchange of gases between the lungs and the blood, and
- understand the mechanisms that control respiration.

The cardiovascular and respiratory systems work in unison to provide oxygen and nutrients to the body under various perturbations such as exercise. In addition, these two systems are instrumental in clearing metabolic by-products (e.g., CO_2) from the muscle. This chapter summarizes the structure and function of both systems.

> The cardiovascular and pulmonary systems work together to deliver important nutrients to the functioning tissues of the body and remove the by-products of metabolism. The two systems are described collectively as the cardiorespiratory system, comprising the heart, blood, blood vessels, and lungs. The system is well integrated with the body and responds accordingly to a change in metabolic demand.

CARDIOVASCULAR ANATOMY AND PHYSIOLOGY

Before discussing the cardiovascular system and gas exchange, it is important to briefly discuss the characteristics of blood, which is involved in transporting oxygen, nutrients, and metabolic by-products throughout the body. Whole blood can be separated into plasma, erythrocytes, and leukocytes and platelets, which compose approximately 55%, 45%, and <1% of whole blood, respectively. In addition, the normal pH range of arterial blood is approximately 7.4, and deviations from this number can be influenced by factors such as exercise, stress, or disease. It should be noted, however, that physiological tolerance for changes in pH for arterial blood and muscle are between 6.9 and 7.5 and 6.6 and 7.1, respectively. Nevertheless, pH is regulated by buffers such as bicarbonate, ventilation, and kidney function.

The authors would like to acknowledge the significant contributions of Mark A. Williams to this chapter.

Oxygen Transport

Oxygen is primarily carried by hemoglobin but is also dissolved within the blood. Oxygen dissolved in the blood accounts for a very small percentage (0.3 ml O_2 per 100 ml of blood, or around 2%), we will focus on hemoglobin (5). **Hemoglobin** is an iron-containing protein within the red blood cells that has the capacity to bind between one and four oxygen molecules. Each gram of hemoglobin can carry approximately 1.39 ml of oxygen. In addition, healthy blood has approximately 15 g of hemoglobin per 100 ml. Therefore, the capacity of healthy blood to carry oxygen approximates to 20.8 ml of oxygen per 100 ml of blood (20.8 ml O_2/100 ml of blood = ~[15 g of Hb/100 ml] × [1.39 ml of O_2]) (4). The average healthy adult who is not anemic has around 5.0 L of blood volume, which accounts for close to 7% of body weight.

Oxygen–Hemoglobin Dissociation Curve

The **oxygen–hemoglobin dissociation curve** illustrates the saturation of hemoglobin at various partial pressures. Partial pressure is essentially the pressure exerted by one gas in a mixture of gases and is calculated as the product of total pressure of a gas mixture and the percent concentration of the specific gas. For example, normal atmospheric pressure is 760 mmHg, whereas the percent concentration of oxygen in the atmosphere is 20.93%. Therefore, the partial pressure of oxygen at sea level is approximately 159 mmHg (760 mmHg × [20.93/100]). As shown in figure 2.1, the relationship between partial pressure of oxygen and oxygen saturation is sigmoidal (S-shaped) as opposed to linear (direct) (2). In part, this is due to **cooperative binding**, which means that as oxygen binds to hemoglobin it facilitates subsequent binding of oxygen molecules (3). That is, binding of the first oxygen molecule to hemoglobin increases hemoglobin's affinity for oxygen such that the fourth oxygen molecule binds to hemoglobin at a much higher affinity than the first oxygen molecule. Therefore, as the oxygen partial pressure increases, hemoglobin becomes saturated, but this saturation begins to plateau. Typically, at around 60 mmHg, the curve beings to become relatively flat, with approximately 90% of hemoglobin saturated with oxygen. The subsequent increase from 60 mmHg to 100 mmHg raises the oxygen saturation of hemoglobin to 98%.

Factors Influencing the Oxygen– Hemoglobin Curve

Various factors can, however, influence the oxygen–hemoglobin curve, thus shifting the curve to the right or left. For example, a decrease in core body temperature shifts the curve toward the left, whereas an increase in temperature shifts the curve toward the right (figure 2.2; 2). Another factor that can cause a leftward or rightward shift in the curve is arterial blood acidity. Blood with low pH (acidic) results in the curve shifting right, whereas blood with high pH (alkalosis) results in the curve shifting left. To apply the oxygen–hemoglobin dissociation curve to a prac-

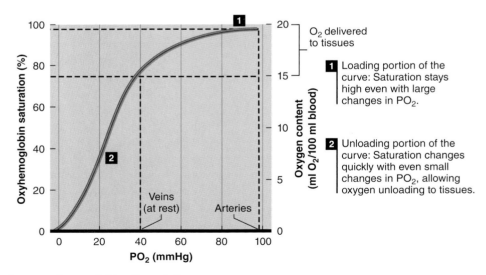

FIGURE 2.1 Oxygen–hemoglobin dissociation curve.

Reprinted by permission from Kenney et al. (2020, p. 189).

tical setting, consider exercise. Typically, exercise increases core body temperature and reduces blood pH, which shifts the curve toward the right. Thus, the affinity of hemoglobin for oxygen has been reduced and oxygen is released more easily at a higher partial pressure. Although reducing the oxygen saturation of hemoglobin may seem counterintuitive, this is a beneficial response because now the oxygen can be used by the working muscles where it is required.

Cardiac Morphology

The heart is composed of four chambers (right atrium, left atrium, right ventricle, and left ventricle) and a layer of cardiac muscle, referred to as the **myocardium**. Cardiac and skeletal muscle are different. For example, skeletal muscle cells are multinucleated and are under the control of the central nervous system. Cardiac muscle cells contain only one nucleus and depolarize action potentials involuntarily (i.e., without central nervous system input) (1). In other words, the heart has its own internal pacemaker and therefore beats automatically. The electrical conduction system of the heart begins with the **sinoatrial (SA) node**, which is the primary intrinsic pacemaker of the heart. The SA node generates an electrical impulse that spreads across the atrium to the **atrioventricular**

(AV) node (figure 2.3; 3a). From there, the impulse continues to spread down through the left and right bundle branches into the Purkinje system. The **Purkinje system** is a series of fibers that surround the ventricles, which then stimulate ventricular contraction. Note that the impulse from the SA node spreads very quickly (~0.08 m/s) across both atria and then slows through the AV node, allowing for a time delay between excitation of the atria and ventricles so the filling can occur. When the impulse reaches the Purkinje fibers, the result is ventricular contraction. The entire time to complete the impulse (SA node → AV node → Purkinje fibers → contraction of ventricles) is approximately 0.2 seconds (1).

As shown in figure 2.4, venous blood (deoxygenated) returns to the right atrium via the superior and inferior vena cava and is delivered to the right ventricle (3a). (A common misconception is that deoxygenated blood has no oxygen, whereas in fact, at rest it is approximately 70% saturated.) The **superior vena cava** returns deoxygenated blood from the head and upper extremities, whereas the **inferior vena cava** returns deoxygenated blood from the trunk and lower extremities. From there, the deoxygenated blood is delivered by the pulmonary artery to the lungs, where gas exchange occurs. That is, the deoxygenated blood is loaded with oxygen while the metabolic by-products

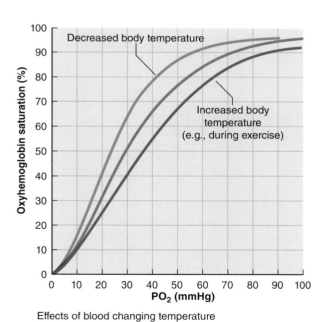

Effects of blood changing temperature

FIGURE 2.2   Shifts in the oxygen–hemoglobin curve with changes in core body temperature.

Reprinted by permission from Kenney et al. (2020, p. 189).

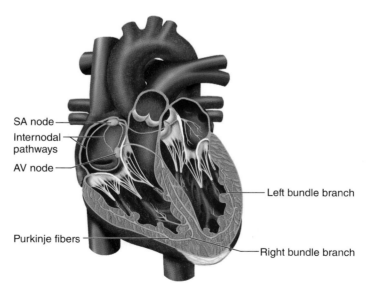

FIGURE 2.3   The conduction system of cardiac muscle.

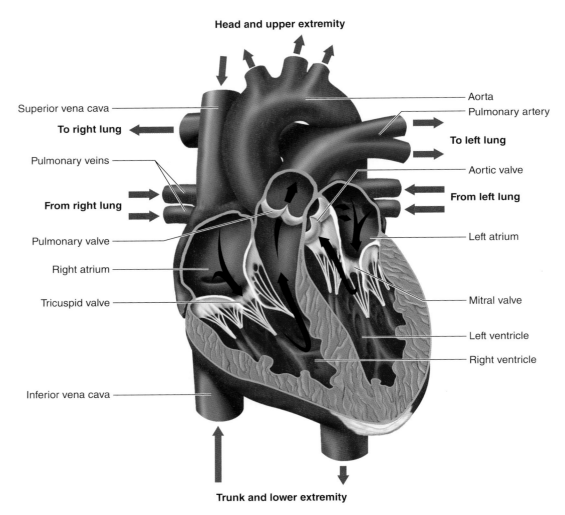

FIGURE 2.4 Structure of the human heart and corresponding blood flow pathway.

are removed. The oxygenated blood now returns to the left atrium via the pulmonary vein and is delivered to the left ventricle. At this point, the oxygen-rich blood is ready to be delivered throughout the body via the **aorta** and thereafter to organs and tissues through miles of vasculature.

> The circulation of the heart and lungs (central circulation) and that of the rest of the body (peripheral circulation) form a single closed-circuit system with two components: an arterial system, which carries blood away from the heart, and a venous system, which returns blood toward the heart.

Electrocardiogram

A way to record the electrical activity of the heart at the surface of the body is to place an array of electrodes on the chest. The electrical impulses generated by the heart (discussed earlier) are detected by the surface electrodes and are presented as distinct patterns called the **electrocardiogram (ECG)**. The ECG has three distinct components: P-wave, QRS complex, and T-wave (1). As shown in figure 2.5, the **P-wave** represents atrial depolarization, occurring when the impulse travels from the SA node to the AV node (3a). The **QRS complex** reflects ventricular depolarization and occurs when the impulse continues from the AV node to the Purkinje fibers throughout the ventricles. The **T-wave** represents electrical recovery (repolarization) of the ventricles. Note that atrial repolarization does occur but cannot be seen

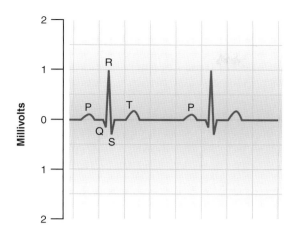

FIGURE 2.5 The various phases of the resting electrocardiogram.

Reprinted by permission from National Strength and Conditioning Association (2016, p. 14).

since it takes place during the QRS complex. Typically, ECGs are obtained during incremental exercise tests in a clinical setting to examine the heart under stress. Abnormal patterns in an ECG cycle, such as ST-segment depression, during an exercise test may indicate the presence of heart disease.

Circulation

The circulation system is composed of **arteries**, which carry blood away from the heart toward the tissues and organs, and **veins**, which carry blood from the tissues and organs back to the heart, with one exception—the **pulmonary veins** carry oxygenated blood from the lungs to the heart. For the systemic circulation, arteries are typically a high-pressure system, ranging from around 100 mmHg in the aorta to approximately 60 mmHg in the arterioles. The veins are characterized by very low pressure relative to the arteries. Because of this low-pressure system, veins have one-way valves and smooth muscle bands that continue moving venous blood toward the heart as we move or contract muscles in our extremities (figure 2.6; 2).

The resistance of the entire systemic circulation is called the **total peripheral resistance**. As blood vessels constrict, peripheral resistance increases, whereas with dilation peripheral resistance decreases. Note, however, that many factors can influence constriction or dilation of vessels, such as type of exercise, sympathetic nervous system stimulation, local muscle tissue metabolism, and environmental stressors (e.g., heat or cold). For example, the sympathetic nervous system constricts arteries that supply blood to nonactive

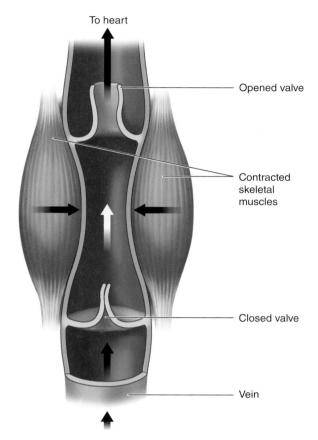

FIGURE 2.6 The muscle pump. As the skeletal muscles contract, they squeeze the veins in the legs and assist in the return of blood to the heart. Valves within the veins ensure the unidirectional flow of blood back to the heart.

> The **autonomic nervous system** controls the activity of internal organs, such as the heart and blood vessels. For example, the two branches of the autonomic nervous system, parasympathetic and sympathetic, act together to regulate heart rate. The parasympathetic system is active during rest by keeping heart rate low. However, the sympathetic system becomes more active during exercise by increasing heart rate. The autonomic nervous system also helps control how much blood is redistributed to active muscle during exercise.

organs, like the liver, during exercise. However, the arterioles that supply blood to active skeletal muscle during exercise vasodilate because the sympathetic nervous system is overridden by the localized release of nitric oxide. Therefore, blood flow to the working muscles is increased. As shown in figure 2.7, during exercise, blood is redistributed from other organs to the muscles used for that particular exercise (2).

Cardiac Cycle

The **cardiac cycle** consists of the events that occur from the start of one heartbeat to the start of another heartbeat. The cardiac cycle, therefore, is composed of periods of relaxation (called **diastole**) and contraction (called **systole**). The diastolic phase allows for the heart to fill with blood. **Systolic blood pressure (SBP)** is the pressure exerted against the arterial walls as blood is forcefully ejected during ventricular contraction (systole). Simultaneous measurement of SBP and heart rate (HR) is useful in describing the work of the heart and can provide an indirect estimation of myocardial oxygen uptake. This estimate of the work of the heart, referred to as the **rate–pressure product (RPP)**, or double product, is obtained with the following equation (1):

$$RPP = SBP \times HR \qquad (2.1)$$

Conversely, **diastolic blood pressure (DBP)** is the pressure exerted against the arterial walls when no blood is being forcefully ejected through the vessels (diastole). It provides an indication of peripheral resistance or vascular stiffness, tending to decrease with vasodilation and increase with vasoconstriction. In addition, the **mean arterial pressure (MAP)** is the mean blood pressure throughout the cardiac cycle, but it should not be mistaken for the average of the systolic and diastolic pressures. The mean arterial pressure is typically estimated with the following equation:

$$MAP = DBP + [0.333 \times (SBP - DBP)] \qquad (2.2)$$

Cardiac Output

Cardiac output ($\dot{Q}$) is defined as the amount of blood pumped by the heart in 1 minute and is represented by the following formula:

$$\dot{Q} = SV \times HR \qquad (2.3)$$

where **SV (stroke volume)** is the amount of blood ejected per heartbeat. Stroke volume is estimated by the following formula:

$$SV = EDV - ESV \qquad (2.4)$$

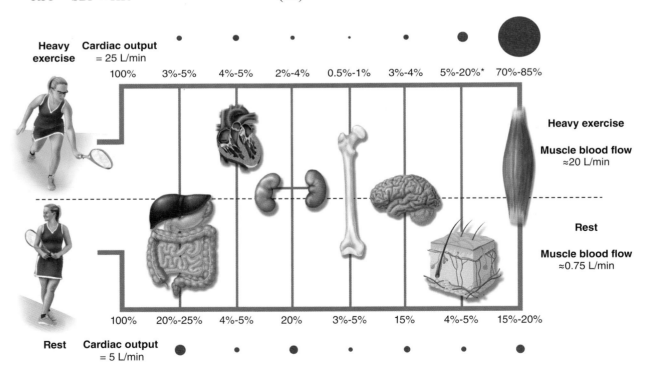

FIGURE 2.7 Redistribution of blood from a resting to a heavy exercise state.

Reprinted by permission from P.O. Åstrand et al. (2003, p. 143).

where **EDV (end-diastolic volume)** is the volume of blood in the ventricles after filling, and **ESV (end-systolic volume)** is the volume of blood in the ventricles after contraction. Therefore, the cardiac output is estimated as

$$\dot{Q} = (EDV - ESV) \times HR \qquad (2.5)$$

The **Frank-Starling principle** indicates that the more the left ventricle is stretched, the more forceful the contraction and thus the greater volume of blood leaving the ventricle. This principle is thus based on the length–tension relationship. An increase in preload (EDV) is directly influenced by the heart volume and the **venous return**, or the flow of blood back to the heart.

RESPIRATORY SYSTEM

The primary function of the respiratory system is the basic exchange of oxygen and carbon dioxide. This section discusses the anatomy and physiology of the lungs as well as gas exchange.

Structure

As air passes through the nose, the nasal cavities perform three distinct functions, which include warming, humidifying, and purifying the air. Air is then distributed to the lungs via the trachea, bronchi, and bronchioles. The trachea is then divided into the left and right bronchi, and each division thereafter is an additional generation. There are approximately 23 generations, finally ending with the alveoli where gas exchange occurs (figure 2.8; 3a) (1).

Inspiration is an active process that involves the diaphragm and external intercostal muscles. Contraction of the diaphragm results in expansion of the thorax and thus lowers air pressure in the lungs. Since gases move from an area of high pressure to one of low pressure, air moves into the lungs. Note, however, that during exercise, other muscles (scalene, sternocleidomastoid, pectoralis major and minor) are involved in inspiration. **Expiration**, at rest, is a passive response and involves no muscular contraction because the external intercostal muscles and the diaphragm relax, resulting in increased pressure in the lungs and exhalation of air. During exercise, however,

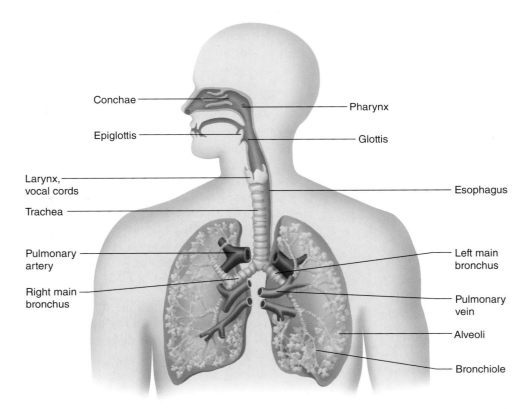

FIGURE 2.8 The respiratory system.

the internal intercostal and abdominal muscles facilitate movement of air in and out of the lungs.

Lung Volumes

Spirometry is a method used in either clinical or research settings to examine static lung volumes. It is the most common pulmonary function test for diagnosing lung disorders, such as asthma and chronic obstructive pulmonary disease. The test measures lung function as the individual breathes into a special tube connected to a spirometer device, measuring the amount and speed of air that is inhaled and exhaled. By comparing the values obtained against normative data, clinicians can determine how well the pulmonary system is performing. Figure 2.9 shows the lung volumes that are measured while breathing through the spirometer. When individuals perform a lung function test, they are asked to breathe normally into a spirometer to measure the amount of air moving into and out of the lungs at rest, known as the **tidal volume**. Thereafter, they are asked to take a deep breath in and fill up their lungs followed by exhaling maximally. These two breathing actions are a measure of **vital capacity** (figure 2.9). If the values obtained from the spirometer test substantially differ from normative data, a lung disorder, such as asthma, may be present. For further information on respiratory conditions and exercise prescription for this population, see chapter 20.

Some descriptions of lung capacities are combinations of various lung volumes. For example, **total lung capacity** is the entire gas volume of a maximally inflated pulmonary system. **Residual volume** is the amount of air left in the lungs after a person consciously exhales as much air as possible (in other words, after performing a vital capacity assessment). **Functional residual capacity**, however, is the amount of air left in the lungs after normal exhalation.

Gas Exchange

The alveolus is covered with **capillaries**, which are the smallest unit of blood vessels within the body and are the site of gas exchange. The movement of gas such as oxygen or carbon dioxide across a cell membrane is called **diffusion** (figure 2.10; 2). Diffusion occurs when there is a **concentration gradient** (i.e., a greater concentration of a gas on one side of the membrane). As mentioned previously, gas moves from an area of high concentration to one of low concentration. At the tissue level, oxygen is used by cells and carbon dioxide is produced. The partial pressures of oxygen and carbon dioxide are different both within the tissue and within the capillaries. As illustrated in figure 2.11, inspired oxygen has a partial pressure of 159 mmHg; however, as it reaches the alveoli the partial pressure is reduced to 100 mmHg because of factors such as humidifying of the air in the respiratory tract (3a). The partial pressure of oxygen and carbon dioxide in the venous blood is approximately 40 and 46 mmHg, respectively. Based on the pressure gradients, gas exchange occurs and thereafter the blood is rich with oxygen (100 mmHg), with a concomitant reduction in carbon dioxide (figure 2.11). Now the oxygen-loaded blood is delivered to the tissue (i.e., working muscle). Similar to gas exchange in the alveolus, gas exchange in the tissue follows the pressure gradient. Thus, oxygen diffuses into the tissue, whereas carbon dioxide diffuses out of the tissue (figure 2.11). The deoxygenated blood (venous blood) is then returned to the alveolus, and the cycle of gas exchange is repeated.

> **With ventilation, oxygen diffuses from the alveoli into the pulmonary blood, and carbon dioxide diffuses from the blood into the alveoli.**

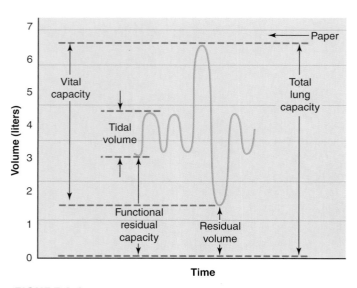

FIGURE 2.9 Various components of pulmonary function. For example, total lung capacity is the sum of vital capacity and residual volume.

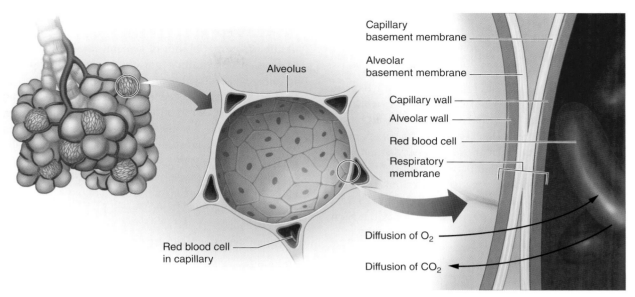

FIGURE 2.10   The anatomy of the respiratory membrane, showing the exchange of oxygen and carbon dioxide between an alveolus and pulmonary capillary blood.

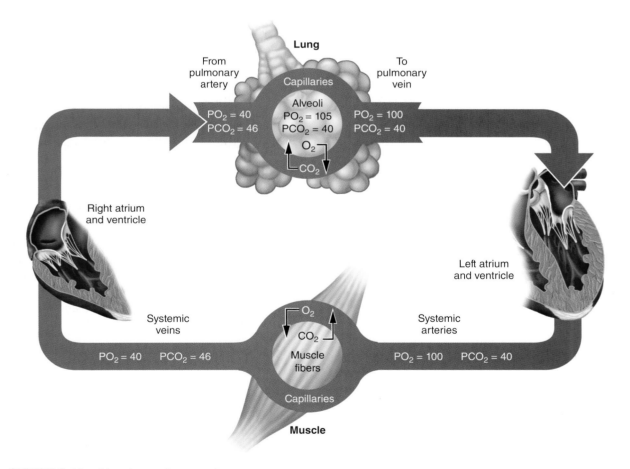

FIGURE 2.11   Alveolus and gas exchange.

Reprinted by permission from National Strength and Conditioning Association (2016, p. 119).

Oxygen Uptake

Oxygen uptake ($\dot{V}O_2$) is the amount of oxygen used by the tissues of the body. Note that the term *oxygen consumption* is used interchangeably with oxygen uptake; however, traditionally *oxygen consumption* is reserved for when the amount of oxygen used by the tissue is directly measured. Typically, $\dot{V}O_2$ in exercise physiology is measured at the mouth using a metabolic cart. $\dot{V}O_2$ is primarily related to the ability of the heart and circulatory system to transport oxygen via blood to the tissues and the ability of the tissues to extract oxygen. The formula that represents $\dot{V}O_2$ is the **Fick equation** (equation 2.6):

$$\dot{V}O_2 = \dot{Q} \times a\text{–}\bar{v}O_2 \tag{2.6}$$

$$\dot{V}O_2 = (HR \times SV) \times a\text{–}\bar{v}O_2 \tag{2.6.1}$$

$$\dot{V}O_2 = (HR) \times (EDV - ESV) \times a\text{–}\bar{v}O_2 \tag{2.6.2}$$

where $\dot{V}O_2$ is the product of cardiac output ($\dot{Q}$, equation 2.3) and a–$\bar{v}O_2$ difference. The **a–$\bar{v}O_2$ difference** is the arterial oxygen content minus the venous oxygen content in milliliters of O_2 per 100 ml of blood. This difference helps us know the amount of oxygen that has been extracted from the transported blood for use in exercise. As shown in table 2.1, oxygen extraction (a–$\bar{v}O_2$) increases with exercise intensity. The following is an example of calculating $\dot{V}O_2$:

$$\dot{V}O_2 = (HR \times SV) \times a\text{–}\bar{v}O_2$$

$$\dot{V}O_2 = (80 \text{ beats/min} \times 65 \text{ ml blood/beat})$$
$$\times (6 \text{ ml } O_2 \text{ ml/100 ml blood})$$

$$\dot{V}O_2 = 312 \text{ ml } O_2/\text{min}$$

This value is in absolute terms (ml O_2/min) but can also be expressed relative to the individual's body mass (ml · kg^{-1} · min^{-1}).

$$\dot{V}O_2 = (312 \text{ ml } O_2/\text{min}) / 75.0 \text{ kg}$$

$$\dot{V}O_2 = 4.16 \text{ ml} \cdot \text{kg}^{-1} \cdot \text{min}^{-1}$$

Maximal oxygen uptake ($\dot{V}O_2$max) is the highest amount of oxygen that can be taken up, transported, and used by the body. This entire process is related to the heart's maximal ability to eject blood (maximal $\dot{Q}$), the maximal ability of skeletal muscle to extract oxygen, and the ability to use it (maximal a–$\bar{v}O_2$ difference) to aerobically produce energy. The process by which $\dot{V}O_2$max is accurately obtained is a **graded exercise test (GXT)** on an aerobic exercise machine, like a treadmill. As the GXT is performed, oxygen consumption is analyzed with a specialized metabolic cart to measure oxygen use. Since oxygen consumption increases with exercise intensity, the metabolic cart is able to estimate the maximal amount of oxygen used by measuring the by-products of aerobic metabolism (e.g., CO_2). In chapter 11, the testing procedures to determine maximal oxygen uptake are discussed along with various field tests that act as surrogates to the laboratory testing procedures. Here, however, we discuss the various components of the Fick equation that contribute to the determination of maximal oxygen uptake.

$\dot{V}O_2$max, or $\dot{V}O_2$peak, is the most accepted measure of aerobic fitness, also known as cardiovascular fitness. It correlates well with the degree of physical conditioning and is related to cardiovascular health. For example, higher $\dot{V}O_2$max values are associated with a lower risk of cardiovascular disease, morbidity, and mortality. Resting $\dot{V}O_2$ is typically estimated at 3.5 ml · kg^{-1} · min^{-1}, whereas $\dot{V}O_2$max has been reported to reach 80 ml · kg^{-1} · min^{-1} or higher in elite aerobic endurance athletes. On the other hand, clinical patients, such as those with heart failure or chronic obstructive pulmonary disease, may have values around 20 ml · kg^{-1} · min^{-1} or lower. $\dot{V}O_2$max for an average person is within a range of 35 to 45 ml · kg^{-1} · min^{-1}.

With aerobic endurance training, $\dot{V}O_2$max can improve by approximately 10% to 15% from baseline. However, this can depend on many factors, such as genetics, training status, nutrition, and recovery. Lower aerobically fit individuals often experience a great percentage increase in $\dot{V}O_2$max with an aerobic exercise program as compared with fitter individuals. The improvement in $\dot{V}O_2$max coincides with increases in both maximal $\dot{Q}$ and maximal a–$\bar{v}O_2$ difference. Maximal $\dot{Q}$ increases as a result of an increased maximal SV; however, maximal HR does not typically change

TABLE 2.1   Relationship Between Exercise Intensity and Oxygen Extraction

Exercise intensity	Arterial side	Venous return	Extraction
Rest	20 ml O_2/100 ml blood	14 ml O_2/100 ml blood	6 ml O_2/100 ml blood
Moderate	20 ml O_2/100 ml blood	10 ml O_2/100 ml blood	10 ml O_2/100 ml blood
High	20 ml O_2/100 ml blood	4 ml O_2/100 ml blood	16 ml O_2/100 ml blood

as a result of training. The physiological adaptations responsible for increases in maximal a–$\bar{v}O_2$ difference after training include an increase in both the number of capillaries around muscle cells and the number of mitochondria within muscle cells. The $\dot{V}O_2$max responses to long-term training are further explained in chapter 6.

> **Aerobic endurance training leads to increased maximal oxygen uptake. The changes are related, in part, to an increase in stroke volume and peripheral adaptations (i.e., increased capillary and mitochondrial density).**

CONCLUSION

Knowledge of the cardiovascular and respiratory systems facilitates understanding of gas exchange at rest and during exercise. The information presented in this chapter can be especially useful because it is incumbent upon personal trainers to explain to clients the underlying physiology related to the conditioning program they are performing.

Study Questions

1. What is the approximate pH of human blood at rest?
    A. 6.6
    B. 7.1
    C. 7.4
    D. 7.9

2. The heart is composed of how many chambers?
    A. 1
    B. 2
    C. 3
    D. 4

3. Which of the following occur to facilitate a redistribution of blood flow at the onset of physical exercise?
    I. skeletal muscle arteriole constriction
    II. skeletal muscle arteriole dilation
    III. nonactive organ arteriole constriction
    IV. nonactive organ arteriole dilation
    A. I and III only
    B. II and IV only
    C. II and III only
    D. I and IV only

4. Which of the following refers to the amount of air moving into and out of the lungs at rest during normal breathing?
    A. vital capacity
    B. tidal volume
    C. residual volume
    D. functional residual capacity

5. Which of the following is *incorrect* regarding maximal oxygen uptake ($\dot{V}O_2$max)?
    A. It relates to the heart's maximal ability to eject blood (maximal $\dot{Q}$).
    B. It represents the maximal ability of skeletal muscle to extract oxygen.
    C. It represents the ability to use maximal a–$\bar{v}O_2$ difference to aerobically produce energy.
    D. Higher $\dot{V}O_2$max values are associated with an increased risk of cardiovascular disease, morbidity, and mortality.

CHAPTER 3

Bioenergetics

Carmine Grieco, PhD, and N. Travis Triplett, PhD

After completing this chapter, you will be able to

- understand the basic terminology of bioenergetics and metabolism related to exercise and training,

- discuss the central role of adenosine triphosphate in muscular activity,

- explain the basic energy systems present in the human body and the ability of each to supply energy for various activities,

- discuss the effects of training on the bioenergetics of skeletal muscle,

- recognize the substrates used by each energy system and discuss patterns of substrate use with various types of activities, and

- develop training programs that demonstrate an understanding of human bioenergetics and metabolism, especially the metabolic specificity of training.

To properly and effectively design exercise and training programs, a personal trainer must know how energy is produced and used in biological systems. After defining essential bioenergetics terminology, including the role of adenosine triphosphate (ATP), this chapter deals with the three basic energy systems that are used to replenish ATP in human skeletal muscle. Then we look at how substrates, or substances that come mainly from the foods we eat, are used for various types of activities, including specifics on how each type of substrate is broken down for energy production and how muscle glycogen is replenished. Finally, we discuss the metabolic specificity of training, which relates to the limitations of each energy system and the contribution of each energy system to physical activity.

ESSENTIAL TERMINOLOGY

The ability or capacity to perform physical work requires energy. In the human body, the conversion of chemical energy to mechanical energy is necessary for movement to occur. **Bioenergetics**, or the flow of energy in a biological system, primarily concerns the conversion of food—or large carbohydrate, protein, and fat molecules that contain chemical energy—into biologically usable forms of energy. The breakdown of chemical bonds in these molecules releases the energy necessary to perform physical activity.

The process of breaking down large molecules into smaller molecules, such as the breakdown of carbohydrates into glucose, is generally accompanied by the release of energy and is termed **catabolic**.

The synthesis of larger molecules from smaller molecules can be accomplished using the energy released from catabolic reactions. This building-up process is termed **anabolic**, and an example is the formation of proteins from amino acids. The human body is in a constant state of anabolism and catabolism, which is defined as **metabolism**, or the total of all the catabolic and anabolic reactions in the body. Energy obtained from catabolic reactions is used to drive anabolic reactions through an intermediate molecule, **adenosine triphosphate (ATP)**. Without an adequate supply of ATP, muscular activity and muscle growth would not be possible. Thus, when designing training programs, personal trainers should have a basic understanding of how exercise affects ATP use and resynthesis.

Adenosine triphosphate is composed of adenine, a nitrogen-containing base; ribose, a five-carbon sugar (adenine and ribose together are called adenosine); and three phosphate groups (figure 3.1; 12b). The removal of one phosphate group yields **adenosine diphosphate (ADP)**; removal of a second phosphate group yields adenosine monophosphate (AMP). Adenosine triphosphate is classified as a high-energy molecule because it stores large amounts of energy in the chemical bonds of the two terminal phosphate groups. The breaking of these chemical bonds releases energy to power various reactions in the body. Because muscle cells store ATP only in limited amounts and activity requires a constant supply of ATP to provide the energy needed for muscle actions, ATP-producing processes must also occur in the cell.

ENERGY SYSTEMS

Three energy systems exist in the human body to replenish ATP:

- Phosphagen system (an anaerobic process, i.e., one that occurs in the absence of oxygen)

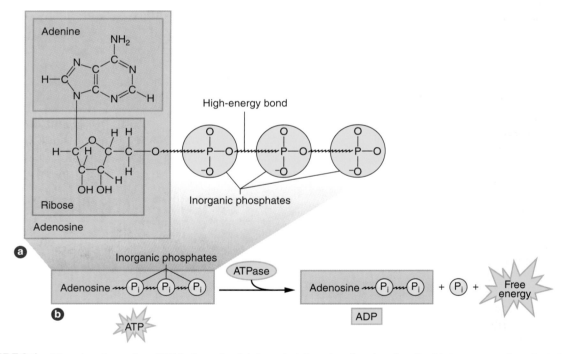

FIGURE 3.1 The structure of an ATP (adenosine triphosphate) molecule, showing the high-energy phosphate bonds.

COMPOSITION OF ADENOSINE TRIPHOSPHATE

- Adenine (a nitrogen-containing base) ———— ■ Together called adenosine
- Ribose (a five-carbon or pentose sugar) ———— ■ Together called triphosphate
- Three phosphate groups ————

- Gylcotic system (two types: fast glycolysis and slow glycolysis; both are also anaerobic)
- Oxidative system (an aerobic process, i.e., one that requires oxygen)

> **Energy stored in the chemical bonds of ATP is used to power muscular activity. The replenishment of ATP in human skeletal muscle is accomplished by three basic energy systems: phosphagen, glycolytic, and oxidative.**

Phosphagen System

The **phosphagen system** is the primary source of ATP for short-term, high-intensity activities (e.g., jumping and sprinting) but is active at the start of all types of exercise regardless of intensity (4). For instance, even during the first few seconds of an easy 5K jog or a moderate-intensity spinning class, the energy for the muscular activity is derived primarily from the phosphagen system. This energy system relies on the chemical reactions of ATP and **creatine phosphate**, both phosphagens, which involve the enzymes myosin adenosine triphosphatase (ATPase) and creatine kinase. **Myosin ATPase** increases the rate of breakdown of ATP to form ADP and inorganic phosphate (P_i) and releases energy, all of which is a catabolic reaction. **Creatine kinase** increases the rate of synthesis of ATP from creatine phosphate and ADP by supplying a phosphate group that combines with ADP to form ATP, which is an anabolic reaction.

These reactions provide energy at a high rate; however, because ATP and creatine phosphate are stored in the muscle in small amounts, the phosphagen system cannot supply enough energy for continuous, long-duration activities. Generally, type II (fast-twitch) muscle fibers contain greater concentrations of phosphagens than type I (slow-twitch) fibers (20).

Creatine kinase activity primarily regulates the breakdown of creatine phosphate. An increase in the muscle cell concentration of ADP promotes creatine kinase activity; an increase in ATP concentration inhibits it (19). At the beginning of exercise, ATP is broken down to ADP, releasing energy for muscular actions. This increase in ADP concentration activates creatine kinase to promote the formation of ATP from the breakdown of creatine phosphate. Creatine kinase activity remains elevated if exercise continues at a high intensity. If exercise is discontinued, or continues at an intensity low enough to allow glycolysis or the oxidative system to supply an adequate amount of ATP for the muscle cells' energy demands, the muscle cell concentration of ATP will likely increase. This increase in ATP then results in a decrease in creatine kinase activity.

Glycolysis

Glycolysis is the breakdown of carbohydrates, either **glycogen** stored in the muscle or glucose delivered in the blood, to produce ATP (4). The ATP provided by glycolysis supplements the phosphagen system initially and then becomes the primary source of ATP for high-intensity muscular activity that lasts up to about 2 minutes, such as keeping a good volley going in a rigorous game of racquetball or running 600 to 800 yards (or meters). The process of glycolysis involves many enzymes controlling a series of chemical reactions (figure 3.2; 12a). The enzymes for glycolysis are located in the cytoplasm of the cells (the sarcoplasm in muscle cells).

Glycolysis is the first step in a multiphase pathway that ultimately converts glucose to ATP, carbon dioxide, and water. As seen in figure 3.2, the process of glycolysis may occur in one of two ways, termed slow (aerobic) and fast (anaerobic) glycolysis. This is not a technically accurate way of describing the bioenergetics of glycolysis because glycolysis itself is not an oxygen-dependent process. Nevertheless, these terms are commonly used to describe the fate of the end products, controlled by cellular energy demands and oxygen availability, when glucose or glycogen is broken down to produce ATP. For example, under conditions of low energy demand (i.e., rest to moderate-intensity exercise), glycolysis will yield three end products: two (glucose) or three (glycogen) ATP molecules, two pyruvate molecules, and two electron transporters (NADH). The ATP can be used immediately for energy, while the pyruvate and NADH enter the mitochondria to continue the process of extracting energy via the Krebs cycle (pyruvate) and electron transport chain (NADH) (figure 3.2). However, during times of intense muscular action, the aerobic system (i.e., oxidative phosphorylation) is not capable of generating a sufficient quantity of ATP to maintain the given activity level or intensity. This

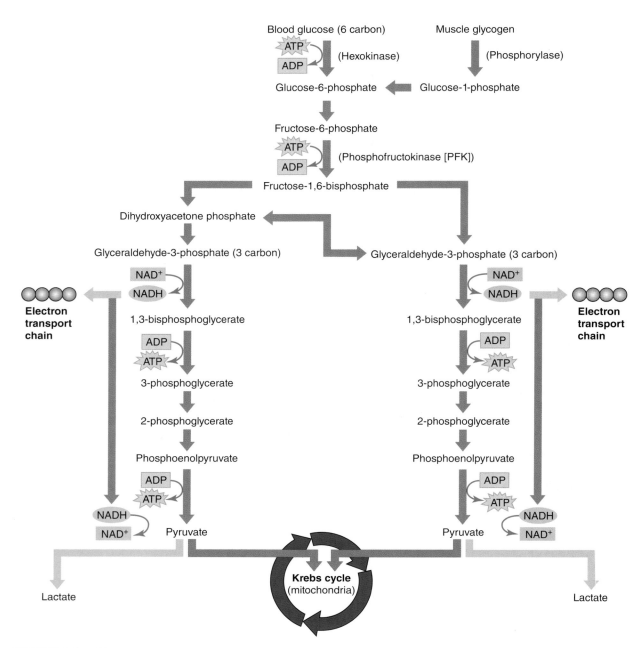

FIGURE 3.2 Glycolysis. ATP = adenosine triphosphate; ADP = adenosine diphosphate; NAD⁺, NADH = nicotinamide adenine dinucleotide.

effectively creates an energetic bottleneck, resulting in pyruvate molecules being converted into lactate via the enzymatic action of lactate dehydrogenase (LDH). Therefore, the end product of fast glycolysis is lactate (equation 3.1), while the end product of slow glycolysis is pyruvate (equation 3.2). The defining factor that differentiates slow from fast glycolysis is whether the resulting pyruvate molecule will be converted to lactate or remain as pyruvate and subsequently enter into the mitochondria.

The net reaction for fast (anaerobic) glycolysis may be summarized as follows:

$$\text{Glucose} + 2\,P_i + 2\,\text{ADP} \rightarrow 2\,\text{lactate} + 2\,\text{ATP} + H_2O \tag{3.1}$$

The net reaction for slow (aerobic) glycolysis may be summarized as follows:

$$\text{Glucose} + 2\,P_i + 2\,\text{ADP} + 2\,\text{NAD}^+ \rightarrow 2\,\text{pyruvate} + 2\,\text{ATP} + 2\,\text{NADH} + 2\,H_2O \quad (3.2)$$

Energy Yield of Glycolysis

Glycolysis produces a net of two molecules of ATP from one molecule of glucose. However, if glycogen (the stored form of glucose) is used, there is a net production of three ATPs because the reaction of phosphorylating (adding a phosphate group to) glucose, which requires one ATP, is bypassed (4) (figure 3.2).

Glycolysis Regulation

Glycolysis is stimulated during intense muscular activity by ADP, P_i, ammonia, and a slight decrease in pH and is strongly stimulated by AMP (3, 4). It is inhibited by the markedly lowered pH that may be observed during periods of inadequate oxygen supply and by increased levels of ATP, creatine phosphate, citrate, and free fatty acids (3, 4) at rest. The phosphorylation of glucose by hexokinase (see figure 3.2) primarily controls glycolysis; but we must also consider the rate of glycogen breakdown to glucose, which is controlled by phosphorylase (figure 3.2), in the regulation of glycolysis (3, 4). In other words, if glycogen is not being broken down into glucose quickly enough and the supply of free glucose has already been depleted, glycolysis will be slowed.

Another important consideration in the regulation of any series of reactions is the **rate-limiting step** (i.e., the slowest reaction in the series). The rate-limiting step in glycolysis is the conversion of fructose-6-phosphate to fructose-1,6-biphosphate (figure 3.2), a reaction controlled by the enzyme phosphofructokinase (PFK). Thus the activity of PFK is the primary factor in the regulation of the rate of glycolysis. Activation of the phosphagen energy system stimulates glycolysis (by stimulating PFK) to contribute to the energy production of high-intensity exercise (4). Ammonia produced during high-intensity exercise as a result of increased AMP or amino acid deamination (removing the amino group of the amino acid molecule) can also stimulate PFK.

Blood Lactate

Fast glycolysis occurs during periods of reduced oxygen availability in the muscle cells, typically during higher-intensity activity, and results in the formation of the end product **lactate**. Lactate is the conjugate base of lactic acid, meaning it has one less hydrogen ion (H^+). There is debate within the scientific community as to whether lactic acid is even produced within the human body as once believed. Thus, muscular fatigue experienced during exercise, previously thought to be associated with high concentrations of lactic acid in the muscle tissue, is actually a result of decreased tissue pH from metabolic by-products, such as H^+ ions, that are acidic in nature as compared with lactate (a base) (3, 18).

As pH decreases (becomes more acidic), it is believed to inhibit glycolytic reactions and directly interfere with muscle action, possibly by inhibiting calcium binding to troponin or by interfering with actin–myosin crossbridge formation (8). Also, the decrease in pH levels inhibits the enzyme activity of the cell's energy systems. The overall effect is a decrease in available energy and muscle force during exercise. Lactate, however, is used as an energy substrate, especially in type I and cardiac muscle fibers (3). It is also used in **gluconeogenesis**, the formation of glucose from non-sugar substances, during extended exercise and recovery (9). Although lactate does not contribute to muscular fatigue, monitoring its clearance from blood can indicate a person's ability to recover. Lactate can be cleared by oxidation within the muscle fiber in which it was produced, or it can be transported in the blood to other muscle fibers to be oxidized (3). Lactate can also be transported in the blood to the liver, where it is converted to glucose via gluconeogenesis. This process is referred to as the **Cori cycle** and is depicted in figure 3.3 (12a).

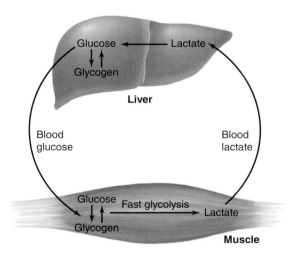

FIGURE 3.3 The Cori cycle.

Normally there is a low concentration of lactate in blood and muscle. The reported normal range of lactate concentration in blood is 0.5 to 2.2 mmol/L at rest (18, 22). Lactate production increases with increasing exercise intensity and appears to depend on muscle fiber type. The higher rate of lactate production by type II muscle fibers may reflect a concentration or activity of glycolytic enzymes that is higher than that of type I muscle fibers (18, 22).

Blood lactate concentrations normally return to preexercise values within an hour after activity (4, 22). Light activity during the postexercise period has been shown to increase lactate clearance rates, with aerobically trained and anaerobically trained individuals having faster lactate clearance rates than untrained people (22). Peak blood lactate concentrations occur approximately 5 minutes after the cessation of exercise, a delay frequently attributed to the time required to transport lactate from the tissue to the blood (22).

It is widely accepted that there are specific inflection points in the lactate accumulation curve (figure 3.4; 7a) as exercise intensity increases (4). The exercise intensity or relative intensity at which blood lactate begins an abrupt increase above the baseline concentration has been termed the **lactate threshold (LT)** (12). The LT represents an increasing reliance on anaerobic mechanisms. The LT typically begins at 50% to 60% of maximal oxygen uptake in untrained subjects and at 70% to 80% in trained subjects (12). A second increase in the rate of lactate accumulation has been noted at higher relative intensities of exercise. This second point of inflection, termed the **onset of blood lactate accumulation (OBLA)**, generally occurs when the concentration of blood lactate is near 4 mmol/L (12). The breaks in the lactate accumulation curve may correspond to the points at which intermediate and large motor units are recruited during increasing exercise intensities. The muscle cells associated with large motor units are typically type II fibers, which are particularly suited for anaerobic metabolism and lactate production.

It has been suggested that training at intensities near or above the LT or OBLA changes the LT and OBLA so that lactate accumulation occurs later at a higher exercise intensity (12). This shift probably occurs as a result of several factors but particularly as a result of the increased mitochondrial content, which allows for greater production of ATP through aerobic mechanisms. The shift allows the individual to perform at higher percentages of maximal oxygen uptake without as much lactate accumulation in the blood (4).

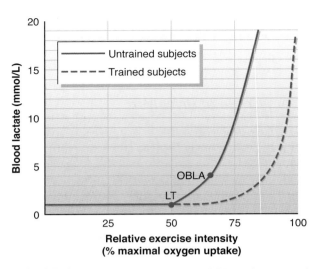

FIGURE 3.4 Lactate threshold (LT) and onset of blood lactate accumulation (OBLA).

Reprinted by permission from National Strength and Conditioning Association (2008, p. 28).

Oxidative (Aerobic) System

The **oxidative system**, the primary source of ATP at rest and during aerobic activities, uses primarily carbohydrates and fats as substrates (4). Clients who are walking on a treadmill, doing water aerobics, or participating in a yoga class are relying primarily on the oxidative system. Protein is normally not metabolized significantly except during long-term starvation and long steady-state bouts (>90 minutes) of exercise (23). At rest, approximately 70% of the ATP produced is derived from fats and 30% from carbohydrates. After the onset of activity, as the intensity of the exercise increases, there is a shift in substrate preference from fats to carbohydrates. During high-intensity aerobic exercise, almost 100% of the energy is derived from carbohydrates if an adequate supply is available. However, during prolonged, submaximal, steady-state work there is a gradual shift from carbohydrates back to fats and protein as energy substrates (4).

Glucose and Glycogen Oxidation

As previously discussed, the oxidative metabolism of blood glucose and muscle glycogen begins with glycolysis. If oxygen is present in sufficient quantities, then the end product of glycolysis, **pyruvate**, is not converted to lactate but is transported to the mitochondria within the cell. When pyruvate enters the mitochondria, it is converted to acetyl-CoA (CoA stands for coenzyme A) and can then enter the **Krebs cycle** for further ATP production. Also transported there are two molecules of NADH produced during the glycolytic reactions. The Krebs cycle, another series of reactions, produces two ATPs indirectly from guanine triphosphate (GTP) for each molecule of glucose (figure 3.5; 12a). Also produced in the Krebs cycle from one molecule of glucose are an additional six molecules of NADH and two molecules of reduced flavin adenine dinucleotide ($FADH_2$). The number of ATPs and amount of NADH and $FADH_2$ are different if fat or protein enters the Krebs cycle, although all of these substrates must be converted to acetyl-CoA before entering the Krebs cycle.

These molecules transport hydrogen atoms to the **electron transport chain (ETC)** to be used to produce ATP from ADP (4). The ETC uses the NADH and $FADH_2$ molecules to rephosphorylate ADP to ATP (figure 3.6; 12a). The hydrogen atoms are passed down the chain, via a series of electron carriers known as **cytochromes**, to form a concentration gradient of protons to provide energy for ATP production, with oxygen serving as the final electron acceptor (resulting in the formation of water). Because NADH and $FADH_2$ enter the ETC at different sites, they differ in their ability to produce ATP. One molecule of NADH can produce three molecules of ATP, whereas one molecule of $FADH_2$ can produce only two molecules of ATP. The production of ATP during this process is referred to as **oxidative phosphorylation**. The oxidative system, beginning with glycolysis, results in the production of approximately 38 ATPs from the degradation of one glucose molecule (4). Table 3.1 summarizes the ATP yield of these processes.

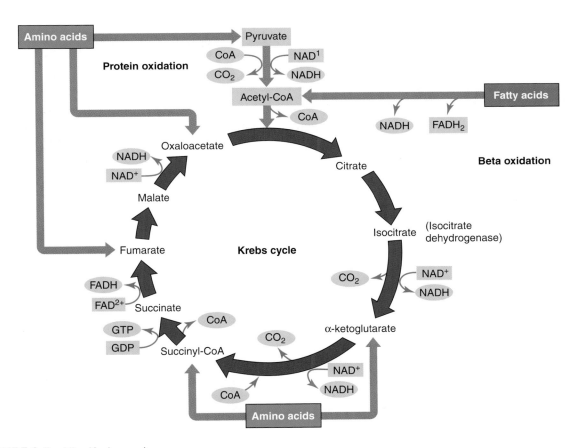

FIGURE 3.5 The Krebs cycle.

CoA = coenzyme A; FAD^{2+}, $FADH_2$ = flavin adenine dinucleotide; GDP = guanine diphosphate; GTP = guanine triphosphate; NAD^+, NADH = nicotinamide adenine dinucleotide.

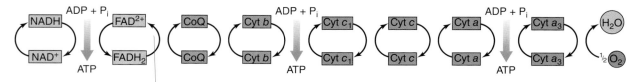

FIGURE 3.6   The electron transport chain.

CoQ = coenzyme Q; Cyt = cytochrome; ATP = adenosine triphosphate; ADP = adenosine diphosphate; P_i = inorganic phosphate; NADH, NAD^+ = nicotinamide adenine dinucleotide; $FADH_2$, FAD^{2+} = flavin adenine dinucleotide; H_2O = water; O_2 = oxygen.

Reprinted by permission from National Strength and Conditioning Association (2016, p. 52).

TABLE 3.1   Total Energy Yield From the Oxidation of One Glucose Molecule

Process	ATP production
SLOW GLYCOLYSIS	
Substrate-level phosphorylation	4
Oxidative phosphorylation: 2 NADH (3 ATP each)	6
KREBS CYCLE (TWO ROTATIONS THROUGH THE KREBS CYCLE PER GLUCOSE)	
Substrate-level phosphorylation	2
Oxidative phosphorylation: 8 NADH (3 ATP each)	24
Via GTP: 2 $FADH_2$ (2 ATP each)	4
Total	**40***

ATP = adenosine triphosphate; NADH = nicotinamide adenine dinucleotide; GTP = guanine triphosphate; $FADH_2$ = flavin adenine dinucleotide.

*Glycolysis consumes 2 ATP (if starting with glucose), so net ATP production is 40 – 2 = 38. This figure may also be reported as 36 ATP depending on which shuttle system is used to transport the NADH to the mitochondria.

Fat Oxidation

Fats can also be used by the oxidative energy system. Triglycerides stored in fat cells can be broken down by an enzyme known as **hormone-sensitive lipase**. This enzyme releases free fatty acids from the fat cells into the blood, where they can circulate and enter muscle fibers (4, 16). Additionally, limited quantities of triglycerides are stored within the muscle, along with a form of hormone-sensitive lipase, to serve as a source of free fatty acids within the muscle (16). Free fatty acids enter the mitochondria, where they undergo **beta oxidation**, a series of reactions in which the free fatty acids are broken down, resulting in the formation of acetyl-CoA and hydrogen atoms (figure 3.5). The acetyl-CoA enters the Krebs cycle directly, and the hydrogen atoms are carried by NADH and $FADH_2$ to the ETC (4). An example of the ATP produced from a typical triglyceride molecule is shown in table 3.2.

Protein Oxidation

Although not a significant source of energy for most activities, protein can be broken down into its constituent amino acids by various metabolic processes. These amino acids can then be converted into glucose (via gluconeogenesis), pyruvate, or various Krebs cycle intermediates to produce ATP (figure 3.5). The contribution of amino acids to the production of ATP has been estimated to be minimal during short-term exercise but may amount to 3% to 18% of the energy requirements during prolonged activity (17). The major amino acids that are oxidized in skeletal muscle appear to be the branched-chain amino acids (leucine, isoleucine, and valine), although alanine, aspartate, and glutamate may also be used (17). The nitrogen-containing waste products of amino acid breakdown are eliminated through the formation of urea and small amounts of ammonia, which end up in the urine. The elimination of ammonia is important because ammonia is toxic and is associated with fatigue (3, 4).

TABLE 3.2 Total Energy Yield From the Oxidation of One (18-Carbon) Triglyceride Molecule

Process	ATP production
One molecule of glycerol	22
18-CARBON FATTY ACID METABOLISM*	
147 ATP per fatty acid × 3 three fatty acids per triglyceride molecule	441
Total	**463**

ATP = adenosine triphosphate.

*Other triglycerides that contain different amounts of carbons will yield more or less ATP.

Oxidative (Aerobic) System Regulation

The rate-limiting step in the Krebs cycle (figure 3.5) is the conversion of isocitrate to a-ketoglutarate, a reaction controlled by the enzyme isocitrate dehydrogenase. Isocitrate dehydrogenase is stimulated by ADP and normally inhibited by ATP. The reactions that produce NADH or $FADH_2$ also influence the regulation of the Krebs cycle. If NAD^+ and FAD^{2+} are not available in sufficient quantities to accept hydrogen, the rate of the Krebs cycle is reduced. Also, when GTP accumulates, the concentration of succinyl CoA increases, which inhibits the initial reaction (oxaloacetate + acetyl-CoA → citrate + CoA) of the Krebs cycle. The ETC is inhibited by ATP and stimulated by ADP (4). Figure 3.7 presents a simplified overview of the metabolism of fat, carbohydrate, and protein (12a).

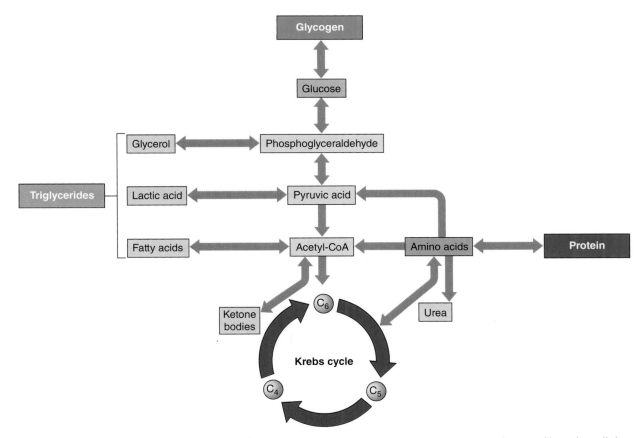

FIGURE 3.7 The metabolism of fat, carbohydrate, and protein share some common pathways. Note that all three are reduced to acetyl-CoA and enter the Krebs cycle.

Reprinted by permission from National Strength and Conditioning Association (2016, p. 54).

> All three energy systems are active at a given time; however, the extent to which each is used depends primarily on the intensity of the activity and secondarily on its duration.

Energy Production and Capacity

The phosphagen, glycolytic, and oxidative energy systems differ in their ability to supply energy for activities of various intensities and durations (tables 3.3 and 3.4). Exercise **intensity** is defined as a level of muscular activity that can be quantified in terms of power output, with **power** defined as the amount of physical work performed for a particular duration of time.

Activities such as resistance training and serving in tennis that are high in intensity, and thus have a high-power output, require rapidly supplied energy and rely almost entirely on the energy supplied by the phosphagen system. Activities that are of lower intensity but longer duration, such as a 10-mile (16.1 km) bike ride or swimming laps in the pool for an hour, require a large energy supply and rely on the energy supplied by the oxidative energy system (table 3.3). The primary source of energy for activities between these two extremes differs depending on the intensity and duration of the event (table 3.4). In general, short, high-intensity activities (e.g., jumping or kicking and punching moves in cardio kickboxing) rely on the phosphagen energy system and fast glycolysis. As the intensity decreases and the duration increases, the emphasis gradually shifts to slow glycolysis and the oxidative energy system (4, 20).

The duration of the activity also influences which energy system is used. Specific exercises within a prescribed program can range in duration from approximately 5 seconds (e.g., one set of bench presses at 90% of the 1RM) to more than an hour (e.g., low-intensity, extended-duration treadmill walking). If an individual makes a best effort (an effort that results in the best possible performance for a given activity), the time considerations shown in table 3.4 are reasonable (4, 10).

At no time, during either exercise or rest, does any single energy system provide the complete supply of energy. During exercise, the degree to which anaerobic and oxidative systems contribute to the energy being produced is determined primarily by the exercise intensity and secondarily by exercise duration (4, 20).

In general, there is an inverse relationship between the relative rate and total amount of ATP that a given energy system can produce. As a result, the phosphagen energy system primarily supplies ATP for high-intensity activities of short duration (e.g., sprinting across a football field), the glycolytic system for moderate- to high-intensity activities of short to medium duration (e.g., running once around a track), and the oxidative system for low-intensity activities of long duration (e.g., completing a 20-mile [32.2 km] bike ride).

> The phosphagen energy system primarily supplies ATP for high-intensity activities of short duration, the glycolytic system for moderate- to high-intensity activities of short to medium duration, and the oxidative system for low-intensity activities of long duration.

TABLE 3.3 Rankings of Rate and Capacity of Adenosine Triphosphate (ATP) Production

System	Rate of ATP production	Capacity of ATP production
Phosphagen	1	5
Fast glycolysis	2	4
Slow glycolysis	3	3
Oxidation of carbohydrate	4	2
Oxidation of fat and protein	5	1

1 = fastest or greatest; 5 = slowest or least; ATP = adenosine triphosphate.

TABLE 3.4   Effect of Event Duration on Primary Energy System Used

Duration of event	Intensity of event	Primary energy system(s)
0 to 6 s	Very intense	Phosphagen
6 to 30 s	Intense	Phosphagen and fast glycolysis
30 s to 2 min	Heavy	Fast glycolysis
2 to 3 min	Moderate	Fast glycolysis and oxidative system
>3 min	Light	Oxidative system

Metabolic Specificity of Training

Appropriate exercise intensities and rest intervals can target specific energy systems during training for specific athletic events or training goals (4). Few sports or physical activities require maximal sustained-effort exercise to exhaustion or near exhaustion. Most sports and training activities (such as football, cardio kickboxing, spinning, and resistance training) are intermittent in nature and therefore produce metabolic profiles that are very similar to that for a series of high-intensity, constant- or near-constant-effort exercise bouts interspersed with rest periods. In this type of exercise, the power output (a measure of exercise intensity) produced during each exercise bout is much greater than the maximal power output that can be sustained using aerobic energy sources. Chapters 15, 16, and 17 discuss training methods that allow appropriate metabolic systems to be stressed.

SUBSTRATE DEPLETION AND REPLETION

Energy **substrates**—molecules that provide starting materials for bioenergetic reactions, including phosphagens (ATP and creatine phosphate), glucose, glycogen, lactate, free fatty acids, and amino acids—can be selectively depleted during the performance of activities of various intensities and durations. Subsequently, the amount of energy that can be produced by the bioenergetic systems decreases. Fatigue experienced during many activities is frequently associated with the depletion of phosphagens (3, 20) and glycogen (3, 4, 11); the depletion of substrates such as free fatty acids, lactate, and amino acids typically does not occur to the extent that performance is limited. Consequently, the depletion and repletion pattern of phosphagens and glycogen after physical activity is important in exercise bioenergetics.

Phosphagens

Fatigue during exercise appears to be at least partially related to the decrease in phosphagens. Phosphagen concentrations in muscle are more rapidly depleted as a result of high-intensity anaerobic exercise than of aerobic exercise (3, 20). Creatine phosphate can decrease markedly (50% to 70%) during the first stage (5-30 seconds) of high-intensity exercise and can be almost eliminated as a result of very intense exercise to exhaustion (3, 6, 14, 19). Muscle ATP concentrations do not decrease by more than about 60% from initial values, however, even during very intense exercise (3). It is also important to note that dynamic muscle actions, such as a complete repetition of a weight training exercise, use more metabolic energy and typically deplete phosphagens to a greater extent than do isometric muscle actions, such as arm wrestling, in which there is no visible shortening of the muscle (3).

Postexercise phosphagen repletion can occur in a relatively short period; complete resynthesis of ATP appears to occur within 3 to 5 minutes, and complete creatine phosphate resynthesis can occur within 8 minutes (3, 19). Repletion of phosphagens occurs largely as a result of aerobic metabolism, although fast glycolysis can contribute to ATP resynthesis after high-intensity exercise (3, 19).

Supplemental strategies can also be used to increase the intramuscular repletion of the phosphagen system. **Creatine**, a naturally occurring organic compound found primarily in red meat, milk, and seafood (7, 14), is one of the most commonly used nutritional ergogenic agents (14).

Glycogen

Limited stores of glycogen are available for exercise. Approximately 300 to 400 g of glycogen is stored in the body's total muscle, and about 70 to 100 g is stored in the liver (13). Resting concentrations of liver and muscle glycogen can be influenced by training and dietary manipulations (13). Research suggests that both anaerobic training, including sprinting and resistance training, and typical aerobic endurance training can increase resting muscle glycogen concentration.

The rate of glycogen depletion is related to exercise intensity (13). Muscle glycogen is a more important energy source than liver glycogen during moderate- and high-intensity exercise; liver glycogen appears to be more important during low-intensity exercise, and its contribution to metabolic processes increases with duration of exercise. Increases in relative exercise intensity of maximal oxygen uptake result in increases in the rate of muscle **glycogenolysis**, which increases available glycogen for the glycolysis pathway (4). Although fat oxidation predominates at rest through light to moderate exercise (1), glycogen becomes the preferred fuel source at intensities above about 60% to 75% of maximal oxygen uptake (21). This phenomenon is referred to as the **crossover concept** (5). Because glycogen (particularly intramuscular glycogen) is the preferred fuel source during high-intensity exercise and is stored in relatively small amounts in the human body, the availability of glycogen (either from intramuscular stores or derived from the liver) can become a limiting factor to exercise and is directly related to fatigue. In fact, nearly all of the glycogen content of some muscle cells can become depleted as a result of a 120-minute cycle session at 65% peak oxygen uptake followed by 1-minute sprints at 120% peak oxygen uptake (11).

Resistance training can also cause substantial depletion of muscle glycogen, with decreases of 24% to 40% (13). As with other types of dynamic exercise, the rate of muscle glycogenolysis depends on duration, intensity, and volume, with higher volumes using moderate loads having the greatest impact, especially in type II fibers (13).

The process of muscle glycogen resynthesis is related to postexercise carbohydrate ingestion, begins immediately after exercise, and is most rapid during the first five to six hours of recovery (11). Some muscle glycogen resynthesis will occur even in the absence of ingested carbohydrate; however, to optimize intramuscular glycogen stores, carbohydrate ingestion during the postexercise period is considered critical. Repletion appears to be optimal if 1.2 g of carbohydrate per kilogram of body weight is ingested approximately every two hours after exercise (2). To optimize glycogen resynthesis, the first feeding should occur at the earliest opportunity postexercise, as a

delay may reduce maximal intramuscular glycogen storage (15). Muscle glycogen may be completely replenished within 24 hours, provided sufficient carbohydrate is ingested (11). However, if the exercise has a high eccentric component (associated with exercise-induced muscle damage), more time may be required to completely replenish muscle glycogen.

> **Glycogen is a vital energy source, particularly for high-intensity exercise. Glycogen storage within the body is limited to about 500 g (about 2,000 kcal), and glycogen depletion is associated with fatigue. Glycogen repletion can occur rapidly but may take up to 24 hours for complete resynthesis.**

OXYGEN UPTAKE AND THE AEROBIC AND ANAEROBIC CONTRIBUTIONS TO EXERCISE

Oxygen uptake (or consumption) is a measure of a person's ability to take in and use oxygen. The higher the oxygen uptake, the more fit the person is thought to be. During low-intensity exercise with a constant power output, oxygen uptake increases for the first few minutes until a steady state of uptake (oxygen demand equals oxygen consumption) is reached (figure 3.8; 12a). At the start of the exercise bout, however, some of the energy must be supplied through anaerobic mechanisms (4, 12). This anaerobic contribution to the total energy cost of exercise is termed the **oxygen deficit**. After exercise, oxygen uptake remains above preexercise levels for a period of time that varies according to the intensity and length of the exercise. Postexercise oxygen uptake has been termed the **oxygen debt**, or the **excess postexercise oxygen consumption (EPOC)**. The EPOC is the oxygen uptake above resting values used to restore the body to the preexercise condition. There are only small to moderate relationships between the oxygen deficit and the EPOC; the oxygen deficit may influence the size of the EPOC, but the two are not equal (4, 12).

Anaerobic mechanisms provide much of the energy for work if the exercise intensity is above the maximal oxygen uptake that a person can attain (figure 3.9; 12a). For instance, if a client who was not used to that type of activity jumped right into an advanced

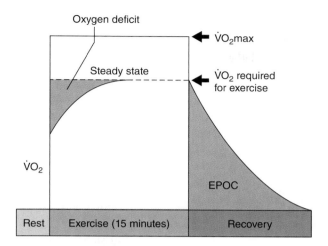

FIGURE 3.8 Low-intensity, steady-state exercise metabolism: 75% of maximal oxygen uptake ($\dot{V}O_2$max). EPOC = excess postexercise oxygen consumption; $\dot{V}O_2$ = oxygen uptake.

Reprinted by permission from National Strength and Conditioning Association (2016, p. 57).

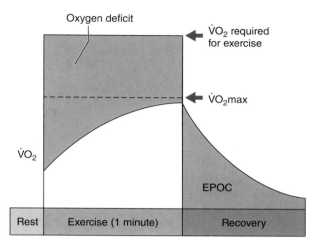

FIGURE 3.9 High-intensity, non–steady-state exercise metabolism (80% of maximum power output). The required $\dot{V}O_2$ here is the oxygen uptake that would be required to sustain the exercise if such an uptake were possible to attain. Because it is not, the oxygen deficit lasts for the duration of the exercise. EPOC = excess postexercise oxygen consumption; $\dot{V}O_2$max = maximal oxygen uptake.

Reprinted by permission from National Strength and Conditioning Association (2016, p. 58).

spinning class, most of the energy would be supplied by anaerobic mechanisms. Generally, as the contribution of anaerobic mechanisms supporting the exercise increases, the exercise duration decreases (4).

PRACTICAL APPLICATION OF ENERGY SYSTEMS

The concept of energy systems can seem very abstract; but with only a basic understanding of the general time frames of energy system use, one can determine the primary energy system that will be taxed in various types of exercise or activities. The main thing to remember is that the higher the exercise intensity, the shorter the amount of time the exercise can be performed and the greater the reliance on the fastest ATP-producing energy systems, which also have the least capacity. The opposite is also true; the lower the exercise intensity, the longer that exercise can be performed, and the greater the reliance on the slower ATP-producing energy systems. In this case, ATP can be produced as long as the body has a good supply of muscle glycogen and fatty acids.

When assessing clients' needs, it is important to consider their training goals from the energy system perspective so that exercise selection and the manner of performing those exercises can be optimized.

Rest periods between sets and exercises also play a factor because longer rest periods allow for more complete ATP resynthesis from the phosphagen system. For example, if a client wants to improve his or her ability to get to the first base marker in the company softball game, repeat activities that stress the phosphagen system are suggested (sprints, intervals on the bike, exercises to improve leg strength, and overall lower body power exercises). If the client wants to train for a 20-mile (32.2 km) hike in the Alps, activities that stress the oxidative system are best, such as work on almost any cardio equipment for extended periods.

> **All three energy systems have the capacity to adapt based on the principle of training specificity. Challenging the glycolytic system via repeated bouts of moderate- to high-intensity activity, for example, will alter lactate production and result in an improvement in lactate threshold (LT).**

CONCLUSION

One can design more productive training programs through an understanding of how energy is produced during various types of exercise and how energy production can be modified by specific training regimens. Which energy system is used to supply energy for muscular action is determined primarily by the intensity and secondarily by the duration of exercise. Metabolic responses and the subsequent training adaptations are largely regulated by those characteristics (i.e., intensity and duration) and form the basis of metabolic specificity of exercise and training. This principle of specificity allows for enhanced physical adaptation and program results through the implementation of precise training programs.

Study Questions

1. Which of the following is *not* a characteristic of bioenergetics?
   A. breakdown of food
   B. conversion of chemical energy to mechanical energy
   C. conversion of mechanical energy to chemical energy
   D. breakdown of chemical bonds

2. How many molecules of ATP are produced from glycolysis of one molecule of glucose *in blood*?
   A. 1
   B. 2
   C. 3
   D. 4

3. Which of the following energy systems is the primary source of energy at rest and during aerobic activities?
   A. phosphagen system
   B. anaerobic glycolysis
   C. oxidative
   D. anaerobic lipolysis

4. Glycogen becomes the preferred fuel source at intensities above about _____ of maximal oxygen uptake.
   A. 30%-40%
   B. 60%-75%
   C. 80%-90%
   D. 90%-100%

5. When relying on the slower ATP-producing energy systems, ATP can be produced as long as the body has a good supply of:_____.
   I. muscle glycogen
   II. fatty acids
   III. protein
   IV. creatine phosphate
   A. I only
   B. III and IV only
   C. I, II and III only
   D. II and IV only

CHAPTER 4

Biomechanics

Douglas W. Powell, PhD, and Megan A. Bryanton Jones, PhD

After completing this chapter, you will be able to

- describe human movements using appropriate anatomical and mechanical terminology,

- apply mechanical concepts to human movement problems,

- understand the factors contributing to human strength and power,

- determine the muscle actions involved in movement tasks, and

- analyze biomechanical aspects of resistance exercises.

Success as a personal trainer requires expertise in a number of scientific subdisciplines. Among these are functional anatomy and biomechanics. In designing exercise programs for performance enhancement and injury prevention, personal trainers must understand human anatomy from a functional perspective and be able to apply biomechanical principles to meet their clients' goals.

Functional anatomy is the study of how body systems cooperate to perform certain tasks (33). Muscles do not always work according to their anatomical classification (36). For example, the quadriceps muscle group is anatomically defined as a knee extensor. However, these muscles actually control movement during the eccentric, or "down," phase of the squat—even though the knee is flexing. To design effective exercise interventions, it is necessary to know which muscles are active during which activities and match them with the appropriate exercises.

Biomechanics is a field of study that applies mechanical principles to understand the function of living organisms and systems. With respect to human movement, several areas of biomechanics are relevant, including movement mechanics, fluid mechanics, material mechanics, and joint mechanics. Although fluid, material, and joint mechanics have important applications to human movement and are mentioned briefly, the focus of this chapter is on movement mechanics and applicable mechanical concepts.

Understanding these concepts is essential for selecting effective exercises. In the first part of the chapter, we define mechanical terms and concepts in an unambiguous way; these definitions may differ from the everyday meanings of the terms. Although the human body acts like a mechanical system during movement, the second part of this chapter examines how our biological structure creates unique mechanical properties. The third part of the chapter combines knowledge of mechanics and anatomy, detailing a formula for determining which muscles are active during a movement. In the last section, the biomechanics of resistance exercise is explored.

The authors would like to acknowledge the significant contributions of William C. Whiting, Sean P. Flanagan, and Everett Harman to this chapter.

MECHANICAL FOUNDATIONS

Mechanics is the branch of physics that deals with the effects of forces and energy on bodies. This section on mechanical foundations focuses on mechanical terminology and concepts that are relevant to human movements involved in strength and conditioning programs.

Mechanical Terminology and Principles

As with every specialized area of study, biomechanics has its own vocabulary. Many of the terms defined and applied here have specific meanings, sometimes different from the meanings of the terms as used by the lay public. Terms such as *strength*, *work*, *power*, and *energy* have common meanings that may differ from scientific definitions and may incorrectly be used interchangeably. The chapter defines each of these terms, along with others.

In biomechanics, for example, the term **body** refers to any collection of matter. Thus in mechanical terms, body may refer to the entire human body, a limb segment (e.g., a thigh or forearm), or some other collection of matter (e.g., a piece of chalk). Mechanically speaking, there are two basic types of movement: **linear motion**, in which a body moves in a straight line (**rectilinear motion**) or along a curved path (**curvilinear motion**), and **angular motion** (also **rotational motion**) in which a body rotates about a fixed line known as the **axis of rotation** (also **fulcrum** or **pivot**). Many human movements (e.g., running, jumping, throwing) involve a combination of linear and angular motion in what is called **general motion**. It is often useful to think about these movements occurring in an anatomical plane (i.e., in the **frontal**, **sagittal**, or **transverse plane**; figure 4.1). Major movements of the joints are presented in figure 4.2 (16), and we will refer to them throughout the chapter.

The study of movement from a descriptive perspective *without* regard to the underlying forces is termed **kinematics**. Kinematic assessment involves the spatial and timing characteristics of movement using five primary variables: timing, or temporal, measurements (e.g., an athlete took 0.8 seconds to lift the barbell); position or location (e.g., a client held his or her arm in 90 degrees of abduction); displacement (e.g., a trainee moved his or her elbow through 60 degrees of flexion); velocity (e.g., a volleyball player extended his

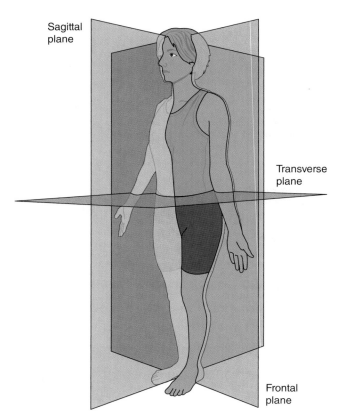

FIGURE 4.1 The three major planes of the human body in the anatomical position.

or her knee at 600 degrees per second while jumping); and **acceleration**, or change in velocity per unit time (e.g., gravity accelerated a jumper's body toward the ground at 9.81 m/s^2).

In contrast to kinematics, movement assessment *with* respect to the forces involved is called **kinetics**. Kinetic assessment involves the characteristics of the forces creating or controlling movement using four primary variables: force production (i.e., the magnitude of resistance overcome during an exercise), the work performed (i.e., the magnitude of force produced over a distance), power (i.e., the rate at which force is applied to the resistance), and torque (i.e., the rotational effect of a force). Forces can be thought of as the causes of motion. Human movement happens as a result of mechanical factors that produce and control movement from the inside (internal forces such as muscle forces) or affect the body from the outside (external forces such as gravity). Many of the mechanical measurements (e.g., force, torque) presented in the next sections are kinetic variables.

Wrist—sagittal
ADL: cooking

Flexion
Exercise: wrist curl
Sport: basketball free throw

Extension
Exercise: wrist extension
Sport: racquetball backhand

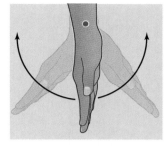
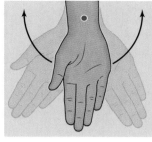

Wrist—frontal
ADL: brushing teeth

Ulnar deviation
Exercise: specific wrist curl
Sport: baseball bat swing

Radial deviation
Exercise: specific wrist curl
Sport: golf backswing

Elbow—sagittal
ADL: feeding oneself

Flexion
Exercise: biceps curl
Sport: bowling

Extension
Exercise: triceps pushdown
Sport: shot put

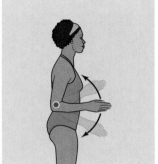
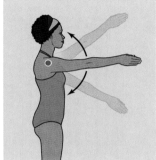

Shoulder—sagittal
ADL: putting dishes away or reaching for an object on a shelf

Flexion
Exercise: front shoulder raise
Sport: boxing uppercut punch

Extension
Exercise: neutral-grip seated row
Sport: freestyle swimming stroke

Shoulder—frontal
ADL: waving hello
or washing windows

Adduction
Exercise: wide-grip lat pulldown
Sport: swimming breast stroke

Abduction
Exercise: wide-grip shoulder press
Sport: springboard diving

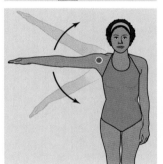
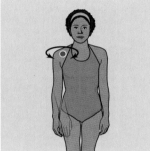

Shoulder—transverse
ADL: turning a doorknob
or screwing in a lightbulb

Internal rotation
Exercise: arm wrestle movement (with dumbbell or cable)
Sport: baseball pitch

External rotation
Exercise: reverse arm wrestle movement
Sport: karate block

Shoulder—transverse
ADL: opening or closing a door
(upper arm to 90° to trunk)

Horizontal adduction
Exercise: dumbbell chest fly
Sport: tennis forehand

Horizontal abduction
Exercise: bent-over lateral raise
Sport: tennis backhand

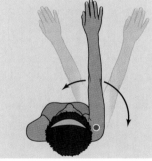
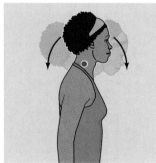

Neck—sagittal
ADL: dressing oneself (buttoning up a shirt or pants) or avoiding an obstacle while walking

Flexion
Exercise: neck machine
Sport: somersault

Extension
Exercise: dynamic back bridge
Sport: back flip

Neck—transverse
ADL: checking the blind spot while driving

Left rotation
Exercise: manual resistance
Sport: wrestling movement

Right rotation
Exercise: manual resistance
Sport: wrestling movement

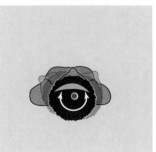
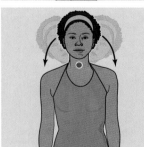

Neck—frontal
ADL: getting out of bed or lifting head off a pillow

Left lateral flexion
Exercise: neck machine
Sport: slalom skiing

Right lateral flexion
Exercise: neck machine
Sport: slalom skiing

FIGURE 4.2 Major body movements. Planes of movement are relative to the body in the anatomical position. The list includes common exercises that provide resistance to the movements and related physical activities.

ADL = activity of daily living.

(continued)

Trunk—sagittal
ADL: bending over
to tie shoes

Flexion
Exercise: sit-up
Sport: javelin throw
follow-through

Extension
Exercise: stiff-leg deadlift
Sport: back flip

Trunk—transverse
ADL: putting on a seatbelt

Left rotation
Exercise: medicine ball side
toss
Sport: baseball batting

Right rotation
Exercise: torso machine
Sport: golf swing

Hip—frontal
ADL: getting out of a vehicle

Adduction
Exercise: standing
adduction machine
Sport: soccer side step

Abduction
Exercise: standing
abduction machine
Sport: rollerblading

Hip—transverse
ADL: getting out of the bathtub
(upper leg to 90° to trunk)

Horizontal adduction
Exercise: adduction machine
Sport: karate in-sweep

Horizontal abduction
Exercise: seated abduction
machine
Sport: wrestling escape

Ankle—sagittal
ADL: pressing the gas
pedal while driving

Dorsiflexion
Exercise: toe raise
Sport: running

Plantar flexion
Exercise: calf (heel) raise
Sport: high jump

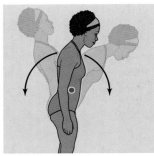
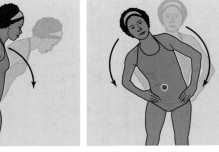

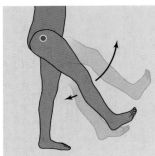

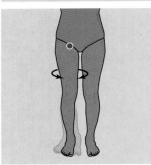

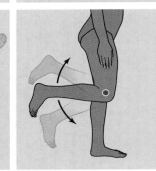

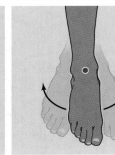

Trunk—frontal
ADL: carrying a suitcase
or grocery bags

Left lateral flexion
Exercise: medicine ball
overhead hook throw
Sport: gymnastics side aerial

Right lateral flexion
Exercise: side bend
Sport: basketball hook shot

Hip—sagittal
ADL: climbing stairs

Flexion
Exercise: leg raise
Sport: American football punt

Extension
Exercise: back squat
Sport: long jump take-off

Hip—transverse
ADL: turning a corner while walking

Internal rotation
Exercise: resisted internal rotation
Sport: basketball pivot movement

External rotation
Exercise: resisted external rotation
Sport: figure skating turn

Knee—sagittal
ADL: moving from sitting
to standing or toileting

Flexion
Exercise: leg (knee) curl
Sport: diving tuck

Extension
Exercise: leg (knee) extension
Sport: volleyball block

Ankle (subtalar)—frontal
ADL: putting on a sock

Inversion
Exercise: resisted inversion
Sport: soccer dribbling

Eversion
Exercise: resisted eversion
Sport: speed skating

FIGURE 4.2 *(continued)* Major body movements. Planes of movement are relative to the body in the anatomical position. The list includes common exercises that provide resistance to the movements and related physical activities.

ADL = activity of daily living.

Adapted by permission from E.A. Harman et al. (1992).

Units of Measure

Before we explore specific mechanical measurements, a few notes are needed on units of measure. Internationally, the standard system of measurement is **le Système International d'Unités** (SI system) (19). In the United States and elsewhere, a traditional (also known as Imperial, British, or English) system is sometimes used. Standard units of measure in each of these systems, along with conversion factors, are presented in t .

We highlight one particular unit of measure, the kilogram, which can be a source of confusion. The potential confusion arises from the relationship between mass (a quantity of matter) and weight (a measure of the effect of gravity on a mass). In the SI system, kilogram (kg) is the unit of mass, with weight measured in newtons (N) of force. Kilogram is also used, however, in some contexts as a unit of force (rather than mass). In the weight room, for example, barbell plates are commonly identified as 10 kg, 20 kg, and so on. In this context, kilogram (kg) is used as a unit measure of force. Thus, the term *kilogram* is used as both a unit of mass (quantity of matter, or kgm) and a unit of force (kg plates in a weight room, or kg).

Force

Force, a fundamental element in human movement mechanics, is defined as a mechanical action or effect applied to a body that tends to produce acceleration. Many forces are relevant to personal trainers as they work with clients. These include internal forces acting inside the body (e.g., muscle, tendon, ligament) and external forces, those acting from the outside (e.g., gravity, **friction**, air resistance).

The effect of forces in producing, controlling, or altering human movement depends on the combined effect of seven force-related factors (34):

- Magnitude (how much force is produced or applied)
- Location (where on a body or structure the force is applied)
- Direction (where the force is directed)
- Duration (during a single force application, how long the force is applied)
- Frequency (how many times the force is applied in a given time period)
- Variability (whether the magnitude of the force is constant or changing over the application period)
- Rate (how quickly the force is produced or applied)

> **Force is the fundamental mechanical element that can produce, change, or stop the motion of a body.**

TABLE 4.1 Units of Measure and Conversions

Quantity	SI (international) unit	Conversion multiplier	Traditional (British) unit	Conversion multiplier	SI (international) unit
Distance	meter	× 3.28 =	foot	× 0.3048 =	meter
Distance	kilometer	× 0.621 =	mile	× 1.61 =	kilometer
Angle	radian	× 57.3 =	degree	× 0.0175 =	radian
Velocity	meters/second	× 2.24 =	miles/hour	× 0.447 =	meters/second
Velocity	kilometers/hour	× 0.621 =	miles/hour	× 1.609 =	kilometers/hour
Force	newton	× 0.225 =	pound	× 4.45 =	newton
Force	kilogram	× 2.205 =	pound	× 0.4535 =	kilogram
Work, energy	joule	× 0.738 =	foot-pound	× 1.356 =	joule
Power	watt	× 0.0013 =	horsepower	× 745.7 =	watt
Torque	newton-meter	× 0.738 =	foot-pound	× 1.356 =	newton-meter

Newton's Laws of Motion

Mechanical analysis of human movement is based largely on the work of Sir Isaac Newton (1642-1727). Most notably, Newton's three laws of motion form the foundation for classical mechanics and provide the rules that govern the physics of human movement. Newton's laws of motion are as follows:

- First law of motion: A body at rest or in motion tends to remain at rest or in motion unless acted upon by an outside force.
- Second law of motion: A net force (ΣF) acting on a body produces an acceleration (a) proportional to the force according to the equation

$$\Sigma F = m \times a \qquad (4.1)$$

(where m = mass). In other words, force equals mass times acceleration.

- Third law of motion: For every action there is an equal and opposite reaction.

Newton's laws of motion apply to all human movements. The first law of motion essentially dictates that forces are required to start, stop, or modify body movements. When a jumper leaves the ground, for example, a force (gravity) slows the upward movement until the jumper reaches his or her peak, and then continues to act in accelerating the jumper's body toward the ground for landing.

Newton's second law of motion is seen when a barbell is lifted off the floor (e.g., a deadlift). The individual must exert enough force to overcome the force of gravity and accelerate the barbell upward. The equation $F = m \times a$ can be used to determine the magnitude of bar acceleration. A greater force (F) will produce a proportionally greater acceleration (a).

Newton's third law of motion says that every force produces an equal and opposite reaction force. In running, for example, at each foot contact, the foot exerts a force on the ground. The ground equally and oppositely reacts against the runner's foot to produce a **ground reaction force**. The magnitude and direction of the ground reaction force determine the runner's acceleration.

Momentum and Impulse

Momentum characterizes a body's quantity of motion. Mechanically, **linear momentum** is the product of mass (m) and velocity (v). Similarly, **angular momen-** tum is the product of moment of inertia (I) and **angular velocity** (v), where I is the resistance of a body to change in angular motion. The moment of inertia depends on two factors: body mass and the distribution of mass relative to the axis of rotation. The effect of mass distribution can be seen in the swinging of a softball bat. The resistance to rotation is greatest when the bat is swung with hands at the handle end of the bat. If the batter "chokes up" on the bat by sliding the hands toward the barrel, it will be easier to swing— even though the mass is the same—because more of the bat's mass is closer to the rotational axis (the hands).

The **transfer of momentum** is an essential mechanism by which momentum is transferred from one body to another. For example, a softball pitcher transfers momentum sequentially from the legs and torso to the arm and hand, and eventually to the ball at pitch release.

To change (either increase or decrease) momentum, a mechanical **impulse** must be applied. Impulse is the product of force (F) multiplied by time (t). Thus, increasing the amount of applied force or the time of force application results in a greater change in momentum.

Torque

Torque (T), or **moment of force** (M), is the rotational effect of a force about an axis. Although there is a technical difference between the two terms, they often are used interchangeably. For simplicity, we will use the term *torque* throughout this chapter.

Torques are evident throughout the human musculoskeletal system. For example, the quadriceps muscle group creates a knee extensor torque, while the hamstrings generate a knee flexor torque.

> **Torque creates an angular acceleration similar to the way force creates a linear acceleration.**

The magnitude of torque (T) is calculated as the mathematical product of force (F) times moment arm (d):

$$T = F \times d \qquad (4.2)$$

Thus, the unit of torque is in newton-meter (N·m).

The **moment arm** is defined as the perpendicular distance (meters) from the fulcrum (axis) to the **line of force action**. In human movement, an **external moment arm** is the perpendicular distance between the external loading imposed on the system and the joint center axis, used to calculate net joint torques. In turn, an **internal moment arm** is the shortest perpendicular distance between the joint axis and the muscle's line of action to determine muscle torques acting on a body segment. As a limb moves through its range of motion about a joint, there is a change in the angle of the directed muscle force. The internal moment arm is largest when the angle of pull on the bone is 90 degrees.

To increase torque, one can increase either the force or the moment arm or both. When a force is applied *through* the axis of rotation, the moment arm is zero and no torque is produced. In human joints, this can result in body tissues (e.g., bone) being subjected to high forces without torque being created. For example, compressive forces acting through the center of a vertebral body will not create vertebral rotation but may subject the vertebral body to an increased risk of injury (23).

Rarely will a single torque be applied in human movement. Therefore, movement is the result of the **net torque**, or the sum of all internal and external torques acting on a limb. For example, a shoulder abduction exercise is completed through the combination of two torques (T_1 and T_2) in opposing directions. T_1 represents the effect of gravity to adduct the glenohumeral joint, while T_2 represents the torque of the abductor muscles (e.g., middle deltoid, supraspinatus). When a person holds a dumbbell with his or her arm in 90 degrees of abduction, gravity acts on both the arm and dumbbell, creating a torque (T_1) about the glenohumeral axis that tends to adduct the arm. If T_1 was the only torque, the arm would adduct under the effect of gravity. To maintain the arm in the abducted position, the abductor muscles (e.g., middle deltoid, supraspinatus) need to create an equal and opposite

torque to oppose the torque created by gravity. This counterbalancing torque (T_2) created by the abductors tends to abduct the arm.

The resulting shoulder movement depends on the relative magnitudes of these two torques (T_1 and T_2). Adding the torques creates a net torque at the joint. If T_1 and T_2 are equal in magnitude (but opposite in direction), the net torque is zero and the arm maintains its abducted position (i.e., isometric action occurs). If the gravitational torque (T_1) is greater than that created by the abductors (T_2), the net torque favors gravity and the arm will adduct (eccentric action). If the torque created by the abductors (T_2) exceeds the gravitational torque (T_1), the net torque favors the muscle action and the arm will further abduct (concentric action).

The relevance of torque-related concepts is of critical importance to the assessment of human movements and the design of exercise programs. This topic will be discussed in further detail later in this chapter.

> **Human movement is produced and controlled by the sum of all internal (muscle) and external (gravity, loading) forces acting on limb segments.**

Lever Systems

With an understanding of the concept of torque, one can visualize joint motion typically resulting from the body's anatomical structures acting as a system of mechanical levers. A **lever** is defined as a rigid structure, fixed at a single point (**fulcrum**, or **axis**), to which two forces are applied (figure 4.3; 22). In terms of human movement, the rigid structure is a

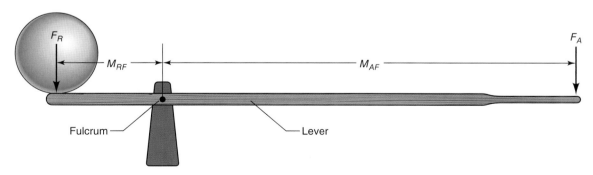

FIGURE 4.3 A lever. Force exerted perpendicular to the lever at one contact point is resisted by another force at a different contact point. F_A = force applied to the lever; $d_{\perp A}$ = moment arm of the applied force; F_R = force resisting the lever's rotation; $d_{\perp R}$ = moment arm of the resistive force.

bone moving about its axis of rotation. One of the forces (F_A) is commonly termed the **applied force** (also **effort force**) and is produced by active muscle. The other force (F_R), referred to as the **resistance force** (also **load**), is produced by the weight being lifted (i.e., gravity) or another external force being applied (e.g., friction, elastic band).

These three lever system components (F_A, F_R, fulcrum) can be spatially arranged in three different configurations. Each of these unique configurations is termed a **lever class**. In a **first-class lever**, the fulcrum is located between the two forces (figure 4.4;22). An example of a first-class lever is the atlanto-occipital joint, between the atlas (C1) and the occiput of the skull). The axis of rotation is the articulation of the occiput on C1; the applied (effort) force is the tension of the neck extensors (posterior to axis); and the resistance force is the center of mass of the head (anterior to axis). A **second-class lever** has F_R located between the fulcrum and F_A (figure 4.5; 22). An example of a second-class lever is the foot and ankle during a calf-raise activity. The axis of rotation is located at the metatarsophalangeal joint (i.e., the ball of the foot); the resistance force is the mass of the body applied downward over the arch of the foot; and the applied (effort) force is the upward force generated by the muscle–tendon unit of the gastrocnemius and Achilles. In a **third-class lever**, F_A lies between the fulcrum and F_R (figure 4.6; 22). An example of a third-class lever is the knee joint during a knee flexion (leg curl)

exercise. The axis of rotation is the knee joint (tibiofemoral); the applied (effort) force is the force of the hamstring muscle group applied to the posterior tibia; and the resistance force is the mass of the shank (lower leg) and any additional resistance (such as weights or bands). Joints in the human body are predominantly third-class levers, with some first-class levers and relatively few second-class levers.

The distances between components are irrelevant in terms of defining the lever class. However, these distances are critically important in determining the mechanical function of a joint. To help illustrate this, we introduce the concept of **mechanical advantage**, which is defined as the ratio $F_R : F_A$ (or alternatively, as the ratio [F_R moment arm : F_A moment arm]). If the mechanical advantage is equal to 1, the moment arms of the resistance force and applied force are

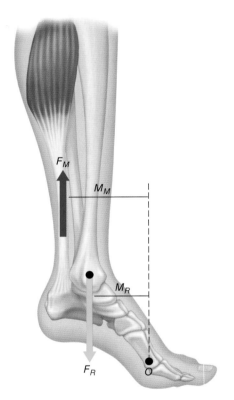

FIGURE 4.5   A second-class lever: the foot during plantar flexion against resistance, as when one is standing up on the toes. F_A = muscle force; F_R = resistive force; $d_{\perp A}$ = moment arm of the muscle force; $d_{\perp R}$ = moment arm of the resistive force. When the body is raised, the ball of the foot, being the point about which the foot rotates, is the fulcrum (O). Because $d_{\perp A}$ is greater than $d_{\perp R}$, F_A is less than F_R.

Reprinted by permission from National Strength and Conditioning Association (2016, p. 22).

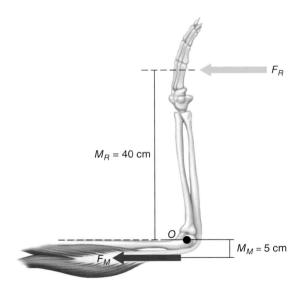

FIGURE 4.4   A first-class lever (the forearm): extending the elbow against resistance.

Reprinted by permission from National Strength and Conditioning Association (2016, p. 21).

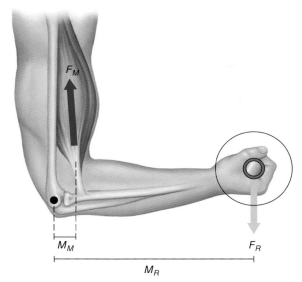

FIGURE 4.6   A third-class lever: the forearm during the biceps curl exercise. F_A = muscle force; F_R = resistive force; $d_{\perp A}$ = moment arm of the muscle force; $d_{\perp R}$ = moment arm of the resistive force. Because $d_{\perp A}$ is much smaller than $d_{\perp R}$, F_A must be much greater than F_R.

Reprinted by permission from National Strength and Conditioning Association (2016, p. 22).

equal, and neither force has an advantage. If the mechanical advantage is less than 1, the resistance force is at an advantage and the applied force will need to be greater than the resistance force to overcome the resistance. Conversely, if the mechanical advantage is greater than 1, the applied force has an advantage over the resistive force. For first-class levers, the force with the longer moment arm will have the mechanical advantage. For second-class levers, the applied force always has the mechanical advantage. For third-class levers, the resistance force always has the mechanical advantage (see the "Moment Arms and Levers of the Human Body" section for a further explanation).

Work

Work is a term with multiple meanings, ranging from a place of employment (e.g., "I'm going to work tomorrow") to physical effort ("I'm working really hard") to energy expenditure ("I worked off 300 calories while cycling"). Mechanically, however, work has a specific definition related to how much force is applied and how far an object moves. **Mechanical work** (W) is defined as the product of force (F) times the distance (d) through which an object moves:

$$W = F \times d \qquad (4.3)$$

The standard unit of work is the joule (1 J = 1 N·m). A person performing a bench press, for example, who lifts 800 N (~180 pounds or ~82 kg) through a distance of 0.5 m (~20 inches) has performed 400 J of mechanical work (figure 4.7).

In a free-weight exercise, the vertical displacement can be measured by the difference in the bar's highest point and its lowest point during each repetition (e.g., d_{AB} in figure 4.7). For a weight stack machine, the high and low points of the stack can be used to measure the vertical displacement.

In addition to the weight being lifted, the portion of the person's body weight that is being moved, or lifted, must be considered. In a squat, for example, the lower extremities are lifting both the barbell and a large portion of the person's own body weight with each repetition. With a leg press machine, the structure and geometry of the device dictate how much of a client's body weight is involved. If a client is pushing horizontally to lift a weight stack, little of his or her body weight is involved. In contrast, in an inclined sled-type leg press device, the amount of body weight being lifted during the exercise varies with the degree of sled inclination.

Power

Mechanical work alone does not always completely describe the mechanics of a particular movement. In the bench press example presented in the previous section, the individual performed 400 J of work during the upward movement phase of each repetition. In a set of 10 repetitions bench-pressing the 800 N weight, the person performs 400 J of work each repetition. If, though, the first repetition takes 1 second to complete and the last repetition takes 2 seconds to complete, there is a mechanical difference between the two repetitions. The difference is not in the *amount* of work performed but in the *rate* at which the work is performed. The rate of work, termed **mechanical power** (P), is calculated as the amount of work (W) divided by the time (t) needed to do the work:

$$P = W / t \qquad (4.4)$$

The standard unit of power is the watt (1 W = 1 J/s). In the bench press example, the upward movement of the first repetition would have a power of 400 W (400 J / 1 second), while the upward movement of the last repetition would have a lower power: 200 W (400 J / 2 seconds). In the traditional (British) system, power is measured in horsepower (hp), where 1 hp = 550 ft-lb/s.

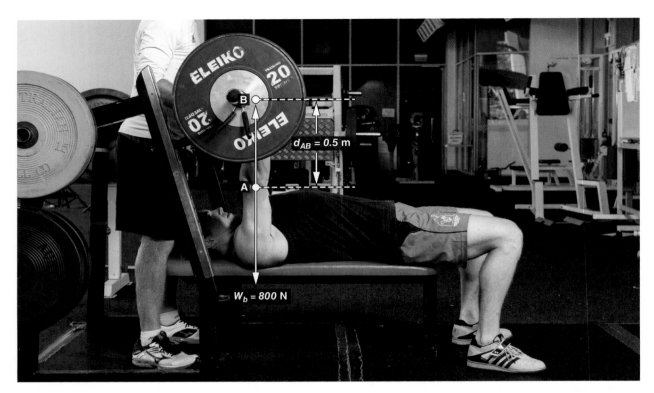

FIGURE 4.7   Calculation of work during resistance exercise.

Power may also be calculated as the product of force (*F*) and velocity (*v*):

$$P = F \times v \qquad (4.5)$$

Many high-speed movement tasks (e.g., jumping, throwing) require high power output. To produce powerful movements and to train for power, a person must generate high forces while moving at a high rate of speed (i.e., high velocity). Many general fitness exercises, such as swimming, walking, and yoga, are performed at relatively slow speeds and therefore are not appropriate for optimizing power. Explosive exercises such as power cleans and snatches, martial arts kicking and punching, and various forms of jumping are much more conducive to power development.

Strength is described as the amount of force (*F*) one can produce during a task. Given that power is the product of force times velocity, strengthening a muscle would allow that muscle to produce more force at any given velocity, or increase movement velocity at a given resistance. Both scenarios would result in increased power output; therefore, increasing strength increases power. As an interesting aside, the sport of powerlifting, despite its name, should be classified as a strength sport, not a power sport. The three events in powerlifting competitions are the squat, bench press, and deadlift. At maximal levels, none of these exercises are performed quickly. Thus, although tremendous strength is certainly required for powerlifting success, the power output is two to three times lower than for the Olympic lifts (e.g., power clean, snatch) (14).

Energy

Energy is another term with multiple meanings. A child, for example, may be very energetic, or a worker at the end of the day may have run out of energy. **Mechanical energy**, however (as is the case with mechanical work), has a specific meaning: the ability, or capacity, to perform mechanical work. Of the many types of energy (e.g., chemical, nuclear, electromagnetic), mechanical energy is the form most commonly used in the description and assessment of human movement. Mechanical energy can be classified as either kinetic energy (energy of motion) or potential energy (energy of position or deformation). Consistent with the two forms of motion, there are two types of kinetic energy.

Linear kinetic energy (LKE) is measured as

$$\text{LKE} = 1/2 \times m \times v^2 \qquad (4.6)$$

where *m* = mass and *v* = linear velocity.

Angular kinetic energy (AKE) is defined as

$$\text{AKE} = 1/2 \times I \times \omega^2 \qquad (4.7)$$

where *I* = moment of inertia and ω = angular velocity.

An important element of these two kinetic energy equations is the squaring of the velocity terms (*v* and ω).

A comparatively small increase in v and ω can result in a considerable increase in kinetic energy. For example, an athlete who increases the vertical velocity of the barbell during a power clean exercise after a period of resistance training will have improved the ability to generate kinetic energy (note the definition of energy as the capacity to do work or apply a force over a distance).

Potential energy can take two forms. The first form, potential energy of position, is termed **gravitational potential energy** and measures the potential to perform mechanical work as a function of a body's height above a reference level (usually the ground). Thus, a barbell held overhead with arms fully extended has more gravitational potential energy than the same barbell held at chest level.

The magnitude of gravitational potential energy (PE) is calculated as

$$PE \times m \times g \times h \qquad (4.8)$$

where m equals mass, g equals gravitational acceleration (~ 9.81 m/s^2), and h equals height (in meters) above the reference level.

The second form of potential energy, termed **deformational** (also **strain**) **energy**, is energy stored within a body when it is deformed (i.e., stretched, compressed, bent, twisted). Examples of deformational energy include a stretched calcaneal (Achilles) tendon, a pole-vaulter's bent pole, and a compressed intervertebral disc. When the force that caused the deformation is removed, the body typically returns to its original (unloaded) shape or configuration and in doing so releases, or returns, some of the stored deformational energy. The stored energy is not totally returned, as some of it is lost as heat energy. Deformational energy storage and return are important in many movement tasks, as illustrated in the stretch–shortening cycle explained later in this chapter.

Mechanical and Movement Efficiency

In biomechanical terms, **efficiency** refers to how much mechanical output (work) can be produced with use of a given amount of metabolic input (energy). The ratio of mechanical output to metabolic input defines the efficiency of a movement task. Human skeletal muscle, for example, is only about 25% efficient. In practical terms, this means that only one-quarter of the metabolic energy involved in muscle activity goes toward performing mechanical work. The remaining

three-quarters is converted to heat or used in energy recovery processes (10).

In addition to the relative inefficiency of muscle in performing mechanical work, several actions or conditions also contribute to movement inefficiency (33). These include

- muscular coactivation (**antagonist** muscle action that works against **agonist** muscle action on the opposite side of a joint),
- jerky movements (alternating changes of direction requiring metabolic energy to accelerate and decelerate limb segments),
- extraneous movements (excessive arm movements during running above and beyond those needed for balance),
- isometric actions (in isometric tasks, there is no displacement, and thus no mechanical work is produced), and
- excessive center of gravity excursions (metabolic energy required to raise and lower the body's center of gravity beyond that minimally required for a given task).

Reducing the contribution of these actions or conditions can improve what is known as **exercise economy**, which can translate to improved performance.

BIOMECHANICS OF HUMAN MOVEMENT

The laws of mechanics govern the way we move. However, personal trainers need to appreciate that humans are biological beings and not machines. Unique characteristics of the muscular system affect how we generate forces and torques. We begin this section by discussing the structure and function of muscle.

Muscle

Skeletal (striated) muscle makes up a substantial portion (40%-45%) of body weight and performs many necessary functions (e.g., movement, protection, heat production). With regard to human movement, muscle generates the forces required to move limb segments at major joints and stabilize body regions. Understanding the roles of muscle is essential to the work of personal trainers.

Muscle tissue has four distinguishing characteristics: **excitability**, the ability to respond to a stimulus;

contractility, the ability to generate a pulling force (also called **tension**); **extensibility**, the ability to lengthen, or stretch; and **elasticity**, the ability to return to its original length and shape when the force is removed. Absence or compromise of any of these properties affects muscle's ability to produce and control human movements.

Muscular action is largely under voluntary control but may also be involved in reflex movements (e.g., rapid response to a painful stimulus) and stereotypical movements (e.g., automatic nonreflex actions such as walking).

Muscle Architecture

Muscle tissue is composed of structural elements that can generate force (**contractile components**), as well as other structures (e.g., connective tissue) that cannot produce force (**noncontractile components**) but are nonetheless important to the proper physiological and mechanical function of muscle. The hierarchical structure of muscle is depicted in figure 1.1 on page 2 of chapter 1, with a single muscle fiber shown in figure 1.2 on page 3. The functional unit for force production within the myofibril is the sarcomere (figure 1.4, p. 4).

The fibers within muscle are arranged in a variety of ways (figure 4.8; 22). In some muscles (e.g., biceps brachii, semitendinosus), the muscle fibers run parallel to a line between the muscle's origin and insertion (line of pull). These muscles are categorized as **fusiform**. In other muscles, the fibers are arranged at an angle (normally <30 degrees) to the line of pull. This angle is termed the **pennation angle**. A unipennate muscle such as the semimembranosus has a single set of fibers, all with the same line of pull. Bipennate muscles such as the rectus femoris have two sets of fibers with different angles. Multipennate muscles (e.g., deltoid) have many sets of fibers acting at a variety of angles. Other muscles, such as the pectoralis major and latissimus dorsi, have a radiating fiber arrangement.

Pennation proves advantageous by allowing more muscle fibers to be packed into a given volume and increasing force production potential by providing a greater functional cross-sectional area than nonpennated muscles. Resistance training cannot change a

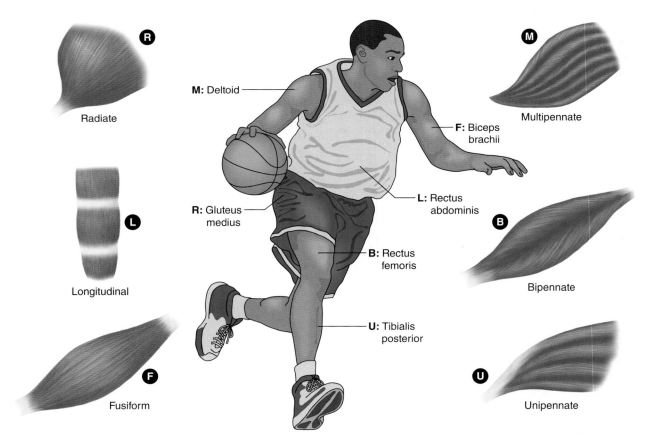

FIGURE 4.8 Muscle fiber arrangements and an example of each.

Reprinted by permission from National Strength and Conditioning Association (2016, p. 31).

muscle's architecture. Understanding structural differences, however, can help personal trainers recognize a muscle's function and potential for injury. The quadriceps group, for example, is designed for force production, whereas the hamstring group is better suited for rapid shortening. These design differences place the two-joint hamstrings (composed of the semitendinosus, semimembranosus, and biceps femoris long head) at greater injury risk than three of the four quadriceps muscles that move one joint (vastus medialis, vastus lateralis, and vastus intermedius) during explosive, high-power tasks such as sprinting and jumping.

Length–Tension

The contractile component (actin-myosin) of muscle generates force. The elements of the noncontractile component (e.g., connective tissue sheaths, tendons, titin proteins) also contribute to the overall force profile of the musculotendinous unit. The combined effect of all the muscle's structural elements is reflected in the **length–tension relationship**, which basically says that the force produced by the musculotendinous unit is determined, in part, by the muscle's length. A schematic length–tension curve is shown in figure 4.9 (33).

The **active component** (shaped like an inverted U) represents the contribution of the sarcomeres in producing force. If a sarcomere is too short, there is complete overlap between the actin filaments, myosin

filament pressure against the Z-lines, and diminished capacity for myosin binding, all resulting in reduced force production. As the sarcomere lengthens, it reaches a range of optimal filament overlap and maximum force production. As the sarcomere further lengthens, actin-filament overlap decreases and force production drops.

The noncontractile component does not contribute to the muscle's force profile until the muscle is stretched past its resting length, as reflected in the right side of the length–tension curve (figure 4.9). In this portion of the curve, the passive, noncontractile elements want to recoil and thus produce resistive tension. The musculotendinous unit's total force production is reflected by the summation of the active contractile and passive noncontractile components.

Clearly there is a limit to the length a muscle can attain, dictated by the range of motion of the joints the muscle crosses. This results in a **functional range** of muscle length as shown in figure 4.9.

Application of the length–tension relationship is readily seen in the following example comparing a calf raise exercise in a standing position to one in a seated position. The gastrocnemius (GA) crosses (i.e., has action at) two joints as a knee flexor and an ankle plantar flexor, whereas the soleus crosses only the ankle joint. In a standing position, the GA assumes a lengthened position and can generate substantially more force than when the knee is flexed in the seated calf raise and the GA is shortened. In the seated calf raise, with the GA's role diminished because of its shorter length, greater demand is placed on the single-joint soleus.

Force–Velocity

In addition to its length, a muscle's ability to generate force depends on its velocity, or speed, of contraction. Each point on a **force–velocity curve** (figure 4.10) represents the maximal force the muscle can produce at the given velocity when the muscle is maximally activated. During concentric muscle actions, faster muscle velocities are associated with lower force production. During isometric muscle actions, more force is produced than at any concentric speed. Muscles are capable of generating more force eccentrically than they can either concentrically or isometrically, and eccentric muscle actions appear to be less affected by movement speed.

The force–velocity relationship can be illustrated using a simple biceps curl exercise. With no weight

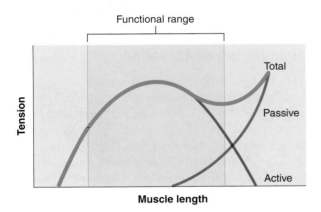

FIGURE 4.9 Length–tension relationship of skeletal muscle measured from the knee extensors of a national-level Olympic weightlifting athlete during an isometric contraction at increasing knee flexion angles (lengthening the muscle).

Adapted by permission from W.C. Whiting and S. Rugg (2006, p. 76).

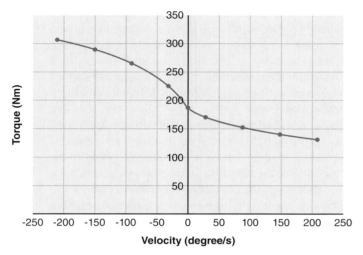

FIGURE 4.10 Force–velocity relationship of skeletal muscle of the knee extensor muscle group in a national-level Olympic weightlifting athlete measured during an isokinetic contraction at increasing knee flexion and extension velocities.

in hand, elbow flexion happens quickly. As successively heavier weights are held, the velocity of flexion decreases. When the weight cannot be moved, the person is at, or very near, his or her isometric maximum. At even higher weights, the muscles cannot lift the weight or even hold it in a set position. They can only control elbow extension in eccentric action consistent with higher forces found in the eccentric portion of the force–velocity curve.

The larger forces generated with eccentric muscle action form the basis for "negative" training. When negatives are performed, either the resistance is increased during the lowering phase or some form of assistance is given during the raising phase. This type of training is an effective means of increasing strength and hypertrophy (17).

Fiber Type and Specific Tension

The maximum force production capability of a muscle is proportional to its cross-sectional area. Theoretically, multiplying the physiological cross-sectional area (cm^2) by the force of contraction per unit area (N/cm^2) would yield the force (N) of the muscle. The force of contraction per unit area is known as **specific tension** (20). Research on isolated motor units has shown that fast-twitch muscle fibers have a higher specific tension (22 N/cm^2) than slow-twitch muscle fibers (15 N/cm^2) (5). Whole muscles have highly variable

specific tensions (21). This finding is not surprising, considering that whole muscles in humans have a mix of fiber types. According to current evidence, muscles that are predominantly fast-twitch will have only a slightly higher specific tension than muscles that are predominantly slow-twitch (20). However, fast-twitch fibers tend to be larger than slow-twitch fibers, so the absolute tension they can develop is greater.

Recruitment

Both intramuscular and intermuscular coordination play a role in the maximum amount of force a muscle can produce. Intramuscularly, or within a muscle, force can be increased by increasing the firing frequency of the motor unit, increasing the number of motor units recruited, and recruiting progressively larger motor units. Intermuscularly, or among more than one muscle, force can be increased by increasing the activation of the agonists and synergists, decreasing the activation of the antagonists, or both. During the first few weeks of training, much of the improvement in strength gains is attributed to these neural adaptations (24) because the increase in strength gains exceeds the increase in muscle fiber size.

Personal trainers need to be cognizant of this fact. A client may be greatly encouraged by large initial increases in strength but become discouraged with the slower rate of improvement that follows. In addition to providing encouragement, the personal trainer should educate the client about how the slower gains due to hypertrophy will result in enhanced strength and improved physical appearance.

Time History of Activation

Muscular force development is not instantaneous; it takes time. Maximal muscle force can take up to 0.5 seconds to develop (32). If an activity lasts less than 0.5 seconds, maximal muscular force will not be attained. In such instances, the rate of force development (RFD) is an important quality in determining performance. **Rate of force development** can be defined as the time rate of change of force, or the ratio of the change in force over the change in time. Rate of force development should not be confused with power. Force can be quickly developed isometrically, for example, yet power would be zero since there is no muscle length change. The RFD can be improved with resistance exercise (32).

Plyometric training enhances RFD by involving the **stretch–shortening cycle (SSC)**. The SSC requires an eccentric muscle action immediately followed by a concentric muscle action. Enhanced force production using the SSC has been attributed to storage of elastic energy and enhanced neural drive (6). During eccentric muscle action, the muscle is developing force, so the muscle does not commence concentric action with zero force. This can be thought of as "pre-forcing" the muscle (36).

This pre-forcing can be seen in the bench press or squat inside a squat rack, when it is harder to lift the bar from the bottom position if it is resting on the supports (with no muscle action). The exercise is slightly easier if the muscles are tensed before lifting the bar (e.g., by holding it above the support) because the muscles are pre-forced, and it is easier still if the bar is quickly reversed at the bottom position thanks to the combined effects of pre-forcing the muscle and the recoil of the elastic components of the muscle–tendon complex.

Moment Arms and Levers of the Human Body

Moment arms can vary considerably among individuals. For example, Bassett and colleagues demonstrated that the standard deviation of the moment arm of the supraspinatus was 52% of the mean (3). This may help explain why two people can have similar muscle sizes but different levels of strength. A person with a larger internal moment arm (tendinous insertions farther away from the joint) can produce more torque for the same level of muscular force. This principle is illustrated in figure 4.11 (22).

Figure 4.11 also demonstrates another important point: Although the distances between a muscle and its tendinous insertions are fixed, the moment arms of that muscle change as a function of joint angle (1). By extension, the torque-producing capability of a muscle also changes as a function of joint angle.

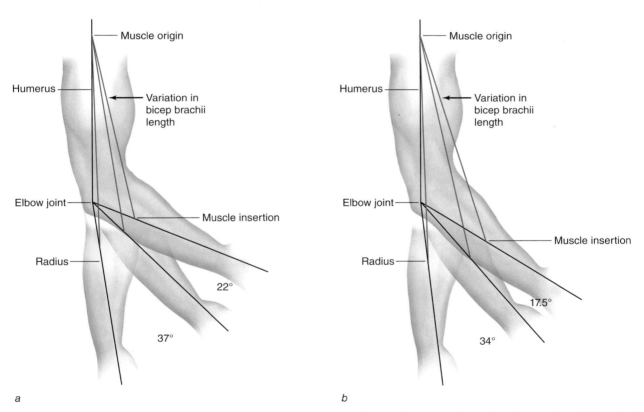

FIGURE 4.11 Changes in joint angle with equal increments of muscle shortening when the tendon is inserted *(a)* closer to and *(b)* farther from the joint center. Configuration *b* has a larger internal moment arm and thus greater torque for a given muscle force, but it has less rotation per unit of muscle contraction and thus slower movement speed.

Reprinted by permission from National Strength and Conditioning Association (2016, p. 24).

Greater torque can be produced at some points in the range of motion than at others.

Recall that there are three classifications of lever systems. The importance of classifying human joints by lever class goes beyond mere application of classical mechanics to anatomical structures. Each lever class has advantages and disadvantages with respect to human movement capabilities. For example, third-class levers in the human body (e.g., biceps brachii acting at the elbow joint) have the applied (muscle) force between the elbow joint axis (fulcrum) and the resistance force (e.g., dumbbell held in the hand). In this structural arrangement, the mechanical advantage (F_A moment arm / F_R moment arm) is much less than 1. In practical terms, this means that given its short moment arm, the muscle must generate a relatively high force to create flexion at the elbow. This apparent disadvantage of an anatomical third-class lever is offset by the joint's ability to increase the effective speed (velocity) of movement. During elbow extension, for example, a given angular displacement produces different linear displacements for points along the forearm and hand. Points farther away from the joint axis move a greater distance along the curved arc than do points closer to the axis. Since all points along the forearm move with the same angular velocity, the more distal points (e.g., dumbbell) have higher linear velocities. This movement advantage is used by baseball pitchers and volleyball spikers to generate high hand velocities before ball release and contact, respectively.

Strength and Sticking Points

With respect to human performance, **strength** generally refers to the ability to exert force. Measurement of strength ranges from simple methods (e.g., how much weight a person can lift) to more complex methods using technological equipment such as force transducers, accelerometers, and isokinetic devices. Given the complexities of muscle force production and given that force generation depends on the speed of muscle action and adaptations to resistance training (2, 12, 27), a more precise definition of strength is the maximal force that a muscle or muscle group can generate at a specified velocity (18). In practical terms, it is not always possible to measure velocity while measuring strength. In such cases, older and simpler methods are still used.

Expressing strength is usually limited to the amount that can be lifted through the weakest point in the range of motion, termed the **sticking point** (or **sticking region**). Determining the sticking point is difficult; it is not simply the point in the range or motion where the external resistance has the largest moment arm (9) because that may also be the same point in the range of motion where the muscle's moment arm is largest. Rather, the sticking point is the point in the range of motion at which the human system is capable of producing the least positive force during a given exercise as a result of mechanical and muscular factors (e.g., moment arm of the resistance, moment arm of the muscle, mechanical advantage of the resistance, length–tension relationship of the muscle, force velocity relationship of the muscle).

Kinematic and Kinetic Chains

In engineering, a series of linkages is referred to as a **kinematic chain**. If the two ends of the series are fixed, the chain is said to be closed. If the terminal end of one link is not fixed, the chain is said to be open. A functional consequence of a closed chain is that movement of one joint will cause every other joint to move in a predictable fashion. Open chains are not subject to these constraints: Movement at one joint will not necessarily cause movement at another joint.

In the mid-1950s, Steindler (29) suggested that the body operates as a kinetic chain. He described an open kinetic chain as "a combination in which the terminal joint is free" and a closed kinetic chain as one "in which the terminal joint meets some considerable external resistance which prohibits or restrains free movement" (p. 63). Steindler noted that a chain is only "strictly and absolutely closed" when no visible motion is produced, yet he believed it was acceptable to "apply the term in all situations in which the peripheral joint of the chain meets with overwhelming external resistance" (p. 63). This is often interpreted as the terminal segment (hand, foot) being fixed.

Note that Steindler used the term *kinetic* (forces), whereas engineers use the term *kinematic* (motion), yet they appear to be talking about the same thing. *Kinetic chain* is not used in engineering or robotics, because kinematic chain is the technically correct description. Yet the term *kinetic chain* is often used in exercise publications, if not interchangeably with *kinematic chain*.

Steindler acknowledged that the chain is rarely "strictly and absolutely closed." This is apparent if we look at the physical description, yet his definition is still confusing because he never described "considerable" external resistance. For example, the squat and leg press are kinematically and kinetically similar

(11), yet the terminal segment (foot) is fixed during the squat and moving during the leg press. Similarly, the bench press and push-up have similar muscle activation patterns throughout the range of motion (4) even when the resistance could hardly be characterized as "considerable."

One could get more out of the terms by looking at the functional consequences rather than physical descriptions of the motion. An open chain is one in which movement of one joint is independent of the other joints in the chain, while a closed chain is one in which movement of one joint causes the other joints in the chain to move in a predictable manner (20). Thus, an open chain movement usually involves a single joint moving against some form of angular resistance (e.g., biceps curl, leg curl). In turn, a closed chain movement typically involves multiple joints moving against a linear resistance (e.g., bench press, squat). However, a distinction should be made between open versus closed kinetic chain and single versus multijoint exercise terminology.

The importance of recognizing a closed chain activity lies in the fact that the motions of multiple joints are coupled (37). For example, during standing in a weight-bearing position and performing a squat motion, flexion of the knee cannot occur without simultaneous flexion of the hip and dorsiflexion of the ankle. A limitation in the range of motion of any one of the joints will affect the range of motion of the entire exercise. Similarly, the torques at the joints are also coupled: As one lowers in the squat position and increases the flexion angles of the joints, all of the muscles in the chain increase their internal torques. Weakness at any one joint will consequently limit performance of the entire movement.

> **The selection of open versus closed kinetic chain exercises is important for transfer ability of an exercise to human movement performance; however, there is no exact consensus on their respective definitions.**

MUSCULAR CONTROL OF MOVEMENT

One of the essential tasks faced by personal trainers when designing and prescribing exercise programs is identifying which specific muscles are active in producing and controlling movements at a particular joint. As discussed earlier, we know that muscles can act in three modes: isometric, concentric, and eccentric. The concentric muscle actions at major joints are listed in table 4.2. A fundamental skill necessary for personal trainers is to determine for a given joint movement both the specific muscles involved and the type of muscle action.

The following muscle control formula provides a step-by-step algorithm for determining muscle involvement and action for any joint movement (33, 35). The formula involves six steps:

Step 1: Identify the joint movement (e.g., abduction, flexion) or position.

Step 2: Identify the effect of the external force (e.g., gravity) on the joint movement or position by asking the question "What movement would the external force produce in the absence of muscle action (i.e., if there were no active muscles)?"

Step 3: Identify the type of muscle action (concentric, eccentric, isometric) using the answers from step 1 (#1) and step 2 (#2) as follows:

  a. If #1 and #2 are in the opposite direction, then the muscles are actively shortening in a concentric action. Speed of movement is not a factor.

  b. If #1 and #2 are in the same direction, then ask, "What is the speed of movement?"

   1. If the movement is faster than what the external force would produce by itself, then the muscles are actively shortening in a concentric action.

   2. If the movement is slower than what the external force would produce by itself, then the muscles are actively lengthening in an eccentric action.

  c. If no movement is occurring yet the external force would produce movement if acting by itself, then the muscles are performing an isometric action.

  d. Movements across gravity (i.e., parallel to the ground) with no other acting external force are produced by a concentric action. When gravity cannot influence the joint movement in question, shortening (concentric) action is needed to pull the segment against its own inertia. The speed of movement is not a factor.

TABLE 4.2 Muscles and Muscle Actions

Hip and knee joint muscle actions			
HIP JOINT			
Extension	**Flexion**	**Abduction**	**Lateral rotation**
Gluteus maximus	Psoas major	Gluteus medius	Gluteus maximus
Semitendinosus	Iliacus	*Gluteus minimus*	Piriformis
Semimembranosus	Pectineus	*Tensor fasciae latae*	Gemellus superior
Biceps femoris (long head)	Rectus femoris	*Gluteus maximus (superior fibers)*	Obturator internus
Adductor magnus (posterior fibers)	*Adductor brevis*	Psoas major	Gemellus inferior
	Adductor longus	*Iliacus*	Obturator externus
	Adductor magnus (anterior upper fibers)	*Sartorius*	Quadratus femoris
	Tensor fasciae latae		*Psoas major*
	Sartorius		*Iliacus*
			Sartorius
Adduction	**Medial rotation**		
Pectineus	Gluteus minimus (anterior fibers)		
	Gluteus medius (anterior fibers)		
Adductor brevis	*Tensor fasciae latae*		
Adductor longus	*Pectineus*		
Adductor magnus	*Adductor brevis*		
Gracilis	*Adductor longus*		
Gluteus maximus (inferior fibers)	*Adductor magnus (anterior upper fibers)*		
Biceps femoris (long head)			
Quadratus femoris			
KNEE JOINT			
Extension	**Flexion**	**Medial rotation**[a]	**Lateral rotation**
Vastus medialis	Semimembranosus	Popliteus	Biceps femoris
Vastus intermedius	Semitendinosus	Semimembranosus	
Vastus lateralis	Biceps femoris	Semitendinosus	
Rectus femoris	*Sartorius*	*Sartorius*	
	Gracilis	*Gracilis*	
	Popliteus		
	Gastrocnemius		
	Plantaris		

Ankle and subtalar joint muscle actions			
ANKLE JOINT		**SUBTALAR JOINT**	
Plantar flexion	**Dorsiflexion**	**Inversion**	**Eversion**
Gastrocnemius	Tibialis anterior	Tibialis anterior	Peroneus longus
Soleus	Extensor digitorum longus	Tibialis posterior	Peroneus brevis
Plantaris	Peroneus tertius	*Flexor hallucis longus*	Peroneus tertius
Tibialis posterior	*Extensor hallucis longus*	*Flexor digitorum longus*	Extensor digitorum longus
Flexor hallucis longus		*Gastrocnemius*	
Flexor digitorum longus		*Soleus*	
Peroneus longus		*Plantaris*	
Peroneus brevis			

Shoulder girdle and shoulder joint muscle actions			
SHOULDER GIRDLE			
Elevation	**Depression**	**Retraction**	**Protraction**
Levator scapulae	Lower trapezius	Rhomboids	Pectoralis minor
Upper trapezius	Pectoralis minor	Middle trapezius	Serratus anterior
Rhomboids		Lower trapezius	
Upward rotation	**Downward rotation**		
Trapezius (upper and lower fibers)	Rhomboids		
Serratus anterior	Levator scapulae		
	Pectoralis minor		
SHOULDER (GLENOHUMERAL) JOINT			
Flexion	**Extension**	**Adduction**	**Abduction**
Pectoralis major (clavicular portion)	Pectoralis major (sternal portion)	Latissimus dorsi	Middle deltoid
Anterior deltoid	Latissimus dorsi	Teres major	Supraspinatus
Biceps brachii (long head)	Teres major	Pectoralis major (sternal portion)	Anterior deltoid
Coracobrachialis	*Posterior deltoid*	*Coracobrachialis*	*Biceps brachii*
	Triceps brachii (long head)		
Medial rotation	**Lateral rotation**	**Horizontal flexion**	**Horizontal extension**
Latissimus dorsi	Teres minor	Pectoralis major	Middle deltoid
Teres major	Infraspinatus	Anterior deltoid	Posterior deltoid
Subscapularis	*Posterior deltoid*	*Coracobrachialis*	Teres minor
Anterior deltoid		*Biceps brachii (short head)*	Infraspinatus
Pectoralis major			*Teres major*
Biceps brachii (short head)			*Latissimus dorsi*

(continued)

TABLE 4.2 *(continued)*

Elbow, radioulnar, and wrist joint muscle actions			
ELBOW JOINT			
Flexion		**Extension**	
Biceps brachii		Triceps brachii	
Brachialis		*Anconeus*	
Brachioradialis			
RADIOULNAR JOINT			
Supination		**Pronation**	
Biceps brachii		Pronator teres	
Supinator		Pronator quadratus	
Brachioradialis[b]		*Brachioradialisb*	
WRIST JOINT			
Flexion	**Extension**	**Radial deviation (abduction)**	**Ulnar deviation (adduction)**
Flexor carpi radialis	Extensor carpi radialis longus	Flexor carpi radialis	Flexor carpi ulnaris
Flexor carpi ulnaris	Extensor carpi radialis brevis	Extensor carpi radialis longus	Extensor carpi ulnaris
Flexor digitorum superficialis	Extensor carpi ulnaris	Extensor carpi radialis brevis	*Extensor digitorum*
Flexor digitorum profundus	*Extensor indicis*		*Flexor digitorum profundus and superficialis*
Palmaris longus	*Extensor digiti minimi*		
	Extensor digitorum		

Vertebral column muscle actions			
VERTEBRAL COLUMN (THORACIC AND LUMBAR REGIONS)			
Flexion	**Lateral flexion**	**Rotation (to the same side)**	**Rotation (to the opposite side)**
Rectus abdominis	External oblique	Internal oblique	External oblique
External oblique	Internal oblique	Erector spinae group	Multifidus
Internal oblique	Quadratus lumborum		
Psoas major (lumbar region)	*Rectus abdominis*		
	Erector spinae group		
Extension			
Erector spinae group	Multifidus		

Note: Nonitalicized muscles are considered prime movers. Italicized muscles represent assistant movers.

[a]Rotation can occur only when the knee is flexed.

[b]Brachioradialis functions to move the forearm to the mid or neutral position.

We have now identified the type of muscle action. Steps 4 through 6 identify which muscles are involved in producing or controlling the movement.

Step 4: Identify the plane of movement (frontal, sagittal, transverse) and the axis of rotation. The purpose of this step is to identify which side of the joint the muscles controlling the movement cross (e.g., flexors cross one side of a joint, while extensors cross the opposite side).

Step 5: Ask, "On which side of the joint axis are muscles lengthening and on which side are they shortening during the movement?"

Step 6: Combine the information from steps 3 and 5 to determine which muscles must be producing or controlling the movement. For example, if a concentric (shortening) action is required (from step 3) and the muscles on the anterior side of the joint are shortening (from step 5), then the anterior muscles must be actively producing the movement. The information in table 4.2 allows us to name the specific muscles (25).

We now apply the muscle control formula to a biceps curl exercise. Consider the simple movement (figure 4.12) of elbow flexion as the person moves the joint from position *a* (elbow fully extended) to position *b* (elbow flexed).

Step 1: The movement is flexion.

Step 2: The external force (gravity) tends to extend the elbow.

Step 3: The movement (flexion) is opposite that created by the external force, so the muscles are actively shortening in concentric action.

Step 4: Movement occurs in the sagittal plane about an axis through the elbow joint.

Step 5: The muscles on the joint's anterior surface are shortening during the movement, while the muscles on the posterior side are lengthening.

Step 6: The muscle action is concentric (from step 3), and muscles on the anterior side of the joint are shortening (from step 5). Thus, the anterior muscles actively produce the movement. Information in table 4.2 identifies the biceps brachii, brachialis, and brachioradialis as the muscles responsible for the movement.

Now consider the reverse movement (figure 4.12) going from position *b* to position *a* as the elbow extends. The movement speed is slow (i.e., the movement

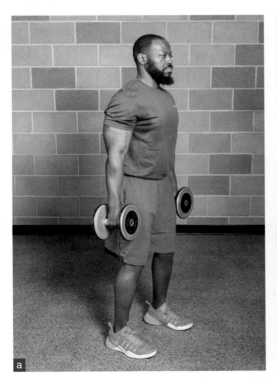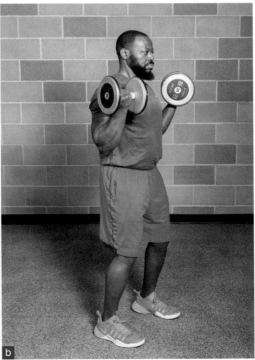

FIGURE 4.12 Biceps curl: elbow flexion from position *a* to *b*; elbow extension from position *b* to *a*.

happens more slowly than it would if the external force were acting by itself in the absence of any muscle action).

Step 1: The movement is extension.

Step 2: The external force (gravity) tends to extend the elbow.

Step 3: The movement (extension) is the same as that created by the external force, so we ask, "What is the speed of movement?" The speed is slow, which dictates that the controlling muscles are actively lengthening in an eccentric action.

Step 4: Movement occurs in the sagittal plane about an axis through the elbow joint.

Step 5: The muscles on the anterior side are lengthening, while the muscles on the posterior side are shortening.

Step 6: The muscle action is eccentric (from step 3), and muscles on the anterior side are lengthening (from step 5). Thus the anterior muscles actively control the movement. Thus, the biceps brachii, brachialis, and brachioradialis are the muscles responsible for controlling the movement. In actions such as this, the muscles normally identified as elbow flexors (biceps, brachialis, brachioradialis) act eccentrically to control elbow extension.

If the elbow extension from position *b* to position *a* occurred quickly (i.e., faster than it would if gravity were acting alone), the muscle control formula would dictate concentric action of the elbow extensors (triceps brachii) as producing the rapid extension.

Space constraints preclude inclusion of more than one example here; however, more examples are described by Whiting and Rugg (33).

When prescribing and evaluating specific exercises, personal trainers should keep in mind that variations in exercise technique can affect muscle recruitment. Consider a few examples:

■ To train the elbow flexors (biceps brachii, brachialis, brachioradialis), many exercises are available (e.g., hammer curl, EZ-bar curl, supinated curl, reverse [pronated] curl). The three elbow flexors are not used equally in each exercise type, largely because forearm position affects the recruitment of the biceps brachii and brachioradialis. For example, hammer curls maximize brachioradialis involvement since the brachioradialis is strongest in midposition (between supination and pronation). Supinated curls target the biceps brachii because the biceps is the strongest supinator of the forearm and in supination it is placed in an advantageous position. In contrast, the brachialis is the prime mover in a reverse curl since its insertion on the ulna means its length and line of pull are unaffected by forearm position. Although the biceps brachii is involved in a reverse curl, the pronated forearm position places the biceps at an anatomical disadvantage to maximize its force contribution.

■ Comparing a flat bench press against an incline bench press shows that the muscle involvement of the pectoralis major differs. In a flat bench press, the primary shoulder motion is horizontal adduction, and the sternal portion of the pectoralis major plays a large role. In an incline bench press, shoulder motion is a combination of horizontal adduction and flexion; and as the incline increases, the sternal portion of the pectoralis major is less involved. The incline press targets the clavicular portion of the pectoralis major because it functions as both a horizontal adductor and flexor. Thus, at steeper inclines, the sternal portion of the pectoralis major becomes less involved, and less weight can be lifted.

■ In a narrow-stance squat, the primary muscle action is provided by the hip extensors. In a wide-stance squat, both the hip extensors and adductors are involved. With more muscle involvement in the wide stance, heavier weights can be lifted.

> **Understanding which muscles are controlling a movement, and how modifying the exercise affects those muscles, is key in selecting appropriate exercises for a given goal.**

BIOMECHANICS OF RESISTANCE EXERCISE

Training to improve motor qualities (such as strength, power, or muscular endurance) requires the application of a progressive overload over time. In many instances, the overload stimulus is provided by some sort of resistance to a particular set of movements. Resistance may be classified as one of three types: constant, variable, or accommodating. Because each type of resistance stresses the body in unique ways, the biomechanics of several different types of resistance are discussed next.

Constant-Resistance Devices

A **constant resistive force** does not change throughout the range of motion. Free weights and certain machines provide a constant-resistance force.

Free Weights

A **free weight** is any object that has a fixed mass and no constraints on its motion. By this definition, barbells, dumbbells, medicine balls, and a person's body (or parts of it) are all considered free weights. A free weight has a force (weight) acting on it by virtue of being in a gravitational field; the force is constant and in the (vertical) direction of the gravity. Thus, the resistance to movement provided by a free weight depends on the direction of movement. In the vertical direction, the resistance provided by the free weight equals the sum of the product of the object's mass times its acceleration and the object's weight (mass times the acceleration due to gravity, -9.81 m/s^2). In all other directions, the resistance equals the product of mass times acceleration. This concept can be expressed as

$$F_R = m \times a + W \qquad (4.9)$$

Note that the object's weight, W, is equal to zero in all directions except the vertical.

To move (accelerate) a free weight, the force must be greater than its weight; otherwise, the weight will not move. The greater the force above this threshold, the faster the weight moves. During a typical exercise repetition, a person starts in a static position (with zero velocity), performs some motion, reverses direction (at which point the velocity is zero), and returns to the starting position (where the velocity is again zero). From this rather simple description, the velocity (and thus acceleration) clearly is not constant but rather changes throughout the movement. However, if the movement speed is sufficiently slow, we tend to approximate the acceleration as zero and state that the resistance provided by free weights is constant and equal to its weight ($m \times g$).

Even if the external forces are constant throughout a movement, the internal forces will not be constant. The reason is that these forces produce torques that must be overcome by the body to move the limbs. Recall that torque is the product of force and its moment arm, and the moment arm is the perpendicular distance from the force to the axis of rotation. During single-joint movements (such as the anatomical illustration of the biceps curl in figure 4.13; 22), the moment arm

of the free weight is constantly changing throughout the range of motion. When the limb is in a horizontal position, the free weight's moment arm will be the greatest and will decrease in both directions until the weight is either directly above or below the joint. At this point, the moment arm will be zero, and consequently the torque will be zero.

One can apply this concept to change the resistance throughout the range of motion by modifying the exercise position. For example, during a leg curl or shoulder lateral raise in the standing position, the moment arm of the weight will be the greatest when the leg or arm is horizontal, which in these cases happens to be at roughly 90 degrees of knee flexion or shoulder abduction, respectively. If the exercise is performed supine (for the leg curl) or side-lying (for the lateral raise), the moment arm of the weight is still greatest when the leg or arm is horizontal, but this is at the starting (neutral) position. Similarly, the forearm is horizontal at 90 degrees of elbow flexion during the biceps curl in the standing position, but

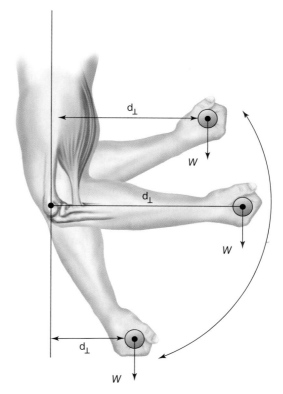

FIGURE 4.13 The horizontal distance ($d_\perp$) from the weight to the elbow changes throughout the biceps curl movement, causing the torque exerted by the weight (W) of the object to change as well.

it is 90 degrees minus the angle of the bench during the preacher curl. Using these concepts, the personal trainer can modify exercises to stress the musculature at different points in the range of motion.

During multijoint movements (such as the squat or bench press), the path of the bar may appear linear, but that linear motion is still produced by angular motion at the joints. The same principle applies: The resistance of a constant weight will be the greatest when the moment arm is the longest. For both the squat and bench press, the moment arm tends to be greatest during the lower part of the movement and decreases as the person moves toward the top of the movement. At the top, the moment arm is essentially zero and the skeletal system is supporting the weight with little muscle action needed.

During multijoint movements, technique variations can shift the demand from the muscles of one joint to another. For example, during the squat exercise, greater forward trunk inclination moves the weight in the anterior direction. This effectively increases the moment arm at the hips and ankles and decreases the moment arm at the knees. Consequently, the muscular demand on the hip extensors and plantar flexors will be greater and the demand on the knee extensors will be less in this position compared with a more upright position.

Certain mechanical constraints during the task should be appreciated as well (37). Because it is necessary to maintain balance throughout an exercise such as the squat, the vertical projection of the combined center of mass of the bar and person must remain within the confines of the base of support created by the feet. If the bar is placed lower on the back, the person has to lean forward to maintain balance. For the reasons just outlined, this increases demand on the hip extensors and plantar flexors and decreases demand on the knee extensors. Similarly, placing the bar in front of the shoulders (e.g., front squat) requires the person to be more upright, increasing the demand on the knee extensors and decreasing the demand on the hip extensors and plantar flexors.

Even within the mechanical constraints of the task, variations in lifting technique can and do occur. In an attempt to lift more weight, clients may adopt subtle or not-so-subtle strategies to shift the demand from relatively weaker muscles to stronger ones. Many factors go into determining if these compensatory strategies are acceptable or not, and they are beyond the scope of this chapter. However, the personal trainer needs to be vigilant in spotting and correcting deviations that could result in injury.

Single- and multijoint movements can complement each other. For example, the demand on the quadriceps during a squat increases as the knee flexion angle increases; the demand is greater at the bottom of the movement where the knee flexion angle is largest and decreases to zero as the knee flexion angle approaches zero (i.e., fully extended knee). Conversely, during a seated knee extension exercise, since the moment arm is largest when the leg is horizontal, the demand on the quadriceps increases as the knee extends. Thus, performing both the squat and knee extension exercise would maximize the demand on the quadriceps throughout the full range of motion and may be beneficial in certain situations (30). The same can be said for other combinations of single- and multijoint movements.

Machines

Unlike a free weight, a machine constrains the motion of the resistance in some way. The path of the resistance can be linear (as with a leg press or Smith machine) or angular (e.g., knee extension or knee curl machine). Although some devices allow pulleys to pivot in many directions, the direction of the resistance must still be in the direction of the cable, and such devices are classified as machines for the purposes of this chapter. A machine with a fixed resistance will constrain movement in some way, but the external resistance will not change. Examples include a pulldown machine using a single pulley, a Smith machine, or any device that uses a pulley with a lever and a fixed axis.

Variable-Resistance Devices

A **variable resistive force** will increase or decrease (or both) throughout the range of motion. Certain machines, elastic bands and tubes, and chains attached to the end of a barbell have this property of variable resistance.

Machines

In a machine with variable resistance, the resistance changes throughout the range of motion. Any machine that loads weight plates to the end of the lever varies its resistance with the changing of the moment arm (similarly to a free weight attached to the end of a limb performing a single-joint exercise). The greatest resistance will occur when the lever is parallel to the floor. The greatest torque-producing capability of a muscle group does not necessarily occur when the distal segment is horizontal. In an effort to match the human strength curve (i.e., the demand is greatest where the torque-producing capability is greatest and lower in other points in the range of motion), machines

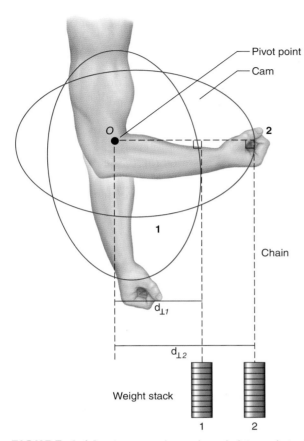

FIGURE 4.14 In cam-based weight-resisted machines, the moment arm ($d_\perp$) through which the weight acts (horizontal distance from chain to pivot point) varies during the exercise movement.

Reprinted by permission from National Strength and Conditioning Association (2008, p. 81).

were developed that had a cam with a variable radius (figure 4.14; 7). The goal of the variable cam was to adjust the moment arm of the weight stack throughout the range of motion, more closely mimicking the torque-producing capabilities of various muscle groups. Since not everyone has the same strength curves for a given joint, this goal was met with limited or no success (13, 15).

Elastic Resistance

The elastic properties of materials can also be used to provide variable resistance. Resistances in this category follow Hooke's law:

$$F_R = -kx \qquad (4.10)$$

Where k is the spring constant (i.e., a measure of the material's stiffness, or resistance to being stretched) and x is the distance the material has been stretched.

Elastic tubing, elastic bands, coils, and springs all have elastic properties that provide resistance. The larger the k, the stiffer the material, with a larger force required to stretch it. The negative sign indicates that the resistance is directed opposite to the direction of the stretch. Unlike the resistance force with a free weight, the resistance force is not constant but increases proportionally with the distance the material is stretched beyond its resting length. Thus, resistance is minimal at the beginning of the exercise and increases as the movement is performed. The resistance is related to the relative change in the original length of the material, not the actual length to which the material stretched (28). For example, stretching a 10-inch (25.4 cm) band from its resting length out to 20 inches (50.8 cm) would result in different forces than stretching that same band from 20 inches out to 40 inches (101.6 cm). Even though the distance the material has been stretched is the same, the resistance would be larger in the second case.

An often overlooked characteristic of elastic materials is their fatigue properties (28). After repeated stretch cycles, a material will lose its ability to provide resistance. Fatigue-related changes happen based on the amount of deformation per stretch cycle and the number of cycles. Investigators found that the resistance provided by tubing and bands decreased between 5% and 6%, and between 9% and 12%, respectively, when deformed to 100% of their initial length for 501 cycles. At 200% deformation, the resistance provided by both tubes and bands decreased by 10% to 15%, with most of the decrease in resistance appearing during the first 50 repetitions (29). These results suggest that elastic materials should be replaced frequently to ensure consistent loading.

Incremental loading also may be problematic. Manufacturers often use color coding to indicate material resistance. Caution is warranted in interpreting color codes because differences can be profound and can vary for bands and tubing. For example, the green band of one manufacturer provides almost twice the resistance of the yellow band, and the black band provides 1.5 times the resistance of the green band. For another manufacturer, green tubing provides 5 times more resistance than yellow tubing, and black tubing provides 1.5 times the resistance of green tubing (28).

Chains

The practice of attaching heavy metal chains to a barbell has been implemented as a method of varying the resistance of an exercise. It is theorized that during exercises with linear movements such as the bench press or squat (without chains), the resistance torque is greatest at the bottom of the movement and progressively decreases as the bar moves to the top position (see earlier discussion). With chains attached to the bar, most of the chain's weight is supported by the floor at the bottom of the movement. As the bar rises, more of the chain lifts off the floor, progressively increasing the resistance. This training method seeks to address the decreasing moment arm (and thus mechanical advantage) of the resistance (bar) by increasing the resistance force with chains. Using chains during exercises with linear movements provides an overload stimulus throughout the entire range of motion. The training advantages are twofold: It improves performance in the terminal range of motion while retaining task specificity, and it increases power and momentum transfer because the client will improve force generation deep in the range of motion to assist in the top-end range of motion.

Accommodating-Resistance Devices

An **accommodating resistive force** will vary depending on the force applied to it. In other words, accommodating resistances provide resistance that is proportional to the client's effort. Accommodating resistances include isokinetic dynamometers, flywheels, and fluid resistance.

Isokinetic Dynamometers

Isokinetic devices control movement speed to provide, at least nominally, constant angular velocity. (*Note:* The term *isokinetic* literally means "same force." Isokinetic devices, however, control the kinematic variable of angular velocity, and thus a more correct term would be *isokinematic*. However, given the pervasive use of *isokinetic*, we ignore the technical discrepancy and use *isokinetic* in this section.) With an isokinetic device, the limb moves at a predetermined speed, anywhere from 0 degrees per second (isometric) up to 300 degrees per second (eccentrically) and 500 degrees per second (concentrically). When the movement of the limb exceeds the predetermined speed, the machine provides an equal and opposite force (torque) to maintain the specified angular velocity (26). This force (torque) is what the individual exerts on the machine.

Flywheels

Flywheels require the person to pull a cord, which in turn rotates a disk. Resistance is provided by the rotating disk through a mass located some distance away from the disk's axis of rotation. The flywheel's resistance increases as its angular acceleration increases. In other words, the harder one pulls on the cord, the greater the resistance to the motion provided by the flywheel (8). Additionally, the kinetic energy of the flywheel is stored (up to 80%, depending on the design). At the end of the pull, the cord will start rewinding, and the person must resist it using eccentric muscle actions.

Fluid Resistance

Hydraulic and pneumatic devices that use some sort of piston to push or pull a fluid (liquid for hydraulic and gas for pneumatic) through a cylinder and movements performed under water have similar biomechanical properties. Fluid resistance follows the form

$$F_R \propto \rho A v^2 \tag{4.11}$$

This means that the resistance force is proportional to the product of ρ (the fluid density), A (the surface area), and v^2 (the square of the movement velocity). With machines, the density of the fluid and the cross-sectional area of the piston are inherent in the design of the equipment and are thus fixed, so the resistance the machine provides to the user increases with the velocity of the movement. A benefit of this type of resistance is there is no external weight that can gain momentum, and thus the client can use very high velocities without a reduction in the force being applied. Note that this is not a linear relationship: Doubling the velocity will increase the resistance fourfold based on the nature of the equation.

Performing Exercises in the Water

When someone exercises in water, a buoyant force acts in the upward direction, in opposition to gravity in the downward direction. When a person floats in water, the buoyant force and gravitational force cancel (i.e., the net vertical force is zero). When a person performs exercises in the shallow end of a pool, the buoyant force depends on how much of the body is submerged. The buoyant force is approximately 50%

when the body is submerged up to the hip (level of the anterior superior iliac spine) but increases up to 90% when the body is submerged to the neck (at the level of C7) (31).

These characteristics can be used to create exercises that are buoyancy supported, buoyancy assisted, or buoyancy resisted (32).

- Buoyancy-supported exercises occur parallel to the bottom of the pool. For example, while the person is performing shoulder horizontal abduction and adduction when submerged up to the neck, the buoyant force helps support the arm, and the resistance will mainly be in the direction of movement.
- Buoyancy-assisted movements occur in the direction of the buoyant force.
- Buoyancy-resisted movements occur in the opposite direction of the buoyant force.

While an individual is submerged up to the neck, the buoyant force assists with the performance of shoulder flexion. Conversely, the buoyant force has to be overcome when the person is reversing directions and performing shoulder extension. Some devices, such as aquatic dumbbells, increase the buoyant force.

When used, they make buoyancy-assisted exercises easier and buoyancy-resisted exercises more difficult.

The resistance force provided by the water, called **drag**, follows the formula discussed previously for hydraulic machines (equation 4.11). As with machines, the force is accommodating and proportional to the velocity squared. Additionally, the surface area, A, can be manipulated to increase or decrease the magnitude of the resistance. Consider performing shoulder flexion and extension underwater. The surface area will be lower if the palm is facing toward the midline as opposed to facing anteriorly (figure 4.15), making the exercise easier. The exercise can be made more difficult if it is performed in the anatomical position using webbed gloves or paddles. Like resistive forces in hydraulic machines, the resistance force provided by water always acts in the direction opposite to the movement. Therefore, the muscle actions required to overcome the force will always be concentric.

> Selection of the type of resistance—constant, variable, or accommodating—is an important factor in designing a safe and effective exercise program.

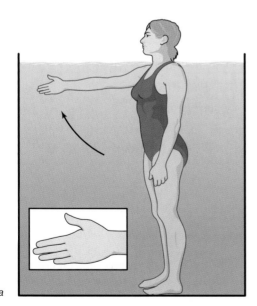 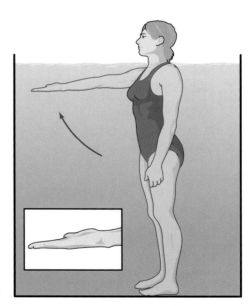

FIGURE 4.15   Shoulder flexion exercise in the water with *(a)* palm facing toward midline and *(b)* palm facing anteriorly.

CONCLUSION

Understanding basic biomechanical principles is important for knowing how exercises elicit desired training effects while minimizing the likelihood of injury. Personal trainers with a solid foundation in biomechanics are better prepared to establish training goals and prescribe exercise programs that effectively and efficiently improve the physical capabilities of their clients.

Study Questions

1. In biomechanics, the term *body* may refer to which of the following?
   I. the human body
   II. limb segment
   III. piece of chalk
      A. I only
      B. II only
      C. III only
      D. I, II, and III

2. Which of the following is the equation that represents work?
      A. force × distance moved
      B. force + distance moved
      C. force − distance moved
      D. force / distance moved

3. Which of the following is *incorrect* regarding rate of force development?
      A. It is the ratio of the change in force over the change in time.
      B. If rate of force development is high, power is also high.
      C. It is time rate of change of force.
      D. It can be improved with resistance training.

4. Which of the following is *incorrect* regarding the use of heavy metal chains on barbells?
      A. They can be used with linear movements.
      B. The chains add resistance throughout the range of motion.
      C. The chains provide a greater resistance at the weakest part of the range of motion.
      D. Chains can be used in exercises such as the squat or bench press.

5. With water resistance, if the surface area is _____, the exercise will be _____.
   I. smaller; easier
   II. larger; easier
   III. smaller; harder
   IV. larger; harder
      A. I only
      B. II only
      C. I and IV only
      D. II and III only

CHAPTER 5

Responses and Adaptations to Resistance Training

Michael D. Roberts, PhD, and Kevin W. McCurdy, PhD

After completing this chapter, you will be able to

- describe the acute responses and chronic adaptations to resistance exercise,

- identify factors that affect the magnitude or rate of adaptations to resistance training,

- design resistance training programs that maximize the specific adaptations of interest,

- design resistance training programs that avoid overtraining, and

- understand the effects of detraining and know how to reduce them.

This chapter explains general adaptations that result from resistance training. These include neurological, muscle and connective tissue, skeletal, metabolic, hormonal, cardiorespiratory, and body composition changes. We also explain the impact of sex, age, and genetics on physiological adaptations. The final sections of the chapter deal with overreaching and overtraining, unwanted physiological responses that must be prevented in the personal training setting, as well as the effects of detraining and how to avoid them. Four prominent themes resonate throughout the chapter, and personal trainers should appreciate these when working with clients.

First, whether a client is novice or advanced, each resistance training bout (if designed properly) is a substantial stressor to the body. The musculoskeletal, endocrine, immune, and cardiorespiratory **stress responses** after each training bout better prepare

the body for subsequent training bouts. Much of this chapter describes intricate musculoskeletal stress responses given that this is the primary site of adaptation, although adaptations in other organ systems are discussed as well. Over time, the summation of these stress responses leads to positive adaptation in the form of muscle growth, increases in bone mineral density, and increases in strength.

Second, **progressive overload** during a training period ensures that the body is adequately stressed. The implementation of progressive overload involves manipulating training volume, intensity, or frequency in order to apply continued stress to the body. Personal trainers should not misapply this concept in the form of overly aggressive programming. In fact, great personal trainers constantly observe clients during training sessions and interpret cues such as prolonged soreness, nagging muscle or joint pain, a loss of enthusiasm for

The authors would like to acknowledge the significant contributions of Joseph P. Weir and Lee E. Brown to this chapter.

training, or plateaus in strength to indicate that the training program is too aggressive or that a deload period (e.g., a recovery week) is needed.

Third, chronic training adaptations occur in phases. The initial and obvious adaptation to resistance training is an increase in strength (within the first month). Visual changes in muscle mass or tone occur as soon as one to two months after initiating a regimented program. Discernable improvements in bone mineral density occur over several months to years. This is critical to appreciate given that each client may have different motivations for training. For instance, client 1 may want to resistance train in order to improve bone mineral density, whereas client 2 may want to resistance train in order to "tone up" for a social event. Personal trainers who understand the time course of each adaptation can clearly communicate this information to clients in order to properly manage expectations.

Finally, every client will respond differently to training. Researchers have observed that people exhibit high, average, and low muscle growth responses to training (60, 92, 113, 122, 128). The causes of these individual responses are multifactorial and can include a person's age, sex, genetics, and environment (e.g., calorie intake, stress levels, sleep patterns). To be certain, researchers posit that only 10% to 20% of individuals are "true" low muscle growth responders, and clients should not be encouraged to assign themselves to this category if they do not visually observe body composition changes within the initial periods of training. However, if the personal trainer has the tools to accurately measure body composition over training periods and suspects that a client is a low muscle growth responder, it is important to consistently encourage the client to adhere to training given that other positive adaptations (e.g., increases in strength) are still taking place (21). Additionally, there is emerging evidence that changing the stimulus (e.g., loading, volume, frequency) can spur results in those who did not respond well to a certain routine.

ACUTE RESPONSES AND CHRONIC ADAPTATIONS TO RESISTANCE TRAINING

In studying the adaptations to resistance training, it is useful to distinguish between acute responses and chronic adaptations. **Acute responses** to exercise are the changes that occur in the body during and shortly after an exercise bout. An example of an acute response is the depletion of fuel substrates in muscle,

such as creatine phosphate (CP), during a short high-intensity exercise bout. In contrast, **chronic adaptations** are changes in the body that occur after repeated training bouts and that persist long after a training session is over. For example, long-term resistance training leads to increases in muscle mass, which play a role in increasing a muscle's force production capability. Two subsequent sections of this chapter address the acute responses and chronic adaptations that typically occur with resistance training.

> **Acute responses are changes that occur in the body during and shortly after an exercise bout. Chronic adaptations are changes in the body that occur after repeated training bouts and that persist long after a training session is over. The summation of acute responses to each training bout catalyzes chronic training adaptations in all the major organ systems (e.g., musculoskeletal, cardiovascular, nervous, endocrine, immune).**

As mentioned previously, the key to inducing increases in muscle size and strength is to strategically stress the system through progressive overload; that is, the neuromuscular system must experience a sufficient and unaccustomed training stress that challenges it in a manner conducive to bringing about such adaptations. The same holds true if one is considering adaptations in bone and connective tissue. If progressive overload is properly implemented over a series of weeks to months, this practice will result in the ability of muscle to handle heavier loads. Again, personal trainers should be aware that the proper implementation of progressive overload in novice or advanced clients does not always translate into having them perform exercises to failure during each training session. In fact, empirical evidence suggests that performing exercises to failure during each training session over a 10-week period may result in artificial strength plateaus (20). Thus, it is crucial that a training program entail a progressive overload scheme; to best promote optimal training adaptations, programming should not have clients perform lifts to failure during every set, and the program should contain interspersed recovery blocks (or deload periods).

A large volume of literature describes the adaptations to resistance training overload. The rapidity with which overload increases the capacity for muscle to handle heavier loads at the start of a training program suggests there is a dramatic increase in the activation of motor units during the initial phases of resistance training. Improvements in strength associated with the first couple of months of resistance training are primarily due to neurological adaptations (6, 33, 74). In addition, during this time the quality of muscle protein (e.g., myosin heavy chains and myosin adenosine triphosphatase [ATPase]) is also altered to allow for more rapid and forceful contractile capabilities (107).

Generally speaking, scientists believe that body size is largely influenced by a person's genetic makeup. Therefore, it makes sense that the potential to gain muscle mass and strength with training is also largely influenced by genetics. As discussed earlier in this chapter, empirical evidence suggests there are low and high muscle growth responders to resistance training (111). A low responder may experience little to no change in whole-body muscle mass or a 5% (marginal) increase in leg muscle thickness in response to 12 weeks of resistance training. On the other hand, a high responder may experience a 10-pound (4.5 kg) increase in whole-body muscle mass, or a 30% increase in leg muscle thickness over this same time course. Researchers are currently searching for genetic and physiological factors that drive these differential responses. However, it is critical for personal trainers and clients to appreciate that only 10% to 20% of individuals are low responders, so this is not a common phenomenon; further, these research studies observed training adaptations over a 12- to 16-week period, and low responders may eventually gain a considerable amount of muscle mass with years of training, particularly when the program is customized to individual needs and abilities. Finally, even low responders experience appreciable increases in strength with resistance training because of neurological adaptations (7, 92).

Differential responses to training aside, it is notable that muscle hypertrophy (i.e., muscle growth) is usually not measurable (although it is still occurring) until four to eight weeks after the initiation of a resistance training program (32, 124). The continued interplay of hypertrophic and neurological adaptations to resistance training continues with long-term training. The impact of long-term training on muscle hypertrophy remains less well studied, but the absolute magnitude of gains in muscle size and strength is lower as clients approach their genetic ceiling. Nevertheless, given that strength decrements later in life are a primary risk factor for frailty, continued training over a client's lifetime helps improve quality of life and minimize the consequences of aging.

A variety of cellular adaptations occur with resistance training programs. These include changes in anaerobic enzyme quantity, changes in stored energy substrates (e.g., glycogen and phosphagens), increased contractile or myofibrillar protein content (i.e., increased actin and myosin proteins), and increased noncontractile muscle proteins. In addition, important changes occur within the central and peripheral nervous systems to aid in the activation of motor units. A variety of changes also occur in other physiological systems (e.g., endocrine, immune, and cardiorespiratory) that support the neuromuscular adaptations to a resistance training program. The summation of these adaptations ultimately harmonizes to support the improvements in force, velocity, and power.

ACUTE RESPONSES TO TRAINING

One exercise training session is a substantial physiological stressor that catalyzes multiple acute physiological responses across numerous organ systems. Akin with the stress theory put forth by the notable physiologist Hans Selye (1907-1982), the acute responses to each training stress that occur in the neuromuscular system during and immediately after a training session likely drive many of the chronic adaptations. This section presents an overview of the major acute responses to resistance exercise (summarized in table 5.1), specifically responses involving the neurological, muscular, and endocrine systems, and personal trainers should appreciate their significance. Just as stock markets respond to cues such as earnings reports and consumer behaviors, each of the physiological cues creates reactions that facilitate chronic adaptations in the body. For example, although the depletion of CP or muscle glycogen during a training bout may seem like a physiological detail that is too nuanced to influence practice, these responses cue muscles to increase the synthesis of enzymes critical for CP and glycogen resynthesis so that the client is more bioenergetically prepared to lift weights as training ensues over weeks to months. Furthermore, different training paradigms differentially affect these responses, which has practical implications as it relates to clients' metabolic conditioning.

Neurological Changes

Resistance training, like all physical activity, requires activation of skeletal muscle. The process of skeletal muscle activation involves action potential generation

TABLE 5.1 Acute Responses to One Bout of Resistance Exercise

Variable	Acute response	
NEUROLOGICAL RESPONSES		
EMG amplitude	Increase	
Number of motor units recruited	Increase	
MUSCULAR CHANGES		
Hydrogen ion concentration	Increase	
Inorganic phosphate concentration	Increase	
Ammonia levels	Increase	
ATP concentration	No change or slight decrease	
CP concentration	Decrease	
Glycogen concentration	Decrease	
ENDOCRINE CHANGES		
Epinephrine concentration	Increase	
Cortisol concentration	Increase	
Testosterone concentration	Increase	
Growth hormone concentration	Increase	

EMG = electromyogram; ATP = adenosine triphosphate; CP = creatine phosphate.

on the muscle cell membrane (sarcolemma) via acetylcholine release from a single alpha motor neuron that innervates (stimulates) a given number of muscle fibers. These fibers contracting together and the innervating neuron are called a **motor unit**. The action potential is manifested as a voltage change on the sarcolemma that can be recorded with either surface or intramuscular electrodes. The technique of recording these electrical events is referred to as **electromyography (EMG)**. The size of an EMG signal varies as a function of muscle force output, but it is also affected by other factors such as fatigue and muscle fiber composition (34). Partly because of these factors, force and EMG measurements are not produced in a perfect linear relationship. Nonetheless, much of what we know about neurological responses and adaptations to resistance training comes from studies using EMG.

Control of muscle force is accomplished by the interplay of two primary factors: motor unit recruitment and rate coding (37). Motor unit **recruitment** refers to the process in which tasks that require more force involve the activation of more motor units. An individual performing a 100-pound (45.4 kg) bench press would need to turn on (or recruit) more motor units than would be required to perform a 50-pound (22.3 kg) bench press. **Rate coding** refers to control of motor unit firing rate (number of action potentials per unit of time). The faster the firing rate, the more force is produced from the unit. Therefore, a motor unit that was activated at a rate of 20 times per second during the 50-pound bench press may be firing at 30 times per second during the 100-pound bench press. As a general rule, small muscles (like those in the hands) that require very precise motor control achieve full recruitment from the available units at relatively low percentages of maximum force output (e.g., 50% of maximum), and after this point they depend entirely on firing rate to increase force production. In contrast, large muscles like those in the quadriceps employ recruitment up to 90% of maximum or more, and maximum firing rates tend to be lower than for the small muscles. Therefore, small muscles typically depend more heavily on firing rate to control force output, while large muscles tend to depend more heavily on recruitment.

During a set of resistance exercise, motor units in the involved muscle or muscles are initially activated at their respective firing rates. Fatigue in the set induces alterations in recruitment and firing rate. Motor unit recruitment increases with fatigue to compensate for the loss in force production capability of the previously activated motor units (94). In addition, motor units that were firing at low rates at the start of the set may have to fire at higher rates (rate coding) as the set progresses in response to the fatigue associated with the task. These changes are detected in the surface EMG signal (23, 94). Specifically, the size of the surface EMG signal gets larger during a set of resistance training exercise (86). This reflects changes in motor unit recruitment and firing rate.

Motor unit recruitment is based on the **size principle** (35) (figure 5.1; 41a). In general, lower-threshold motor units innervate fewer muscle fibers than do higher-threshold motor units. Lower-threshold motor units are typically activated during tasks that do not demand a high amount of force output (e.g., maintenance of posture or walking). However, as the demand for force output increases (e.g., during a sprint or maximal leg exercise on a resistance-loaded device), low-threshold and high-threshold motor units (and muscle fibers innervated by these motor units) are simultaneously recruited to meet this demand (36). In essence, the size principle describes this orderly manner of motor unit recruitment during muscular contraction.

> **Recruitment of motor units for force production follows the size principle, meaning that lower-threshold motor units are recruited at lower force levels and both lower- and higher-threshold motor units are recruited at higher force levels.**

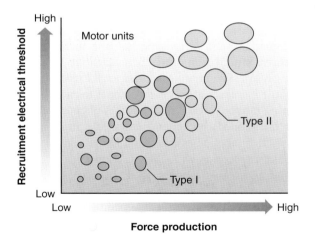

FIGURE 5.1 Graphic representation of the size principle.

Reprinted by permission from National Strength and Conditioning Association (2016, p. 91).

Muscular Changes

As previously noted, muscles can experience fatigue during a set of resistance exercise. Although fatigue is a highly complex phenomenon, it is clear that the acute changes in muscle cells include an accumulation of **metabolites** (i.e., substances [such as lactate]

formed during metabolic reactions) and depletion of fuel substrates (28). The factors involved are tied to the metabolic pathways that are primarily stressed during anaerobic activities (like resistance training), specifically the phosphagen system and glycolysis. Metabolites that accumulate include lactate, hydrogen ions (H^+, resulting in a decrease in muscle pH), inorganic phosphate (P_i), and ammonia (84). All of these metabolites have been studied as potential causes of muscle fatigue, but researchers are now beginning to appreciate their roles in promoting long-term adaptation. For instance, petri dish and rodent experiments have shown that chronic lactate administration increases muscle cell hypertrophy in the absence of exercise (99, 100), whereas phosphate administration increases the cellular process of autophagy, which can potentially be leveraged to remove cellular structures affected by exercise-induced muscle damage (142). Although these data are preliminary and more studies are needed to validate findings in humans, the studies conceptually illustrate that skeletal muscle adaptation is likely facilitated through a plethora of mechanisms.

Also noted earlier, CP can become depleted during resistance exercise, reflecting the reliance on the phosphagen system during typical resistance training. CP is important for phosphorylation of adenosine diphosphate (ADP) to adenosine triphosphate (ATP) during high-intensity exercise, and depletion of CP likely leads to decreased power production. Although complete muscle glycogen depletion is unlikely to occur with resistance training, glycogen breakdown is an important factor in the supply of energy for this type of training (110). In fact, it has been estimated that over 80% of the ATP production during bodybuilding-type resistance training comes from glycolysis (80). Therefore, glycogen levels decrease in response to high-intensity resistance training, and this points to the importance of adequate dietary carbohydrate for those who perform intensive resistance training.

Endocrine Changes

Hormones are blood-borne molecules that are produced in the endocrine glands. There are two primary types of hormones: protein and peptide hormones and steroid hormones. Two examples of protein and peptide hormones are growth hormone and insulin. Steroid hormones are all derived from a common precursor (cholesterol) and include hormones such as testosterone (the primary male sex hormone) and estrogen (the primary female sex hormone).

Many hormones have effects on either the growth or the degradation of tissue such as skeletal muscle.

Anabolic hormones such as testosterone, growth hormone (GH), insulin, and insulin-like growth factor-1 (IGF-1) stimulate growth processes, while catabolic hormones such as cortisol promote protein degradation to help maintain blood glucose homeostasis. To facilitate a biological response, hormones must bind to a hormone-specific receptor in a target tissue. For example, testosterone affects muscle cells at the molecular level by binding to androgen receptors. The interaction of testosterone with androgen receptors then signals the muscle to upregulate the production of a variety of contractile and noncontractile proteins (i.e., increase **muscle protein synthesis**, a process critical for skeletal muscle hypertrophy that will be discussed in greater detail later in this chapter). Muscle protein synthesis rates are determined by the sum of noncontractile protein (e.g., mitochondrial or sarcoplasmic) and myofibrillar protein (e.g., actin and myosin) synthesis rates.

Additionally, **net protein balance** in muscle (or any given tissue) is the sum of protein synthesis and protein breakdown rates. Under normal physiological conditions (i.e., well-nourished, nondiseased states), muscle protein breakdown rates are relatively stable, and a bout of resistance exercise increases net protein balance by elevating muscle protein synthesis rates. However, research suggests that the initial phases of training (i.e., first three or four weeks) involve concomitant increases in muscle protein synthesis and breakdown rates after each exercise bout (31), and increases in breakdown rates after each bout become more subdued as an individual continues training. Over time, these acute responses lead to the net accretion of more contractile and noncontractile muscle proteins, resulting in skeletal muscle hypertrophy. These topics are revisited later in the chapter.

An acute bout of exercise affects the blood concentrations of many hormones. Indeed, changes in some hormone concentrations are needed to support the metabolic response to exercise. For example, exercise increases epinephrine concentrations. Epinephrine binds to adrenergic receptors to increase fat and carbohydrate breakdown by the cell so that more ATP will be available for muscle contraction. Epinephrine also has effects on the central nervous system, which may facilitate motor unit activation.

Testosterone and GH concentrations are also transiently elevated in males during and after a bout of resistance exercise (56, 77, 79, 119), and both hormones stimulate increases in skeletal muscle protein synthesis. These associations have led many to speculate that anabolic hormones (e.g., testosterone, GH, and IGF-1), more specifically the summation of postexercise increases in these hormones, likely promote muscle mass increases with longer-term resistance training. However, although repeated increases in anabolic hormone concentrations after multiple training bouts may lead to training adaptations, there has been considerable debate on this topic. Scientists have determined that postexercise increases in blood testosterone, GH, or IGF-1 concentrations within 60 minutes after the first session of a 16-week resistance training intervention were not associated with muscle fiber hypertrophy (91). Instead, research has suggested that intrinsic mechanotransduction signaling in skeletal muscle primarily facilitates resistance training adaptations. Simplistically, **mechanotransduction** is the process where protein signals in muscle increase in response to a resistance exercise bout (69). These signals ultimately converge to activate the mammalian target of rapamycin signaling complex 1 (mTORc1) to increase muscle protein synthesis.

The aforementioned 16-week training study revealed that pre- to postintervention increases in muscle androgen receptor concentrations were significantly associated with increases in muscle fiber size (91), and other research supports these findings (3). Thus, these data indeed suggest that anabolic hormones promote skeletal muscle adaptations to training. Chronic resistance training adaptations are likely facilitated through various mechanisms including the repetitive stimulation of mechanosensitive signaling pathways in skeletal muscle after each exercise bout, pulsatile increases in certain hormones to each bout of training (although the impact of this phenomena has been questioned), and enhanced skeletal muscle sensitivity to anabolic hormones via increased hormone receptor expression with chronic training.

The hormonal response to resistance exercise is dependent on the characteristics of the training bout. As a general rule, bouts that have higher volume and shorter rest periods elicit stronger endocrine responses than do bouts with lower volume and longer rest periods (78), although the differences between protocols may diminish with prolonged training. Similarly, large muscle mass exercises promote greater increases in anabolic hormones than do small muscle mass exercises (78). Other factors such as sex and age can affect the acute endocrine response. Males tend to have larger acute changes in anabolic hormone concentrations than do females (78). Similarly, elderly individuals tend to exhibit an attenuated anabolic hormonal response to training relative to younger individuals (78). However, again, these pulsatile postexercise increases in hormones appear to play a limited role in the adaptive response to training. Alternatively stated, higher-volume exercise may promote greater skeletal muscle growth than higher-load, lower-volume resistance training because of intrinsic adaptations that occur in skeletal muscle fibers.

CHRONIC ADAPTATIONS

Chronic adaptations are long-term changes in the structure and function of the body as a consequence of exercise training. With respect to resistance training, the general adaptations that one experiences after prolonged resistance training are increases in strength and muscle mass. Increases in strength are influenced by changes in neurological function as well as changes in muscle mass. In addition, changes in muscle enzyme and substrate concentrations may influence muscular endurance. These chronic adaptations are summarized in table 5.2.

TABLE 5.2   Chronic Adaptations to Resistance Training

Variable	Chronic adaptation
MUSCLE PERFORMANCE	
Muscular strength	Increase
Muscular endurance	Increase
Power	Increase
MUSCLE ENZYMES	
Phosphagen system enzyme concentrations	May increase
Phosphagen system enzyme absolute levels	Increase
Glycolytic enzyme concentrations	May increase
Glycolytic enzyme absolute levels	Increase
MUSCLE SUBSTRATES	
ATP concentration	May increase
ATP absolute levels	Increase
CP concentration	May increase
CP absolute levels	Increase
ATP and CP changes during exercise	Decrease
Lactate increase during exercise	Decrease
MUSCLE FIBER CHARACTERISTICS	
Type I CSA	Increase (<type II)
Type II CSA	Increase (>type I)
% Type IIa	Increase
% Type IIx	Decrease
% Type I	No change
BODY COMPOSITION	
% Fat	Likely decrease
Fat free mass	Increase
Metabolic rate	Likely increase
NEUROLOGICAL CHANGES	
EMG amplitude during MVC	Likely increase
Motor unit recruitment	Likely increase
Motor unit firing rate	Increase
Cocontraction	Decrease
STRUCTURAL CHANGES	
Connective tissue strength	Likely increase
Bone mass and density	Likely increase

ATP = adenosine triphosphate; CP = creatine phosphate; CSA = cross-sectional area; EMG = electromyogram; MVC = maximal voluntary contraction.

Neurological Changes

Increases in strength occur rapidly during the early stages of a resistance training program, and they are larger than can be accounted for by changes in muscle size. These early strength gains are often attributed to so-called neural factors (93), and several studies indicate that strength increases consequent to resistance training are influenced by increases in neural drive (33, 74). The assumption that neural factors are involved is based not only on the discrepancy between hypertrophic and strength increases early in a training program but also on increases in EMG amplitude measured during maximal contractions (74).

The influence of neural factors on strength gains is believed to be dominant in the early phases of a training program (one to two months), and thereafter hypertrophy begins to significantly contribute to strength gains (figure 5.2; 132a). Much of the improvement seen early in training is likely due to improvements in performing the resistance exercises, especially in individuals who are using free-weight exercises requiring balance and efficiency of movement. However, some evidence suggests this effect is partly due to changes in motor unit recruitment and firing rate. With respect to motor unit recruitment, the argument is that many untrained individuals are

unable to activate all the available motor units, and resistance training may increase their ability to activate high-threshold, fast-twitch motor units, leading to an increase in force production capability that is independent of muscle hypertrophy. We should note, however, that according to some studies untrained individuals are able to recruit all available motor units (10, 88). In addition, not all studies show an increase in EMG amplitude following resistance training programs (49, 136), indicating increased strength may be a result of improvement in neural sequencing. Evidence suggests that resistance training can also increase maximal motor unit firing rates (33), and this adaptation would theoretically increase muscle force production capability independent of hypertrophy.

In addition to changes in motor unit recruitment and firing rate, other neurological adaptations have been reported in the literature. **Cocontraction** (or **coactivation**) refers to the simultaneous activation of an agonist and an antagonist during a motor task. As an example, during knee extension exercise, the quadriceps muscles are the agonists (prime movers) while the hamstrings are the antagonist muscles. Several studies have shown significant cocontraction during isometric and isokinetic actions of the knee joint (101, 109, 134), primarily to provide joint stabilization. Decreased cocontraction would reduce the antagonist torque that must be overcome by the agonist during a muscle action, thus enhancing the expression of strength. There appear to be decreases in cocontraction after isometric resistance training without compromised joint stabilization through improved skill of the exercise and neurological recruitment patterns (6). Whether similar changes in cocontraction occur during dynamic exercise, such as with free weights, is unknown but appears likely. Other research has shown changes in motor neuron excitability (115) and, as noted earlier, increases in motor unit synchronization after resistance training (90). The contribution of neural factors to strength improvement has also been inferred from observations that unilateral resistance training improves strength in the untrained limb (i.e., cross-education effect) (135, 136), as well as from observations that isometric resistance training at one joint angle results in strength increases that are larger at the trained angle than at other joint angles (129, 136).

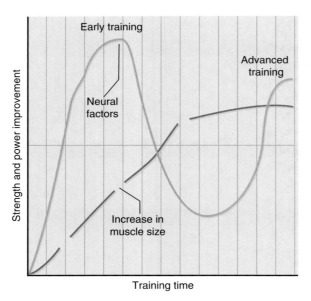

FIGURE 5.2 The contributions of neural factors and muscular size to improvements in strength. Neural factors include those related to improved skill, motor recruitment, and firing rate.

Reprinted by permission from National Strength and Conditioning Association (2000).

Muscle Tissue Changes

Resistance training results in adaptations in muscles, tendons, and ligaments. The most obvious adaptation in skeletal muscle is **hypertrophy** in the form of increased muscle size (cross-sectional area and volume). Resistance training also increases the cross-sectional area of both type I and type II muscle fibers. However, type II fibers typically show a greater degree of hypertrophy compared with type I fibers (41), and type II fibers are also susceptible to a greater degree of atrophy following detraining (70). Although definitive reasons for this are currently unknown, emerging evidence suggests that overload-induced hypertrophy in rodents elicits greater type II versus type I fiber hypertrophy owing to more robust increases in muscle protein synthesis, greater decrements in muscle proteolysis, and greater increases in muscle ribosomes, which are the macromolecules that facilitate muscle protein synthesis (112).

Given that muscle cells volumetrically contain ~70% of contractile protein in the form of myofibrils (62), it has been speculated that the increase in muscle fiber cross-sectional area is due to a proportional increase in the number of myofibrils within a given muscle fiber. Alternatively stated, if an individual experiences a 30% increase in muscle fiber size with resistance training, this is likely due to a 30% increase in the number of myofibrils within the hypertrophied muscle fibers. The increase in myofibril number is likely caused by the pulsatile increases in myofibrillar protein synthesis rates stimulated by each training bout as well as the possible splitting of existing myofibrils into separate "daughter" myofibrils (62). **Hyperplasia**, or the increase in number of muscle fibers, has not been definitively shown to occur in humans, but there is evidence that hyperplasia occurs in animals that undergo extreme loading models to induce supraphysiological hypertrophy (5). The net result of an increase in muscle cross-sectional area, and the associated increase in myofibrils containing actin and myosin filaments, is an increase in the force and power production capability of the muscle.

> **The primary adaptation of skeletal muscle to long-term resistance training is hypertrophy, or increased cross-sectional area of the muscle fiber, resulting in increased force and power production capability.**

With respect to muscle fiber types, resistance training induces a fiber subtype shift from type IIx to type IIa muscle fibers (54, 121, 132). These subtype shifts are observable after just a few training sessions (120) and likely reflect a change in the myosin heavy chain composition of the muscle cell. Therefore, resistance training alters not only the quantity of muscle tissue (hypertrophy) but also the quality of contractile proteins within individual fibers. It has been heavily debated as to whether resistance training can induce a shift from slow- to fast-twitch fibers or vice versa. However, some researchers have posited that years of resistance training may eventually promote the transition of some type I fibers to type II fibers (140). In support of this argument, several human biopsy studies have revealed that type IIa and IIx fibers are more prominent in individuals who engage in long-term resistance training, whereas type I fibers are prominent in individuals who engage in long-term aerobic endurance training (24, 25, 47, 48, 108). Additionally, a case study on monozygotic twins with discordant lifelong exercise training habits (i.e., one twin was aerobic endurance-trained, and the other was not) reported that the lifelong aerobic endurance-trained twin expressed 55% more type I fibers compared with the untrained twin (8). Thus, there is compelling evidence suggesting significant fiber type transitions can occur with long-term aerobic endurance training (and likely resistance training).

As mentioned previously, the hypertrophic response to resistance training is the net result of an increase in protein synthesis relative to protein breakdown in muscle fibers, and protein synthesis clearly increases after a bout of resistance training (82). A bout of resistance training also increases the rate of muscle protein degradation, but this response is less robust in magnitude as an individual becomes more trained (31). Increased protein degradation with a bout of resistance exercise is likely a consequence of muscle damage that has occurred during training via primarily eccentric contractions, and there is some speculation that the damage may be a stimulus for hypertrophy. In support of this notion, researchers have shown that training responses are enhanced when eccentric actions are included in the training, as occurs during typical resistance training, and eccentric actions are primarily implicated in the development of delayed-onset muscle soreness and muscle damage. There is evidence, however, that concentric-only training causes skeletal muscle hypertrophy (38, 124). Thus, it is likely that the magnitude or volume of loading, rather than eccentric muscle damage, is a more important determinant of muscle growth with resistance training.

In addition to increasing the contractile protein content of skeletal muscle, resistance training appears to increase cytoskeletal and structural proteins. These proteins help give skeletal muscle cells shape and structural integrity. They are also involved in force transmission from the myofibrils to the extracellular matrix and in the storage of elastic energy as occurs in stretch–shortening cycle activities. The study of adaptations in skeletal muscle cytoskeleton proteins to resistance training is newer and less developed than work on contractile protein changes. Nonetheless, there is clear evidence that the content of cytoskeletal proteins increases in response to resistance training (104, 141). Strength and power athletes have also been shown to have higher levels of the protein titin (87), a large elastic structural protein, which may enhance elastic energy storage. Interestingly, resistance training has not been shown to affect expression of the key protein dystrophin (104, 141), which suggests that the synthesis of specific structural proteins is stimulated by resistance training.

Skeletal Changes

It is tempting to conceptualize the skeletal system as an inert framework comprising simply a set of levers that muscles act upon to create movement. However, bone tissue is dynamic and very much alive. In addition to its role in movement and protection, bone serves as a depot for important minerals, most notably calcium. **Osteoporosis** is the consequence of long-term net demineralization of bone. Resistance training has been studied for its possible influence on bone mineral density (BMD). Bone tissue is significantly influenced by strain; that is, deformation (bending) of bone rapidly stimulates bone cells to begin activities that stimulate bone formation (68). Therefore, it seems logical to examine the effects of resistance training on bone formation, especially in the context of osteoporosis. Because osteoporosis is mainly, though not exclusively, a condition associated with postmenopausal women, most research has focused on women. Specifically, researchers have focused on the effect of resistance training on the accumulation of bone tissue before menopause (peak bone mass is typically achieved before age 40) (30), as well as on the effect of resistance training on the decline in bone mass associated with aging and menopause. Menopause is particularly critical in the development of osteoporosis because hormones like estrogen, which facilitate bone formation, markedly decline after menopause. The greater the bone mass before menopause, the less severe the consequences of loss of bone mass.

The research literature has shown quite clearly that, in cross-sectional studies, stronger women tend to have thicker and stronger bones. However, selection bias may influence such studies (1). Scholarly position stands and reviews of the scientific literature suggest resistance training can positively affect BMD and be used as a countermeasure to offset the progression of osteoporosis (9, 85, 130). However, outcomes likely vary in the literature owing to differences in study length, characteristics (e.g., intensity, volume, type of exercises) of the training programs, sample sizes, the extent of bone demineralization before training, sex, and age. Although the presence of an overload stimulus is likely required to produce bone adaptation, overload may be walking or jogging for sedentary individuals or heavy resistance exercise for athletes. A meta-analysis has reported that high-intensity resistance training can significantly increase lumbar spine BMD, but not BMD of the femoral neck, in premenopausal women (85). What has not been examined in depth is the effect of explosive and plyometric types of training on BMD. Both strain magnitude and strain rate affect the stimulus for bone formation (131), and these would be expected to be higher with explosive and plyometric training (74). In addition to the obvious effects of resistance training on muscle mass and strength, resistance training may lead to decreased risk for osteoporosis, fractures, and falls in later life.

> The greater the bone mass before menopause, the less severe the consequences of loss of bone mass. Resistance training may lead to decreased risk for osteoporosis, fractures, and falls in later life.

Tendon and Ligament Changes

Tendons and ligaments can also undergo adaption through prolonged resistance training. These connective tissues, made up primarily of bundles of fibrous collagen, have relatively few cells in their structure, so they do not require much blood, oxygen, or nutrients. Consequently, they also have poor vascular supplies, which increases the time it takes them to recover from injuries. Notwithstanding, an acute bout of resistance exercise stimulates collagen turnover and net collagen production (81, 89). Research has consistently shown that tendons can adapt to the loads applied during training, but there is little data on the specific effects of training on ligaments.

Research employing ultrasound and magnetic resonance imaging technology (MRI) has found changes in tendon size and mechanical properties associated with physical activity. For example, one study showed that male distance runners have thicker Achilles tendons than do kayakers (76), while another showed that elite fencers and badminton players have significantly greater patellar tendon cross-sectional areas (and thigh-muscle cross-sectional area and strength) in the lead leg compared with the trail leg (27). Notably, both fencing and badminton involve unilateral lunging motions that place high eccentric loads on the lead leg. Thus, as in muscle, these data suggest eccentric loading also stimulates tendon adaptations in spite of connective tissue's much lower supply of blood and nutrients. Other research has suggested that the specific effects of physical activity on tendon size may vary according to sex.

One study found that female distance runners do not exhibit greater cross-sectional area of either the Achilles or patellar tendons relative to female controls and that female runners have markedly lower tendon cross-sectional areas relative to male distance runners (138). The study's authors suggested that sex differences in tendon size might be due to endocrine differences between males and females because estrogen and progesterone receptors are present in fibroblasts of ligaments, and estrogen has been shown to inhibit collagen synthesis. This interpretation is supported by data showing suppressed rates of postexercise collagen synthesis in women taking oral contraceptives (59).

Longitudinal training studies have shown that resistance training may alter the mechanical properties of tendons. For example, increased tendon stiffness (amount of force per unit of tendon length change under load) has been shown to occur after 10 weeks of resistance training (137). However, a meta-analysis indicates that years of resistance training, while increasing tendon cross-sectional area, does not affect mechanical properties (139). Thus, further research is necessary to delineate the training variables (e.g., type, load, volume, frequency) that maximize the training benefits to tendons and determine how this affects injury risk and rehabilitation.

Cartilage Changes

Resistance and aerobic training are currently accepted as an effective treatment for osteoarthritis (OA) patients, but appropriate exercise prescription for those with OA is yet to be determined. Consensus from research reveals resistance exercise can improve strength, increase joint function, and reduce pain in sufferers of hip and knee OA (50, 64, 65); still, consistent application of resistance training principles (specificity, overload, and progression) considering age, sex, and level of disease is needed to better understand a dose–response relationship.

Being avascular, cartilage relies on diffusion of nutrients; consequently, vertebral discs have demonstrated greater nutrient transport during dynamic loading replicating stair climbing versus static loading (116). Further, in vitro evidence shows that human cartilage responds to mechanical stimulation of dynamic compressional loads via upregulation of gene expression, resulting in increased production of the structural components of cartilage (glycosaminoglycan and collagen) with no change in markers of hypertrophy (96). Although a wide range of resistance training methods are safe and beneficial for at-risk and OA patients (73), the effects of training on cartilage composition, thickness, and volume are currently inconclusive from findings of both positive (11, 114) and nonsignificant improvement (98). A conservative approach to increasing intensity is warranted when applying the principle of overload in OA patients to minimize the risk of further degeneration (105); still, a spectrum of intensities (ranging from 30% of 1RM to near-maximal loads) can provide adequate resistance for strength improvement with a high level of effort, resulting in sets nearing or ending in repetition failure (117). A training program designed to improve strength is beneficial in OA clients and may be a requisite to augment morphology and composition.

Longitudinal studies investigating the effect of resistance exercise on healthy cartilage are limited and do not support morphological improvement above normal levels (26). Yet professional weightlifters and sprinters have demonstrated greater patellar cartilage thickness compared with untrained participants (52). With significant loss of cartilage and function found during periods of immobilization (97), the data indicate that the primary benefit of physical activity is to either maintain healthy cartilage thickness and composition or minimize loss from genetic predisposition (125). Although some evidence indicates that resistance exercise strengthens cartilage structure and function, more training studies are needed to establish appropriate guidelines across all types of resistance exercise for specific populations ranging from healthy to various levels of arthritic disease.

Metabolic Changes

Research has shown that chronic resistance training induces a variety of cellular changes that affect the metabolism of skeletal muscle. All studies of metabolic adaptations to resistance training are complicated by the fact that cellular expansion during hypertrophy likely dilutes certain enzyme and substrate levels so that changes in absolute levels may result in no change of relative levels (e.g., concentration per unit of muscle mass). In addition, relative decreases in enzyme or substrate concentrations may simply reflect hypertrophy. As an example, if an individual displays a 30% average increase in muscle fiber size following 12 weeks of resistance training and no change in the relative amount of muscle glycogen, these outcomes indicate that the absolute amount of glycogen increased, given that glycogen levels were not diluted as the cell expanded. Many studies have concluded that hypertrophy as a result of resistance training dilutes skeletal muscle mitochondria since the relative levels (per milligram of muscle mass) decrease (55). However, this does not indicate that mitochondria are lost with training; rather, the expansion of the muscle cell occurred at a greater rate relative to the creation of new mitochondria. In fact, given that skeletal muscle mitochondria are critical for aerobic capacity (i.e., $\dot{V}O_2$max) and resistance training does not change or may even enhance $\dot{V}O_2$max (42, 106), certain forms of resistance training (while diluting mitochondrial content within muscle fibers) may promote favorable mitochondrial adaptations (e.g., an increase in mitochondrial enzymes used for ATP synthesis).

Resistance training primarily stresses anaerobic metabolism, and therefore one should expect that any enzymatic or substrate adaptations would involve anaerobic metabolism. Anaerobic metabolism is typically thought of as having two components: the phosphagen system and glycolysis. Conflicting data exist regarding whether anaerobic substrate and enzyme concentrations increase or decrease with resistance training. With respect to the phosphagen system, some evidence suggests that resistance training does not result in increased concentration of ATP or CP in skeletal muscle, although equivocal evidence also exists (83, 127). Similarly, some data suggest that the enzymes involved in this system, creatine kinase and myokinase, have decreased in concentration after six months of resistance training (126), although again, there is equivocal evidence suggesting these enzymes increase in response to six weeks of very-high-volume resistance training (61).

With respect to glycolytic activity, research has typically shown that key enzymes involved in the glycolytic pathway (e.g., phosphofructokinase, lactate dehydrogenase) are not found in higher concentrations after resistance training (126). However, these results may be specific to the type of resistance training performed, since bodybuilders who perform higher-volume training with shorter rest periods than powerlifters have glycolytic enzyme concentrations similar to those of aerobic endurance athletes such as swimmers (127a). Further, the aforementioned study implementing very-high-volume resistance training loads over a six-week period revealed that although muscle glycogen concentrations were unaffected by training, numerous glycolytic enzymes were upregulated (61). Differences in outcomes between studies likely reflect differences in training mode and volume and indicate the importance of designing programs to meet the specific needs of individual clients. However, it is likely that higher-volume resistance training upregulates creatine kinase as well as various glycolytic enzymes, whereas low-volume, high-load training has marginal effects.

From a practical perspective, the endurance capacity of muscle to lift weights for more repetitions typically increases with resistance training (16), and this is likely due to increases in creatine kinase as well as glycolytic enzyme levels.

Endocrine Changes

Although resistance training can cause large changes in hormone concentrations during and after a bout of training, the long-term effects of resistance training on resting hormone concentrations are less clear. Also, understanding of these effects is complicated by the fact that overreaching or overtraining can cause changes in hormone concentrations that are different from those seen during normal training situations. That said, some evidence suggests that prolonged resistance training results in chronically elevated testosterone concentrations (57, 58); however, it is difficult to discern if this modest increase in serum testosterone further facilitates muscle growth. In contrast, other studies show no changes in resting testosterone concentrations with months of resistance training (4, 92). There does not appear to be a chronic training effect on resting GH concentrations (56, 58).

As alluded to previously, chronic resistance training may also affect the magnitude of the endocrine response and the sensitivity of tissues to a hormone. For instance, and as mentioned earlier in the chapter, there are multiple lines of evidence to suggest months of resistance training upregulates skeletal muscle androgen receptor content (3, 91). Thus, the effect of testosterone on skeletal muscle may be amplified because of increased hormone-receptor interaction.

Cardiorespiratory Changes

Resistance training places a markedly different stress on the cardiorespiratory system than does aerobic endurance exercise such as running or cycling, and therefore the effects on the cardiorespiratory system are quite different. With respect to aerobic endurance performance, a meta-analysis examining 17 studies indicated that only 3 of the reviewed studies showed resistance training was capable of increasing peak $\dot{V}O_2$ max in young adults (20-40 years) (102). An important caveat to this study, however, is that resistance training typically increases $\dot{V}O_2$ max in older subjects (>60 years). Moreover, the authors speculated that resistance training better increases $\dot{V}O_2$ max in both younger and older individuals with low aerobic fitness levels. It is important for personal trainers to understand that aerobic fitness adaptations from resistance training are likely dependent on the age and pre-existing fitness levels of the client.

Although resistance training programs do not typically improve maximal oxygen consumption to the extent seen with other modes of aerobic endurance training (e.g., running, cycling), they augment the development of cardiovascular endurance performance and improve running efficiency while not causing any negative effects on the development of maximal oxygen consumption (66, 67, 103). Therefore, although resistance training does not directly increase peak $\dot{V}O_2$, it can serve as an important adjunct to aerobic endurance training. Nonetheless, to achieve optimal results in increasing the aerobic endurance capabilities of a client requires aerobic endurance–specific training. Chapter 16 provides the details of such programs for improving maximal oxygen consumption and discusses the effects of such training on strength gains.

> **Increasing aerobic endurance capabilities requires aerobic endurance–specific training to achieve optimal results; however, resistance training can augment aerobic endurance performance and running efficiency by increasing muscular strength and power.**

As noted previously, resistance training depends primarily on anaerobic metabolism to generate ATP for muscle actions. Therefore, it is not surprising that resistance training does not appear to improve skeletal muscle cellular aerobic function as assessed by oxidative enzyme activity and capillary density. However, resistance training likely does increase the formation of new muscle capillaries, or capillarization, so that capillary number per muscle fiber and muscle blood flow are maintained in spite of increased muscle size (54). As stated previously, mitochondrial density also generally decreases with resistance training. However, again, this indicates that the rate of cellular growth outpaces the intracellular accretion of mitochondria and does not indicate that resistance training leads to a loss of this organelle.

Despite the lack of improvement in skeletal muscle cellular aerobic function, normal increases in muscle size (i.e., hypertrophy) with resistance training do not reduce muscular endurance. On the contrary, increases in muscle size and strength due to resistance training increase local muscular endurance (16). That is, a hypertrophied muscle, with the corresponding increases in strength and volume of metabolic enzymes and substrates (but not necessarily a higher density), can perform more work over time.

Body Composition Changes

A variety of models have been developed to quantify body composition. For the personal trainer, the model that best relates to the needs of clients is the two-component model, which segregates the body into fat mass and fat free mass (FFM). The FFM is composed of tissues such as muscle, bone, and connective tissue. As noted previously, resistance training can affect all of these components, so it follows that a resistance training program inducing hypertrophy will directly affect body composition. Increases in FFM independent of changes in fat mass will decrease body fat percentage. As an example, an individual who begins training with 140 pounds (63.5 kg) of FFM and 30 pounds (13.6 kg) of fat mass has a body fat percentage of 17.6% (30 pounds of fat mass ÷ 170 pounds of total body mass). If this individual subsequently gains 5 pounds (2.3 kg) of muscle during a four-month training period without losing fat, then the new body composition value is 17.1% (30 pounds of fat mass ÷ 175 pounds of total body mass). According to several studies, resistance training increases FFM and decreases body fat percentage in men (12a), women (29), and the elderly (14a).

All of this is not to say, however, that resistance training is not capable of promoting fat loss. In fact, long-term resistance training may decrease fat mass over time given that the act of lifting weights expends calories to fuel muscle contraction. Resistance training also elevates calorie expenditure during the recovery period between training sessions in order to replenish fuel substrate in muscle used during training (118). Notwithstanding, there are several misnomers in regard to resistance training, calorie expenditure, and fat loss. For instance, "gym talk" and internet threads have notoriously propagated a longstanding myth that one added pound of muscle from resistance training increases resting energy expenditure (REE) by 50 kcal/day. A well-controlled study determined that this is an erroneous suggestion (17); instead, the authors reported an increase in REE of <10 kcal/day per pound of added muscle.

Additionally, although some studies have shown that resistance exercise can increase resting metabolic rate, others have not. However, a higher-volume bout of full-body resistance exercise expends ~200 to 300 calories during the bout and another 100 calories over the remainder of the day (63). Hence, an individual who full-body trains using higher volumes (e.g., 3 sets of 10 repetitions with multiple exercises) can expect to expend ~900 to 1,200 calories per week, which, over time, may promote potential decreases in fat mass assuming dietary intakes remain relatively constant. Notably, these calculations apply to higher-volume lifting; training that involves lower volumes (e.g., 4 sets of 3-5 repetitions per set) expend fewer calories (by comparison) during and after exercise. It also remains questionable as to whether the magnitude of increased caloric expenditure from resistance training continues over time, as attenuation of muscle damage from consistent training reduces the energy-intensive muscle protein synthesis response to subsequent exercise bouts (31).

FACTORS THAT INFLUENCE ADAPTATIONS TO RESISTANCE TRAINING

A variety of factors affect the adaptations to resistance training described in the previous sections. These include **specificity** (i.e., the ability of the body to make adaptations that uniquely enhance performance in activities that are most similar to the exercise stressor), sex, age, and genetics. These factors affect the magnitude and rate of long-term adaptations that occur in the body. The following subsections explore these topics.

Specificity

The effects of exercise training have been shown to be highly specific. That is, the body adapts to exercise in such a way that it can perform optimally in relation to a particular type of exercise stressor, but not necessarily other types of exercise. For instance, distance running has little to no positive effect on bench press performance. However, specificity also influences resistance exercise adaptations. In terms of resistance exercises, the correlations between static and dynamic performance are poor. Many studies have examined the effect of one type of resistance training on performance of other types of resistance exercise. In general, strength increases are larger in modes of exercise similar to those used during training. For example, resistance training with weights results in much larger performance increases in tests that involve free weights versus laboratory tests such as knee torque assessment using isokinetic dynamometers (133). Isometric exercise training has also been shown to have little to no effect on muscular strength tests implementing free-weight exercises that involve the same muscle groups. Thus, it appears that the effects of resistance training are specific to the muscle action mode in which the exercise was performed.

Resistance training adaptations are also specific with respect to the velocity with which muscle actions have been performed in training. That is, strength increases tend to be greater when individuals are tested in situations that involve muscle actions occurring at velocities similar to those experienced during training (133). Further, plyometric-type training is more effective than relatively slow-velocity heavy resistance exercise in improving force production at higher velocities (132). Therefore, for athletes who are participating in resistance exercise to improve athletic performance, the sport performance coach or personal trainer should tailor the training program, as much as possible, to include similar muscle actions experienced in the athletic competition. Likewise, although all clients will benefit from a well-rounded resistance training program, an older client desiring the muscular strength and endurance to carry heavy bags of groceries long distances would benefit from walking with hand weights, and a client desiring the strength to do home improvement projects such as pounding fence posts would benefit from more explosive pushing and pulling exercises.

Sex

Males and females respond to resistance training in much the same way, yet they show significant quantitative differences in strength, muscle mass, and hormone levels. With respect to muscular strength, much of the difference between the sexes is attributable to differences in body size and body composition. Specifically, men tend to be larger than women, and the associated differences in muscle mass contribute to strength differences. Similarly, women tend to have a higher percentage of body fat than men; therefore, most women have less muscle per pound of body weight. These differences in body size and body composition are largely driven by differences in hormone levels between men and women, most notably testosterone and estrogen. For example, adult male athletes have approximately 10 times the testosterone concentration of comparable female athletes (19). Interestingly, sex-related differences in strength are larger in the upper body than in the lower body (13), which likely reflects sex differences in the distribution of muscle mass. That is, women and men tend to exhibit similar relative lower body strength, whereas men typically have much greater upper body strength than do women.

When one considers strength per pound of fat free mass, strength differences between the sexes are marginalized (13), and when assessed per unit of muscle cross-sectional area, sex differences are negligible (72). Furthermore, muscle architecture characteristics are similar between males and females (2). Thus, it appears that the force production capability of a given amount of muscle is not affected by whether one is male or female.

> The force production capability of a given amount of muscle is not affected by a person's sex.

Age

The process of aging produces a variety of changes in all body systems. Starting as early as the age of 30 or so, muscle mass begins to decline progressively with time in sedentary individuals (14). This age-related loss of muscle mass is referred to as **sarcopenia**. In addition to the loss in muscle mass, some evidence suggests that muscle quality also declines with age (44). That is, for a given amount of muscle, the amount of force that can be generated by that muscle declines. Aging skeletal muscle experiences muscle loss more severely in the higher-threshold motor units (123). Therefore, as individuals age, they see declines in both their ability to produce force and their ability to produce force rapidly. These aging effects on skeletal muscle affect performance in physical tasks such as those required for everyday activities and may be associated with the increased incidence of falls that occurs with age.

Fortunately, these deleterious effects of aging can be significantly moderated or even reversed with a program of high-intensity resistance training. It is well recognized that resistance training can increase muscle mass and strength in persons who are elderly. In addition, the training can result in significant improvements in muscle function in particular and also general motor performance (e.g., walking, stair climbing) (40). With low initial baseline levels, relative strength gains can be dramatic (upwards of 200% for knee extension strength), and increases in muscle size may occur in both type I and type II muscle fibers (43). Elderly populations can also increase BMD with resistance training as stated earlier in this chapter. Chapter 18 presents a more comprehensive overview of resistance training in older adults.

> As individuals age, they see declines in both their ability to produce force and their ability to produce force rapidly.

Genetics

Since the discovery of the DNA structure by renowned geneticists Watson, Crick, and Franklin in the 1950s, predisposition toward certain traits (e.g., body fatness or even certain behaviors) has been largely attributed to genetics. The potential adaptations to resistance training are also believed to have a genetic basis (15). Comprehensively outlining how genetics may affect training responsiveness is a complex topic and well beyond the scope of this chapter. However, effectively communicating how genetics may play a partial role in exercise training responsiveness can help empower and motivate clients.

> Just as with sex, scientists hypothesize that a person's genetics undoubtedly play a role in the ability to adapt to resistance training. This is a complex issue, given that numerous genes as well as environmental factors (e.g., nutrition, stress, and sleep) influence resistance training outcomes. Knowing how genetics may play a partial role in exercise training responsiveness can empower and motivate clients.

Simply stated, the body is made up of trillions of cells, and each one of these cells contains a nucleus that houses DNA; as an aside, muscle cells have hundreds of nuclei interspersed across the entire cell, which makes them unique from other cell types. Within an individual, the DNA (or base pair) code across all cells is exactly the same, and the full complement of DNA within each cell's nucleus contains two copies of over 20,000 genes—one copy inherited from each biological parent (15). These 20,000 genes are used by cells to make proteins (e.g., enzymes, transporters, contractile proteins, mitochondrial proteins). There are several genes in the human genome that direct cells to synthesize contractile proteins, and these genes are "turned on" in muscle cells to a greater extent relative to other cell types (e.g., fat or endocrine cells).

Other genes are responsible for making enzymes that store fat, and these genes are "turned on" in fat cells to a greater extent than in other cell types (e.g., brain or kidney cells). Individual genetic potential in regard to gaining muscle mass, increasing strength, or losing fat is largely dictated by slight differences in genetic code, or **gene variants**, that exist across multiple genes. A prominent example in exercise science research involves the **alpha actinin-3 (ACTN3) gene**, which has been coined the "strength and power" or "athletic" gene by mainstream entities. The ACTN gene is responsible for producing a structural Z-line protein found mainly in type II muscle fibers. Individuals who possess two versions of the ACTN gene containing the X alleles (termed the ACTN XX genotype) make a partial version of the ACTN protein that cannot function properly, whereas individuals possessing the ACTN RX or RR genotype have muscle cells that synthesize functional ACTN 3 protein. Unlike various mutations in the dystrophin gene, which can lead to lethal muscular dystrophies, being a carrier of the ACTN XX genotype does not present deleterious health consequences.

Multiple studies suggest that >90% of elite power-lifters do not carry the ACTN XX genotype (111). This has led many scientists and practitioners to believe that individuals who carry the ACTN XX genotype were not born to be elite-level power athletes. Given that commercial DNA testing companies commonly let people know whether they possess the ACTN XX genotype, personal trainers may be faced with the conundrum of having this conversation with a knowing ACTN XX client. However, a well-controlled scientific study suggested ACTN XX carriers respond just as well to resistance training in terms of increasing muscle size and strength relative to RX and RR carriers (22). There are other gene variants that may also marginally affect resistance training adaptations, such as bradykinin type 2 receptor (B2BRK), myostatin (MSTN), and IGF-1 (111).

Again, even carriers of the unfavorable versions of these genes have been shown to gain muscle mass and strength with resistance training. Collectively, the aforementioned studies point toward genetics' potential influence on resistance training outcomes. However, this is a very complex and scientifically unresolved issue, and a client should not be led to believe that possessing a certain genotype will deter him or her from experiencing the numerous positive benefits that resistance training offers. In fact, pointing an ACTN XX client to this portion of the chapter and challenging him or her to defy the ACTN XX stereotype can serve as a powerful source of motivation for exercise adherence.

OVERTRAINING

Although physical adaptations are best brought about by increases in training volume and intensity, at certain points in a training program, more is not better. Inappropriate levels of volume or intensity can lead to a phenomenon known as overtraining. As the term suggests, **overtraining** is a condition in which an individual trains excessively, resulting in staleness and general fatigue. The overtraining condition does not enhance strength and power levels in the client but leads to decreased performance. A detailed discussion of the many aspects of resistance exercise overtraining (e.g., metabolic, neuromuscular, endocrine) as both a physical and a psychological phenomenon is beyond the scope of this chapter, and the reader is referred to other detailed scientific review articles on the topic (18, 45, 51). Because of the danger of overtraining, the tolerance of and recovery from resistance exercise stress are crucial factors that must be monitored carefully in every resistance training program.

Overtraining in resistance exercise has received much less attention than aerobic endurance overtraining, as significantly fewer studies have been reported. These studies make it clear that established markers of overtraining in aerobic endurance exercise are not always representative of overtraining in resistance exercise. It appears that the two primary contributors to overtraining in response to resistance training are too much intensity and too much volume (45). Yet each variable has been difficult to study. However, it is clear that resistance exercise overtraining can lead to decreases in neuromuscular performance (45). It is interesting to note that, at least in experimental situations, inducing an overtraining state requires a very severe exercise intervention but can be accomplished through repeated bouts of high-intensity exercise (~100% of the 1RM [1-repetition maximum]) with relatively low volume (46). Many overtraining syndromes are a function of the rate of progression (i.e., attempting to do too much, too soon before the body's physiological adaptations can cope with the stress). This typically results in extreme soreness or injury.

Individuals may fall into either or both of two overtraining scenarios: overuse injury of a joint or muscle and overtraining of the body, which can lead to changes in mood profile, lethargy, and premature strength plateaus. Both scenarios are common, and many people experience both. As alluded to earlier, overtraining is most often a result of increasing the volume of the program at too rapid a pace. In addition, some people may maintain too many days at high intensity without varying their load or taking a rest. Effective program design includes increasing and decreasing the total volume of the workout and using the concepts of periodization to plan changes in volume, intensity, and recovery (75) (see chapter 23). The difficulty in dealing with real overtraining and the symptoms that may develop is that there is no 100% accurate measurement for the onset of overtraining. Generally, once symptoms develop, overtraining is certain and strength gains are attenuated. Once symptoms have developed, the most effective cure is rest, which can vary from days to weeks of not training until the symptoms improve.

Some programs use short periods of overwork followed by rest or reduced training to achieve the benefits of a rebound, or supercompensation, in physical strength and power. This process of **overreaching** is best used only by elite athletes under the direction of experienced coaches; most clients would be best served by more moderate training regimens.

SYMPTOMS OF OVERTRAINING FROM RESISTANCE EXERCISE

- Plateau followed by decrease of strength gains
- Sleep disturbances
- Decrease in lean body mass (when not dieting)
- Decreased appetite
- A cold that just will not go away
- Persistent flu-like symptoms
- Loss of interest in the training program
- Mood changes
- Excessive muscle soreness

DETRAINING

Detraining refers to the physiological and performance adaptations that occur when an individual ceases an exercise training program. These changes are the exact opposite of what occurs during training programs, and the individual regresses toward his or her condition before starting the program. Specifically, there is a loss of muscle mass (i.e., **atrophy**) (95), and the changes in neurological function (e.g., recruitment, rate coding, cocontraction) that occurred with training dissipate (70). Thus, the muscle becomes weaker and less powerful. Skeletal muscle atrophy appears to occur faster in the fast-twitch muscle fibers (95).

There is relatively little research on the detraining process with resistance training as compared with the training process, so the rapidity of the detraining process is poorly understood. However, short-term detraining (14 days) appears to have little effect on muscular strength and explosive power in experienced resistance-trained athletes and individuals who do resistance training on a recreational basis, suggesting the effects are relatively slow (95). Extended detraining (48 weeks) has been shown to result in significant decreases in muscular strength in older males who resistance trained 24 weeks prior (39). Interestingly, however, this depended on the loads used during training. In this regard, participants who routinely lifted with higher training loads (~80% of the 1RM) lost less strength than the other participants who trained with lighter loads (~55% of the 1RM).

Given that the effects of detraining have been found to be significantly reduced with the incorporation of just one training session per week (53), clients with unexpectedly busy or difficult schedules may maintain a certain level of strength by training only once per week. It should be noted, however, that while muscle gains experienced from a resistance training program can be maintained with markedly reduced volumes of training, older individuals appear to require somewhat higher volumes for maintenance (12). Thus, certain clients may maintain strength by training one day per week, while some older clients may have to train at least two times per week.

CONCLUSION

Resistance training is a very potent physiological stimulus. It has substantive effects on almost every component of the body, including muscle, bone, nerve tissue, hormones, and connective tissue. Although resistance training is not a panacea, its effects are almost universally positive, and personal trainers should encourage all clients to engage in an appropriate level of resistance training. Benefits include improved physical function and capacity, self-efficacy, physical appearance, body composition, muscular strength, power, muscular endurance, and bone and connective tissue strength. These changes can improve quality of life and may have significant health benefits, including the attenuation of the deleterious effects of sarcopenia during aging and possibly attenuation of the effects of osteoporosis. In addition, the increased muscle performance (strength, endurance, power) will likely improve the performance of activities of daily living, so that tasks like carrying groceries and changing a tire are more easily accomplished.

Study Questions

1. Which of the following is *incorrect* regarding stress responses to resistance exercise?
   - A. can lead to increases in bone mineral density
   - B. is a negative response that inhibits adaptation
   - C. leads to muscle growth
   - D. results in increased strength

2. Which of the following is *not* a steroid hormone?
   - A. testosterone
   - B. growth hormone
   - C. estrogen
   - D. any hormone derived from cholesterol

3. Which of the following is *incorrect* regarding endocrine adaptations to resistance exercise?
   - A. Testosterone has been shown to increase.
   - B. Chronic changes to hormones are *greater* than acute changes.
   - C. Resistance exercise leads to upregulation of androgen receptor content.
   - D. Growth hormone does *not* appear to increase.

4. Which of the following is *incorrect* regarding individuals who possess the ACTN XX genotype?
   - A. They respond less well to resistance training.
   - B. Commercial DNA testing companies can inform individuals if they possess it.
   - C. The ACTN gene is responsible for producing a structural Z-line protein found mainly in type II muscle fibers.
   - D. Being a carrier of the ACTN XX genotype does not present deleterious health consequences.

5. Approximately how often does resistance exercise need to be performed to prevent detraining?
   - A. 3 sessions per week
   - B. 1 or 2 sessions per week
   - C. 1 session every 2 weeks
   - D. 1 session per month

CHAPTER 6

Responses and Adaptations to Aerobic Endurance Training

Don Melrose, PhD, and David J. Heikkinen, PhD

After completing this chapter, you will be able to:

- identify acute physiological responses to aerobic exercise,

- identify chronic physiological adaptations to aerobic endurance training,

- understand the factors that influence adaptations to aerobic endurance training,

- understand and identify the physiological factors associated with overtraining, and

- identify the physiological consequences of detraining.

The primary purpose of this chapter is to discuss the effects of aerobic exercise on the body's physiological systems and to explain the adaptations that occur. Acute responses occur immediately during a single exercise bout, whereas chronic training adaptations occur through a series of repeated exercise bouts. The effects of aerobic exercise are regulated by the intensity, duration, and frequency of the activity. Paramount among these is intensity (e.g., %HRmax [% maximal heart rate]). Specifically, the body adapts to an acute exercise stressor in proportion to that stressor. In general, exercising at a greater heart rate during aerobic exercise will induce greater training adaptations than exercising at a lower heart rate. Of course, this assumes that frequency and duration are constant across training sessions. It is the interplay of these components that results in aerobic physiological adaptations. With aerobic endurance training, the body responds through alterations in many physiological processes and systems. The sections that follow explain in further detail exactly how these changes occur. The overall adaptation to recurring aerobic exercise is a more efficient body, resulting in less effort by all organs at the same exercise work rate.

ACUTE RESPONSES TO AEROBIC ENDURANCE EXERCISE

This section describes the acute effects of aerobic exercise on the cardiovascular, respiratory, and endocrine systems as well as its effects on metabolism. These responses are summarized in table 6.1; responses for most physiological variables (e.g., oxygen consumption [$\dot{V}O_2$], heart rate [HR]) are strongly related to exercise intensity.

The authors would like to acknowledge the significant contributions of John P. McCarthy, Jane L.P. Roy, Lee E. Brown, and Matthew J. Comeau to this chapter.

TABLE 6.1 Summary of Acute Responses to Aerobic Endurance Training

Variable	Response
CARDIOVASCULAR	
Heart rate	Increase
Stroke volume	Increase
Cardiac output	Increase
Total peripheral resistance	Decrease
Blood flow to coronary vasculature	Increase
Skeletal muscle blood flow	Increase
Splanchnic blood flow	Decrease
Mean arterial pressure	Increase
Systolic blood pressure	Increase
Diastolic blood pressure	No change or slight decrease
Rate–pressure product	Increase
Plasma volume	Decrease
Hematocrit	Increase
RESPIRATORY	
Pulmonary minute ventilation	Increase
Breathing rate	Increase
Tidal volume	Increase
RER or RQ	Increase
METABOLIC	
Oxygen consumption	Increase
Arteriovenous oxygen (a–$\dot{v}O_2$) difference	Increase
Blood lactate	Increase
Blood pH	Decrease
ENDOCRINE	
Catecholamines	Increase
Glucagon	Increase
Insulin	Decrease
Cortisol	Decrease—low to moderate intensity
	Increase—moderate to high intensity (>60% $\dot{V}O_2$max)
Growth hormone	Increase

RER = respiratory exchange ratio; RQ = respiratory quotient.

Cardiovascular Responses

The cardiovascular system consists of two components, the heart and the vasculature (i.e., blood and blood vessels). For specific information on the cardiovascular system's structure and function, refer to chapter 2. During aerobic exercise, an increased stimulation or excitation of the heart occurs in order to supply blood to the exercising skeletal muscle. Although not the only reason for an increase in blood flow, a simple explanation is an increase in stimulation of the heart by the sympathetic nervous system and, at the same time, a reduction in parasympathetic nervous system stimulation. Because of the effect of the nervous system, the HR and **stroke volume (SV,** amount of blood ejected per beat from the left ventricle) increase during exercise. The increase in HR and SV ultimately increases the cardiac output ($\dot{Q}$). The following formula helps identify the relationship between HR and SV in determining $\dot{Q}$:

$$\dot{Q} \text{ (L/min)} = \text{HR (beats/min)} \times \text{SV (L/beat)} \quad (6.1)$$

Stroke volume has been shown to increase to maximal levels at 40% to 60% of maximal oxygen consumption ($\dot{V}O_2$max) and plateau long before exhaustion (29). This finding is not conclusive; other studies indicate that SV continues to rise more linearly until exhaustion (66). During exercise, an increase in venous filling of the heart contributes to an increased pressure and stretching of the walls of the heart, resulting in an increase in elastic contractile force that is independent of neural and humoral factors. This is one explanation for why more blood is ejected from the left ventricle (increasing SV), and it is known as the **Frank-Starling mechanism** (60, 64); that is, the stroke volume of the heart increases proportionally to the volume of blood filling the heart.

As aerobic exercise intensity increases from a resting state to maximal exercise, there is a 50% to 60% reduction in **total peripheral resistance (TPR,** resistance to blood flow in the systemic vascular system). This reduction in TPR is due to vasodilation that occurs in an effort to supply the working skeletal muscle with blood (37). During exercise, a greater proportion of blood is shunted to the exercising skeletal musculature where it is needed (45). At the same time, blood flow to other areas of the body, such as the splanchnic region, is decreased. Several mechanisms account for the changes in peripheral vasculature in

response to aerobic exercise, but explaining them is beyond the scope of this chapter.

Blood pressure (BP, mmHg) is the force exerted by the blood on the vessels to drive blood through the circulatory system. Measurements of systolic blood pressure (SBP) and diastolic blood pressure (DBP) represent the pressure exerted on the vessels during ventricular systole (contraction) and diastole (relaxation), respectively. During aerobic endurance exercise involving large muscle groups, such as walking, jogging, cycling, and swimming, there is a linear increase in SBP in direct proportion to the exercise intensity and cardiac output and a negligible change in DBP. Total peripheral resistance also decreases (but $\dot{Q}$ increases to a greater extent) as the exercise intensity increases and has a major effect on blood pressure. As a result, mean arterial pressure (MAP) increases during exercise and can be expressed quantitatively by the following two formulas:

$$\text{MAP} = \text{DBP} + [0.333 \times (\text{SBP} - \text{DBP})] \quad (6.2)$$

$$\text{MAP} = \dot{Q} \times \text{TPR} \quad (6.3)$$

During exercise, the increase in BP helps facilitate the increase in blood flow through the vasculature and also the amount of plasma forced from the blood into the intercellular space (becoming part of the interstitial fluid). Thus, during exercise, a decrease in plasma volume and an increase in **hematocrit** (proportion of blood that consists of red blood cells) occur, even though the total number of red blood cells does not change (39, 65).

Coronary vasculature, composed of the right and left coronary arteries, dilates (vasodilation) during exercise as a result of the increased oxygen demand placed on the heart muscle. The **rate–pressure product (RPP)** indicates how much oxygen the heart needs. It is a fairly easy measurement to take and provides a good noninvasive index of how hard the heart is working (48). It is expressed quantitatively by the following formula:

$$\text{RPP} = \text{HR} \times \text{SBP} \quad (6.4)$$

> ▶ **Cardiac output, heart rate, stroke volume, mean arterial blood pressure, coronary artery diameter, and rate pressure product increase during exercise.**

Respiratory Responses

Pulmonary minute ventilation ($\dot{V}_E$) is the product of breathing rate (BR) and tidal volume (TV) and represents the amount of air moved into or out of the lungs in 1 minute. During exercise, $\dot{V}_E$ increases because of the body's increased oxygen requirement and consumption.

$$\dot{V}_E \text{ (L/min)} = \text{BR} \times \text{TV} \qquad (6.5)$$

The **respiratory quotient (RQ)** is the ratio of the volume of carbon dioxide production ($\dot{V}CO_2$) to oxygen consumption ($\dot{V}O_2$) at the cellular level. RQ cannot feasibly be measured at the level of the cell, but the CO_2 and O_2 ratio is commonly assessed via expired gases from the mouth, termed the **respiratory exchange ratio (RER)**. Despite subtle differences, the RQ and RER are calculated by the same formula:

$$\text{RQ or RER} = \dot{V}CO_2 / \dot{V}O_2 \qquad (6.6)$$

Essentially, the RER and RQ estimate the proportion of fat, carbohydrate, and protein used during rest and exercise. However, since the ratio involves the measurement of O_2 use, the contribution of anaerobic processes (i.e., phosphocreatine and glycolysis) is not included. If measured at the cellular level, the RQ scale ranges between 0.7 and 1.0. Because many factors can alter the exchange of oxygen and carbon dioxide in the lungs, the RQ does not fully explain all the contributing factors in the calculation of metabolism. Among the other factors that affect resting RER are diet and whether a person is fed or fasted. The average RER in a fed, nonketogenic individual is 0.82 (approximately 60% of energy derived from fat and 40% derived from carbohydrate) (48). As exercise intensity increases, both RQ and RER approach 1.0, and the proportion of energy derived from carbohydrate increases (table 6.2; 39).

Because the RQ is measured at the cellular level, it cannot exceed 1.0; however, since RER is assessed via expired gases from the mouth, it can increase to levels greater than 1.0. This typically occurs during high-intensity exercise from the rapid breathing rate (i.e., hyperventilation) and the increased buffering of hydrogen ions. The increase in hydrogen ions is accompanied by an associated increase in acidity that is neutralized by buffers, such as bicarbonate, which are eventually removed as CO_2 during respiration. Thus, a greater presence of buffers increases the amount of CO_2 expired in comparison with the amount of O_2 consumed, driving the RER value above 1.0. At this point, the RER no longer reflects carbohydrate metabolism. Alternatively, RER values that exceed 1.0 are often seen as an indicator of exercise intensity and fatigue as well as a criterion measure for attaining $\dot{V}O_2$max during a progressive exercise test (39, 48, 60).

> ▶ **Ventilation, breathing rate, tidal volume, RER, and RQ increase during exercise.**

Metabolic Responses

Aerobic exercise in an untrained person beginning an exercise program is inefficient. Limitations in the cardiovascular and respiratory systems impose a limit

TABLE 6.2 Caloric Equivalence of the Respiratory Exchange Ratio (RER) and % kcal From Carbohydrates and Fats

% kcal from		Energy	
Carbohydrate	Fat	RER	kcal/L O_2
0	100	0.71	4.69
16	84	0.75	4.74
33	67	0.80	4.80
51	49	0.85	4.86
68	32	0.90	4.92
84	16	0.95	4.99
100	0	1.00	5.05

Reprinted by permission from W.E. Kenney et al. (2020, p. 126).

on the metabolic processes that take place in order to allow aerobic exercise to occur. Poor performance for a short time is the ultimate result. During exercise, the demand for adenosine triphosphate (ATP) is higher, causing the body to consume more oxygen. The difference between the amount of oxygen in the arterial and mixed venous blood is the **arteriovenous oxygen difference (a–$\bar{v}O_2$ difference)**, representing the extent to which oxygen is removed from the blood as it passes through the body. Normal values for resting arterial and venous oxygen per 100 ml of blood are 20 and 14 ml, respectively, and the normal resting a–$\bar{v}O_2$ difference is approximately 6 ml of oxygen per 100 ml of blood. This value increases almost linearly with exercise intensity and can reach approximately 18 ml of oxygen per 100 ml of blood at $\dot{V}O_2$max (39). The volume of oxygen consumed ($\dot{V}O_2$) is determined as the product of $\dot{Q}$ and the a–$\bar{v}O_2$ difference, which is known as the **Fick equation**:

$$\dot{V}O_2 \text{ (L/min)} = \dot{Q} \times \text{a–}\bar{v}O_2 \text{ difference} \qquad (6.7)$$

During aerobic exercise the body's metabolism is increased, producing more CO_2 and lactate (which results in higher concentrations of H^+ ions) than at rest. At high exercise intensities, there is an increased reliance on the anaerobic pathways for energy production. As with the RER when it exceeds 1.0, hydrogen ions accumulate in the active muscles, causing a marked increase in blood acidity (a decrease in pH) (19). In response to the increase in blood acidity, bicarbonate ions (HCO_3^-) are released, resulting in greater CO_2 expiration. See chapter 3 for a review of the energy systems as they pertain to aerobic exercise.

Endocrine Responses

In response to a bout of aerobic exercise, a major purpose of the endocrine system is to facilitate metabolism by maintaining the availability of carbohydrates (glucose) and fats (free fatty acids) that are needed to meet increased energy demands. Catecholamines also facilitate cardiovascular responses to enhance the delivery of oxygen and nutrients and the removal of waste products. Glands of major concern with regard to aerobic exercise include the pancreas, adrenal cortex, and adrenal medulla. The endocrine system is complex, and this section contains only basic information related to acute responses.

The **pancreas** is an endocrine gland that plays a major role in acute exercise metabolism because of the production and release of glucagon and insulin.

These hormones release or uptake glucose from the tissues, which is vital to the survival of the body. Plasma **glucagon** stimulates an increase in plasma glucose concentration, whereas **insulin** facilitates glucose transport into the cells of the body. Because of the increased metabolic demands of acute exercise, glucagon secretion is increased whereas insulin secretion is decreased. An increase in plasma glucagon stimulates the conversion of glycogen to glucose, thus increasing the plasma glucose concentration so that more glucose is available to be transported into cells. During exercise, insulin plasma concentration decreases, insulin sensitivity is improved, and non–insulin-mediated glucose transport into cells is increased (7, 54). The increased glucagon release (and reduced insulin release) during acute exercise enhances fat breakdown in tissue (**lipolysis**) and triggers an increase in plasma fatty acids, making more fat available as a fuel for exercise.

Cortisol is the only substance released from the adrenal cortex that plays a direct role in metabolism. It is responsible for stimulating the conversion of proteins to be used by aerobic systems and in glycolysis. As well, cortisol plays a role in the maintenance of normal blood sugar levels; it also promotes the use of fats. Exercise intensity affects the level of cortisol secretion; plasma levels of cortisol have been shown to decrease with low-intensity exercise and increase with moderate- to high-intensity exercise (12, 36). During exercise, growth hormone is secreted from the anterior pituitary, which assists cortisol and glucagon in making more fat and carbohydrate available in the plasma for the increased metabolism of exercise (48, 71).

The **catecholamines** (epinephrine and norepinephrine) are the "flight-or-fight hormones" released from the adrenal medulla when it is acted upon by the sympathetic nervous system during stressful situations. The adrenal medulla perceives exercise as a stressor and releases additional catecholamines during exercise. Catecholamine plasma concentration increases during exercise because these hormones help the body deliver blood and oxygen to the working muscles (e.g., by increasing heart rate and blood pressure) (39).

In general, during exercise of increasing intensity, progressive elevations in plasma hormone concentrations of glucagon, cortisol, growth hormone, epinephrine, and norepinephrine occur (48, 60). These changes are accompanied by a progressive decrease in insulin. Similar progressive changes in these hormones also occur as exercise of moderate intensity continues for a long duration (60).

CHRONIC ADAPTATIONS TO AEROBIC EXERCISE

In addition to understanding how the body's systems respond during bouts of aerobic exercise, personal trainers need to understand how the different body systems adapt to chronic aerobic exercise training. This section describes the chronic effects of aerobic training on the cardiovascular, respiratory, and endocrine systems as well as the effects on skeletal muscle, bone and connective tissue, metabolism, body composition, and performance. To facilitate understanding of these training adaptations, three summary tables are provided. Table 6.3 provides an overview of chronic adaptations at rest and during submaximal and maximal exercise for key cardiorespiratory and metabolic variables. Table 6.4 provides typical baseline and post-training values for an initially inactive male, as well as comparison values for a male world-class aerobic endurance runner (39). Table 6.5 summarizes other chronic physiological and performance adaptations.

Cardiovascular Adaptations

Several terms are used to refer to maximal aerobic power, a key component for improving aerobic exercise performance. It is also known as $\dot{V}O_2$max, **maximal oxygen uptake**, maximal oxygen consumption, and **aerobic capacity**. Increasing maximal aerobic power relies greatly on the effective function and integration of the cardiovascular and respiratory systems. Oxygen uptake can be expressed by the Fick equation (6.7), presented earlier. The equation indi-

cates that maximal aerobic power is dependent on the body's ability to deliver (i.e., cardiac output) and use (i.e., a–$\bar{v}O_2$ difference) oxygen. One of the hallmark adaptations to chronic aerobic training is an increase in maximal cardiac output, resulting primarily from an increase in stroke volume (48) (see figures 6.1 and 6.2; 39). Aerobic endurance training does not affect maximal heart rate or decreases it slightly (see figure 6.3; 39). Maximal cardiac output correlates closely with maximal aerobic power; the higher the cardiac output, the higher the aerobic power. In response to aerobic endurance training, cardiac output remains essentially unchanged at rest and is either unchanged or slightly decreased at any fixed submaximal exercise intensity (48). At rest and at any fixed submaximal exercise intensity, adaptations include a decrease in heart rate and an increase in stroke volume (table 6.3). A training-induced reduction in heart rate has been shown to occur in two weeks (11), but depending on the intensity, duration, and frequency of training, may take up to 10 weeks (63). This response is believed to come from an increased parasympathetic influence, decreased sympathetic influence, and lower intrinsic heart rate (39).

 Aerobic endurance training increases $\dot{V}O_2$max, which is generally regarded as the single best measure of aerobic fitness.

Long-term aerobic exercise training leads to moderate cardiac hypertrophy characterized by left ventricular cavity enlargement and increased myocardial

---

TABLE 6.3 Chronic Cardiorespiratory and Metabolic Adaptations to Aerobic Endurance Training at Rest and During Exercise

Variable	Rest	Fixed submaximal exercise*	Maximal exercise
Heart rate	Decrease	Decrease	No change or slight decrease
Stroke volume	Increase	Increase	Increase
Cardiac output	No change	No change or slight decrease	Increase
Systolic blood pressure	Decrease	Decrease	Little or no change
Diastolic blood pressure	Decrease	Decrease	Little or no change
Pulmonary ventilation	No change	Decrease	Increase
Oxygen consumption	No change	No change or slight decrease	Increase
Arteriovenous oxygen difference	No change	No change or slight increase	Increase

*Responses in the fixed submaximal exercise column indicate adaptations comparing post- and pretraining responses at the same absolute (fixed) work rate.

TABLE 6.4   Effects of Aerobic Endurance Training in a Previously Inactive Man Along With Values for a Male World-Class Endurance Athlete

Variable	Pretraining, sedentary male	Posttraining, sedentary male	World-class endurance athlete
CARDIOVASCULAR			
HRrest (beats/min)	75	65	45
HRmax (beats/min)	185	183	174
SVrest (ml/beat)	60	70	100
SVmax (ml/beat)	120	140	200
$\dot{Q}$ at rest (L/min)	4.5	4.5	4.5
$\dot{Q}$max (L/min)	22.2	25.6	34.8
Heart volume (ml)	750	820	1,200
Blood volume (L)	4.7	5.1	6.0
Systolic BP at rest (mmHg)	135	130	120
Systolic BPmax (mmHg)	200	210	220
Diastolic BP at rest (mmHg)	78	76	65
Diastolic BPmax (mmHg)	82	80	65
RESPIRATORY			
$\dot{V}_E$ at rest (L/min)	7	6	6
$\dot{V}_E$max (L/min)	110	135	195
TV at rest (L)	0.5	0.5	0.5
TVmax (L)	2.75	3.0	3.9
VC (L)	5.8	6.0	6.2
RV (L)	1.4	1.2	1.2
METABOLIC			
a–$\bar{v}O_2$ diff at rest (ml/100 ml)	6.0	6.0	6.0
a–$\bar{v}O_2$ diff max (ml/100 ml)	14.5	15.0	16.0
$\dot{V}O_2$ at rest (ml · kg^{-1} · min^{-1})	3.5	3.5	3.5
$\dot{V}O_2$max (ml · kg^{-1} · min^{-1})	40.7	49.9	81.9
Blood lactate at rest (mmol/L)	1.0	1.0	1.0
Blood lactate max (mmol/L)	7.5	8.5	9.0
BODY COMPOSITION			
Weight (kg)	79	77	68
Fat weight (kg)	12.6	9.6	5.1
Fat free weight (kg)	66.4	67.4	62.9
Fat (%)	16.0	12.5	7.5

HR = heart rate; SV = stroke volume; $\dot{Q}$ = cardiac output; BP = blood pressure; $\dot{V}_E$ = ventilation; TV = tidal volume; VC = vital capacity; RV = residual volume; a–$\bar{v}O_2$ diff = arterial–mixed venous oxygen difference; $\dot{V}O_2$ = oxygen consumption.

TABLE 6.5 Selected Chronic Adaptations to Aerobic Endurance Training

Variable	Chronic adaptation
HEART	
Left ventricular end-diastolic chamber diameter	Increase
Left ventricular muscle thickness	Increase
Coronary arteriole densities, diameters, or both	Increase
Myocardial capillary density	No change or increase
BLOOD	
Blood volume	Increase
Plasma volume	Increase
Red blood cell volume	Increase
RESPIRATORY SYSTEM	
Ventilatory muscle endurance	Increase
Respiratory muscle aerobic enzymes	Increase
SKELETAL MUSCLE	
Whole muscle cross-sectional areas	No change
Type I fiber cross-sectional areas	No change or small increase
Type IIa fiber cross-sectional areas	No change
Type IIx fiber cross-sectional areas	No change
Capillary density	Increase
Mitochondria density	Increase
Myoglobin	Increase
Glycogen stores	Increase
Triglyceride stores	Increase
Oxidative enzymes	Increase
METABOLIC	
Lactate threshold	Increase
SKELETAL SYSTEM	
Bone mineral density	No change or increase
BODY COMPOSITION	
Body mass	Decrease
Fat mass	Decrease
Fat free mass	No change
% Body fat	Decrease
PERFORMANCE	
Aerobic endurance performance	Increase
Muscular strength	No change
Vertical jump	No change
Anaerobic power	No change
Sprint speed	No change

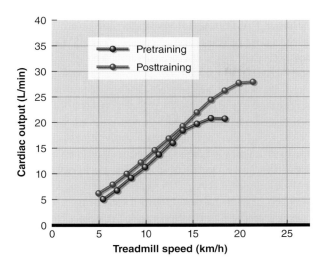

FIGURE 6.1 Changes in cardiac output with aerobic endurance training during walking, then jogging, and finally running on a treadmill as velocity increases.

Reprinted by permission from W.E. Kenney et al. (2020, p. 273).

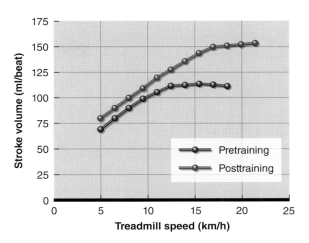

FIGURE 6.2 Changes in stroke volume with aerobic endurance training during walking, jogging, and running on a treadmill at increasing velocities.

Reprinted by permission from W.E. Kenney et al. (2020, p. 273).

wall thickness (2, 48). The increased left ventricular volume, along with increased ventricular filling time resulting from training-induced bradycardia (slower heart rate), and improved cardiac contractile function are major factors accounting for chronic stroke volume increases (48, 53). An increase in blood volume occurs very quickly as an adaptation to aerobic endurance training and contributes to ventricular cavity enlargement and improvements in $\dot{V}O_2max$ (65). Blood volume can be broken down into the two components of plasma volume and red blood cell volume. Aerobic exercise training induces a very rapid increase in plasma volume (a measurable change occurs within 24 hours), but the increase in red blood cell volume takes a few weeks (65).

Many studies have investigated the effects of chronic aerobic endurance training on resting blood pressure. For individuals with normal BP, SBP/DBP values average only 3/2 mmHg lower with chronic aerobic endurance training; in people with hypertension (SBP >140 or DBP >90 mmHg), greater reductions are noted, with an average of 7/6 mmHg (58). Immediate reductions in resting blood pressure occur after a bout of aerobic exercise in both normotensive and hypertensive individuals, which may persist for up to 22 hours (40, 58). The term **postexercise hypotension** is used to describe these changes. At the same submaximal exercise work rate, chronic

aerobic training also results in a decrease in SBP (18, 48). Since both SBP and HR are reduced at a given level of submaximal exercise with aerobic endurance training, it should be obvious that the RPP is also decreased, indicating a reduction in myocardial oxygen consumption and reduced workload on the heart (18, 48).

In trained peripheral skeletal muscle, prolonged aerobic training leads to an increase in the density of capillaries per unit of muscle (41). This allows for improved oxygen and substrate delivery and a decrease in diffusion distance between blood and exercising muscle. Based on animal studies, it is also apparent that aerobic exercise training is linked with adaptations in the cardiac muscle vasculature, including increases in arteriole densities, arteriole diameters, or both (16). Myocardial capillary density has been shown to increase with swim training in young male rats; in larger animals (i.e., dogs and pigs) undergoing treadmill training, the number of capillaries increases in proportion to the added ventricular mass, and thus no change in capillary density occurs (16).

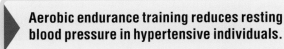

Aerobic endurance training reduces resting blood pressure in hypertensive individuals.

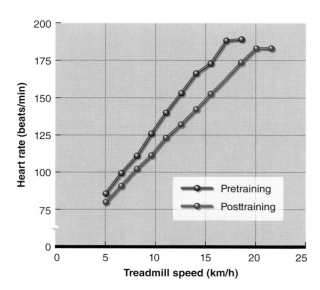

FIGURE 6.3 Changes in heart rate with aerobic endurance training during walking, jogging, and running on a treadmill at increasing velocities.

Reprinted by permission from W.E. Kenney et al. (2020, p. 275).

Respiratory Adaptations

With the respiratory system's large capacity to increase ventilation in response to exercise, as well as the relatively low oxygen (or energy expenditure) cost of breathing in terms of percentage of total body oxygen cost, the demands of aerobic endurance training on the human respiratory system are not as great as they are for other systems. Consequently, chronic aerobic training produces considerably less adaptation than occurs in the cardiovascular system and skeletal muscle (18, 48). For the great majority of healthy adults, the respiratory system is also not a limiting factor for performing maximal exercise (13, 39, 48). There are, however, several important adaptations in the respiratory system that relate to aerobic performance enhancement.

Adaptations in pulmonary minute ventilation ($\dot{V}_E$) in response to chronic aerobic training occur during submaximal and maximal exercise, with no changes at rest. With aerobic endurance training, V_E values during a standardized submaximal work rate test may decrease by as much as 20% to 30% (39); in contrast, during maximal exercise, $\dot{V}_E$ may increase 15% to 25% or more (18). With aerobic endurance training, adaptations during submaximal exercise generally include an increase in tidal volume and a decrease in breathing frequency, while during maximal exercise both tidal volume and breathing frequency increase.

During moderate-intensity aerobic exercise, the oxygen cost of breathing averages 3% to 5% of total body oxygen cost and increases to 8% to 10% of total body cost at $\dot{V}O_2$max (14). With standardized submaximal exercise, after aerobic endurance training the percentage of the total body oxygen cost for breathing is reduced and the ventilatory equivalent for oxygen ($\dot{V}_E/\dot{V}O_2$) is lowered, indicating improvements in ventilatory efficiency (18, 48). This reduced oxygen cost for breathing enhances aerobic endurance performance by freeing more oxygen for use by exercising skeletal muscle (22) and by reducing the fatiguing effects of exercise on the diaphragm muscle (70). Specificity in respiratory training adaptations also occurs as can be illustrated through comparison of arm and leg aerobic training. Individuals performing arm training show an improvement in $\dot{V}_E/\dot{V}O_2$ with arm exercise but not with leg exercise; and the opposite occurs in individuals training with leg cycling (61). It thus appears that local adaptations in trained muscle are responsible for adaptations in $\dot{V}_E/\dot{V}O_2$.

> **Ventilatory efficiency improves with aerobic endurance training; pulmonary minute ventilation decreases during submaximal exercise and increases during maximal exercise.**

Skeletal Muscle Adaptations

Aerobic endurance training consists of a large number of rather continuous low-level muscle actions and thus elicits specific marked adaptations within trained skeletal muscle. Chronic aerobic training does not affect muscle size at the macroscopic level (whole muscle) and has little, if any, effect at the microscopic level (specific fiber type cross-sectional areas) (31, 50, 62). Aerobic exercise recruits predominantly type I (slow-twitch) muscle fibers, and the low-level muscle actions elicit either no change or small increases in cross-sectional areas of these fibers. Cross-sectional areas of both type IIa and IIx (fast-twitch) fibers do not change with aerobic endurance training. Small changes in fiber type distribution may occur in response to chronic aerobic training that shifts the distribution toward a larger percentage of more oxidative fibers, and this may translate into improved aerobic endurance performance (39, 60). One study, with a rather large sample size, showed that after 20 weeks of three days per week of aerobic training, percent distribution of type IIx fibers decreased by 5%; there was no change in type IIa fibers, while the percentage of type I fibers increased by 4% (62).

Major changes with aerobic endurance training in skeletal muscle that directly relate to enhanced aerobic endurance performance include an increase in capillary supply, an increase in mitochondrial density, and an enhancement in the activity of oxidative enzymes. With chronic aerobic exercise, capillary supply to the trained muscle increases, expressed as either the number of capillaries per muscle fiber or the number of capillaries per unit of cross-sectional area of muscle (capillary density) (62). More capillaries enable an improved exchange of oxygen, nutrients, and waste products between the blood and working muscle (39). Mitochondria, the energy powerhouses within cells, produce over 90% of the body's ATP (48). With chronic aerobic endurance training, both the number and size of mitochondria increase, as well as the activity of important oxidative enzymes (e.g., citrate synthase and succinate dehydrogenase) within the mitochondria that speed up the breakdown of nutrients to form ATP (39, 48, 62). Oxidative enzyme activity increases rapidly in response to aerobic endurance training; and with intense regular training, enzyme activity levels may double or triple (30, 39, 48).

Intramuscular stores of glycogen are increased with chronic aerobic training (17, 48, 59). Fatigue from prolonged lower body aerobic exercise is associated with glycogen depletion in leg muscle type I and type IIa fibers (30, 48). The enhanced glycogen stores, together with the mitochondrial adaptations just mentioned, result in slower depletion of muscle glycogen stores, which generally translates into improved aerobic endurance performance. Myoglobin is an iron-containing protein that provides intramuscular oxygen stores, with higher concentrations in type I fibers than in type II fibers. Myoglobin oxygen stores are released to the mitochondria during the transition from rest to exercise and during intense exercise, when oxygen needs of the mitochondria greatly increase (39, 48). Aerobic endurance training has been shown to increase muscle myoglobin stores by up to 80% (28, 39).

> In skeletal muscle, aerobic endurance training induces three major changes that directly relate to enhanced aerobic endurance performance: an increase in capillary density; an increase in mitochondrial density; and an enhancement in oxidative enzyme activity.

Metabolic Adaptations

In response to chronic aerobic training, the integration of the cardiovascular, respiratory, and skeletal muscle adaptations already discussed is reflected in adaptations in metabolism (39). The major metabolic adaptations are an increased reliance on fat as energy (and a coupled reduction in use of carbohydrates during submaximal exercise), an increase in lactate threshold, and an increase in maximal oxygen consumption. These changes translate into a greater capacity to perform at higher exercise intensities for prolonged periods.

Enhancement in blood supply (oxygen delivery) and increases in mitochondrial content (and mitochondrial density) and aerobic enzymes in trained muscle greatly enhance the ability to produce ATP aerobically. These changes facilitate increased fatty acid use for energy during submaximal exercise (32, 35). They also conserve glycogen stores (less use of carbohydrates), which are very important for maintaining high-intensity prolonged aerobic exercise (39, 48). The training adaptations in fat and carbohydrate metabolism are also reflected in decreases in the respiratory quotient at both fixed and relative submaximal exercise intensities (39).

Similar patterns for lactate production and accumulation are present in untrained people and those who have undergone aerobic endurance training, except that the threshold for lactate accumulation (blood lactate threshold) occurs at a higher percentage of a trained person's aerobic capacity. Untrained individuals with a lactate threshold occurring at 50% to 60% of maximal aerobic capacity can increase their threshold to a range of 70% to 80%, while an aerobic endurance athlete who undertakes fairly intense training, and perhaps with favorable genetic factors, may have a lactate threshold in the range of 80% to 90% of aerobic capacity (48). Since a trained person's $\dot{V}O_2$max also increases with chronic aerobic training, the enhancement in percentage of capacity where lactate threshold occurs effectively translates into a substantially higher work rate for sustained aerobic endurance performance.

Adaptations in resting, submaximal exercise, and maximal oxygen consumption are somewhat different in response to chronic aerobic training. Resting oxygen consumption (also known as resting metabolic rate) generally does not change (39, 72). After training, there is either no change or a slight decrease in submaximal exercise oxygen consumption at a fixed work rate. An improvement in exercise economy (i.e., performing the same amount of work at a lower energy cost) can account for a decrease in oxygen consumption at the same fixed work rate posttraining (39, 48). In response to 6 to 12 months of aerobic training, a wide range of percent improvements have been reported in maximal oxygen consumption (related to differences in training intensity, duration, or frequency and initial fitness levels or some combination of these); but the great majority of improvements fall in the range of 10% to 30% (18, 20).

Arteriovenous oxygen difference is a variable that could fall under cardiovascular, respiratory, or metabolic adaptation categories. As expressed by the Fick equation (6.7), a $\bar{v}O_2$ difference can be a major contributor to improvement in $\dot{V}O_2$max. With chronic aerobic training, a $\bar{v}O_2$ difference increases, particularly at maximal exercise. This increase is accomplished by both adaptations in skeletal muscle, which enhance extraction of oxygen during exercise, and a more effective distribution of blood flow toward active tissue and away from inactive tissue (48).

Endocrine Adaptations

Aerobic endurance training generally leads to a blunted response in hormone release at the same absolute level of submaximal exercise. Comparisons between pre- and posttraining at the same absolute level of submaximal exercise represent a comparison of responses to aerobic exercise performed at any specific fixed (or absolute) submaximal work rate (such as a specific speed of running on a level treadmill). Training causes a reduction in the rise of plasma epinephrine, norepinephrine, glucagon, cortisol, and growth hormone in a person who performs the same absolute level of submaximal exercise posttraining as compared with pretraining (23, 48, 60, 73). Plasma insulin levels also decrease less in a trained person during submaximal exercise. At the tissue level, effects of exercise on insulin sensitivity are particularly important considering the high and increasing prevalence of diabetes in our society. An acute bout of moderate or intense exercise improves insulin sensitivity and decreases plasma glucose levels in persons with type 2 diabetes (8, 25, 27, 42, 48). These favorable changes usually deteriorate within 72 hours of the last exercise session. With regular exercise, the acute effects of enhanced insulin sensitivity can improve long-term glucose control. However, it appears that this enhanced long-term glucose control is not a consequence of chronic adaptation in muscle tissue function (8, 25, 48).

Bone and Connective Tissue Adaptations

Chronic aerobic training that incorporates moderate to high bone-loading forces can play a significant role in maximizing bone mass in childhood and early adulthood, maintaining bone mineral content through middle age, and attenuating bone mineral loss in older age (43). **Bone mineral density (BMD)**, which is the amount of mineral content per unit area or volume of bone, is the most common measure used to assess bone strength. The basic principles of specificity and progressive overload are particularly important with respect to adaptations in bone with exercise training. Only bone that is subjected to chronic loading will undergo changes. Changes will occur only when the stimulus is greater than what the bone is accustomed to. Continued improvement also requires a progression in overload. Considering these principles, aerobic endurance training that incorporates moderate to high bone-loading forces likely induces the most beneficial effects (43, 55, 59). Indeed, although walking training programs of up to one year in duration are not effective in preventing bone loss with aging (6), jogging, with its higher-intensity bone-loading forces, has been shown to attenuate bone loss with aging (43, 52). Keep in mind that since BMD decreases in middle-aged and older adults, exercise that attenuates this loss should be viewed as beneficial (33, 43). Results are equivocal in a number of studies assessing the effect of aerobic and other types of training on BMD (43, 55, 59). Studies that report an increase in BMD favor relatively high-intensity weight-bearing aerobic exercise, plyometric or jump training, resistance training, or some combination of these (43, 55, 59). A combination of weight-bearing aerobic exercise (including jogging at least intermittently if walking is the main mode of exercise) and activities that involve jumping and resistance training (incorporating exercises that load all major muscle groups) is the recommended standard for maintaining bone health in adulthood (43).

There has been less research on the effects of aerobic endurance training on tendon, ligament, and cartilage than there has on the skeletal or cardiovascular systems, and the research that has been done has focused primarily on animals (38). Tendons, ligaments, and articular cartilage appear, like bone, to remodel in response to the mechanical stress placed on them (5, 56). Tendons and ligaments become stronger and stiffer when stressed with increased overload and weaker and less stiff with decreased overload (5, 38).

Articular cartilage has been shown to become thicker with moderate volumes of running in young dogs (5). Tendons, ligaments, and cartilage have relatively few living cells dispersed within an abundance of nonliving extracellular material. This characteristic, along with a poorer blood supply to these tissues, prolongs the time for training adaptations as compared with other types of tissue (38, 47).

Body Composition Adaptations

Since more than 66% of adults in the United States are either overweight or obese and multiple chronic diseases are associated with excess fatness, the effect of exercise on body composition is an important public health issue (57). Results from a number of studies with a wide range in months of physical activity intervention indicate that moderate-intensity aerobic activity of less than 150 minutes per week induces minimal weight loss; greater than 150 minutes per week of moderate activity for a duration of 12 weeks induces a modest weight loss of about 4.4 to 6.6 pounds (2-3 kg); and moderate aerobic activity for 225 minutes per week for 16 months duration induces an 11-pound (5 kg) weight loss, while 420 minutes per week for a duration of 3 months induces an 16.5-pound (7.5 kg) weight loss (15). Thus, evidence supports a dose–response relationship between the amount of the aerobic activity performed and the amount of weight loss. A benefit of aerobic endurance training regarding body composition is that it induces reductions in fat mass while having a minimal effect on (or preserving) fat free mass (4, 49, 68). Aerobic endurance training alone or in combination with an energy-restricted diet induces a greater loss in fat mass than an energy-restricted diet alone since the exercise promotes conservation of fat free mass (48, 68).

> **Health-related benefits of aerobic endurance exercise include enhanced insulin sensitivity, reduced body fat, and favorable effects on bone mineral density.**

Performance Adaptations

Considering the physiological adaptations just discussed and keeping in mind that aerobic endurance training consists of fairly continuous low-level muscle actions, the effects of this type of training on specific types of performance should be evident. Aerobic endurance training is particularly effective in enhancing aerobic endurance performance, although it generally has no effect on types of performance that involve high levels of muscle activation or anaerobic metabolism. Thus, chronic aerobic endurance training generally does not improve muscular strength (26, 44, 49), vertical jump performance (26, 34, 49), anaerobic power (44), or sprint speed (26) in young adults. Although not discussed in this chapter, chronic aerobic training also has many health-related benefits for a number of chronic visceral diseases and physical disabilities (24).

FACTORS THAT INFLUENCE ADAPTATIONS TO AEROBIC ENDURANCE TRAINING

The physiological adaptations to aerobic endurance training addressed in this chapter are influenced by a number of individual factors. These include the types of activity the person engages in (i.e., specificity), genetics, sex, and age. All these factors play a role in determining the success one may see with aerobic endurance training.

Specificity

The effects of exercise are all subject to the rule of **specificity**. This means that adaptations occur as a consequence of the training and in a fashion specifically related to the training. In short, if the exercise involves cycling, then the training adaptations will be most closely related to cycling performance. This is true also for running, swimming, or training on an ergometer or treadmill. The body seeks to adapt to the stress it encounters in as specific a manner as possible, a principle that has obvious implications for the design of training programs. Although programming is beyond the scope of this chapter, it is important for the personal trainer to bear in mind that any exercise program will produce adaptations very closely related to the specific activities in which the client engages.

Genetics

It is safe to say that people are born with a theoretical ceiling of human performance. This ceiling is not absolute but rather falls within a range of values that is dependent on training stimulus and motivation levels.

However, there appears to be an absolute level that may not be exceeded based on genetic factors inherited from our ancestors. There is a saying that the best training begins with choosing the right parents. Although this is obviously an uncontrollable factor, it does play a major role in development. However, research has also shown that the body is not completely unchangeable. For example, people who undertake extended aerobic exercise make changes to their fast-twitch muscle fibers. These fibers take on characteristics similar to those of slow-twitch muscle fibers, resulting in improved aerobic performance. It has been estimated that genetic factors account for 20% to 30% of differences between individuals in maximal aerobic capacity and for about 50% of differences in maximal heart rate (3, 48).

Sex

The physiological changes due to aerobic exercise are similar for males and females. However, some basic differences affect the absolute amounts of the changes. Women on average have less muscle mass and more body fat than their male counterparts. They also have smaller hearts and lungs and an overall smaller blood volume. Research has shown that when males and females are matched for age, females typically have a lower cardiac output, stroke volume, and oxygen consumption than males when exercising at 50% of $\dot{V}O_2$max. Considering that females generally start an aerobic training program with smaller physiological values, they generally show smaller absolute adaptations than males but very similar relative (percent) adaptations (39).

Age

As children mature, levels of absolute maximal aerobic power (L/min) increase. Females tend to reach their highest values for $\dot{V}O_2$max (L/min) between 12 and 15 years of age, while males do not reach their highest $\dot{V}O_2$max until 17 to 21 years of age (39). This period is followed by a plateau and then a gradual decrease as we age. Much of the decline can be negated through continued training regimens. Aerobic endurance–trained athletes who are older exhibit only slight declines during the fifth and sixth decades when they maintain training, whereas those who stop training show declines similar to those in untrained individuals. In five middle-aged men, 100% of the age-related decline in aerobic power that had occurred over 30

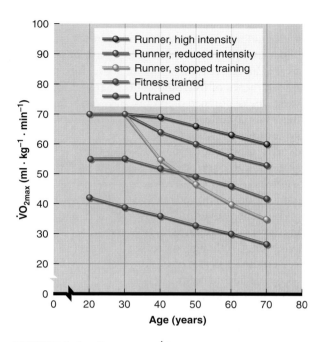

FIGURE 6.4 Changes in $\dot{V}O_2$max with age for trained and untrained men.

Reprinted by permission from W.E. Kenney et al. (2015, p. 471).

years was reversed by six months of aerobic endurance training (51). Figure 6.4 depicts changes in $\dot{V}O_2$max with age in both trained and untrained men (39a).

OVERTRAINING

When intensity, duration, frequency of training, or any combination of these factors exceeds an individual's capacity for adaptation, overreaching and overtraining may occur. Exceeding adaptation capacity without sufficient recovery normally leads to decrements in physical performance due to complex interactions among several biological systems and psychological influences (1, 21, 46, 48, 69). **Overreaching** refers to short-term training, without sufficient recuperation, that exceeds an individual's capacity. Successful recovery from overreaching can occur within a few days or up to two weeks with an adequate recovery intervention (1, 48). Although some authorities view overreaching as an unplanned and undesirable consequence of strenuous training, others view it as a training technique to enhance performance (1, 39). Short-term overreaching results in a decrement in performance, but when it is followed with appropriate recovery periods the result may be enhanced performance as compared against baseline. **Overtraining** syndrome is more serious and results from untreated overreaching that produces long-term impairments in performance and other conditions that may require medical intervention.

Two types of overtraining have been theorized to exist; the difference is in the predominance of either the sympathetic or the parasympathetic nervous system (1, 39, 46). Apparently, aerobic endurance overtraining results predominantly from an excessive volume overload (parasympathetic dominant), whereas anaerobic or resistance overtraining (sympathetic dominant) primarily results from excessive high-intensity overload. These two types of overtraining have been reported to have different signs and symptoms, although performance decrements are a key common aspect of both. Discussion of the many complicated and not fully understood aspects of overtraining is beyond the scope of this chapter, and the reader is referred to other sources for more complete information on these concepts (1, 21, 46, 69).

Researchers have identified multiple markers for overreaching and overtraining. See the sidebar for a list of some of the most common markers (i.e., signs and symptoms) of aerobic endurance overreaching, overtraining, or both (1, 21, 46, 48, 69).

There is a high degree of variability between individuals with regard to developing overtraining. Training practices that cause some individuals to thrive lead to overtraining in others. Unfortunately, there are also highly individualized responses and symptoms for overreaching and overtraining that make them difficult for clients and personal trainers to recognize (1, 39, 49).

Besides a decrement in performance, people generally exhibit only a few, if any, of the other signs and symptoms. Being familiar with each client's progression through training is essential for preventing overtraining. A decline in performance coupled with one or more of the easily recognizable markers (i.e., fatigue, malaise, loss of enthusiasm for training, increased soreness) should lead to suspicion of this condition. Checking the heart rate response to a standardized submaximal exercise load would be another appropriate method to monitor clients undergoing strenuous aerobic endurance training. For prevention of overtraining, an important component would be a properly planned periodization program. It is critical for the client to have sufficient rest between training days to facilitate the recovery process. The amount of rest, however, depends on the duration and intensity of the training program and should be individualized for each client. Periods of high-volume or high-intensity training especially require sufficient recovery. Keep in mind that individuals undergoing strenuous and frequent aerobic endurance training also need sufficient carbohydrate intake to maintain muscle glycogen stores. Successive days of training can gradually reduce glycogen levels and impair performance (39, 48).

DETRAINING

How the body responds to **detraining** is analogous to how it responds to training. Once training is stopped, muscular endurance decreases after only two weeks.

COMMON MARKERS OF AEROBIC ENDURANCE OVERREACHING OR OVERTRAINING

- Decreased performance
- Decreased maximal oxygen uptake
- Earlier onset of fatigue
- General malaise
- Loss of interest or enthusiasm for training
- Disturbed psychological mood states (increased depression, anxiety, fatigue or decreased vigor, or a combination of these changes)
- Increased muscle soreness
- Decreased resting and maximal heart rate
- Increased submaximal exercise heart rate
- Decreased submaximal exercise plasma lactate concentration
- Increased sympathetic stress response
- Decreased catecholamine levels

After four weeks, one study showed reductions in the trained muscles' respiratory ability, decreases in glycogen levels, and increases in lactate production, demonstrating obvious changes in the muscle metabolism (9). Another study showed a 7% decline in both $\dot{V}O_2$max and maximal cardiac output, as well as 17% to 19% decreases in aerobic enzyme levels, after training was stopped for only 12 days (10). Another investigation demonstrated that when aerobically trained rats stopped training, there was a site-specific decrease in the BMD of the tibia (67).

CONCLUSION

The interest in and understanding of the physiology of aerobic endurance training has greatly expanded in the last few decades. Aerobic endurance training is a potent stimulus to physiological changes in the cardiovascular, respiratory, skeletal muscle, metabolic, endocrine, and skeletal systems and has substantial effects on body composition and performance. To be a highly effective personal trainer, it is crucial to have a clear understanding of both the acute responses and chronic adaptations of the many physiological systems of the human body. Understanding how the body adapts to the overload of aerobic exercise is critical for designing effective exercise training programs, monitoring exercise responses and progress, and assessing training outcomes. The personal trainer must also recognize the effects that genetics, sex, age, specificity, overtraining, and detraining have on physiological responses and adaptations.

Study Questions

1. Which of the following increases during an aerobic exercise bout?
   - A. respiratory exchange rate
   - B. blood pH
   - C. insulin
   - D. plasma volume

2. Which of the following represents the Fick equation?
   - A. $\dot{V}O_2$ (L/min) = $\dot{Q} \times$ a–$\bar{v}O_2$ difference
   - B. $\dot{V}O_2$ (L/min) = $\dot{Q}$ / a–$\bar{v}O_2$ difference
   - C. $\dot{V}O_2$ (L/min) = $\dot{Q}$ + a–$\bar{v}O_2$ difference
   - D. $\dot{V}O_2$ (L/min) = $\dot{Q}$ – a–$\bar{v}O_2$ difference

3. Which of the following is incorrect regarding skeletal muscle adaptations to chronic aerobic exercise training?
   - A. decreased intramuscular glycogen stores
   - B. increased muscle myoglobin stores
   - C. no change in type II muscle fiber cross-sectional area
   - D. little to no change in type I muscle fiber cross-sectional area

4. Which of the following is incorrect regarding age differences in maximal aerobic power?
   - A. Females tend to reach their maximal aerobic power at 12-15 years of age.
   - B. Men tend to reach their maximal aerobic power at 17-21 years of age.
   - C. In adults, maximal aerobic power gradually decreases with age without regular training.
   - D. Maximal aerobic power substantially decreases in the fifth and sixth decade even when training is maintained.

5. Approximately how soon after aerobic training is stopped does muscular endurance decrease?
   - A. 3 days
   - B. 1 week
   - C. 2 weeks
   - D. 6 weeks

CHAPTER 7

Nutrition Concepts and Strategies

Eric R. Helms, PhD, and Brian St. Pierre, MS, RD

After completing this chapter, you will be able to

- identify a personal trainer's scope of practice and know when to refer clients to a nutrition professional;

- review a client's diet and estimate energy and nutrient requirements;

- understand the changes in a client's nutritional and fluid requirements due to exercise;

- advise clients on guidelines and behavior change for weight gain, weight loss, health, and performance; and

- recognize the role and appropriateness of dietary supplementation.

Nutrition and physical activity should be addressed in conjunction with one another. Focusing on one at the exclusion of the other will yield less than optimal results for clients. Personal trainers can enhance their overall effectiveness by maintaining a core knowledge of nutrition and by individualizing their nutrition advice. Nutrition assessment and recommendations should match the needs and goals of the client and will vary accordingly. Finally, personal trainers should know when they need to refer a client to a dietitian because the client's needs are outside of their scope of expertise or practice (61).

ROLE OF THE PERSONAL TRAINER REGARDING NUTRITION

Websites, social media, television, newspapers, and magazines are the major sources of nutrition information for most people. Nutrition information communicated as sound bites and advertisements can lead to consumer confusion. Personal trainers have the opportunity to help clear the confusion by serving as a source of credible nutrition information.

The authors would like to acknowledge the significant contributions of Marie Spano and Kristin J. Reimers to this chapter.

It is well within the personal trainer's scope of practice to address misinformation and to give general advice related to nutrition for physical performance, disease prevention, weight loss, and weight gain. A personal trainer would be conveying general nutrition knowledge by saying, for example, "According to the American Heart Association, omega-3 fatty acids from fatty fish like salmon or mackerel may benefit those who are at risk of developing cardiovascular disease." An important part of the core knowledge, from the standpoint of both ethics and safety, is the ability to recognize more complicated nutrition issues and know who to refer clients to.

Referral to a nutrition professional is indicated when the client has a disease state (e.g., diabetes, heart disease, gastrointestinal disease, eating disorder, osteoporosis, elevated cholesterol) that is affected by nutrition. This type of nutrition information is called **medical nutrition therapy** and falls under the scope of practice of a licensed nutritionist, dietitian, or registered dietitian (RD) (depending on the country and in the United States, on the state's licensure laws) (4). Referral is also indicated when the complexity of the nutrition issue is beyond the competence of the personal trainer, which will vary. Personal trainers should find several nutrition professionals they feel comfortable referring their clients to and with whom they can communicate about clients. In the United States and Canada, registered dietitians can be located through state dietetic organizations; the Academy of Nutrition and Dietetics (AND) website, www.eatright.org; the Sports, Cardiovascular and Wellness Nutrition website (SCAN, a dietetic practice group of the AND), www.scandpg.org; and Dietitians of Canada, www.dietitians.ca. The European Federation of the Association of Dietitians, www.efad.org, provides links to each country's dietitian organization. The website of Sports Dietitians Australia provides a tool to locate a local sports dietitian: www.sportsdietitians. com.au. In other countries, personal trainers will want to consult local dietetic organizations or national websites. To facilitate communication, the client should sign a release of information form so that the personal trainer and the nutrition professional can communicate about the client's training program and general nutrition needs.

> Personal trainers should refer clients to a dietitian when the client has a disease state, such as cardiovascular disease, that has a dietary component or when the complexity of the nutrition issue is beyond the competence of the personal trainer.

WHO CAN PROVIDE NUTRITION COUNSELING AND EDUCATION?

Before assessing a client's diet, personal trainers should turn to their state dietetic licensing board or to their country's organization for dietetic regulations to find out the laws within their particular region that govern the provision of nutrition advice. In the United States, each state regulates the provision of nutrition information through licensure, statutory certification, or registration. According to the Academy of Nutrition and Dietetics (formerly known as the American Dietetic Association; 4), definitions for these terms are as follows:

- *Licensing:* Statutes include an explicitly defined scope of practice, and performance of the profession is illegal unless a license has been obtained from the state.

- *Statutory certification:* Limits use of particular titles to persons meeting predetermined requirements, while persons not certified can still practice the occupation or profession.

- *Registration:* This is the least restrictive form of state regulation. As with certification, unregistered persons are permitted to practice the profession. Typically, exams are not given and enforcement of the registration requirement is minimal.

At the time of this writing, the scope of nutrition practice in Alabama is clearly defined, and specific guidance on a person's diet is allowed only by a registered dietitian or nutritionist (2). But in Arizona, for example, no licensure law exists, and any professional can offer nutrition advice (39). Various states and countries have different regulations governing whether or not personal trainers can provide dietary advice, and personal trainers should follow these guidelines. With that said, regardless of the varying regulations from state to state, a personal trainer can be held accountable for negligence, or misinformation provided to a client, which may result in civil action (and perhaps criminal charges) in extreme cases. Thus, it is extremely important that personal trainers know their limitations.

DIETARY ASSESSMENT

Should a client seek nutrition information that is within the scope of the personal trainer's practice, the personal trainer may want to assess the client's diet. If the request is out of the scope of the personal trainer's practice, he or she can work alongside a dietitian who assesses the client's diet.

A complete nutrition assessment includes dietary data, anthropometric data, biochemical data (lab tests), and a clinical examination (condition of skin, teeth, and so on). Although personal trainers are usually not involved in the comprehensive assessment, they may want to be familiar with the individual components of a comprehensive dietary assessment so they can work with the dietitian to provide their clients the best service possible. (*Note:* The term **diet** as used throughout this chapter refers to the usual eating pattern of an individual, not a restrictive weight loss plan.)

Dietary Intake Data

Before the personal trainer can give valid nutrition advice, gleaning some information about the client's current diet is imperative. How complete is the client's current diet? Is the client allergic or intolerant to certain foods? Is the client following a specific diet (e.g., vegetarian, ketogenic)? Restricting food groups? Dieting to lose weight? Is the client a sporadic eater? Has the individual just adopted a new way of eating? The answers to these questions and others may influence the personal trainer's advice to the client.

Gathering dietary intake data is a simple concept, but it is extremely complex to do. Most people have difficulty recalling fully and accurately what they ate in a given day. Research shows there is a tendency to underestimate or underreport actual intake, sometimes significantly, especially in persons who are overweight (71). Keeping in mind these general shortcomings, personal trainers, again if under the scope of practice as allowed in their state, can choose from three methods for gathering dietary intake data:

- Diet recall
- Diet history
- Diet record

In a **diet recall**, clients report what they have eaten in the past 24 hours. With a **diet history**, clients answer questions about usual eating habits, likes and dislikes, eating schedule, medical history, weight history, and so forth. The **diet record** is typically a log, filled out for three days, in which the client records everything consumed (foods, beverages, and supplements).

The three-day diet record is considered the most valid of the three methods for assessing the diet of an individual. However, a valid record requires scrupulous recording as well as scrupulous analysis. The pitfall of this method is that recording food intake usually inhibits regular eating patterns, and recorded intake thus underestimates true intake. To get useful data, the personal trainer should ask only the most motivated clients to complete this process. The diet recall or diet history is more appropriate for many clients. To facilitate better tracking, and in the cases where a diet history or recall is used, diet tracking apps may be useful because they can be used on the go, as the individual consumes food, and sometimes have features such as food barcode scanning.

The personal trainer should never make assumptions about a client's eating habits. Assessing the client's diet is essential before one makes dietary recommendations.

Evaluating the Diet

When the personal trainer has successfully gathered dietary intake data, there are several options for evaluating the information. One way is to compare a client's diet with the recommendations given in the country's general dietary guidelines. In the United States, the U.S. Department of Agriculture (USDA) created MyPlate (73). For clients who are keenly interested in nutrition, a more detailed analysis of the diet using diet analysis software may be indicated. Both methods are reviewed here.

MyPlate

The USDA **MyPlate** is a tool that helps people find and build a healthy eating style throughout their lifetimes. The *my* in *MyPlate* signifies the importance of personalizing the recommendations to one's lifestyle, while the familiar plate symbol provides a visual representation of how much of one's diet should be made up of the following food groups:

- Fruits
- Vegetables
- Grains
- Protein foods
- Dairy

Each food group in MyPlate provides key nutrients that are more difficult to acquire in the diet if that group is omitted.

The USDA's website for MyPlate provides messages to help Americans build a healthy eating style (73):

All food and beverage choices matter—focus on variety, amount, and nutrition.

- Focus on making healthy food and beverage choices from all five food groups including fruits, vegetables, grains, protein foods, and dairy to get the nutrients you need.

- Eat the appropriate number of calories based on your age, sex, height, weight, physical activity level, and goals. Building a healthier eating style can help you avoid overweight and obesity and reduce your risk of diseases such as heart disease, diabetes, and cancer.

Choose an eating style low in saturated fat, sodium, and added sugars.

Use Nutrition Facts labels and ingredient lists to find amounts of saturated fat, sodium, and added sugars in the foods and beverages you choose. Look for food and drink choices that are lower in saturated fat, sodium, and added sugar. Eating fewer calories from foods high in saturated fat and added sugars can help to manage your calories and prevent overweight and obesity. Most people eat too many foods that are high in saturated fat and added sugar. Eating foods with less sodium can reduce your risk of high blood pressure.

Make small changes to create a healthier eating style.

- Make half your plate fruits and vegetables.
  - Focus on whole fruits.
  - Vary your veggies.
- Make half your grains whole grains.
- Move to low-fat or fat-free milk or yogurt.
- Vary your protein routine, choosing leaner cuts when eating meat.

Support healthy eating for everyone.

- Create settings where healthy choices are available and affordable to you and others in your community.

- Professionals, policymakers, partners, industry, families, and individuals can help others in their journey to make healthy eating a part of their lives.

> **The USDA has identified specific goals that relate to each of the main food groups. For instance, consumers are told to eat at least half their grains as whole grains, vary their vegetable intake, focus on whole fruits, choose lower-fat dairy foods, and eat a variety of protein-rich foods.**

The older MyPyramid and MyPlate versions provided guidelines for "discretionary" and "empty" calories, respectively. However, the current MyPlate guidelines focus on practical solutions to help limit sodium, saturated fats, and added sugars (73):

Tips for Salt and Sodium

- Many processed foods contain high amounts of sodium. Choose fresh vegetables, meats, poultry, and seafood when possible.

- Using spices or herbs, such as dill, chili powder, paprika, or cumin, and lemon or lime juice, can add flavor without adding salt.

Tips for Saturated Fats

- Keep it lean and flavorful. Try grilling, broiling, roasting, or baking—they do not add extra fat.

- Simple substitutions can help you stay within your saturated fat limit. Try using nonfat Greek yogurt when you make tuna or chicken salad.

Tips for Added Sugars

- Split the sweet treats and share with a family member or friend.

- Cut calories by drinking water or unsweetened beverages. Soda, energy drinks, and sports drinks are major sources of added sugars.

The MyPlate website (www.ChooseMyPlate.gov) is an interactive tool that clients can use on their own or with a personal trainer's assistance. Along with providing useful educational material, the website allows visitors to create customized meal plans, analyze their diets, and track their physical activity. The *Plan a Healthy Diet* function allows users to enter data about their age, weight, height, sex, and physical activity level in order to receive individualized directions for meeting their daily nutrition goals (see table 7.1a through 7.1c for examples). If users click on a food category, they will be given more specific information on how to integrate that food group into their diets (73).

Computerized Diet Analysis

Computerized analysis can provide a snapshot of a client's diet, including vitamin and mineral intake. However, it is important that the client accurately and completely record usual intake for at least three days.

TABLE 7.1a Sample Menu Plan 1

Food group	Daily serving
Grains	10 oz (300 g)
Vegetables	3.5 cups (875 ml)
Fruits	2.5 cups (625 ml)
Dairy	3 cups (750 ml)
Protein foods	7 oz (200 g)

Menu plan is for a 22-year-old, 5 ft 6 in. (167.6 cm), 140 lb (63.5 kg) male who exercises more than 60 min on most days of the week.

TABLE 7.1b Sample Menu Plan 2

Food group	Daily serving
Grains	6 oz (175 g)
Vegetables	2.5 cups (625 ml)
Fruits	1.5 cups (375 ml)
Dairy	3 cups (750 ml)
Protein foods	5 oz (150 g)

Menu plan is for a 45-year-old, 5 ft 4 in. (162.6 cm), 165 lb (74.8 kg) female who exercises less than 30 min on most days of the week.

TABLE 7.1c Sample Menu Plan 3

Food group	Daily serving
Grains	9 oz (275 g)
Vegetables	3.5 cups (875 ml)
Fruits	2 cups (500 ml)
Dairy	3 cups (750 ml)
Protein foods	6.5 oz (185 g)

Menu plan is for a 60-year-old, 6 ft (182.9 cm), 235 lb (106.6 kg) male who exercises between 30 and 60 min on most days of the week.

The client should input the amount of each food and beverage, specify how it was cooked, and give the brand name versus the generic term (e.g., Wheaties vs. just bran flakes).

> **Analyzing a client's diet is a detailed, time-consuming process that requires expertise. The personal trainer should consider referring the analysis to a dietitian or referring the client to self-directed diet analysis.**

Even if the diet is recorded perfectly, the analysis will not be completely accurate because all software programs have shortcomings. For some foods in the database, values for certain vitamins and minerals are missing, meaning the analysis for those nutrients is also missing, which will result in an erroneously low intake value. Additionally, without fail, some foods the client eats are not in the database, necessitating substitutions or typing in the actual food data (and for processed foods, the results may not include values for all vitamins and minerals since this is not a requirement for food labels).

Before asking clients to assess their diets, it is helpful for personal trainers to complete a computerized diet analysis on themselves to recognize the bias that recording can impose on true habits. Additionally, analyzing one's own diet makes one aware of the level of detail needed to accurately assess a diet.

In many cases, the personal trainer does not have the training, time, knowledge, or resources to complete a computerized dietary analysis. This is an area in which many personal trainers turn to dietitians for assistance. Another option is to refer motivated clients to websites or apps where they can enter their own diet and receive feedback (see the "Diet Analysis Websites and Apps" sidebar). These tools are excellent resources because they put the responsibility on the client. Additionally, some clients feel more comfortable asking questions and reporting intake in private situations. One drawback is that most of these websites and apps do not have the extensive database that comes with food analysis programs, and they typically do not analyze food intake for all vitamins, minerals, types of fat, and so on. Instead, most tell the user only the number of calories consumed, along with grams of fat, carbohydrate, and protein. A second drawback is that these sites cannot calculate calorie needs with the precision of a professional dietitian.

ENERGY

Energy is commonly measured in kilocalories (kcal). A kilocalorie equates to the heat required to raise the temperature of 1 kg of water 1 °C (or 2.2 pounds of water 1.8 °F). The general public refers to this as a **calorie**. (The terms *calorie* and *energy* are used interchangeably in this chapter.)

Factors Influencing Energy Requirements

Three factors make up the energy requirement of adults: resting metabolic rate, physical activity, and the thermic effect of food. Each of these factors can be affected directly or indirectly by age, genetics, body size, body composition, environmental temperature, training conditions, nontraining physical activity, and calorie intake. For infants, children, and teens, growth is another variable that increases the energy requirement.

Resting metabolic rate (RMR) is the largest contributor to total energy requirement, accounting for approximately 60% to 75% of daily energy expenditure in all but manual laborers and athletes undergoing heavy training periods. It is a measure of the calories required for maintaining normal body functions such as respiration, cardiac function, and thermoregulation (i.e., the energy a person would expend while lying down, awake, and resting). Factors that increase RMR include gaining lean body tissue, young age, growth, abnormal body temperature, menstrual cycle, and hyperthyroidism. Factors that decrease RMR include low caloric intake, loss of lean tissue, and hypothyroidism. All things equal, RMR can vary up to 20% between individuals because of normal genetic variations in metabolism.

The second largest component of energy requirement is physical activity. Of all components, it is the most variable. The amount of energy needed for physical activity depends on the intensity, duration, and frequency of training. It also depends on the environmental conditions; that is, extreme heat or cold increases calorie expenditure. When estimating how physically active a client is, the personal trainer needs to determine how physically active the client is aside from structured exercise. Even if people have an exercise routine, those with the sedentary lifestyle of a desk job and sedentary leisure activities may be con-

sidered only lightly active. Additionally, non-exercise activity's contribution to energy expenditure is variable between individuals and occurs through both conscious (more easily modifiable) and subconscious (less easily modifiable) means (77). For example, behavior change can result in increased activity (e.g., taking the stairs rather than the elevator, walking to the store instead of driving, or taking a short walk or stretching breaks during extended periods of sitting), but other factors such as habitual posture or fidgeting are difficult to modify.

The **thermic effect of food** is the increase in energy expenditure above the RMR that can be measured for several hours following a meal. It is the energy needed to digest and assimilate foods, approximately 7% to 10% of a person's total energy requirement. One of the main determinants of the thermic effect of food is the proportion of daily calories from protein. Protein has the highest thermic effect of the macronutrients, and an intake that is appropriately high in protein (such as the recommended range mentioned later in this chapter for those with resistance training–specific goals) will lead to a higher thermic effect within the given percentage range.

DIET ANALYSIS WEBSITES AND APPS

- *www.myfitnesspal.com:* This website and app tracks food intake and exercise to determine calorie and macronutrient needs, along with tracking progress toward weight loss or muscle gain goals. The app uses a database of over five million foods, although there are user-entered records that often have missing data.

- *www.loseit.com:* LoseIt is an app focused on weight loss. It allows users to track food intake, exercise activity, and more. It connects to many wearable devices and suggests specific calorie and macronutrient intakes to reach goals.

- *www.sparkpeople.com:* This website and app offers a food tracker, personalized meal plans, customized fitness plan, recipes, articles, and message boards.

- *www.ChooseMyPlate.gov:* The MyPlate website allows users to track diet and physical activity and energy balance; in addition, it provides an analysis of food intake and physical fitness.

Estimating Energy Requirements

A true estimation of energy requirement (i.e., energy expended in a day) is difficult to obtain directly. Therefore, surrogate methods are often used. One such method is to measure calorie intake. This method is valid if the client is maintaining a stable body weight, because a stable body weight indicates that energy intake generally equals energy expenditure. For the motivated client who accurately records intake, the best way to determine energy requirement using this method is to assess the calorie intake from the three-day food log. If that is not possible, mathematical equations can roughly estimate caloric expenditure. However, it is difficult to calculate energy needs because of the many variables affecting caloric requirements and the significant inter- and intraindividual variation. These equations are only estimates and are meant as a frame of reference. Actual energy expenditure of individuals will vary widely. Table 7.2 lists factors that can be used for energy requirement estimation. For example, for a male who weighs 170 pounds (77.1 kg) and is highly physically active, the requirement would be 3,910 kcal (23×170).

Another method for calculating energy expenditure is to first calculate **resting energy expenditure (REE)**—which is synonymous with RMR—then multiply it by a factor based on activity level. Several equations for estimating REE exist. One set of REE equations, developed by the Food and Agriculture Organization (20), is shown in table 7.3.

The result is the number of calories the person is likely to expend in an average day. Clients wishing to maintain current body weight would need to consume the same number of calories that they expend.

> It is difficult, if not impossible, to obtain an accurate estimate of a client's energy expenditure. The personal trainer can help the client base the estimation on intake or use an equation such as those provided in this chapter. Regardless of the method, these are rough estimates of the actual expenditure.

Energy Availability

Just because a client may be eating enough calories to maintain a desired body mass, this does not necessarily mean he or she is getting an adequate energy intake for health. The term **energy availability** refers to whether or not sufficient energy is available to meet the energy demands not only of exercise but also of physiological function. Specifically, a client may present a stable body mass—and therefore is consuming a maintenance energy intake—yet be in a state of relative energy deficiency, where reproductive and metabolic function are downregulated to maintain energy balance. This often occurs in aesthetic, aerobic endurance, and weight-class athletes who attempt to improve their performance through energy restriction in an effort to lose body mass, while concurrently expending a substantial amount of energy in training. Likewise, relative energy deficiency can occur in clients seeking weight loss who consume a relatively low number of calories while exercising. As a natural physiological response to an energy deficit, **adaptive thermogenesis** (the downregulation of multiple components of energy expenditure, often called metabolic

TABLE 7.2 Estimated Daily Calorie Needs of Males and Females by Activity Level

Activity level	Male (kcal/pound)	Male (kcal/kg)	Female (kcal/pound)	Female (kcal/kg)
Light[a]	17	38	16	35
Moderate[b]	19	41	17	37
Heavy[c]	23	50	20	44

[a]Light activity level: Walking on a level surface at 2.5 to 3.0 mph (4-5 km/h), garage work, electrical trades, carpentry, restaurant trades, housecleaning, child care, golf, sailing, table tennis.
[b]Moderate activity level: Walking 3.5 to 4.0 mph (5.5-6.5 km/h), gardening, carrying a load, cycling, skiing, tennis, dancing, water aerobics, yoga.
[c]Heavy activity level: Walking with load uphill, tree felling, heavy manual labor, basketball, climbing, football, soccer, running, swimming laps, jumping rope, aerobics, hockey.

TABLE 7.3   Estimated Daily Calorie Needs Based on Resting Energy Expenditure (REE) and Activity Level

1. To calculate REE, choose one of these eight formulas:	
Age and sex	**kcal per day**
Males 10-18 years	(17.686 × weight in kg) + 658.2
Males 19-30 years	(15.057 × weight in kg) + 692.2
Males 31-60 years	(11.472 × weight in kg) + 873.1
Males >60 years	(11.711 × weight in kg) + 587.7
Females 10-18 years	(13.384 × weight in kg) + 692.6
Females 19-30 years	(14.818 × weight in kg) + 486.6
Females 31-60 years	(8.126 × weight in kg) + 845.6
Females >60 years	(9.082 × weight in kg) + 658.5
2. Then multiply the REE by a factor to account for physical activity level (PAL) to estimate daily calorie needs:	
Level of activity	**PAL value (× REE)**
Sedentary or light activity lifestyle	1.40-1.69
Active or moderately active lifestyle	1.70-1.99
Vigorous or vigorously active lifestyle	2.00-2.40*

*PAL values greater than 2.40 are difficult to maintain for a long period.

Adapted from Food and Agriculture Organization (14).

adaptation in fitness circles) can occur depending on the amount of weight lost and the magnitude of, and time spent in, an energy deficit (50). This adaptive response to an energy deficit is normal and can result in a cessation of weight loss, but in some cases—especially if weight loss is achieved with low energy availability—the reduction in energy expenditure can include downregulation of metabolic, hormonal, and other physiological functions (49).

The state of maintaining weight while experiencing these physiological adaptations is a condition proposed by the International Olympic Committee (IOC) known as **relative energy deficiency in sport**, or **RED-S** (56). Energy availability can be mathematically conceptualized as the energy left over after exercise expenditure is subtracted from energy intake, available for physiological function. This calculated value is expressed relative to lean mass. As an example, a 248-pound (112.5 kg) client with 20% body fat (198 pounds [89.8 kg] of lean mass) consuming 3,000 kcal and expending 400 kcal on average through exercise (2,600 kcal left over), is said to have an energy availability of 13.1 kcal/pound (2,600 kcal divided by 198 pounds), or 29 kcal/kg (2,600 kcal divided by 89.8 kg). Risk factors, signs, and symptoms of RED-S include but are not limited to (76) the following:

- Eating disorders and disordered eating
- Extreme weight loss methods (e.g., crash diets, dehydration, vomiting, laxative use)
- Very low resting heart rate or blood pressure
- Loss of 10% of body mass or more in a single month
- Changes in menstrual cycle regularity, or loss of menstrual cycle not associated with menopause
- Low markers for iron status
- Low bone mineral density
- BMI of 17.5 or lower

Importantly, the presence of even multiple signs does not necessarily indicate the presence of RED-S. Additionally, although symptoms of RED-S can occur when energy availability calculations fall below the threshold value of 30 kcal/kg (13.6 kcal/pound) of lean mass proposed by the IOC (49), the point at which RED-S occurs differs from person to person based on genetic makeup, lifestyle, history, and habitual non-exercise activity levels (14).

Thus, simple mathematical calculations are inappropriate for screening RED-S in clients. Furthermore, RED-S often occurs as a consequence of or alongside eating disorders and the female athlete triad, and only health care professionals should attempt to diagnose or treat this condition. Although personal trainers can advise clients to follow a given energy intake consistent with their activity level and body mass, if concerns arise related to the possible occurrence of RED-S, a qualified health care practitioner (e.g., a registered dietitian or primary care physician) should be consulted.

NUTRIENTS

Once the personal trainer knows a client's dietary intake and energy requirements, it is possible to assess general nutritional needs. To understand the relationship between the body and food, as well as to provide nutrition guidance, it is important to have an understanding of the six nutrients: protein, carbohydrate, fat, vitamins, minerals, and water.

Protein

For centuries, protein was considered the staple of the diet and the source of speed and strength for athletic endeavors. Although we now know that carbohydrates are the main energy source for sport, protein remains a main nutrient of interest, especially for those who wish to improve adaptations to resistance training, increase lean muscle mass, or lose body fat.

When determining how much protein a client needs, the personal trainer must consider a number of factors, including energy intake, activity level, the type of exercise performed, the body composition of the client, and in some cases, the source of protein. Protein is primarily used to repair and build tissue, but some is oxidized for energy. The proportion of protein used for energy increases when fewer calories are consumed than are expended and when body fat or levels of **glycogen** (stored carbohydrate primarily in muscle and liver) are low (26). Thus, when caloric intake or stored energy goes down, the protein requirement goes up. Importantly, protein intake recommendations by health and government organizations are based on providing an adequate intake to prevent amino acid deficiency and subsequent declines in health; they are not intended to improve fitness, health, or body composition. Additionally, protein requirements are based on the assumption that "reference proteins" such as meat, fish, poultry, dairy products, and eggs—which are considered high-quality proteins—are consumed. If the goal is to improve adaptations to exercise for health, performance, or body composition, or in clients whose dietary protein comes mostly from plants, the requirement is higher (37). The U.S. Recommended Dietary Allowance (RDA) for protein for healthy, sedentary adults is 0.8 g/kg of body weight for both men and women (52). The World Health Organization identifies the **safe intake level**, an amount that is sufficient for 97.5% of the population, at 0.83 g of protein/kg per day. At the safe level there is a low risk that needs will not be met, but this level also ensures there is no risk to individuals from excess protein intake up to amounts considerably higher than 0.83 g/kg (82).

Although the intake set by both of these organizations may be sufficient for nonactive healthy, young adults consuming reference protein sources, for clients who have greater protein needs, it is not enough to offset protein–amino acid oxidation during exercise, repair muscle damage, and build lean tissue (28). A general recommendation for athletes is 1.4 to 2.0 g/kg per day depending on the sport, training intensity, total calorie intake, and overall health (15). Further, if the goal is to enhance adaptations to resistance training—either strength or muscle mass gain—evidence indicates 1.6 g/kg per day will optimize outcomes for most individuals. An upper-end recommendation of 2.2 g/kg per day may be appropriate for individuals with the specific goal of maximizing strength or muscle mass (48). Likewise, as mentioned previously, this upper-end recommendation may be useful for clients with fat loss goals in a caloric deficit (78), not only for the previously mentioned reasons but also because some data suggest higher-protein diets can blunt the desire to eat (59) and may enhance fat loss, possibly owing to an increased thermic effect of food and improved satiety (5).

The personal trainer should be aware that excessively high protein intakes (e.g., greater than 4 g/kg body weight per day) are not indicated for clients with impaired renal function, those with low calcium intake, or those who are restricting fluid intake. These situations could be exacerbated by a high protein intake. For the most part, however, concerns about potential negative effects of high protein intakes are unfounded, especially in healthy individuals (55). Proteins consumed in excess of amounts needed for the synthesis of tissue are converted to other substrates and used for energy. Thus, if excess total calories are consumed, even on a high-protein diet, fat storage can occur. Although protein itself is unlikely to be converted to body fat and stored, more of the other substrates will be stored because they will not be needed for energy.

Carbohydrate

As mentioned before, carbohydrate is the primary fuel for athletic performance. Because dietary carbohydrate replaces muscle and liver glycogen used during high-intensity physical activity, a high-carbohydrate diet (up to 60%-70% of total calories) is commonly recommended for physically active individuals (63). However, a variety of diets, with various carbohydrate, protein, and fat mixtures, have been shown to be equally effective in supporting training and performance. Which diet is appropriate depends on a client's goals, training regimen, personal preference, and fitness level (11, 12, 54, 56). Some physically active individuals may benefit from a high-carbohydrate diet, but others do not benefit and may experience negative effects such as an increase in serum triglycerides or weight gain. Individualizing carbohydrate intake based on the training program, individual genetics, and how the client has historically responded is imperative.

One important factor to consider when determining carbohydrate intake is the training program. If a client is an aerobic endurance athlete (e.g., a distance runner, road cyclist, triathlete, or cross-country skier who trains aerobically for 90 minutes or more daily), he or she should replenish glycogen levels by consuming approximately 7 to 10 g/kg body weight per day (30, 64, 65). This is equivalent to 600 to 750 g of carbohydrate (2,400-3,000 kcal from carbohydrate) per day for an individual weighing 165 pounds (74.8 kg). This amount has been shown to adequately restore skeletal glycogen within 24 hours (1, 16, 35, 43, 57). In cases where performance depletes glycogen and an additional glycogen-depleting workout or performance is required (such as when training more than once per day, or during multistage aerobic endurance events), strategies of carbohydrate timing may take on increased importance (69).

However, the majority of physically active individuals do not train aerobically for more than an hour each day. Research on the carbohydrate needs of these individuals is sparse. Moderately low carbohydrate intake and muscle glycogen levels seem to have a minor impact, if any, on resistance training performance (47, 70, 74). Intake of approximately half of that recommended for aerobic endurance exercise appears adequate to support training and performance of strength, sprint, and skill exercise; thus an intake of 5 to 6 g/kg body weight per day is reasonable (13, 64)—with the caveat that for clients with fat loss goals who must be in a caloric deficit, this amount may not be possible while consuming appropriate amounts of protein and fat. In such cases, clients should simply consume their remaining calories from carbohydrate after establishing an appropriate intake of dietary protein and fat (25).

Roughly 50 to 100 g of carbohydrate (the equivalent of three to five pieces of bread) per day prevents **ketosis** (high levels of ketones in the bloodstream), which results from the incomplete breakdown of fatty acids (79). Beyond that basal requirement, the role of carbohydrate is to provide fuel for energy, and thus the amount of carbohydrate needed by clients depends on their total energy requirement. However, diets that severely restrict carbohydrate—known as ketogenic diets—to leverage ketones as a more dominant metabolic substrate have become popular in the fitness industry and have also been investigated in research. It seems that very-low-carbohydrate diets in the 50 to 100 g range are likely safe (21) and clinically equivalent for fat loss (72) and retention of maximal strength (24) in comparison with higher-carbohydrate diets. Further, they may increase satiety more than higher-carbohydrate diets even when protein is matched (31). With that said, carbohydrate restriction is not necessary for fat loss, and following a ketogenic diet forces one to avoid the consumption of almost all carbohydrate sources. Restricting commonly consumed food sources such as bread can reduce dietary adherence (42), and a "good-food, bad-food" mindset of rigid dietary restraint is associated with poor food and body relationships, attenuated weight loss, and weight regain (80). Finally, there is some evidence that a ketogenic diet may be suboptimal for the purposes of muscle gain (33, 75).

Dietary Fat

The human body has a low requirement for dietary fat. It is estimated that individuals should consume at least 3% of energy from omega-6 (linoleic) fatty acids and 0.5% to 1% from omega-3 (alpha linolenic acid) fatty acids to prevent true deficiency (17). Even though the requirement is low, inadequate fat intake is a potential problem for otherwise healthy individuals who overly restrict dietary fat. Very-low-fat diets, such as those sometimes prescribed for patients with severe heart disease, are not recommended for healthy, active individuals. Diets with less than 15% fat may decrease testosterone production and thus negatively affect metabolism and muscle development (76). And very-low-fat diets may impair the absorption of fat-soluble vitamins.

Personal trainers need to be aware of their clients' perceptions about dietary fat and provide education on the importance of essential fatty acids (omega-3 and omega-6 fats). It is, of course, the overconsumption rather than the underconsumption of fat that has held the attention of scientists, health care providers, and the general public for the past several decades, specifically with respect to the relationship between dietary fat and cardiovascular disease.

Approximately 34% of calories in the typical American diet are consumed as fat (18). Dietary intake in most European countries is similar, with 34% of calories from fat in women and 36% in men (41). The recommendation for the general public from most health organizations is that fat should contribute 30% or less of the total calories consumed. It is recommended that 20% of the total calories (or two-thirds of the total fat intake) come from monounsaturated or polyunsaturated sources, that less than 10% come from saturated fats (one-third of total fat intake), and that minimal manufactured trans fats from partially hydrogenated oils be consumed.

Just as a diet very low in carbohydrate forces a more restrictive diet, the same can be said for a diet that is very low in fat. Thus, it is advisable for a personal trainer to consider multiple factors before making recommendations about decreasing dietary fat (see the sidebar "When Should the Client Decrease Dietary Fat?").

> **Protein, carbohydrates, and fats are all important nutrients in a balanced diet to support fitness and health, both physically and in terms of having a healthy relationship with food. The personal trainer should help clients stay focused on the quality and quantity of the overall dietary pattern, not any individual food or nutrient.**

Vitamins and Minerals

Dietary Reference Intakes (DRIs), which are used in the United States and Canada, are recommendations of the Food and Nutrition Board for the intake of vitamins and minerals, to be used for planning and assessing diets for healthy people (table 7.4; 52).

The DRIs are based on life stage groups that take into account age, sex, pregnancy, and lactation. A personal trainer who has the computerized analysis of a client's diet can assess actual vitamin and mineral

intake compared against the DRIs. Starting in 1997 the DRIs replaced the Recommended Dietary Allowances that had been published since 1941. Dietary Reference Intakes represent a different approach, with the emphasis on long-term health instead of deficiency diseases. The DRIs are split into four categories:

1. **Recommended Dietary Allowance (RDA)** is the intake that meets the nutrient needs of almost all (97%-98%) healthy individuals in a specific age and sex group.

2. **Adequate Intake** is a goal intake when sufficient scientific information is unavailable to estimate the RDA.

3. **Estimated Average Requirement** is the intake that meets the estimated nutrient needs of half the individuals in a specific group.

4. **Tolerable Upper Intake Level** is the maximum intake that is unlikely to pose risks of adverse health effects in almost all healthy individuals in a group.

Instead of being published in one volume as were the RDAs, the DRIs have been published as separate nutrient groups, each group having its own volume. The first book was published in 1997; several more have followed. The reader is referred to the National Academies Press website at www.nap.edu, where DRI tables and links to the full texts of the reports are freely available. It is important to remember that the recommendations for nutrient intakes represent the state of the science at the time, and as such, continue to evolve.

Historically, focus has been on inadequate nutrient intake. However, both inadequate intakes and excessive intakes are problematic. Accordingly, the DRIs include an upper limit, or the amount of a nutrient that may cause negative side effects. Excessively high vitamin and mineral intakes are unnecessary and can even be harmful in some instances.

The European Food Safety Authority (EFSA) developed the **Dietary Reference Values** for nutrients. At the time of this writing, the dietary reference values are current with the 2018 EFSA guidelines for vitamins and minerals. Personal trainers can find up-to-date information concerning Dietary Reference Values at www.efsa.europa.eu.

Water

Fluid intake is a nonissue for some and an obsession for others. Surprisingly little research exists on

TABLE 7.4 Dietary Reference Intakes for Individuals in Life Stage Group 19 to 30 Years

Specific vitamin or mineral	Males	Females	Tolerable upper limit
Vitamin A (µg/day)	**900**	**700**	3,000
Vitamin C (mg/day)	**75**	**75**	2,000
Vitamin D (µg/day)	**15**	**15**	100
Vitamin E (mg/day)	**15**	**15**	1,000
Vitamin K (µg/day)	120	90	ND
Thiamin (mg/day)	**1.2**	**1.1**	ND
Riboflavin (mg/day)	**1.3**	**1.1**	ND
Niacin (mg/day)	**16**	**14**	35
Vitamin B$_6$ (mg/day)	**1.3**	**1.3**	100
Folate (µg/day)	**400**	**400**	1,000
Vitamin B$_{12}$ (µg/day)	**2.4**	**2.4**	ND
Pantothenic acid (mg/day)	5	5	ND
Biotin (µg/day)	30	30	ND
Choline (mg/day)	550	425	3,500
Calcium (mg/day)	**1,000**	**1,000**	2,500
Chromium (µg/day)	35	25	ND
Copper (µg/day)	**900**	**900**	10,000
Fluoride (mg/day)	4	3	10
Iodine (µg/day)	**150**	**150**	1,100
Iron (µg/day)	**8**	**18**	45
Magnesium (mg/day)	**400**	**310**	350
Manganese (mg/day)	2.3	1.8	11
Molybdenum (µg/day)	**45**	**45**	2,000
Phosphorus (mg/day)	**700**	**700**	4,000
Selenium (µ/day)	**55**	**55**	400
Zinc (mg/day)	**11**	**8**	40

Note: This table (taken from the Dietary Reference Intake reports, see www.nap.edu) presents Recommended Dietary Allowances **(RDAs) in bold type** and adequate intakes (AIs) in ordinary type. RDAs are set to meet the needs of almost all (97%-98%) individuals in a group. The AI is believed to cover needs of all individuals in each group (i.e., adult males and females), but lack of data does not allow specifying the percentage of individuals covered by this intake.

ND = not determined.

Adapted from The National Academy of Sciences and The National Academies (33).

WHEN SHOULD THE CLIENT DECREASE DIETARY FAT?

In general, there are three reasons for individuals to reduce dietary fat:

1. Need to increase carbohydrate intake to support training (see the earlier section on carbohydrate). In this case, to ensure adequate protein provision, fat is the nutrient to decrease so that caloric intake can remain similar while the person is increasing carbohydrate.

2. Need to reduce total caloric intake to achieve weight loss. Achieving a negative calorie balance is the only way to reduce body fat. Fat can be a source of excess calories because it is energy dense (fat has 9 kcal/g vs. 4 kcal/g in carbohydrate and protein). Studies also suggest that the good flavor of high-fat foods (particularly high-fat foods that are also rich in refined carbohydrates) increases the likelihood of overeating these foods. Thus, decreasing excess dietary fat can help reduce caloric intake. (The recommendation to reduce dietary fat should not be made before assessment of dietary intake. The individual may already have a low-fat diet.)

3. Need to decrease elevated blood cholesterol. Manipulation of fat and carbohydrate may be medically indicated for clients who have high blood cholesterol levels or a family history of heart disease. This diet therapy should be provided only by a registered dietitian.

---

the water requirements of humans, setting the stage for confusion about how much and what to drink. Research that does exist is primarily limited to hospitalized patients, soldiers, or serious athletes in hot environments. Assumptions that thirst will drive adequate water intake and the kidneys will do their job have largely led scientists to overlook the issue of hydration in healthy individuals.

General Fluid Intake Guidelines

Unlike the situation with many other nutrients, it is impossible to set a general requirement for water. Common knowledge and folklore have put the requirement at anywhere from 64 ounces (1.9 L) per day to 2 gallons (7.6 L). Both could be appropriate, depending on the situation. The reality is that water requirements change based on a variety of factors including environment, sweating, body surface area, calorie intake, body size, and lean muscle tissue, leading to tremendous inter- and intraindividual variation. Instead of looking at prescriptive amounts to be consumed each day, it is important for personal trainers to assess each client's situation and attempt to individualize recommendations.

The basic goal of fluid intake is to prevent dehydration (i.e., to maintain fluid balance). Fluid balance exists when the water that is lost from the body through urine, through insensible loss from skin and lungs, and through feces is replaced. The kidneys dilute or concentrate urine to keep the body's internal milieu unchanged regardless of significant changes in intake. Thirst is triggered at about 1% dehydration. Thus, encouraging fluid intake based on thirst works quite well to maintain fluid balance for healthy adult

individuals in temperature-controlled environments who are sedentary and who have plenty of fluid readily available.

The average fluid intake needed to offset fluid losses in sedentary adults may range from 1.5 to 2.7 quarts (1.4-2.6 L) per day. People often ask whether higher fluid intakes are healthful. The answer is unclear, but an emerging area of study on the relationship between disease prevention and fluid intake indicates that higher fluid intakes may be preventive against bladder cancer, kidney stones, gallstones, and colon cancer (10, 36, 46, 62).

> It is impossible to set a generic water recommendation, such as eight glasses of water a day. Each individual's water requirement varies over time, as do requirements among various populations.

Fluid Intake and Exercise

Although the answers regarding general fluid intake in sedentary conditions are unclear, more is known about fluid intake and exercise. Guidelines have been developed for individuals before, during, and after exercise.

Before Exercise Approximately 5 to 7 ml of fluid per kilogram body weight should be consumed at least 4 hours prior to exercise. Additional fluid should be consumed 2 hours prior to exercise, approximately 3 to 5 ml/kg body weight if urine is dark and scant (62).

During Exercise Preventing dehydration can be difficult for physically active people exercising in a warm environment. Continuous sweating during prolonged exercise can exceed 1.9 quarts (1.8 L) per hour, increasing water requirements significantly. Unless sweat losses are replaced, body temperature rises, leading to heat exhaustion, heatstroke, and even death. Paradoxically, during exercise, humans do not adequately replace sweat losses when fluids are consumed at will. In fact, most individuals replace only about two-thirds of the water they sweat off during exercise. Personal trainers must be aware of this tendency and make their clients aware of it as well. During times of high sweat loss under physical stress, a systematic approach to water replacement is necessary because thirst is not a reliable indicator of fluid needs in these situations.

After Exercise Slight dehydration is common in almost all physical endeavors, and therefore rehydration is necessary. However, preventive maintenance is also important. Starting exercise in a hydrated state, as well as consuming fluids during activity, is a very important part of the systematic approach to hydration. After exercise, the main goal is to replace any fluid and electrolyte losses.

Clients should monitor sweat loss by checking body weight before and after physical activity (removing sweaty clothes before weighing, for accuracy). Clients should drink 20 to 24 ounces (about 600 to 700 ml) of fluids for every pound lost (62). Sodium-rich foods or a sport drink should be used to stimulate thirst, replace lost electrolytes, and enhance rehydration. During the rehydration process, urine is produced before full rehydration occurs (66). Ideally, the amount of fluid clients need to replace should be measured into water bottles, pitchers, and so forth so that rehydration is not left to chance.

Clients who have a goal of weight loss may misperceive acute weight loss during a workout as loss of fat and therefore see it as positive. It is important for personal trainers to clarify with clients that the acute weight loss during a workout is water, not fat, and must be replaced by hydrating (preferably with the inclusion of sodium-rich foods or an electrolyte-enhanced sport beverage).

Monitoring Hydration Status

Although not as sensitive as weight change, other indicators of hydration status can be useful monitoring tools. Signs of dehydration include dark yellow, strong-smelling urine; decreased frequency of urination; rapid resting heart rate; and prolonged muscle soreness (3). Normal urine production for adults is about 1.2 quarts (1.1 L) per day, or 8 to 10 fluid ounces (~240-300 ml) per urination four times per day. Normal urine is the color of light lemon juice, except in clients who are taking supplemental vitamins, which tend to make the urine bright yellow.

What to Drink Before and After Activity

All fluids, from beverages and from food, contribute to the body's fluid requirement. Juice and soft drinks are 89% water; milk is 90% water, and even pizza is 50% water. Before and after physical activity, water or other beverages such as milk, juice, carbonated or uncarbonated soft drinks, and sport drinks are suitable choices for fluid replacement. For clients who eat many fruits, vegetables, and soups, much of their water requirement may be coming from foods.

Whether consuming caffeine-containing beverages causes dehydration is a frequently asked question. Data show that tolerance to caffeine occurs in one to four days and that people who are tolerant do not experience increased urine output. Thus, caffeine-containing beverages contribute to hydration (22).

When significant sweating has occurred, consumption of sodium chloride (salt) in the form of beverages or food minimizes urine output and hastens recovery of water and electrolyte balance (44, 45). In practical terms, this means that consuming a wide variety of beverages and foods after training is important. In fact, most fluid consumption occurs during and around mealtimes.

What to Drink During Activity

The goal of fluid replacement during exercise is to move the fluid from the mouth, through the gut, and into circulation rapidly and to provide a volume that matches sweat losses. The way to achieve this is to provide fluids that are absorbed rapidly and that the client finds palatable. A variety of fluids can serve as effective fluid replacement during exercise (27). Cool water is ideal except during long-duration activity (e.g., aerobic endurance exercise, multiple games in a day)—when replacing sodium becomes very important to prevent a dangerous drop in blood sodium levels, called **hyponatremia**. Other options include commercial sport drinks or homemade sport drinks, such as diluted juice or diluted soft drinks. Although plain water can meet fluid requirements in most cases, some people find flavored drinks more palatable than water and consequently drink more (81). During aerobic endurance training, carbohydrate along with water intake can be helpful for activities lasting more than 60 to 90 minutes (9).

Commercial sport drinks contain water, sugars, and electrolytes (usually sodium, chloride, and potassium). The sugar content of sport drinks is slightly less than the amount in most soft drinks and juices. The carbohydrate concentration of commercial sport drinks ranges from 6% to 8%, a solution that tends to be rapidly absorbed.

Clients who are monitoring calorie intake in an effort to maintain or lose weight may be averse to consuming the extra calories in sport drinks. In this case, the cost to benefit of consuming carbohydrate must be examined. It is worth remembering that the benefits of carbohydrate during aerobic endurance training are important for competitive clients wanting to increase speed and aerobic endurance but might be less so for a client who is training primarily for health and fitness and interested in weight loss.

WEIGHT GAIN

There are two reasons clients may attempt to gain weight: to improve physical appearance or enhance athletic performance. For weight gain in the form of muscle mass, a combination of diet and progressive resistance training is essential. However, genetic predisposition, body type, and compliance determine the client's progress. Muscle tissue is approximately 75% water, 20% protein, and 5% fatty acids, minerals, metabolites, and glycogen. When viewing protein as simply a sum of its parts, a 1-pound (0.5 kg) quantity of muscle tissue contains only 500 to 600 kcal. Thus, if aiming to gain 1 pound of muscle mass per week, one might think an energy surplus of less than 100 kcal per day would be all that is needed. However, this does not account for the energy required to fuel tissue synthesis, the energy expended during resistance training, increases in the thermic effect of food, and adaptive increases in energy expenditure. Thus, an intake of 350 to 500 kcal above nonresistance training energy requirements for maintenance may be needed to support a 1-pound (0.5 kg) weekly gain in lean tissue (68), with the caveat that experienced trainees who have already gained a large amount of muscle mass may benefit from a smaller energy surplus and slower rate of weight gain to prevent excess body fat accumulation (29).

To accomplish increased caloric intake, it is recommended that clients eat larger portions of foods at mealtime, eat more total calories at each meal, eat frequently, and choose higher-calorie foods. To accommodate frequent eating, meal replacement drinks can come in handy, especially when a person is not hungry.

Muscle is gained more efficiently when sufficient protein is consumed. An intake of at least 1.6 g/kg body weight per day is recommended, and potentially higher if the client's primary source of protein is plant based. Plant proteins contain a lower amount of the amino acids related to muscle protein synthesis (e.g., leucine).

> The two primary nutrition principles for weight gain are to increase calorie intake and to ensure sufficient protein intake (or maintain an adequate level if already at 1.6 g/kg body weight per day or higher).

WEIGHT LOSS

People who have weight loss as a goal, specifically fat loss, can be split into two general groups: those who are normal weight but want to lose body fat for aesthetic reasons and those who are overweight or obese—that is, they have a body mass index (BMI) greater than 25 or 30, respectively. The following are general principles to be considered when a client embarks on a weight loss regimen:

- The ability to achieve and maintain minimal body fat is to some extent genetic.
- Whether clients can gain muscle and lose body fat simultaneously depends on their training status, training program, and nutrition intake. Previously untrained clients can lose body fat and gain lean body mass as a result of caloric restriction and training; however, it becomes increasingly difficult for trained persons who already possess a low percentage of body fat to achieve body fat reduction without losing some lean body mass.
- An average loss of 1 to 2 pounds (0.5-0.9 kg) per week represents a daily caloric deficit of approximately 500 to 1,000 kcal, which can be achieved through a combination of dietary restriction and exercise. Faster rates of weight loss can lead to dehydration and decrease vitamin and mineral

status as a result of the decreased food intake (23). Substantial weight loss by caloric restriction will result in decreases in performance (19) and loss of marked amounts of lean body mass (77). Fat loss rates vary depending on body composition, food intake, and training program. A rate of loss of 0.5% to 1% total body weight per week is a common guideline. For example, losing at a rate of 1%, a 110-pound (49.9 kg) client would strive for about a 1-pound (0.5 kg) weight loss per week, while a 331-pound (150.1 kg) client would aim to lose about 3 pounds (1.4 kg) per week.

- The diet should be composed of food low in energy density. **Energy density** refers to the calories per weight or volume of food. Examples of foods with low energy density are broth-based soup, salad greens, vegetables, and fresh fruits. In general, foods with low energy density contain a high proportion of water and fiber. These are foods that people can eat in large portions without consuming excess calories. This can help control hunger and lower caloric intake (60).

- The diet should be nutritionally balanced and should provide a variety of foods.

- The diet should contain at least 1.6 g/kg body weight per day of protein, and possibly more (as high as 2.2 g/kg), to help aid satiety and muscle retention and perhaps increase energy expenditure to a small degree.

> The guiding principle for weight loss is to help clients achieve a negative energy balance. Many clients think the issue is more complex than that, so the personal trainer should keep them focused on this principle, or more importantly, help them adopt habits that result in a negative energy balance.

EVALUATING WEIGHT LOSS DIETS

The array of popular weight loss diet plans is virtually endless—high protein, low fat, low carbohydrate, this shake, that bar, fat burners, do not eat at night, eat six times a day, eat one time a day—and the list goes on and on. What makes things confusing is that every client can name at least one person for whom at least one of these diets has worked. In addition, each client can think of many people for whom nothing seems to work. The truth is, *any* dietary regimen will lead to weight loss if, and only if, the person achieves a negative calorie balance. As personal trainers answer their clients' questions about diets they read about or see on TV, it is essential to keep in mind that people need to expend more calories than they consume for fat loss to occur.

Clearly, it is impossible to keep up with every new diet, and a personal trainer does not need to. Instead, one evaluates a diet not on the claims it makes but by the foods (and therefore nutrients) that are included and excluded. Personal trainers can help clients spot fad diets by checking for signs like the following:

- The diet excludes one or more groups of foods, which means it may be deficient in certain nutrients or too restrictive for clients to stay on for the long term.

- It overemphasizes one particular food or type of food. The Cabbage Soup Diet is an example.

- It is very low in calories. Very-low-calorie diets can lead to higher loss of lean tissue, are limited in nutrients, and may decrease compliance.

- The advocates discourage physical activity or indicate that it is not necessary.

- The diet promises quick weight loss.

Last but not least, personal trainers need to talk to clients about what they are really doing, not what the diet plan says. Often, the two are different. Personal trainers can decipher nutrition misinformation by taking a close look at the source of the information and cross-referencing the information with trusted websites or sport nutrition experts.

The personal trainer should examine whether a diet plan includes dietary supplements. Stimulants are commonly added to weight loss supplements. These types of supplements are generally contraindicated in individuals with high blood pressure or other medical conditions. Stimulants for weight loss should be used only under the supervision of a physician. In many cases, clients are not aware of all the ingredients in the supplement they ingest. The personal trainer can ask the client to bring in the container so they can review the contents together. At this time the personal trainer can gather information on any questionable ingredients and provide relevant guidance.

DIETARY SUPPLEMENTS

Dietary supplements cover the spectrum from traditional vitamin and mineral tablets to prohormones such as androstenedione. Because of the diversity of dietary supplements, it is difficult to give blanket recommendations or guidelines about them. The following is a brief overview of the science and regulation of dietary supplements.

Dietary Supplement Regulation

In the United States, dietary supplements are regulated under the Dietary Supplement Health and Education Act of 1994 (DSHEA). This act was a landmark law, affirming the status of dietary supplements as a category of food, not drugs, and defining **dietary supplements** as products "intended to supplement the diet." The ingredients of a supplement include vitamins, minerals, herbs or botanicals, amino acids, a substance that increases the total dietary intake, or variations and combinations thereof.

In January of 2000, the U.S. Food and Drug Administration ruled that supplement manufacturers can make claims on the label about the body's structure or function affected by the supplement but cannot claim to diagnose, prevent, cure, or treat disease. In other words, it is permissible to say that a calcium supplement will "help maintain bone health" but not permissible to say that calcium will "help prevent osteoporosis."

Although the Food and Drug Administration does not have the resources to monitor and test individual supplements, a few independent organizations offer quality testing and approval. One independent company, ConsumerLab.com, tests supplements for quality and purity and provides the results on its website. Supplements that pass the test can carry the ConsumerLab-approved quality product seal on the label. An independent voluntary organization called United States Pharmacopeia (USP) created their Dietary Supplement Certification Program. The acronym USP on the label is meant to assure the consumer that the label information is accurate and that the company follows good manufacturing practices. The World Anti-Doping Agency, the National Sport Foundation (NSF), and Informed Choice also test supplements for banned substances.

Evaluating Supplement Regimens

It is estimated that 48% of U.S. adults take some kind of dietary supplement. Vitamin and mineral supplements are the most commonly used. Although vitamin and mineral supplements are perceived to be without risk, excess intake of vitamins and minerals is not beneficial and, depending on the circumstance, potentially harmful. For example, excess iron can be dangerous for those with the genetic disorder called **hemochromatosis**, in which the body absorbs and stores excess iron in tissues, leading to multiorgan failure.

When evaluating a client's supplement regimen, it is important to evaluate all sources of the nutrient. Because vitamins and minerals are often added to supplements (e.g., shakes, powders) as well as breakfast cereal, sport bars, and energy drinks, the likelihood of excessive intakes is increasing. Excessive intakes, especially of iron, calcium, zinc, magnesium, niacin, B_6, and vitamin A, should be corrected through changes in the supplement regimen.

A common finding is that the individual's supplementation choices do not match the inadequacies of the diet, causing excess intakes of some nutrients without correcting the low intake of others. Helping a client adjust food and supplement choices to optimize the vitamin and mineral intake is a useful function of diet analysis.

Besides questions about vitamins and minerals, clients may have questions about other types of supplements such as creatine or amino acids. One way to make sense of the wide array of supplements is to categorize them. Most supplements fit into the categories shown in table 7.5. Evaluation of the particular supplement for a client depends on the individual's goals and situation. For example, meal replacement drinks and bars can be an excellent snack for busy people. Protein supplements can round out protein needs in those who don't eat enough dietary protein. If a client participates in National Collegiate Athletic Association, United States Olympic Committee, or other competitions where drug testing occurs, it is important to know that some supplements contain banned substances that could lead to a positive drug test. Opting for brands with certification from Informed Choice or NSF on the label can help ensure that the supplement is not tainted with banned substances.

TABLE 7.5 Selected Dietary Supplement Categories

Category	Examples
Protein sources	Drinks, powders, and bars including whey, casein, egg, soy, peas, plant blends, milk blends, collagen
Meal replacements	Drinks and bars
Amino acids	Glutamine, tyrosine, BCAAs, EAAs, leucine, arginine, glutamine, tyrosine, lysine
Carbohydrate sources	Sport drinks, energy drinks, bars, gels, powders
Pre- and prohormones*	Androstenedione, DHEA
Biochemicals or energy metabolites	Creatine, citrulline, beta-alanine, HMB, pyruvate, CLA
Herbs	Ginseng, St. John's wort, guarana

BCAAs = branched-chain amino acids; EAAs = essential amino acids; DHEA = dehydroepiandrosterone; HMB = beta-hydroxy-beta-methylbutyrate; CLA = conjugated linoleic acid.

*Pre- and prohormones are precursors to or enhancers of hormone production. The products attempt to mimic anabolic steroids, sometimes with problematic outcomes.

It is outside the scope of practice for a personal trainer to recommend supplements. Rather, it is the duty of the personal trainer to aid clients as consumers, ensuring they are informed of the safety and scientific legitimacy of products and know how to assess whether a supplement company follows best practices. Competitive athletes need to check with their sponsoring organizations for guidelines to ensure compliance with their sporting body. Further, any time a client decides to use a dietary supplement, he or she should be guided to consult a registered dietitian— ideally trained in sport nutrition—to ensure there are no potential complications from existing medical conditions, drug interactions, or other issues within the scope of an allied health professional.

Although the scope for recommending supplements is outside the purview of most personal trainers, they should be equipped to provide scientific information and resources on the topic because, inevitably, clients will come to them for guidance. More than half of U.S. adults use dietary supplements, with multivitamin and -mineral, calcium, and fish oil supplements being the most prevalent. However, less than a quarter of these U.S. adults use supplements based on the recommendation of a health care provider (6). A review of the position stands of the International Society of Sports Nutrition (ISSN) on specific supplements, published in its open-access journal, is a useful resource for personal trainers. The review includes a comprehensive analysis on the efficacy and safety of various ergogenic aids; see "ISSN Exercise & Sport Nutrition Review: Research & Recommendations" (www.jissn. com/content/7/1/7).

THE ART OF MAKING DIETARY RECOMMENDATIONS

When a personal trainer is evaluating a client's eating habits and giving advice, it is important to keep a few things in mind. First, nutritional status is influenced by intake over a relatively long period. Short-term dietary inadequacies or excesses will typically have a minimal impact on long-term status. Additionally, the body can obtain the nutrients it needs through countless combinations of foods consumed over time. There is no "right way to eat" or "best diet" that applies to everyone. Generally speaking, an adequate diet provides nutrients the body needs, other components from food that promote health or prevent disease, and calories at the level necessary to achieve desired body weight; and it does so in a way that matches the individual's preferences, lifestyle, training goals, and budget (58). As outlined previously, having clients track their intake via a diet recall, food journal, website, or app can give the personal trainer a clear indication of current food intake, areas of success, and areas of concern.

Closely tracking intake is not appropriate for all clients, however. Although many personal trainers and their clients successfully use food tracking to be healthy, fit, and lean, there are potential downsides of consistent tracking. Growing evidence demonstrates a potential link between the use of macronutrient, calorie, and weight tracking apps and websites with both attitudinal and behavioral eating disorder symptoms as well as increased psychological stress (38, 40, 53,

67). However, other experimental evidence shows tracking and regular weigh-ins do not result in greater occurrence or symptoms of negative food attitudes or eating disorders (32). With this in mind, it would be wise for most clients to closely track their intake only temporarily to gain an awareness of their food consumption and nutritional status, better understand portion sizes, read nutrition labels and understand the nutrients in food, assess how well they are following the agreed-on action steps, and give the personal trainer the information needed to make appropriate recommendations.

After this learning phase, the emphasis should be on nontracking, habit-based strategies focused on internal cues (hunger and satiety), with detailed tracking used only if progress is not made. For clients with more advanced performance or physique goals, the potential risks of tracking are usually outweighed by the benefits of such close monitoring of intake for achieving aesthetic goals. Consistent tracking is therefore often warranted in populations where becoming extremely lean is the main goal.

To help clients achieve their goals, it is necessary to help them change their habits and behaviors systematically over time. Research in psychology and behavior change shows many successful processes for facilitating change that can also be implemented when coaching nutrition. Here are some of the most beneficial core concepts:

- *Be client centered, not coach centered.* A client-centered coach respects their clients' values, priorities, and goals by putting their clients' agenda first. In the client-centered approach, the coach is a guide and collaborator, working in partnership with clients to help them change. The personal trainer should aim to build strong coaching relationships by showing compassion, respecting client autonomy, and being nonjudgmental and genuine (8).

- *Focus on solutions rather than on problems.* Instead of focusing on the things clients are doing "wrong" or poorly (i.e., their problems), the personal trainer should focus on the things clients are already doing well and encourage them to do more of these positive habits. For example, perhaps a client eats a good amount of protein and vegetables at dinner but not lunch. The personal trainer and client can work together to discover what makes dinner different and determine how the client can use this knowledge to consume enough protein and vegetables at lunch. Or the personal trainer can leverage skills the client already has to help him or her eat better. Maybe the client is highly organized or has strong cooking skills. The client can use those skills to his or her advantage to improve nutritional intake (34).

- *Add before taking away.* The personal trainer can have clients add more minimally processed, nutrient-rich whole foods that they like or are willing to try before having them remove energy-dense, highly processed foods. This shift helps prevent the feelings of deprivation, increases intake of nutrient-rich but calorie-sparse whole foods, better manages appetite, and displaces energy-dense processed foods.

Helping clients build skills and develop healthy eating habits requires a systematic process that is repetitive and cyclical to continually help clients progress toward their goals. The following five-step process can be employed to enhance success:

Step 1: Assess and gather data about goals, current intake, anthropometrics, and health status. This provides baseline information to see how clients are progressing across many domains—food intake, weight, body composition, health markers, performance, and so on.

Step 2: Collaboratively create a solution-focused action plan and outline possible next steps. What are they already doing well? How can they do more of that? What skills do they already have that can be leveraged?

Step 3: Collaboratively choose some next steps and have the client implement them. Prioritize the next steps from Step 2 and choose the next few the client will tackle. Agree together on how to assess their consistency with those actions.

Step 4: Observe and monitor outcomes of those steps. Were they consistently able to implement the chosen actions? Did those chosen actions lead to progress toward their goals?

Step 5: Assess and gather data about behaviors and outcomes (then repeat Steps 2 through 5). If clients weren't able to consistently implement the chosen actions, why not? What got in their way? If they were able to do it sometimes, what was different about those times? How can they do more of that? If those actions did not lead them toward their goals, do the actions need to change?

CONCLUSION

From a nutrition standpoint, the most important thing for personal trainers is to operate under their scope of practice. Before assessing a client's diet, personal trainers should first turn to their dietetic licensing board to find out the laws within their particular state, province, or country that govern the provision of nutrition advice. Because nutrition is a complex field, just like personal training, the personal trainer can benefit from collaborating with a dietitian who specializes in sport nutrition.

The personal trainer can benefit from three fundamental tools when discussing nutrition with clients. One is factual information, such as that provided in this book, on which to base assessments and recommendations. The second tool is the individualized approach. Personal trainers are likely to find themselves recommending something to one client and advising the next client against the same thing (if they can make individual recommendations under their local dietitian or nutritionist licensure laws). The ability to match the recommendations to the individual's situation enhances the personal trainer's effectiveness exponentially. The third tool is a network of knowledgeable professionals to consult or refer to when clients have nutrition issues outside the scope of the personal trainer's expertise. With these three tools, the personal trainer can help nutrition work for, not against, clients' health and fitness goals.

Study Questions

1. Which of the following is within the personal trainer's scope of practice regarding providing nutrition information to a client?

   A. Help a client with a disease state affected by nutrition.

   B. Convey general nutrition knowledge.

   C. Offer medical nutrition therapy.

   D. None; nutrition is outside the scope of practice for a personal trainer.

2. Which of the following is *not* realistically attainable by a personal trainer to estimate energy requirements of a client?

   A. direct measurement of energy expenditure of all physical activity

   B. log of all food and drink intake

   C. estimated activity level

   D. estimated resting energy expenditure

3. Which of the following is defined as "the average daily nutrient requirement adequate for meeting the needs of most healthy people within each life stage and sex"?

   A. Estimated Average Requirement

   B. Recommended Dietary Allowance

   C. Adequate Intake

   D. Dietary Reference Intake

4. An intake of _____ kcal above nonresistance training energy requirements for maintenance may be needed to support a 1-pound (0.5 kg) weekly gain in lean tissue.

   A. 100

   B. 200-300

   C. 350-500

   D. 600-800

5. Which of the following is *not* a suggested dietary recommendation?

   A. Focus on solutions rather than problems.

   B. Commit to long-term dietary tracking.

   C. There is no "right way to eat".

   D. The diet should match the individual's preferences, lifestyle, training goals, and budget.

CHAPTER 8

Exercise Psychology, Goal Setting, and Motivation

E. Whitney G. Moore, PhD, and Brian T. Gearity, PhD

After completing this chapter, you will be able to

- understand the psychological benefits of exercise,
- work with a client to set effective exercise goals,
- recognize the value of motivation, and
- implement methods to motivate a client.

Participation in physical activity results in desirable health consequences in terms of both acute responses and chronic adaptations in the physiological and psychological domains (81). Despite the well-known benefits of exercise, current estimates from the National Center for Health Statistics indicate that approximately 40% of American men and women are sedentary during their leisure time (11). According to one study, fewer than 50% of those who begin a program of regular physical activity will continue their involvement after six months (11). In addition, for those who do adhere, the level of improvement in muscular strength, cardiovascular fitness, and other fitness-related goals may be compromised by a lack of intensity and effort.

Thus for many people, the benefits of exercise remain elusive, and lack of compliance with programs offered by personal trainers results in a less than satisfactory experience for both the client and the personal trainer. Although the promotion of exercise behavior presents a significant challenge, understanding and implementing fundamental motivational principles can improve participation and program adherence as well as the intensity of effort during training sessions. Although it might appear that some individuals are naturally more motivated toward achievement than others, in actuality, those motivated individuals are likely employing their own motivational strategies. If personal trainers can elicit a client's specific mental strategy for summoning motivation and can stimulate a client to employ that strategy, it is possible to turn on motivation in much the same way one flips a switch on the wall to illuminate a room. This approach may lead to the realization of exercise and nutrition goals.

The first section of this chapter considers the psychological benefits of physical activity, including the **anxiolytic** (i.e., anxiety reducing) and anti-depressive effects of exercise, as well as the cognitive benefits, especially for persons who are older. Thus, the notion that exercise is essential "medicine" is supported, with some men and women deriving greater psychological and physiological benefit from exercise than others.

The authors would like to acknowledge the significant contributions of Bradley D. Hatfield and Phil Kaplan to this chapter.

Educating clients about these benefits could provide additional motivation or energy for exercise. The second section deals with goals, goal orientations, and effective goal setting. The final sections cover motivation, reinforcement, the development of self-efficacy or confidence, and practical instructions for motivational techniques. Here the personal trainer will find specific steps to help clients minimize procrastination, overcome false beliefs, identify and modify self-talk, and employ mental imagery.

MENTAL HEALTH ASPECTS OF EXERCISE

In addition to the desirable physiological consequences of physical activity, there is ample scientific evidence that participation in physical activity has significant mental health benefits. Further, people who are aware of such benefits may be encouraged to increase commitment to regular exercise. Notable among the mental health benefits are a reduction of anxiety and depression (28), decreased reactivity to psychological stress (8, 37, 56), and enhanced cognition (71). In this section, we discuss the psychological impact of exercise in order to help the personal trainer communicate such benefits to the client for educational and motivational purposes.

Stress Reduction Effects of Exercise: Evidence and Mechanisms

It is estimated that 7.3% (48, 49) to 8.5% (31a) of the American population have anxiety-related disorders to the extent that treatment is warranted. In addition, most people experience episodic, and sometimes extended, stress-related symptoms during their lives. Regular physical exercise relieves both state and trait anxiety–related symptoms (64); state anxiety refers to short-term stress-related processes while trait anxiety refers to long-term processes. For many people, the alleviation of anxiety through physical activity likely provides a strong rationale for maintaining participation.

State anxiety can be defined as the actual experience of anxiety that is characterized by feelings of apprehension or threat and accompanied by increased physiological arousal, particularly as mediated by the autonomic nervous system (41, 77). State anxiety can largely be characterized by the flight-or-fight response

first described by Cannon in 1929 (13)—relatively uncontrolled elevations in heart rate, blood pressure, and activity in the hypothalamic-pituitary-adrenal (HPA) axis, with heightened stress hormones such as cortisol. On the other hand, **trait anxiety** is a dispositional factor relating to the probability that a given person is likely to perceive situations as threatening (41, 77). Typically, both forms of anxiety are measured by self-report scales such as the State-Trait Anxiety Inventory (77) or in terms of physiological variables such as muscle tension, blood pressure, or brain electrical activity. Clearly, both acute (i.e., state) and chronic (i.e., trait) anxiety represent negative psychological variables that one would want to avoid, and participation in physical activity effectively alleviates the symptoms associated with anxiety (64).

According to a review of the literature (49), there have been well over 100 scientific studies on the anxiety-reducing effects of exercise. Such a volume of research can be overwhelming, especially when some of the investigations provide contradictory conclusions. Consequently, personal trainers may feel uncertain about their knowledge of the anxiety-reducing effects of exercise, but clarification has been provided by meta-analytic (i.e., broad and integrative) research reviews based on quantitative summaries of the relevant literature. Meta-analytic reviews suggest general patterns of the collective findings in the research literature, as opposed to highlighting individual studies, such that the personal trainer can see the "forest" instead of the "trees."

Small to moderate reductions in anxiety with physical activity have been consistently reported in the exercise psychology literature for over 30 years (12, 45, 50, 52, 55, 64, 86, 87). These effects are typically observed for aerobic forms of exercise across a wide range of intensities, although low-intensity and higher-volume resistance training appears to be efficacious as well (4). Further, researchers have found that individuals who did a combination of resistance, flexibility, and aerobic exercises had significantly greater reductions in their depression than individuals who completed only aerobic exercise (18). Exercise helps individuals with both clinical and nonclinical depression and anxiety (18, 43).

As one would expect, higher-intensity exercise (i.e., above ventilatory threshold) does not seem to provide immediate stress reduction benefits or enjoyment, although some people who are extremely well conditioned may derive a cathartic release from this type of activity (31). Such an effect may be explained by the opponent-process theory of emotion advanced by Solomon and Corbit (76), which posits a rebound expression of positive affect on termination of a high-intensity exercise bout after the uncomfortable feelings and strain during exertion. The rebound "feel-better" effect following intense exercise may be due to the unmasking of physiological coping responses such as the release of beta-endorphin and mood-altering central neurotransmitters (e.g., serotonin), which attenuate the stress of exercise during exertion but are no longer opposed by the stress processes once the work and effort stop (5). In this regard, the release of beta-endorphin manages or economizes the hormonal response to work, as well as the ventilatory or breathing activity involved during exercise, which is a primary input to perceived exertion or the effort sense (37). The maintenance of these counteractive physiological responses—which manage exercise-induced strain—beyond the period of exertion may explain why the trained exercise participant derives a sense of satisfaction and substantial positive affect once a challenging and demanding workout is completed. Furthermore, a continually growing body of exercise psychology studies has revealed the majority of general population exercisers do not respond positively to training at or above the ventilatory threshold (30, 31). The intensity difference between individuals enjoying aerobic exercise during and after the exercise bout versus not enjoying their exercise bout was just 10 heartbeats per minute (30).

There are several possible explanations for the anxiety-reducing effects of exercise (37). One possibility is the rhythmic nature of many forms of physical activity and many exercise routines. People find that walking, running, or cycling at a steady pace promotes mental and physical relaxation. Stair stepping and aerobic dance routines are often performed to a cadence or in time to music. The calming psychological effects of rhythmic exercise may be due to biological processes. It is possible that cerebro-cortical arousal is inhibited by a volley of afferent rhythmic impulses from the skeletal muscles during the exercise that provide feedback to an inhibitory, or relaxation, site in the brain stem, and this causes a "quieting" of the cognitive activity associated with anxiety or stress states (8, 37, 56). Interestingly, many workout routines are rhythmic in nature.

In addition, studies have revealed that exercise alters the activity of the frontal region of the brain such that left frontal activation of the cerebral cortex is elevated relative to right-side activation after exertion (63). On the basis of a number of investigations, Davidson (21) has clearly described the phenomenon of frontal asymmetry and provided evidence that relative left frontal activation (i.e., greater than right-side activation), which can be measured with technologies such as brain electrical activity or electroencephalography (EEG), underlies positive affect and motivation to engage one's environment, while right frontal activation underlies negative affect and withdrawal-oriented motivation. Some investigators have argued that the physiological changes experienced systemically during exercise reflexively influence the central nervous system and the brain, resulting in desirable changes in frontal asymmetry and mood (86, 87).

Another possible reason for the stress reduction effect of exercise is the **thermogenic effect** (37, 64). According to this model based on work with animals (83), the metabolic inefficiency of the human body results in heat production during exercise that causes a cascade of events culminating in relaxation. The part of the brain known as the hypothalamus detects the elevation in the body's temperature and consequently promotes a cortical relaxation effect in an attempt to maintain homeostasis. This results in decreased activation of efferent (motor) nerve fibers—specifically the alpha and gamma motor neurons to the extrafusal and intrafusal muscle fibers, respectively—leading to reduced muscle tension and less sensitivity of the muscle spindles to stretch. This "calming down" effect results in less afferent (sensory) nerve stimulation or feedback to the brain stem arousal center (i.e., the reticular activating formation) and subsequently promotes a relaxation state.

As described earlier in relation to the opponent-process theory, the effects from the natural release of beta-endorphin during exercise stress are maintained for some time after the cessation of exercise. In concert with the calming effects of rhythmic activity and the thermogenic effects of exercise, these collective effects may underlie the altered state of mental and physical tension people typically experience immediately after working out.

It is also important to remember that exercise may take place either in a social context or in relative independence from others. In both cases, the exercise session may provide a diversion or time-out from daily concerns that occupy the participant's mind and cause stress (2). Intervention research in exercise settings has shown clients feel more competent when their leaders make them feel safe, welcomed, and valued (i.e., **caring**), as well as when their leaders emphasize individual effort and mastery and treat mistakes as learning opportunities (i.e., **task-involving**) (10). Caring and task-involving leader behaviors fostered greater connection between the clients and the exercise leaders (e.g., personal trainer or group exercise instructor) (10). As a result of the clients' increased connection and competence, their intrinsic motivation, commitment to continue exercising, and life satisfaction were all increased (10). Furthermore, studies have shown that youth and young adult group exercise participants perceived being less stressed, and they produced less cortisol (i.e., stress hormone) when they experience a caring, task-involving climate (38, 39). Therefore, a safe, welcoming, and respectful environment where clients get technical, informative, and positive reinforcement feedback can reduce clients' stress, thus promoting positive exercise experiences, including social connections, exercise competence, intrinsic motivation, and likelihood to continue.

Finally, accomplishing the exercise goal may promote a significant sense of mastery or self-efficacy that can also alter how a person feels after exercise. Overall, the change in psychological state from exercise is referred to as the feel-better phenomenon (58) and may result from a complex interaction of social and psychobiological factors that come together to change the overall psychological state of the exercise participant.

Anti-Depressive Effects of Exercise

As with anxiety, research evidence clearly and consistently reveals that physical exercise yields statistically significant and moderate effect sizes (i.e., reductions) both for men and women who are clinically depressed and for those experiencing less severe forms of depression, with the effects being somewhat larger for people with clinical (i.e., more severe) depression (20, 61). Although depression is commonly treated by physicians with psychiatric intervention or psychotherapy, exercise would seem to be a desirable alternative given its relative cost-effectiveness and lack of unwanted side effects. In addition, physical exercise appears to be as effective as medication in men and women experiencing clinical depression (7, 18, 28). Such efficacy of exercise to alleviate depression relative to pharmacological treatment is highly desirable in light of the negative side effects of drug treatment including cost, potential weight gain, and suicidal thoughts, as well as several other physiological effects such as muscle spasm and heart arrhythmias. In contrast, the side effects of exercise are generally, if not universally, desirable; these include reductions in body fat, cardio-vascular disease, high blood pressure, certain cancers, and arthritis, as well as reductions in dementia and Alzheimer's disease. Because many people have episodic bouts of depression over stressful events in their lives, exercise appears to offer an appropriate and effective means of coping and feeling better.

As in the case of anxiety, exercise alleviates depression through several mechanisms. Two related possibilities center on the release of biogenic amines in the brain. Central levels of **serotonin**, an important neurotransmitter with antidepressant effects, are elevated during and after physical activity (16), as are dopamine and its receptor-binding sensitivity, thus reducing the likelihood of both depression and Parkinson's disease (78). There is strong evidence that physical activity maintains **dopamine** (an essential neurotransmitter involved in motor control processes) in the central nervous system (78). In addition, research reveals that this neurotransmitter is essential to the learning of motor skills and to mental health (i.e., protection against depression) (78). Levels of norepinephrine, another neurotransmitter that is lowered during bouts of depression, are also increased with exercise (24).

Beyond the biogenic amine hypothesis, it is also likely that some people benefit from the social interaction that occurs in many exercise settings or from the sense of accomplishment or enhanced self-efficacy that stems from greater strength and flexibility in performing daily activities. This effect may be particularly important for people in older age groups, who may gain a sense of independence and experience decreased feelings of helplessness as a result of being physically fit. Such a perception, along with attendant elevations in muscular strength and endurance, may contribute to increased life satisfaction and opportunity to sustain independent living in the elderly. Research has also shown that, after controlling for depressive symptoms, adolescents' use of positive coping skills increased with their perception of the physical education class climate as task-involving (40).

Cognitive Benefits

In addition to the emotional (**affective**) benefits, exercise confers cognitive benefits. **Cognition** consists of memory, analytical thinking, planning, focus, concentration, and decision making. People who are physically fit seem to function more effectively than less physically active people on tasks involving cognitive demands (71). The outcomes are particularly impressive in men and women in older age groups (i.e., 55 and older), who typically show some degree of cognitive decline in some functions due to the aging process. In an early study demonstrating the advantageous effects of physical activity on the aging brain, the typical age-related increase in reaction time (RT) was moderated in physically active men compared with those who were less physically active (71). This effect was even more pronounced for choice (complex) RT. Sedentary men showed large age-related increases in these RTs, whereas physically active men showed little change (by way of correlation not causation). Importantly, RT has been described as a fundamental index of the overall integrity of the central nervous system (CNS) (78).

Beyond the basic index of reaction time, improved mental performance has been linked to higher levels of physical fitness. In one study, men in their 60s who were physically fit achieved better mental performance on a complex battery of cognitive challenges than did sedentary men (29). In fact, the older men who were physically fit performed similarly to a group of younger college-aged men while also outperforming the sedentary men.

GOAL SETTING

As described in the previous sections, physical activity and physical fitness confer substantial psychological and physiological benefits. However, the motivation and energy to engage in activity and exercise are critical elements in the achievement of such benefits. **Goal setting** is a powerful strategy for increasing the level of participation in exercise programs. This technique can be defined as a strategic approach to behavioral change by which progressive standards of success (i.e., goals) are set in an attempt to increasingly approximate a desired standard of achievement (i.e., the long-term goal). Importantly, systematic goal setting fosters a sense of mastery and success as people pursue the desired standard or target of achievement. Feelings of success and competency promote commitment and help maintain exercise behavior. Personal trainers can be instrumental in helping clients set goals that prove to be compelling and achievable.

Goal setting is not a one-size-fits-all endeavor. Rather than simply extracting information from an assessment and imposing goals on the client, it is important for the personal trainer to identify the client's true wants and needs and to act as a facilitator in uncovering the goals that the client is most compelled to achieve (35). Then, together, through directed conversation, the personal trainer and the client should identify goals that are measurable, achievable, and consistent with one another. In this manner, the goals or standards of successive achievement represent a series of attainable steps framed within a long-term goal that provides personal meaning to the participant.

Setting Goals for Feedback and Reinforcement

Feedback and reinforcement are critical to the success of a goal-setting program as each progressive goal is sought. For example, a client may want to change body composition by reducing the percentage of fat. The long-term goal could be to shed 60 pounds (27.2 kg) or achieve a target percentage of body fat. This could be accomplished by a series of short-term weight reduction goals to be achieved in specified time frames (19). **Feedback**, or knowledge of results, is inherent in the completion of or progress toward the short-term goal and leads to the cognitive evaluation of success or failure. Importantly, the realization of success or failure also invokes a corresponding emotional or affective state. Although the client may be far from the ultimate goal of losing 60 pounds, the positive mood, or affective state, that results from reaching the short-term goal will enhance commitment. Goals that are challenging but nearer to the present ability level of the client are superior to too-easy or very difficult goals to effecting behavior change (46).

> **Goal setting is not a one-size-fits-all endeavor. Rather than simply extracting information from an assessment and imposing goals on the client, it is important to identify the client's true wants and needs.**

The purpose of a **long-term goal** is to provide a meaningful pursuit for the client. Additionally, a personal trainer can assume that a goal selected by the client has a high level of meaning and purpose because it sets the direction of the short-term goals and provides a destination that the client values. Thus, it is prudent to conduct initial interviews with clients to assess not just their short-term needs but also their core values. Clients are much more likely to pursue and maintain purposeful and meaningful physical activity over a lifetime than they are to maintain activity without purpose or meaning (59). For example, some people perceive themselves as runners and are so deeply committed to the activity that they are likely to maintain it indefinitely barring injury or chronic health problems.

A **short-term goal** provides a strategy to achieve the long-term goal via attainable steps. Challenging short-term goals are an effective tool to elicit the effort and intensity from the client that will result in a meaningful physiological and psychological change. A challenging goal is one that has about a 50% chance of success. Thus, a well-constructed short-term goal represents a compromise between guaranteeing success, as in the case of a goal that is too easy and requiring too much effort. Short-term goals are meaningless if they are not reasonably difficult; they will lead to going through the motions as opposed to investing real effort. If clients do not achieve a short-term goal initially, they will likely continue to attempt to achieve it or maintain the behavior (e.g., caloric restriction and walking activity in the case of weight reduction) in order to obtain the desired reinforcement. If a short-term goal is not attained in the specified time period, then it needs to be adjusted or replaced with another.

The power of behavioral reinforcement can be explained on both a psychological and a neurobiological level. Psychologically, the client may experience an increase in self-esteem or self-efficacy (3). Reinforcement on a neurobiological level consists of the release of dopamine, which strengthens synaptic pathways involved in learning a behavior (3, 11). In fact, the two concepts may be inherently linked. Accordingly, feedback and the associated reinforcement are critical to effective goal setting, but feedback cannot reliably occur when short-term goals are vague. Thus, it is best to identify objective or highly quantifiable goals so that clients can target effort toward a clear standard resulting in unambiguous knowledge of results. The following sections deal with specific characteristics that enhance the effectiveness of goals.

> An effective, challenging goal is one that has about a 50% chance of success.

Types of Goals

The specifics of long-term and short-term goals vary according to the client. For example, the number of short-term goals needed to achieve the same desired long-term goal for two clients depends on their initial fitness level and training experience. Another general characteristic of goals concerns the amount of control that a client can exert over their attainment. Goals can be categorized as process, performance, and outcome goals depending on the level of personal control the client has over them. **Process goals** are goals that clients have a high degree of personal control over, whereas **outcome goals** are ones the client has little control over. **Performance goals** fall in between in relation to personal control.

Process Goals

The amount of effort applied during a workout is an example of a process goal. Other examples are exercise form and technique, positive attitude during an exercise routine, and number of days per week the client engages in physical activity outside of exercising with a personal trainer. Regardless of the difficulty of the short-term goal, clients can experience success with a high degree of effort if they set a process goal. As success or goal accomplishment defined in other ways (i.e., outcome goals) becomes increasingly difficult, process goals may be very important for maintenance of exercise behavior, since failure could result in the client dropping out.

Outcome Goals

For some clients, process goals alone may not be fulfilling; some want to compare themselves socially. For example, they may want to be the fastest walker in the neighborhood walking group or the strongest lifter at the gym. Outcome goals are exemplified by social comparison such as winning or beating an opponent in a race. Such goals can be highly arousing and can induce great intensity of effort for individuals who like to compare themselves against others. However, outcome goals present less probability of success than do process goals: Clients can guarantee the effort they give to achieve an advantage over an "opponent" but they cannot guarantee the outcome itself.

Performance Goals

Performance goals are more difficult to achieve than process goals and are typically stated in terms of a self-referenced personal performance standard for the client rather than in comparison to another client or an opponent. Performance goals are intermediate on the continuum of personal control ranging from low (outcome) to high (process). An example of personalized performance goals that challenge the client to focus on self-improvement in a personally meaningful way is based on the notion of a range or **interval goal** (62). For example, during a periodized resistance training program, a client may want to improve maximal strength in the squat or bench press exercise. Interval goals are calculated from the client's recent performance history in which a range of success is identified. The limits of the goal are established in the form of a lower (most attainable) and an upper (most challenging) boundary of success. The lower boundary is defined as the client's previous best 1-repetition maximum (1RM) performance. To determine the upper boundary, the average of recent performances (three to five) is calculated to determine the difference between the average and previous best performance. This difference yields an estimate of the client's performance variability. The difference is then added to the previous best to generate a highly challenging self-referenced level of success.

Performance goals can be calculated with the client so the client knows how the goal was determined and can develop additional process goals. Personal trainers can also calculate performance goals based on how much their client is expected to improve during the current phase of training. This can help a client hold reasonable expectations during different training phases, such as for hypertrophy compared with maximal strength or muscular endurance.

Overall, it seems appropriate to set a variety of goals or diversify the goal-setting strategy to balance the client's underlying reasons for exercise, while maintaining a reasonable probability of success and reinforcement.

Diversified Goal Setting

A successful goal-setting program should include a variety of goals just as financial success entails a diversified financial portfolio (19). In addition, such diverse goals need to be formed within the context of a sound scientific strategy for long-term goal attainment. Thus, the personal trainer needs to incorporate and integrate knowledge from the psychological, biomechanical, physiological, nutritional, and other relevant scientific domains.

As an example of a diversified goal-setting approach, think of a middle-aged client who wishes to run a 10 km (6.2 mile) race in a time he or she can feel proud of. The long-term goal should be clearly stated in the form of a desired result that will be personally meaningful. Assume this client has the talent and the ability to achieve the performance goal if he or she trains in a sound, strategic manner with optimal effort. However, a number of motivational problems are bound to occur during the training of any client who is striving

for a challenging standard of behavior. To overcome the disappointments that can occur if the client focuses on a single performance goal such as "finishing the race in less than an hour," the client should also set short-term goals using a goal diversification strategy in the context of a well-designed training program. Well-developed, shorter-term performance goals can be established for the client to attain in preparation for achieving the long-term goal of running the 10K in less than 60 minutes. One short-term performance goal sequence can focus on achieving the pace the client must be able to run every two to four weeks in order to run the necessary pace (i.e., 9:40 minutes/mile or 6 minutes/km). A second short-term performance goal can focus on increasing running distance each week until the race distance has been achieved.

The following are process goals the client may use on different training days to connect the training to the long-term race goal. On some training days, the client may set the goal of proper form during footstrike and mechanically sound arm swing and stride length. On other days, the client may stress resistance training goals to facilitate the strength and power of the lower extremities to develop hill running and sprinting speed (e.g., at the start and finish). And still, on other days, he or she may concentrate on psychological goals such as positive focus and self-talk during a training run. Positive feedback from the attainment of such process and short-term performance goals can perpetuate the sense of desire and commitment to the long-term goal. Again, the principle is that a variety of goals associated with varying levels of personal control may well sustain commitment and adherence to the physical training program.

A successful goal-setting program should include a diverse combination of short-term and long-term goals.

Goal Orientations

Consideration of individual differences in clients' perceptions of achievement situations helps increase the effectiveness of goal setting (26, 66, 68). For example, clients who gauge their performance improvement on the basis of previous ability level are said to be **task-involved** (27). On the other hand, **ego-involved** or other-referenced clients base their sense of improvement on comparison with the performance of one or more others (27, 67). Everyone holds each of these goal orientations or definitions of success to some degree (27).

It is important to understand how these goal orientations can affect a client's motivation. When clients perceive their own ability or fitness level to be high and are highly ego-involved (i.e., comparative with others), then they are highly aroused by social comparison and put forth greater effort in a situation that permits social comparison (27). Not everyone feels highly capable when it comes to exercise. Luckily, personal trainers can help promote clients' focus on task-involved goals using caring and task-involving climate behaviors (33, 57). Task-involved goals are self-referenced goals. In other words, goals that are relative to the client and the client's prior performance. Clients who are already task-involved may become discouraged if inappropriate emphasis is placed on comparisons of their achievements with those of others. Promoting self-referenced goals and recognizing (i.e., praising) when a client's goals are achieved helps emphasize goals that are achievable by the client and fosters their task involvement. To be effective in goal setting, personal trainers want to include the type of goals that fit their clients' goal orientations and perceived ability.

Tips for Effective Goal Setting

The following suggestions may help the personal trainer develop an effective goal-setting strategy. "Practical Principles of Effective Goal Setting" on page 131 summarizes the primary research-based elements of goal setting.

- Determine the client's perceived needs and desires and agree on and plan the long-term goals.

- Figure out the steps and the short-term goals that will lead to long-term achievement. If the goal is to run a marathon and the client has never run even 5 miles (8 km), the first goal might be to develop the habit of training four times per week (i.e., a process goal); the second might be to run 2 miles (3.2 km; a performance goal); and the third might be to run in a 10K (6.2 mile) race (i.e., a performance goal). The short-term goals should progress from there, ultimately leading up to the point that the client can complete a marathon.

- When starting out with a new client, clarify a preliminary goal based more on process than

on performance. For example, one could set the process goal of showing up at the gym three times per week for the first two weeks, or the process goal of eating a healthy breakfast every morning. By beginning with goals that are simple to achieve and are free of the pressure of potential impending failure, the personal trainer creates a task-involved mindset of success and helps build a client's self-efficacy. Once the client begins accumulating small successes, additional goals, including more challenging performance goals, may be added.

- Both the personal trainer and client should recognize that absence of required knowledge can hinder the achievement of long-term goals. Evaluating the client's present level of knowledge will help set a complementary knowledge-based goal, which might be to learn the names and functions of the major muscle groups or to read a series of recommended nutrition books.

- As time progresses and the client proves to be committed to the sessions and the results, it is appropriate to set more aggressive process and performance goals. Examples of such performance goals include "to bench press 200 pounds [90 kg]," "to walk 3 miles [5 km]," or "to lose 15 pounds [7 kg] of fat." These goals should be set in measurable terms and with realistic time frames so the personal trainer and client can easily discern the moment of achievement.

- Once measurable goals are clarified, attach a time frame to each goal. It is important to recognize that if a goal is not achieved by the assigned date, reevaluation and adjustment of action will move the client closer to the goal. Goals can and should be evaluated and adjusted at regular intervals, perhaps every two weeks or monthly.

- Agree on a way to recognize whether the program is working. If a goal is to reduce waist girth, some clients may want to use a tape measure, whereas others may find it psychologically more helpful to gauge progress by occasionally trying on a pair of pants they have not worn in years.

- After setting goals, always check to make certain the client believes they are attainable. If not, work on adjusting the client's belief (i.e., by educating the client) or adjusting the goal.

- Examine the goals to make sure they are compatible with one another. If goals conflict, the client's chance for success may be compromised.

PRACTICAL PRINCIPLES OF EFFECTIVE GOAL SETTING

1. Make goals specific, measurable, and observable.
2. Clearly identify time constraints.
3. Set moderately difficult goals (46).
4. Record goals and monitor progress.
5. Diversify process, performance, and outcome goals.
6. Set short-term goals to achieve long-term goals.
7. Make sure goals are internalized (clients should participate or set their own).

Adapted from Cox (19).

The acronym SMART helps capture these essential points:

Specific

Measurable

Action oriented

Realistic

Time bound

■ Goals should be prioritized. If a client comes up with a long list of goals, it is best to first isolate three, for example, that are most important and then to put those three in order of importance.

> Attach a time frame to each goal and note if a goal is not achieved by the assigned date. Goals can and should be evaluated and adjusted at regular intervals.

MOTIVATION

According to its basic definition, **motivation** is a psychological construct that arouses and directs behavior (47). A **construct** is simply an internal drive or neural process that cannot be directly observed but must be indirectly inferred from observation of outward behavior. For example, a person who rises every day at dawn and works intensely at his or her job is considered to be highly motivated. There are many other examples of constructs in psychology, such as personality, ambition, and assertiveness. Although not directly observable, they yield powerful influence on behavior.

The basic definition suggests that motivation has two dimensions: a directional aspect that influences the choices clients make about their time and commitment, and the intensity with which they pursue those choices. Such a definition helps clarify the concept of motivation but falls short of offering a strategy or clue

regarding how to change behavior. Because regular exercise involvement is a problem in our society, the following psychological principles are offered as a strategy to increase the level of participation.

Positive and Negative Reinforcement and Punishment

The use of goal setting is related to the concept of behaviorism. To clarify the philosophy of motivational practices, it is helpful to define the basic concepts used in behavioral, or operant, conditioning. Formalized by B.F. Skinner (73, 74), **behaviorism** as a view of learning holds that behavior is molded or shaped by its consequences. Accordingly, personal trainers can significantly influence exercise adherence by their reactions to a client's behaviors.

A **target behavior** (e.g., completing 45 minutes of a step aerobics class) is termed an operant, and the probability that an operant will be repeated in the future increases when the behavior is reinforced. On the other hand, the likelihood of a behavior being repeated decreases when it is punished. **Reinforcement** is any act, object, or event that increases the likelihood of future operant behavior when the reinforcement follows the target behavior; and **punishment** is any act, object, or event that decreases the likelihood of future operant behavior when the punishment follows that behavior. Understanding behaviorism can help personal trainers clarify their own leadership philosophies and understand how they relate to enhancing client motivation.

> **Reinforcement increases the likelihood that a behavior will be repeated, and punishment decreases the likelihood that a behavior will be repeated.**

The terms **positive reinforcement** and **negative reinforcement** are often confused. Both terms refer to consequences that increase the probability of occurrence of a desired behavior or operant; but positive reinforcement "gives" something to the client in response to the behavior, while negative reinforcement "takes away" something (54). In essence, something aversive is removed in order to reward behavior. An example of positive reinforcement is social approval or congratulations given to a client for completing a workout. Specifically, giving a client a high five to acknowledge his or her training effort or improvement at an exercise is a positive reinforcement. Providing positive reinforcement and technical, instructional feedback to address client mistakes promotes a task-involving climate (75). An example of negative reinforcement is relieving the client of a disliked chore, such as mopping accumulated sweat from the floor around the exercise equipment, after successful completion of a workout. Another example is a client who dislikes running on a treadmill to increase heart rate during a training session. If the client is able to maintain the target heart rate at the other circuit stations, then he or she will not have to perform the treadmill session.

Conversely, a personal trainer who focuses on the shortcomings or deficiencies of the client subscribes to a punishing style of motivation since punishment after a behavior, by definition, decreases the probability of the client engaging in that behavior again. **Positive punishment** implies presentation of something aversive such as disapproval, while **negative punishment** implies removal of something valued by the client in order to decrease the operant (unwanted behavior). Criticism of a client for poor exercise technique is an example of positive punishment. Removal of a privilege because of poor exercise technique or failure to complete an exercise goal is an example of negative punishment. Although it might seem appropriate for personal trainers to resort to reasonable forms of disapproval or punishment in the case of poor effort, this approach often results in disengagement by the client. Personal trainers modify clients' behavior more successfully by using a reinforcing style of leadership by providing instructional feedback and reinforcement of the client's progress.

Self-Determination Theory

Although new routines, new music, or a new piece of equipment can help a client continue to want to exercise, motivation runs deeper in the client's psyche. People are driven to act based on one of two possible stimuli. They either feel a compulsion to move toward a desire (pleasure) or feel a need to move away from pain. *Pain* does not mean only physical pain, although sometimes that may be an element to be considered; more commonly it means emotional pain. When a situation becomes increasingly uncomfortable, a client's motivation to move away from the discomfort will increase.

Intrinsically motivated behavior is engaged in for the sense of enjoyment derived from it, while extrinsically motivated behavior is engaged in to achieve another goal or outcome. Rephrased, **intrinsic motivation** implies a true love for the experience of exercise and a sense of fun during its performance. **Extrinsic motivation**, on the other hand, implies a desire to engage in a behavior to get an external reward. Although originally conceived as independent, intrinsic and extrinsic motivation are tied together by the concept of self-determination, or internalization (22, 23). In essence, **self-determination** implies that the individual is participating in the activity for his or her own fulfillment as opposed to trying to meet the expectations of others (which would be a type of extrinsic motivation). As such, intrinsic and extrinsic motivation represent important landmarks on a motivational continuum, or range.

> **An intrinsically motivated client truly loves to exercise, whereas an extrinsically motivated client typically exercises only to achieve an external reward.**

Clients who initially exhibit intrinsic motivation are more likely to maintain their exercise behavior than those who lack intrinsic motivation (69). Therefore, awareness of a client's location on the motivation continuum holds implications for the type of motivational approach that will enhance enjoyment of an exercise program. Major points along the self-determination continuum have been identified (82) and can be summarized (19) as follows:

1. **Amotivation**: The client has a total lack of intrinsic or extrinsic motivation.

2. **External regulation**: The client engages in behavior to avoid punishment, not for personal satisfaction. An example is a client who starts exercising to avoid judgement or lectures from his or her physician.

3. **Introjected regulation**: These clients exercise because they feel obligated to exercise. In other words, they feel bad or guilty if they do not exercise; they are not exercising because they inherently want to.

4. **Identified regulation**: The client values exercise and its benefits. These clients exercise because they view themselves as healthy and active people.

5. **Integrated regulation**: The client personally values exercise behavior, internalizes it, and freely engages in it. These clients have incorporated exercising into who they (e.g., they describe themselves as "a runner," "a weightlifter," "a regular exerciser").

6. **Internal regulation**: Many personal trainers' motivation is within this internal regulation category. Individuals with internal regulation for exercise engage because they enjoy exercising, in the moment. It is important to recognize that although personal trainers may be intrinsically motivated, their clients often are not.

Clients develop greater commitment to their exercise goals if they are intrinsically motivated because they possess the desire to be competent and committed to achieving goals in which they have a personal stake (22). Although some people may be able to maintain their exercise behavior based solely on extrinsic reinforcement, the more clients move toward being intrinsically motivated, the more likely they are to continue their exercise behavior and at least gain an enjoyment and appreciation of the benefits of exercise, even if they never truly enjoy themselves during an exercise session. Thus, clients may have different preferences regarding involvement in goal setting, and the personal trainer can determine whether their participation is appropriate. That is, some individuals prefer goals formulated by the personal trainer, while others desire to actively participate in the goal-setting process. In general, consideration of client input in the goal-setting process seems well founded.

Effect of Rewards on Intrinsic Motivation

External rewards can play a role in increasing intrinsic motivation and exercise adherence. Although the personal trainer should not count solely on the value of ongoing extrinsic rewards, the promise of a T-shirt, a dinner gift certificate, or a 30-day complimentary health club membership can facilitate early compliance and follow-through. Given this, personal trainers might logically assume they could enhance intrinsically motivated behavior by giving a client even more rewards. For example, if a client derives great satisfaction from running in 10K races, it might seem that a trophy or financial reward for each performance would result in even greater satisfaction. In actuality, external rewards or recognition can reduce intrinsic motivation (22). In a meta-analysis of over 125 studies, Deci, Koestner, and Ryan (21a) demonstrated that extrinsic motivation, in the form of tangible rewards, expected rewards, or performance-, competition-, and engagement-contingent rewards reduced an individual's intrinsic motivation whereas, simply giving positive feedback increased intrinsic motivation and interest. This meta-analysis highlights results observed in studies since the early 1970's explaining that external rewards reduce intrinsic motivation by shifting an individual's focus from an inherent enjoyment and interest in an activity to receiving external rewards. Thus, external rewards undermine intrinsic motivation for the activity, which is entirely self-referenced. Just as positive experiences (e.g., sense of success, competence, self-referenced achievement or improvement, enjoyment, positive reinforcement) promote intrinsic motivation, external rewards promote external, controlled forms of motivation.

A well-known example (72) is the story of a retired psychology professor in need of peace and quiet who was disturbed by the sound of children playing on his lawn. Instead of punishing the playful (i.e., intrinsically motivated) behavior of the children, he gave each child 50 cents and heartily thanked them for the "entertainment" they had afforded him. The children looked forward to returning the next day. At the end of their next romp on the man's lawn, he told them he was short of money but that he was able to give them 25 cents. A little disappointed, the children returned on a third day and were even more disappointed when they learned the man had no money to give. Alas, they never returned to play on the man's lawn again! What happened? Exactly what the professor had hoped! If a strong dependency is formed between behavior and reward, removal of the reward is likely to result in a lessening of the behavior. In this scenario, the reward is perceived as controlling (22). Rewards can be viewed as controlling if the recipient perceives a contingency or connection between the behavior and the reward.

When to Intervene With Motivational Efforts

To be the most effective at motivating a client, the personal trainer needs to be aware of the client's **stage of readiness** for exercise participation. The **transtheoretical model** suggests the process a client goes through as he or she "gets ready to start exercise" (6, 65):

1. **Precontemplation**: The person does not intend to increase physical activity and is not thinking about becoming physically active.

2. **Contemplation**: The person intends to increase physical activity and is giving it a thought now and then but is not yet physically active.

3. **Preparation**: The person is engaging in some activity, accumulating at least 30 minutes of moderate-intensity physical activity at least one day per week, but not on most days of the week.

4. **Action**: The person is accumulating at least 30 minutes of moderate-intensity physical activity on five or more days of the week but has done so for less than six months.

5. **Maintenance**: The person is accumulating at least 30 minutes of moderate-intensity physical activity on five or more days of the week and has been doing so for six months or more.

Having identified the client's stage of readiness, the personal trainer can apply the appropriate processes for change or interventions in order to move the client to the next level, with the ultimate goals of action and maintenance. The transtheoretical model may appear to be only common sense, but surveying prospective clients to individualize interventions may be helpful. The Stage of Exercise Scale (SES) (14) can be used to conveniently capture the stage of a prospective client. In general, research has supported the efficacy of this approach (1, 15, 17, 53).

Self-Efficacy: Building Confidence

To have a truly successful experience with a client, it is important to consider the client's motivation in conjunction with his or her confidence about achieving the desired behaviors. For example, there are people who have a poor self-concept or social physique anxiety and therefore lack the confidence to engage in an exercise program (36). In his social cognitive theory, Bandura (3) described **self-efficacy** as a person's confidence in his or her own ability to perform specific actions leading to a successful behavioral outcome. Exercise self-efficacy is a powerful predictor of exercise behavior. Self-efficacy is characterized by the degree to which the client is confident about performing the task and by the maintenance of that belief in the face of failure or obstacles. In other words, self-efficacy is related to persistence in striving for goal achievement. Four types of influences affect or build self-efficacy:

1. Performance accomplishments
2. Modeling effects
3. Verbal persuasion
4. Physiological arousal or anxiety

The successful performance of a behavior or of successive approximations of that behavior has the most powerful influence on enhancing self-efficacy for future behavior, and in that sense underscores the relationship of goal accomplishment to building confidence. For example, performing a power clean correctly can enhance a client's belief in continuing to perform proper exercise technique for this exercise and others.

Observing others perform a target behavior can also increase self-efficacy by enhancing imitative behavior. For example, some clients may be more confident of effecting a significant behavioral change such as weight loss if they see others similar to themselves in age, sex, and body type reach the same goal. Another example of modeling effects is demonstrating exercise technique for a client.

Another positive influence on self-efficacy is verbal persuasion from a respected source. A person who is respected and who is known to possess expertise in a given area (e.g., strength development or bodybuilding) can significantly influence a client's self-efficacy by offering encouragement and stating, for example, that the client "has potential." Researchers have shown that individuals who receive positive reinforcement and encouraging feedback from a certified professional have increased self-efficacy for performing that exercise (85). Simply providing clients with encouraging, reinforcing, praising, or informative feedback about their performance has been shown to increase their self-efficacy (60, 79). When individuals have higher self-efficacy, their performance increases on their next attempt of that same exercise (32, 84).

Finally, the client's own interpretation of his or her physiological state before or during exercise also exerts an influence on self-efficacy and can effectively decrease or increase confidence. For example, before performing a multiple-repetition maximum test to estimate 1RM strength in the bench press, the client may judge his or her level of arousal negatively ("I'm too nervous") or positively ("I'm ready"). Personal trainers can help their clients take a positive interpretation of this arousal (e.g., increased heart, respiratory, and sweat rate) by reminding them that this is the body's way of preparing for the maximal effort they are about to give during the bench press test.

PRACTICAL MOTIVATIONAL TECHNIQUES

1. Have the client use an exercise log or journal to document baseline measurements and the details of each workout. Teach the client to use the journal not only as a report card for exercise sessions but also for recording emotions, meals, and perspectives on progress.

2. Begin clients with exercise sessions that involve familiar activities. Lack of familiarity with an exercise or exercise mode can frustrate clients and decrease their desire to continue exercising.

3. Whenever possible, offer choices. Keep the client involved in decisions by offering choices that are equally beneficial. Rather than having the client question whether he or she should exercise at all that day, change the decision to "Would you rather do your warm-up on the elliptical climber or the exercise bike today?"

4. Provide feedback often. Look for small achievements. The personal trainer can notice and comment on increases in aerobic capacity, increases in strength, and decreases in body fat while providing exercise assistance. If, for example, the client moves up 5 pounds (2.5 kg) in a specific resistance training exercise, make it clear that progress is taking place.

5. Model the appropriate behavior for a fitness lifestyle. One of the best things a personal trainer can do for clients is to act as a role model and set an example of exercise commitment.

6. Prepare the client for periods during which adherence may be disrupted. If the client understands that even the most dedicated individuals lower the intensity of their training occasionally, those unavoidable or undesired lapses are less likely to result in program abandonment. For example, when a client is going to be traveling, discuss the client's exercise goals for the trip ahead of time and ways to achieve those goals while in unfamiliar locations. The client may want to do less or different types of exercise while on vacation or traveling, which is acceptable.

7. Use social support resources. The personal trainer can check on a client's moods, responses, and adherence by tactful telephone calls, text messaging, e-mail correspondence, and sharing educational resources or motivational information. If possible, conversations with family members regarding the desired outcome and course of action can contribute to motivation and adherence by providing a stronger support network at home. Clients can find it difficult to make changes if those they live with are unsupportive. Helping to find activities clients can do with others at home or determining how clients can explain the importance of their exercise routines to those they live with may be necessary.

8. Let the past go. If a client feels as if he or she failed to obtain the benefits of an exercise program in the past, focus instead on future goals.

9. Use a "do your best" outlook instead of a "be perfect" attitude. Clients who strive for perfection are guaranteed to hit a point of perceived failure. Teach clients to understand that giving effort and commitment is the equivalent of excellence.

10. Agree on a motivational affirmation and have the client write it down.

METHODS TO MOTIVATE A CLIENT

Sometimes a particular psychological method is helpful in motivating a client. This section offers techniques for minimizing procrastination, overcoming false beliefs, identifying and modifying self-talk, and using mental imagery.

Minimizing Procrastination

The 14th-century philosopher Jean Buridan told the story of a mule that starved to death trying to decide between two equidistant bales of hay. The bales of hay were equally desirable, so the mule could not decide which way to go. The fable presents a valuable analogy for human indecision. Health and fitness are attributes most desire, but only a disappointing margin of our population manages to commit to and maintain an exercise lifestyle. If people believe they have too many options to choose from—diets, devices, or personal trainers—the decision-making process itself often leads to stagnation. Personal trainers have to think beyond the personal training session and toward influencing clients to exercise not only today, or next week, but for the long haul. When clients procrastinate, they are weighing options, possibly left in a frozen state of indecision, instead of taking any action that will reap some benefits.

Identifying False Beliefs

Because quick fixes are so often positioned as solutions, many clients have allowed flawed and misleading information into their belief systems. If, for example, a client believes that weight loss can be achieved only by severely restricting food intake, he or she is going to block out the personal trainer's suggestions of a more appropriate and sustainable caloric intake. Further, many people have been socialized to believe that exercise is not for them or that their bodies will not respond to exercise as the bodies of others do. "No pain, no gain" is another flawed belief. This belief increases a person's tendency to overtrain, which can sabotage the potential for results.

Before attempting to instill new, empowering beliefs, the personal trainer has to first identify, and then work to change, limiting false beliefs. The first step, therefore, in opening a clear and effective line of communication between the personal trainer and client must involve a questioning process that includes

> ## QUESTIONS TO HELP IDENTIFY FALSE BELIEFS
>
> To identify false beliefs, personal trainers can ask clients questions such as the following:
>
> - What is your ideal approach to getting in shape?
> - What have you tried in the past to achieve the fitness results you want?
> - What exercise and nutrition strategies do you feel are important?
> - What do you feel you need to do to reshape your body and improve your health and fitness?

discussion of the client's present beliefs about fitness and exercise. With education, reasoning, and reinforcement, the personal trainer can then help the client understand why the false beliefs are in fact deceptive and limiting. With that understanding, the false beliefs are weakened and ultimately dismissed, allowing the client to learn new, correct information.

Identifying and Modifying Self-Talk

Each client has an "internal voice." Sometimes this is a source of motivation, but if this **self-talk** is negative, a person is less likely to accept even the most positively directed affirmations. Over time, strong and repetitive external encouragement can change a client's negative self-talk, but positive affirmations will have more effect if the client changes the negative self-talk first. The following are four simple exercises to identify and modify potentially negative self-talk:

1. Ask the client simply to notice self-talk throughout the day and realize that what he or she thinks creates mental pictures, words, and feelings.

2. Once the client has an awareness of the inner voice, direct him or her to identify it at the same point in time each day, ideally just before the scheduled personal training session, so the personal trainer can review and potentially modify the self-talk with the client. For example, if a client has a 5 p.m. personal training appointment each day, ask the client to write down his or her self-talk at 4:45 p.m. to prepare for the workout.

3. Ask the client to draw a line down the middle of a sheet of paper and on the left-hand side write down precisely his or her self-talk. The client should then write down on the right-hand side what the self-talk *could* say that would be supportive or motivating instead. After the client has done this at a given time each day, encourage him or her to identify self-talk at several pertinent times each day (such as on waking or before going to bed), along with what the self-talk could say.

4. After identifying three common self-talk phrases, the client should write three corresponding positive self-talk phrases (affirmations) and privately recite the positive phrases, at first, aloud five or six times each minute at the particular time of day the encouragement is desired to instill the habit of vocalizing the "better" words. Once the personal trainer helps the client create this habit, the client can shift to mentally "speaking" the words instead. With practice, clients' positive self-talk will motivate them toward success and achievement. Positively worded affirmations such as "I can do squats well" or "I like doing squats" are stronger than the negatively worded "I am not afraid of doing squats".

Mental Conditioning

At the 1988 Olympic Games in Seoul, track and field athletes who had qualified for the Olympic trials participated in a survey (34). The survey showed that 83% of the athletes had practiced mental conditioning exercises. Since then, the popularity of mental imagery has grown immensely. The recognized value of mental conditioning for optimal performance is not limited to athletes. Mental conditioning is valuable in music (51), in military training (25), and in rehabilitation (70)—all arenas in which consistency of effort is required for excellence.

Mental Imagery

Mental imagery, or mental rehearsal, involves using the ability of the brain to "draw" and "recall" mental images to help a client learn how to create positive emotional responses and improve motivation and exercise technique execution. The following are mental imagery exercises that can be performed in a relaxed state:

- *Witnessing a past success:* If a client has experienced an achievement or witnessed his or her own excellence, the belief that such a performance is possible becomes concrete. Since the mind and nervous system are closely linked, perception of a remembered event might have the same "belief" power as an actual achievement. For example, clients can image their prior exercise performance, such as proper execution of a back squat. They can also focus on the cues they need to remember and how it felt when performed properly.

- *Witnessing a success yet to be:* Even if a client has not yet achieved the desired goal or performance, with strong imagination skills he or she can create a mental movie of success as if it has already happened. For example, a client can imagine properly executing a box jump before the first attempt.

- *Witnessing the value:* Immediately before, during, or after a workout, the client mentally "sees" the result or valued outcome. This will greatly enhance the client's desire to achieve the outcome. Clients may want to image how their training will result in successfully completing a race, for example.

As a client's imagery becomes more powerful, the sensations the mental images bring about will become more powerful. Each time clients mentally see themselves achieving a goal, lifting the weight, transforming their bodies, or crossing the finish line, that vision will be accompanied by the feelings of winning and achievement.

Relaxation and Deep Breathing

Mental imagery should be performed in a relaxed, tension-free state. Sport psychologists use several techniques to facilitate a state of relaxation. Progressive relaxation, developed by Jacobson (42), is one technique that can be used to prepare for mental imagery. In progressive relaxation, the individual is asked to tighten each muscle group, one group at a time, and to follow each contraction with full relaxation. Another technique often used to prepare for mental imagery, as well as to relieve tension in general, is deep breathing. Deep breathing emphasizes diaphragmatic breathing (breathing with one's diaphragm) rather than shallow breathing, which uses only the upper portion of the lungs (44). Clients can use deep breathing on its own to help relieve tension by completing up to five deep breaths before starting their training program or a particular exercise. Physiological effects of deep breathing include a lower heart rate and blood pressure (9). With practice, clients can complete a deep, cleansing breath during cardiovascular exercise. This can be a good habit to develop to remind clients to continue breathing fully with their lungs rather than taking shallow, short breaths that can result in tightening chest, shoulder, or neck muscles (80).

There are multiple deep breathing techniques. A simple procedure for learning and continuing to practice deep breathing is for clients to breathe in for 4 to 5 seconds (focusing on belly or diaphragmatic inflation rather than chest expansion), hold that breath for 4 seconds, and then exhale completely over 4 to 5 seconds. Clients should continue this cycle for 1 minute to build their capacity for deep breathing, reduce muscular tension, and improve their relaxation. This technique can be done while lying down, sitting, or standing. When lifting, clients can use this deep breathing technique while completing repetitions, particularly of large muscle, multijoint exercises.

CONCLUSION

The mental health aspects of exercise come from its anxiety-reducing and antidepressive benefits, both of which have special applications to new clients and individuals who are older. One method of encouraging regular participation in exercise is for the personal trainer and client to collectively set goals that are specific, measurable, action oriented, realistic, and time bound. Further, one of the roles of a personal trainer is to motivate clients expediently toward their established goals while minimizing delays, misconceptions, and negative self-talk via methods that include education, positive self-talk, and mental imagery.

Study Questions

1. _____ anxiety is the actual experience of apprehension and uncontrolled arousal, and _____ anxiety is a personality characteristic, which represents a latent disposition to perceive situations as threatening.
   - A. Somatic; cognitive
   - B. Trait; state
   - C. Cognitive; somatic
   - D. State; trait

2. Which of the following is *incorrect* regarding *process* goals?
   - A. Positive attitude during an exercise routine is an example of a process goal.
   - B. Clients can experience success with a high degree of effort if they set a process goal.
   - C. As success or goal accomplishment defined in other ways becomes increasingly difficult, process goals may be very important for maintenance of exercise behavior.
   - D. Process goals generally have a low degree of success.

3. Which of the following is *incorrect* regarding a psychological construct?
   - A. is an internal drive
   - B. is directly observable
   - C. examples include ambition and assertiveness
   - D. is a neural process

4. Which of the following is *not* recommended as a practical motivational technique?
   - A. whenever possible, offer choices
   - B. begin with familiar activities
   - C. model the appropriate behavior for a fitness lifestyle
   - D. do not allow for adherence to be disrupted

5. Which of the following is *incorrect* regarding mental imagery?
   - A. emphasizes diaphragmatic breathing
   - B. helps to keep neck, shoulders and chest muscles engaged
   - C. can lower heart rate and blood pressure
   - D. remind clients to continue breathing fully with their lungs rather than taking shallow, short breaths

CHAPTER 9

Client Consultation and Health Appraisal

Robert Linkul, MS, and Chat Williams, MS

After completing this chapter, you will be able to

- conduct an initial client interview to assess compatibility, develop goals, and establish a client–personal trainer agreement;

- understand the process of a preparticipation health appraisal screening;

- identify positive coronary risk factors associated with cardiovascular disease;

- evaluate and classify the health status of potential clients; and

- recognize individuals requiring referral to health care professionals.

The scope of practice of the personal trainer involves the responsibility of interviewing potential clients to gather pertinent information regarding their personal health, lifestyle, and exercise readiness. The consultation process is a vital screening mechanism that is instrumental in appraising health status and developing comprehensive programs of exercise to meet the participant's individual objectives safely and effectively. This chapter covers the client consultation; preparticipation health screening; evaluation of coronary risk factors, disease, and lifestyle; interpretation of results; the referral process; and medical clearance.

PURPOSE OF CONSULTATION AND HEALTH APPRAISAL

The NSCA-Certified Personal Trainer Job (Task) Analysis Committee has defined **scope of practice** for the personal training profession by characterizing personal trainers as follows:

Personal trainers are health/fitness professionals who use an individualized approach to assess, motivate, educate, and train clients regarding their health and fitness needs. They design safe and effective exercise programs and provide the guidance to help clients achieve their personal goals. In addition, they respond appropriately in emergency situations. Recognizing their area of expertise, personal trainers refer clients to other health care professionals when appropriate (37).

The most important principle underlying the client consultation and health appraisal process is to screen participants for risk factors and symptoms of chronic cardiovascular, pulmonary, metabolic, and orthopedic diseases to optimize safety during exercise testing and participation. Thus, this chapter focuses on assessing health status and classifying risk as a basis for referral to health care professionals.

The authors would like to acknowledge the significant contributions of Tammy K. Evetovich, Kristi R. Hinnerichs, and John A.C. Kordich to this chapter.

DELIVERY PROCESS

Because the health and fitness industry is diverse, there is no specific standardized process for implementing the client consultation and health appraisal mechanism. However, typically, delivery of the process is predicated on four factors that dictate implementation:

1. Credentials of the personal trainer
2. Site of delivery
3. Specific population served
4. Legal statutes

Because of the differences in credentials, delivery sites, populations served, and legal issues, the "Steps of the Client Consultation and Health Appraisal" sidebar provides an example of the steps that may be involved in the delivery of the consultation and preparticipation health appraisal screening process.

CLIENT CONSULTATION

Even though no recognized uniform process of administration appears to exist, there is agreement about the value of an initial interview as the first step in the client consultation to obtain and share essential information associated with the program delivery process (12, 26). The **initial interview** is a scheduled appointment intended as a mutual sharing of information with the expected outcomes of assessing client–personal trainer compatibility, discussing goals, and developing a client–personal trainer agreement.

> During the initial interview, the personal trainer and client assess compatibility, develop goals, and establish a client–personal trainer agreement.

Assessing Client–Personal Trainer Compatibility

As the first step in determining personal trainer–client compatibility, the personal trainer provides a detailed description of the services available. Important information to convey to the potential client includes an explanation of the personal trainer's formal education, professional experience, certifications, and expertise or specializations, as well as the mission statement, success rate, and unique features of the program deliv-

ery system. Other important components that may affect suitability include logistical aspects regarding where and when services are available.

The personal trainer may also need to evaluate the level of exercise readiness by assessing the motivation and commitment of the individual. An attempt to predict compliance may begin with a discussion of past experiences, appreciation for exercise, availability of support, time management and organizational skills, and potential obstacles that may affect exercise adherence. Paper tests are available that are sensitive to predicting levels of exercise readiness and compliance. An attitudinal assessment form is shown starting on page 157.

The last step in determining compatibility is to assess suitability and appropriateness. It is important that the personal trainer and potential client agree to boundaries, roles, resources, and expectations and address concerns related to any of the issues or information discussed in the initial interview.

If facts are discovered during the initial interview that would establish incompatibility, it is important for the personal trainer to provide the person with an option to receive services through a referral process.

Discussion of Goals

If compatibility and suitability are established, the next step may be a discussion of goals. The main function of identifying objectives is to provide and define direction as it relates to purpose and motivation. Developing goals that are specific, measurable, action oriented, realistic, and time sensitive (SMART) is a vital element of the training process. Goal setting is discussed in chapter 8.

STEPS OF THE CLIENT CONSULTATION AND HEALTH APPRAISAL

1. Schedule interview appointment.
2. Conduct interview.
3. Implement and complete health appraisal forms.
4. Evaluate for coronary risk factors, diagnosed disease, and lifestyle.
5. Assess and interpret results.
6. Refer to an allied health professional when necessary.
7. Obtain medical clearance and program recommendations.

Establishing the Client–Personal Trainer Agreement

After the personal trainer and client have identified and clarified goals, the next step may be to finalize the client–personal trainer agreement. Entering into an agreement under the elements of contract law requires a formal process that in most cases is legally driven. Components of a contract include written documentation describing the services, parties involved, expectations of those parties, timeline of delivery, cost structure, and a payment process. Language of the contract should also cover the cancellation policy, termination of contract, and circumstances that would render the document void. An opportunity for discussion regarding the content of the contract should be provided during the consultation. The personal trainer should document and clarify questions and issues concerning the agreement before receipt of acknowledgment of acceptance. The contract becomes valid when signed by both parties, assuming appropriate legal age and competency (21). An example of a personal training contract/agreement is provided starting on page 162. Personal training professionals should consult with an attorney to make sure their contract or agreement is in accordance with their local city and state laws.

Establishing the Client– Personal Trainer Fitness Facility Agreement

After the personal trainer and the client have entered into the client–personal trainer agreement, they must then enter an agreement to validate the safe use of the facility. This form is an agreement of facility permissions, indicating what the personal trainer and client are permitted to use while inside the facility. Examples include the use of the restrooms, locker rooms, strength equipment, cardio equipment, and multipurpose spaces. Also discussed in this form is the explanation of liability between the personal trainer, the client, and the facility itself. If the personal trainer is a self-employed independent contractor, this form will explain what the facility is liable for and what it is not. This form typically indicates that the facility is not responsible for injuries, broken equipment, accidents, and so on because the independent contractor is operating as an independent business within the walls of the fitness facility, and the independent contractor is the responsible party accepting liability under his or her own insurance during the client's training session.

Personal trainers hired as employees should have a similar form provided by the facility explaining what responsibilities the facility has. This can include providing safe and well-maintained equipment; providing a clean training space; and ensuring a safe environment to exercise and work in. This form will also indicate what, if any, responsibility the facility will take in case of an accident. Typical agreements such as these ask that participants waive all liability, indicating they are choosing to participate in activities inside the facility fully understanding they have waived their liability.

In most cases, the employee-based personal trainer is covered under the facility's liability insurance and will need to abide by the rules and regulations dictated under that umbrella. This agreement requires a signature from all three parties involved: the client, the personal trainer, and the facility manager. All three parties sign under their own free will with a full understanding of the agreed-on terms to use the facility.

PREPARTICIPATION HEALTH APPRAISAL SCREENING

The purpose of the **preparticipation health appraisal** is to identify known diseases and risk factors associated with cardiovascular disease, assess lifestyle factors that may require special considerations, and identify individuals who may require medical referral before starting an exercise program.

The first step in the preparticipation health appraisal screening process is to ask the client to complete relevant forms. The personal trainer should review the completed forms before services are provided and any activity occurs. It is essential that the process be cost-effective and time efficient to avoid unnecessary barriers to exercise for individuals who do not need a medical clearance to participate (35).

Health appraisal instruments are tools by which information is collected and evaluated to assess appropriateness for various levels of exercise and referral. The two instruments that are commonly used are the PAR-Q+ and a health/medical questionnaire.

Physical Activity Readiness Questionnaire for Everyone

Abbreviated **PAR-Q+**, the **Physical Activity Readiness Questionnaire for Everyone** is a tool developed in Canada that consists of questions requiring self-recall of observations and signs and symptoms experienced by the client, in addition to confirmation of diagnosis by a physician (52). The PAR-Q+ form starts on page 163.

The advantages of the PAR-Q+ are that it is cost-effective, easy to administer, and sensitive in that it identifies individuals who require additional medical screening while not excluding those who would benefit from participation in low-intensity activity (6). The PAR-Q+ appears to have limitations in that it was designed essentially to determine the safety of exercise and not necessarily the risk for cardiovascular disease. Because of the limitations of the PAR-Q+ with respect to identifying coronary risk factors, medications, and contraindications to exercise, it is advisable for personal trainers to use an additional health appraisal instrument for more effective identification of these critical elements.

The **health/medical questionnaire** is an effective tool for assessing the appropriateness of moderate and vigorous levels of exercise in that it can identify positive coronary risk factors associated with cardiovascular disease, sudden cardiac death risk factors, existing diagnosed pathologies, orthopedic concerns, recent operations, personal history of suggested signs and symptoms, medications, supplements, and lifestyle management. A sample health/medical questionnaire starts on page 167.

Information gathered from both health appraisal tools is instrumental in identifying risk factors and determining the appropriateness of testing and exercise. Reasons for which clients must seek a physician's clearance before exercise testing or participation are discussed later in this chapter.

Additional Screening

Additional screening forms that provide an opportunity to gather and exchange valuable information include lifestyle inventories, informed consent forms, and assumption of risk agreements.

Lifestyle Questionnaires

Lifestyle questionnaires vary in their format, substance, and depth. However, they usually consist of questions to evaluate personal choices and patterns related to dietary intake, management of stress, level of physical activity, and other practices that may affect the person's health. Although the specific benefits of the questionnaire results may be unclear, there appears to be some value in qualitatively and quantitatively assessing behaviors that may have a positive or nega-

tive impact on facilitating change in an individual's health and fitness. A personal trainer may use a lifestyle questionnaire to augment previously gathered health- and fitness-related information to clarify and confirm personal issues possibly perceived as assets or obstacles to the client's success. In addition, the results of the questionnaire may provide valuable information for use in developing goals.

Most of the existing standard lifestyle questionnaire assessments were developed for the average, apparently healthy population. Persons with existing health-related conditions who have been previously diagnosed by a physician may not obtain valid and reliable information from the results of the questionnaires and therefore should rely on diagnostic information from their physicians for guidance. The health risk analysis form that begins on page 169 is an example of a lifestyle questionnaire.

Informed Consent

The **informed consent form** gives clients information about the content and process of the program delivery system. The essential elements of an informed consent include a detailed description of the program, the risks and the benefits associated with participation, a confidentiality clause, responsibilities of the participant, and documentation of acknowledgment and acceptance of the terms described within the form. It has been commonly accepted that the information on this form should be conveyed both verbally and in writing to the client before any testing or participation to ensure that the participant knows and understands the risks and circumstances associated with the program. See chapter 25 for a discussion of legal issues regarding informed consent. An example of an informed consent form begins on page 676.

Assumption of Risk or Waiver

An **assumption of risk** or **waiver** is an agreement by a client, before beginning participation, to give up, relinquish, or waive the participant's rights to legal remedy (damages) in the event of injury, even when such injury arises because of provider negligence (3). The legal implications associated with the implementation and execution of the assumption of risk agreement appear to be unclear at best because of the various legal interpretations associated with waiver documents (see chapter 25). An assumption of risk agreement needs to identify the potential risks associated with participation and establish that the potential client understands those risks and voluntarily chooses to assume the responsibility. A signed assumption of risk agreement may limit liability. If a personal trainer needs to prove in court that a participant was aware of how to avoid risks and assumed the risk of an activity, this type of document may prove helpful. However, acknowledgment of the content and authorization of this form does not relieve the personal trainer of the duty to perform in a competent and professional manner. An example of an assumption of risk agreement appears on page 169.

Preparticipation Documents for Children

As the number of overweight and obese children continues to grow, parents are employing personal trainers to help their children lose weight, increase their fitness level, and increase their self-esteem. In addition, some parents are enlisting the help of personal trainers to improve their child's sport performance. Unfortunately, little has been written about the medical and legal considerations for the participation of children in a training program. Parents or legal guardians should fill out a health history questionnaire for their child before he or she begins participation. A preparticipation physical evaluation form has been approved by the American Academy of Pediatrics and the American Academy of Family Physicians as well as other organizations (41). This form may be helpful in determining whether a child should visit and get the permission of a physician before participation in a physical activity program. It is not so clear, however, whether waivers, parental consent forms, or assumption of risk documents for this age group are helpful and thus should be administered. Regarding assumption of risk or waiver agreements, parents do not have the right to execute such waivers on behalf of their children (20). Thus, it is difficult to free the personal trainer from liability in the event of an injury or claim. In fact, according to laws in many states, "children of particular ages (generally 7-14 years) are incapable of self-negligence" (20, p. 77). Thus, a child's self-negligence is not sufficient to bar or limit any award of damages.

Given these concerns, it goes without saying that personal trainers of children need to be knowledgeable about safe and effective training methods and be aware of the unique psychological and physiological characteristics of younger populations. Although personal training for children involves unique legal and medical considerations, the benefits of physical activity in this age group are vast (14). If personal trainers follow established training guidelines and safety procedures, they can decrease the risk of injury and protect themselves from liability.

Record Keeping

The personal trainer needs to develop a strategy to collect, organize, and store the vital information and materials obtained through the initial interview process. A record-keeping system to verify the completion and receipt of forms, along with other documentation concerning the status of the client, is instrumental in allowing one to move on to the next step of the preparticipation health appraisal screening process. The personal trainer needs to follow **HIPAA (Health Insurance Portability and Accountability Act) protocols** with sensitive client material pertaining to personal and private health information. Health care providers, insurance companies, and health care clearinghouses are required by law to follow a national set of standards. The national set of security standards were established to protect hard copies and electronically transferred copies of personal information. Following these standards ensures the confidentially and integrity of the client–personal trainer relationship.

> The scope of practice of the personal trainer involves the responsibility to interview potential clients to gather and assess pertinent information about their personal health, medical conditions, and lifestyle to meet their individual health and fitness objectives safely and effectively.

EVALUATION OF CORONARY RISK FACTORS, DISEASE, AND LIFESTYLE

Once the appropriate forms are completed and the documentation is reviewed, it is necessary to evaluate the content of the information to identify any potential risks associated with the client's current health status so he or she can be referred to a physician, as necessary. The key areas to evaluate include risk factors associated with cardiovascular disease (CVD), medical conditions and diagnosed disease, and current lifestyle.

Cardiovascular Disease Risk Factors

Cardiovascular disease (CVD) is the leading cause of mortality in Western society (51). **Atherosclerosis** is a progressive degenerative process associated with CVD through which the endothelial lining of the arterial walls becomes hardened and the walls consequently lose elasticity. Over time, deposition of fat and plaque buildup occur, and the artery wall narrows, which in turn occludes blood flow through the vascular system to the heart, causing heart tissue to die or leading to a **myocardial infarction** (heart attack).

Identifiable positive risk factors are associated with the potential to acquire CVD. A **positive risk factor** may be defined as "an attribute or exposure that is associated with an increased probability of a specified outcome, such as the occurrence of a disease" (27, p. 218). It is necessary to evaluate positive risk factors associated with CVD to identify individuals who may be at higher risk during exercise.

Positive Coronary Risk Factors

Epidemiological research suggests that a person's potential risk for developing CVD is associated with the positive coronary risk factors the person possesses. The greater the number and severity of those risk factors, the greater probability of CVD (51). The eight identifiable positive CVD risk factors relate to age, family history, cigarette smoking, physical inactivity, body mass index and waist circumference, blood pressure (i.e., hypertension), blood lipid levels, and blood glucose levels (table 9.1; 4).

Age The probability of developing CVD increases with age. Although CVD is the leading cause of death in both men and women in the United States, males are more likely to develop CVD at younger ages; as a result, the prevalence of CVD is greater in males (51). Reaching the threshold of 45 years for men and 55 years for women is a positive risk factor for CVD (4).

TABLE 9.1 Cardiovascular Disease (CVD) Risk Factors and Defining Criteria

Positive risk factors[a]	Defining criteria
Age	Men ≥45 years; women ≥55 years (17)
Family history	Myocardial infarction, coronary revascularization, or sudden death before 55 years of age in biological father or other male first-degree relative, or before 65 years of age in biological mother or other female first-degree relative (35a)
Cigarette smoking	Current cigarette smoker or someone who quit within the previous 6 months, or exposure to environmental tobacco smoke (35a, 50)
Physical inactivity	Not meeting the minimum threshold of 500-1,000 MET–min of moderate-to-vigorous physical activity or 75-150 min/week of moderate-to-vigorous intensity physical activity (39, 49)
Body mass index/waist circumference	Body mass index of ≥30 kg/m² or waist girth of >102 cm (40 in.) for men and >88 cm (35 in.) for women (23)
Blood pressure	Systolic blood pressure ≥130 mmHg and/or diastolic ≥80 mmHg, based on an average of ≥2 readings obtained on ≥2 occasions, *or* on antihypertensive medication (5a)
Blood lipid levels	Low-density lipoprotein cholesterol (LDL-C) ≥130 mg/dl (3.37 mmol/L) *or* high-density lipoprotein cholesterol (HDL-C) of <40 mg/dL (1.04 mmol/L) in men and <50 mg/dL in women, or non-HDL-C[b] ≥160 (4.14 mmol/L) or on lipid-lowering medication. If total serum cholesterol is all that is available, use ≥200 mg/dl (5.18 mmol/L) (22a)
Blood glucose levels	Fasting plasma glucose ≥100 mg/dl (5.5 mmol/L) or 2 h plasma glucose values in oral glucose tolerance test ≥140 mg/dl (7.77 mmol/L) or HbA1C ≥5.7% (5)
Negative risk factors	**Defining criteria**
HDL-C[c]	≥60 mg/dl (1.55 mmol/L) (22a)

[a]If the presence or absence of a CVD risk factor is not disclosed or is not available, that CVD risk factors should be counted as a risk factor.
[b]Equal to total cholesterol minus HDL-C.
[c]If high-density lipoprotein (HDL-C) cholesterol is high, one positive risk factor is subtracted from the sum of positive risk factors.

Reprinted by permission from American College of Sports Medicine (2022, p. 47).

Family History Cardiovascular disease appears to have a predisposing genetic connection and a tendency to be familial. Although it is difficult to ascertain whether a genetic code or an environmental influence is involved, it may be safe to speculate that people with a documented family history are more susceptible to CVD (24). Thus, people with a family history possess a risk factor if a myocardial infarction, coronary revascularization, or sudden death occurred before 55 years of age in their biological father or another male **first-degree relative** (sibling or child), or before 65 years of age in their biological mother or other female first-degree relatives (4, 35a).

Cigarette Smoking Overwhelming empirical evidence identifies cigarette smoking as a major positive risk factor for CVD (4, 18, 50). A linear relationship also appears to exist between the risk for cardiovascular disease and the volume of cigarette smoking and number of years a person smoked (28). The chemical makeup of cigarettes accentuates risk by elevating myocardial oxygen demand and reducing oxygen transport, causing the cardiovascular system to work harder to obtain a sufficient oxygen supply (9). In addition, cigarette smoking lowers high-density lipoprotein (HDL) cholesterol, which accelerates the atherosclerotic process (9). Persons who currently smoke cigarettes, and those who previously smoked but who have quit within the last six months, or those individuals exposed to environmental tobacco smoke have a greater potential risk for CVD and have this risk factor (4, 35a, 50).

Physical Inactivity Physical inactivity is recognized as a leading contributing factor to morbidity and mortality. In contrast, physical activity has beneficial effects on other CVD risk factors (e.g., by decreasing resting systolic and diastolic blood pressures, reducing triglyceride levels, increasing serum HDL-cholesterol levels, and enhancing glucose tolerance and insulin sensitivity) (4, 15). For health benefits, adults should perform at least 150 minutes a week of moderate-intensity or 75 minutes of vigorous-intensity physical activity (4, 49).

Physical inactivity and sedentary lifestyle are not the same and the terms should not be used interchangeably. Physical inactivity specifically refers to low levels of moderate-to-vigorous physical activity. Sedentary behavior refers to a lifestyle of a very low intensity activity level (sitting or reclining). It is possible to be physically inactive but not sedentary, or both sedentary and physically active (e.g., work a desk job for 10 hours a day but still meeting the physical activity guidelines by performing 30 minutes of exercise each weekday).

Body Mass Index and Waist Circumference Obesity is the accumulation and storage of excess body fat. The prevalence of obesity in the United States has reached epidemic proportions. An analysis of the relationship between obesity and CVD is confounded because of the connection between obesity and other risk factors such as physical inactivity, hypertension, hypercholesterolemia, and diabetes. However, evidence has suggested that obesity in and of itself may be considered an independent risk factor for CVD (22). In addition to the risk associated with accumulation of excess body fat, there may be an increased risk related to the location and deposition of stored visceral fat. Individuals who store or accumulate excess body fat in the central waist or abdominal area appear to be at greater risk for CVD (13). The assessments and values associated with obesity as a positive risk factor include a body mass index (BMI) equal to or greater than 30 kg body weight per height in meters squared (i.e., 30 kg/m^2) or a waist girth >40 inches (102 cm) for men and >35 inches (88 cm) for women (4, 23). Refer to chapter 11 for instructions on how to calculate BMI and measure waist girth.

Blood Pressure **Hypertension** is chronic, persistent sustained elevation of blood pressures (see table 11.2 on page 244). Most individuals who are clinically diagnosed have essential hypertension, which cannot be attributed to any specific cause. Secondary hypertension refers to elevated blood pressures caused by specific factors such as kidney disease and obesity (54).

Regardless of the etiology, hypertension is believed to predispose individuals to CVD through the direct vascular injury caused by high blood pressure and its adverse effects on the myocardium. These include increased wall stress, which dramatically increases the workload of the heart in pumping blood required to overcome peripheral vascular resistance (11). In general, the higher the blood pressure, the greater the risk for CVD.

Blood Lipid Levels **Cholesterol** is a fatlike substance found in the tissues of the body that performs specific metabolic functions in the human organism. Cholesterol is carried in the bloodstream by molecular proteins known as **high-density lipoproteins (HDLs)** and **low-density lipoproteins (LDLs)**. Evidence suggests that the LDL molecules release cholesterol, which penetrates the endothelial lining of the arterial wall and in turn contributes to the atherosclerotic plaque buildup that eventually leads to vascular occlusion and heart attacks, strokes, and peripheral artery disease (13). HDLs act as a protective mechanism by transporting cholesterol through the bloodstream to the liver, where it is metabolized and eliminated.

According to a report by the National Cholesterol Education Program, epidemiological research has identified a strong relationship between high levels of total cholesterol, high LDL-cholesterol, and low HDL-cholesterol and a higher rate of CVD in both men and women (13). Individuals who have low-density lipoprotein cholesterol (LDL-C) ≥130 mg/dl (3.37 mmol/L) or non-high-density lipoprotein cholesterol (HDL-C) ≥160 (4.14 mmoL/L), *or* men with HDL-C of <40 mg/dL (1.04 mmol/L) or women with HDL-C <50 mg/dL (1.04 mmoL/L), or individuals who are on lipid-lowering medication have a greater risk for CVD (4, 22a). If total serum cholesterol is all that is available, the marker is ≥200 mg/dl (5.18 mmol/L) (4, 22a). It is important to note that the LDL may be more predictive of CVD risk than total cholesterol levels. In any event, people who have these values have a positive risk factor for CVD.

Blood Glucose Levels Fasting blood glucose levels are markers used to assess the body's metabolic function. Elevated levels of circulating glucose in the bloodstream—that is, fasting plasma glucose levels of ≥100 mg/dl (5.5 mmol/L), plasma glucose values from an oral glucose tolerance test of ≥140 mg/dl (7.77 mmol/L), or an HbA1C of ≥5.7% (4, 5)—cause a chemical imbalance that impedes the use of lipids. Individuals with this metabolic imbalance are more susceptible to atherosclerosis and have an increased risk for CVD (5).

Negative CVD Risk Factors

A **negative CVD risk factor** suggests a favorable influence that may contribute to the development of a protective cardiovascular benefit (38). High-density lipoproteins appear to provide a protective mechanism against CVD by removing cholesterol from the body and preventing plaque from forming in the arteries. Research suggests that increases in HDLs are consistent with decreased risk for CVD (22a, 36). Thus, individuals who have a serum HDL-cholesterol of ≥60 mg/dl can subtract one risk factor from the sum of positive risk factors shown in table 9.1, thereby decreasing the risk of CVD (4, 22a).

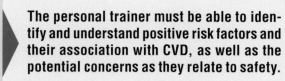

The personal trainer must be able to identify and understand positive risk factors and their association with CVD, as well as the potential concerns as they relate to safety.

Identification of Medical Conditions and Diagnosed Disease

Identifying and understanding positive risk factors and their association with CVD, as well as the potential concerns that exist when these risk factors are present, is an important responsibility of the personal trainer in the screening process. However, more critical is the ability to identify signs and symptoms of various chronic cardiovascular, pulmonary, metabolic, and orthopedic diseases that may contraindicate exercise and could potentially exacerbate an existing condition, thus leading to an adverse impact on the individual's health. Individuals who have evidence of a known disease, have symptoms of CVD, or are presently on medications to control CVD require special attention because of the increased risk.

Cardiovascular and Pulmonary Disease

Personal history plays a fundamental role in the process of early detection of CVD. Signs and symptoms suggestive of CVD are important guides in identifying individuals who are at higher risk for the future development of disease. People who exhibit signs and symptoms of CVD present special safety concerns as to the appropriateness of participating in an exercise program. The health appraisal screening mechanisms mentioned earlier are intended to initially identify signs and symptoms that have been previously diagnosed or personally detected. However, the personal trainer needs to use enhanced observation throughout the client consultation and health appraisal process to identify and assess signs and symptoms suggestive of cardiovascular and pulmonary disease that the client may exhibit. The major signs or symptoms suggestive of cardiovascular and pulmonary disease are as follows:

- Pain or discomfort (or other anginal equivalent) in the chest, neck, jaw, arms, or other areas that may be due to **ischemia** (lack of blood flow)
- Shortness of breath at rest or with mild exertion

- Dizziness or **syncope** (fainting)
- **Orthopnea** (the need to sit up to breathe comfortably) or **paroxysmal** (sudden, unexpected attack) **nocturnal dyspnea** (shortness of breath at night)
- Ankle **edema** (swelling, water retention)
- Palpitations or **tachycardia** (rapid heart rate)
- Intermittent **claudication** (cramp-like pain during exercise that disappears after exercise cessation)
- Known heart murmur
- Unusual fatigue or shortness of breath with usual activities

Adapted from American College of Sports Medicine (4).

It is important for personal trainers to understand that these signs and symptoms must be interpreted in a clinical setting for diagnostic purposes and that they are not all specific to cardiovascular, pulmonary, and metabolic disease (7). However, if an individual exhibits these signs or symptoms, it is the role and responsibility of the personal trainer to take appropriate action by referring the client to a physician for a medical examination.

Various pulmonary diseases affect the respiratory system's ability to transport oxygen during exercise to the tissue level via the cardiovascular system. The systematic breakdown that occurs because of inadequate oxygen supply creates a greater than normal demand on the cardiorespiratory system, in some cases markedly reducing exercise tolerance. Chronic bronchitis, emphysema, and asthma are syndromes associated with chronic obstructive pulmonary disease (COPD) and are the most commonly diagnosed diseases related to respiratory dysfunction. **Chronic bronchitis** is an inflammatory condition caused by persistent production of **sputum** (a mixture of coughed up saliva and mucus) owing to a thickened bronchial wall, which in turn creates a reduction of airflow. **Emphysema** is a disease of the lung that affects the small airways. An enlargement of air spaces accompanied by the progressive destruction of alveolar-capillary units leads to elevated pulmonary vascular resistance, which in most cases can contribute to heart failure. **Asthma** is mostly due to a spasmodic contraction of smooth muscle around the bronchi that produces swelling of the mucosal cells lining the bronchi and an excessive secretion of mucus. Constriction of airway paths associated with asthma results in attacks that may be caused by allergic reactions, exercise, air quality factors, and stress (8). (Chapter 20 provides detailed information.)

Risk of Sudden Cardiac Death

Sudden cardiac death related to exercise is caused by cardiac arrest that occurs instantaneously with an abrupt change in an individual's preexisting clinical state or within a few minutes of that change. Exercise does not typically provoke cardiovascular events in healthy individuals with normal cardiovascular systems (16). In fact, regular physical activity is strongly advocated by the medical community, in part because substantial epidemiological, clinical, and basic scientific evidence suggests that physical activity and exercise training delay the development of atherosclerosis and reduce the incidence of coronary heart disease events (16). However, vigorous physical activity can acutely and transiently increase the risk of acute myocardial infarction and sudden cardiac death in susceptible individuals (16).

Both younger (<35 years) and older populations are at risk of sudden cardiac death. However, the underlying causes vary. Among young individuals, the most frequent cardiovascular abnormalities leading to sudden cardiac death include hypertrophic cardiomyopathy, coronary artery anomalies, aortic stenosis, aortic dissection and rupture (typically related to Marfan syndrome), mitral valve prolapse, various heart arrhythmias, and myocarditis. In all these conditions except Marfan syndrome, where aortic rupture is often the cause, ventricular arrhythmias are the immediate cause of death (16). Older, previously asymptomatic individuals who experience sudden cardiac death often show evidence of acute coronary artery plaque disruption with acute thrombotic occlusion (16).

A thorough history as part of the health/medical questionnaire (page 167) can help the personal trainer identify potential risks for sudden cardiac death. Identification of one or more of the following conditions should warrant a referral for a cardiovascular examination.

- Chest pain or discomfort with physical exertion
- Excessive exertional dyspnea
- Syncope
- Family history of sudden and unexpected death before age 50 in more than one relative
- Family history of disability from heart disease before age 50 in a close relative

Adapted from Maron et al. (32).

Sudden cardiac death from genetic or congenital heart diseases is more common in young people not engaged in competitive sports programs than it is in competitive athletes (31, 33). A health/medical questionnaire that includes family history questions may be used to screen both competitive athletes and the general population for CVD (32).

Signs and symptoms must be interpreted in a clinical setting for diagnostic purposes, and they are not all specific to sudden cardiac death. However, if an individual identifies one or more of these risk factors, it is the role and responsibility of the personal trainer to take appropriate action through the referral process by recommending a medical examination by a physician before initiating any type of activity (16).

Personal trainers must keep in mind that the causes of exercise-related sudden cardiac death events are not strictly separated by age. Younger individuals may exhibit signs of early onset of cardiovascular disease, while older individuals may present with structural congenital cardiac abnormalities (16). It is important to understand the potential risk factor or factors for each individual. For those with or at risk for coronary heart disease, the benefits of regular physical activity outweigh the risks of sudden cardiac death. However, for individuals with diagnosed or difficult-to-detect cardiac diseases, the health risks of vigorous physical activity almost always exceed the benefits (16).

Sudden cardiac death in any population is an uncommon yet catastrophic event. Just one death is still one too many if it could have been prevented. An absolute rate of exercise-related death among younger competitive athletes has been estimated to be 1 per 185,000 in men and 1 per 1,500,000 in women (30). These estimates include all sport-related nontraumatic deaths and are not restricted to cardiovascular events. The rate of sudden cardiac death occurs every 1.5 million episodes of vigorous physical activity in men (1) and every 36.5 million hours of moderate to vigorous physical activity in women (53). Sudden cardiac death, especially in the younger population, has stirred quite a controversy regarding preparticipation screening guidelines (40). It is important for the personal trainer to include sudden cardiac death risk factors in the health/medical questionnaire to identify individuals who may be at risk for sudden cardiac death. It is also important to advance all clients according to individual readiness. Sudden cardiac death at all ages is more prevalent in those who perform activity that they are not accustomed to (16).

Metabolic Disease

As mentioned earlier, an impaired fasting glucose level has been identified as a positive risk factor for CVD and a potential predictor for the development of diabetes. **Diabetes mellitus**, a metabolic disease, affects the body's ability to metabolize blood glucose properly. The disease is characterized by hyperglycemia resulting from defects in insulin secretion (type 1), insulin action (type 2), or both. Persons with **type 1 diabetes** are insulin dependent, meaning they require insulin injections to metabolize glucose. Persons with **type 2 diabetes** in most cases can produce insulin, but the tissue is insensitive to it, and consequently glycemic control is inadequate. Diabetes is known to be an independent contributing factor in the development of CVD, increasing the potential for developing CVD, peripheral vascular disease, and congestive heart failure (19). Although physical activity and exercise along with dietary modifications and prescribed medications appear to have an impact on the regulation of glucose levels, diabetes still requires ongoing medical attention and warrants precautions (5). Chapter 19 provides information on working with clients who have diabetes.

Orthopedic Conditions and Disease

Even though orthopedic limitations and disease do not appear to present the same relative risk as those associated with cardiovascular function, musculoskeletal concerns are an important factor for the personal trainer to consider in assessing an individual's functional capacity and may require a physician's referral before initiation of a program. Common musculoskeletal concerns related to acute trauma, overuse, osteoarthritis, and lower back pain present issues and challenges that may need to be assessed on a case-by-case basis. Although these conditions may limit performance and are important to the personal trainer, dealing with individuals who have rheumatoid arthritis, who have had recent surgery, or who have diagnosed degenerative bone disease may involve greater concerns because of the potential implications regarding advanced complications. Issues related to orthopedic replacements, recent surgical procedures, osteoporosis, and rheumatoid arthritis may require communication with a physician and in most cases medical clearance.

Medications

Individuals being treated by a physician on an ongoing basis may be taking prescribed medications as a therapeutic measure to manage a diagnosed condition or disease. The chemical reactions that occur in the body may influence physiological responses during activity. Various medications may alter heart rate, blood pressures, cardiac function, and exercise capacity. It is important for the personal trainer to understand the classes of commonly used drugs and their effects. For example, medications commonly prescribed for persons with high blood pressure (e.g., β-blockers) may affect normal increases in heart rates during exercise; as a result, people will have difficulty obtaining, and should not strive to achieve, training heart rates. In addition, monitoring intensity of exercise by using heart rates may be inappropriate because of the masking effect of the medications on heart rates, and therefore rating of perceived exertion would be a more effective mechanism for regulating intensity levels of exercise (42).

Lifestyle Evaluation

Identifying an individual's behavioral patterns concerning choices about dietary intake, physical activity, and stress management provides additional information for assessing potential health risks associated with current lifestyle. Evidence clearly suggests a strong relationship between lifestyle choices regarding dietary intake, physical activity, and the management of stress on the one hand and the potential risk of CVD and other leading causes of morbidity and premature mortality on the other (55).

Dietary Intake and Eating Habits

Because of the significant contributory impact of nutritional habits on health and performance, the personal trainer should consider encouraging clients to evaluate their current dietary intake. Identifying, quantifying, and assessing a person's daily dietary intake gives the personal trainer valuable information for assessing overconsumption, underconsumption, and caloric imbalances that may be contributing factors in the development of disease. There is a solid link between dietary intake and disease. The most evident connection is between dietary saturated fat and cholesterol and the development of atherosclerosis (44), although this relationship remains a topic of controversy (29). Alcohol consumption has also been associated with an increased risk for atrial fibrillation (25), and diets high in sodium can lead to chronic elevation of systolic blood pressure or, more importantly, can result in worsening of heart failure (11). Overconsumption of calories may contribute to obesity and diabetes; and underconsumption may lead to muscle loss, degenerative bone diseases, and psychological health issues related to disordered eating.

An analysis of a typical dietary intake through documentation of a three-day or seven-day dietary record may be a starting point for assessing the health-related value of the individual's eating habits. A dietary recall or diet history, as discussed in chapter 7, may also be used. The information obtained through these methods is part of a collective process for identifying potential concerns in relation to disease risk. See chapter 7 for detailed guidance about seeking information on and evaluating clients' nutrition habits. In addition, strategies have been developed for recognizing and referring individuals who exhibit signs and symptoms related to disordered eating (see chapter 19).

Exercise and Activity Pattern

Identifying patterns of physical activity and exercise helps the personal trainer to recognize individuals with little or no history of physical activity or exercise. As discussed earlier, physical inactivity is a major contributing positive risk factor associated with the development of CVD and requires evaluation to assess potential concerns and level of risk. An evaluation of physical activity and exercise patterns should include identifying the specific activity and the frequency, volume, and level of intensity (moderate or vigorous) of that activity, as well as documenting signs or symptoms associated with the activity, particularly shortness of breath or chest pains. Any musculoskeletal concerns related to joint discomfort or chronic pain should also be identified.

Stress Management

Epidemiological studies provide evidence that stress is related to the risk for CVD (10, 46, 48). In addition, type A behavior patterns may contribute to the overall risk for developing CVD (34). Type A behavior pattern characteristics include hostility, depression, social isolation, and chronic stress produced by situations involving high demand and low control (2, 43). These lifestyle stress–related characteristics can be measured psychosocially and physiologically through emotional stress inventories and standard exercise testing (47). Because of the implications of stress and its impact on developing CVD, it is important for the personal trainer to be able to identify the common signs and symptoms of stress overload and to develop intervention strategies to reduce health risks. The health risk analysis form on page 169 can be used to assess a client's potential for stress and response to stressors. This inventory is to be completed during the preparticipation health screening.

> Once the preparticipation health appraisal screening is complete, the personal trainer should evaluate the client's positive risk factors associated with CVD, medical conditions and diagnosed disease, and current lifestyle.

INTERPRETATION OF RESULTS

After the preparticipation health appraisal screening process has taken place and a review and evaluation of coronary risk factors, disease, and lifestyle are complete, the next step in the screening process is to identify individuals who may be at increased risk and to classify that risk. Classifying risk for potential health-related concerns is a preliminary step in determining the appropriateness of activity and identifying clients who require referral before beginning an exercise program. To meaningfully interpret the results obtained through the screening process, the personal trainer should use the PAR-Q+ results to identify people who have a greater potential for risk and may require referral and a clearance from a physician.

PAR-Q+

As mentioned earlier, the PAR-Q+ is easy to administer and is a cost-effective mechanism for initially screening individuals who are apparently healthy and want to engage in regular low-intensity exercise. The PAR-Q+ is useful for referring individuals who require additional medical screening while not excluding those who may benefit from exercise. After eliciting objective *yes* or *no* answers to seven questions related to signs and symptoms associated with CVD, orthopedic concerns, and diagnosis by a physician, the self-administered questionnaire form provides direction based on interpretation of the results and specifies recommendations as to the appropriateness of activity and the referral process. Specific recommendations related to this form are discussed later in this chapter in the "Referral Process" section.

American College of Sports Medicine Preparticipation Screening Algorithm

The **ACSM preparticipation screening algorithm** determines a person's preparedness to begin an exercise program using current exercise status, known cardio-vascular, metabolic, or renal disease, and personal signs and symptoms (4). Figure 9.1 is divided into two subsets: individuals who do not participate in regular exercise and individuals who do. Participants are grouped into one of the following six categories:

1. Apparently healthy participants who do not currently exercise and have no history, signs, or symptoms of cardiovascular, metabolic, or renal disease

2. Participants who do not exercise and have a known cardiovascular, metabolic, or renal disease and are asymptomatic

3. Individuals with any signs or symptoms suggestive of disease regardless of disease status who do not currently exercise

4. Apparently healthy participants who currently exercise and have no history, signs, or symptoms of cardiovascular, metabolic, or renal disease

5. Individuals who currently exercise and have a known history of cardiovascular, metabolic, or renal disease but have no current signs or symptoms

6. Individuals who currently exercise and experience signs or symptoms suggestive of cardiovascular, metabolic, or renal disease

Personal trainers should monitor their clients for changes while they are participating in a fitness program and make appropriate recommendations within the categories of the screening algorithm.

Case study 9.1 (page 155) illustrates how the personal trainer might categorize an individual using the ACSM preparticipation screening algorithm. The personal trainer might obtain the relevant information during the preparticipation health appraisal screening interview.

REFERRAL PROCESS

The processes described so far (i.e., preparticipation health appraisal screening; evaluation of coronary risk factors, disease, and lifestyle; and interpretation of the information obtained through the initial interview and client consultation process) are intended to help identify individuals who will need a referral to a health care professional for medical clearance before participating in activity. The following referral processes may be implemented to assess readiness and appropriateness for exercise.

Medical Examinations

Regular medical examinations to evaluate health status are normally encouraged for preventive purposes for

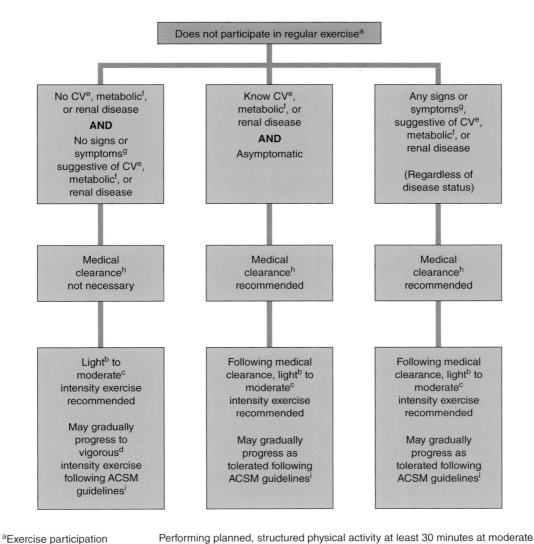

Does not participate in regular exercise[a]

No CV[e], metabolic[f], or renal disease **AND** No signs or symptoms[g] suggestive of CV[e], metabolic[f], or renal disease	Know CV[e], metabolic[f], or renal disease **AND** Asymptomatic	Any signs or symptoms[g], suggestive of CV[e], metabolic[f], or renal disease (Regardless of disease status)
Medical clearance[h] not necessary	Medical clearance[h] recommended	Medical clearance[h] recommended
Light[b] to moderate[c] intensity exercise recommended May gradually progress to vigorous[d] intensity exercise following ACSM guidelines[i]	Following medical clearance, light[b] to moderate[c] intensity exercise recommended May gradually progress as tolerated following ACSM guidelines[i]	Following medical clearance, light[b] to moderate[c] intensity exercise recommended May gradually progress as tolerated following ACSM guidelines[i]

[a]Exercise participation — Performing planned, structured physical activity at least 30 minutes at moderate intensity on at least 3 days · week[-1] for at least the last 3 months

[b]Light intensity exercise — 30%–39% HRR or $\dot{V}O_2R$, 2–2.9 METs, RPE 9–11, an intensity that causes slight increases in HR and breathing

[c]Moderate intensity exercise — 40%–59% HRR or $\dot{V}O_2R$, 3–5.9 METs, RPE 12–13, an intensity that causes noticeable increases in HR and breathing

[d]Vigorous intensity exercise — ≥60% HRR or $\dot{V}O_2R$, ≥6 METs, RPE ≥14, an intensity that causes substantial increases in HR and breathing

[e]Cardiovascular (CV) disease — Cardiac, peripheral vascular, or cerebrovascular disease

[f]Metabolic disease — Type 1 and 2 diabetes mellitus

[g]Signs and symptoms — At rest or during activity. Includes pain, discomfort in the chest, neck, jaw, arms, or other areas that may result from ischemia; shortness of breath at rest or with mild exertion; dizziness or syncope; orthopnea or paroxysmal nocturnal dyspnea; ankle edema, palpitations or tachycardia; intermittent claudication; known heart murmur; unusual fatigue or shortness of breath with usual activities.

[h]Medical clearance — Approval from a health care professional to engage in exercise

[i]ACSM guidelines — See the most current edition of *ACSM's Guidelines for Exercise Testing and Prescription*

(continued)

FIGURE 9.1   ACSM's Preparticipation Screening Algorithm.

ACSM, American College of Sports Medicine; HR, heart rate; HRR, heart rate reserve; METs, metabolic equivalents; RPE, rating of perceived exertion; $\dot{V}O_2R$, oxygen uptake reserve.

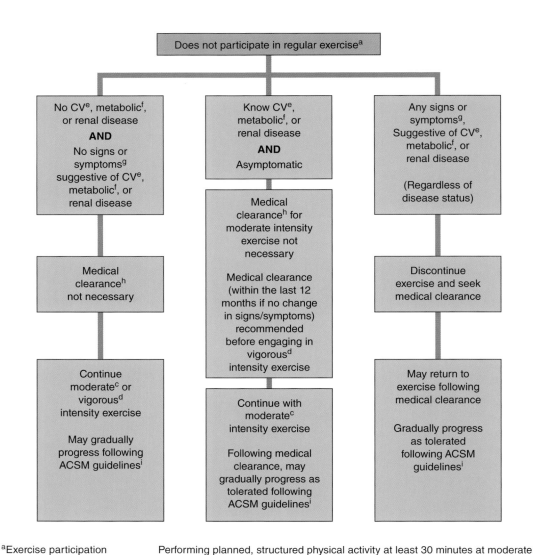

[a]Exercise participation	Performing planned, structured physical activity at least 30 minutes at moderate intensity on at least 3 days · week[-1] for at least the last 3 months
[b]Light intensity exercise	30%–39% HRR or $\dot{V}O_2R$, 2–2.9 METs, RPE 9–11, an intensity that causes slight increases in HR and breathing
[c]Moderate intensity exercise	40%–59% HRR or $\dot{V}O_2R$, 3–5.9 METs, RPE 12–13, an intensity that causes noticeable increases in HR and breathing
[d]Vigorous intensity exercise	≥60% HRR or $\dot{V}O_2R$, ≥6 METs, RPE ≥14, an intensity that causes substantial increases in HR and breathing
[e]Cardiovascular (CV) disease	Cardiac, peripheral vascular, or cerebrovascular disease
[f]Metabolic disease	Type 1 and 2 diabetes mellitus
[g]Signs and symptoms	At rest or during activity. Includes pain, discomfort in the chest, neck, jaw, arms, or other areas that may result from ischemia; shortness of breath at rest or with mild exertion; dizziness or syncope; orthopnea or paroxysmal nocturnal dyspnea; ankle edema, palpitations or tachycardia; intermittent claudication; known heart murmur; unusual fatigue or shortness of breath with usual activities.
[h]Medical clearance	Approval from a health care professional to engage in exercise
[i]ACSM guidelines	See the most current edition of *ACSM's Guidelines for Exercise Testing and Prescription*

FIGURE 9.1 *(continued)*   ACSM's Preparticipation Screening Algorithm.

ACSM, American College of Sports Medicine; HR, heart rate; HRR, heart rate reserve; METs, metabolic equivalents; RPE, rating of perceived exertion; $\dot{V}O_2R$, oxygen uptake reserve.

everyone. It is also reasonable to recommend that persons beginning a new program of activity or exercise consult with a physician before participation.

PAR-Q+ Recommendations

After a client has completed the PAR-Q+, the personal trainer can derive recommendations from the seven-question form through the following analysis. If the client gave a *yes* answer to one or more questions (related to signs and symptoms associated with CVD, orthopedic concerns, and diagnosis by a physician), it is recommended that the individual contact his or her physician and tell the physician which questions elicited *yes* answers before increasing physical activity and taking part in a fitness appraisal or assessment. The client should seek recommendations from the physician regarding the level and progression of activity and restrictions associated with his or her specific needs. If the client gave *no* answers to all questions, there is reasonable assurance that it is suitable for him or her to engage in a graduated exercise program and a fitness appraisal or assessment. Also note the PAR-Q+ recommendation that a client who is or may be pregnant should talk with her doctor before she starts becoming more active. Chapter 18 provides guidance about conditions in which pregnant women should cease exercising or seek physician advice.

Recommendations for Current Medical Examinations and Exercise Testing

Suggested guidelines have been developed for determining when a diagnostic medical examination and submaximal or maximal exercise tests are appropriate before participation in moderate and vigorous exercise, and when a physician's supervision is required to monitor these tests. The sidebar, "Preparticipation and Physical Examination Components", provides the American College of Sports Medicine's recommendations for current medical examinations and exercise testing before participation and physician supervision of exercise tests (4).

Components that can be evaluated during a preparticipation examination include but are not limited to the following: body weight, body composition, pulse rate, blood pressure, heart sounds and breath sounds (auscultation), palpation of the major arteries, and the skin on the feet and legs of clients with diabetes mellitus. See the sidebar "Preparticipation Physical Examina-

tion Components" for a complete list (4). Depending on the health status of the client, laboratory tests may be administered, including total cholesterol and fasting blood glucose levels. A resting 12-lead ECG, Holter monitoring, cardio echocardiography, chest radiography, pulmonary function, and oximetry may also be performed if a client has known cardiovascular or pulmonary disease or is exhibiting symptoms.

MEDICAL CLEARANCE

In the cases in which referral is considered necessary, it is the personal trainer's responsibility to encourage medical clearance as a reasonable and safe course of action. A recommendation to consult with a physician before participation in an exercise program should not be considered an abdication of responsibility by the personal trainer, but rather a concerted effort to obtain valuable information and professional guidance to ensure safety and protection of the individual's health.

Physician Referral

Once medical clearance is recommended, the personal trainer should give the client a physician's referral form to obtain the necessary information about health status, physical limitations, and restrictions that would be required in order to make future fitness program recommendations. An example of a physician's referral form appears on page 174. The physician's referral form includes assessment of the individual's functional capacity, classification of ability to participate based on the evaluation, identification of preexisting conditions that may be worsened by exercise, prescribed medications, and fitness program recommendations. Chapter 25 includes discussion of the personal trainer's scope of practice as related to referral.

Program Recommendations

The physician recommendations provide the personal trainer with guidance and directions regarding what specific concerns and needs the individual has and which programs are appropriate. On the basis of results obtained during the diagnostic medical examination and exercise tests, a physician may recommend an unsupervised, supervised, or medically supervised exercise program.

- An **unsupervised program** is commonly recommended for people who are apparently healthy or presumably healthy with no apparent risks. This

PREPARTICIPATION PHYSICAL EXAMINATION COMPONENTS

Appropriate components of the physical examination may include the following:

- Body weight; in many instances determination of body mass index, waist girth, or body composition (percent body fat) is desirable
- Apical pulse rate and rhythm
- Resting blood pressure: seated, supine, and standing
- Auscultation of the lungs with specific attention to uniformity of breath sounds in all areas (absence of rales, wheezes, and other breathing sounds)
- Palpation of the cardiac apical impulse and point of maximal impulse
- Auscultation of the heart with specific attention to murmurs, gallops, clicks, and rubs
- Palpation and auscultation of carotid, abdominal, and femoral arteries
- Evaluation of the abdomen for bowel sounds, masses, visceromegaly, and tenderness
- Palpation and inspection of lower extremities for edema and presence of arterial pulses
- Absence or presence of tendon xanthoma and skin xanthelasma
- Follow-up examination related to orthopedic or other medical conditions that would limit exercise testing
- Tests of neurological function including reflexes and cognition (as indicated by history)
- Inspection of the skin, especially of the lower extremities in known patients with diabetes mellitus

Reprinted by permission from American College of Sports Medicine (2022, p. 54).

type of program recognizes the positive health-associated benefits that regular activity provides in relation to the relatively low risk involved in participation. These programs may be designed and initiated with the support of a personal trainer, the intended long-term eventual outcome being a combination of consistent weekly training sessions conducted by the personal trainer and other sessions that are self-directed and unsupervised.

- A **supervised program** may be recommended for people who have limitations or preexisting conditions that would restrict involvement but not limit participation. These programs are usually directed by a certified fitness professional, such as a certified personal trainer, who monitors intensity and modifies activity to meet the special concerns of the participant.
- A **medically supervised program** may be recommended for individuals who present a higher potential risk because of a predisposed condition, multiple risk factors, or an uncontrolled disease. These programs

are directed and monitored by allied health professionals in clinical settings with immediately accessible emergency response capabilities.

Since there is no guarantee that the initial program recommendation resulting from a physician referral will meet the client's specific goals, it is important for those involved in the referral and recommendation process to monitor and readjust the program to ensure it will be both safe and effective for the client.

CONCLUSION

The client consultation and health appraisal process is directly in line with the scope of practice of the personal trainer to motivate, assess, train, educate, and refer when necessary. To develop programs of exercise that will safely and effectively meet the individual's objectives, the personal trainer needs to gather pertinent information and documentation that will be used to assess health status, evaluate potential for risk, and refer for medical clearance when necessary.

CASE STUDY 9.1

IDENTIFYING CVD RISK FACTORS: RALPH D.

Presentation

Ralph is a physically inactive 36-year-old male tool and die engineer. His father survived a heart attack at age 70. Ralph reports that his blood pressure has been recorded at 136/86 mmHg and that his total cholesterol is 250 mg/dl, with an HDL of 45 mg/dl. His BMI has recently been measured at 30, his hip circumference is 40 inches (101.6 cm), and his waist girth is 47 inches (119.4 cm). Ralph reports no signs or symptoms and indicates that he quit smoking seven months ago.

Analysis

An evaluation of this scenario leads to the conclusion that Ralph presently has four positive coronary risk factors: hypertension (systolic blood pressure ≥130 mmHg and diastolic ≥80 mmHg), hypercholesterolemia (total cholesterol >200 mg/dl), inactive lifestyle, and obesity (waist girth >40 inches or 102 cm; BMI of 30). Consequently, Ralph would be considered asymptomatic, and light- to moderate-intensity exercise is recommended after receiving medical clearance, as per the ACSM preparticipation screening algorithm.

CASE STUDY 9.2

IDENTIFYING CVD RISK FACTORS: MARTHA G.

Presentation

Martha is a 56-year-old secretary. Her father died of a myocardial infarction (MI) at the age of 45. Martha reports that her LDL-cholesterol has been recorded at 125 mg/dl. Her BMI is 25. She reports that she has an active lifestyle that includes golf, tennis, and a daily walking routine.

Analysis

Martha has two positive coronary risk factors: age (over 55) and family history (her father died of an MI before the age of 55). Using the ACSM preparticipation screening algorithm, Martha may begin moderate-intensity exercise without medical clearance, and may continue to gradually progress following ACSM guidelines.

CASE STUDY 9.3

IDENTIFYING CVD RISK FACTORS: KATHLEEN K.

Presentation

Kathleen is a 47-year-old inactive female. Kathleen reports a total cholesterol of 210 mg/dl with an HDL-cholesterol reading of 68 mg/dl. She stands 5 feet, 2 inches (157.5 cm) tall, and her body weight is 110 pounds (49.9 kg) with a BMI of 20. Her blood pressure taken on two separate occasions is recorded as 120/80 mmHg. She reports that she was diagnosed with type 1 diabetes in early childhood.

Analysis

A review of the scenario shows that Kathleen has three positive coronary risk factors: an inactive lifestyle, elevated blood pressure (diastolic BP ≥80 mmHg), and hypercholesterolemia (total cholesterol level >200 mg/dl). However, she presents an HDL-cholesterol level of 68 mg/dl, which gives her a negative risk factor (HDL-cholesterol >60 mg/dl) that cancels one of the positive risk factors—leaving her with two total positive risk factors. It would initially appear that her age (younger than 55) and two risk factors would classify her at a lower risk. However, the fact that she has been diagnosed with a metabolic disease (type 1 diabetes) would warrant recommended medical clearance before she begins a light- to moderate-intensity exercise program using the ACSM preparticipation screening algorithm.

CASE STUDY 9.4

EFFECTS OF FAMILY HISTORY: ALEX M.

Presentation

Alex is a 20-year-old active male. He enjoys cycling, snow skiing, hiking, and running. On two separate occasions, Alex's blood pressure has been recorded as 145/85 mmHg. He stands 6 feet, 1 inch (185.4 cm) tall, and his body weight is 176 pounds (79.8 kg) with a BMI of 23. He reports that his uncle died suddenly of unknown causes at the age of 34. Physicians determined that the cause of death was related to an unidentified heart condition. Alex's grandfather also died suddenly of unknown causes at the age of 47. No cause was ever determined.

Analysis

A review of the scenario shows that Alex has two risk factors for sudden cardiac death: blood pressure of 145/85 mmHg and a family history of sudden and unexpected death in two close family members before age 50, resulting from either a heart condition or unknown causes. Alex has a healthy BMI, an active lifestyle, and only one positive risk factor (high blood pressure) so can continue current activity without medical clearance per the ACSM preparticipation screening algorithm.

Study Questions

1. What is the *most* important principle underlying the client consultation?

    A. Assess goals.

    B. Motivate the client.

    C. Screen participants for risk factors.

    D. Educate the client.

2. Which of the following is *incorrect* regarding the assumption of risk or waiver?

    A. It is an agreement by a client, before beginning participation, to give up, relinquish, or waive the participant's rights to legal remedy in the event of injury.

    B. The document typically includes waiving rights even in the case of provider negligence.

    C. The legal implications associated with the implementation and execution of the assumption of risk agreement are clear.

    D. If a personal trainer needs to prove in court that a participant was aware of how to avoid risks and assumed the risk of an activity, this type of document may prove helpful.

3. Which of the following is *incorrect* regarding blood lipids?

    A. Cholesterol is carried in the blood by HDL and LDL.

    B. LDL may be more predictive of CVD than total cholesterol.

    C. HDL molecules release cholesterol.

    D. HDLs act as a protective mechanism.

4. Which of the following is *incorrect* regarding stress and CVD?

    A. Stress is related to the risk for CVD.

    B. Type B behavior patterns may contribute to the overall risk for developing CVD.

    C. Risk factors can be measured through emotional stress inventories.

    D. The personal trainer should be able to identify signs and symptoms of stress overload.

5. Which of the following programs are likely to be recommended by a physician for a person who has limitations or preexisting conditions that would restrict involvement but not limit participation?

    A. No program recommended.

    B. An unsupervised program.

    C. A supervised program.

    D. A medically supervised program.

THE ATTITUDINAL ASSESSMENT

The initial assessment should be viewed not only as an assessment of physical condition but also as a gauge of attitude, outlook, and perspective. For each question, ask the client to rate him- or herself on a scale of 1 to 4. The first time you go through this exercise, your client might want to answer only the first section for each question (denoted with an asterisk [*]). You might come back whenever you feel the client is ready and complete the rest of each question. In the first part of each question, the assessment of where the client stands right now, the most motivated and driven athletes would likely have at least seven ratings of a 4 and not a single rating below a 3. Clients with three or more questions for which the answer is a 1 will need extra assistance to develop proper goals and may require frequent rewards, discussion, and education.

1. What would you consider your present attitude toward exercise?

1. I can't stand the thought of it.
2. I'll do it because I know I should, but I don't enjoy it.
3. I don't mind exercise, and I know it is beneficial.
4. I am motivated to exercise.

*Your answer: _____

How would you like to feel about exercise, if you could change your feelings?

Your answer: _____

Describe why and any specifics of how you would like to change your feelings about exercise and how those feelings might bring about positive change in your life:

_____

_____

_____

2. What would you consider your present attitude toward goal achievement?

1. I feel that whatever happens, happens, and I'll roll with the punches.
2. I set goals and believe it adds clarity and gives me some control over my outcome.
3. I write down my goals and believe it is a very valuable exercise in determining my future performance and achievement.
4. I have written goals and I review them often. I believe I have the power to achieve anything I desire and know that setting goals is a vital part of achievement.

*Your answer: _____

How would you like to feel about goal achievement, if you could change your feelings?

Your answer: _____

Describe why and any specifics of how you would like to change your feelings about goal achievement and how those feelings might bring about positive change in your life:

_____

_____

_____

(continued)

THE ATTITUDINAL ASSESSMENT   *(continued)*

   3. How important to you are the concepts of health and well-being?

   1. I don't need to put any effort into bettering my health.

   2. I make certain I devote some time and effort into bettering my physical body.

   3. I am committed to maintaining and working to improve my health and physical well-being.

   4. My health and well-being are the foundation of all that I achieve, and they must remain my top priorities.

   *Your answer: _____

How would you like to feel about the concepts of health and well-being, if you could change your feelings?

Your answer: _____

Describe why and any specifics of how you would like to change your feelings about the concepts of health and well-being and how those feelings might bring about positive change in your life:

_____

_____

_____

_____

   4. How strong and driving is your desire for improvement?

   1. I'm really pretty satisfied with the way things are. Striving for improvement might leave me frustrated and disappointed.

   2. I'd like to improve but don't know that it's worth all the work involved.

   3. I love feeling as if I've bettered myself and am open to any suggestions for improvement.

   4. I'm driven to excel and am committed to striving for consistent and ongoing improvement.

   *Your answer: _____

How strong and driven would you like to feel about improvement?

Your answer: _____

Describe why and any specifics of how you would like to change your feelings about improvement and how those feelings might bring about positive change in your life:

_____

_____

_____

_____

   5. How do you feel about yourself and your abilities (self-esteem)?

   1. I am not comfortable with the way I look, feel, or perform in most situations.

   2. I would love to change many things about myself although I am proud of who I am.

   3. I'm very good at the things I must do, I take pride in many of my achievements, and I am quite able to handle myself in most situations.

   4. I have great strength, ability, and pride.

   *Your answer: _____

How would you like to feel about yourself and your abilities, if you could change your feelings?

Your answer: _____

Describe why and any specifics of how you would like to change your feelings about yourself and your abilities and how those feelings might bring about positive change in your life:

_____

_____

_____

_____

6. How do you feel about your present physical condition in terms of the way you look?

   1. I would like to completely change my body.

   2. There are many things about my reflection in the mirror that I'm not comfortable with.

   3. For the most part I look OK, and I can look really good in the right clothing, but I do feel uncomfortable with a few things about my physical appearance.

   4. I am proud of my body and am comfortable in any manner of dress in appropriate situations.

*Your answer: _____

How would you like to feel about the way you look, if you could change your feelings?

Your answer: _____

Describe why and any specifics of how you would like to change your feelings about the way you look and how those feelings might bring about positive change in your life:

_____

_____

_____

_____

7. How do you feel about your present physical condition in terms of overall health?

   1. I wish I felt healthy.

   2. I feel healthy for my age compared to most people I meet.

   3. I maintain a high level of health.

   4. I am extremely healthy.

*Your answer:_____

How would you like to feel about yourself and your abilities, if you could change your feelings?

Your answer: _____

Describe why and any specifics of how you would like to change your feelings about yourself and your abilities and how those feelings might bring about positive change in your life:

_____

_____

_____

_____

(continued)

THE ATTITUDINAL ASSESSMENT *(continued)*

8. How do you feel about your physical condition in terms of your performance in any chosen physical fields of endeavor (sports, training, etc.)?

    1. I feel as if I'm in very poor condition and am uncomfortable when faced with a physical challenge.

    2. I am not comfortable with my performance abilities; however, I am comfortable training to improve.

    3. I feel pretty good about my ability to perform physically although I would like to improve.

    4. I have exceptional physical abilities and enjoy being called upon to display them.

*Your answer: _____

How would you like to feel about your performance, if you could change your feelings?

Your answer: _____

Describe why and any specifics of how you would like to change your feelings about your performance and how those feelings might bring about positive change in your life:

_____

_____

_____

_____

9. How strongly do you believe that you can improve your body?

    1. I believe most of my physical shortcomings are genetic, and most efforts to change would be a waste of time.

    2. I've seen many people change their bodies for the better and am sure with enough effort I can see some improvement.

    3. I strongly believe the proper combination of exercise and nutrition can bring about some improvement.

    4. I know without question that with the proper combination of exercise and nutrition I can bring about dramatic changes in my body.

*Your answer: _____

How would you like to feel about your ability to improve your body, if you could change your feelings?

Your answer: _____

Describe why and any specifics of how you would like to change your feelings about your ability to improve your body and how those feelings might bring about positive change in your life:

_____

_____

_____

_____

10. When you begin a program or set a goal, how likely are you to follow through to its fruition?

1. I've never been good at following things through to the end.

2. With the right motivation and some evidence of results I think I might stick to a program.

3. I have the patience and ability to commit to a program and will give it a chance in order to assess its value.

4. Once I set a goal, there's no stopping me.

*Your answer:_____

How would you like to feel about following through on goals, if you could change your feelings?

Your answer:_____

Describe why and any specifics of how you would like to change your feelings about following through on goals and how those feelings might bring about positive change in your life:

_____

_____

_____

_____

From *NSCA's Essentials of Personal Training,* 3rd ed., edited for the National Strength and Conditioning Association by B. Schoenfeld and R. Snarr (Champaign, IL: Human Kinetics, 2022).

PERSONAL TRAINING CONTRACT/AGREEMENT

Congratulations on your decision to participate in an exercise program! With the help of your personal trainer, you greatly improve your ability to accomplish your training goals faster, safer, and with maximum benefits. The details of these training sessions can be used for a lifetime.

To maximize your progress, it will be necessary for you to follow program guidelines during supervised and (if applicable) unsupervised training days. Remember, exercise and healthy eating are *equally* important! During your exercise program, every effort will be made to assure your safety. However, as with any exercise program, there are risks, including increased heart stress and the chance of musculoskeletal injuries. In volunteering for this program, you agree to assume responsibility for these risks and waive any possibility for personal damage. You also agree that, to your knowledge, you have no limiting physical conditions or disability that would preclude an exercise program.

By signing below, you accept full responsibility for your own health and well-being *and* you acknowledge an understanding that no responsibility is assumed by the leaders of the program.

It is recommended that all program participants work with their personal trainer three (3) times per week. However, because of scheduling conflicts and financial considerations, a combination of supervised and unsupervised workouts is possible.

PERSONAL TRAINING TERMS AND CONDITIONS

1. Personal training sessions that are not rescheduled or canceled 24 hours in advance will result in forfeiture of the session and a loss of the financial investment at the rate of one session.

2. Clients arriving late will receive the remaining scheduled session time, unless other arrangements have been previously made with the personal trainer.

3. The expiration policy requires completion of all personal training sessions within 120 days from the date of the contract. Personal training sessions are void after this time period.

4. No personal training refunds will be issued for any reason, including but not limited to relocation, illness, and unused sessions.

Description of program (number of sessions purchased, monthly membership dues, etc.):

_____

_____

Total investment: _____ Method of payment: _____

Participant's name (please print clearly):

_____ Date: _____

Participant's signature:

_____ Date: _____

Parent/guardian's signature (if needed):

_____ Date: _____

Witness's signature: _____

From *NSCA's Essentials of Personal Training,* 3rd ed., edited for the National Strength and Conditioning Association by B. Schoenfeld and R. Snarr (Champaign, IL: Human Kinetics, 2022).

PHYSICAL ACTIVITY READINESS QUESTIONNAIRE FOR EVERYONE (PAR-Q+)

2021 PAR-Q+

The Physical Activity Readiness Questionnaire for Everyone

The health benefits of regular physical activity are clear; more people should engage in physical activity every day of the week. Participating in physical activity is very safe for MOST people. This questionnaire will tell you whether it is necessary for you to seek further advice from your doctor OR a qualified exercise professional before becoming more physically active.

GENERAL HEALTH QUESTIONS

Please read the 7 questions below carefully and answer each one honestly: check YES or NO.	YES	NO
1) Has your doctor ever said that you have a heart condition ☐ **OR** high blood pressure ☐ ?	☐	☐
2) Do you feel pain in your chest at rest, during your daily activities of living, **OR** when you do physical activity?	☐	☐
3) Do you lose balance because of dizziness **OR** have you lost consciousness in the last 12 months? Please answer **NO** if your dizziness was associated with over-breathing (including during vigorous exercise).	☐	☐
4) Have you ever been diagnosed with another chronic medical condition (other than heart disease or high blood pressure)? **PLEASE LIST CONDITION(S) HERE:** _____	☐	☐
5) Are you currently taking prescribed medications for a chronic medical condition? **PLEASE LIST CONDITION(S) AND MEDICATIONS HERE:** _____	☐	☐
6) Do you currently have (or have had within the past 12 months) a bone, joint, or soft tissue (muscle, ligament, or tendon) problem that could be made worse by becoming more physically active? Please answer **NO** if you had a problem in the past, but it **does not limit your current ability** to be physically active. **PLEASE LIST CONDITION(S) HERE:** _____	☐	☐
7) Has your doctor ever said that you should only do medically supervised physical activity?	☐	☐

✔️ **If you answered NO to all of the questions above, you are cleared for physical activity.**
Please sign the PARTICIPANT DECLARATION. You do not need to complete Pages 2 and 3.

▶ Start becoming much more physically active – start slowly and build up gradually.

▶ Follow Global Physical Activity Guidelines for your age (https://www.who.int/publications/i/item/9789240015128).

▶ You may take part in a health and fitness appraisal.

▶ If you are over the age of 45 yr and NOT accustomed to regular vigorous to maximal effort exercise, consult a qualified exercise professional before engaging in this intensity of exercise.

▶ If you have any further questions, contact a qualified exercise professional.

PARTICIPANT DECLARATION
If you are less than the legal age required for consent or require the assent of a care provider, your parent, guardian or care provider must also sign this form.

I, the undersigned, have read, understood to my full satisfaction and completed this questionnaire. I acknowledge that this physical activity clearance is valid for a maximum of 12 months from the date it is completed and becomes invalid if my condition changes. I also acknowledge that the community/fitness center may retain a copy of this form for its records. In these instances, it will maintain the confidentiality of the same, complying with applicable law.

NAME _____ DATE _____

SIGNATURE _____ WITNESS _____

SIGNATURE OF PARENT/GUARDIAN/CARE PROVIDER _____

⬤ **If you answered YES to one or more of the questions above, COMPLETE PAGES 2 AND 3.**

⚠️ **Delay becoming more active if:**

✓ You have a temporary illness such as a cold or fever; it is best to wait until you feel better.

✓ You are pregnant - talk to your health care practitioner, your physician, a qualified exercise professional, and/or complete the ePARmed-X+ at www.eparmedx.com before becoming more physically active.

✓ Your health changes - answer the questions on Pages 2 and 3 of this document and/or talk to your doctor or a qualified exercise professional before continuing with any physical activity program.

2021 PAR-Q+

FOLLOW-UP QUESTIONS ABOUT YOUR MEDICAL CONDITION(S)

1. **Do you have Arthritis, Osteoporosis, or Back Problems?**

If the above condition(s) is/are present, answer questions 1a-1c   If **NO** ☐ go to question 2

1a. Do you have difficulty controlling your condition with medications or other physician-prescribed therapies? (Answer **NO** if you are not currently taking medications or other treatments)   YES ☐ NO ☐

1b. Do you have joint problems causing pain, a recent fracture or fracture caused by osteoporosis or cancer, displaced vertebra (e.g., spondylolisthesis), and/or spondylolysis/pars defect (a crack in the bony ring on the back of the spinal column)?   YES ☐ NO ☐

1c. Have you had steroid injections or taken steroid tablets regularly for more than 3 months?   YES ☐ NO ☐

2. **Do you currently have Cancer of any kind?**

If the above condition(s) is/are present, answer questions 2a-2b   If **NO** ☐ go to question 3

2a. Does your cancer diagnosis include any of the following types: lung/bronchogenic, multiple myeloma (cancer of plasma cells), head, and/or neck?   YES ☐ NO ☐

2b. Are you currently receiving cancer therapy (such as chemotheraphy or radiotherapy)?   YES ☐ NO ☐

3. **Do you have a Heart or Cardiovascular Condition? This includes Coronary Artery Disease, Heart Failure, Diagnosed Abnormality of Heart Rhythm**

If the above condition(s) is/are present, answer questions 3a-3d   If **NO** ☐ go to question 4

3a. Do you have difficulty controlling your condition with medications or other physician-prescribed therapies? (Answer **NO** if you are not currently taking medications or other treatments)   YES ☐ NO ☐

3b. Do you have an irregular heart beat that requires medical management? (e.g., atrial fibrillation, premature ventricular contraction)   YES ☐ NO ☐

3c. Do you have chronic heart failure?   YES ☐ NO ☐

3d. Do you have diagnosed coronary artery (cardiovascular) disease and have not participated in regular physical activity in the last 2 months?   YES ☐ NO ☐

4. **Do you currently have High Blood Pressure?**

If the above condition(s) is/are present, answer questions 4a-4b   If **NO** ☐ go to question 5

4a. Do you have difficulty controlling your condition with medications or other physician-prescribed therapies? (Answer **NO** if you are not currently taking medications or other treatments)   YES ☐ NO ☐

4b. Do you have a resting blood pressure equal to or greater than 160/90 mmHg with or without medication? (Answer **YES** if you do not know your resting blood pressure)   YES ☐ NO ☐

5. **Do you have any Metabolic Conditions? This includes Type 1 Diabetes, Type 2 Diabetes, Pre-Diabetes**

If the above condition(s) is/are present, answer questions 5a-5e   If **NO** ☐ go to question 6

5a. Do you often have difficulty controlling your blood sugar levels with foods, medications, or other physician-prescribed therapies?   YES ☐ NO ☐

5b. Do you often suffer from signs and symptoms of low blood sugar (hypoglycemia) following exercise and/or during activities of daily living? Signs of hypoglycemia may include shakiness, nervousness, unusual irritability, abnormal sweating, dizziness or light-headedness, mental confusion, difficulty speaking, weakness, or sleepiness.   YES ☐ NO ☐

5c. Do you have any signs or symptoms of diabetes complications such as heart or vascular disease and/or complications affecting your eyes, kidneys, **OR** the sensation in your toes and feet?   YES ☐ NO ☐

5d. Do you have other metabolic conditions (such as current pregnancy-related diabetes, chronic kidney disease, or liver problems)?   YES ☐ NO ☐

5e. Are you planning to engage in what for you is unusually high (or vigorous) intensity exercise in the near future?   YES ☐ NO ☐

2021 PAR-Q+

6.   Do you have any Mental Health Problems or Learning Difficulties? This includes Alzheimer's, Dementia, Depression, Anxiety Disorder, Eating Disorder, Psychotic Disorder, Intellectual Disability, Down Syndrome

If the above condition(s) is/are present, answer questions 6a-6b   If **NO** ☐ go to question 7

6a.	Do you have difficulty controlling your condition with medications or other physician-prescribed therapies? (Answer **NO** if you are not currently taking medications or other treatments)	YES☐ NO☐
6b.	Do you have Down Syndrome **AND** back problems affecting nerves or muscles?	YES☐ NO☐

7.   Do you have a Respiratory Disease? This includes Chronic Obstructive Pulmonary Disease, Asthma, Pulmonary High Blood Pressure

If the above condition(s) is/are present, answer questions 7a-7d   If **NO** ☐ go to question 8

7a.	Do you have difficulty controlling your condition with medications or other physician-prescribed therapies? (Answer **NO** if you are not currently taking medications or other treatments)	YES☐ NO☐
7b.	Has your doctor ever said your blood oxygen level is low at rest or during exercise and/or that you require supplemental oxygen therapy?	YES☐ NO☐
7c.	If asthmatic, do you currently have symptoms of chest tightness, wheezing, laboured breathing, consistent cough (more than 2 days/week), or have you used your rescue medication more than twice in the last week?	YES☐ NO☐
7d.	Has your doctor ever said you have high blood pressure in the blood vessels of your lungs?	YES☐ NO☐

8.   Do you have a Spinal Cord Injury? This includes Tetraplegia and Paraplegia

If the above condition(s) is/are present, answer questions 8a-8c   If **NO** ☐ go to question 9

8a.	Do you have difficulty controlling your condition with medications or other physician-prescribed therapies? (Answer **NO** if you are not currently taking medications or other treatments)	YES☐ NO☐
8b.	Do you commonly exhibit low resting blood pressure significant enough to cause dizziness, light-headedness, and/or fainting?	YES☐ NO☐
8c.	Has your physician indicated that you exhibit sudden bouts of high blood pressure (known as Autonomic Dysreflexia)?	YES☐ NO☐

9.   Have you had a Stroke? This includes Transient Ischemic Attack (TIA) or Cerebrovascular Event

If the above condition(s) is/are present, answer questions 9a-9c   If **NO** ☐ go to question 10

9a.	Do you have difficulty controlling your condition with medications or other physician-prescribed therapies? (Answer **NO** if you are not currently taking medications or other treatments)	YES☐ NO☐
9b.	Do you have any impairment in walking or mobility?	YES☐ NO☐
9c.	Have you experienced a stroke or impairment in nerves or muscles in the past 6 months?	YES☐ NO☐

10.   Do you have any other medical condition not listed above or do you have two or more medical conditions?

If you have other medical conditions, answer questions 10a-10c   If **NO** ☐ read the Page 4 recommendations

10a.	Have you experienced a blackout, fainted, or lost consciousness as a result of a head injury within the last 12 months **OR** have you had a diagnosed concussion within the last 12 months?	YES☐ NO☐
10b.	Do you have a medical condition that is not listed (such as epilepsy, neurological conditions, kidney problems)?	YES☐ NO☐
10c.	Do you currently live with two or more medical conditions?	YES☐ NO☐

PLEASE LIST YOUR MEDICAL CONDITION(S) AND ANY RELATED MEDICATIONS HERE: _____

_____

GO to Page 4 for recommendations about your current medical condition(s) and sign the PARTICIPANT DECLARATION.

2021 PAR-Q+

 If you answered NO to all of the FOLLOW-UP questions (pgs. 2-3) about your medical condition, you are ready to become more physically active - sign the PARTICIPANT DECLARATION below:

- ▶ It is advised that you consult a qualified exercise professional to help you develop a safe and effective physical activity plan to meet your health needs.
- ▶ You are encouraged to start slowly and build up gradually - 20 to 60 minutes of low to moderate intensity exercise, 3-5 days per week including aerobic and muscle strengthening exercises.
- ▶ As you progress, you should aim to accumulate 150 minutes or more of moderate intensity physical activity per week.
- ▶ If you are over the age of 45 yr and **NOT** accustomed to regular vigorous to maximal effort exercise, consult a qualified exercise professional before engaging in this intensity of exercise.

⬤ **If you answered YES to one or more of the follow-up questions** about your medical condition:

You should seek further information before becoming more physically active or engaging in a fitness appraisal. You should complete the specially designed online screening and exercise recommendations program - the **ePARmed-X+ at www.eparmedx.com** and/or visit a qualified exercise professional to work through the ePARmed-X+ and for further information.

⚠ **Delay becoming more active if:**

 You have a temporary illness such as a cold or fever; it is best to wait until you feel better.

 You are pregnant - talk to your health care practitioner, your physician, a qualified exercise professional, and/or complete the ePARmed-X+ **at www.eparmedx.com** before becoming more physically active.

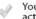 Your health changes - talk to your doctor or qualified exercise professional before continuing with any physical activity program.

- ⬤ You are encouraged to photocopy the PAR-Q+. You must use the entire questionnaire and NO changes are permitted.
- ⬤ The authors, the PAR-Q+ Collaboration, partner organizations, and their agents assume no liability for persons who undertake physical activity and/or make use of the PAR-Q+ or ePARmed-X+. If in doubt after completing the questionnaire, consult your doctor prior to physical activity.

PARTICIPANT DECLARATION

- ⬤ All persons who have completed the PAR-Q+ please read and sign the declaration below.
- ⬤ If you are less than the legal age required for consent or require the assent of a care provider, your parent, guardian or care provider must also sign this form.

I, the undersigned, have read, understood to my full satisfaction and completed this questionnaire. I acknowledge that this physical activity clearance is valid for a maximum of 12 months from the date it is completed and becomes invalid if my condition changes. I also acknowledge that the community/fitness center may retain a copy of this form for records. In these instances, it will maintain the confidentiality of the same, complying with applicable law.

NAME _____ DATE _____

SIGNATURE _____ WITNESS _____

SIGNATURE OF PARENT/GUARDIAN/CARE PROVIDER _____

─── **For more information, please contact** ───
www.eparmedx.com
Email: eparmedx@gmail.com

Citation for PAR-Q+
Warburton DER, Jamnik VK, Bredin SSD, and Gledhill N on behalf of the PAR-Q+ Collaboration. The Physical Activity Readiness Questionnaire for Everyone (PAR-Q+) and Electronic Physical Activity Readiness Medical Examination (ePARmed-X+). Health & Fitness Journal of Canada 4(2):3-23, 2011.

Key References
1. Jamnik VK, Warburton DER, Makarski J, McKenzie DC, Shephard RJ, Stone J, and Gledhill N. Enhancing the effectiveness of clearance for physical activity participation; background and overall process. APNM 36(S1):S3-S13, 2011.
2. Warburton DER, Gledhill N, Jamnik VK, Bredin SSD, McKenzie DC, Stone J, Charlesworth S, and Shephard RJ. Evidence-based risk assessment and recommendations for physical activity clearance; Consensus Document. APNM 36(S1):S266-s298, 2011.
3. Chisholm DM, Collis ML, Kulak LL, Davenport W, and Gruber N. Physical activity readiness. British Columbia Medical Journal. 1975;17:375-378.
4. Thomas S, Reading J, and Shephard RJ. Revision of the Physical Activity Readiness Questionnaire (PAR-Q). Canadian Journal of Sport Science 1992;17:4 338-345.

The PAR-Q+ was created using the evidence-based AGREE process (1) by the PAR-Q+ Collaboration chaired by Dr. Darren E. R. Warburton with Dr. Norman Gledhill, Dr. Veronica Jamnik, and Dr. Donald C. McKenzie (2). Production of this document has been made possible through financial contributions from the Public Health Agency of Canada and the BC Ministry of Health Services. The views expressed herein do not necessarily represent the views of the Public Health Agency of Canada or the BC Ministry of Health Services.

─── Copyright © 2021 PAR-Q+ Collaboration **4/ 4**
01-11-2020

HEALTH/MEDICAL QUESTIONNAIRE

Date: _____

Name: _____ Date of birth: _____

Address:

Street: _____ City: _____ State: _____ Zip: _____

Phone (H): _____ (W): _____

E-mail address: _____

In case of emergency, whom may we contact?

Name: _____ Relationship: _____

Phone (H): _____ (W): _____

Personal Physician

Name: _____ Phone: _____

Present/Past History

Have you had OR do you presently have any of the following conditions? (Check if yes.)

- ❏ Rheumatic fever
- ❏ Recent operation
- ❏ Edema (swelling of ankles)
- ❏ High blood pressure
- ❏ Injury to back or knees
- ❏ Low blood pressure
- ❏ Seizures
- ❏ Lung disease
- ❏ Heart attack
- ❏ Fainting or dizziness with or without physical exertion
- ❏ Diabetes
- ❏ High cholesterol
- ❏ Orthopnea (the need to sit up to breathe comfortably) or paroxysmal (sudden, unexpected attack) nocturnal dyspnea (shortness of breath at night)
- ❏ Shortness of breath at rest or with mild exertion
- ❏ Chest pains
- ❏ Palpitations or tachycardia (unusually strong or rapid heartbeat)
- ❏ Intermittent claudication (calf cramping)
- ❏ Pain, discomfort in the chest, neck, jaw, arms, or other areas with or without physical exertion
- ❏ Known heart murmur
- ❏ Unusual fatigue or shortness of breath with usual activities
- ❏ Temporary loss of visual acuity or speech, or short-term numbness or weakness in one side, arm, or leg of your body
- ❏ Other conditions: _____

(continued)

HEALTH MEDICAL QUESTIONNAIRE *(continued)*

Family History

Have any of your first-degree relatives (parent, sibling, or child) experienced the following conditions? (Check if yes.) In addition, please identify at what age the condition occurred.

- ❏ Heat arrhythmia
- ❏ Heart attack
- ❏ Heart operation
- ❏ Congenital heart disease
- ❏ Premature death before age 50
- ❏ Significant disability secondary to a heart condition
- ❏ Marfan syndrome
- ❏ High blood pressure
- ❏ High cholesterol
- ❏ Diabetes
- ❏ Other major illness: _____

Explain checked items: _____

_____

_____

_____

Activity History

1. How were you referred to this program? _____
2. Why are you enrolling in this program? _____
3. Are you presently employed? Yes_____ No_____
4. What is your present occupational position? _____
5. Name of company: _____
6. Have you ever worked with a personal trainer before? Yes _____ No_____
7. Date of your last physical examination performed by a physician:_____
8. Do you participate in a regular exercise program at this time? Yes_____ No_____ If yes, briefly describe:_____
9. Can you currently briskly walk for 30 minutes without fatigue? Yes_____ No_____
10. Have you ever performed resistance training exercises in the past? Yes_____ No_____
11. Do you have injuries (bone or muscle) that may interfere with exercising? Yes _____No_____ If yes, briefly describe:_____
12. Do you smoke? Yes_____ No _____ If yes, how much per day and what was your age when you started? Amount per day:_____ Age:_____
13. What is your body weight now?_____ What was it one year ago?_____ At age 21?_____
14. Do you follow or have you recently followed any specific dietary intake plan, and in general how do you feel about your nutritional habits? _____
15. List the medications you are presently taking: _____
16. List in order your personal health and fitness objectives:_____

HEALTH RISK ANALYSIS FORM

This health risk analysis form helps to identify positive and negative aspects of health behavior. Although many of the effects are based on real findings from large epidemiological investigations, the estimates are generalized and should not be taken too literally. Accurately predicting how long you will live or when you will die is impossible.

Plus one (+1) represents a positive effect that could add a year to your life or life to your years, and minus one (–1) indicates a loss in the quantity or quality of life. A zero (0) indicates no shortening or lengthening of your longevity. If none of the categories listed for a factor apply to you, enter 0. Complete each section and record the totals in section VIII.

SECTION I: CARDIOVASCULAR DISEASE (CVD) RISK FACTORS

Cholesterol or total cholesterol to HDL ratio					Score
<160	160-200	200-240	240-280	>280	
<3	3-4	4-5	5-6	>6	
+2	+1	−1	−2	−4	

Blood pressure (choose your highest number for either value)					Score
<110	110-120	120-150	150-170	170	
<60	60-80	80-90	90-100	>100	
+1	0	−1	−2	−4	

Smoking					Score
Never	Quit	Smoke cigar or pipe or close family member smokes	One pack of cigarettes daily	Two or more packs daily	
+1	0	−1	−3	−5	

Heredity					Score
No family history of CHD	One close relative over 60 with CHD	Two close relatives over 60 with CHD	One close relative under 60 with CHD	Two or more close relatives under 60 with CHD	
+2	0	−1	−2	−4	

Body mass index (BMI, use table 11.7 on page 247)					Score
<19	19-24	24-29	30-39*	>40*	
+2	0	−1	−3	−5	

*If waist is under 40 in. (102 cm) subtract one less (e.g., −2 or −4)

Sex					Score
Female under 55 years	Female over 55 years	Male	Stocky male	Bald, stocky male	
0	−1	−1	−2	−3	

Stress					Score
Phlegmatic, unhurried, generally happy	Ambitious but generally relaxed	Sometimes hard-driving, time-conscious, competitive	Hard-driving, time-conscious, competitive (type A)	Type A with repressed hostility	
+1	0	0	−1	−3	

Physical activity					Score
High intensity, 60 min most days	Moderate, 30 min most days	Moderate, 20-30 min, 3-5 times per week	Light, 10-20 min,1 or 2 times per week	Little or none	
+3	+2	+1	−1	−3	

TOTAL: I. CVD risk factors					

(continued)

HEALTH RISK ANALYSIS FORM *(continued)*

SECTION II: HEALTH HABITS (RELATED TO GOOD HEALTH AND LONGEVITY)

Breakfast					Score
Daily	Sometimes	None	Coffee	Coffee and pastry	
+1	0	−1	−2	−3	
Regular meals					**Score**
Three or more	Two daily	Not regular	Fad diets	Starve and stuff	
+1	0	−1	−2	−3	
Sleep					**Score**
7-8 h	8-9 h	6-7 h	>9 h	<6 h	
+1	0	0	−1	−2	
Alcohol					**Score**
None	Women 3/week	Men 1-2 daily	3-6 daily	>6 daily	
+1	+1	+1	−2	−4	
TOTAL: II. Health habits					

SECTION III: MEDICAL FACTORS

Medical exam and screening tests (blood pressure, diabetes, glaucoma)					Score
Regular tests, see doctor when necessary	Periodic medical exam and selected tests	Periodic medical exam	Sometimes get tests	No tests or medical exams	
+1	+1	0	0	−1	
Heart					**Score**
No history of problems, self or family	Some history	Rheumatic fever as child, no murmur now	Rheumatic fever as a child, have murmur	Have ECG abnormality or angina pectoris	
+2	0	−1	−2	−3	
Lung (including pneumonia and tuberculosis)					**Score**
No problem	Some past problem	Mild asthma or bronchitis	Emphysema, severe asthma, or bronchitis	Severe lung problems	
+1	0	−1	−1	−3	
Digestive tract					**Score**
No problem	Occasional diarrhea, loss of appetite	Frequent diarrhea or stomach upset	Ulcers, colitis, gall bladder, or liver problems	Severe gastrointestinal disorders	
+1	0	−1	−2	−3	
Diabetes					**Score**
No problem or family history	Controlled hypoglycemia (low blood sugar)	Hypoglycemia and family history	Mild diabetes (diet and exercise)	Diabetes (insulin)	
+1	0	−1	−2	−4	
Drugs					**Score**
Seldom take	Minimal but regular use of aspirin or other drugs	Heavy use of aspirin or other drugs	Regular use of mood-altering or psychogenic drugs	Heavy use of mood-altering or psychogenic drugs	
+1	0	−1	−2	−3	
TOTAL: III. Medical factors					

SECTION IV: SAFETY FACTORS

Driving in car					Score
<7,000 miles (11,000 km) per year, mostly local	7,000-10,000 miles (11,000-16,000 km) per year, local and some highway	10,000-15,000 miles (16,000-24,000 km) per year, local and highway	>15,000 miles (24,000 km) per year, highway and some local	>15,000 miles (24,000 km) per year, mostly highway	
+1	0	0	−1	−2	
Using seat belts					**Score**
Always	Most of time (>75%)	On highway only	Seldom (<25%)	Never	
+1	0	−1	−2	−4	
Risk-taking behavior (motorcycle, skydive, mountain climb, fly small plane, etc.)					**Score**
Some with careful preparation	Never	Occasional	Often	Try anything for thrills	
+1	0	−1	−1	−2	
TOTAL: IV. Safety factors					

SECTION V: PERSONAL FACTORS

Diet					Score
Low fat, low calories, fruits and vegetables	Balanced with complex carbohydrate	High protein, limited fat	Extra calories, low carbohydrate	Fad diets and fat	
+2	+1	0	−1	−2	
Longevity					**Score**
Grandparents lived past 90, parents past 80	Grandparents lived past 80, parents past 70	Grandparents lived past 70, parents past 60	Few relatives lived past 60	Few relatives lived past 50	
+2	+1	0	−1	−3	
Love and marriage					**Score**
Happily married	Married	Unmarried	Divorced	Extramarital relationship(s)	
+2	+1	0	−1	−3	
Education					**Score**
Postgraduate or master craftsman	College graduate or skilled craftsman	Some college or trade school	High school graduate	Grade school graduate	
+1	+1	0	−1	−2	
Job satisfaction					**Score**
Enjoy job, see results, room for advancement	Enjoy job, see some results, able to advance	Job OK, no results, nowhere to go	Dislike job	Hate job	
+2	+1	0	−1	−3	
Social					**Score**
Have some close friends	Have some friends	Have no good friends	Stuck with people I don't enjoy	Have no friends at all	
+1	0	−1	−2	−3	
Race					**Score**
White or Asian	Black or Hispanic	American Indian			
0	−1	−2			
TOTAL: V. Personal factors					

(continued)

HEALTH RISK ANALYSIS FORM *(continued)*

SECTION VI: PSYCHOLOGICAL FACTORS

Outlook					Score
Feel good about present and future	Satisfied	Unsure about present or future	Unhappy in present, don't look forward to future	Miserable, rather not get out of bed	
+2	+1	0	−1	−3	
Depression					**Score**
No family history of depression	Some family history, feel OK	Family history and mildly depressed	Sometimes feel life isn't worth living	Thoughts of suicide	
+1	0	−1	−2	−3	
Anxiety					**Score**
Seldom anxious	Occasionally anxious	Often anxious	Always anxious	Panic attacks	
+1	0	−1	−2	−3	
Relaxation					**Score**
Relax or meditate daily	Relax often	Seldom relax	Usually tense	Always tense	
+1	0	−1	−2	−3	
TOTAL: VI. Psychological factors					

SECTION VII: FOR WOMEN ONLY

Health care					Score
Regular breast and Pap tests	Occasional breast and Pap tests	Never have exams	Treated disorder	Untreated cancer	
+1	0	−1	−2	−4	
Birth control pill					**Score**
Never used	Quit 5 years ago	Still use, under 30 years	Use pill and smoke	Use pill, smoke, over 35	
+1	0	0	−2	−3	
TOTAL: VII. For women only					

SECTION VIII: SCORING SUMMARY

You can now estimate your longevity. Add your total score from the previous sections to your normal life expectancy (from the chart below) to find your longevity estimate. If you would like to improve your longevity estimate, go back and decide on some lifestyle areas you would like to improve.

Category	Score (+ or − from previous sections)
I. CVD risk factors	_____
II. Health habits	_____
III. Medical factors	_____
IV. Safety factors	_____
V. Personal factors	_____
VI. Psychological factors	_____
VII. For women only	_____
Total _____	_____ + _____ = _____
	(Total from sections I-VII) **(Life expectancy** *from the following table***)**

LIFE EXPECTANCY

| Nearest age | EXPECTANCY (ALL RACES) | |
	Male	Female
30	77.1	81.5
35	77.5	81.7
40	77.8	81.9
45	78.3	82.2
50	79.0	82.7
55	79.9	83.2
60	80.9	83.9
65	82.2	84.9
70	83.7	86.0
75	85.6	87.5
80	87.9	89.9

From *NSCA's Essentials of Personal Training,* 3rd ed., edited for the National Strength and Conditioning Association by B. Schoenfeld and R. Snarr (Champaign, IL: Human Kinetics, 2022). Adapted by permission from Sharkey and Gaskill (2013, pp. 397-401).

PHYSICIAN'S REFERRAL FORM PERTAINING TO A FITNESS EVALUATION AND PREVENTIVE PROGRAM OF EXERCISE

Dear Doctor: _____

Your patient _____ has contacted us regarding the fitness evaluation conducted by_____ . The program is designed to evaluate the individual's fitness status prior to embarking on an exercise program. From this evaluation, an exercise prescription is formulated. In addition, other parameters related to a health improvement program are discussed with the participant. It is important to understand that this program is preventive and is not intended to be rehabilitative in nature. The fitness testing includes:

_____

A comprehensive consultation will be provided to the participant that serves to review the test results and explain recommendations for an individualized fitness program. A summary of test results and our recommendations will be kept on file and may be made available to you upon request. In the interest of your patient and for our information, please complete the following:

Has this patient undergone a physical examination within the last year to assess functional capacity to perform exercise?

Yes ____ No____

I consider this patient (please check one):

____ Class I: presumably healthy without apparent heart disease; eligible to participate in an unsupervised program

____ Class II: presumably healthy with one or more risk factors for heart disease; eligible to participate in a supervised program

____Class III: patient not eligible for this program; a medically supervised program is recommended

Does this patient have any preexisting medical/orthopedic condition(s) requiring continued or long-term medical treatment or follow-up?

Yes ____ (Please explain: _____) No ____

Are you aware of any medical condition(s) that this patient may have or may have had that could be worsened by exercise?

Yes ____ No____

Please list any currently prescribed medication(s): _____

Please provide specific recommendations and/or list any restrictions concerning this patient's present health status as it relates to active participation in a fitness program: _____

_____

_____

Referring physician's signature: _____

Date:_____ Client's name:_____

Phone (H): _____ (W): _____

Address:_____

From *NSCA's Essentials of Personal Training,* 3rd ed., edited for the National Strength and Conditioning Association by B. Schoenfeld and R. Snarr (Champaign, IL: Human Kinetics, 2022).

CHAPTER 10

Fitness Evaluation, Selection, and Administration

Robert Lockie, PhD, and Laura Kobar, MS, MC

After completing this chapter, you will be able to

- explain the purposes of performing physical assessments on a client;

- evaluate a test's validity and reliability;

- determine the factors that contribute to cardiovascular disease to determine suitability for specific tests, ability to begin exercise, or need for medical clearance; and

- select appropriate tests for individual clients.

After conducting the client consultation and health appraisal, the personal trainer needs to gather more information about the client's level of fitness and skills before developing a program. There is no one-size-fits-all test or battery of assessments that will suit each client and circumstance. Selecting appropriate physical assessments requires thoughtful consideration of the client's health and exercise history, the client's personal goals, and the personal trainer's own experience and training in conducting various assessments. Choosing valid and reliable tests suitable for individual clients and conducting them accurately requires practice on the part of the personal trainer. The availability and appropriateness of equipment and facilities, environmental factors, and the client's preassessment preparation influence test selection and implementation. Having determined the assessment protocols, the personal trainer must conduct them accurately, record and manage the data, and interpret the results. Developing an individualized program that incorporates the client's goals and interests is the "personal" in personal training. Implementation of the program requires formative and summative evaluation of the plan, reassessment of the client's fitness levels and goals, and subsequent adjustments to the program in an ongoing cycle.

PURPOSES OF ASSESSMENT

The purposes of assessment are to gather baseline data and to provide a basis for developing goals and effective exercise programs. Gathering and evaluating the various pieces of information give the personal trainer a broader perspective of the client. The process and the data collected assist the personal trainer in identifying potential areas of injury and reasonable starting points for recommended intensities and volumes of exercise based on the goals and fitness outcomes.

The authors would like to acknowledge the significant contributions of Sharon Rana, Jason B. White, John A.C. Kordich, and Susan L. Heinrich to this chapter.

Gathering Baseline Data

There are many valid reasons for administering assessments to clients. The data collected provide

- a baseline for future comparisons of improvement or rate of progress;

- identification of current strengths and weaknesses that may affect program emphasis on specific components;

- assistance in establishing appropriate intensities and volumes of exercise;

- assistance in clarification of short-, intermediate-, and long-term goals;

- identification of areas of potential injury or contraindications before program initiation, which may lead to referral to a physician or other health care professionals; and

- a record demonstrating prudent judgment and appropriate scope of practice in program design should client injuries occur after a program has begun (22, 35).

The assessment process may fall within the services typically provided to all clients, may constitute an additional revenue stream for the personal trainer, or may do both. However, subjecting clients to a seemingly endless barrage of assessments that have little or no relevance to their program goals is a violation of the trust the client places in the personal trainer to gather necessary information to design a program.

Goal and Program Development

The personal trainer can use physical assessment information in conjunction with personal information gathered about the client to plan a time-efficient, specific program that will help the client achieve desired goals. Understanding personal characteristics and current lifestyle factors about the client helps the personal trainer plan sessions that are reasonable in length, frequency, intensity, and complexity so that the client is more likely to continue adhering to the program. Developing goals with a client is critical for both program design and motivation. (Refer to chapter 8 for more details on motivating clients.)

When possible and appropriate, choosing specific tests that are congruent with clients' goals or preferred mode of exercise may give them a clearer picture of their progress and may be more motivating. For highly trained clients, choosing an exercise ergometer that most closely matches their mode of exercise (treadmill, cycle, swim flume) leads to a more accurate assessment of their performance (19, 58). For average or deconditioned clients, the type of test is not as important when assessing aerobic function; however, a treadmill test will usually produce the highest maximal $\dot{V}O_2$ scores (37, 38). Clients who seldom if ever ride a bike may experience local muscular fatigue and as a result achieve a lower estimated $\dot{V}O_2$max value on a bike test compared with a treadmill test (21, 36). In addition, if clients are tested on a cycle ergometer but will not be riding a bike in their program, they may overlook some of the indicators of their improved performance during the training period.

A timed mile can be easily repeated on occasion during a walking program; if clients can cover the distance more quickly or easily with a lower exercise heart rate or rating of perceived exertion (RPE), they know immediately that they are making progress. In this instance an appropriate test may match the type of activity the client enjoys doing. However, for clients who are overweight or who have lower body joint issues that make weight-bearing activities painful, the advantages of a non–weight-bearing cycle test may override any concerns about slightly lower estimates of maximal oxygen consumption. Additionally, since cycling tests give results independent of body weight, they are more accurate indicators of progress for a person on a weight loss program than a treadmill test, whose results are directly related to an individual's body weight (33, 58). Assessment of health- or skill-related fitness components, or both, provides the personal trainer and client with baseline information that will be used to develop safe, effective, and appropriately challenging goals.

CHOOSING APPROPRIATE ASSESSMENTS

A primary duty of the personal trainer is to facilitate improvements in the client's physical well-being without causing harm. With the exception of assessing factors that could contribute to cardiovascular disease, there is no standardized battery of tests one can give each client before designing an appropriate program (2, 33, 45). The first step in individualizing the personal trainer's approach to each client is determining the specific tests to give to measure various parameters of health- and skill-related fitness. These decisions should be based on the client's apparent health and potential for an adverse cardiovascular event as well as the desired program outcomes expressed by the client. In order for the personal trainer to conduct meaningful assessments, appropriate tests must be chosen. Given the wide range of fitness tests available, it is wise for the personal trainer to become educated about which assessments provide the best information for a given client. Assessment is the act of measuring a specific component using a well-constructed, valid, and reliable test and then evaluating and interpreting the results (37). If the evaluation is carried out in accordance with the client's goals, the results will be more meaningful to the client. Assessment can be formal, following specific test protocols, or informal, through observation of the client performing specific activities and exercises.

Formative and Summative Evaluation

There are two ways of looking at assessments—as formative or summative evaluations. **Formative evaluations** include formal assessment with a specified **test protocol**, as well as the subjective observations the personal trainer makes during each interaction with the client. The formative assessments take place before a program begins and periodically throughout the training period. They offer the personal trainer opportunities to formulate or plan a program, give the client feedback, and make modifications to the program while it is still in progress.

Although this chapter covers selecting the specific assessment instruments, it is important to keep in mind that every observation of a client provides important data that the personal trainer must consider in designing, implementing, and modifying that client's program. Subjective observations are variable between evaluators and might include noticing posture, gait, exercise technique, response to cardiovascular exercise, comments or body language relating to specific exercises or suggestions, and daily energy levels in each exercise session. These provide immediate opportunities for the personal trainer to focus on educating, motivating, and modifying activities for the client. Data from specific test protocols provide objective evidence that the personal trainer can compare against relevant standards to interpret the client's performance.

Summative evaluations are made when a client completes a specified training period, class, or season. They represent the sum total of what has been accomplished in a given period. The same assessments used

at the beginning and midpoint of an exercise program can and generally should be used to provide the final evaluation, but how the results are used will differ. For example, if a client has a flexibility goal for a specific joint, the formative evaluation would have included an initial measurement of the range of motion in the joint and a realistic goal for improved flexibility of that joint. The program might include a variety of stretching techniques for that joint with periodic repetitions of the test so the client knows the amount of progress being made toward the goal. At the end of the specified period, the same test is repeated under similar conditions, and the client and personal trainer can determine whether the stated goals were achieved in that time: This evaluation is a summary of what was achieved during the specified training period.

Assessment Terminology

Before selecting tests to use with a specific client, the personal trainer must have an understanding of the terminology specific to tests, measurements, and evaluation, and to some extent, the process by which tests are developed. The purpose of this chapter is not to list or explain all the possible choices of assessment instruments available for each health- and skill-related component and each type of client (sedentary, athletic, healthy, or medically compromised). As new research and tests are reported, personal trainers need to evaluate new information and decide whether it has a place in the battery of tests used for their particular clientele. A test may be excellent in terms of validity and reliability but still not be appropriate for a specific client—for example, a near-maximal exertion running test would not be appropriate for a deconditioned adult (25, 41). Additionally, although some tests may be excellent for measuring a specific component or trait, they may require equipment, facilities, or expertise that the personal trainer does not have (e.g., hydrostatic weighing). Conversely, the fact that a particular piece of equipment or computer-generated test battery is available does not make it appropriate for all clients. For example, if a client is visibly obese, it might not be necessary or accurate to assess body composition via the skinfold method, but it would be fine to simply use body mass index until weight loss occurs.

The personal trainer must sort through the information and select tests appropriate to each client while recognizing that some clients will be more interested in personal progress than in multiple formal assessments. The objective of the personal trainer in selecting assessments for the client is to reduce error and increase the accuracy of the assessment. Questions to answer in attempting to improve the accuracy of a test include the following:

- How reliable and objective was the assessment?
- Was it valid?
- Was the equipment calibrated, and did it produce accurate results?
- Was the subject physically or emotionally influenced by anything before or during the test that may have affected the results?
- Was the test protocol followed carefully and were data collected accurately?

When these factors receive adequate attention, the personal trainer may confidently and accurately interpret data and apply the results.

Reliability and Objectivity

Reliability is a measure of repeatability or consistency of a test or an observation (37). To determine if a measurement is reliable, one must measure the same trait under the same conditions, with no intervention (e.g., physical conditioning, diet) before a subsequent measurement is performed. If the results of the test are the same from one trial to another, the test is reliable. A common method of determining reliability of a test is the **test–retest method**. This is when a test is repeated with the same individual or group within one to three days, and sometimes up to one week later if the test is particularly strenuous (52). In order for a test to be reliable, the person conducting the test must be consistent when administering it. This is called intrarater reliability and can be determined as just described. However, a personal trainer could be consistent but not accurate. Therefore, scores collected by different personal trainers on the same client without intervention should be compared in order to determine interrater reliability or objectivity (7, 37, 52). If more than one personal trainer can consistently get the same result from a client, the test is objective rather than subjective. It is not practical to test a client multiple times per day or week on the same assessment, so the personal trainer must look for assessments that were found to have good reliability when they were developed. However, the fact that an assessment has good reliability is meaningless if the personal trainer does not take the time to practice giving the assessment under very strict and standardized conditions (35). Factors affecting reliability will be discussed later in the chapter; those that relate to the personal

trainer can include competence, confidence, concentration on the task, familiarity with the instrument, and motivation (8).

Validity

Validity indicates that a test measures what it is supposed to measure (52). In other words, is the test score truthful (37)? Does the assessment instrument really test what it claims to be testing? For example, when selecting a test for aerobic capacity, one must choose a test that is long enough and is sufficiently intense to require provision of energy primarily from the aerobic system. Therefore, the 50-yard or -meter sprint would not give a valid or truthful measure of aerobic capacity ($\dot{V}O_2$max). For a test to be valid, it must also be relevant (37). The relevance indicates how well the test matches the objectives of testing. In the example just mentioned, a test of speed is not relevant for assessing aerobic capacity. A body mass index (BMI) measurement is a relevant indicator of overweight status in a fairly sedentary population, but it is not relevant to a group of athletes with increased lean muscle mass and a low percentage of body fat (23, 26, 42). **Face validity**, then, means the test appears to test what it is supposed to test (35, 52). In this sense, a 1RM test is a valid measure of muscular strength but not muscular flexibility. A related term is **content validity**, which indicates an expert has determined that a test covers all topics or abilities it should (35, 52). For example, a volleyball athlete should be tested on more than just jumping ability in order to cover all skills performed in that particular sport (18, 53).

Construct validity is a theoretical concept meaning a test is able to differentiate between performance abilities. In other words, if a test is to measure sport skills, those with the relevant skills should score better on the test than those who take the test without having previously acquired the skills (25, 37, 52).

Criterion-related validity allows personal trainers to use tests in the field or in the fitness center instead of tests that can be performed only in a laboratory setting or with expensive equipment, because the laboratory test results and field test results have been statistically compared with each other (37). A maximal-exertion stress test should be given only in a controlled environment, and depending on the client, with medical personnel and equipment on hand (2, 41, 44). Since that is not practical in a fitness center setting, personal trainers can select a submaximal cardiovascular endurance test, such as a treadmill test, a step test, or a cycle ergometer test that has been statistically correlated to the maximal exertion tests on the basis of certain assumptions. The assumptions are that the more fit the individual is, the more work he or she should be able to do at a given heart rate and the more total work he or she should be able to perform before reaching maximal heart rate (43). The results on the submaximal tests are not precisely the same as those on the maximal test, nor will the estimated $\dot{V}O_2$ max score on different types of submaximal tests identically match each other. However, if the margin of error between the submaximal and maximal tests is small and the test is reliable and valid, then it is a good test. The following should serve as an example of these points.

Hydrostatic weighing is an **indirect measure** or estimate of body fatness, based on the assumption that the body is made up of fat mass and fat free mass (23, 57). An autopsy is a **direct measure**, but because it cannot be used on living individuals it is not a useful measure. Other common methods (field methods) of assessing body composition such as skinfold assessments, bioelectrical impedance (BIA), near-infrared interactance (NIR), or anthropometric measures are doubly indirect (14). This means the statistical relationship is with hydrostatic weighing, and the standard error of estimating body composition is established against hydrostatic weighing, not against the direct method. The error involved in assessing body composition with a doubly indirect test may be higher than with an indirect test. Also, when a specific test is selected to assess a client, the same test should be used for any further testing of the given fitness component. A skinfold estimate of body fatness cannot be reliably compared against an estimate made by means of BIA or NIR, for example (20). (See chapter 11 for further discussion.)

> A valid test is one that measures what it purports to measure. A reliable test is one that can be repeated with accuracy by the same tester or another. A good assessment instrument is both valid and reliable.

Factors That Affect Reliability and Validity

All tests have a **standard error of measurement**, which is the difference between a person's observed score—what the result was—and that person's true score, a theoretically errorless score. For example, when choosing to assess body composition using the skinfold technique, a personal trainer must understand that this measurement will involve some error. A skinfold can only estimate the percent fat (observed score); it cannot measure the client's actual percent fat (true score). Empirically any test result consists of a true score and error. All test results contain the true value of the factor being measured as well as the errors associated with the test itself. Measurement error can arise from several sources, including the client, the personal trainer, the equipment, or the environment (35, 37).

Client Factors

To select appropriate tests, the personal trainer must consider several factors that may influence client performance and subsequently have an impact on the validity and reliability of the assessment results. These key client factors include health status and functional capacity, age, sex, and pretraining status.

Health Status and Functional Capacity The health status and functional capacity of a client dictate which assessments are appropriate. Information gathered during the preparticipation screening process (see chapter 9) should be used to identify potential physical limitations. Understanding those limits provides a context for selecting assessments that will reasonably match the capabilities of the individual. As an example, if an individual is sedentary, over the age of 60, and has a functional aerobic capacity of 5 METs (MET = **metabolic equivalent**; 1 MET is equal to an oxygen consumption of 3.5 ml · kg⁻¹ · min⁻¹ and is an estimate of a person's oxygen consumption at rest), it may be unreasonable for that person to perform the YMCA step test or 1.5-mile (2.4 km) run. Both of these assessments may require a greater metabolic level of performance than 5 METs and in some instances may be considered near-maximal tests for deconditioned individuals (2, 4, 25). Also, client fatigue (and motivation), whether a function of recent activities, food and fluid intake, or sleeping patterns, or due to the number and physical demands of the assessments being administered in one session, will influence the assessment outcomes (9).

Age Chronological age and maturity may influence testing performance. For example, the 1.5-mile (2.4 km) run is considered a standard field test to measure aerobic capacity for apparently healthy college-age men and women. However, this same assessment will not appropriately measure aerobic ability of preadolescents, primarily because of the immature physical development of the cardiovascular system and the experiential maturity needed to cover the distance by pacing (13). A better choice for children may be the timed 1-mile (1.6 km) run, the 9-minute run for distance, or the PACER (9, 34, 54); and for older clients the 1-mile walk has been recommended as a safer field test (40).

Sex Sex-specific biological factors may influence performance in a variety of activities or assessments such as the chin-up, push-up, and bench press to assess muscular endurance of the upper extremities. Several differences between men and women appear to influence performance: Women tend to have more body fat and less muscle, plus a smaller shoulder structure that supports less muscle tissue, and as a result less of a mechanical advantage for muscles working at the shoulder (30, 55). For example, the chin-up test appears to provide reliable results for males; however, it may in some cases fail to differentiate between strength and muscular endurance for females. As a result, the flexed arm hang is sometimes used as an alternative method to assess muscular endurance, through a static rather than a dynamic muscular action, by measuring the length of time the flexed elbow hang position can be sustained. Also, push-up tests to measure dynamic muscular fitness of the upper body include a variation to accommodate for the differences in upper body strength; this modification uses the same standard military push-up position as for men with the exceptions that the knees are flexed, the lower legs are in contact with the testing surface, and the ankles are plantar flexed (2, 29). In addition, the YMCA fixed-load bench press test provides different fixed loads for men and women (35 pounds [16 kg] for women and 80 pounds [36 kg] for men), illustrating the sex-specific differences related to client factors that should be considered when selecting appropriate tests (20). (See chapter 11 for the complete procedures for these tests.)

Pretraining Status The pretraining status of the client may affect test selection when the skills required for the test and the relative level of exertion are considered. Caution should be emphasized in assessment of untrained, deconditioned individuals, even when they express a desire to achieve high performance levels. For example, the 1.5-mile (2.4 km) run test and the 12-minute run test are considered near-maximal-exertion tests, as they require the individual to cover distance as quickly as possible (2, 4, 25, 39). A deconditioned client should have a period of at least four to six weeks of aerobic conditioning before participating in either of these assessments (41). Clients who are unaccustomed to pacing themselves may do better on subsequent trials of a 1-mile (1.6 km) walk test as they learn to adjust their initial pace with a practice trial (37, 39). Similarly, clients who do not have an opportunity to practice a footwork pattern for an agility test may not get an accurate score. Allowing the client time to practice the movement pattern will yield a better indication of the person's agility (37).

Likewise, a 1-repetition maximum (1RM) test in the squat movement may be appropriate for a conditioned individual who has previous experience with that free-weight movement pattern. However, for someone with no pretraining experience, the lack of motor skill and the intensity required for the exercise may create an unacceptably high risk for injury (15, 27, 32). The greater the load, the more stress the joints, muscles, bones, and connective tissues experience (5, 6, 48). In order to improve safety and reliability, it may be necessary to modify the test to one that estimates maximal strength with a submaximal load, such as a 10RM (32). One or more practice sessions of the specific exercise with a lighter load to learn the proper technique may be necessary. For the untrained person, adaptations in the coordination of the neuromuscular system may account for most of the initial strength gains in a resistance training program (5, 15, 36). Even so, a familiarization period may be prudent to acquaint the untrained individual with the new skill involved in the movement and to protect the person from injury. The length of the familiarization period varies by client and the relative intensity required by the strength test chosen.

Some muscular endurance tests may involve resistances heavy enough that untrained clients can perform only a limited number of repetitions. For example, clients with weak or smaller upper body muscles (e.g., younger and older clients, some women, sedentary clients) will not be able to complete very many repetitions (i.e., <6) in the push-up test because their body weight—even using the modified body position—is simply too heavy. For these clients, the push-up test can be used to assess muscular strength, and another test of upper body muscle endurance would be more appropriate, such as the YMCA bench press test, which will be more accurate if the client has experience with lifting.

Personal Trainer Factors

The level of experience and training of the personal trainer has an impact on the selection of assessments. To maintain objectivity and reduce intrarater error, testing protocols that require adept technical skills need to match the abilities of the personal trainer. As an example, theoretical prediction errors of ±3.5% or less body fat are considered acceptable on various equations and combinations of skinfold measurements to assess body composition (23), but tester error may account for 3% to 9% variability between raters (interrater reliability) (23). Errors can be further compounded by failure to follow a protocol, inaccurate identification of measurement sites, improperly calibrated equipment, and the choice of prediction equations (23). Taking accurate skinfold measurements is a complicated skill that requires about 100 practice opportunities on different clients in order for the personal trainer to gain adequate proficiency (23). To develop intrarater consistency, the personal trainer should perform the measurements on different sites and body types (23).

The relative test difficulty and the type of measurement required can affect outcomes. It is not reasonable to expect a personal trainer to read through a protocol, administer an assessment to a client, and get good results without practice. Some tests require quite a bit more skill and practice than others. For example, relatively little skill is required to manage a

> **Personal trainers who are unfamiliar with administration of an assessment should not select it but should continue their professional development by taking time to practice administration of the assessment for use with future clients.**

stopwatch and monitor heart rate for a timed 1-mile (1.6 km) walk or run test. On the other hand, the skills required to get reliable results on a noncomputerized cycle ergometer test are much more complex (e.g., monitoring and adjusting the workload and pedal cadence on the ergometer; obtaining heart rates every minute of the test) (24, 45).

Equipment Factors

Any mechanism or device used to measure work, performance, or physiological response requires **calibration**, or the adjusting of the device to ensure precision, in order to accurately measure the specific trait being assessed. Through calibration one checks the accuracy of a measuring device to provide an accurate reading. Reliability, validity, and objectivity of the assessment are directly affected by the accuracy of the measurement tool. Common mechanisms and devices used in the assessment process that require calibration are cycle, stepping, and treadmill ergometers; blood pressure sphygmomanometers; skinfold calipers and body composition mechanisms; metronomes; and other electronic devices used to measure time, distance, and power. To ensure the accuracy of equipment, it is important to institute a scheduled plan for checking and calibrating mechanisms and devices according to manufacturer specification and based on warranty recommendations (2, 25).

Environmental Factors

Climatic elements and the physical setting of the environment present potential concerns that may influence client performance and safety. Consequently when the personal trainer is selecting and administering tests, it is necessary to consider environmental planning and quality control assurance related to weather, altitude, air pollution, and the physical setting of a facility.

Temperature and Humidity   The environment poses challenges related to physiological responses that may have an impact on test administration and performance. High heat and humidity and cold weather exposure need to be considered in the selection of assessments. High ambient temperatures in combination with high humidity inhibit the body's thermoregulatory system from dissipating heat, which impedes physical endurance performance, poses health risks, and affects test results. The personal trainer should be aware of the thresholds of a combined temperature and humidity above which participation in continuous activity may increase the risk of heat injury and also affect performance (12). For example, between 65 and 72 °F (18.4-22.2 °C) and 65.1% and 72% humidity, the risk of exertional heatstroke begins to rise (3, 12). Geographic areas that experience high temperatures along with high humidity may not be suitable for outdoor tests to assess aerobic endurance since performance may be affected. Furthermore, a period of acclimatization to higher temperatures (and humidity) may be necessary for testing in an area with seasonal fluctuations in temperatures (51).

Exposure to cold temperatures, less than 25 °F (-4 °C), may not have a significant impact on the performance and health of younger, apparently healthy individuals; however, older people and those who have cardiovascular and circulatory disorders and respiratory problems may need to use caution. Cold exposure may stimulate the sympathetic nervous system, which can affect total peripheral resistance, arterial pressure, myocardial contraction, and cardiac work (41, 56). Of particular concern are outdoor performances that require significant effort of the upper extremities. Clients with respiratory conditions, particularly asthma, may also be more prone to problems in cold temperatures, as cold air may trigger a bronchial spasm (2, 50).

Altitude Altitude can also impair aerobic endurance performance. Tests to measure aerobic endurance may not correlate with normative performance data when assessment takes place at altitudes higher than 1,900 feet (~580 m) (17). In addition, individuals not acclimated to altitude changes may require an adaptation period of 7 to 12 days before engaging in aerobic endurance assessments (2).

Air Pollution Another environmental consideration is the **air quality index (AQI)**. This is a measure of air quality as it relates to pollutants. Pollution can have a negative effect on performance and health by decreasing the ability of the blood to transport oxygen, by increasing the resistance in the airways, and by altering the perception of effort for a given task (16, 41). The AQI is usually reported in local weather forecasts, and the personal trainer should become knowledgeable about which groups of individuals are sensitive to given levels of the AQI (41). See table 10.1 for more information regarding AQI and health concerns (1).

Test Setting Issues associated with health and environmental control are important factors related to assessment validity and reliability. To minimize external distractions and the potential anxiety related to the assessment process, the testing area should be quiet and private. The personal trainer should project a positive, relaxed, confident demeanor; and the process should be clearly explained and not rushed. The testing room should be well equipped with comfortable furnishings and standardized and calibrated testing devices. The room temperature should be set at 68 to 72 °F (20-22 °C), with 60% or less humidity and adequate air flow (2). Physical facilities must be inspected for deficiencies, and safety procedures need to be clearly documented and posted. Appropriate emergency equipment must be operable and immediately available in the event that an incident requires an emergency response (10). (See chapter 25 for more details about recommended facility characteristics.)

> **The integrity of the assessment process depends on the validity and reliability of the assessments selected and proper administration by a trained fitness professional. Personal trainers should take care to enhance reliability by consistently attending to controllable factors related to the client, personal trainer, equipment, and environment.**

ASSESSMENT CASE STUDIES

The most important required assessments for initiating and designing an exercise program are of the client's risk factors for cardiovascular disease and the potential contraindications for specific activities because of known musculoskeletal limitations or diseases. The outcome of the health screening process dictates the selection and administration of all other assessments. Before selecting the assessment instruments for each client, the personal trainer must also consider other factors, including the client's exercise goals, exercise history, and attitudes about assessments; his or her own experience and skill in performing the assessments; and the equipment and facilities available. In most cases, more than one assessment instrument may be used to collect the information needed to design a program.

> **Selecting valid, reliable, and safe assessments that will provide meaningful results requires an understanding of the health status, risk factors for cardiovascular disease, and goals of the client; a high level of experience of the personal trainer; the availability of relevant equipment; and knowledge of the specific test characteristics associated with the assessment.**

TABLE 10.1   Air Quality Index Levels

AQI levels of health concern	Numerical value	Meaning
Good	0-50	Air quality is considered satisfactory, and air pollution poses little or no risk.
Moderate	51-100	Air quality is acceptable; however, for some pollutants there may be a moderate health concern for a very small number of people who are unusually sensitive to air pollution.
Unhealthy for sensitive groups	101-150	Members of sensitive groups may experience health effects. The general public is not likely to be affected.
Unhealthy	151-200	Everyone may begin to experience health effects. Members of sensitive groups may experience more serious health effects.
Very unhealthy	201-300	Health alert: Everyone may experience more serious health effects.
Hazardous	>300	Health warnings of emergency conditions. The entire population is more likely to be affected.

Reprinted from AirNow (1).

MARIA G.

Maria G. is a 57-year-old grandmother of four who has been active most of her life. She is 5 feet, 5 inches (165.1 cm) tall and weighs 144 pounds (65.5 kg). She participated in step aerobics and spinning classes three or four times per week at her old club before she moved to be closer to her daughters' families. She is planning on resuming those activities at her new club. She also enjoys occasional games of recreational tennis and golf with her friends. She would like to increase her strength because she is helping more with the toddlers and finds carrying them and their gear tiring. She has never been a smoker, although her husband still smokes a pack a day. Her father died at age 73 in a car accident, and her 82-year-old mother is still alive.

Last month, a local hospital sponsored a health fair, and Maria took full advantage of the screening opportunities. Her average blood pressure was 129/79 mmHg. Her total cholesterol was 231 mg/dl, with a low-density lipoprotein (LDL) count of 150 mg/dl and a high-density lipoprotein (HDL) score of 65 mg/dl. Her fasting glucose was 93 mg/dl. She also had her body fat tested with a handheld BIA device and was told she was 28% fat. She has no other health problems. See the "Individual Assessment Recording Form for Maria" for a summary of the assessment findings.

Health Screening Analysis for Exercise Participation

Do the results indicate Maria requires a medical clearance? Maria currently participates in regular physical activity; has no known cardiovascular, renal, or metabolic disease; and has no signs or symptoms of disease. Although the results from Maria's health screening report borderline total cholesterol levels (above 200 mg/dl) and LDL level (above 130 mg/dl), she does not require medical clearance to continue exercise participation.

Assessment Recommendations

What assessment recommendations would be appropriate for this client? For assessment of cardiovascular endurance, the personal trainer has several choices of activities. Since Maria has been consistently active in aerobic exercise, she would be a candidate for one of the tests that require some preconditioning (e.g., 1.5-mile [2.4 km] run test, 12-minute run test, and the multistage YMCA cycle ergometer test) (2, 25). Single-stage or graded treadmill tests, walking tests, cycling tests, and step tests (12-inch or 30 cm step, or lower) would be acceptable choices since she has no joint complaints and used to participate in two of the three activities.

Since Maria has not been performing a resistance training program, maximal (1RM) strength tests are not recommended. Performing a muscular endurance test such as the YMCA fixed-weight bench press test may pose no problem since she has been active, but the exercises are unfamiliar to Maria. It would be best to wait until she is comfortable with the mechanics of performing the exercises and becomes better trained to perform standardized strength assessment. However, because of her relatively weak upper body, the personal trainer could choose to use a submaximal load on the bench press to estimate Maria's 1RM and thus her relative strength in order to assess baseline upper body strength. The personal trainer could allow the client to practice the bench press movement before performing the submaximal test so the results would be more valid, as long as full rest is given between the practice and the actual assessment.

If Maria had expressed concerns related to body weight or body size, it would be prudent to repeat a test for body composition under the prescribed conditions to get the baseline data for future comparisons, since the testing conditions at the health fair are unknown. For measures of body fat, it is recommended that the same test be administered under the same conditions by the same tester (20). Therefore, Maria could be retested with, for example, skinfold calipers if the personal trainer is skilled in using this tool. Circumference measures, especially around the waist, would also provide baseline data for health risks related to excess abdominal fat and allow Maria to track changes in her body after participating in an exercise program. (See chapter 11 for further discussion of how to perform these anthropometric measurements.)

Maria has not expressed a desire to improve athletic performance, and therefore tests for agility, speed, and power are not necessary at this time. Balance, reaction time, and coordination issues related to her activities of daily living may become more apparent and require further investigation or programming in the future. If the client continues to participate in tennis and golf, she may welcome some activities related to improved performance after the personal trainer has designed a program to meet her current goal of increased functional strength.

Pretest / Posttest (circle one)

Client's name: Maria G.   **Age:** 57

Goals: Increase muscular strength; maintain aerobic capacity and body composition; improve balance and blood lipid profile.

Preparticipation screening notes: Maria is physically active and asymptomatic with no known cardiovascular, metabolic, or renal disease and therefore may continue her usual exercise and progress gradually as tolerated.

Assessment dates: 8/9/21; 8/11/21

Comments: Will reevaluate % body fat using skinfold calipers; she previously was active but has not exercised recently; wants to begin aerobic classes again; recently completed lipid screening (cholesterol: 231 mg/dl; LDL: 150 mg/dl; HDL: 65 mg/dl; fasting glucose: 93 mg/dl); husband is smoker.

Vital signs	Score or result	Classification[a]	Examples and norm- and criterion-referenced standards (see chapter 11)
Resting blood pressure	129/79	Elevated	Table 11.2
Resting heart rate	72 beats/min	Average	Table 11.1
Body composition measures	**Score or result**	**Classification[a]**	
Height	5 ft 5 in. (165.1 cm)	Percentile: ~75th	Table 11.6
Weight	144 lb (65.5 kg)	--	--
Body mass index (BMI)	24.0	Normal (healthy)	Table 11.7
Waist circumference	29 in. (73.7 cm)	Under the 88 cm (35 in.) cutoff	Table 11.4
Hip circumference	36 in. (91.4 cm)	--	--
Waist-to-hip ratio	0.81	Moderate risk	Table 11.11
Percent body fat Method: BIA	28%	Percentile: ~50th Criterion: leaner than average	Percentile: table 11.10 Criterion: table 11.10
Cardiovascular endurance	**Score or result**	**Classification[a]**	
Åstrand-Rhyming cycle test initial work rate: 450 kg · m⁻¹ · min⁻¹	28.64 ml · kg⁻¹ · min⁻¹	Criterion: good	Criterion: table 11.18
Muscular endurance	**Score or result**	**Classification[a]**	
YMCA bench press test weight: 35 lb (16 kg)	9 reps at 35 lb (16 kg)	Percentile: 50th	Table 11.25
Muscular strength	**Score or result**	**Classification[a]**	
Estimate a 1RM bench press with a submaximal load	1RM estimated as 60 lb (27 kg), which is ~42% of body weight	Percentile: ~90th	Table 11.23
Flexibility	**Score or result**	**Classification[a]**	
YMCA sit-and-reach test	13 in. (33 cm)	Percentile: 30th	Table 11.28
Other tests	**Score or result**	**Classification[a]**	
Thomas hip range of motion test[b]	Both tested legs remained on floor	Adequate hip flexor flexibility	--
One-foot stand test, eyes open[c]	Right: 6 s Left: 9 s	Below average	--

[a]Classification refers to either the norm- or criterion-referenced standard, depending on the test and protocol. Refer to the examples and the norm and criterion-referenced standards provided in chapter 11 for a further explanation of how the classification labels were assigned to Maria's results.

[b]Protocol and normative data in Howley and Franks (25).

[c]Protocol and normative data in Springer et al. (47).

CASE STUDY 10.2

PAUL C.

Paul C. is a 28-year-old accountant in a very busy office. He is 6 feet (182.9 cm) tall and weighs 260 pounds (117.9 kg) and has never smoked or used tobacco products. Paul's father had two heart attacks prior to his death at age 47, and Paul's 34-year-old brother recently underwent triple-bypass surgery after experiencing chest pains. His mother has type 2 diabetes, which is under control. Paul has not had his fasting blood glucose measured. During the initial interview, his blood pressure measured 150/96 mmHg; his percentage of body fat was 30, and his waist measurement was 41 inches (104.1 cm) compared with a hip measurement of 44 inches (111.8 cm). His last cholesterol test was over six months ago, and he does not recall the numbers but states, "The doctor didn't say anything, so I guess it was okay." Paul has developed asthma, induced by seasonal allergies and exercise. He has an inhaler of albuterol and finds that activity easily winds him, sometimes precipitating an asthma attack. He also reports some intermittent pain in his left knee, probably related to a fall several months ago. He has not had the knee examined by the doctor. Paul has come in at his wife's insistence because she is concerned that he is as much a candidate for a heart attack as his brother was. He has never been active or enjoyed exercise and is concerned about how to fit activity into his busy work schedule.

Health Screening Analysis for Exercise Participation

Do the results indicate Paul requires medical clearance? Paul has never been active, and he reports possible symptoms of cardiovascular, metabolic, or renal disease. There is family history of cardiovascular disease, with both his father and brother having experienced heart attacks or cardiovascular disease before age 55. His BMI is 35.3, which places him in obesity class II (very high risk) (see table 11.4 on page 245). The other anthropometric measures also support excess visceral fat, which puts Paul at high risk of cardiovascular disease. Notably, Paul's body fat is ≥30% (see table 11.10 on page 250), his waist circumference is >40 inches (102 cm), and his waist-to-hip ratio is 0.93 (see table 11.11 on page 251). Paul has intermittent pain in his left knee, which may be due to the reported fall several months ago; however, it may also suggest intermittent claudication beginning in the thigh. He reports developing asthma from seasonal allergies and exercise, but he also becomes easily winded from activity, which may be a sign or symptom of cardiovascular disease. The results indicate Paul should seek medical clearance before beginning an exercise program.

Assessment Recommendations

Given Paul's situation, his physician may choose to perform a diagnostic stress test. If that is the case and Paul is released for a program of limited activity, the personal trainer can use the maximal heart rate and maximal oxygen consumption data from the stress test to design the exercise program. If Paul is not stress tested and is released for moderate exercise, the assessment of cardiovascular function will be submaximal, with a bike test as possibly the most appropriate since it is non–weight bearing and may put the least stress on his left knee. Additional consideration needs to be given to some of the other information provided by this client. He is not an active person, does not particularly enjoy exercise, and is already erecting roadblocks in terms of finding time to exercise. He appears to be in the contemplation, or possibly preparation, stage of readiness for lifestyle change. (See chapter 8 for more information about psychological readiness for exercise.) Also, the personal trainer could have Paul complete "The Attitudinal Assessment" form (see chapter 9, p.157), which gauges attitudes toward exercise. While awaiting the physician's release, Paul may benefit from a consultation with a nutrition specialist as well as sessions to discuss goal setting, his readiness to change lifestyle behaviors, and strategies to enhance his adherence to a program.

ADMINISTRATION AND ORGANIZATION OF FITNESS ASSESSMENTS

Administration of a fitness assessment requires advanced preparation and organization to ensure psychometrically sound results and safe outcomes. When organizing and administering the fitness assessment process, the personal trainer must pay close attention to factors that will have an impact on obtaining safe, accurate, and meaningful results.

Test Preparation

Appropriate and valuable test outcomes are predicated on the ability of the personal trainer to prepare clients by educating them as to the content of the test, pretest requirements, and expectations of the assessment process. Preparation to evaluate someone's level of fitness requires the personal trainer to execute preassessment screening procedures, review safety considerations, select appropriate assessments, select facilities and verify accuracy of equipment, and perform record-keeping responsibilities. Review the "Test Preparation and Implementation Checklist" located at the end of this chapter.

Conduct Preassessment Screening Procedures and Review Safety Considerations

A fitness assessment procedure should be implemented only after a thorough preactivity screening that includes an initial interview, execution of a health appraisal tool, completion of appropriate forms, and, when required, recommendations from a physician regarding the management of medical contraindications (see chapter 9). Documented risks are associated with exercise testing; however, evidence suggests that complications are relatively low (e.g., 0.06%, or 6 per 10,000) (2).

Verify Appropriateness of Selected Assessments

Selecting valid, reliable, and safe assessments that will provide meaningful results requires an understanding of the goals and health status of the client, level of experience of the personal trainer, and the specific test characteristics associated with the assessment.

Select Facilities and Verify Accuracy of Equipment

Ease of administration, cost-effectiveness, availability of equipment, and the facility setting influence the selection and implementation of the assessment process. Two types of assessments, laboratory tests and field tests, may be administered to yield valuable results; but in most situations they are administered under different conditions. **Laboratory tests**, in most cases, are performed in clinical facilities using specialized diagnostic equipment to assess an individual's maximal functional capacity. Examples of laboratory tests include the use of a metabolic cart to measure oxygen consumption and hydrostatic weighing to measure body composition. Testing is relatively complex, and direct-measurement tools are used to reduce data error and quantify results based on physiological responses. Because of the diagnostic capabilities of the tests and the high risk of cardiac complications, allied health professionals are responsible for administering the assessment and evaluation process of laboratory tests. For these tests, it is helpful to have equipment such as the following:

- Bicycle ergometer or treadmill
- Equipment for measuring body composition (e.g., skinfold calipers)
- Equipment for measuring flexibility (e.g., goniometer or sit-and-reach box)
- Equipment for measuring the force of muscular contraction (e.g., dynamometer)
- Perceived exertion chart
- Stopwatch
- Metronome
- Sphygmomanometer
- Stethoscope
- Tape measure
- Bodyweight scale
- First aid kit
- Automated external defibrillator (AED) (11)

Field tests are practical assessments that are inexpensive, are easy to administer, require less equipment, are less time consuming, can be performed at various venues, and may be more efficient for evaluating large groups. Examples of field tests include walk/run tests, agility tests, and 1RM tests. The assessments may be submaximal or maximal and are usually administered by a certified fitness professional. These assessments, which are not diagnostic, use indirect measurements to quantify and extrapolate performance results. The major concerns with the maximal assessments are the potential risks that exist as a result of an individual's putting forth a maximal effort without being monitored with diagnostic devices. Because of the cost of laboratory equipment and the consideration of ease of administration, it may not be practical or appropriate for the personal trainer to implement laboratory testing. In any case, one can use field tests effectively and efficiently to obtain the information needed to assess performance and compare against norm- or criterion-referenced standards.

Instruct Client on Preassessment Protocols

An appointment for the assessment should be scheduled in advance in order for the client to adequately prepare mentally and physically for the event. The client should receive pretest instructions in preparation for the assessment. These include

- adequate rest (e.g., 6 to 8 hours the night before and no vigorous exercise 24 hours preceding the test);
- moderate food intake (e.g., a light meal or snack 2 to 4 hours before the test);
- adequate hydration

- abstinence from chemicals that accelerate heart rate (with the exception of prescribed medications);
- proper attire (e.g., loose-fitting clothing; sturdy athletic shoes);
- specific testing procedures and expectations before, during, and after the test; and
- conditions for terminating a test.

It is important for clients to be told that they may terminate a test for any reason at any time. Also, occasionally it may be necessary, for safety reasons, for the personal trainer to terminate a test before its completion. Reasons for stopping a test when performed without direct involvement of a physician or electrocardiographic monitoring are listed in "General Indications for Stopping an Exercise Test" (2). If a test must be terminated abruptly, it should be followed by a 5- to 15-minute cooldown period, when possible.

Prepare Record-Keeping System

An organized method to collect, record, and store data is critical in reducing the incidence of error and is instrumental to the evaluation and interpretation of testing results. Creating a systematic method for collecting and storing data is one of the professional responsibilities associated with the role of the personal trainer. In addition, documentation may provide evidence of reasonable and prudent care in the event that the standard of care is questioned and litigation is pursued (46).

GENERAL INDICATIONS FOR STOPPING AN EXERCISE TEST

- Onset of angina or angina-like symptoms
- Drop in systolic BP of ≥10 mmHg with an increase in workload, or if SBP decreases below the value obtained in the same position prior to testing
- Excessive rise in BP: systolic pressure >250 mmHg and/or diastolic pressure >115 mmHg
- Shortness of breath, wheezing, leg cramps, or claudication
- Signs of poor perfusion (e.g., light-headedness, confusion, ataxia, pallor, cyanosis, cold or clammy skin, or nausea)
- Failure of HR to rise with increased exercise intensity
- Noticeable change in heart rhythm by palpation, auscultation, or ECG
- Client requests to stop
- Physical or verbal manifestations of severe fatigue
- Failure of the testing equipment

Adapted from American College of Sports Medicine (2).

A systematic approach to data collection would include manual recording forms or software programs that allow documentation of raw scores expressed in specific units of measurement. Recording devices should also contain vital client information related to the assessment process and provide space for comments pertaining to the collection of data during the process. In addition, the data collection system should be organized so that testing results can be retrieved from it in a time-efficient manner. This feature is especially important when one is making pretest-to-posttest comparisons during the reassessment process. The system should also have a protective mechanism to ensure confidentiality. See the blank copy of the "Individual Assessment Recording Form" (used in case study 10.1) as an example of an assessment recording form that you may use.

Test Implementation

Organizing and implementing an assessment procedure requires the personal trainer's detailed attention to a number of tasks: identifying the sequence of the assessments, defining and following testing protocols, collecting and interpreting data, and scheduling a review of the results. Refer to the "Test Preparation and Implementation Checklist" on page 192.

Determine Sequence of Assessments

When organizing a testing protocol, the personal trainer must determine the proper order of testing to ensure optimal performance and adequate rest and recovery. Test order is influenced by many factors including the number of clients to be tested, components to be evaluated, skill involved, energy system demand, time available, and specific goal of the client. Many clients do not require a battery of tests as inclusive as the lists that follow. There are multiple strategies for ordering tests; however, the following are examples of logical sequences for clients with general fitness or athletic performance–related goals (35):

General Fitness

1. Resting tests (e.g., resting heart rate, blood pressure, height, weight, body composition)
2. Nonfatiguing tests (e.g., flexibility, balance)
3. Muscular strength tests (e.g., 10RM bench press)
4. Local muscular endurance tests (e.g., YMCA bench press test, partial curl-up test)

5. Submaximal aerobic capacity tests (e.g., step test, Rockport walking test, Åstrand-Rhyming cycle ergometer test, 1.5-mile [2.4 km] run, 12-minute run/walk)

Athletic Performance

1. Resting tests (e.g., resting heart rate, blood pressure, height, weight, body composition)
2. Nonfatiguing tests (e.g., flexibility, vertical jump)
3. Agility tests (e.g., T-test)
4. Maximum power and strength tests (e.g., 3RM power clean, 1RM bench press)
5. Sprint tests (e.g., 40-yard [36.6 m] sprint)
6. Local muscular endurance tests (e.g., 2-minute sit-up test, 1-minute push-up test)
7. Anaerobic capacity tests (e.g., 300-yard [274.3 m] shuttle run, Wingate anaerobic test)
8. Maximal or submaximal aerobic capacity tests (e.g., maximum treadmill test, 1.5-mile [2.4 km] run, YMCA cycle ergometer test)

If possible, it is more appropriate to schedule assessments to measure maximum anaerobic (e.g.. repeat-sprint or shuttle tests, exhaustive sprint tests such as the Wingate anaerobic test) and aerobic capacity (e.g.. aerobic tests to failure) on a separate day. However, if all assessments are performed on the same day, the personal trainer should ideally follow the order of tests presented earlier. This should ensure that clients complete any physically demanding tests to the best of their ability and produce accurate results for the personal trainer to process. McGuigan (35) has provided some practical examples that have application for the personal trainer. A test that maximally taxes the phosphagen energy system (e.g., maximal sprint tests) should have 3 to 5 minutes of rest to allow the client to recover. Any tests that require actions requiring high skill, such as change-of-direction speed or agility tests, should be administered before fatigue-inducing tests such as maximal aerobic tests. Maximal tests of anaerobic glycolytic capacity (e.g., repeat-sprint tests, Wingate, even maximal aerobic tests) require at least 60 minutes rest for complete recovery. Nonetheless, and where possible, maximal aerobic tests should be scheduled last in a testing session, as they will generally induce the greatest fatigue in a client.

Define and Follow Test Protocols

Individuals should receive precise test instructions before the scheduled assessment appointment. The clarity and simplicity of instructions have a direct impact on the reliability and objectivity of a test (7). Test instructions should define the protocols, including the purpose of the test, directions on implementation, performance guidelines regarding technique and disqualification, test scoring, and recommendations for maximizing performance. The personal trainer should also provide a demonstration of appropriate test performance and should give the client an opportunity to practice and ask questions about the protocol.

It is the responsibility of the personal trainer to ensure that testing protocols are followed safely and efficiently. To enhance reliability, strict standardized procedures should be followed with each client every time the test is administered. Also, the test selected for the pretest should be repeated as the posttest so that a reliable comparison of scores can be made. The personal trainer should institute an adequate warm-up and cooldown procedure when warranted and implement spotting practices when required by the testing protocol.

> Administration of the assessments should follow a standardized procedure including mentally and physically preparing the client, verifying the accuracy of the equipment, applying the specific test protocol, ensuring safety throughout the process, and performing record-keeping responsibilities.

INTERPRETATION AND REVIEW OF RESULTS

The data collected through the assessment process provide baseline information for the client. The interpretation of the baseline data is dependent on the specific purpose of the assessment and the goals of the client. Common ways to explain data to a client are through norm-referenced and criterion-referenced standards (see chapter 11).

Norm-Referenced Standards

The two reference perspectives for comparison of data are norm-referenced standards and criterion-referenced standards. **Norm-referenced standards** are used to compare the performance of an individual against the performance of others in a like category. Chapter 11 provides several tables demonstrating **percentile** values for various fitness measures. The results show how the men and women in the study performed. In other words, the percentile scores compare the actual "best, worst, and in-between" performance scores of each participant. Table 11.28 on page 265, for example, compares a client's score in the YMCA sit-and-reach test against all the other participants of the same sex. The highest and lowest scores were off the respective ends of this chart, and the rest were statistically divided into percentile rankings. Some clients may confuse percentile scores with percent scores, such as those they may have received in school, with 70% generally being a passing grade. Therefore, a personal trainer should be able to interpret the test results for clients and educate them on the relative value of their scores. For example, a score at the 50th percentile is an average performance (meaning the person performed better than roughly half of the performers and was outperformed by half).

Many clients are content to know their raw (performance) score and whether they get stronger, faster, or more flexible after training. Clients who are very unfit or who have had negative experiences with fitness testing in the past may have no interest in knowing how poorly they performed compared with others. Other clients feel more motivated with use of the normative data to articulate performance goals and feel a sense of achievement as they "climb the chart." Although using the normative approach may provide positive feedback related to performance, it does not address the health-related status of the individual based on desirable health standards.

Criterion-Referenced Standards

What norm-referenced standards do not do is let the client know whether the performance met a health standard. A **health standard** could be defined as the lowest performance that would allow an individual to maintain good health and lessen the risk of chronic diseases (41). Another way of stating this is to say that a criterion is a specific, minimal standard—one that theoretically each person can strive for because it is not compared with how other individuals perform. **Criterion-referenced standards** are set against a combination of normative data and the best judgment of the experts in a given field to identify a specific level of achievement (37). Criterion-referenced standards that have been matched to healthy levels of fitness provide reasonable goals for most people to achieve for improved health. For example, table 11.4 on page 245 provides a classification of overweight and obesity based on waist circumference and BMI. If a female client had a waist circumference greater than 35 inches (88 cm) and also was in the overweight category according to BMI, she would have a high risk of diseases such as diabetes or coronary heart disease. As another example, table 11.2 on page 244 demonstrates the criterion-referenced standards for blood pressure, or whether a client would be considered hypertensive, elevated, or normal.

Unfortunately, there is disagreement on the exact level of performance that accurately reflects a health standard (37). For example, among the various criterion-referenced health-related fitness batteries of tests that are given to school-age children in the United States, each has a different criterion denoting acceptable performance levels for health (28, 37). There is no consensus on what determines minimal health standards for adults in all areas, either (37). Does this mean, then, that a client achieving a score at a certain percentile on a fitness test is considered *healthy*? Not necessarily. The problem is that exact cutoffs for health for each component of fitness for all segments of the adult population have not been identified and universally accepted. This limitation can be an issue for a deconditioned client who scores at or near the bottom of a column on a norm-referenced table; the results may be demoralizing if the client thinks, mistakenly, that he or she must score at or near the top to be healthy.

Where they exist, criterion-referenced data can provide a reasonable estimate of the level of fitness that can then be associated with health. In the absence of criterion-referenced data for a test chosen for a particular client, the best way to use the normative tables is to encourage clients with goals related to health to strive for fitness improvements until they reach the "average" or higher levels for a given component, and then to maintain their level of performance (25). Clients with average or higher levels of performance initially or after training may have already achieved a healthy level of fitness but may be motivated to improve both health and performance by setting higher performance goals using the norm-referenced tables (25).

The personal trainer should schedule a review of results immediately or shortly after the assessment process. The client should receive an illustrated summary of the test results, along with an explanation of personal strengths and areas identified that may have room for improvement. It is important to note that testing data are neither good nor bad—they are baseline data to provide a foundation for positive change.

REASSESSMENT

Once the assessments are complete and the personal trainer has reviewed the results with the client, the program is designed and implemented based on the client's goals. The initial assessments, intermediate assessments (repetitions of some or all of the initial assessments), anecdotal records, and exercise logs documenting client progress are all part of the formative evaluation of the client, providing frequent opportunities for feedback and guidance. A time frame for accomplishing goals is set, and posttests are scheduled. The date scheduled for a posttest may be eight or more weeks from program initiation. The personal trainer should keep in mind that reassessments performed too frequently may disclose a learning effect by the client rather than true physiological changes. The summative evaluation should be scheduled just after the posttesting is complete to discuss the degree to which goals were achieved, review the strengths and weaknesses of the initial program, and modify the program where appropriate in order to set new goals.

It is important to keep in mind that formative evaluations are a measure of progress toward a goal, and the summative evaluation is a measure of the degree of attainment of a stated goal. For most clients, regardless of whether norm- or criterion-referenced standards are used, it is more appropriate to have them compare their own performances over time than against the skills or fitness levels of others.

CONCLUSION

If the personal trainer is truly providing individualized programming for his or her clients, the process begins with a thoughtful evaluation of the client's total circumstances—age, health, past experiences with exercise, current training status, exercise readiness, personal interests, and goals. Once these are identified, the personal trainer must consider the appropriateness of various valid and reliable tests that will yield meaningful baseline data from which a program can be developed. The personal trainer must further consider his or her own skills, equipment availability and appropriateness, and environmental factors in selecting the assessments to gather these data. A system of record keeping and storage must be developed to facilitate communication with the client after the initial testing and subsequent follow-up assessments. The entire process is part art and part science. It takes energy and initiative to continually search for assessment protocols relevant to one's clientele and to practice administering and interpreting them correctly. The personal trainer who does so will increase his or her knowledge, skills, and confidence; and both the personal trainer and the clients will benefit from the effort.

Study Questions

1. Which of the following is *incorrect* regarding gathering baseline data?

   A. They establish a baseline for future comparisons of improvement or rate of progress.

   B. Personal trainers should conduct all tests available to them.

   C. They provide assistance in clarification of short-, intermediate-, and long-term goals.

   D. They help to identify of areas of potential injury or contraindications before program initiation.

2. If an expert has determined that a test covers all of the topics that it should, it is said to have which of the following?

   A. reliability

   B. construct validity

   C. content validity

   D. face validity

3. Which of the following devices do *not* typically require calibration?

   A. sphygmomanometers

   B. skinfold calipers

   C. stopwatches

   D. treadmills

4. When preparing the client for a battery of fitness testing, the personal trainer should recommend that the client consume a light snack or meal approximately how long before the test?

   A. 30 minutes

   B. 1 hour

   C. 2-4 hours

   D. 8 hours

5. Which of the following would be the *most* appropriate amount of time following an initial test of strength to schedule a reassessment?

   A. 1 week

   B. 2 weeks

   C. 8 weeks

   D. 16 weeks

TEST PREPARATION AND IMPLEMENTATION CHECKLIST

Client's name: _____

Personal trainer's name: _____

Test preparation	√	Date/comments
1. Verify appropriateness of selected assessments:		
a. Identify and evaluate client's specific goals.		
b. Assess professional expertise associated with the tests to determine appropriateness of current skill level to obtain accurate results.		
c. Evaluate the characteristics of tests to determine congruency with client's goals and to assess the risk-to-benefit relationship.		
2. Review safety considerations:		
a. Conduct a preparticipation health appraisal screening.		
b. Obtain a physician referral, medical clearance, or both.		
c. Distribute and collect completed informed consent and screening forms.		
d. Review emergency procedures.		
3. Select facilities and verify accuracy of equipment:		
a. Identify tests that are easy to administer and are cost-effective.		
b. Select appropriate equipment and confirm availability.		
c. Calibrate equipment.		
d. Provide a testing atmosphere that is calm, private, and relaxed.		
e. Make sure the assessment area is safe, clean, set up, and ready for testing.		
f. Evaluate room temperature and humidity (68-72 °F [20-22 °C]; 60% humidity).		
4. Instruct client on preassessment protocols:		
a. Provide clients with pretest instructions. Adequate rest (6-8 h the night before testing) Moderate dietary intake (including adequate hydration) Abstinence from chemicals that accelerate heart rates (except for presently prescribed medications) Appropriate attire (loose-fitting clothing and sturdy shoes)		
b. Explain conditions for starting and stopping procedures of the protocol.		
5. Prepare record-keeping system:		
a. Create and supply a recording form or system.		
b. Develop a storage and retrieval system for data that is secure and confidential.		

Test implementation	√	Date/comments
1. Determine sequence of assessments:		
a. Establish an organized and appropriate testing order.		
b. Develop an appointment schedule for testing.		
2. Define and follow test protocols:		
a. Provide written test directions and guidelines to client.		
b. Explain technique, reasons for disqualification, and test scoring.		
c. Demonstrate test performance and allow time to practice.		
d. Provide an opportunity for client to ask questions regarding the tests.		
e. Implement an adequate warm-up and cooldown procedure.		
f. Spot the client when appropriate.		

From *NSCA's Essentials of Personal Training,* 3rd ed., edited for the National Strength and Conditioning Association by B. Schoenfeld and R. Snarr (Champaign, IL: Human Kinetics, 2022).

INDIVIDUAL ASSESSMENT RECORDING FORM

Pretest   Posttest   (circle one)

Client's name: _____ **Age:** _____

Goals: _____

_____

Preparticipation screening notes: _____

_____

_____

Assessment dates: _____

Comments: _____

_____

Vital signs	Score or result	Classification
Resting blood pressure		
Resting heart rate		
Body composition measures	**Score or result**	**Classification**
Height		
Weight		
Body mass index (BMI)		
Waist circumference		
Hip circumference		
Waist-to-hip ratio		
Percent body fat (method: _____)		
Cardiovascular endurance	**Score or result**	**Classification**
$\dot{V}O_2$max		
Other: _____		
Muscular endurance	**Score or result**	**Classification**
YMCA bench press		
Partial curl-up		
Prone double straight-leg raise		
Other: _____		
Muscular strength	**Score or result**	**Classification**
1RM bench press		
1RM leg press		
Other: _____		
Flexibility	**Score or result**	**Classification**
Sit-and-reach		
Other: _____		
Other tests	**Score or result**	**Classification**
Other: _____		
Other: _____		
Other: _____		

From *NSCA's Essentials of Personal Training*, 3rd ed., edited for the National Strength and Conditioning Association by B. Schoenfeld and R. Snarr (Champaign, IL: Human Kinetics, 2022).

CHAPTER 11

Fitness Evaluation Protocols and Norms

David H. Fukuda, PhD, and Kristina L. Kendall, PhD

After completing this chapter, you will be able to

- understand the protocols for selected fitness evaluations,

- correctly administer the selected fitness evaluations,

- attain valid and reliable measurements of clients' fitness levels and select appropriate tests for individual clients, and

- compare clients' results with normative data.

As discussed in chapter 10, personal trainers must choose valid and reliable fitness evaluations that are suitable for an individual client. To do this effectively, the personal trainer must administer assessments accurately and record and interpret the results. This chapter describes the most frequently used and widely applicable fitness testing protocols for assessing a client's vital signs, training load, body composition, cardiovascular endurance, speed, agility, muscular strength, muscular power, muscular endurance, flexibility, postural alignment, and movement assessment. Specific descriptive or normative data are also provided for each protocol. More fitness evaluation protocols are available, but many do not have associated descriptive and normative data and thus are not included here.

The authors would like to acknowledge the significant contributions of Eric D. Ryan, Joel T. Cramer, and Jared W. Coburn to this chapter.

Fitness Evaluation Protocols

VITAL SIGNS

Many of the assessments that a personal trainer performs during a fitness evaluation involve two basic tasks: taking the client's pulse and blood pressure. Sometimes these assessments are performed with the client in a resting state (e.g., measuring resting heart rate); but monitoring heart rate and blood pressure changes with exercise—especially aerobic exercise—is an effective method to determine appropriate exercise intensity (i.e., keeping the client's exercise heart rate in the prescribed target zone).

HEART RATE

Most adults have a resting heart rate (HR), or pulse, between 60 and 80 beats per minute (beats/min); however, a normal resting heart rate can be anywhere between 60 and 100 beats/min. On average, the HR for females is 7 to 10 beats/min greater than that for males (26). Those slower than 60 beats/min are classified as bradycardia and those higher than 100 beats/min as tachycardia (26). Table 11.1 (page 244) provides resting HR norm values (28). Three commonly used field techniques for assessing resting HR may be particularly useful for personal trainers: palpation, auscultation, and heart rate monitors.

Equipment

Depending on the specific procedure used to assess HR, any one or a combination of the following devices may be necessary.

- Stopwatch
- Stethoscope
- Heart rate monitor

Palpation Procedure

Palpation is probably the most common and certainly the most cost-effective method for assessing both resting and exercise HR.

1. Use the tips of the index and middle fingers to palpate the pulse. Avoid using the thumb because its inherent pulse may be confusing and potentially confounding. Any one of the following anatomical landmarks can be used to palpate the pulse:

   - *Brachial artery:* the anterior–medial aspect of the arm just distal to the belly of the biceps brachii muscle, 1 inch (2.5 cm) superior to the antecubital fossa (26).

   - *Radial artery:* on the anterior–lateral surface of the wrist, in line with the base of the thumb (26). This position is illustrated in figure 11.1*a*.

   - *Carotid artery:* on the anterior surface of the neck just lateral to the larynx (26). This position is illustrated in figure 11.1*b. Note:* Avoid applying too much pressure to this location when palpating for HR. Baroreceptors located in the arch of the aorta and the carotid sinuses can sense increases in applied pressure and will feed back to the medulla to decrease HR. Thus, use of the carotid site for measuring HR, if done incorrectly, can result in artificially low HR values.

   - *Temporal artery:* the lateral side of the cranium on the anterior portion of the temporal fossa, usually along the hairline at the level of the eyes.

2. If using a stopwatch to keep the time while counting beats, and if the stopwatch is started simultaneously with the first beat, count the first beat as zero. If the stopwatch has been running, count the first beat as one (26). The HR should be counted for 6, 10, 15, 30, or 60 seconds.

3. If the HR is counted for less than a full minute, use the following multipliers to convert the measurement to beats per minute: × 10 for 6 seconds; × 6 for 10 seconds; × 4 for 15 seconds; and × 2 for 30 seconds.

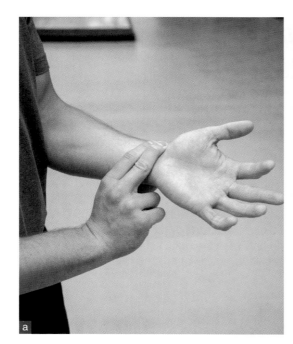 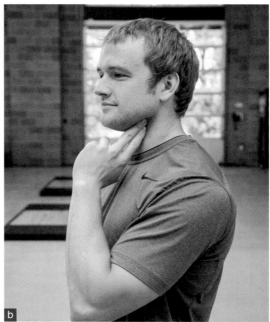

FIGURE 11.1 *(a)* Radial pulse determination and *(b)* carotid pulse determination.

Typically, the shorter-duration HR counts (6, 10, and 15 seconds) are used during exercise and postexercise conditions (26). Shorter-duration HR counts are more time efficient, and they may also provide a more accurate representation of momentary HR because of the immediate fluctuations that often occur with changes in exercise intensity. Resting HR, however, is generally assessed with the longer-duration HR counts (30 and 60 seconds) to reduce the risk of miscounts and measurement error.

Auscultation Procedure

Auscultation requires the use of a stethoscope. The bell of the stethoscope should be placed directly on the skin over the third intercostal space just left of the sternum (26). The sounds heard from the heart beating should be counted for either 30 or 60 seconds (26). Refer to previously given instructions for the correct conversion factor for the 30-second HR count.

LOCATING THE PULSE

Radial Pulse

- Flex the elbow with the arm at the side. The palm of the hand should be up.
- The radial artery is located on the inside of the wrist near the base of the thumb.
- Using the middle (long) and index (pointer) fingers, gently feel for the radial artery.

Carotid Pulse

- Using the middle (long) and index (pointer) fingers, gently feel the carotid artery on either side of the neck, in the space between the windpipe (trachea) and muscle (right or left sternocleidomastoid), beneath the lower jawbone.
- *Caution:* Some pressure needs to be applied to allow one to feel the pulse, but too much pressure may cause reduced blood flow to the head. Therefore, it is important to be careful not to press too hard on the artery and not to press on both arteries at the same time.

Heart Rate Monitor Procedure

Digital display HR monitors are becoming increasingly popular because of their validity, stability, and functionality (51). One drawback, however, is the cost of HR monitoring equipment. Nevertheless, personal trainers may find these monitors a very efficient and convenient way to assess HR at rest and during exercise.

EXAMPLE 11.1

Converting Pulse Measurements

12 heartbeats counted during a 6-second period:

$$12 \text{ beats per 6 s} \times 10 = 120 \text{ beats/min}$$

18 heartbeats counted during a 10-second period:

$$18 \text{ beats per 10 s} \times 6 = 108 \text{ beats/min}$$

24 heartbeats counted during a 15-second period:

$$24 \text{ beats per 15 s} \times 4 = 96 \text{ beats/min}$$

41 heartbeats counted during a 30-second period:

$$41 \text{ beats per 30 s} \times 2 = 82 \text{ beats/min}$$

FACTORS AFFECTING HEART RATE ASSESSMENT

- Smoking and tobacco products (↑resting HR; ↑ or ↔ exercise HR)
- Caffeine (↑ or ↔ resting and exercise HR—responses to caffeine consumption are quite variable and depend on previous exposure or consumption; therefore, caffeine consumption should be avoided before HR measurements)
- Environmental temperature extremes (↑ resting and exercise HR in hot environmental temperatures; HR responses can be quite variable in cold environmental temperatures and largely dependent on a client's body composition, acclimatization, and metabolism)
- Altitude (↑ HR at altitudes greater than approximately 4,000 feet [1,200 m])
- Stress (↑ resting and exercise HR)
- Food digestion (↑ resting and exercise HR)
- Body position (↓ HR when supine, ↑ HR from supine to seated position or standing position)
- Time of day (↓ HR first thing in the morning, ↑ or ↔ during afternoon or evening hours)
- Medications (↑, ↔, or ↓ resting and exercise HR—responses to medications are quite variable and contingent on the specific medication)

Note: ↑ = increase; ↓ = decrease; ↔ = no significant change.

Reprinted by permission from J.A. Kordich (2002).

BLOOD PRESSURE

Blood pressure (BP) can be defined as the forces of blood acting against vessel walls (6). The sounds that are emitted as a result of these vibratory forces are called **Korotkoff sounds**. The detection and disappearance of Korotkoff sounds under controlled pressure environments are the basis of most BP measurement methods. Although there are various invasive and noninvasive techniques for determining BP (6), **sphygmomanometry** is the most commonly used field technique and as such gives personal trainers a convenient tool for evaluating their clients' BP. One can also use a mercury or an aneroid sphygmomanometer. However, both of these require the use of an inflatable air bladder–containing cuff and a stethoscope to auscultate the Korotkoff sounds; thus this procedure is also commonly referred to as the cuff or auscultatory method (6).

Repeated BP measurements are important for detecting hypertension (table 11.2, page 244; [84]) and for monitoring the antihypertensive effects of an exercise program or dietary changes (6). When assessing BP, it is imperative to use calibrated equipment that meets certification standards (70) and to follow standardized protocol (10a). It is recommended that BP readings be taken with a mercury sphygmomanometer. However, recently calibrated aneroid sphygmomanometers or validated electronic devices are being used more frequently, although their accuracy has been questioned compared with that of traditional mercury sphygmomanometers (67).

Equipment

- Mercury or aneroid sphygmomanometer
- Air bladder–containing cuff
- Stethoscope

Procedure

1. Instruct the client to refrain from smoking or ingesting caffeine at least 30 minutes prior to BP measurements (10a).

2. Have the client sit upright in a chair that supports the back with either the right or the left arm and forearm exposed, supinated, and supported at the level of the heart (differences between right and left arm BP measurements are marginal). *Note:* If exposing the arm by rolling or bunching up the sleeves of clothing causes any occlusion of circulation above the cuff site, ask the client to remove the constricting clothing articles (26).

3. Select the appropriate cuff size for the client. See table 11.3 on page 244 for the correct cuff size based on the client's arm circumference (67). To determine the arm circumference, have the client stand with arms hanging freely at the sides, and take the arm circumference measurements midway between the acromion process of the scapula and the olecranon process of the ulna (26), roughly midway between the shoulder and elbow.

4. Begin BP measurements only after the client has rested for a minimum of 5 minutes in the position described in step 2 (67).

FACTORS AFFECTING BLOOD PRESSURE ASSESSMENT

- Smoking and tobacco products (↑ resting and exercise)
- Caffeine (BP responses to caffeine consumption are quite variable and depend on previous exposure and consumption; therefore, caffeine consumption should be avoided prior to BP measurements)
- Stress (↑ resting and exercise)
- Body position (↓ when supine, ↑ from supine to seated position or standing position)
- Time of day (↓ first thing in the morning, ↑ or ↔ during afternoon or evening hours)
- Medications (↑, ↔, or ↓ resting and exercise BP—responses to medications are quite variable and contingent on the specific medication)

Note: ↑ = increase; ↓ = decrease; ↔ = no significant change.

Reprinted by permission from J.A. Kordich (2002).

5. Place the cuff on the arm so that the air bladder is directly over the brachial artery (some cuffs have a line indicating the specific placement over the brachial artery). The bottom edge of the cuff should be 1 inch (2.5 cm) above the antecubital space (6).

6. With the client's palm facing up, place the stethoscope firmly, but not hard enough to indent the skin, over the antecubital space (6). *Note:* Most personal trainers find it easier to use their dominant hand to control the bladder airflow by placing the air bulb in the palm and using the thumb and forefinger to control the pressure release. The nondominant hand is then used to hold the stethoscope (6).

7. Position the sphygmomanometer so that the center of the mercury column or aneroid dial is at eye level and the air bladder tubing is not overlapping, obstructing, or being allowed to freely contact the stethoscope head or tubing (26). See figure 11.2 for common errors in performing a BP assessment.

8. Once the cuff, stethoscope, and sphygmomanometer are in place, quickly inflate the air bladder either to 160 mmHg or to 20 mmHg above the anticipated systolic BP. Upon maximum inflation, turn the air release screw counterclockwise to release the pressure slowly at a rate of 2 or 3 mmHg per second (6).

9. Record both systolic blood pressure (SBP) and diastolic blood pressure (DBP) measurements in even numbers using units of millimeters of mercury (mmHg) to the nearest 2 mmHg on the sphygmomanometer. To do this, it is necessary during cuff deflation to make a mental note of the pressure corresponding with the first audible detection of Korotkoff sounds via auscultation, or SBP. The pressure at which the Korotkoff sounds disappear is the DBP (6). *Note:* Traditionally, Korotkoff sounds occur as sharp "thud" noises that can be similar to the sounds of gentle finger tapping on the stethoscope head (bell). Consequently, Korotkoff sounds are also similar to the extraneous noises often made when the air bladder tubing is allowed to bump against the stethoscope bell, so it is important to take great care to avoid these erroneous and potentially confusing noises (26).

10. Upon the disappearance of the Korotkoff sounds, carefully observe the manometer for an additional 10 to 20 mmHg of deflation to confirm the absence of sounds. Once the absence of sounds is confirmed, release the remaining pressure rapidly and remove the cuff (6).

11. After a minimum of 2 minutes' rest, measure BP again using the same technique. If the two consecutive measurements of either the SBP or the DBP differ by more than 5 mmHg, take a third BP measurement and record the average of the three SBP and the average of the three DBP measurements as the final scores (see example 11.2 on page 202, client A). If the consecutive measurements of neither the SBP nor the DBP differ by more than 5 mmHg, average the two SBP scores and average the two DBP scores to determine the final BP (see example 11.2 on page 202, client B) (6).

12. Once a client's BP has been determined, it can be classified from table 11.2 on page 244.

FIGURE 11.2 Common errors for blood pressure measurement.

1. The stethoscope is put on backward resulting in the earpieces not pointing toward the personal trainer's ear canals.

2. The measurement dial is not at the personal trainer's eye level.

3. The bell of the stethoscope is under the blood pressure cuff.

4. The blood pressure cuff is placed too close to the bend in the client's elbow (termed the antecubital space or fossa).

5. The blood pressure cuff is either too large or small for the client's arm.

6. The blood pressure cuff is not inflated enough to correctly capture the first Korotkoff sound.

7. The air is released out of the blood pressure cuff either too quickly or too slowly.

TIPS FOR BLOOD PRESSURE MEASUREMENT

1. The client should be seated comfortably with the back supported and the legs not crossed.
2. The upper arm should be bare and have no restrictive clothing.
3. The client's arm should be completely relaxed and supported at approximately heart level.
4. The bladder of the cuff should cover at least 80% of the client's upper arm.
5. The cuff should be deflated at 2 or 3 mm/s, with the first and last audible sounds taken as the SBP and DBP, respectively.
6. Both the client and tester should remain quiet during testing.

Adapted from Pickering et al. (67).

EXAMPLE 11.2

Measuring Blood Pressure

Client A	SBP (mmHg)	DBP (mmHg)
Trial 1	132	78
Trial 2	126	80
Difference	*6*	*2*
Trial 3 (*required*)	130	78
Averaged final score	**129**	**79**

Client B	SBP (mmHg)	DBP (mmHg)
Trial 1	110	68
Trial 2	114	66
Difference	*4*	*2*
Trial 3 (*not required*)	–	–
Averaged final score	**112**	**67**

TRAINING LOAD

Training load reflects the relative balance between the various stressors imposed on the body via exercise, termed **external training load**, and the body's physiological response to exercise, termed **internal training load** (21, 59). Knowledge of a client's specific external and internal training loads over time can aid in day-to-day decision making as well as inform long-term program design (figure 11.3; 21). For example, positive physiological adaptations may be present if a client displays relatively low internal training load values (e.g., decreased perceived exertion or increased wellness ratings) with a high external training load (e.g., increased physical activity or exercise intensity). Conversely, negative adaptations may be present if internal training loads are high (e.g., increased perceived exertion or decreased wellness ratings) despite relatively low external training loads (e.g., decreased physical activity or exercise intensity). Furthermore, relatively low or high values for both internal and external training load may warrant quicker or slower progressions in the training program, respectively.

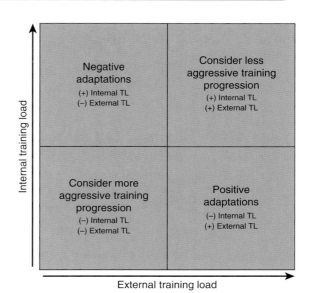

FIGURE 11.3 Decision matrix for the balance between external and internal training loads.

Adapted from Gabbett et al. (21).

EXTERNAL TRAINING LOAD

The process of calculating training volume, or monitoring training activities, over time can be used as an indicator of external training load. From a resistance exercise perspective, this can be accomplished by tracking the total number of repetitions (i.e., sets × repetitions) or volume load (sets × repetitions × load [in lb or kg]) for a given training session. From an endurance- or team-sport perspective, this can be accomplished by tracking the total distance covered or the number and intensity of shorter-distance runs during a training session.

INTERNAL TRAINING LOAD

The most straightforward method of evaluating internal training load involves determining the client's rating of perceived exertion or perceptual well-being. Rating of perceived exertion (RPE) values provided by the client allow for the subjective evaluation of a training session (figure 11.4), which can be multiplied by the duration of the session or the number of repetitions completed to determine session RPE. For example, if a client provides an RPE value of 6 for a 30-minute training session, the session RPE would be 180. The process of determining perceptual well-being relies on the consistent recording of any number of factors that may reflect how the client is responding to the training program. For instance, extraneous lifestyle factors, such as sleep quality and stress related to school, work, or interpersonal relationships, contribute to the physiological adaptations to exercise (39, 59). An example containing individual ratings for sleep, muscle soreness, general stress, and fatigue is provided in figure 11.5 (16a). Perceptual well-being ratings and session-RPE values can provide an overall indicator of internal training load that can then be compared over time to better quantify training sessions and examine the influence of external training load.

FIGURE 11.4 Sample rating of perceived exertion (RPE) scale.

Rating	Description
1	Nothing at all (lying down)
2	Extremely little
3	Very easy
4	Easy (could do this all day)
5	Moderate
6	Somewhat hard (starting to feel it)
7	Hard
8	Very hard (making an effort to keep up)
9	Very, very hard
10	Maximum effort (cannot go any further)

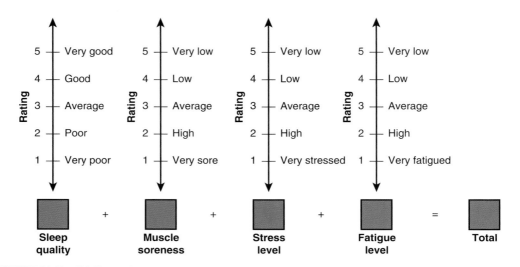

FIGURE 11.5 Wellness inventory for sleep quality, muscle soreness, stress level, and fatigue level.

From *NSCA's Essentials of Personal Training*, 3rd ed., edited for the National Strength and Conditioning Association by B. Schoenfeld and R. Snarr (Champaign, IL: Human Kinetics, 2022). Reprinted by permission from Fukuda (2019, p. 267).

BODY COMPOSITION

The measurement of body composition is of great interest to personal trainers and their clients. A variety of methods are available, each with its own advantages and disadvantages. Regardless of the method chosen, the personal trainer must be meticulous in following the appropriate protocol and must take great care in measuring and evaluating clients to avoid unreliable and inaccurate values.

ANTHROPOMETRY

Anthropometry, which is the science of measurement applied to the human body, generally includes measurements of height, weight, and selected body girths. Measurement of height requires a flat wall against which the client stands, a measuring tape attached or unattached to the wall, and a rectangular object placed concurrently against both the client's head and the wall. More detailed instructions for measuring height are given later in this section.

The most accurate body mass or bodyweight measurement is performed with a certified balance beam scale (of the type normally found in physicians' offices), which is generally more reliable than a spring scale and should be calibrated on a regular basis. A calibrated electronic scale is an acceptable alternative. Clients should be weighed while wearing minimal dry clothing (e.g., gym shorts and T-shirt, no shoes). For comparison measurements at a later date, they should dress similarly and be weighed at the same time of day. The most reliable body mass (weight) measurements are made in the morning upon rising, after elimination and before ingestion of food or fluids. Level of hydration can result in variability of body mass (weight). Thus, clients should be encouraged to avoid eating salty food (which increases water retention) the day before weighing and to go to bed normally hydrated.

The most reliable girth measurements are usually obtained with the aid of a flexible measuring tape equipped with a spring-loaded attachment at the end that, when pulled out to a specified mark, exerts a fixed amount of tension on the tape (e.g., a Gulick tape). Girth measurements can be made at the beginning of a training or incentive period for comparison with subsequent measurements.

BODY MASS INDEX

Personal trainers often use the body mass index (BMI) to examine body mass related to stature. To calculate BMI, it is necessary to have the client's height and weight.

$$\text{BMI (kg/m}^2\text{)} = \text{Body weight (kg)} \div \text{Height}^2 \text{ (m}^2\text{)} \tag{11.1}$$

Once a client's BMI has been determined, this value can be compared with those in table 11.4 (page 245) (66). Note that BMI does not take into account the relative composition of an individual (i.e., fat mass versus fat free mass). For example, for individuals possessing greater amounts of muscle mass (e.g., athletes), BMI may inaccurately classify the individual as overweight or obese, despite a low percentage of actual body fat. Alternatively, individuals with a greater accumulation of body fat and lower volume of muscle mass may be classified as "normal," despite an increased health risk for obesity-related diseases. Thus, BMI alone should not be used to monitor weight loss or program success.

HEIGHT

Height is a basic anthropometric measurement for which **stature** is a more accurate term (6). Although stature can be measured in several different ways, the two most common techniques involve using a stadiometer, typically located on the upright of a standard platform scale and simply having a client stand with the back against a flat wall. The anthropometer method is convenient but requires access to a standard platform scale. The use of a wall is cost-effective but requires a right-angled device to simultaneously slide against the wall and contact the top of the client's head (crown). Regardless of the specific technique used, the following standard protocol is recommended for assessing a client's stature (6).

Equipment

Depending on the procedure used to assess a client's stature, one of the following devices is necessary.

- Standard platform scale with stadiometer
- Flat, ridged, right-angled device (to simultaneously slide against a wall and rest on top of client's crown)

Procedure

1. Ask the client to remove all footwear.
2. Instruct the client to stand as erect as possible, with feet flat on the floor and heels together facing away from wall or stadiometer.
3. Instruct the client to look straight ahead. Make sure the lowest point of the orbit of the eye is horizontally aligned with the opening of the ear.
4. Immediately before taking the measurement, instruct the client to take a deep breath and hold until the measurement has been taken.

5. Rest the anthropometer arm or measurement angle gently on the crown of the client's head.

6. Mark the wall or stabilize the anthropometer and record the measurement to the nearest centimeter. If only inches are available as a unit of measure, then record the value to the nearest 1/4 to 1/2 inch and convert the measurement in inches to centimeters.

7. Once a client's height has been measured, the value can be compared with those in tables 11.5 and 11.6 on pages 246-247 (57).

EXAMPLE 11.3

Calculating BMI

Client A

A female client is measured with a height of 65 inches and a weight of 145 pounds.

Stature	=	65 in. × 0.0254 = 1.651 m
Mass	=	145 lb ÷ 2.2046 = 65.8 kg
BMI	=	65.8 ÷ (1.651 × 1.651) = 65.8 ÷ 2.726
	=	**24.1**

From table 11.4, a BMI of 24.1 is normal.

Client B

A male client is measured with a height of 69 inches and a weight of 214 pounds.

Stature	=	69 in. × 0.0254 = 1.753 m
Mass	=	214 lb ÷ 2.2046 = 97.1 kg
BMI	=	97.1 ÷ (1.753 × 1.753) = 97.1 ÷ 3.073
	=	**31.6**

From table 11.4, a BMI of 31.6 is consistent with class I obesity.

FACTORS AFFECTING BODY MASS ASSESSMENT

- Previous meals (↑ after meal consumption)
- Time of day (↓ first thing in the morning, ↑ during afternoon or evening hours)
- Hydration status (↓ when dehydrated; body mass will ↓ postexercise because of sweat loss)

Note: ↑ = increase; ↓ = decrease.

WEIGHT

The term **weight** is defined as the mass of an object under the normal acceleration due to gravity; therefore, a more accurate term to characterize body weight is **body mass** (6). An accurate measurement of body mass can be taken only with a calibrated and certified scale. One of the types of scales most commonly used is the platform-beam scale. The personal trainer should adhere to the following standard protocol when assessing a client's body mass (6).

Equipment

Calibrated and certified scale

Procedure

1. Ask the client to remove as much clothing and jewelry as feasible.
2. Instruct the client to step gently onto the scale and remain as still as possible throughout the measurement.
3. Record the weight to the nearest 1/4 pound or, when a sensitive metric scale is available, to the nearest 0.02 kg (6).
4. Convert the measurement in pounds to kilograms using the following equation:

pounds (lb) ÷ 2.2046 = kilograms (kg)   (11.2)

5. Bodyweight measurements can be compared with the values in table 11.7 on page 247 (35). For example, for a 36-year-old female client who is 60 inches (152.4 cm) tall and weighs 135 pounds (61.2 kg), table 11.7 indicates that she is classified as overweight based on her BMI.

SKINFOLDS

Skinfolds (SF) indirectly measure the thickness of subcutaneous fat tissue. Sum of SF measurements are highly correlated with body density (Db) measurements from underwater weighing when using population-specific SF equations. Population-specific, or linear, equations are developed for homogenous populations and are valid only for individuals who display similar characteristics such as age, sex, ethnicity, or physical activity level. Using these equations in clients not representative of the sample used to develop the equation can lead to inaccurate estimates of body fat (42). Therefore, it is recommended to use generalized prediction equations, which use a quadratic regression model, when estimating body fat in individuals varying in age (18-60 years) and body fatness (up to 45% body fat) (36).

Most equations use multiple SF sites to predict Db, which can then be converted to percent body fat (%BF) using the appropriate prediction equation (table 11.8 on page 248; 23). Using these equations, Db and %BF can be estimated within acceptable values (±0.0080 g/cc or ±3.5% body fat) for most individuals (52).

The accuracy of SF measurements can be affected by the skill level of the technician, the type of caliper used, client factors, and the prediction equation used to estimate %BF. Inter- and intrarater reliability can be improved when technicians follow standardized testing procedures. Inconsistencies of the anatomical location and direction of the SF can also lead to a lack of agreement between technicians. To improve intrarater reliability, it is recommended that personal trainers practice SF measurements on 50 to 100 clients in order to develop a high degree of skill and proficiency (43). Given that the type of caliper used is a potential source of error, using the same caliper when monitoring changes in SFs is recommended, as well as periodically checking the accuracy of the caliper and calibrating it as needed.

Equipment

- Skinfold caliper
- Nonelastic (i.e., plastic or metal) tape measure
- Pen or other marking device

General Considerations for Skinfold Testing

- Take all skinfold measurements on the right side of the body.
- Take the skinfold measurements when the client's skin is dry and free of lotion. In addition, skinfold measurements should always be taken before exercise. Exercise-induced changes in the hydration status of different body tissues can significantly affect the thickness of a skinfold.
- Carefully identify, measure, and mark the skinfold site.

- Grasp the skinfold firmly between the thumb and fingers. The placement of the thumb and fingers should be at least 1 cm (0.4 inches) away from the site to be measured.
- Lift the fold by placing the thumb and index finger approximately 8 cm (~3 inches) apart on a line that is perpendicular to the long axis of the skinfold. The long axis is parallel to the natural cleavage lines of the skin. The thicker the fat tissue layer, the greater the separation between the thumb and finger as the fold is lifted.
- Keep the fold elevated while taking the measurement.
- Place the jaws of the caliper perpendicular to the fold, 1 cm (0.4 inches) away from the thumb and index finger, and release the jaw pressure slowly.
- Record the skinfold measurement after 1 to 2 seconds (but within 4 seconds) after the jaw pressure has been released.
- If the caliper is not equipped with a digital display (Skyndex II), read the dial of the caliper to the nearest 0.2 mm (Harpenden), 0.5 mm (Lange or Lafayette), or 1 mm (Slim Guide, The Body Caliper, or Accu-Measure). Studies have been conducted to compare skinfold measurements and body composition estimates from different types of calipers (14a, 60a). The practical implications, however, regarding any potential variations among skinfold calipers are marginal.
- Take a minimum of two measurements at each site. If the values vary by more than 2 mm or 10%, take an additional measurement.

From Harrison et al. (32).

Procedure for Specific Skinfold Sites

1. Select an appropriate combination of skinfold sites, based on the body density equations in table 11.8 on page 248, for the client from the following list.
   - Chest
   - Midaxillary
   - Triceps
   - Subscapular
   - Abdominal
   - Suprailiac
   - Thigh
   - Medial calf

2. Carefully identify and mark the appropriate skinfold sites. All measurements should be made on the right side of the body with the client standing upright.
   - *Chest:* Take a diagonal fold half the distance between the anterior axillary line (imaginary line extending from the front of the armpit downward) and the nipple for men (figure 11.6*a*), and one-third of the distance from the anterior axillary line to the nipple for women.
   - *Midaxilla:* Take a vertical fold on the midaxillary line (imaginary line extending from the middle of the armpit downward; it divides the body into front and back halves) at the level of the xiphoid process (bottom of the sternum) (figure 11.6*b*). An alternate method is a horizontal fold taken at the level of the xiphoid/sternal border on the midaxillary line.
   - *Triceps:* Take a vertical fold on the posterior midline of the upper arm (over the triceps muscle), halfway between the acromion (top of shoulder) and olecranon processes (elbow); the elbow should be extended and relaxed so that the arm hangs freely to the side of the body (figure 11.6*c*).
   - *Subscapula:* Take a fold on a 45° diagonal line coming from the vertebral (medial) border to 1 to 2 cm (0.4-0.8 inches) from the inferior angle (bottommost point) of the scapula (figure 11.6*d*). (*Note:* The model has a small scapula, so the fold appears to be higher than where it was actually located.)
   - *Abdomen:* Take a vertical fold at a lateral distance of approximately 2 cm (1 inch) from the umbilicus (figure 11.6*e*).
   - *Suprailium:* Take a diagonal fold above the crest of the ilium (top of the pelvis) in line with the natural angle of the iliac crest at the spot where an imaginary line would come down from the anterior axillary line (figure 11.6*f*).

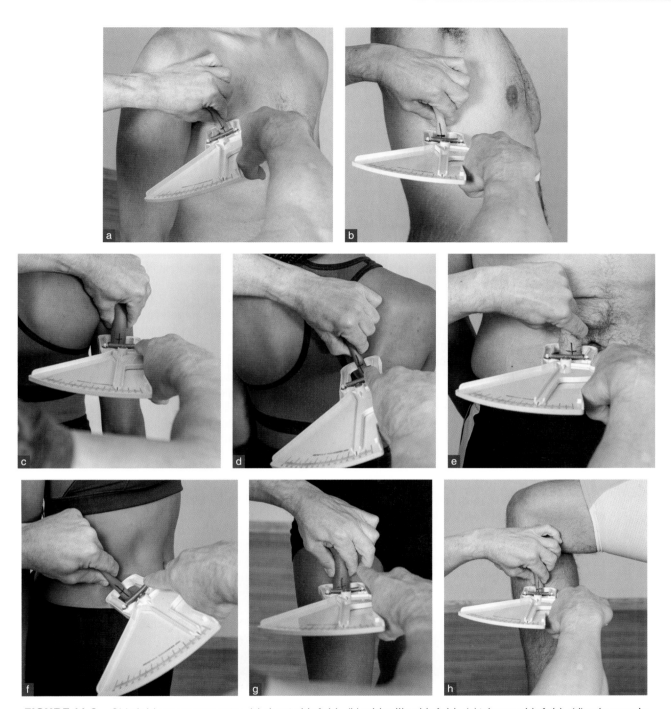

FIGURE 11.6   Skinfold measurements: *(a)* chest skinfold, *(b)* midaxilla skinfold, *(c)* triceps skinfold, *(d)* subscapula skinfold, *(e)* abdomen skinfold, *(f)* suprailium skinfold, *(g)* thigh skinfold, and *(h)* medial calf skinfold.

- *Thigh:* Take a vertical fold on the anterior aspect of the thigh midway between the hip and knee joints (figure 11.6*g*).
- *Medial calf:* Have the client place the right leg on a bench with the knee flexed at 90 degrees. On the midline of the medial border, mark the level of the greatest calf circumference. Raise a vertical skinfold on the medial side of the calf 1 cm (0.4 inches) above the mark, and measure the fold at the maximal girth (figure 11.6*h*).

Adapted from American College of Sports Medicine (1).

3. Using the appropriate population-specific equation from table 11.8 on page 248 (23), calculate the estimated body density from the skinfold measurements.

4. Enter the body density into the appropriate population-specific equation from table 11.9 on page 249 (36) to calculate the percent body fat.

5. Compare the percent body fat against the normative values in table 11.10 on page 250 (28).

BIA TECHNIQUES FOR MEASURING BODY COMPOSITION

Bioelectrical impedance analysis (BIA) is a noninvasive, relatively inexpensive method for measuring body composition. BIA works via measurement of the amount of impedance or resistance to a small, painless electrical current passed through the body between two electrodes, which are often placed on the wrist and ankle (14). Total body water (TBW) is estimated from the impedance measurement because electrolytes in the body's water are excellent conductors of electrical current. Impedance measures are higher in individuals with large amounts of body fat because of the low water content in adipose tissue. Conversely, individuals with larger amounts of fat free mass (FFM) have less resistance to the current flowing through their bodies because the water content of FFM is relatively large (~73% water). Some authors have suggested that BIA methods for determining body composition are roughly as accurate as skinfold techniques, reporting typical prediction errors (SEE) ranging from 2 to 4 pounds (0.9-1.8 kg) TBW, 4.4 to 6.6 pounds (2-3 kg) FFM, and 3.0% to 4.0% body fat in adults (41).

The variety of BIA devices, both single- and multifrequency, include hand-to-hand, foot-to-foot, and hand-to-foot systems. Single-frequency BIA devices operate at a frequency of 50 kHz, whereas multifrequency BIA and bioelectrical impedance spectroscopy devices use a wide range of frequencies (ranging from 1 kHz to 500 kHz), allowing for the measurement of TBW, intracellular water, extracellular water, fat mass, and FFM. Inexpensive lower body (foot-to-foot) and upper body (hand-to-hand) BIA devices have become available for home and commercial use. They provide estimates of %BF and FFM using proprietary equations developed by the manufacturers. For healthy clients with normal fluid balance, these analyzers provide reasonably accurate estimates of FFM, reporting small prediction errors (SEE = 4.9 to 8.6 pounds, or 2.2 to 3.9 kg), depending on the model used) when compared with underwater weighing (8, 22, 80). In certain clinical populations with abnormal fluid distribution, multifrequency approaches are recommended for measuring and monitoring changes in TBW and body fat.

BIA measurements can be easily and significantly affected by factors such as hydration status, racial characteristics, and the prediction equation used (56). Eating, drinking, dehydration, exercise, and menstrual cycle phase can affect total body resistance and the estimate of FFM. Therefore, it is important to follow pretesting guidelines to ensure accuracy when using the BIA method. Furthermore, there is a tendency for BIA to overestimate body fat in lean individuals and underestimate body fat in obese individuals, with individual error rates as high as 11 pounds (5 kg). BIA equations should be selected based on the client's age, sex, ethnicity, physical activity level, and level of body fatness (16, 75, 81). Ethnic differences in fat patterning and body proportions can affect the validity of generalized equations, with the majority of studies indicating that the BIA method is not accurate when a generalized equation is applied to different ethnic groups, including African Americans, Asians, and Hispanics (13, 36, 82).

BIA PRETESTING GUIDELINES

- Refrain from eating or drinking within four hours of the test.
- No exercise within 12 hours of the test.
- No alcohol consumption within 48 hours of the test.
- No diuretic medications within seven days of the test.
- Do not test female clients who perceive they are retaining water during their menstrual cycle.
- Ask clients to void their bladder within 30 minutes of the test.

Source: Heyward and Wagner (36).

WAIST-TO-HIP GIRTH RATIO

Although not truly a measure of body composition per se, measurement of the waist-to-hip ratio is a valuable tool for assessing relative fat distribution and risk of disease. Individuals with a larger accumulation of fat in the trunk, particularly abdominal region, are at increased risk for a variety of cardiovascular and metabolic diseases (1).

Equipment

Nonelastic (i.e., plastic or metal) tape measure

Procedure

1. Place the tape measure around the girth of the waist (smallest girth around the abdomen) and hip (largest girth measured around the buttocks). See figures 11.7 and 11.8.

2. Hold the zero end of the tape in one hand, positioned below the other part of the tape, which is held in the other hand.

3. Apply tension to the tape so that it fits snugly around the body part but does not indent the skin or compress the subcutaneous tissue.

4. Align the tape in a horizontal plane, parallel to the floor. (*Note*: Some protocols state that the client's arms should hang relaxed at the sides. For either position, be sure to have the client get into the same position for a retest as what was used for the initial test.)

5. To determine the waist-to-hip ratio, divide the waist circumference by the hip circumference.

6. Use table 11.11 on page 251 (7) to assess risk.

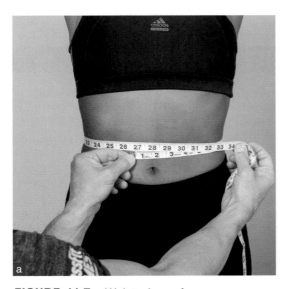

FIGURE 11.7 Waist circumference measurement.

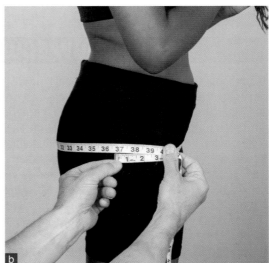

FIGURE 11.8 Hip circumference measurement.

ASSUMPTIONS AND SOLUTIONS FOR SUBMAXIMAL EXERCISE TESTS

Assumption 1: Heart rate measurements must be steady state.

Solution: Heart rate can fluctuate dramatically with sudden changes in work rate. To ensure that HR has achieved steady state, personal trainers should record HR values at the end of a constant work-rate stage or after 2 or 3 minutes of exercise at a constant work rate (6). Steady-state HR is defined as two consecutive HR measurements that are within five beats/min of each other (1).

Assumption 2: True maximal HR for a given age must be the same for all clients.

Solution: For any given age, maximal HR can vary as much as ±10 to 12 beats/min across individuals (1); therefore, the typical equation to calculate age-predicted maximal HR can introduce an unknown error into the model for submaximal estimation of $\dot{V}O_2$max.

$$\text{Age-predicted maximal HR (beats/min)} = 220 - \text{Age (years)} \qquad (11.3)$$

(See table 16.2 on page 429 for alternative formulas for estimating maximal heart rate.)

Assumption 3: The relationship between HR and work rate must be strong, positive, and linear.

Solution: The positive relationship between HR and workload is most linear between 50% and 90% of maximal HR (6). One should consider this when extrapolating HR versus work-rate data points. In example 11.4 on page 215, only the HR values at stages 2, 3, and 4 should be used to estimate $\dot{V}O_2$ max since those HR values are between 50% and 90% of the age-predicted maximal HR.

Assumption 4: Mechanical efficiency ($\dot{V}O_2$ at a given work rate) is the same for all clients.

Solution: Personal trainers should choose a test that is specific to the client's existing cardiovascular exercise mode(s), daily activities, or both. For example, if a client typically goes for long walks three or four times per week, the Rockport walking test or a submaximal treadmill walking test might be the best indicator of that client's $\dot{V}O_2$ max.

CARDIOVASCULAR ENDURANCE

The personal trainer can use submaximal cardiovascular endurance tests to attain a reasonably accurate estimation of a client's $\dot{V}O_2$max (1). Submaximal exercise tests are used most often because of high equipment expenses, the personnel needed, and the increased risks associated with maximal tests. See "General Indications for Stopping an Exercise Test" on page 188 of chapter 10 for a list of indicators a personal trainer should look for that would require immediate termination of an exercise test. The concept behind a submaximal test is to monitor HR, BP, or rating of perceived exertion (RPE)—or some combination of these—during exercise until a predetermined percentage of the client's predicted maximal HR is achieved, at which point the test is terminated. To get a true measure of a client's cardiovascular endurance, one would need to conduct a maximal test, taking the client to his or her extreme limits of HR and oxygen consumption rate ($\dot{V}O_2$max). Maximal tests, however, are not safe or necessary for many clients and sometimes cannot be conducted without physician supervision; thus, submaximal tests are used instead. By their very nature, submaximal tests provide estimations of a client's $\dot{V}O_2$max. However, most submaximal exercise testing protocols, such as those presented in this chapter, provide a valid, reliable, specific, and sensitive estimation of $\dot{V}O_2$max. As with many estimation techniques, however, certain assumptions must be considered. Refer to the previous sidebar to understand the basic assumptions underlying a submaximal exercise test as well as some potential solutions the personal trainer should consider. Due to the distinct differences in $\dot{V}O_2$max values between the treadmill and cycle ergometer), normative data for each mode has been provided in table 11.13 and table 11.14, respectively (44a, 44b).

GENERAL PROCEDURES FOR CYCLE ERGOMETER TESTING

1. Ensure that the cycle ergometer has been recently and correctly calibrated.
2. Adjust the seat height so there is a slight flexion at the knee joint (about 25 degrees) at maximal leg extension (lowest pedal position) when the ball of the foot is on the pedal (24).

3. The client should be seated on the cycle ergometer in an upright position with the hands properly positioned on the handlebars (24). Ask the client to maintain the same grip and posture throughout the duration of the test.

4. Establish the pedaling cadence before setting the resistance (24). If a metronome is necessary to set the pedaling cadence, set it at twice the desired cadence so that one full pedal revolution occurs for every two metronome beats (e.g., set the metronome at 100 for a test requiring a pedaling cadence of 50 revolutions per minute [rpm]) (24).

5. Set the workload. The workload on a cycle ergometer usually refers to the work rate. Work rate is defined as a power output and is measured in units of kilogram-meters per minute ($kg \cdot m \cdot min^{-1}$) or watts (W). It can be calculated with the following equation:

$$\text{Work rate } (kg \cdot m \cdot min^{-1}) = \text{Resistance (kg)} \times \text{Distance (m)} \times \text{Cadence (rpm)} \qquad (11.4)$$

where *resistance* = the amount of friction placed on the flywheel (usually in kilograms or kiloponds), *distance* = the distance the flywheel travels as a result of one pedal revolution (meters), and *cadence* = the pedaling cadence (revolutions per minute).

The work rate in watts can now be calculated by the following equation:

$$\text{Work rate (W)} = \text{Work rate } (kg \cdot m \cdot min^{-1}) \div 6.12 \qquad (11.5)$$

- Setting the work rate on an electronically braked cycle ergometer is usually simple because these expensive ergometers often have computer- or digitally interfaced work-rate settings that automatically adjust the resistance based on the pedaling cadence to maintain a predetermined work rate.

- On a mechanically braked ergometer, maintaining a work rate is more difficult. Mechanically braked cycle ergometers have a flywheel "braked" by a belt that adds resistance by friction as it is tightened. Since the work rate is controlled by the resistance and the pedaling cadence, both must remain constant to maintain the work rate.

6. Check the resistance setting frequently during the test to prevent the unexpected increases or decreases that are common with use of mechanically braked cycle ergometers (24).

7. Continuously monitor the appearance and symptoms of the client (see "General Indications for Stopping an Exercise Test" on page 188 of chapter 10) for a list of general indications for stopping an exercise test in low-risk adults (1).

8. During multistage tests (e.g., the YMCA cycle ergometer test):

- Assess HR near the end of each stage or until steady-state HR is achieved. For example, if the client is working through a 3-minute stage, measure HR during the final 15 to 30 seconds of the second and third minutes. If the consecutive HR measurements are not within five beats/min of each other, continue the stage for one more minute and measure HR again (see HR testing protocol [(1)]).

- Assess BP near the end of each stage and repeatedly in the case of a hypo- or hypertensive response (see BP testing protocol [(1)]).

- Assess RPE near the end of each stage using either the 6 to 20 or the 0 to 10 RPE scale (6).

9. After terminating the test, initiate an appropriate cooldown. The cooldown can be an active recovery period consisting of light pedaling at a resistance equal to or less than the starting resistance. Or if the client is uncomfortable or is experiencing signs and symptoms (see "General Indications for Stopping an Exercise Test" on page 188 of chapter 10), a passive recovery may be necessary (1).

10. During the cooldown, monitor HR, BP, and signs and symptoms regularly for at least 4 minutes. If unusual or abnormal responses occur, further monitoring of the recovery period will be necessary (1).

YMCA CYCLE ERGOMETER TEST

The YMCA cycle ergometer test is a submaximal, multistage exercise test for cardiovascular endurance. This popular test is designed to progress clients to 85% of their predicted maximal HR using 3-minute stages of increasing work rate.

Equipment

- Mechanically or electrically braked cycle ergometer
- Metronome (if the cycle ergometer does not have an rpm gauge)
- Stopwatch
- Heart rate and BP measurement equipment (see "Heart Rate" and "Blood Pressure" sections earlier in this chapter)
- Rating of perceived exertion scale

Procedure

1. Instruct the client to begin pedaling at 50 rpm and maintain this cadence throughout the duration of the test.
2. Set the work rate for the first 3-minute stage at 150 kg · m · min^{-1} (0.5 kg at 50 rpm).
3. Measure the client's HR during the final 15 to 30 seconds of the second and third minutes of the first stage; if they are not within six beats/min of each other, continue the stage for one more minute.
4. See table 11.12 on page 251 for directions on how to set the work rate for the remaining stages. If the client's HR at the end of the first stage is

   - <80 beats/min, set the work rate for the second stage at 750 kg · m · min^{-1} (2.5 kg at 50 rpm)
   - 80 to 89 beats/min, set the work rate for the second stage at 600 kg · m · min^{-1} (2.0 kg at 50 rpm)
   - 90 to 100 beats/min, set the work rate for the second stage at 450 kg · m · min^{-1} (1.5 kg at 50 rpm)
   - >100 beats/min, set the work rate for the second stage at 300 kg · m · min^{-1} (1.0 kg at 50 rpm)

5. Measure the client's HR during the final 15 to 30 seconds of the second and third minutes of the second stage; if they are not within five beats/min of each other, continue the stage for one more minute.
6. Set the third and fourth 3-minute stages (if required) according to table 11.12 (work rates for the third and fourth stages are located in the rows below the second stage). Be sure to measure the client's HR in the final 15 to 30 seconds of the second and third minutes of each stage; if they are not within five beats/min of each other, continue each stage for one more minute.
7. Terminate the test when two steady state HRs between 110 beats/min and 85% age-predicted maximal HR are achieved, the client reaches 85% of his or her age-predicted maximal HR, or if the client meets one of the criteria listed in "General Indications for Stopping an Exercise Test" on page 188 of chapter 10.

Adapted from American College of Sports Medicine (1) and Golding (28).

Estimating V̇O$_2$max From the YMCA Cycle Ergometer Test

When the test is complete, the personal trainer should have the following data:

- Body weight (kg)
- Age-predicted maximal HR
- At least two steady state HR measurements between 110 beats/min and 85% age-predicted maximal HR at two different work rates
- A BP measurement at each work rate
- An RPE assessment at each work rate

To attain an estimation of the client's V̇O$_2$max:

1. Plot the HR (Y-axis in beats/min) versus work rate (X-axis in kg · m · min^{-1} or W) on a graph (see example 11.4 on page 215.
2. Construct a horizontal line at the age-predicted maximal HR value (A in figure 11.9).

3. Extrapolate the data by drawing a line of best fit for the HR values between 110 bpm and 85% of the age-predicted maximal HR (B in figure 11.9).

4. Continue the line of best fit (B) beyond the final data point until it crosses the horizontal line (A) representing the age-predicted maximal HR. Construct a vertical line from the intersection (C in figure 11.9) of the line of best fit and the horizontal age-predicted maximal HR line. Extend the vertical line to the X-axis and record the corresponding work-rate value (D in figure 11.9). This X value is the predicted maximal work rate that will be used to calculate the estimated $\dot{V}O_2$max (E in figure 11.9).

5. If the predicted maximal work rate is in kg · m · min^{-1}, it will need to be converted to watts (W). Use equation 11.5 to convert the kg · m · min^{-1} value to W.

6. Use the following equation (from [2]) to calculate the predicted $\dot{V}O_2$max value in milliliters per kilogram per minute (ml · kg^{-1} · min^{-1}):

$$\dot{V}O_2\text{max (ml · kg}^{-1} \cdot \text{min}^{-1}) = [(10.8 \times W) \div BW] + 7 \tag{11.6}$$

where W = the predicted maximal work rate (in watts) and BW = body weight (kg).

7. Once a client's $\dot{V}O_2$max has been estimated (ml · kg^{-1} · min^{-1}), use table 11.14 on page 252 (44b) to rank the client's $\dot{V}O_2$max using a cycle ergometer based on age. For example, if the $\dot{V}O_2$max has just been estimated to be 36.7 ml · kg^{-1} · min^{-1} for a 46-year-old male client, that client would rank just below the 90th percentile on a cycle ergometer when compared with others his age. In other words, one can say that 90% of men his age have a lower $\dot{V}O_2$max, while 10% have a higher $\dot{V}O_2$max.

EXAMPLE 11.4

YMCA Cycle Ergometer Test

Client A, a 23-year-old male client who weighs 181 pounds (82.1 kg), has just completed a YMCA cycle ergometer test with the following data:

Resting HR = 62 beats/min

Resting BP = 124/78 mmHg

Age-predicted maximal HR = 197 beats/min = 220 – 23 = 197 beats/min (from equation 11.3; see table 16.2 on page 429 for alternative formulas).

85% age-predicted maximal HR = 0.85 × 197 beats/min = 167 beats/min

Stage	Work rate	Elapsed time	HR	Average HR*	BP	RPE
1	150 kg · m · min^{-1}	2:00	88 beats/min			
1	150 kg · m · min^{-1}	3:00	88 beats/min	88 beats/min*	134/82 mmHg	9
2	600 kg · m · min^{-1}	5:00	132 beats/min			
2	600 kg · m · min^{-1}	6:00	136 beats/min	134 beats/min*	148/76 mmHg	13
3	750 kg · m · min^{-1}	8:00	153 beats/min			
3	750 kg · m · min^{-1}	9:00	159 beats/min	156 beats/min*	152/80 mmHg	15
4	900 kg · m · min^{-1}	11:00	166 beats/min			
4	900 kg · m · min^{-1}	12:00	168 beats/min	167 beats/min*	160/82 mmHg	17

*Average HR was calculated by averaging the two consecutive HR values at each work rate.

Step 1: Plot all of the average HR measurements (Y-axis) versus the corresponding work rates (X-axis) on a graph.

Step 2: Construct a horizontal line (A in figure 11.9) at 197 beats/min (the age-predicted maximum HR).

Step 3: Construct a line of best fit (B in figure 11.9) for the plotted data points (from step 1) and extend the line beyond the horizontal line at 197 beats/min (A in figure 11.9).

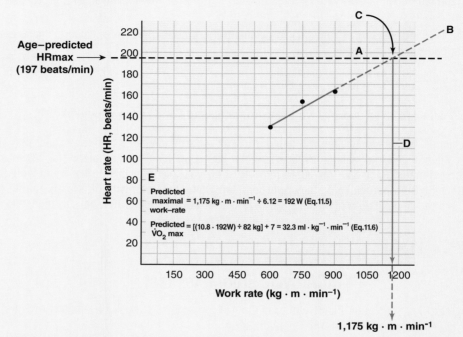

FIGURE 11.9 Using data from example 11.4, this figure illustrates how to graph a client's submaximal YMCA test data and how to construct the horizontal line for predicted maximal HR (A), extrapolate the line of best fit (B), identify the intersection (C), construct a vertical line for predicted maximal work rate (D), and use equations 11.5 and 11.6 to determine the predicted $\dot{V}O_2$max (E).

Step 4: Construct a vertical line (D in figure 11.9) from the intersection (C in figure 11.9) of lines A and B that extends to the X-axis.

Step 5: Identify the X-axis value that corresponds with the vertical line D. This value is the predicted maximal work rate that will be used to calculate the estimated $\dot{V}O_2$max (E in figure 11.9). In this example, it is 1,175 kg · m · min⁻¹.

Step 6: Use equation 11.5 to convert the kg · m · min⁻¹ value to watts.

Work rate (W) = Work rate (kg · m · min⁻¹) ÷ 6.12 (11.5)

From step 5, predicted maximal work rate (kg · m · min⁻¹) = 1,175 kg · m · min⁻¹

Predicted maximal work rate (W) = 1,175 kg · m · min⁻¹ ÷ 6.12 = 192 W

Step 7: Use equation 11.2 to convert the client's body weight in pounds to kilograms.

pounds (lb) ÷ 2.2046 = kilograms (kg) (11.2)

Body weight (lb) = 181 lb

181 lb ÷ 2.2046 = 82 kg

> *Step 8:* Use equation 11.6 (from [2]) to determine the predicted $\dot{V}O_2$max score in ml · kg^{-1} · min^{-1}.
>
> $$\dot{V}O_2\text{max (ml · kg}^{-1} \cdot \text{min}^{-1}) = [(10.8 \times W) \div BW] + 7 \qquad (11.6)$$
>
> From step 6, predicted maximal work rate (W) = 192 W
>
> Body weight (kg) = 82 kg
>
> $$\dot{V}O_2\text{max (ml · kg}^{-1} \cdot \text{min}^{-1}) = [(10.8 \times 192) \div 82] + 7 = 32.3 \text{ ml · kg}^{-1} \cdot \text{min}^{-1}$$
>
> *Step 9:* Use table 11.14 on page 252 (44b) to compare this client's predicted $\dot{V}O_2$max of 32.3 ml · kg^{-1} · min^{-1} to normative values; 32.3 ml · kg^{-1} · min^{-1} for a 23-year-old male ranks at less than the 20th percentile on a cycle ergometer. Therefore, more than 80% of the population have higher $\dot{V}O_2$max scores, while less than 20% have a lower $\dot{V}O_2$max.
>
> From Golding (28).

ÅSTRAND-RHYMING CYCLE ERGOMETER TEST

The Åstrand-Rhyming cycle ergometer test is a single-stage test (4). Total duration of the test is 6 minutes.

Equipment

- Mechanically or electrically braked cycle ergometer
- Metronome (if the cycle ergometer does not have an rpm gauge)
- Stopwatch

Procedure

1. Set the pedaling cadence at 50 rpm.
2. Set the work rate. Work rates used for the Åstrand-Rhyming test are chosen based on sex and fitness level (6). Note that for estimating a client's fitness level (unconditioned vs. conditioned) before the Åstrand-Rhyming test to determine the starting work rate, the recommendation is to always choose the more conservative work rate (unconditioned) if there is any question about the client's status.

    - *Males, unconditioned:* 300 or 600 kg · m · min^{-1}
    - *Males, conditioned:* 600 or 900 kg · m · min^{-1}
    - *Females, unconditioned:* 300 or 450 kg · m · min^{-1}
    - *Females, conditioned:* 450 or 600 kg · m · min^{-1}

3. Instruct the client to begin pedaling. Once the proper cadence is achieved, start the stopwatch. After 2 minutes, take a HR measurement.

    - If the HR is ≥120 beats/min, have the client continue the selected work rate throughout the 6-minute test duration.
    - If the HR after 2 minutes is <120, increase the resistance to the next highest increment or until the HR measurement is ≥120 beats/min after 2 minutes of riding at a constant work rate.

4. Take HR measurements at the end of the fifth and sixth minutes of the test, average them, and use this average value to estimate $\dot{V}O_2$max in liters per minute (L/min) from table 11.15 on page 252 (3) for males and table 11.16 on page 253 (3) for females.

5. Once the $\dot{V}O_2$max is estimated, it must be corrected for the age of the client. To obtain the age-corrected $\dot{V}O_2$max estimation, multiply the unaltered $\dot{V}O_2$max value (L/min) from table 11.15 or table 11.16 by the appropriate age correction factor in table 11.17 on page 254 (3).

6. After age correction of the $\dot{V}O_2$max estimation (L/min), it can be converted to $ml \cdot kg^{-1} \cdot min^{-1}$ by the following equation:

$$\dot{V}O_2max \ (ml \cdot kg^{-1} \cdot min^{-1}) = \dot{V}O_2max \ in \ L/min \times 1,000 \div BW \qquad (11.7)$$

where BW = body weight in kilograms (kg).

7. Compare the age-corrected $\dot{V}O_2$max estimations ($ml \cdot kg^{-1} \cdot min^{-1}$) from the Åstrand-Rhyming test against the normative values listed in table 11.18 on page 254 (6).

EXAMPLE 11.5

Åstrand-Rhyming Cycle Ergometer Test

A 57-year-old female client who weighs 145 pounds (65.8 kg) has just completed the Åstrand-Rhyming cycle ergometer test. The following data were recorded:

Work rate = 600 kg · m · min⁻¹

Heart rate after second minute = 122 beats/min

Heart rate after fifth minute = 129 beats/min

Heart rate after sixth minute = 135 beats/min

Step 1: (129 beats/min + 135 beats/min) ÷ 2 = 132 beats/min average.

Step 2: Estimated $\dot{V}O_2$max value from table 11.16 for an average HR of 132 beats/min and a work rate of 600 kg · m · min⁻¹ = 2.7 L/min.

Step 3: Age correction factor from table 11.17 for a 57-year-old client = 0.70.

Step 4: 2.7 L/min × 0.70 age correction factor = 1.89 L/min.

Step 5: (1.89 L/min × 1,000) ÷ 66 kg = 28.64 ml · kg⁻¹ · min⁻¹.

Step 6: Aerobic fitness category from table 11.18 for 28.64 ml · kg⁻¹ · min⁻¹ for a 57-year-old female = good.

Step 7: Percentile rank on a cycle ergometer from table 11.14 for 28.64 ml · kg⁻¹ · min⁻¹ for a 57-year-old female is greater than 90%.

YMCA STEP TEST

The YMCA step test is a basic, inexpensive cardiovascular endurance test that can be easily administered individually or to large groups. This test classifies fitness levels based on the postexercise HR response but does not provide an estimation of $\dot{V}O_2$max. The objective of the YMCA step test is to have the client step up and down to a set cadence for 3 minutes and to measure the HR recovery response immediately after the test.

Equipment

- 12-inch or 30 cm step bench or box
- Metronome set at 96 beats/min
- Stopwatch

Procedure

1. For familiarization, the client should listen to the cadence before stepping.
2. Instruct the client to step "up, up, down, down" to a cadence of 96 beats/min, which allows 24 steps per minute. It does not matter which foot leads or if the foot lead changes during the test.

3. Have the client continue stepping for 3 minutes.

4. Immediately after the final step, help the client sit down and, within 5 seconds, measure the HR for 1 minute.

5. Compare the 1-minute recovery HR value against the normative values in table 11.19 on page 255 (61).

DISTANCE RUN AND WALK TEST CONSIDERATIONS

Distance run tests are based on the assumption that a more "fit" client will be able to run a given distance in less time or run a greater distance in a given period of time. These tests are practical, inexpensive, less time consuming than other tests, and easy to administer to large groups. They also can be used to classify the cardiovascular endurance level of healthy men under 40 years of age and healthy women under 50 years of age. The personal trainer cannot, however, use field tests to detect or control for cardiac episodes because HR and BP are typically not monitored during the performance of these tests.

These field tests are effort-based assessments and are suited for clients who can run (or walk briskly) for either 12 minutes, 1.5 miles (2.4 km), or 1 mile (1.6 km). Examples of clients for whom these tests are appropriate are those who have been training for several weeks and those who regularly use running or fast walking as a mode of cardiovascular exercise. Other tests for $\dot{V}O_2$max such as the Åstrand-Rhyming cycle ergometer test or the YMCA step test are recommended for clients who do not meet these criteria.

From Golding (28).

12-MINUTE RUN/WALK

The 12-minute run/walk test is a field test designed to measure the distance traveled over 12 minutes of running, walking, or a combination of both. After distance is recorded as the test score, it is used in a regression equation (equation 11.8) to estimate $\dot{V}O_2$max.

Equipment

- 400-meter (437-yard) track or flat course with measured distances so that the number of laps completed can be easily counted and multiplied by the course distance
- Visible place markers—may be necessary to divide the course into predetermined section lengths (e.g., every one-fourth or one-half of a lap) so that the exact distance covered in 12 minutes can be determined quickly
- Stopwatch

Procedure

1. Instruct the client to run as far as possible during the 12-minute duration. Walking is allowed; however, the objective of this test is to cover as much distance as possible in 12 minutes.

2. Record the total distance completed in meters. For example, a client has just completed five full laps and one-fourth of the last lap (5.25 laps). Since there are 400 meters per lap, the client completed 2,100 meters (5.25 laps × 400 m = 2,100 m).

3. Use the following equation (from [(28)]) to estimate the client's $\dot{V}O_2$max (ml · kg^{-1} · min^{-1}):

$$\dot{V}O_2\text{max (ml} \cdot \text{kg}^{-1} \cdot \text{min}^{-1}) = (0.022351 \times D) - 11.3 \tag{11.8}$$

where D = distance completed in meters.

4. Compare the estimated $\dot{V}O_2$max score against the normative values on a treadmill listed in table 11.13 (44a).

> ## EXAMPLE 11.6
>
> ### 12-Minute Run/Walk
>
> A 31-year-old female client who weighs 128 pounds (58.1 kg) has just completed the 12-minute run. The following data were recorded:
>
> 12-min run distance = 1.16 miles (6,109 feet; 1,862 m)
>
> 1. $[0.022351 \times (1,862 \text{ m})] - 11.3 = 30.32 \text{ ml} \cdot \text{kg}^{-1} \cdot \text{min}^{-1}$.
>
> 2. Percentile rank on a treadmill from table 11.13 for $30.32 \text{ ml} \cdot \text{kg}^{-1} \cdot \text{min}^{-1}$ for a 31-year-old female is just about the 50th percentile.

1.5-MILE RUN

The 1.5-mile run is a field test designed to measure the time it takes for a client to run 1.5 miles (2.4 km). Once the time is recorded as the test score, it is used in a regression equation (equation 11.9) to estimate $\dot{V}O_2$max.

Equipment

- 400-meter (437-yard) track or flat course with the 1.5-mile (2.4 km) distance measured (to measure the course, use an odometer or measuring wheel [(28)])
- Stopwatch

Procedure

1. Instruct clients to cover the 1.5-mile (2.4 km) distance in the fastest possible time. Walking is allowed, but the objective is to complete the distance in as short a time as possible.

2. Call out or record the elapsed time (in minutes and seconds, 00:00) as the client crosses the finish line.

3. Convert the seconds to minutes by dividing the seconds by 60. For example, if a client's time for the test is 12:30, the run time is converted to 12.5 minutes (30 ÷ 60 seconds = 0.5 minutes).

4. Use the following equation (from [(28)]) to estimate the client's $\dot{V}O_2$max ($\text{ml} \cdot \text{kg}^{-1} \cdot \text{min}^{-1}$):

$$\dot{V}O_2\text{max (ml} \cdot \text{kg}^{-1} \cdot \text{min}^{-1}) = 88.02 - (0.1656 \times BW) \tag{11.9}$$
$$- (2.76 \times \text{time} + (3.716 \times \text{sex}^*)$$

  where *BW* = body weight in kilograms (kg) and *time* = 1.5-mile run time to completion (to the nearest hundredth of a minute, 0.00 min).

  *For sex, substitute 1 for males and 0 for females.

5. Estimated $\dot{V}O_2$max scores can be compared against the normative values using a treadmill listed in table 11.13 on page 251 (44a).

EXAMPLE 11.7

1.5-Mile Run

A 28-year-old male client who weighs 171 pounds (77.6 kg) has just completed the 1.5-mile (2.4 km) run. The following data were recorded:

1.5-mile run time = 8:52 min:s

1. 52 s ÷ 60 s = 0.87 min, so 8:52 min:s = 8.87 min.
2. 88.02 − [0.1656 × (77.6)] − [2.763 (8.87)] + [3.716 × (1 for males)] = 54.40 ml · kg^{-1} · min^{-1}.
3. Percentile rank from table 11.13 for 54.40 ml · kg^{-1} · min^{-1} for a 28-year-old male is just below the 75th percentile on a treadmill.

ROCKPORT WALKING TEST

The Rockport walking test has been developed to estimate $\dot{V}O_2$max for men and women ages 18 to 69 years (47). Because this test requires only walking at a fast pace, it is useful for testing older or sedentary clients.

Equipment

- Stopwatch
- Measured 1-mile (1.6 km) walking course that is flat and uninterrupted (preferably an outdoor track)

Procedure

1. Instruct the client to walk 1 mile (1.6 km) as briskly as possible.
2. Immediately after the test, calculate the client's HR (in beats per minute) using a 15-second HR count duration (see "Heart Rate" section earlier in this chapter).
3. Convert the seconds to minutes by dividing the seconds by 60 (see step 3 for the 1.5-mile run procedure).
4. Estimate the client's $\dot{V}O_2$max (ml · kg^{-1} · min^{-1}) using the following equation (from [(49)]):

$$\dot{V}O_2\text{max (ml · kg}^{-1} \cdot \text{min}^{-1}) = 132.853 - (0.0769 \times BW) - (0.3877 \times age) \tag{11.10}$$
$$+ (6.315 \times sex^*) - (3.2649 \times time) - (0.1565\ 3\ HR)$$

where *BW* = body weight in pounds, *age* = age in years, *time* = 1-mile walk time to completion (to the nearest hundredth of a minute, 0.00 minutes), and *HR* = heart rate in beats per minute.

*For sex, substitute 1 for males and 0 for females.

5. Estimated $\dot{V}O_2$max scores can be compared against the normative values using a treadmill listed in table 11.13 (44a).
6. 1-mile walk times can also be compared against the normative values listed in table 11.20 on page 255 (61).

EXAMPLE 11.8

Rockport Walking Test

A 52-year-old male client who weighs 228 pounds (103.4 kg) has just completed the Rockport walking test. The following data were recorded:

Posttest HR = 159 beats/min

1-mile walk time = 10:35 min:s

1. 35 s ÷ 60 s = 0.58 min; 10:35 min:s = 10.58 min.
2. 132.853 − [0.0769 × (228 lb)] − [0.3877 × (52)] + [6.315 × (1 for males)] − [3.2649 × (10.58 min)] − [0.1565 × (159)] = 42.05 ml · kg⁻¹ · min⁻¹.
3. Percentile rank from table 11.13 for 42.05 ml · kg⁻¹ · min⁻¹ for a 52-year-old male is between the 80th and 90th percentiles on a treadmill.
4. Rating from table 11.20 for 10:35 min:s = good.
5. Percentile rank from table 11.20 for 10:35 min:s = over 90th percentile.

1-MILE RUN

The 1-mile run has been developed to estimate cardiovascular endurance for children ages 6 to 17 years (61).

Equipment

- Stopwatch
- A flat and uninterrupted 1-mile (1.6 km) course (e.g., an outdoor track)

Procedure

1. Instruct clients to cover the 1-mile (1.6 km) distance in the fastest possible time. Walking may be interspersed with running, but the client should try to complete the distance in the fastest time possible.
2. Record the elapsed time (in minutes and seconds, 00:00) as the client crosses the finish line.
3. Convert the seconds to minutes by dividing the seconds by 60 (see step 3 for the 1.5-mile run procedure).
4. Compare the recorded time against the normative values listed in table 11.21 on page 256 (69).

NON–EXERCISE-BASED ESTIMATION OF $\dot{V}O_2$MAX

Non–exercise-based equations have been developed by Malek and colleagues (54, 55) to estimate a client's $\dot{V}O_2$max from various demographic and descriptive variables. These equations have been used to provide reasonable estimates of $\dot{V}O_2$max for both trained and untrained men and women. In addition, the errors associated with these equations range between ±10% to 15% of $\dot{V}O_2$max, which are similar to the errors often encountered with exercise-based estimates of $\dot{V}O_2$max (54, 55). Overall, non–exercise-based equations for the prediction of $\dot{V}O_2$max can be very useful, especially when the risk of conducting an exercise-based $\dot{V}O_2$max assessment is too high or unknown for clients who may be susceptible to exercise-induced stress.

Equipment

- Standard platform scale with anthropometer arm or flat, ridged, right-angled device (to simultaneously slide against a wall and rest on top of client's crown)
- Calibrated and certified scale
- Rating of perceived exertion scale

Procedure

1. Record the client's height in centimeters, body weight in kilograms, and age in years.
2. Estimate the typical intensity of training using the Borg RPE scale (e.g., 6-20).
3. Indicate the number of hours per week the client exercises.
4. Indicate the number of years the client has been training consistently with no more than one month without exercise.
5. Determine the natural log of the years of training. That is, enter the client's years of training and then hit "LN," or the natural log, on a handheld calculator.
6. Determine $\dot{V}O_2$max in L/min using the equations in table 11.22 on page 265 (54, 55).
7. Calculate $\dot{V}O_2$max in ml · kg^{-1} · min^{-1} using equation 11.7.
8. Compare the client's scores to the cycle ergometer data from table 11.14 on page 252.

SPEED AND AGILITY

Because of their commonalities with sporting activities, particularly with team sports, speed and change-of-direction tests are popular in athletic evaluation settings. Maximal speed and the time required to achieve maximal speed are typical outcomes of sprint tests, while agility tests provide an indication of planned or unplanned change-of-direction speed using a variety of movement patterns. Although tests focused primarily on athletic performance are included here, numerous assessments are available that provide invaluable information for older adults and those engaged in the process of physical rehabilitation.

STRAIGHT-LINE SPRINT TESTS

Straight-line sprint tests assess maximal speed and acceleration. The starting body position (e.g., standing two-point stance, kneeling three- or four-point stance), the use of static or running (or "flying") starts, and distance covered will depend on the goals or activities of the clients. The total sprinting distance can be separated into shorter split distances if appropriate timing equipment is available. A 40-yard (36.6 m) sprint test with a static start from a standing two-point stance will be described.

Equipment

- Measuring tape
- Cones, markers, adhesive tape, or field paint
- Timing device

Procedure

1. Have the client complete a standardized warm-up with several moderate-intensity running trials.
2. Designate the start and finish lines 40 yards (36.6 meters) apart, as well as any intermediate lengths for relevant split distances (e.g., 10 yards or meters), using cones, markers, tape, or paint (figure 11.10; 16a).
3. Ask the client to stand with the front foot behind the start line and, on the signal to begin, to increase speed as quickly as possible and maintain maximal speed until approximately 5 yards (or meters) beyond the finish line (a second set of cones can be placed 5 yards or meters after the finish line to encourage this).
4. Record the sprint time (in seconds to the nearest 0.1 s) as the shortest time between the starting signal and the client's reaching the finish line (and relevant split distances) from at least three attempts separated by approximately 3 to 5 minutes.
5. Compare the client's score against the values for youth (figure 11.11 on page 256; 30) or college-age individuals (figure 11.12 on page 257; 64).

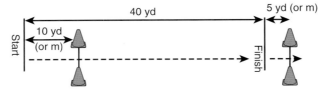

FIGURE 11.10   Setup for a 40 yd (36.6 m) straight-line sprint test.

300-YARD SHUTTLE

The 300-yard (274.3 m) shuttle provides an indicator of anaerobic capacity through a combination of sustained sprinting and change-of-direction abilities.

Equipment

- Measuring tape
- Cones, markers, adhesive tape, or field paint
- Timing device

Procedure

1. Have the client complete a standardized warm-up with several moderate-intensity running trials and change-of-direction movements.

2. Designate the start/finish and turning lines 25 yards (22.9 meters) apart using cones, markers, tape, or paint (figure 11.13; 16a).

3. Ask the client to stand with the front foot behind the start line and face the turning line. On the signal to begin, the client will sprint to the far line, make foot contact with it, then turn and sprint back to the start line. This down-and-back pattern will be repeated a total of six times.

4. Record the 300-yard shuttle time (in seconds to the nearest 0.1 s) as the shortest time to complete the series of shuttles out of two attempts separated by approximately 3 to 5 minutes.

5. Compare the client's score against the categories for NCAA Division I athletes (figure 11.14 on page 257; 37) or various populations (figure 11.15 on page 257; 58).

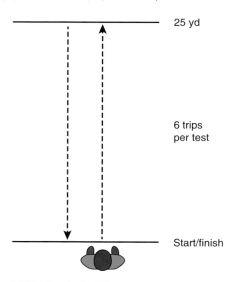

FIGURE 11.13 Setup for the 300 yd (274.3 m) shuttle run.

T-TEST

The T-test reflects speed and agility using planned change-of-direction ability and varied movement patterns (sprinting, side-shuffling, and backpedaling).

Equipment

- Measuring tape
- Cones or markers
- Timing device

Procedure

1. Have the client complete a standardized warm-up with several moderate-intensity running trials and change-of-direction movements.

2. Align the cones or markers in a T configuration, with the start/finish (marker A) located 10 yards (9.1 m) from marker B. Markers C and D should be placed 5 yards (4.6 m) from marker B in a straight line and perpendicular to the straight line formed by marker B and marker A (figure 11.16; 16a).

3. Ask the client to stand with the front foot behind marker A looking toward marker B. Once the signal is given by the test administrator, the client will sprint toward marker B and touch the base of the cone with the right hand.

4. Next, the client will side-shuffle to the left, not crossing the feet, for 5 yards until touching the base of marker C with the left hand.

5. The individual will then side-shuffle to the right, not crossing the feet, for 10 yards to marker D, touching the base with the right hand.

6. The client will then side-shuffle back to the left for 5 yards, touch the base of marker B with the left hand, then proceed to backpedal as fast as possible past marker A.

7. Record the T-test time (in seconds to the nearest 0.1 s) as the shortest time to complete the planned movement out of at least three attempts separated by approximately 3 to 5 minutes.

8. Compare the client's score against the values in figure 11.17 on page 258 (64).

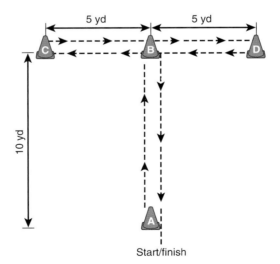

FIGURE 11.16   Setup for the T-test.

PRO AGILITY (20-YARD SHUTTLE RUN, OR 5-10-5 TEST)

The pro agility test reflects planned change-of-direction ability and speed during several short sprints separated by quick turning movements.

Equipment

- Measuring tape
- Cones, markers, or field paint
- Timing device

Procedure

1. Have the client complete a standardized warm-up with several moderate-intensity running trials and change-of-direction movements.
2. Using the cones, markers, or field paint, create three parallel lines separated by 5 yards (15 ft; 4.6 m) (figure 11.18; 16a).
3. Ask the client to stand straddling the middle line looking straight head. Once the signal is given by the test administrator, the client will turn to the right and sprint until touching the line with the right hand.
4. Next, the client will turn to the left and sprint 10 yards (30 ft; 9.1 m) past the middle line until touching the far left line with the left hand.
5. The individual will then turn to the right and sprint as fast as possible past the middle line to finish the test.
6. Record the pro agility test time (in seconds to the nearest 0.1 s) as the shortest time to complete the planned movement out of at least three attempts separated by approximately 3 to 5 minutes.
7. Compare the client's score to the values in figure 11.19 on page 258 (38).

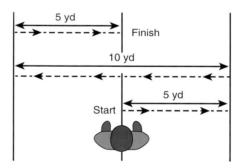

FIGURE 11.18   Setup for the pro agility test.

MUSCULAR STRENGTH

Muscular strength is an important component of physical fitness. A minimal level of muscular strength is needed to perform daily activities, especially as one ages, and to participate in recreational or occupational activities without undue risk of injury. Strength may be tested as 1-repetition maximum (1RM) or multiple-repetition maximum and expressed either as absolute strength or as relative strength. **Absolute strength** is simply the raw strength score a person achieves, while **relative strength** is usually expressed relative to body weight. For example, a 175-pound (79.4 kg) client with a 1RM bench press of 225 pounds (102.1 kg) would have an absolute strength score of 225 pounds and a relative strength score of 1.3 (225-pound 1RM absolute strength divided by 175 pounds of body weight). Many personal trainers prefer not to have their clients perform 1RM testing because of safety or technique concerns. Fortunately, it is possible to estimate a client's 1RM from a submaximal resistance (74, 83). This involves having the client perform multiple-repetition maximum testing.

MULTIPLE-REPETITION MAXIMUM BENCH PRESS

A multiple-repetition maximum (e.g., 5RM) bench press test may be used to measure upper body strength. Because free weights are used, this test requires skill on the part of the client being tested.

Equipment

- Adjustable barbell and weight plates that allow resistance increments of 5 to 90 pounds (~2.5-40 kg).

Procedure

Provide a spotter and closely observe technique. See page 348 for proper bench press technique. Then, follow these steps for determining a 5RM:

1. Instruct the client to warm up with a light resistance that easily allows 8 to 10 repetitions.
2. Provide a 1-minute rest period.
3. Estimate an additional warm-up load that the client will use to complete 6 to 8 repetitions by adding as follows:
   - *Upper body exercise:* 5- to 10-pound increase (~2.5-5 kg)
   - *Lower body exercise:* 15- to 20-pound increase (~7.5-10 kg)
4. Provide a 2- to 4-minute rest period.
5. Make a load increase:
   - *Upper body exercise:* 5- to 10-pound increase (~2.5-5 kg)
   - *Lower body exercise:* 15- to 20-pound increase (~7.5-10 kg)
6. Instruct the client to attempt a 5RM.
7. If the client was successful, provide a 2- to 4-minute rest period and go back to step 5. If the client failed, provide a 2- to 4-minute rest period and decrease the load as follows:
   - *Upper body exercise:* 2.5- to 5-pound decrease (~1.25-2.5 kg)
   - *Lower body exercise:* 5- to 10-pound decrease (~2.5-5 kg), or 5%-10%

   Then go back to step 6.

8. Continue increasing or decreasing the load until the client can complete 5 repetitions with proper exercise technique. Note that load increases may need to be adjusted depending on the strength or experience level of the individual; a lower initial load and subsequently lower increments should be used if 10RM maximum testing is preferred. Ideally, the client's multiple-repetition maximum value will be measured within 3 to 5 testing sets.
9. Record the 5RM value as the maximum weight lifted (i.e., the client's absolute strength) for the last successful attempt.

Once these steps are completed, either record the multiple-repetition maximum strength values or use the conversion nomograms in figure 11.20 on page 259 to estimate 1RM strength (83). You can also divide the estimated 1RM value by the client's body weight to determine relative strength for comparison against values provided in table 11.23 on page 260 (23). The process for estimating starting loads for a resistance training program is described in chapters 15 and 23.

MULTIPLE-REPETITION MAXIMUM LEG PRESS

The multiple-repetition maximum leg press may be used to measure lower body strength. Chapter 13 provides a detailed account of client and spotter responsibilities during most lower body exercises. Personal trainers should be familiar with the guidelines in chapter 13 before attempting multiple-repetition maximum trials.

Equipment

- Universal leg press machine. This resistance training device is less common than many others and therefore may be difficult to find. The personal trainer can instead opt to use a different exercise such as an angled hip sled or horizontal leg press to assess a client's lower body muscular strength. Note, however, that the normative data shown in table 11.24 on page 261 (23) will apply only if a Universal leg press machine is used.

Procedure

1. Have the client sit in the seat of the leg press machine and place the feet on the upper pair of foot plates.
2. Adjust the seat to standardize the knee angle at approximately 120 degrees.
3. Follow the steps for determining a 5RM described in the "Multiple-Repetition Maximum Bench Press" section to assess the client's leg press 5RM (58, 77).
4. Either record the multiple-repetition maximum strength values or use the conversion nomograms in figure 11.20 to estimate 1RM strength (83).
5. If the Universal leg press machine was used, the estimated 1RM can also be divided by the client's body weight to determine relative strength for comparison to values in table 11.24 (23).

From Baumgartner, Jackson, Mahar, and Rowe (5).

MUSCULAR POWER

Muscular power is the ability to produce force (i.e., muscular strength) within a short time. In athletic settings, power is often referred to as **explosiveness** and may be a better indicator of performance than strength or speed alone. This physical quality also plays a role in occupational settings and activities of daily living by allowing individuals to quickly move their bodies or objects (e.g., getting up from a chair or lifting a suitcase into a vehicle) and safely navigate their environments (e.g., avoiding an oncoming cyclist or climbing a flight of stairs). When assessing muscular power, fitness professionals must consider the joints being used, the planes of movement, and the skill and technique required to successfully, and safely, complete the selected tests.

VERTICAL JUMP TEST

The vertical jump test evaluates muscular power in the vertical plane, primarily using the lower body with assistance from the trunk and upper body (i.e., momentum). The version described here uses a countermovement jump; however, the test may be performed without the rapid eccentric prejump movement by starting from a static partial squat position, termed a squat jump.

Equipment

- Wall with high ceiling
- Chalk
- Measuring tape
- Alternative equipment: vertical jump measurement device (e.g., Vertec, switch mat)

Procedure

1. Have the client complete a standardized warm-up with three to five practice jumps at ~50% of perceived maximal effort.
2. Ask the client to place chalk on the fingertips of the dominant hand and stand with the dominant side of the body about 6 inches (15 cm) from the wall (figure 11.21a).
3. With both feet flat on the ground, the client reaches as high as possible with the dominant hand and marks the wall with the chalk. Record this value as standing reach height (in centimeters or inches) (figure 11.21b).

4. Once standing height is recorded (figure 11.22*a*) , instruct the client to perform a quick partial squat (countermovement) by flexing at the hips and knees while swinging the arms backward (figure 11.22*b*) . This movement is quickly followed by a maximal vertical jump with the goal of making a chalk mark as high as possible on the wall with the outstretched dominant arm (figure 11.22*c*). Stress the importance of a safe, controlled landing after the jump.

5. Record the vertical height (in centimeters or inches) as the distance between the standing reach height and the highest chalk mark out of at least three jump attempts separated by ~60 seconds.

6. Compare the client's score against the values in figure 11.23 or figure 11.24 on page 262 (38, 63).

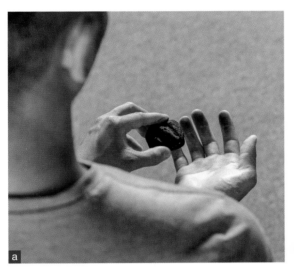
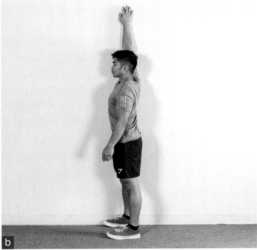

FIGURE 11.21   *(a)* Placement of chalk on fingers; *(b)* determining standing reach height with chalked hand.

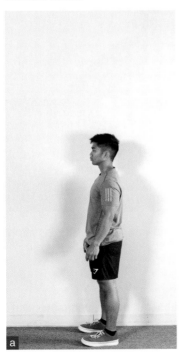
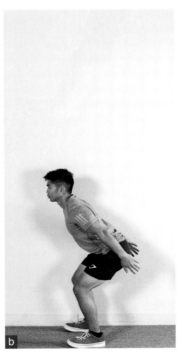
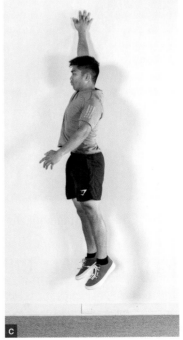

FIGURE 11.22   Vertical jump test: *(a)* beginning position, *(b)* countermovement, and *(c)* maximal jump.

STANDING LONG JUMP TEST

The standing long jump (or broad jump) test evaluates muscular power in the horizontal plane, primarily using the lower body with assistance from the trunk and upper body.

Equipment

- Adhesive tape or field paint
- Measuring tape

Procedure

1. Have the client complete a standardized warm-up with three to five broad jumps for practice at ~50% of perceived maximal effort.
2. Ask the client to stand with toes on the start line, marked by a strip of adhesive tape or field paint on the ground.
3. From a standing position with both feet on the floor and arms at the side, the client performs a quick partial squat (countermovement) (figure 11.25*a*) followed by a maximal jump as far forward as possible in a straight line (figure 11.25*b*). Stress the importance of a safe, controlled landing on the feet after the jump and of remaining in the landing position until the measurement is completed (figure 11.25*c*).
4. Record the standing long jump as the distance between the starting line and the back of the client's rearmost heel.
5. The best trial, to the nearest 0.5 inches or 1 cm, out of three maximal jumps is recorded and compared against the values in figure 11.26 on page 262 or figure 11.27 on page 263 (11, 78).

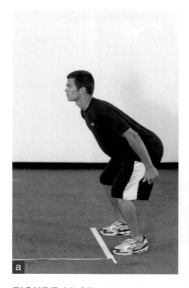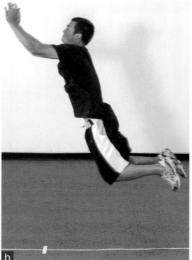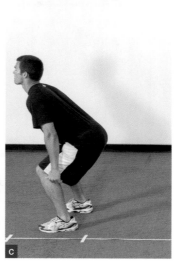

FIGURE 11.25 Standing long jump test: *(a)* beginning position, *(b)* mid-jump, and *(c)* end position.

MEDICINE BALL CHEST PASS TEST

The medicine ball chest pass test evaluates muscular power using an upper body pushing movement.

Equipment

- Incline bench at a 45-degree angle
- Medicine ball (6 kg [13.2 lb] for females, 9 kg [19.8 lb] for males)
- Measuring tape

Procedure

1. Have the client complete a standardized warm-up with three to five practice throws at ~50% of perceived maximal effort.

2. Secure the measuring tape with its zero end underneath the front support beam and extend it out at least 25 feet (7.6 m) in a straight line.

3. Ask the client to sit on the bench, making contact with the back and head, feet flat on the floor, and holding the medicine ball against the chest with hands on the sides of the ball (figure 11.28*a*).

4. Next, instruct the individual to maximally throw the medicine ball as far forward as possible along the measuring tape (figure 11.28*b*) .

5. Record the throwing distance (in centimeters or inches) along the measuring tape as the longest of at least three attempts separated by approximately 2 minutes.

6. Compare the client's score against the values in figure 11.29 on page 263 (12).

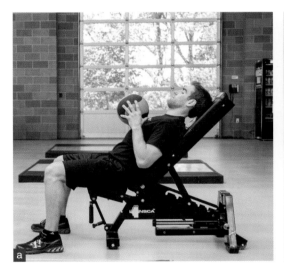 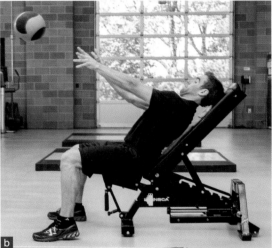

FIGURE 11.28 Medicine ball chest pass: *(a)* beginning position and *(b)* end position.

MUSCULAR ENDURANCE

Muscular endurance is the ability of a muscle or muscle group to exert submaximal force for extended periods. Along with muscular strength, muscular endurance is important for performing the activities of daily living, as well as in recreational and occupational pursuits. Muscular endurance may be assessed during static and dynamic muscle actions.

YMCA BENCH PRESS TEST

The YMCA bench press test is used to measure upper body muscular endurance. This is a test of absolute muscular endurance; that is, the resistance is the same for all members of a given sex.

Equipment

- Adjustable barbell and weight plates
- Metronome

Procedure

1. Spot the client and closely observe the technique.

2. Set the resistance at 80 pounds (36 kg) for male clients, 35 pounds (16 kg) for female clients.

3. See page 348 for proper bench press technique.

4. Set the metronome cadence at 60 beats/min to establish a rate of 30 repetitions per minute.

5. Have the client, beginning with the arms extended and a shoulder-width grip, lower the weight to the chest. Then, without pausing, the client should raise the bar to full arm's length. The movement should be smooth and controlled, with the bar reaching its highest and lowest positions with each beat of the metronome.

6. Terminate the test when the client can no longer lift the barbell in cadence with the metronome.

7. Compare the client's score against values in table 11.25 on page 264 (28).

SIT-UP TEST

The sit-up test is a two-minute assessment designed to measure localized endurance of the abdominal muscles. While multiple variations of this test exist (e.g., partial curl-up or plank) widely accepted normative data is still needed in order to accurately assess and compare individuals.

Equipment

- Mat

Procedure

1. Direct the client to assume a supine position on a mat with the knees at 90 degrees and the arms crossed across the chest, hands on shoulders, with the elbows pointing toward the thighs (figure 11.30a).

2. Have a partner kneel on the ground facing the client and hold the client's feet or ankles to keep them stationary during the test.

3. Have the client perform controlled sit-ups by using the abdominal muscles to lift the shoulder blades and torso off the mat until the elbows touch the thighs (figure 11.30b). The torso and shoulder blades should return to the ground in a controlled manner, avoiding momentum, prior to beginning the next repetition.

4. Encourage the client to perform as many sit-ups as possible for a period of two minutes.

5. Compare the client's score against table 11.26 on page 264 (38a).

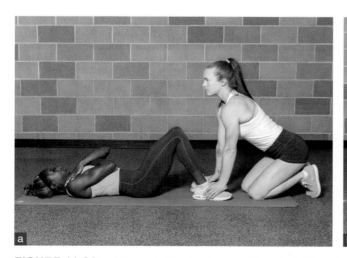 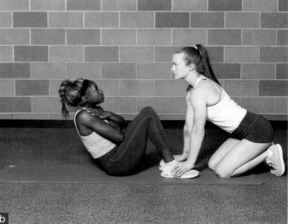

FIGURE 11.30 Sit-up: *(a)* beginning position and *(b)* end position.

PRONE DOUBLE STRAIGHT-LEG RAISE TEST

The prone double straight-leg raise is useful for examining low back muscular endurance and predicting potential low back pain (15, 60).

Equipment

- A mat or massage table

Procedure

1. Have the client begin the test in the prone position, legs extended, hands underneath the forehead, and forearms perpendicular to the body (figure 11.31*a*).
2. Instruct the client to raise both legs to the point of knee clearance from the table or floor (figure 11.31*b*).
3. Monitor the test by sliding one hand under the thighs.
4. Record the test duration in seconds.
5. Terminate the test when the client can no longer maintain knee clearance from the table or floor.
6. Compare the client's score against the values in table 11.27 on page 264 (60).

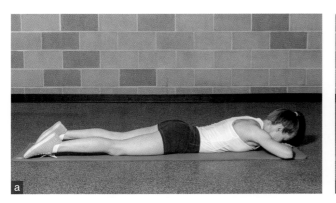
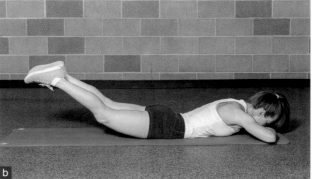

FIGURE 11.31   Prone double straight-leg raise: *(a)* beginning position and *(b)* legs raised position.

FLEXIBILITY

Flexibility refers to the range of motion (ROM) around a joint (e.g., shoulder) or a series of joints (e.g., vertebral column). It is believed to be related to the development of a number of musculoskeletal disorders (e.g., low back pain). There is no single test that can measure whole-body flexibility. Separate tests need to be administered for each area of interest. Traditionally, personal trainers have focused on tests that measure the flexibility of joints believed to be associated with risk of developing low back pain.

SIT AND REACH

The sit-and-reach test is often used to measure hip and low back flexibility. Although the sit-and-reach test is commonly seen as an indicator of previous back discomfort, its ability to predict the incidence of low back pain is limited (25, 29). Nonetheless, a lack of hip and low back flexibility, along with poor muscular strength and endurance of the abdominal muscles, is believed to be predictive of low back pain.

Equipment

- Yardstick or sit-and-reach box
- Adhesive tape
- Measuring tape

Procedure

1. Have the client warm up and perform some moderate stretching before the test. All testing should be done without shoes. The test should be performed with slow, controlled stretches.

2. For the YMCA sit-and-reach test, place a yardstick on the floor and place tape across the yardstick at a right angle to the 15-inch (38.1 cm) mark (see figure 11.32a). The client then sits with the yardstick between the legs, extending the legs at right angles to the taped line on the floor. The heels should touch the edge of the taped line and should be about 10 to 12 inches (25-30 cm) apart. If a sit-and-reach box is used, the heels should be placed against the edge of the box (see figure 11.33a).

3. Have the client reach forward slowly with both hands, moving as far as possible and holding the terminal position. The fingers should overlap and should be in contact with the yardstick (figure 11.32b) or sit-and-reach box (figure 11.33b).

4. The score is the most distant point reached. Use the best of two trials as the score. The knees must stay extended throughout the test, but the tester should not press the client's legs down.

5. Compare the test results using either table 11.28 on page 265 for the YMCA sit-and-reach (28) or tables 11.29 and 11.30 on pages 265 and 266 for the sit-and-reach box (9). Note that the norms for the YMCA sit-and-reach test use a "zero point" (the zero point is the point at which the client reaches the toes) of 15 inches (38.1 cm), while the sit-and-reach box typically uses a zero point set at 26 cm (10.2 inches). When using a different zero point, be sure to adjust the client's score before using the norm tables. For example, if the box has a zero point of 23 cm (9.1 inches), add 3 cm (1.2 inches) to the client's score before consulting table 11.29 or table 11.30 (or subtract 3 cm from the norms in the table before comparing the client's score to table 11.29 or table 11.30).

Adapted from American College of Sports Medicine (2).

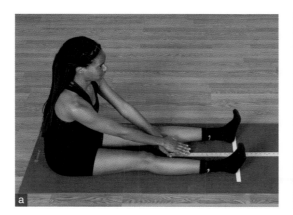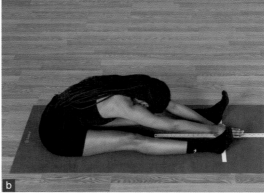

FIGURE 11.32   Sit-and-reach positioning with a yardstick: *(a)* beginning position and *(b)* end position.

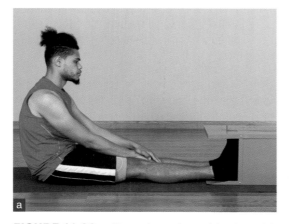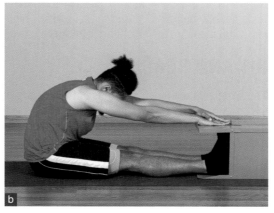

FIGURE 11.33   Sit-and-reach positioning with a sit-and-reach box: *(a)* beginning position and *(b)* end position.

BACK SCRATCH TEST

The back scratch test is used as an indication of upper body flexibility and shoulder range of motion, which contribute to the ability to complete activities of daily living (e.g., changing a shirt, reaching into a cupboard) and a variety of overhead movements related to exercise.

Equipment

- Measuring tape or ruler

Procedure

1. Have the client complete a standardized warm-up including various shoulder movements (e.g., forward and rearward arm circles).

2. While in a standing position, the client raises the right arm overhead, bends the elbow, and places the palm of the hand along the spine on the upper back (see figure 11.34a).

3. Next, reaching behind the back, the client places the left hand, with the palm facing outward, along the spine on the lower back (with the left elbow pointed downward) (figure 11.34b).

4. Direct the client to slowly slide each hand along the spine while attempting to overlap the fingertips as far as possible (while avoiding unusual compensation strategies such as overarching the back or contorting the shoulders) and to hold this position for approximately 2 seconds.

5. Using the measuring tape or ruler, measure any overlap between the fingertips as a positive value or gap as a negative value (to the nearest centimeter or quarter inch).

6. Ask the client to complete the procedure with the palm of the left hand along the spine on the upper back (with the left elbow pointed upward) and the back of the right hand along the spine on the lower back (with the right elbow pointed downward) (not seen in figure 11.34).

7. Repeat measurements on each side several times and record the highest values, which can be evaluated individually (left and right) or calculated as an average [(left + right) ÷ 2].

8. Compare the client's score against the values in figures 11.35 through 11.38 on pages 266-268 (10, 46).

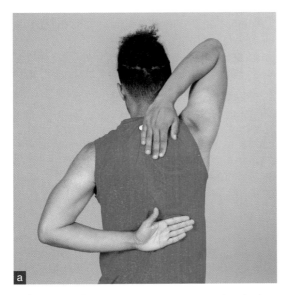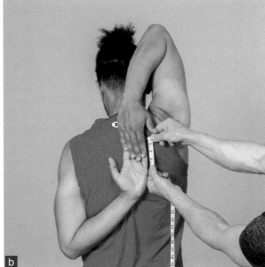

FIGURE 11.34   Back scratch test (*a*) beginning position; (*b*) fingers overlapping.

POSTURAL ALIGNMENT AND MOVEMENT ASSESSMENTS

Postural alignment and movement assessments provide the opportunity for fitness professionals to evaluate potential inherent physical limitations or functional imbalances that may impede the ability of clients to engage in the training process. Although these assessments are often qualitative or subjective in nature, they may be useful with the appropriate combination of human anatomy knowledge, experience, and training.

PLUMB LINE ASSESSMENT

The plumb line assessment is often used as a reference of alignment for the body when examining static posture (44, 45). It is made up of a hanging line (string, rope, or cord) attached to a small weight and suspended in front of a postural grid (or body diagram). The plumb line provides a vertical line of reference by which anatomical landmarks can be assessed.

Equipment

- A string suspended overhead with a small weight at the bottom (plumb line)
- A body diagram to show plumb line alignment (optional)

Procedure

1. The client is in a standing position and wearing tight-fitting clothing to ensure a clear view of the anatomical landmarks used for reference (figure 11.39).

2. Starting with the lateral view, instruct the client to stand behind the plumb line and take a few steps in place before standing still. Ask the client to assume a comfortable and relaxed position, looking straight ahead with the feet hip-width apart, arms relaxed at the sides with the palms facing in. The plumb line should fall in line with the client's earlobe and just anterior to the lateral malleolus (or through the greater trochanter).

3. From an anterior view, the feet should be equal distance from the plumb line, with the plumb line intersecting the midline of the nose, the midline of the sternum, and through the umbilicus.

4. From a posterior view, the feet should be equal distance from the plumb line, with the plumb line evenly bisecting the client's sacrum and falling midway between the heels.

5. Postural examination is most commonly performed by assessing the client's body in a lateral view first, followed by anterior and posterior views. Refer to the description of common faults provided in table 11.31 (44).

Posture is evaluated in accordance with the guidelines given by Kendall (45), in the form of ideal plumb alignment from each view. A disadvantage of this method is results are subjective and cannot produce quantifiable data; however, postural faults can be used as guidelines for identifying alterations in muscle and ligament lengths. This may occur when a muscle, or group of muscles, becomes tight because of occupation, injury, disease, or disuse. Synergistic muscles around a joint may also be unbalanced.

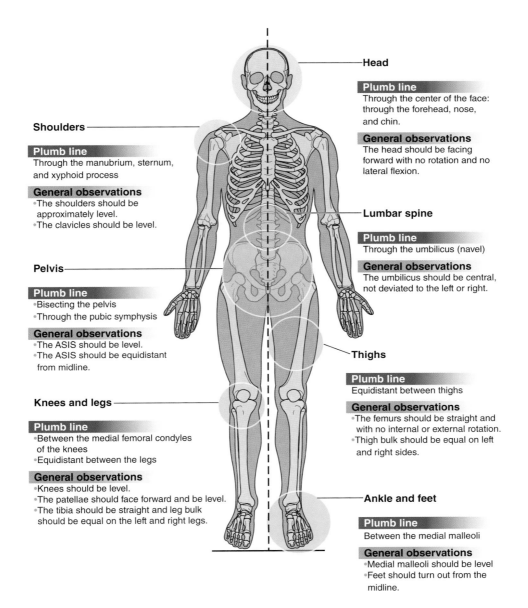

Standard anterior alignment

Head

Plumb line
Through the center of the face: through the forehead, nose, and chin.

General observations
The head should be facing forward with no rotation and no lateral flexion.

Shoulders

Plumb line
Through the manubrium, sternum, and xyphoid process

General observations
• The shoulders should be approximately level.
• The clavicles should be level.

Lumbar spine

Plumb line
Through the umbilicus (navel)

General observations
The umbilicus should be central, not deviated to the left or right.

Pelvis

Plumb line
• Bisecting the pelvis
• Through the pubic symphysis

General observations
• The ASIS should be level.
• The ASIS should be equidistant from midline.

Thighs

Plumb line
Equidistant between thighs

General observations
• The femurs should be straight and with no internal or external rotation.
• Thigh bulk should be equal on left and right sides.

Knees and legs

Plumb line
• Between the medial femoral condyles of the knees
• Equidistant between the legs

General observations
• Knees should be level.
• The patellae should face forward and be level.
• The tibia should be straight and leg bulk should be equal on the left and right legs.

Ankle and feet

Plumb line
Between the medial malleoli

General observations
• Medial malleoli should be level
• Feet should turn out from the midline.

FIGURE 11.39 *(a)* Plumb line positioning from the anterior view.

(continued)

Standard posterior alignment

Head

Plumb line
Through midline of the skull

General observations
The head should be facing forward with no rotation and no lateral flexion.

Shoulders

Plumb line
Equidistant between the medial borders of the scapulae

General observations
The height of the shoulders should be approximately level. However, the shoulder of the dominant hand may be lower than the shoulder of the non-dominant hand.

Pelvis and thigh

Plumb line
Through the midline of the pelvis

General observations
•The posterior superior iliac spines (PSIS) should be equidistant from the spine and be level.
•The greater trochanters of the femurs should be level.
•The buttock creases should be level and equal.

Knees and legs

Plumb line
Between the knees

General observations
•The legs should be straight and equidistant from the plumb line with no genu varum or genu valgum.
•Calf bulk should be equal on the left and right legs.

Neck

Plumb line
Through midline of all cervical vertebrae

General observations
The neck should appear straight with no lateral flexion.

Upper limbs

General observations
•The arms should hang equidistant from the trunk, palms facing the sides of the body.
•The elbows should be level.
•The wrists should be level.

Thorax and scapulae

Plumb line
Through midline of all thoracic vertebrae

General observations
•The scapulae should be equidistant from the spine, the medial borders of each approximately 1.5 to 2 inches (3.8 to 5 cm) from the spine.
•The scapulae should lie flat against the rib cage with no anterior tilting.
•The inferior angles of the scapulae should be level, with no evidence of elevation, depression, or scapular rotation.
•Flare in the rib cage should be symmetrical left and right.

Lumbar spine

Plumb line
Through midline of all lumbar vertebrae

General observations
The lumbar spine should be straight with no curvature to the right or left.

Ankle and feet

Plumb line
Between the medial malleoli

General observations
•The lateral malleoli should be level.
•The medial malleoli should be level.
•The Achilles tendon should be vertical.
•The calcaneus should be vertical.
•The feet should be turned out slightly.

FIGURE 11.39 *(b)* Plumb line positioning from the posterior view.

Standard lateral alignment

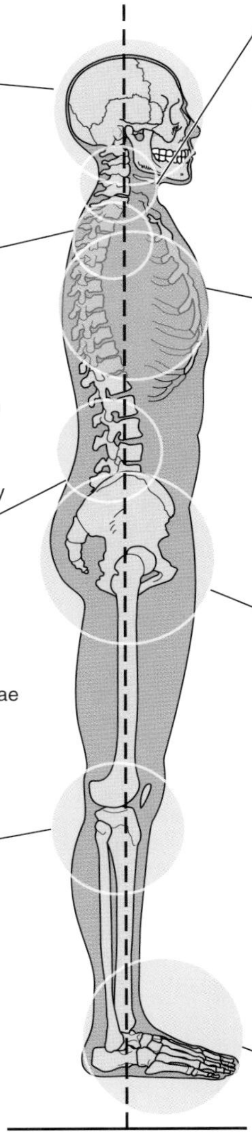

Head

Plumb line
Through the earlobe

General observations
The head should appear positioned over the thorax—neither pushed forward with chin out nor pulled back.

Shoulders

Plumb line
Through the shoulder joint: specifically, through the acromion process (not shown on this illustration)

General observations
The shoulders should be neither internally nor (in rare cases) externally rotated.

Lumbar spine

Plumb line
Through the bodies of the lumbar vertebrae

General observations
The lumbar spine should have a normal lordotic curve that is neither exaggerated nor flattened.

Knees and legs

Plumb line
Slightly anterior to the knee joint

General observations
There should be neither flexion nor hyperextension at this joint in standing.

Neck

Plumb line
Through the bodies of most of the cervical vertebrae

General observations
•The cervical spine should have a normal lordotic curve that is neither exaggerated nor flattened.
•There should be no deformity at the cervicothoracic junction such as a dowager's hump.

Thorax and scapulae

Plumb line
Midway through the trunk

General observations
•There should be a normal kyphotic curve in this region that is neither exaggerated nor flattened.
•The chest should be held comfortably upright and not excessively elevated (military posture) nor depressed.

Pelvis and thigh

Plumb line
Through the greater trochanter of the femur

General observations
•The pelvis should be in a neutral position. That means the anterior superior iliac spine (ASIS) is in the same vertical plane as the pubis.
•The ASIS and the PSIS should be approximately in the same plane. There should be no anterior or posterior pelvic tilt.
•Gluteal and thigh muscle bulk should appear equal on both the left and right sides.

Ankle and feet

Plumb line
Slightly anterior to the lateral malleolus

General observations
There should be normal dorsi-flexion at the ankle.

FIGURE 11.39 *(c)* Plumb line positioning from the lateral view.

TABLE 11.31 Description of Common Faults Identified Using Plumb Line Assessment

Anatomical markers	Lateral view	Posterior view	Anterior view	Causes of common faults
Head and neck	Plumb line: falls through the earlobe to the acromion process Common faults: forward head, lordotic cervical curve	Plumb line: midline bisects the head through the external occipital protuberance Common faults: head tilt, head rotated	Plumb line: bisects the head at the midline into equal halves Common faults: lateral tilt, head rotation, mandibular asymmetry	Excessive cervical lordosis; tight cervical muscles; elongated levator scapulae muscles; compression and rotation of the vertebrae
Shoulder	Plumb line: falls through the acromion process Common faults: forward shoulders and lumbar lordosis	Plumb line: falls midway between shoulders (examine to see if shoulder levels are even bilaterally) Common faults: dropped or elevated shoulders, medial or lateral rotation of the shoulders, adducted or abducted scapulae	Plumb line: vertical line bisects sternum and xiphoid process (examine to see if shoulder levels are even bilaterally) Common faults: dropped or elevated shoulders, clavicle asymmetry	Tight pectoralis muscles, serratus anterior, latissimus dorsi, rhomboid muscles, intercostal muscles
Thoracic and lumbar vertebrae	Plumb line: falls midway between the abdomen and back, and anterior to the sacroiliac joint Common faults: kyphosis, barrel chest, funnel chest, lordosis, sway back, flat back	Plumb line: bisects the spinous process of the thoracic and lumbar vertebrae Common faults: lateral deviation (scoliosis)	Plumb line: bisects the pectoral muscles and umbilicus; arms should lie next to sides, with palms facing in toward thighs Common faults: palms in front of thighs and facing posteriorly, internal rotation of the shoulders	Stretched thoracic extensors, middle and lower trapezius muscles, and posterior ligaments; tightness of upper abdominal muscles, shoulder adductors, pectoralis muscles, and intercostal muscles; compression of vertebrae posteriorly; tightness of posterior longitudinal ligaments, lower back extensors, and hip flexor muscles
Pelvis and hip	Plumb line: falls anterior to sacroiliac joint, posterior to hip joint, and through the greater trochanter Common faults: anterior pelvic tilt, posterior pelvic tilt	Plumb line: bisects the gluteal cleft; iliac crests, gluteal folds, and greater trochanters are all level Common faults: lateral pelvic tilt, pelvic rotation, abducted hip	Plumb line: bisects the pelvic girdle and falls midway between the left and right iliac crest Examine the anterior superior iliac spines bilaterally to determine if they are level Common faults: uneven hip height, lateral or medial rotation of the femur causing the knees to angle out or face in	Stretched hip flexors, lower abdominal muscles, and joint capsule; tightness of hamstring and hip abductor muscles
Knee	Plumb line: slightly anterior to the midline of the knee Common faults: hyperextended knee, flexed knee	Plumb line: lies equidistant between the knees Common faults: bowleggedness, knee valgus	Plumb line: legs are equidistant from a vertical line through the body Common faults: excess rotation of tibia	Tightness of quadriceps, gastrocnemius, soleus, and hamstring muscles
Ankle and foot	Plumb line: lies anterior to the lateral malleolus, aligned with 5th metatarsal Common faults: forward posture	Plumb line: lies equidistant from the malleoli Common faults: feet are overly pronated or supinated	Plumb line: lies equidistant from the malleoli Common faults: lateral deviation of the first digit; hyperextension of the joints	Tightness of dorsal and adductor hallucis musculature; elongated posterior tibialis muscle; elongated peroneal and lateral ligaments

Adapted from Johnson (44).

CLOSED KINETIC CHAIN UPPER EXTREMITY STABILITY (CKCUES) TEST

The closed kinetic chain upper extremity stability (CKCUES) test is an assessment tool for upper limb function and stability. It can also be used for assessing risk of injury to the shoulder and upper extremities. It is easy to administer, is cost-effective, and has been validated by peak torque during internal and external shoulder rotation (isokinetic dynamometer) and maximum grip strength (hand dynamometer) (50, 76). The test requires the client to assume a push-up position and, while alternating hands, tap a piece of tape on the floor next to the opposite hand as many times as possible within 15 seconds.

Equipment

- Measuring tape
- Adhesive tape
- Stopwatch

Procedure

1. Place two pieces of tape parallel to each other on the floor 36 inches (91.4 cm) apart.
2. To begin the test, have the client assume a push-up (male) or modified push-up (female) position, with one hand on each piece of tape (figure 11.40a).
3. Instruct the client to use one hand to reach across the body and touch the opposite hand (figure 11.40b).
4. After touching the opposite hand, the client returns the hand to the starting position and repeats the movement with the other hand.
5. Touches are counted every time the hand reaches across the body and touches the back of the other hand.
6. Have the client perform a warm-up round before completing three trials, each lasting 15 seconds with 45 seconds of rest in between.
7. Average the scores from the three trials to use for data analysis.
8. Compare the client's score against the values in table 11.32 on page 269 (79a).

If the client is unable to perform the test properly, stop the test, wait for 45 seconds, and start the test again. For a trial to be counted as successful, the client must keep the back in a neutral position, with the arms staying perpendicular to the floor and the knees not touching the floor (males).

Data analysis for this test can occur in one of three ways. First, the number of touches can be counted. Second, a normalized value can be obtained by dividing the number of touches by the client's height. Third, a power score can be developed by multiplying the average number of touches by 68% of the client's body weight in kilograms (which equals the approximate weight of the arms, head, and trunk) divided by 15 (duration of the test in seconds). The power score reflects the amount of work performed in a unit of time.

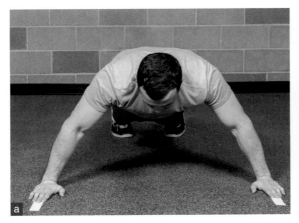 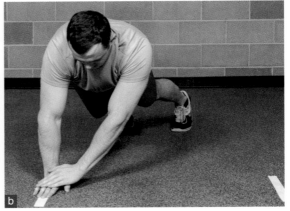

FIGURE 11.40 Closed kinetic chain upper extremity stability (CKCUES) test.

SINGLE-LEG SQUAT AND FORWARD STEP-DOWN TESTS

The single-leg squat and forward step-down movements are used to assess movement quality in the lower limb. They require strength, proprioception, neuromuscular control, and adequate range of motion at the hip, knee, and ankle joints. During these tests, the quality of the movement is observed and assessed using a qualitative assessment tool developed specifically for lower limb tasks (33, 34). The forward step-down procedure provides an alternative for less conditioned individuals and those unable to perform a single-leg squat.

Procedure

1. Instruct the client to take a single-leg stance on the leg to be tested. The client should be looking straight ahead, with the arms held straight out in front and the hands clasped together.

2. Have the client squat to at least 45-degree knee flexion, but no greater than 60 degrees, for 5 seconds.

3. Allow two or three practice trials to ensure the individual is comfortable and familiar with the movement.

4. Do not count trials if the client is unable to squat within the desired degrees of knee flexion or is unable to maintain balance for the duration of the test.

5. If the individual is unable to perform a single-leg squat, a forward step-down test can be performed.

6. Have the client stand on a 6-inch (15.2 cm) box with both feet. Instruct the client to step forward to tap the nontesting leg on the ground in front of the step, while keeping the tested leg on the step, before returning to the starting position.

7. Movement patterns to be observed during the descent phase are the same for both tests: flexion at the knee, hip, and trunk; pelvic tilt; hip adduction; and internal rotation and abduction of the knee.

8. Each repetition should be evaluated as positive or negative with respect to the potential errors outlined in table 11.33 (34). For the client to pass, five of the six specific criteria must be negative.

TABLE 11.33 Qualitative Analysis of Single-Leg Loading or Forward Step-Down Tasks

Movement category	Potential errors	Optimal example	Suboptimal example
Arm strategy	Excessive arm movement to assist with balance		
Trunk alignment	Excessive lean in any direction		
Pelvic plane	Loss of horizontal plane, or excessive tilt or rotation		
Thigh motion	Weight-bearing thigh moves into hip adduction, or non–weight-bearing thigh not held in neutral		
Knee position	Noticeable valgus of the weight-bearing knee		
Steady stance	Noticeably wobbly weight-bearing leg, or client touches down with non–weight-bearing foot		

Adapted by permission from Herrington and Munro (2014).

CONCLUSION

Typically the personal trainer has the challenge of working with clients who have a broad spectrum of fitness or exercise capabilities. To gather baseline assessments, the personal trainer may test for a variety of fitness parameters such as HR, BP, training load, body composition, cardiovascular endurance, muscular strength, muscular endurance, muscular power, speed, agility, flexibility, postural alignment, and movement assessment and then make comparisons against established sets of descriptive or normative data. The resulting conclusions can then form the basis for the client's exercise prescription.

Study Questions

1. Which of the following is *incorrect* regarding vital signs?
   A. Vital signs include heart rate.
   B. Vital signs include blood pressure.
   C. A personal trainer will only measure them in the rested state.
   D. They can be used to determine exercise intensity.

2. All of the following skinfold sites are appropriate for performing a three-site skinfold for a 45-year-old male client *except*
   A. chest
   B. suprailium
   C. abdomen
   D. thigh

3. Which of the following is *incorrect* regarding the T-test?
   A. The first 10 yards is a forward sprint.
   B. Crossing of the feet during the shuffle is allowed.
   C. The client shuffles to the left for a *total* of 10 yards.
   D. The client shuffles to the right for a *total* of 10 yards.

4. Which of the following terms is used to refer to the range of motion around a joint or a series of joints?
   A. flexibility
   B. laxity
   C. dynamic stability
   D. stiffness

5. Which of the following is *incorrect* regarding single-leg squat and forward step-down tests?
   A. The number of repetitions performed are used to score the test.
   B. Used to assess movement quality in the lower limb.
   C. The forward step-down procedure provides an alternative for less conditioned individuals.
   D. They require strength, proprioception, neuromuscular control, and adequate range of motion.

TABLE 11.1 Norms for Resting Heart Rate (beats/min)

| | Age (years) | | | | | | | | | | | |
| | 18-25 | | 26-35 | | 36-45 | | 46-55 | | 56-65 | | >65 | |
Rating	M	F	M	F	M	F	M	F	M	F	M	F
Excellent	40-54	42-57	36-53	39-57	37-55	40-58	35-56	43-58	42-56	42-59	40-55	49-59
Good	57-59	59-63	55-59	60-62	58-60	61-63	58-61	61-64	59-61	61-64	57-61	60-64
Above average	61-65	64-67	61-63	64-66	62-64	65-67	63-65	65-69	63-65	65-68	62-65	66-68
Average	66-69	68-71	65-67	68-70	66-69	69-71	66-70	70-72	68-71	69-72	66-69	70-72
Below average	70-72	72-76	69-71	72-74	70-72	72-75	72-74	73-76	72-75	73-77	70-73	73-76
Poor	74-78	77-81	74-78	77-81	75-80	77-81	77-81	77-82	76-80	79-81	74-79	79-83
Very poor	82-103	84-103	81-102	84-102	83-101	83-102	84-103	85-104	84-103	84-103	83-103	86-97

Adapted from Golding (28).

TABLE 11.2 Classification of Blood Pressure for Adults[a]

Systolic BP (mmHg)[b]	Category	Diastolic BP (mmHg)[b]
<120	Normal	<80
120-129	Elevated	<80
130-139	Stage 1 hypertension	80-89
≥140	Stage 2 hypertension	≥90

[a]Based on average of two or more readings on two or more occasions.

[b]When systolic and diastolic pressures fall into different categories, use the higher category for classification.

Data from Whelton et al. (84).

TABLE 11.3 Recommended Cuff and Bladder Sizes for Arm Circumferences

Client or patient	Arm circumference (cm)	Bladder width × length (cm)
Older child	NR	9 × 18
Small adult	22-26	12 × 22
Adult	27-34	16 × 30
Large adult	35-44	16 × 36
Obese adult or high upper body muscularity (thigh cuff)	45-52	16 × 42

NR = not reported.

Data from Pickering et al. (67).

TABLE 11.4 Classification of Overweight and Obesity by Body Mass Index (BMI), Waist Circumference, and Associated Disease Risks

	BMI (kg/m²)	Obesity class	Disease* risk relative to normal weight and waist circumference	
			Men ≥102 cm (≥40 in.) Women ≥88 cm (≥35 in.)	Men >102 cm (>40 in.) Women >88 cm (>35 in.)
Underweight	<18.5		–	–
Normal	18.5-24.9		–	–
Overweight	25.0-29.9		Increased	High
Obesity	30.0-34.9	I	High	Very high
	35.0-39.9	II	Very high	Very high
Extreme obesity	≥40.0	III	Extremely high	Extremely high

*Disease risk for type 2 diabetes, hypertension, and coronary heart disease.

Data from Pi-Sunyer et al. (66).

TABLE 11.5 Average Stature and Percentiles for American Men (cm)

Race, ethnicity, and age	Mean	Percentile								
		5th	10th	15th	25th	50th	75th	85th	90th	95th
ALL RACES AND ETHNICITIES										
20 years and over	176.3	163.6	166.6	168.4	171.3	176.3	181.5	184.4	186.0	188.7
20-29 years	177.6	164.2	167.1	169.3	172.3	177.8	183.0	185.3	186.8	190.1
30-39 years	176.4	162.7	165.9	167.9	171.4	176.4	181.5	184.6	186.4	189.6
40-49 years	177.1	165.6	168.2	169.8	172.3	177.0	181.8	184.6	186.2	188.0
50-59 years	176.6	165.1	167.2	168.8	171.4	176.6	181.5	184.6	186.5	189.1
60-69 years	175.4	163.1	166.2	167.8	170.5	175.3	180.7	182.7	184.8	187.2
70-79 years	173.8	162.1	164.1	166.3	168.6	174.0	178.5	180.4	182.9	185.7
80 years and over	170.7	159.2	161.7	163.4	166.4	170.7	175.0	177.8	179.0	181.2
NON-HISPANIC WHITE										
20 years and over	177.5	166.0	168.5	170.2	172.6	177.4	182.4	184.9	186.5	189.1
20-39 years	178.9	167.4	170.1	171.9	174.4	178.9	183.4	185.7	187.7	190.3
40-59 years	178.0	167.3	169.2	170.8	173.1	177.9	182.8	185.2	186.6	188.8
60 years and over	174.6	162.6	165.2	167.1	169.8	174.6	179.7	182.2	183.7	186.4
NON-HISPANIC BLACK										
20 years and over	177.2	165.4	167.8	169.8	172.3	177.0	181.9	184.7	186.4	189.6
20-39 years	178.0	166.3	167.9	170.1	173.1	177.7	183.0	185.2	187.1	190.6
40-59 years	177.4	166.0	168.6	170.3	172.7	177.2	181.6	184.5	186.6	189.0
60 years and over	174.3	163.0	164.7	166.8	169.4	174.0	179.1	181.8	183.5	185.7
MEXICAN AMERICAN										
20 years and over	170.3	158.7	161.1	163.0	165.2	170.4	174.9	177.0	178.9	182.0
20-39 years	170.6	158.3	161.2	163.3	165.3	170.6	175.2	177.6	180.5	183.7
40-59 years	170.2	159.4	161.4	163.3	165.6	170.8	174.9	176.3	178.1	180.1
60 years and over	167.8	157.7	159.4	160.8	163.4	167.8	172.4	173.7	175.1	176.9

Reprinted from McDowell et al. (57).

TABLE 11.6 Average Stature and Percentiles for American Women (cm)

Race, ethnicity, and age	Mean	Percentile								
		5th	10th	15th	25th	50th	75th	85th	90th	95th
ALL RACE AND ETHNICITY GROUPS										
20 years and over	162.2	150.7	153.3	154.9	157.7	162.2	166.7	169.1	170.8	173.1
20-29 years	163.2	152.2	154.8	156.5	158.7	163.0	167.9	169.8	171.4	172.8
30-39 years	163.2	152.4	154.4	156.2	158.9	163.0	167.6	170.4	172.0	174.2
40-49 years	163.1	152.1	153.9	155.8	158.5	163.1	167.6	169.8	171.9	174.0
50-59 years	162.2	150.7	153.3	155.4	158.1	162.1	166.8	168.7	170.3	172.4
60-69 years	161.8	151.9	153.8	155.1	157.6	161.9	165.9	168.0	170.0	171.5
70-79 years	159.2	149.0	150.9	152.6	155.0	159.0	163.7	165.5	167.4	169.4
80 years and over	156.0	146.2	148.0	149.4	151.7	155.8	159.7	162.3	164.3	166.1
NON-HISPANIC WHITE										
20 years and over	163.0	152.1	154.4	156.3	158.7	163.0	167.5	169.7	171.3	173.6
20-39 years	164.8	154.7	157.2	158.6	160.7	164.7	168.9	171.1	172.4	174.4
40-59 years	163.6	152.6	155.5	157.5	159.4	163.4	167.7	169.9	171.8	174.0
60 years and over	160.2	149.7	152.0	153.6	155.9	159.8	164.5	166.7	168.6	170.5
NON-HISPANIC BLACK										
20 years and over	162.7	151.5	153.9	155.5	158.2	162.7	167.0	169.6	171	173.8
20-39 years	163.2	151.6	154.7	156.3	158.5	163.0	167.3	170.1	171.8	174.5
40-59 years	163.2	152.2	154.1	155.9	158.7	163.5	167.5	169.7	171.2	173.7
60 years and over	160.6	150.0	152.6	153.6	156.2	160.5	165.2	166.8	169.0	170.5
MEXICAN AMERICAN										
20 years and over	157.8	147.3	149.8	151.1	153.6	157.8	161.9	164.3	166.2	168.1
20-39 years	158.7	148.2	150.7	152.5	154.6	159.0	162.6	165.0	166.6	168.9
40-59 years	157.7	˙	149.9	151.1	153.5	157.6	161.7	164.0	165.8	˙
60 years and over	153.9	144.9	145.9	147.4	150.1	154.0	158.1	159.7	161.6	164.3

˙Value does not meet standards of reliability.

Reprinted from McDowell et al. (57).

TABLE 11.7 Body Mass Index Chart

BMI	Normal (healthy) weight						Overweight					Obese					
	19	20	21	22	23	24	25	26	27	28	29	30	31	32	33	34	35
Height (in.)	**Body weight (lb)**																
58	91	96	100	105	110	115	119	124	129	134	138	143	148	153	158	162	167
59	94	99	104	109	114	119	124	128	133	138	143	148	153	158	163	168	173
60	97	102	107	112	118	123	128	133	138	143	148	153	158	163	168	174	179
61	100	106	111	116	122	127	132	137	143	148	153	158	164	169	174	180	185
62	104	109	115	120	126	131	136	142	147	153	158	164	169	175	180	186	191
63	107	113	118	124	130	135	141	146	152	158	163	169	175	180	186	191	197
64	110	116	122	128	134	140	145	151	157	163	169	174	180	186	192	197	204
65	114	120	126	132	138	144	150	156	162	168	174	180	186	192	198	204	210
66	118	124	130	136	142	148	155	161	167	173	179	186	192	198	204	210	216
67	121	127	134	140	146	153	159	166	172	178	185	191	198	204	211	217	223
68	125	131	138	144	151	158	164	171	177	184	190	197	203	210	216	223	230
69	128	135	142	149	155	162	169	176	182	189	196	203	209	216	223	230	236
70	132	139	146	153	160	167	174	181	188	195	202	209	216	222	229	236	243
71	136	143	150	157	165	172	179	186	193	200	208	215	222	229	236	243	250
72	140	147	154	162	169	177	184	191	199	206	213	221	228	235	242	250	258
73	144	151	159	166	174	182	189	197	204	212	219	227	235	242	250	257	265
74	148	155	164	171	179	186	194	202	210	218	225	233	241	249	256	264	272
75	152	160	168	176	184	192	200	208	216	224	232	240	248	256	264	272	279
76	156	164	172	180	189	197	205	213	221	230	238	246	254	263	271	279	287

Reprinted from Heyward and Gibson (35).

TABLE 11.8 Skinfold Prediction Equations

SKF sites	Population	Equation	Ref
Σ7SKF (chest + abdomen + thigh + triceps + subscapular + suprailiac + midaxilla)	Black or Hispanic women, 18-55 years	Db (g · cc^{-1}) = 1.0970 – 0.00046971 (Σ7SKF) + 0.00000056 (Σ7SKF)^2 – 0.00012828 (age)	[1]
	Black men or male athletes, 18-61 years	Db (g · cc^{-1}) = 1.1120 – 0.00043499 (Σ7SKF) + 0.00000055 (Σ7SKF)^2 – 0.00028826 (age)	[2]
Σ4SKF (triceps + anterior suprailiac + abdomen + thigh)	Female athletes, 18-29 years	Db (g · cc^{-1}) = 1.096095 – 0.0006952 (Σ4SKF) + 0.0000011 (Σ4SKF)^2 – 0.0000714 (age)	[1]
Σ3SKF (triceps + suprailiac + thigh)	White or anorexic women, 18-55 years	Db (g · cc^{-1}) = 1.0994921 – 0.0009929 (Σ3SKF) + 0.0000023 (Σ3SKF)^2 – 0.0001392 (age)	[1]
Σ3SKF (chest + abdomen + thigh)	White men, 18-61 years	Db (g · cc^{-1}) = 1.109380 – 0.0008267 (Σ3SKF) + 0.0000016 (Σ3SKF)^2 – 0.0002574 (age)	[2]
Σ3SKF (abdomen + thigh + triceps)	Black or white collegiate athletes, 18-34 years	%BF = 8.997 + 0.2468 (Σ3SKF) – 6.343 (sex[a]) – 1.998 (race[b])	[3]
Σ2SKF (triceps + calf)	Black or white boys, 6-17 years	%BF = 0.735 (Σ2SKF) + 1.2	[4]
	Black or white girls, 6-17 years	%BF = 0.610 (Σ2SKF) + 5.1	

ΣSKF = sum of skinfolds (mm). Use population-specific conversion formulas to calculate %BF (percent body fat) from Db (body density).

[a]Male athletes = 1; female athletes = 0.

[b]Black athletes = 1; white athletes = 0.

[1] Jackson et al., 1980. Generalized equations for predicting body density of women. *MSSE* 12: 175-182. [2] Jackson and Pollock. 1978. Generalized equations for predicting body density of men. *Brit J Nutr* 40: 497-504. [3] Evans et al. 2005. Skinfold prediction equation for athletes developed using a four-component model. *MSSE* 37: 2006-2011. [4] Slaughter et al.1988. Skinfold equations for estimation of body fatness in children and youth. *Hum Biol* 60: 709-723.

Reprinted by permission from Gibson et al. (2019, p. 249).

TABLE 11.9 Population-Specific Equations for Calculating the Estimated Percent Body Fat From Body Density (Db)

Population	Age (years)	Sex	%BF[a]	FFB$_d$ (g · cc^{-1})[b]
RACE AND ETHNICITY				
African American	9-17	Female	(5.24/Db) – 4.82	1.088
	19-45	Male	(4.86/Db) – 4.39	1.106
	24-79	Female	(4.85/Db) – 4.39	1.106
American Indian	18-62	Male	(4.97/Db) – 4.52	1.099
	18-60	Female	(4.81/Db) – 4.34	1.108
Asian: Japanese Native	18-48	Male	(4.97/Db) – 4.52	1.099
	18-48	Female	(4.76/Db) – 4.28	1.111
	61-78	Male	(4.87/Db) – 4.41	1.105
	61-78	Female	(4.95/Db) – 4.50	1.100
Asian: Singaporean (Chinese, Indian, Malay)		Male	(4.94/Db) – 4.48	1.102
		Female	(4.84/Db) – 4.37	1.107
White	8-12	Male	(5.27/Db) – 4.85	1.086
	8-12	Female	(5.27/Db) – 4.85	1.086
	13-17	Male	(5.12/Db) – 4.69	1.092
	13-17	Female	(5.19/Db) – 4.76	1.090
	18-59	Male	(4.95/Db) – 4.50	1.100
	18-59	Female	(4.96/Db) – 4.51	1.101
	60-90	Male	(4.97/Db) – 4.52	1.099
	60-90	Female	(5.02/Db) – 4.57	1.098
Hispanic		Male	NA	NA
	20-40	Female	(4.87/Db) – 4.41	1.105
ATHLETES				
Resistance trained	24 ± 4	Male	(5.21/Db) – 4.78	1.089
	35 ± 6	Female	(4.97/Db) – 4.52	1.099
Endurance trained	21 ± 2	Male	(5.03/Db) – 4.59	1.097
	21 ± 4	Female	(4.95/Db) – 4.50	1.100
All sports	18-22	Male	(5.12/Db) – 4.68	1.093
	18-22	Female	(4.97/Db) – 4.52	1.099
CLINICAL POPULATIONS				
Anorexia nervosa	15-44	Female	(4.96/Db) – 4.51	1.101
Obesity	17-62	Female	(4.95/Db) – 4.50	1.100
Spinal cord injury (paraplegic or quadriplegic)	18-73	Male	(4.67/Db) – 4.18	1.116
		Female	(4.70/Db) – 4.22	1.114

%BF = percent body fat; Db = body density; NA = no data available for this population subgroup; FFB$_d$ = fat free body density.

[a]Multiply value by 100 to calculate %BF.

[b]FFB$_d$ based on average values reported in selected research articles.

Reprinted by permission from Heyward et al. (2004, p. 9).

TABLE 11.10 Criterion Scores and Normative Values for Percent Body Fat for Males and Females

Score or value	Age (years)						
MALE RATING (CRITERION SCORES)[a]							
	6-17[b]	18-25	26-35	36-45	46-55	56-65	66+
Very lean	<5 (not recommended)	3-7	4-10	5-13	8-16	11-17	12-18
Lean (low)	5-10	8-10	11-13	15-17	17-19	19-21	19-20
Leaner than average	—	11-12	14-16	18-20	20-22	22-23	21-22
Average (mid)	11-25	13-15	17-19	21-22	23-24	24-25	23-24
Fatter than average	—	16-18	20-22	23-25	25-27	26-27	25-26
Fat (upper)	26-31	19-21	23-26	26-28	28-30	28-29	27-29
Overfat (obesity)	>31	23-35	27-38	29-39	31-40	31-40	30-39
MALE PERCENTILES (NORMATIVE REFERENCES)[c]							
		20-29	30-39	40-49	50-59	60-69	70-79
90		7.9	12.5	15.0	17.0	18.1	17.7
80		10.5	14.9	17.5	19.4	20.2	20.2
70		12.6	16.8	19.3	21.0	21.7	21.6
60		14.8	18.4	20.8	22.3	23.0	22.9
50		16.7	20.0	22.1	23.6	24.2	24.1
40		18.6	21.6	23.5	24.9	25.6	25.2
30		20.7	23.2	24.9	26.3	27.0	26.3
20		23.3	25.1	26.6	28.1	28.8	28.0
10		26.6	27.8	29.1	30.6	31.2	30.6
FEMALE RATING (CRITERION SCORES)[a]							
	6-17[b]	18-25	26-35	36-45	46-55	56-65	66+
Very lean	<12 (not recommended)	9-17	7-16	9-18	12-21	12-22	11-20
Lean (low)	12-15	18-19	18-20	19-22	23-25	24-26	22-25
Leaner than average	—	20-21	21-22	23-25	26-28	27-29	26-28
Average (mid)	16-30	22-23	23-25	26-28	29-30	30-32	29-31
Fatter than average	—	24-26	26-28	29-31	31-33	33-35	32-34
Fat (upper)	31-36	27-30	29-32	32-35	34-37	36-38	35-37
Overfat (obesity)	>36	32-43	34-46	37-47	39-50	39-49	38-45
FEMALE PERCENTILES (NORMATIVE REFERENCES)[c]							
		20-29	30-39	40-49	50-59	60-69	70-79
90		15.2	15.5	16.8	19.1	20.1	18.8
80		16.8	17.5	19.5	22.3	23.2	22.6
70		18.6	19.2	21.6	24.7	25.5	24.5
60		20.0	21.0	23.6	26.6	27.5	26.3
50		21.8	22.9	25.5	28.3	29.2	27.8
40		23.5	24.8	27.4	30.0	30.8	30.0
30		25.6	26.9	29.5	31.7	32.5	31.6
20		28.6	29.6	31.9	33.8	34.4	33.6
10		33.8	33.6	35.0	36.0	36.6	36.1

When personal trainers assess a client's body composition, they must account for a standard error of the estimate (SEE) and report a range of percentages that the client falls into. Note that the minimum SEE for population-specific skinfold equations is ±3% to 5%. Therefore, if a 25-year-old male client's body fat is measured at 24%, there is a minimum of a 6% range (21%-27%) that suggests a criterion-reference score of "fat." Note that reporting a client's body fat percentage with an SEE range can also cover any gaps and overlaps in the criterion-referenced norms shown. For example, what is the criterion score for a 30-year-old male with 29% body fat? The minimum SEE of ±3% places this client between 26% and 32% and therefore would suggest a criterion-reference score of "fat-overfat" or "borderline overfat."

[a]Data for male and female rating (criterion scores), ages 18 to 66+, are adapted from Morrow et al. (61).

[b]Data for male and female rating (criterion scores), ages 6 to 17, are adapted from Lohman et al. (53).

[c]Data for male and female percentiles (normative references) are reprinted from ACSM 2022 (1).

TABLE 11.11 Waist-to-Hip Circumference Ratio Norms for Men and Women

Age (years)	Risk			
	Low	Moderate	High	Very high
MEN				
20-29	<0.83	0.83-0.88	0.89-0.94	>0.94
30-39	<0.84	0.84-0.91	0.92-0.96	>0.96
40-49	<0.88	0.88-0.95	0.96-1.00	>1.00
50-59	<0.90	0.90-0.96	0.97-1.02	>1.02
60-69	<0.91	0.91-0.98	0.99-1.03	>1.03
WOMEN				
20-29	<0.71	0.71-0.77	0.78-0.82	>0.82
30-39	<0.72	0.72-0.78	0.79-0.84	>0.84
40-49	<0.73	0.73-0.79	0.80-0.87	>0.87
50-59	<0.74	0.74-0.81	0.82-0.88	>0.88
60-69	<0.76	0.76-0.83	0.84-0.90	>0.90

Reprinted by permission from Gibson et al. (2019, p. 274). Adapted from Bray and Gray (7).

TABLE 11.12 YMCA Cycle Ergometry Protocol

First stage	150 kg · m · min^{-1} (0.5 kg)			
	HR <80 beats/min	HR 80-89 beats/min	HR 90-100 beats/min	HR >100 beats/min
Second stage	750 kg · m · min^{-1} (2.5 kg)*	600 kg · m · min^{-1} (2.0 kg)	450 kg · m · min^{-1} (1.5 kg)	300 kg · m · min^{-1} (1.0 kg)
Third stage	900 kg · m · min^{-1} (3.0 kg)	750 kg · m · min^{-1} (2.5 kg)	600 kg · m · min^{-1} (2.0 kg)	450 kg · m · min^{-1} (1.5 kg)
Fourth stage	1,050 kg · m · min^{-1} (3.5 kg)	900 kg · m · min^{-1} (3.0 kg)	750 kg · m · min^{-1} (2.5 kg)	600 kg · m · min^{-1} (2.0 kg)

*Resistance settings shown here are appropriate for an ergometer with a flywheel that is geared to travel 6 m (19.7 ft) per pedal revolution.

Adapted from American College of Sports Medicine (1) and Golding (28).

TABLE 11.13 Percentile Values for Maximal Aerobic Power ($\dot{V}O_2$max; ml · kg^{-1} · min^{-1}) on a Treadmill

Percentile	Age (years)						Percentile	Age (years)					
	20-29	30-39	40-49	50-59	60-69	70-79		20-29	30-39	40-49	50-59	60-69	70-79
MALES							**FEMALES**						
95	66.3	59.8	55.6	50.7	43.0	39.7	95	56.0	45.8	41.7	35.9	29.4	24.1
90	61.8	56.5	52.1	45.6	40.3	36.6	90	51.3	41.4	38.4	32.0	27.0	23.1
75	55.2	49.2	45.0	39.7	34.5	30.4	75	44.7	36.1	32.4	27.6	23.8	20.8
50	48.0	42.4	37.8	32.6	28.2	24.4	50	37.6	30.2	26.7	23.4	20.0	18.3
25	40.1	35.9	31.9	27.1	23.7	20.4	25	30.5	25.3	22.1	19.9	17.2	15.6
10	32.1	30.2	26.8	22.8	19.8	17.1	10	23.9	20.9	18.8	17.3	14.6	13.6
5	29.0	27.2	24.2	20.9	17.4	16.3	5	21.7	19.0	17.0	16.0	13.4	13.1

Adapted by permission from Kaminsky et al. (2015).

TABLE 11.14 Percentile Values for Maximal Aerobic Power ($\dot{V}O_2$max; ml · kg⁻¹ · min⁻¹) on a Cycle Ergometer

Percentile	Age (years) 20-29	30-39	40-49	50-59	60-69	Percentile	Age (years) 20-29	30-39	40-49	50-59	60-69
	MALES						FEMALES				
90	55.5	41.7	37.1	34.0	29.9	90	42.6	30.0	26.2	22.6	20.5
80	51.4	36.2	34.2	30.7	26.7	80	38.8	26.0	23.4	20.7	18.8
70	47.9	33.9	30.4	28.2	24.5	70	35.6	24.2	22.0	19.3	17.8
60	44.5	31.1	28.6	26.3	23.2	60	33.6	22.5	20.7	18.2	16.7
50	41.9	30.1	27.1	24.8	22.4	50	31.0	21.6	19.4	17.3	16.0
40	38.3	28.1	25.4	23.6	21.4	40	28.1	20.1	18.4	16.6	15.4
30	36.2	26.9	24.0	22.6	20.2	30	25.6	18.8	17.1	15.7	14.7
20	33.2	25.4	22.2	21.5	19.0	20	21.6	17.0	15.8	14.9	14.0
10	29.5	21.8	20.6	20.4	17.3	10	19.3	20.9	14.6	13.7	13.0

Reprinted by permission from Kaminsky et al. (2015).

TABLE 11.15 Prediction of Maximal Oxygen Consumption (L/min) From Heart Rate and Cycling Power in Men

HR (beats/min)	Power (kg · m · min⁻¹; watts) 300; 50	600; 100	900; 150	1,200; 200	1,500; 250	HR (beats/min)	Power (kg · m · min⁻¹; watts) 600;100	900; 150	1,200; 200	1,500; 250
120	2.2	3.5	4.8			146	2.4	3.3	4.4	5.5
121	2.2	3.4	4.7			147	2.4	3.3	4.4	5.5
122	2.2	3.4	4.6			148	2.4	3.2	4.3	5.4
123	2.1	3.4	4.6			149	2.3	3.2	4.3	5.4
124	2.1	3.3	4.5	6.0		150	2.3	3.2	4.2	5.3
125	2.0	3.2	4.4	5.9		151	2.3	3.1	4.2	5.2
126	2.0	3.2	4.4	5.8		152	2.3	3.1	4.1	5.2
127	2.0	3.1	4.3	5.7		153	2.2	3.0	4.1	5.1
128	2.0	3.1	4.2	5.6		154	2.2	3.0	4.0	5.1
129	1.9	3.0	4.2	5.6		155	2.2	3.0	4.0	5.0
130	1.9	3.0	4.1	5.5		156	2.2	2.9	4.0	5.0
131	1.9	2.9	4.0	5.4		157	2.1	2.9	3.9	4.9
132	1.8	2.9	4.0	5.3		158	2.1	2.9	3.9	4.9
133	1.8	2.8	3.9	5.3		159	2.1	2.8	3.8	4.8
134	1.8	2.8	3.9	5.2		160	2.1	2.8	3.8	4.8
135	1.7	2.8	3.8	5.1		161	2.0	2.8	3.7	4.7
136	1.7	2.7	3.8	5.0		162	2.0	2.8	3.7	4.6
137	1.7	2.7	3.7	5.0		163	2.0	2.8	3.7	4.6
138	1.6	2.7	3.7	4.9		164	2.0	2.7	3.6	4.5
139	1.6	2.6	3.6	4.8		165	2.0	2.7	3.6	4.5
140	1.6	2.6	3.6	4.8	6.0	166	1.9	2.7	3.6	4.4
141		2.6	3.5	4.7	5.9	167	1.9	2.6	3.5	4.4
142		2.5	5.5	4.6	5.8	168	1.9	2.6	3.5	4.3
143		2.5	3.4	4.6	5.7	169	1.9	2.6	3.5	4.3
144		2.5	3.4	4.5	5.7	170	1.8	2.6	3.4	4.3
145		2.4	3.4	4.5	5.6					

Adapted by permission from Åstrand (1960).

TABLE 11.16 Prediction of Maximal Oxygen Consumption (L/min) From Heart Rate and Cycling Power in Women

| HR (beats/min) | Power (kg · m · min⁻¹; watts) | | | | | HR (beats/min) | Power (kg · m · min⁻¹; watts) | | | |
	300; 50	600; 100	900; 150	1,200; 200	1,500; 250		600; 100	900; 150	1,200; 200	1,500; 250
120	2.6	3.4	4.1	4.8		146	1.6	2.2	2.6	3.2
121	2.5	3.3	4.0	4.8		147	1.6	2.1	2.6	3.1
122	2.5	3.2	3.9	4.7		148	1.6	2.1	2.6	3.1
123	2.4	3.1	3.9	4.6		149		2.1	2.6	3.0
124	2.4	3.1	3.8	4.5		150		2.0	2.5	3.0
125	2.3	3.0	3.7	4.4		151		2.0	2.5	3.0
126	2.3	3.0	3.7	4.4		152		2.0	2.5	2.9
127	2.2	2.9	3.5	4.2		153		2.0	2.4	2.9
128	2.2	2.8	3.5	4.2		154		2.0	2.4	2.8
129	2.2	2.8	3.4	4.1		155		1.9	2.4	2.8
130	2.1	2.7	3.4	4.0	4.7	156		1.9	2.3	2.8
131	2.1	2.7	3.4	4.0	4.6	157		1.9	2.3	2.7
132	2.0	2.7	3.3	4.0	4.5	158		1.8	2.3	2.7
133	2.0	2.6	3.2	3.8	4.4	159		1.8	2.2	2.7
134	2.0	2.6	3.2	3.8	4.4	160		1.8	2.2	2.6
135	2.0	2.6	3.1	3.7	4.3	161		1.8	2.2	2.6
136	1.9	2.5	3.1	3.6	4.2	162		1.8	2.2	2.6
137	1.9	2.5	3.0	3.6	4.2	163		1.7	2.2	2.6
138	1.8	2.4	2.9	3.5	4.1	164		1.7	2.1	2.5
139	1.8	2.4	2.8	3.5	4.0	165		1.7	2.1	2.5
140	1.8	2.4	2.8	3.4	4.0	166		1.7	2.1	2.5
141	1.8	2.3	2.8	3.4	3.9	167		1.6	2.1	2.4
142	1.7	2.3	2.8	3.3	3.9	168		1.6	2.0	2.4
143	1.7	2.2	2.7	3.3	3.8	169		1.6	2.0	2.4
144	1.7	2.2	2.7	3.2	3.8	170		1.6	2.0	2.4
145	1.6	2.2	2.7	3.2	3.7					

Adapted by permission from Åstrand (1960).

TABLE 11.17 Age Correction Factors (CF) for Age-Adjusted Maximal Oxygen Consumption

Age	CF	Age	CF	Age	CF	Age	CF	Age	CF	Age	CF
15	1.10	25	1.00	35	0.87	45	0.78	55	0.71		
16	1.10	26	0.99	36	0.86	46	0.77	56	0.70		
17	1.09	27	0.98	37	0.85	47	0.77	57	0.70		
18	1.07	28	0.96	38	0.85	48	0.76	58	0.69		
19	1.06	29	0.95	39	0.84	49	0.76	59	0.69		
20	1.05	30	0.93	40	0.83	50	0.75	60	0.68		
21	1.04	31	0.93	41	0.82	51	0.74	61	0.67		
22	1.03	32	0.91	42	0.81	52	0.73	62	0.67		
23	1.02	33	0.90	43	0.80	53	0.73	63	0.66		
24	1.01	34	0.88	44	0.79	54	0.72	64	0.66		

Adapted by permission from Åstrand (1960).

TABLE 11.18 Norms for Evaluating Åstrand-Rhyming Cycle Test Performance

Age (years)	Aerobic fitness categories					
	Very high	High	Good	Average	Fair	Low
	Maximal oxygen consumption (ml · kg^{-1} · min^{-1})					
MEN						
20-29	>61	53-61	43-52	34-42	25-33	<25
30-39	>57	49-57	39-48	31-38	23-30	<23
40-49	>53	45-53	36-44	27-35	20-26	<20
50-59	>49	43-49	34-42	25-33	18-24	<18
60-69	>45	41-45	31-40	23-30	16-22	<16
WOMEN						
20-29	>57	49-57	38-48	31-37	24-30	<24
30-39	>53	45-53	34-44	28-33	20-27	<20
40-49	>50	42-50	31-41	24-30	17-23	<17
50-59	>42	38-42	28-37	21-27	15-20	<15
60-69	>39	35-39	24-34	18-23	13-17	<13

Reprinted by permission from W.C. Beam and G.M. Adams (2014).

TABLE 11.19 Male and Female Norms for Recovery Heart Rate Following the 3-Minute Step Test (beats/min)

Rating	18-25	26-35	36-45	46-55	56-65	66+
			Age (years)			
			MALE			
Excellent	70-78	73-79	72-81	78-84	72-82	72-86
Good	82-88	83-88	86-94	89-96	89-97	89-95
Above average	91-97	91-97	98-102	99-103	98-101	97-102
Average	101-104	101-106	105-111	109-115	105-111	104-113
Below average	107-114	109-116	113-118	118-121	113-118	114-119
Poor	118-126	119-126	120-128	124-130	122-128	122-128
Very poor	131-164	130-164	132-168	135-158	131-150	133-152
			FEMALE			
Excellent	72-83	72-86	74-87	76-93	74-92	73-86
Good	88-97	91-97	93-101	96-102	97-103	93-100
Above average	100-106	103-110	104-109	106-113	106-111	104-114
Average	110-116	112-118	111-117	117-120	113-117	117-121
Below average	118-124	121-127	120-127	121-126	119-127	123-127
Poor	128-137	129-135	130-138	127-133	129-136	129-134
Very poor	142-155	141-154	143-152	138-152	142-151	135-151

Reprinted by permission from Morrow et al. (2011, p. 200).

TABLE 11.20 Norms for the Rockport Walk Test

Clients aged 30-69 years (min:s)		
Rating	Males	Females
Excellent	<10:12	<11:40
Good	10:13-11:42	11:41-13:08
High average	11:43-13:13	13:09-14:36
Low average	13:14-14:44	14:37-16:04
Fair	14:45-16:23	16:05-17:31
Poor	>16:24	>17:32

Clients aged 18-30 years (min:s)		
Percentile	Males	Females
90	11:08	11:45
75	11:42	12:49
50	12:38	13:15
25	13:38	14:12
10	14:37	15:03

Reprinted by permission from Morrow et al. (2011, p. 200).

TABLE 11.21 Norms for th e 1-Mile Run (min:s)

Age (years)	Boys 85	Boys 50	Boys 15	Girls 85	Girls 50	Girls 15
6	10:15	12:36	16:30	11:20	13:12	16:45
7	9:22	11:40	15:00	10:36	12:56	16:00
8	8:48	11:05	14:10	10:02	12:30	15:19
9	8:31	10:30	12:59	9:30	11:52	14:57
10	7:57	9:48	13:07	9:19	11:22	14:00
11	7:32	9:20	12:29	9:02	11:17	14:16
12	7:11	8:40	11:30	8:23	11:05	14:12
13	6:50	8:06	10:39	8:13	10:23	14:10
14	6:26	7:44	10:18	7:59	10:06	12:56
15	6:20	7:30	9:34	8:08	9:58	13:33
16	6:08	7:10	9:22	8:23	10:31	14:16
17	6:06	7:04	8:56	8:15	10:22	13:03

Data from The President's Council on Fitness, Sports and Nutrition (69).

TABLE 11.22 Equations for Predicting $\dot{V}O_2$max (L/min) for Specific Populations

Population	Equation for predicting $\dot{V}O_2$max (L/min)
Untrained males	$(0.046 \times H) - (0.021 \times A) - 4.31$
Untrained females	$(0.046 \times H) - (0.021 \times A) - 4.93$
*Aerobically trained males	$(27.387 \times BW) + (26.634 \times H) - (27.572 \times A) + (26.161 \times D) + (114.904 \times I) + (506.752 \times Y) - 4609.791$
*Aerobically trained females	$(18.528 \times BW) + (11.993 \times H) - (17.197 \times A) + (23.522 \times D) + (62.118 \times I) + (278.262 \times Y) - 1375.878$

H = height in cm; A = age in years; BW = body weight in kg; D = duration of training in hours per week; I = intensity of training using the Borg scale; Y = natural log of years training.

Aerobically trained is defined as having participated in continuous aerobic exercise for a minimum of 1 h per workout session, three or more sessions per week, for at least the last 18 months.

Adapted from Malek et al. (54) and Malek et al. (55).

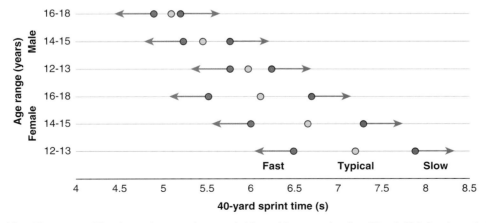

FIGURE 11.11 Time classifications for youths aged 12 to 18 years in the 40 yd (36.6 m) sprint: fast—70th percentile; typical—50th percentile; slow—30th percentile.

Reprinted by permission from Fukuda (2019, p. 123). Data from Haff and Dumke (31).

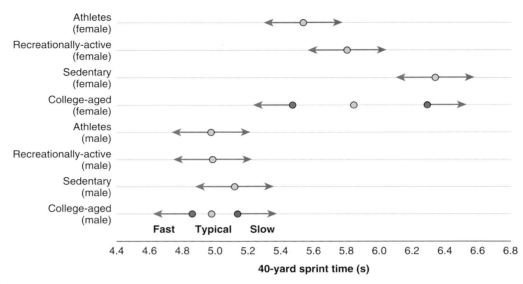

FIGURE 11.12 Time classifications for college-age individuals in the 40 yd (36.6 m) sprint: fast—75th percentile; typical—50th percentile; slow—25th percentile.

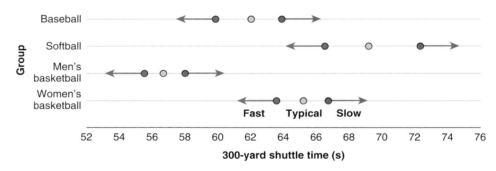

FIGURE 11.14 Classification values for the 300 yd (274.3 m) shuttle run for NCAA Division I athletes.

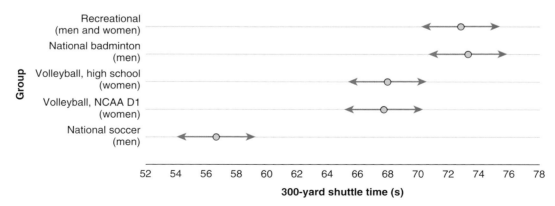

FIGURE 11.15 Descriptive (average) values for the 300 yd (274.3 m) shuttle run in various populations.

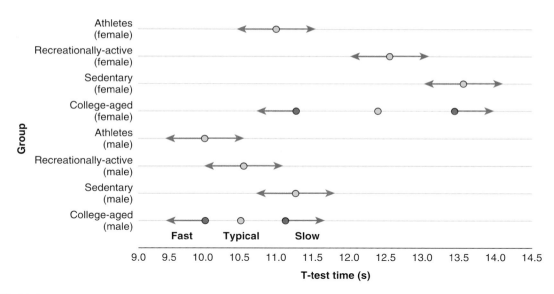

FIGURE 11.17 Time classifications for college-age individuals in the T-test: fast—75th percentile; typical—50th percentile; slow—25th percentile.

Reprinted by permission from Fukuda (2019, p. 112). Data from Pauole et al. (64).

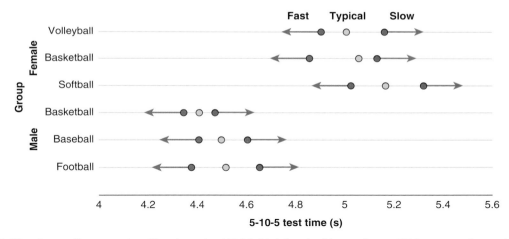

FIGURE 11.19 Pro agility test classifications for NCAA Division I athletes: fast—75th percentile; typical—50th percentile; slow—25th percentile.

Reprinted by permission from Fukuda (2019, p. 109). Data from Hoffman (38).

Bench press or back squat

Bench press or back squat

Leg press

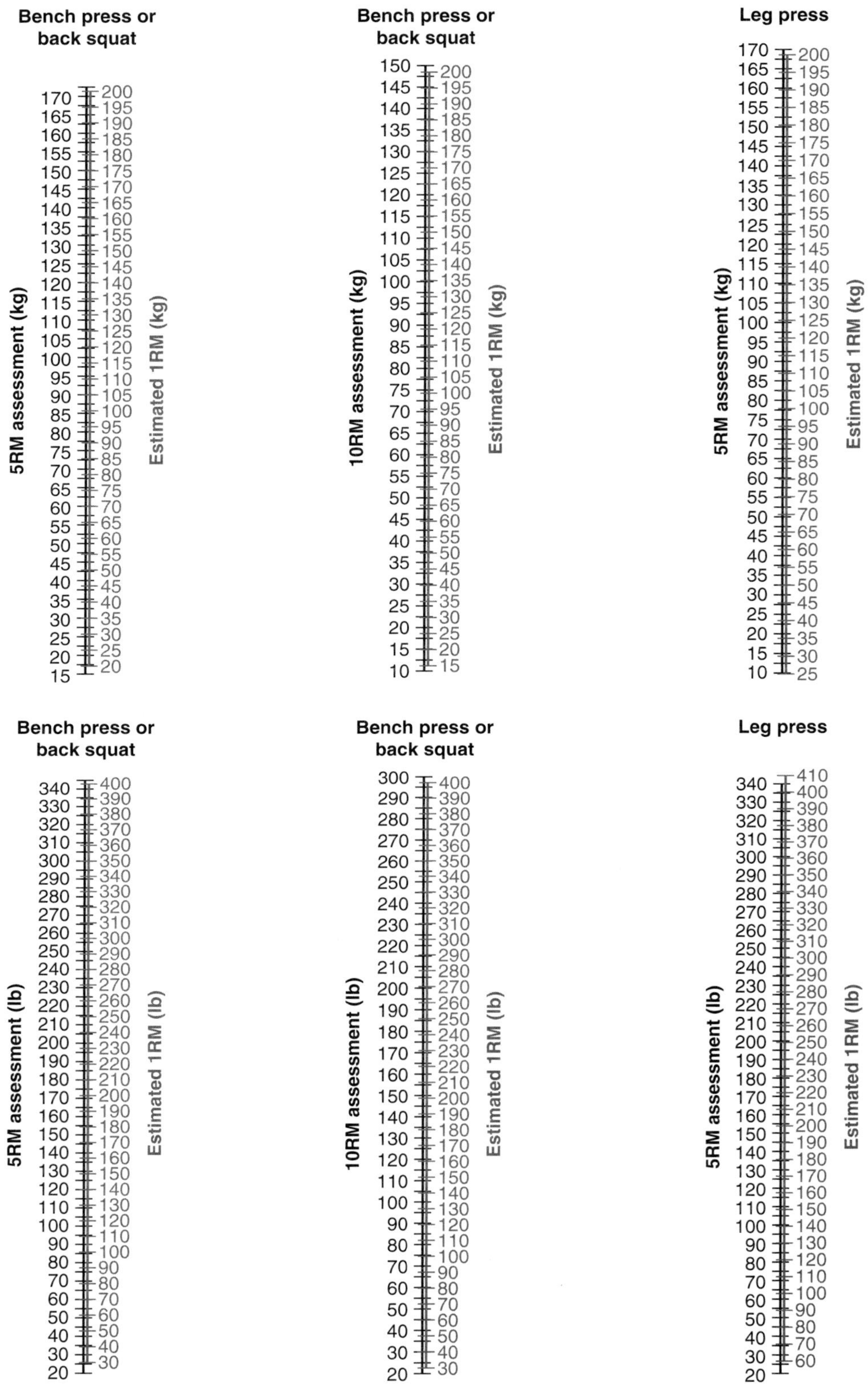

FIGURE 11.20 Conversion nomograms for estimating 1RM strength from 5RM and 10RM bench press or back squat and 5RM leg press assessments.

From *NSCA's Essentials of Personal Training,* 3rd ed., edited for the National Strength and Conditioning Association by B. Schoenfeld and R. Snarr (Champaign, IL: Human Kinetics, 2022).

TABLE 11.23   Relative Strength Norms for 1RM Bench Press

Percentile rankings* for men	Age (years)					
	20-29	30-39	40-49	50-59	60+	
90	1.48	1.24	1.10	0.97	0.89	
80	1.32	1.12	1.00	0.90	0.82	
70	1.22	1.04	0.93	0.84	0.77	
60	1.14	0.98	0.88	0.79	0.72	
50	1.06	0.93	0.84	0.75	0.68	
40	0.99	0.88	0.80	0.71	0.66	
30	0.93	0.83	0.76	0.68	0.63	
20	0.88	0.78	0.72	0.63	0.57	
10	0.80	0.71	0.65	0.57	0.53	
Percentile rankings* for women	**Age (years)**					
	20-29	30-39	40-49	50-59	60-69	70+
90	0.54	0.49	0.46	0.40	0.41	0.44
80	0.49	0.45	0.40	0.37	0.38	0.39
70	0.42	0.42	0.38	0.35	0.36	0.33
60	0.41	0.41	0.37	0.33	0.32	0.31
50	0.40	0.38	0.34	0.31	0.30	0.27
40	0.37	0.37	0.32	0.28	0.29	0.25
30	0.35	0.34	0.30	0.26	0.28	0.24
20	0.33	0.32	0.27	0.23	0.26	0.21
10	0.30	0.27	0.23	0.19	0.25	0.20

Norms were established using a Universal bench press machine.

*Descriptors for percentile rankings: 90 = well above average; 70 = above average; 50 = average; 30 = below average; 10 = well below average.

Data for men provided by the Cooper Institute for Aerobics Research, the Physical Fitness Specialist Manual, the Cooper Institute, Dallas, TX, 2005.

Data for women provided by the Women's Exercise Research Center, the George Washington University Medical Center, Washington, D.C., 1998.

Reprinted by permission from Gibson et al. (2019, p. 168).

TABLE 11.24 Relative Strength Norms for 1RM Leg Press

Percentile rankings* for men	Age (years)				
	20-29	30-39	40-49	50-59	60+
90	2.27	2.07	1.92	1.80	1.73
80	2.13	1.93	1.82	1.71	1.62
70	2.05	1.85	1.74	1.64	1.56
60	1.97	1.77	1.68	1.58	1.49
50	1.91	1.71	1.62	1.52	1.43
40	1.83	1.65	1.57	1.46	1.38
30	1.74	1.59	1.51	1.39	1.30
20	1.63	1.52	1.44	1.32	1.25
10	1.51	1.43	1.35	1.22	1.16

Percentile rankings* for women	Age (years)					
	20-29	30-39	40-49	50-59	60-69	70+
90	2.05	1.73	1.63	1.51	1.40	1.27
80	1.66	1.50	1.46	1.30	1.25	1.12
70	1.42	1.47	1.35	1.24	1.18	1.10
60	1.36	1.32	1.26	1.18	1.15	0.95
50	1.32	1.26	1.19	1.09	1.08	0.89
40	1.25	1.21	1.12	1.03	1.04	0.83
30	1.23	1.16	1.03	0.95	0.98	0.82
20	1.13	1.09	0.94	0.86	0.94	0.79
10	1.02	0.94	0.76	0.75	0.84	0.75

Norms were established using a Universal leg press machine.

*Descriptors for percentile rankings: 70 = above average; 50 = average; 30 = below average; 10 = well below average.

Data for men provided by the Cooper Institute for Aerobics Research, the Physical Fitness Specialist Manual, the Cooper Institute, Dallas, TX, 2005.

Data for women provided by the Women's Exercise Research Center, the George Washington University Medical Center, Washington, D.C., 1998.

Reprinted by permission from Gibson et al. (2019, p. 169).

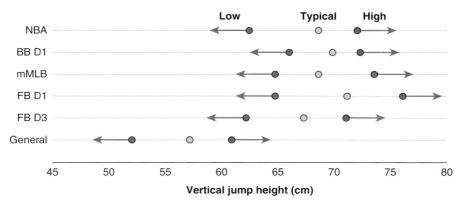

FIGURE 11.23 Vertical jump classifications for the male general adult population (general, 21-25 years old), National Collegiate Athletic Association (NCAA) Division I (FB D1) and III (FB D3) football players, minor and major league professional baseball players (mMLB), and NCAA Division (BB D1), and professional National Basketball Association (NBA) basketball players: high—70th percentile; typical—50th percentile; low—30th percentile.

Reprinted by permission from Fukuda (2019, p. 139). Data from Hoffman (38) and Patterson and Peterson (63).

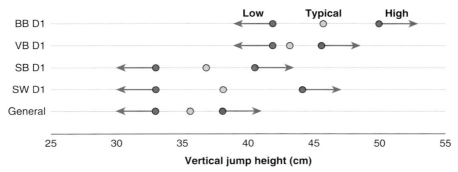

FIGURE 11.24 Vertical jump classifications for the female general adult population (general, 21-25 years old) and NCAA Division I swimming (SW D1), softball (SB D1), volleyball (VB D1), and basketball (BB D1) athletes: high—70th percentile; typical—50th percentile; low—30th percentile.

Reprinted by permission from Fukuda (2019, p. 139). Data from Hoffman (38) and Patterson and Peterson (63).

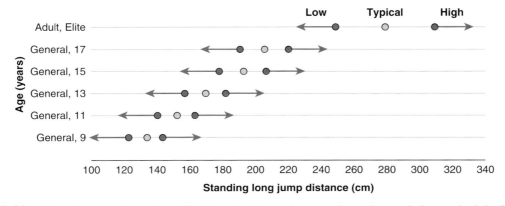

FIGURE 11.26 Standing long jump classifications for the male general youth population and adult elite athletes: high—70th percentile; typical—50th percentile; low—30th percentile.

Reprinted by permission from Fukuda (2019, p. 142). Data from Chu (11) and Tomkinson et al. (78).

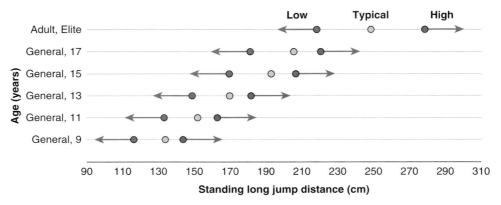

FIGURE 11.27 Standing long jump classifications for the female general youth population and adult elite athletes: high—70th percentile; typical—50th percentile; low—30th percentile.

Reprinted by permission from Fukuda (2019, p. 143). Data from Chu (11) and Tomkinson et al. (78).

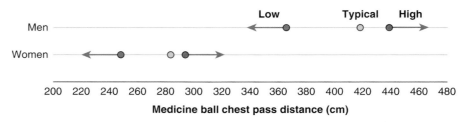

FIGURE 11.29 Medicine ball chest pass classifications for college-age men and women: high—70th percentile; typical—50th percentile; low—30th percentile. A 6 kg (13.2 lb) medicine ball was used for females, and a 9 kg (19.8 lb) medicine ball was used for males.

Reprinted by permission from Fukuda (2019, p. 148). Data from Clemons et al. (12).

TABLE 11.25 YMCA Bench Press Norms

Percentile	Age (years)											
	18-25		26-35		36-45		46-55		56-65		66+	
	M	F	M	F	M	F	M	F	M	F	M	F
90	44	42	41	40	36	33	28	29	24	24	20	18
80	37	34	33	32	29	28	22	22	20	20	14	14
70	33	28	29	28	25	24	20	18	14	14	10	10
60	29	25	26	24	22	21	16	14	12	12	10	8
50	26	21	22	21	20	17	13	12	10	9	8	6
40	22	18	20	17	17	14	11	9	8	6	6	4
30	20	16	17	14	14	12	9	7	5	5	4	3
20	16	12	13	12	10	8	6	5	3	3	2	1
10	10	6	9	6	6	4	2	1	1	1	1	0

Note: Score is number of repetitions completed in 1 minute using 80 lb (36 kg) barbell for men and 35 lb (16 kg) barbell for women.

Adapted from Golding (28).

TABLE 11.26 Ratings by Age Groups and Sex for Sit-Ups Completed in Two Minutes

Rating	Age (years)				
	17-19	20-29	30-39	40-49	50+
MEN					
Outstanding	88	84	75	73	68
Excellent	72	68	54	48	45
Good	60	50	40	35	33
Satisfactory	45	40	32	29	27
WOMEN					
Outstanding	86	84	74	72	67
Excellent	67	61	54	48	45
Good	52	45	39	34	32
Satisfactory	40	33	27	24	22

Adapted from Hodgdon (38a).

TABLE 11.27 Normative Percentile Data in Seconds for Prone Double Straight-Leg Raise

Percentile	Age (years)									
	19-29		30-39		40-49		50-59		60+	
	M	F	M	F	M	F	M	F	M	F
75	130	126	123	111	95	87	80	83	60	40
50	88	74	73	73	55	45	48	37	22	23
25	55	49	45	45	35	29	22	18	11	7

Reprinted from McIntosh et al. (60).

TABLE 11.28 Percentiles by Age Groups and Sex for YMCA Sit-and-Reach Test (inches)

Percentile	Age (years)											
	18-25		26-35		36-45		46-55		56-65		>65	
	M	F	M	F	M	F	M	F	M	F	M	F
90	22	24	21	23	21	22	19	21	17	20	17	20
80	20	22	19	21	19	21	17	20	15	19	15	18
70	19	21	17	20	17	19	15	18	13	17	13	17
60	18	20	17	20	16	18	14	17	13	16	12	17
50	17	19	15	19	15	17	13	16	11	15	10	15
40	15	18	14	17	13	16	11	14	9	14	9	14
30	14	17	13	16	13	15	10	14	9	13	8	13
20	13	16	11	15	11	14	9	12	7	11	7	11
10	11	14	9	13	7	12	6	10	5	9	4	9

These norms are based on a yardstick placed so that the zero point is set at 15 in. (38.1 cm).

Adapted from Golding (28).

TABLE 11.29 Fitness Categories by Age Groups for Trunk Forward Flexion Using a Sit-and-Reach Box (cm): Ages 20 to 69

Rating	Age (years)									
	20-29		30-39		40-49		50-59		60-69	
	M	F	M	F	M	F	M	F	M	F
Excellent	40	41	38	41	35	38	35	39	33	35
Very good	39	40	37	40	34	37	34	38	32	34
	34	37	33	36	29	34	28	33	25	31
Good	33	36	32	35	28	33	27	32	24	30
	30	33	28	32	24	30	24	30	20	27
Fair	29	32	27	31	23	29	23	29	19	26
	25	28	23	27	18	25	16	25	15	23
Needs improvement	24	27	22	26	17	24	15	24	14	22

These norms are based on a sit-and-reach box in which the zero point is set at 26 cm (10.2 in.). When using a box in which the zero point is set at 23 cm (9.1 in.), subtract 3 cm (1.2 in.) from each value in this table.

Source: CSEP Physical Activity Training for Health (CSEP-PATH®), 2nd Edition, 2019. Reprinted with permission of the Canadian Society for Exercise Physiology.

TABLE 11.30 Fitness Categories by Age Groups for Trunk Forward Flexion Using a Sit-and-Reach Box (cm): Ages 5 to 17+

	Percentile					
	Boys			Girls		
Age (years)	85	50	15	85	50	15
5	30	25	21	31	27	22
6	31	26	20	32	27	22
7	30	25	19	32	27	22
8	31	25	20	33	28	21
9	31	25	20	33	28	21
10	30	25	18	33	28	21
11	31	25	18	34	29	22
12	31	26	18	36	30	22
13	33	26	18	38	31	22
14	36	28	21	40	33	24
15	37	30	22	43	36	28
16	38	30	21	42	34	26
17+	41	34	25	42	35	28

Data from The President's Council on Fitness, Sports and Nutrition (69).

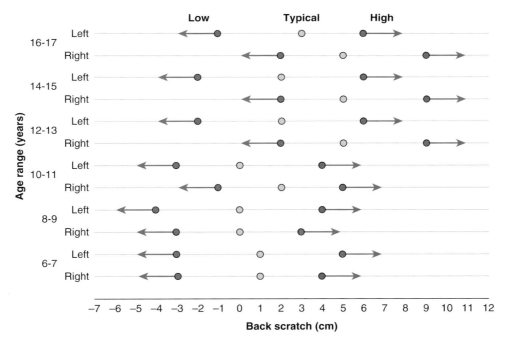

FIGURE 11.35 Back scratch classifications for boys (left and right side): low—30th percentile; typical—50th percentile; high—70th percentile.

Reprinted by permission from Fukuda (2019, p. 83). Data from Castro-Piñero et al. (10).

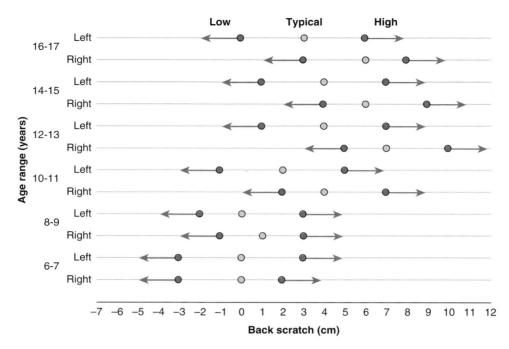

FIGURE 11.36 Back scratch classifications for girls (left and right side): low—30th percentile; typical—50th percentile; high—70th percentile.

Reprinted by permission from Fukuda (2019, p. 83). Data from Castro-Piñero et al. (10).

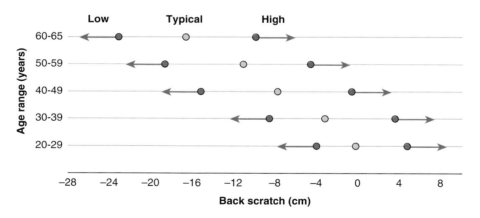

FIGURE 11.37 Back scratch classifications across the lifespan for men: low—25th percentile; typical—50th percentile; high—75th percentile.

Reprinted by permission from Fukuda (2019, p. 83). Data from Kjaer et al. (46).

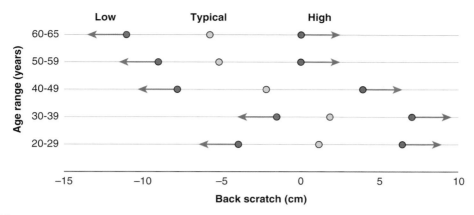

FIGURE 11.38 Back scratch classifications across the lifespan for women: low—25th percentile; typical—50th percentile; high—75th percentile.

TABLE 11.32 Normative Values for Closed Kinetic Chain Upper Extremity Stability (CKCUES) Test

	Number of touches	Power	Normalized score
Sedentary males	23.99	88.40	0.35
Sedentary females	26.53	67.90	0.42
Active males	25.96	88.63	0.40
Active females	29.97	77.81	0.48

Adapted from Tucci et al. (79a).

Flexibility and Warm-Up Concepts and Bodyweight and Stability Ball Exercise Technique

Nick Tumminello, Jonathan Mike, PhD, and Jay Dawes, PhD

After completing this chapter, you will be able to

- describe the benefits of participating in a flexibility training program,
- understand the factors that affect flexibility,
- explain the value of warming up before participating in flexibility training,
- list and explain the various types of flexibility training,
- supervise a flexibility training program emphasizing a combination of dynamic and static stretching, and
- supervise exercises using body weight only, suspension training, manual resistance, and stability balls.

This chapter covers four major topics. The first is flexibility training, which forms an important part of an overall conditioning program. The second topic is warm-up, with discussion of both its importance and the techniques used for warming up before physical activity. This is followed by a discussion of training methods using body weight, suspension training systems, manual resistance, and stability balls, highlighting the potential benefits of each. Finally, the chapter presents detailed instructions for recommended static and dynamic flexibility movements and proper exercise techniques for the resistance training methods discussed.

The authors would like to acknowledge the significant contributions of Allen Hedrick to this chapter.

DEFINING FLEXIBILITY

Those involved in supervising conditioning or rehabilitation programs typically use some form of stretching with their clients or patients. Despite this, there can be confusion about the notion that people must achieve extreme levels of flexibility to reduce the chance of injury and to improve movement capabilities. This does not accurately represent the role that flexibility plays in training. Flexibility is an important piece of the training puzzle; but like other aspects of training, it must be based on the needs of the individual. Thus, it is imperative that personal trainers be aware of factors that influence range of motion and focus on systematic, safe, and effective applications of stretching techniques to enhance flexibility. Typically, these specific applications require actively moving the joints through progressively greater ranges of motion.

According to a common definition, **flexibility** is the range of motion of a joint or a series of joints (48, 79). For personal trainers, who are concerned with improving clients' movement performance and mitigating injury, a more relevant definition might be the ability of a joint to move freely through the full normal range of motion (ROM) (48, 79).

FLEXIBILITY TRAINING AS PART OF THE TOTAL EXERCISE PROGRAM

Although a later section of the chapter discusses warm-up in more detail, it is important to note here that each training session should begin with a warm-up designed to elevate core temperature. After completing the warm-up session, the client may or may not need to immediately participate in flexibility training, depending on the nature of the activity to follow. For example, if clients are going to participate in a dynamic activity (e.g., basketball, racquetball) after the warm-up, they need to engage in flexibility training (e.g., dynamic flexibility or elastic elongation) first. If they are going to participate in a less dynamic activity (e.g., stationary bike, stair climber), they can work on flexibility after the training session is complete.

> ▶ **Every workout should be preceded by a warm-up session. However, the ideal time to perform flexibility training is dependent on the nature of the activity that is to take place during the workout.**

BENEFITS OF FLEXIBILITY TRAINING

Developing or maintaining flexibility is an important goal of many training programs. Achieving optimal flexibility helps improve movement efficiency by allowing joints to move freely through a full normal ROM, and it also reduces the risk of musculoskeletal injuries (60, 62); prevents the development of muscular imbalances; and improves posture, strength, range of motion, and power (11, 43, 64). Improving flexibility is a fundamental element of any training program. However, although more elite athletes may have above-average flexibility, this may not be why they are successful. The ability to move effectively depends on strength and coordination, and being flexible may enhance this ability. Therefore, the goal of flexibility training should be to optimize flexibility based on the clients' specific goals and to improve coordination and motor control.

Flexibility training is also important for injury prevention (2, 6). Among the more common problems seen in individuals with poor flexibility is lower back pain potentially resulting from tight quadriceps, iliopsoas, and back muscles (and possibly a corresponding weakness in the abdominal muscles and hamstrings) (73). A lack of flexibility may also increase the incidence of muscle tears resulting from tight muscles on one or both sides of a joint (6). The accepted belief regarding the role of flexibility in terms of injury prevention is that a normal ROM (i.e., the ROM common to most individuals) in each joint will reduce injury potential (6). If a client is involved in a sport or activity that requires greater than normal ROM (e.g., hurdlers, golfers, Olympic weightlifters), then a greater emphasis should be placed on increasing flexibility to help protect against injury.

Because of these important benefits, it is recommended that personal trainers supervise stretching just as they would any other part of the training session. Doing this communicates the importance of the warm-up and stretching period and may encourage clients to prioritize this portion of the training session.

> ▶ **Flexibility training is important because of the role that flexibility plays in improving movement performance and reducing the opportunity for injury.**

FACTORS AFFECTING FLEXIBILITY

Several physiological, lifestyle, and environmental factors influence flexibility. Although some of these are out of the client's control, such as joint structure, age, and sex, factors like muscle and connective tissue elasticity, core temperature, activity level, and the client's training program can have a profound influence on ROM, and these can be influenced by training (22, 60).

Joint Structure

One of the primary limiting factors in static ROM is the structure of the joint itself. Because of joint structure, there is a limit to how much movement is available. Joint structures vary between individuals, and the personal trainer must consider this variation when evaluating flexibility.

Joint structure also varies between joints. Some joints offer a reduced ROM compared with others by virtue of their construction. The hinge-type joints of the knee and elbow allow movements almost entirely in the sagittal plane (i.e., flexion and extension), so knee and elbow ROM is significantly less than that of the shoulder or hip (60). The ball and socket joints of the hip and shoulder allow movements in all anatomical planes and have the greatest ROM of all joints (60).

Flexibility is joint specific. That is, it is relatively common to have above-average flexibility in one joint and below-average ROM in another. Thus, flexibility should be thought of as a characteristic specific to a particular joint and joint action rather than a general trait. For this reason, it is incorrect to think that a single flexibility test can provide an accurate measure of overall flexibility (6).

Muscle and Connective Tissue

Connective tissue (muscles, ligaments, and tendons) is the area of emphasis during ROM exercise. This is because, under normal circumstances, connective tissues are the major structures limiting joint ROM. These connective tissue structures include ligamentous joint capsules, tendons, and muscles (48, 60). Although muscle itself is not usually thought of as a connective tissue structure, when a relaxed muscle is stretched during ROM exercise, most of the resistance to the stretch comes from the extensive connective tissue framework and sheathing within and around the muscle (48, 60).

Most of the differences between individuals in static ROM are due to the elastic properties of the muscle and tendons attached across the joints. "Stiff" muscles and tendons reduce ROM, while "compliant" muscles and tendons increase ROM. It is these elastic properties that are altered from stretching exercises. When a muscle is held at a fixed length while under tension in a static stretch, the **passive tension** [i.e., the amount of external force required to lengthen the relaxed muscle (49)] declines. This is called a **viscoelastic stress relaxation response** (39, 56). Obviously, the more pliable the muscle, the less external force is required. The increased pliability lasts up to 20 minutes after the stretching session, even after very high volumes of passive stretching (e.g., 8 minutes of stretching for a single muscle group) (55).

Hyperlaxity

Although it is uncommon, some individuals are born with a tissue structure that predisposes them to **hyperlaxity**. Hyperlaxity allows the joints of the body to achieve a ROM that exceeds what is considered normal (54). If it has been determined that a client has joint hyperlaxity, the personal trainer should use caution when implementing a stretching program and should ensure that the client has been assessed by an appropriate health care professional. It is important that the client avoid overstretching and creating even greater levels of laxity within the joint. Poor selection of stretching exercises may also cause problems because excessive ROM in the joint may increase the opportunity for injury (22) and may have a negative effect on performance.

Age

The biological age of an individual can have a significant impact on flexibility. Although flexibility tends to diminish as one ages, this reduction may be partially attributable to a decrease in overall physical activity throughout the life span (41, 42). However, a well-designed flexibility training program is effective for increasing joint ROM among older adults (44). Because of the wide range of intervention protocols, body parts studied, and functional measurements, conclusive recommendations regarding flexibility training and functional outcomes for older adults remain limited (70).

Sex

Sex may also have a significant impact on flexibility levels. It is well known that the connective tissues of men and women differ physiologically (34), although the mechanisms contributing to these differences are not well understood. Estrogen may play a role in flexibility because estrogen receptors are present in fibroblasts of tendons and ligaments, which may affect collagen synthesis or alter tissue behavior (14). Eiling and colleagues (22) found significant decreases in musculotendinous stiffness of the knee flexors during the ovulatory phase, when estrogen and progesterone are elevated. Males generally also have greater muscle mass compared with women, which may contribute to the higher musculotendinous stiffness values observed for males versus females. Indeed, after accounting for body weight, body mass, and limb size, sex-related differences in musculotendinous stiffness are inconsequential (10).

Temperature

ROM is positively affected by an increase in either core temperature or external temperature (21, 51). The positive effect of increased core temperature on ROM points to the importance of warming up before participating in flexibility training. Warm-up is discussed later in the chapter.

Activity Level

As would be expected, people who are physically active tend to be more flexible than inactive individuals (9). The decrease in flexibility in inactive individuals primarily occurs because connective tissues may become less pliable when exposed only to limited ROMs (9). A decrease in activity level will typically result in an increase in percent body fat and a decrease in the pliability of connective tissue (15, 33).

Resistance Training

A well-designed and properly executed resistance training program using exercises that are performed through a full range of motion can also increase flexibility. Resistance training programs should be designed to develop both agonist and antagonist muscles, and all exercises should be performed through the full available ROM of the involved joints (64). Although improper resistance training can impair flexibility, the reason is not usually that the person has become too muscular, or "muscle bound." Instead, the decrease occurs because of the improper development of a muscle or a group of muscles around a joint, resulting in a restriction of motion at that joint (64). For example, a person with large biceps and deltoids may have difficulty stretching the triceps, racking a power clean, or holding a bar while performing the front squat (64). This is another reason resistance training programs should be designed to develop both agonist and antagonist muscles and to take all the involved joints through the full available ROM.

> Flexibility is influenced by a variety of factors. Some of these factors (e.g., joint structure, age, and sex) cannot be influenced by training. However, core temperature during flexibility training, overall activity level, participation in a well-designed resistance training program, and stretching on a regular basis can all affect flexibility and can be positively influenced by the personal trainer.

ELASTICITY AND PLASTICITY

Flexibility training targets two different tissue adaptations: elasticity and plasticity. **Elasticity** refers to the ability to return to original resting length after a passive stretch (64). Thus, elasticity provides a temporary change in length. In contrast, **plasticity** refers to the tendency to assume a new and greater length after a passive stretch, even after the load is removed (46).

Ligaments and tendons have both plastic and elastic properties. When connective tissue is stretched, some of the elongation occurs in the elastic tissue elements and some occurs in the plastic elements. When the stretch is removed, the elastic deformation recovers, but the plastic deformation remains (46). The specific stretching techniques used by the personal trainer should be designed to produce a plastic elongation if a permanent increase in ROM is the goal (46). During stretching, the proportion of elastic and plastic deformation can vary, depending on the conditions in which the flexibility training occurs.

TYPES OF FLEXIBILITY TRAINING

Several stretching techniques can be used to maintain or increase flexibility. The most common of these methods are ballistic, dynamic, static, and various proprioceptive neuromuscular facilitation (PNF) techniques (1, 3, 5, 19).

Flexibility training can be further categorized into active and passive stretching exercises. **Active stretching** occurs when the person who is stretching supplies the force of the stretch. For example, during the sitting toe touch, the client supplies the force for the forward lean that stretches the hamstrings and low back. In contrast, **passive stretching** occurs when a partner or stretching device provides the force for the stretch (48).

The most important aspect of designing an effective flexibility training program is to ensure correct performance of exercises, regardless of the flexibility training method. For example, one technique commonly used to stretch the hamstrings is the toe touch stretch. However, this position involves low back flexion, which posteriorly rotates the pelvis, decreasing the effectiveness of the stretch for the hamstrings. A better method to stretch the hamstrings is to place one foot slightly in front of the other, leaning forward from the hips and keeping a neutral spine. Supporting upper body weight with the hands on the rear leg, the client should feel the stretch in the front leg. This position ensures that the pelvis remains tilted forward, keeping the hamstrings optimally lengthened (44). Good technique is necessary to bring about optimal increases in flexibility.

Ballistic Stretching

Ballistic stretching involves continuous, rapid bouncing movements at the end ROM where the muscle is at maximal length. It is generally no longer considered an acceptable method for increasing ROM because there is an increased risk of injury to the muscles and connective tissues associated with these types of movements, especially in joints where there has been a previous injury (7, 79). The most frequently cited reason for this is that ballistic stretching involves rapid stretching of the muscle, which may activate the muscle spindle and prevent adequate muscle relaxation before the subsequent stretch. Therefore, ballistic stretching has three distinct disadvantages:

1. Increased danger of exceeding the extensibility limits of tissues involved

2. Greater energy requirements

3. Activation of the stretch reflex

Two of the sensory organs within skeletal muscle that function as protective mechanisms against injury during passive and active stretching are the **muscle spindles**, which are located within the center of the muscle (48), and the **Golgi tendon organ**, which is located at the musculotendon junction. Muscle spindles initiate the stretch reflex, while the Golgi tendon organ initiates the Golgi tendon reflex.

The **stretch reflex** occurs in response to the extent and rapidity of a muscle stretch. When the muscle spindles are not stimulated, the muscle remains fully relaxed, allowing a greater stretch. During a rapid stretching movement, however, the sensory neuron from the muscle spindle excites a motor neuron in the spine that innervates muscle fibers in the stretched muscle. Thus, excitation of the motor neuron then causes contraction of the previously stretched extrafusal muscle fibers. When the client bounces, for instance, the stretch reflex is initiated and causes the muscles to contract to protect themselves from overstretching. Thus, internal tension develops in the muscle and prevents it from being fully stretched. A familiar example of this reflex is the knee jerk response. When the patellar tendon is struck, the tendon, and consequently the quadriceps muscle, experiences a slight but rapid stretch. The induced stretch results in activation of muscle spindle receptors within the quadriceps, causing the lower leg to jerk. Since motion is limited by this reflexive muscle action, stimulation of the muscle spindle and the subsequent activation of the stretch reflex should be avoided during stretching.

In addition to the stretch reflex, when excessive force is generated in the muscle, the Golgi tendon organ causes a reflex opposite that of the muscle spindle by inhibiting muscle contraction and causing the muscle to relax. This reflex helps prevent injury by decreasing muscle activity, thereby keeping the muscle from developing too much force or tension during active stretching (62).

Static Stretching

The most used method of increasing flexibility is **static stretching**. A slow, constant speed is used, with the stretched position held for approximately 30 seconds (79). Static stretching involves relaxation and simultaneous lengthening of the stretched muscle. Because of the slow speed of the stretches, static stretching does not activate the stretch reflex of the muscle. Thus, the risk for injury is lower than during ballistic stretching (79). Although injury to muscles or connective tissue may result if the static stretch is too intense, there are no real disadvantages to static stretching in terms of injury potential if proper technique is used. However, research indicates that static and ballistic stretching can interfere with exercise and athletic performance, and their effects seem to depend on the stretching method employed (1, 3, 5, 19, 29). For example, the acute effects of static, PNF, and ballistic stretching can negatively affect sprint performance (although sprint performance is less affected after ballistic stretching than after static or PNF) (1, 23). Note, however, that if stretching is performed before a sport-specific warm-up or if enough time is allowed to elapse between stretching and actual performance (as in most sport performance settings), then there is very likely no residual negative effect of stretching on performance (31, 63).

Individuals beginning a flexibility program may find it challenging to hold a stretched position for longer durations. Therefore, the personal trainer may initially decrease the duration of the stretch and progress to longer time intervals as tolerance improves (e.g., 15-30 seconds). As previously mentioned, when performing a static stretch the movement should occur slowly and only to the point of minor discomfort. As the stretched position is held, the feeling of tension should diminish at a given ROM as the number of repetitions increases. This specific technique of static stretching should help eliminate activation of the stretch reflex.

> **To prevent activation of the stretch reflex, the client should move into the final static stretch position slowly and only to a point of minor discomfort. As the stretched position is held, the feeling of tension should diminish; if it does not, the stretched position should be slightly reduced.**

Proprioceptive Neuromuscular Facilitation

Proprioceptive neuromuscular facilitation (PNF) stretching was originally developed as a technique to relax muscles that demonstrated increased tone or activity. It has since expanded to the conditioning of both athletes and the general population as a method of increasing ROM.

RECOMMENDATIONS FOR STATIC STRETCHING

The following recommendations can be made to clients who are implementing a static flexibility training program (48):

- Stretching should be preceded by a warm-up of 5 to 15 minutes, until a light sweat appears.

- Emphasize slow, smooth movements and coordinate deep breathing. Have clients inhale deeply and then exhale as they stretch to the point of mild discomfort. Then, have them ease back slightly and hold the stretch for 30 seconds as they breathe normally. Finally, have clients exhale as they slowly stretch farther, again to the point of mild discomfort. Repeat three times and emphasize the importance of staying relaxed.

- Properly performed stretches should cause no more than mild discomfort. If clients feel pain, they are stretching too far.

- Ensure that clients do not lock their joints.

- To reduce the chance of activating the stretch reflex, discourage bouncing.

- Large muscle groups should be stretched first, and the same routine should be repeated every training day. As areas that are less flexible become apparent, a greater emphasis can be placed on performing additional stretches for those muscle groups and joints.

- Stretches should be done at least three times per week and, to track performance improvements, should be done at the same time of day. Clients are least flexible in the morning because core temperature is the lowest at that time, so stretching early in the morning without first elevating core temperature is not advantageous in enhancing flexibility.

- The ideal time to stretch is after aerobic activity or resistance training, when core temperature is maximally elevated.

RECOMMENDATIONS FOR DYNAMIC STRETCHING

The following are recommendations for implementing a dynamic flexibility training program (48).

- Moderation and common sense are important. Flexibility is just one component of fitness and should not be overemphasized.
- The stretch should never be forced. If the stretch hurts, it should be discontinued.
- Flexibility training should be combined with resistance training.
- Flexibility should be joint specific based on the needs of the client and the requirements of the activity.
- Ballistic stretching should be avoided.
- Stretching movements that position the body in the most functional stance possible, relative to the involved joints and musculature to be stretched and the activity requirements of the client, should be emphasized.
- It is important to make use of gravity, body weight, and ground reaction forces when stretching. Further, changes in planes and proprioceptive demand should be considered to further enhance improvements in flexibility.

- The dynamic flexibility training program should be specific to the demands of the sport or activities the client takes part in. The individual flexibility requirements of the client are also an important consideration.
- Improvements in flexibility can occur from day to day. Additionally, once increases in ROM have occurred, it is easy to maintain that ROM. Maintaining flexibility requires less work than improving it does.
- Clients should stretch the large muscle groups first and repeat the same routine every training day. As areas that are less flexible become apparent, a greater emphasis can be placed on performing additional stretches for those muscle groups and joints.
- Train for dynamic flexibility at least three times per week or along with each exercise session. To track performance improvements, clients should be consistent with the time of day they perform dynamic flexibility training, remembering they are least flexible in the morning.
- Stretching should take place after the core temperature has been elevated.

Proprioceptive neuromuscular facilitation is widely accepted as an effective method of increasing ROM (23, 25, 62). These techniques are normally performed with a partner and make use of both passive movement and active (i.e., concentric and isometric) muscle actions. There are a variety of PNF techniques, but perhaps the most common method (i.e., the **hold-relax method**) involves taking the muscle or joint into a static stretch position while keeping the muscle relaxed. After this static stretch position is held for about 10 seconds, the muscle is contracted for 6 seconds with a strong isometric contraction against an external fixed object (i.e., a force acting in the direction of the stretch). The partner should not allow the client to have any movement in the joint. After a very brief (1-2 second) rest, another passive stretch is performed for 30 seconds, potentially resulting in a greater stretch. The isometric contraction will result in stimulation of the Golgi tendon organs; this may help maintain low muscle tension during the second stretching maneuver, allowing connective tissue to further lengthen and resulting in increased ROM (62).

Proprioceptive neuromuscular facilitation stretching may be superior to other stretching methods because it assists muscular relaxation, potentially assisting in increased ROM (23, 25, 62). Despite this, some PNF methods may have limited application in personal training settings. Because a partner is needed, PNF can be more time consuming than other methods, and the partner must be careful not to overstretch the muscle. Practically, though, because static and dynamic flexibility methods are effective at increasing flexibility and because most clients do not need to achieve superior flexibility levels, PNF methods are not generally needed.

Dynamic Stretching

Dynamic and ballistic stretching are similar in that both allow for faster movements to occur during training. However, **dynamic stretching** avoids bouncing and includes movements specific to a sport or movement pattern. An example of a dynamic stretch is a lunge walk in which the client exaggerates the length of the stride and flexes the back leg so that he or she ends up in a position in which the front knee is over the toe (but not in front of it) and the back knee is just off the floor, with the torso held in an upright position. With reference to the principle of specificity, dynamic stretching more closely simulates movements that occur in sport- and exercise-related activities and activities of daily living (ADL). An example is the everyday movement of reaching for an item on the top shelf at the grocery store, at home, or in the workplace. Dynamic arm circles, which are done with fluidity of movement, may more closely resemble reaching overhead in everyday life than would a position in which the arms are held statically over the head.

Dynamic stretching emphasizes functionally based movements. As training progresses, advancing from a standing position to a walk or a skip can enhance the specificity of dynamic stretching exercises. Adjusting from static stretching to dynamic exercises is not difficult. Often the stretching exercise is the same but is preceded and followed by some form of movement.

Personal trainers who wish to implement dynamic flexibility training in a client's program should begin dynamic stretches with low volume and low intensity because dynamic flexibility exercises require balance and coordination. Furthermore, dynamic flexibility training may lead to soreness for a short period of time when introduced because it represents a new stress to the body.

Many of the guidelines established for static flexibility training programs are also applicable to dynamic flexibility training. As already discussed, a warm-up period should occur before any flexibility training. Frequency should be two to five times per week, depending on the flexibility requirements of the activities the client is preparing for and his or her flexibility. Because dynamic flexibility training uses movement, each stretch should be repeated over 20 to 25 yards or meters.

As the client becomes better able to perform each drill, the exercises can be performed in combinations. For example, a knee tuck and a lunge walk can be combined, alternating legs after performance of each movement. The possible combinations of exercises are nearly limitless. There are two primary advantages of combining movements. First, the variety is greater, so the program is less likely to become monotonous. Second, combining stretches is more time efficient because the client is stretching a larger number of muscle groups rather than duplicating the same stretch repeatedly. This is important because many clients have limited time to devote to their training programs.

A later section of this chapter describes and illustrates common dynamic flexibility exercises. Since dynamic flexibility exercises are based on movements that occur both in sport and in everyday life, this selection of exercises does not represent an all-inclusive list of dynamic stretches. The number and types of dynamic stretches that can be used is limited only by the creativity of those designing the programs.

> **Dynamic and PNF stretching may be the most appropriate types of flexibility training for improving movement capability before a workout. If additional flexibility work is needed, performance of static flexibility exercises after the workout is effective.**

RECOMMENDED FLEXIBILITY ROUTINE AND GUIDELINES

A combination of dynamic and static flexibility training is recommended when the goal of training is increased ROM. Dynamic flexibility training is often associated with training athletes. However, dynamic flexibility training can also be successfully used in a non-athletic population. Increasing flexibility is of value during any type of movement regardless of whether that movement is occurring during an athletic competition or during performance of the multitude of movements that occur during daily life. The more functional the training, the more benefit it provides to those taking part in the training program.

Using dynamic flexibility alone can have limitations, however. Some of the dynamic stretches require a significant level of strength and mobility. This may preclude clients from performing some of the more demanding dynamic flexibility exercises. Further, some joints (e.g., neck, shoulders) and muscle groups may be more effectively stretched using static stretching techniques as compared with dynamic flexibility techniques.

WARM-UP

Clients should regularly perform preparatory exercises before undertaking vigorous activities. These preparatory exercises or movements are generally referred to as a **warm-up**.

Warm-up and stretching are not the same thing. Warm-up is an activity that raises the total body temperature, as well as temperature of the muscles, to prepare the body for vigorous exercise (48, 53). Warming up is a part of the foundation of a successful practice session. Getting fully warmed up, mentally and physically, is a key aspect of attaining the training intensity required to achieve optimal results. A warm-up period is also important for increasing core temperature, thus improving the pliability of the muscles (4). Further, a warm-up increases flexibility because muscle elasticity is dependent on the temperature of the muscle tissue (4). Unfortunately, many clients attempt to take shortcuts in the warm-up procedure, which may translate into poor performance and increased injury risks. Although the psychological aspects of the warm-up have not yet been adequately investigated, research indicates that individuals who perform a warm-up before their main activity tend to be more mentally tuned or prepared (36, 50).

Most research indicates that the major benefits of warm-up are related to temperature-dependent physiological processes. The increase in tissue temperature that occurs during warm-up is the result of the friction of the sliding filaments during muscular action, the metabolism of fuels, and the dilation of intramuscular blood vessels (4, 32). An adequate warm-up does the following:

■ Increases blood flow to the muscles

■ Increases the sensitivity of nerve receptors

■ Increases the disassociation of oxygen from hemoglobin and myoglobin

■ Increases the speed of nerve impulse transmissions

■ Reduces muscle viscosity

■ Lowers the energy rates of metabolic chemical reactions

Range of motion is increased after a warm-up period because elevated core temperatures lower muscle, tendon, and ligament viscosity (6). This decrease in viscosity enables achievement of the best possible results and reduces the potential risk of stretching-induced injuries. It also reduces muscle and joint stiffness and provides protection against sudden, unexpected movements (4). It has been reported that excessive stretching when the tissue temperatures are relatively low increases the risk of connective tissue damage (4).

Unfortunately, many clients' preactivity warm-up program consists primarily of static stretching. There are three distinct disadvantages to using static stretching to increase core temperature (7).

1. Because static stretching is a passive activity, minimal friction of the sliding filaments occurs.

2. There is little, if any, increase in the rate of fuels being metabolized.

3. There is no need for the intramuscular blood vessels to dilate in response to static stretching.

For these reasons, clients who begin exercise sessions with static stretching experience only a minimal increase in core body temperature (6, 32) and are thus missing out on the benefits of an increased core temperature and decreased muscle viscosity. Warming up, mentally and physically, is a key aspect of reaching a training intensity required to achieve optimal results.

> **Flexibility exercises should not be used as the sole method of warming up. Instead, they should be performed after core temperature has been elevated to a point that the client is beginning to perspire.**

Types of Warm-Up

Regardless of the warm-up method chosen, the general purpose of warming up before physical activity is to increase muscle temperature. There are four types of warm-up methods—passive, general, specific, and RAMP.

Passive Warm-Up

Passive warm-up involves such methods as hot showers, heating pads, or massage. Research studies (24, 63, 72) have shown that passive warm-up methods can contribute to increases in muscle tissue temperature. One obvious advantage of a passive warm-up is that it does not fatigue a client before an exercise session; once elevated temperatures are achieved, the increase in temperature can be preserved before physical activity with minimal energy expenditure (74). Unfortunately, passive warm-up procedures (e.g., a moist heat pack) may not be practical in many settings.

General Warm-Up

A **general warm-up** consists of basic activities requiring movement of the major muscle groups, such as jogging, cycling, or jumping rope, causing increases in heart rate, blood flow, deep muscle temperature, respiration rate, viscosity of joint fluids, and perspiration (4, 32, 53). Thus, a general warm-up seems more appropriate than a passive warm-up when the goal is preparing the body for demanding physical activity.

Specific Warm-Up

Unlike general warm-up, **specific warm-up** includes movements that are an actual part of the activity, such as slow jogging before going out on a run or lifting lighter loads in the bench press exercise before progressing to the workout weight (4). A specific warm-up appears to be the most desirable method because it increases the temperature of the same muscles that will be used in subsequent, more strenuous activity and may also serve as a mental rehearsal of the event, allowing complex skills to be performed more effectively.

RAMP Warm-up

The **RAMP warm-up** is a systematic method of preparing the body for more vigorous activity. It consists of three main phases: raise, activate and mobilize, and potentiation (32). The goal of this approach is to prepare clients physically and psychologically for the training session while emulating specific movement patterns and skills clients may perform in daily activities or their respective sports. The RAMP approach lets the client prepare for exercise while simultaneously improving movement skill and efficiency. For example, a client might perform a single-leg hip bridge and a lunge walk to activate and mobilize a portion of the lower body in preparation for a lower body training day. (For more information, see reference 31.)

Warm-Up Guidelines

The amount, intensity, and duration of the warm-up should ideally be adjusted to every individual depending on his or her level of fitness. The length of the warm-up period depends on climate and physical conditioning level. In general, the warm-up activity should last approximately 5 to 15 minutes, long enough for the individual to break into a light sweat (48).

As conditioning improves, the intensity and duration of the warm-up need to increase to bring about the desired increase in core temperature, again demonstrated by the client's breaking into a slight sweat. Compared with a less conditioned person, a well-conditioned individual probably requires a longer or more intense warm-up, or one that is both longer and more intense, to achieve an optimal level of body temperature (32, 48, 53).

The warm-up should not create significant fatigue. Rather, this portion of the workout should serve as a transition stage that helps the client feel more physically prepared to perform a training session. Fatiguing the client during the warm-up portion of the training session may not only hinder performance but also increase injury risk depending on the training status of the client (53, 76).

BODYWEIGHT AND STABILITY BALL EXERCISES

Personal trainers may work with a client who does not have access to traditional weight training equipment or simply prefers not to train in a health club setting. This does not mean the client cannot perform resistance training activities, but it does mean the personal trainer will need to take a creative approach.

One possible solution is to have the client perform a series of bodyweight exercises or stability ball exercises. If the stress of the exercise is of an appropriate intensity, the body will adapt by increasing muscle size or strength. Further, caloric expenditure will occur during activity; and as the intensity of the activity increases, so will the rate of caloric expenditure.

It is important to remember that the mode of exercise is not the most important variable in this setting. For example, clients can train the pectoralis and triceps muscle groups by performing a free-weight bench press, a bench press on a selectorized machine, or push-ups on the floor or on a stability ball. If the intensity is at the necessary threshold, adaptation will occur in the working muscle groups, regardless of the mode of training.

Bodyweight Training

Bodyweight training is simply a mode of resistance training in which the resistance is provided by the body rather than by an external weight such as a barbell or the weight stack of a selectorized machine. In cases in which no equipment is available or if the client prefers this type of training, bodyweight training is a viable option. The personal trainer needs to be aware that clients will not develop maximal strength or power with bodyweight training because it cannot provide the intensity necessary to develop these physiological adaptations. However, if the goal of training is to develop basic strength levels or muscular endurance or both, bodyweight training is acceptable. To gain maximal benefits from this type of training, the emphasis must be on performing each exercise in a slow, controlled manner with perfect technique.

Suspension Training

Suspension training describes a specific type of bodyweight training that uses adjustable straps suspended from an overhead anchor point (e.g., wall, squat rack, door jam, or ceiling) (40). The straps generally hang perpendicular to the floor, with handles or foot straps attached at the ends. When clients hold the straps, or position their feet in the foot cradles, they can hang from this device and manipulate the position of their center of mass to adjust exercise intensity. There are several potential benefits to this method of training. First, it allows the client to overload specific muscle groups and exercises, and second, it allows for a range of intensities that may be difficult to accomplish via traditional calisthenic bodyweight training.

The degree of resistance varies depending on the individual's center of mass in relation to the anchor point. In general, the farther the center of mass is from the anchor point, the less resistance the individual will encounter. For example, Melrose and Dawes (40) reported that the average resistance for individuals performing an inverted row while using a suspension training system was approximately 50% to 79% of total body mass. Additionally, the least amount of resistance was encountered when the center of mass was farthest away from the anchor point. As individuals (and their center of mass) moved closer to the anchor point (i.e., the torso was brought closer to the floor), the intensity, or the percentage of body mass they were required to lift, increased. However, these researchers did not investigate sex-related differences in body mass distribution, which may affect the total amount of resistance encountered. Regardless, suspension training allows the personal trainer to make acute manipulations in training load based on the client's capabilities and specific training goals (i.e., muscular endurance, hypertrophy, strength, power).

Several investigations have shown that using a suspension training system may increase muscle activation of the upper body and core muscles for numerous exercises (e.g., push-ups, planks, and bridges) (12, 27, 65, 66, 67, 68). However, although muscle activity is increased in some muscle groups, it may be reduced in others. For instance, Harris and colleagues (27) found that when individuals performed a floor row exercise on a suspension device, muscle activity significantly increased in the middle deltoid, rectus abdominis, and obliques compared with a traditional floor row. However, although not statistically significant, there were reductions in muscle activity within the serratus anterior, rhomboids, and middle trapezius. As such, personal trainers must be aware of these potential tradeoffs and program accordingly based on the needs and goals of the client as well as the intended muscle groups they wish to emphasize.

The intensity of many upper body pulling exercises, such as a suspension row, increases when using a single-arm variation. In contrast, for many upper body pushing exercises, using a single-arm variation may actually reduce the amount of force one can produce because of greater amounts of instability (e.g., a single-arm push-up while holding a strap). Indeed, it is important that the personal trainer understand how each exercise and its variations may affect stability, balance, and force production and select exercise based on the physiological attributes they are targeting.

Like other forms of bodyweight exercise, the total volume load for suspension training is difficult to quantify. Therefore, the total volume of suspension training exercises is calculated by multiplying the number of sets by the number of repetitions performed. Furthermore, to ensure the target training goals (e.g., muscular endurance, strength) are being met, the personal trainer should manipulate the intensity of a suspension training exercise so that the ranges for the repetition maximum or the repetitions in reserve corresponding to these specific goals are consistent with the resistance training guidelines found in chapter 15. For example, if muscular endurance is the primary training goal, repetition ranges of 10 or greater would be appropriate. However, if muscular strength is the primary training goal, the load lifted would need to be increased so that fewer repetitions could be performed before volitional fatigue (e.g., ≤6 repetitions). For this reason, suspension training may not be the most appropriate form of training for all training goals and all situations because stronger individuals may have a difficult time overloading the targeted musculature using this modality. However, the addition of other devices, such as weighted vests, can safely increase the training load of many suspension training exercises.

> **The degree of resistance when performing a suspension training exercise varies depending on the individual's center of mass in relation to the anchor point.**

RECOMMENDATIONS FOR SUSPENSION TRAINING

The following are recommendations for implementing suspension training exercises in a client's training program (20).

- Securely anchor the suspension training system to a stable object.
- Adjust the length of the straps based on the exercise and desired intensity level.
- After adjusting the strap length, the personal trainer should make sure the straps are even in length.
- Make certain the handles and foot cradles are secured and do not slip when load (i.e., the client's body mass) is applied.
- Make certain the client has a firm, closed grip of the suspension trainer handles when using the straps for support.
- Ensure the feet are securely in the foot cradles before the client begins exercises aimed at developing the legs or trunk.
- When performing suspension training exercises that involve holding onto the handles: To increase the difficulty, clients lower the body closer to the floor by stepping toward the anchor point. To decrease the difficulty, clients step away from the anchor point.
- To emphasize balance and stability, the foot position can be made narrower (i.e., feet together to hip width). To increase stability and force production, the base should be wider (i.e., hip to shoulder width).
- Allow time for the client to become familiar with each suspension trainer exercise. This is accomplished by using lower resistances and practicing the exercise to build comfort and competency in each movement before increasing intensity.
- Emphasize correct technique, which will limit client fatigue. Limiting fatigue with newer clients allows them to enhance corrective approaches to an exercise while keeping injury risk to a minimum.

Manual Resistance Training

Manual resistance training involves the application of an external resistance, applied by a partner or personal trainer via manual muscle force, through a full or partial range of motion for an exercise (16). This external resistance may be applied directly to a body part (e.g., wrist, ankle) or via an implement (e.g., towel, dowel rod). This form of training provides a very versatile modality for the personal trainer when space and equipment are an issue.

There are several proposed physiological benefits of manual resistance training. According to Chulvi-Medrano and colleagues (16), one of the major benefits is that it allows a personal trainer to use an accommodating, rather than a constant, resistance throughout the full range of an exercise. This permits the personal trainer to reduce any biomechanical advantages that may occur through the varying joint ROM during an exercise. Manual resistance training is also an effective training strategy for isometric muscle actions of the trunk, in addition to other muscle groups.

Research indicates that manual resistance training is a viable method of improving muscular strength and muscular endurance in recreationally trained individuals (16). However, to experience these improvements in muscular fitness, the training load applied must be commensurate with the recommended loads, repetition ranges, and rest periods for these specific goals. For these reasons, it is essential that the personal trainer be familiar with these guidelines and apply them in the context of this training modality to ensure clients' goals are being met.

> **Manual resistance training can be a viable method of developing muscular fitness if the acute training variables of resistance training (i.e., intensity, volume, and rest) are appropriately applied.**

Stability Ball Training

The use of stability balls has increased significantly (30, 69). Initially, stability balls were used primarily by individuals with low back problems in physical therapy clinics (38). However, stability balls are now

RECOMMENDATIONS FOR MANUAL RESISTANCE TRAINING

The following are recommendations for implementing manual resistance training exercises in a client's training program:

- For manual resistance exercises that require the personal trainer to lay hands on the client, the client should be informed beforehand about the procedures and provide consent.

- Check for damage to any equipment being used to apply manual resistance to make certain it does not create a safety risk (e.g., tears in towels; cracks or splinters on a dowel rod).

- When applying manual resistance, adjust the training load based on the number of goal repetitions to achieve the desired muscular adaptation (e.g., muscular strength or endurance).

- The amount of resistance applied should be consistent throughout the entire range of motion for the exercise selected.

- In general, applying resistance to the distal end of a segment is more challenging than when this resistance is applied more proximal.

- Clients should maintain correct form though the entire exercise movement.

---

more commonly used in orthopedic rehabilitation programs, with the physically active in fitness centers, in physical education classes, and with special needs populations and the elderly. Many fitness and rehabilitation facilities incorporate stability balls into their training programs, and the use of stability balls has expanded into sport conditioning programs (80).

The primary motivation for the use of stability balls in these applications is the belief that an unstable surface will provide a greater challenge to the trunk muscles, increase dynamic balance, and possibly help stabilize the spine to prevent injuries. Additionally, although a primary emphasis with stability balls has been and continues to be trunk training, it is now common to see stability balls used in conjunction with resistance training for multiple muscle groups, not just the trunk (80).

Research Findings

Training on an unstable surface has been proposed to enhance sport-specific training through increased activation of stabilizers and trunk muscles (38, 80). Further, several practitioners have suggested that stability ball exercises are most effective for training core stability. Research on the use of unstable platforms and their effects on force and muscle activation of the upper body musculature has produced mixed results, warranting further investigation to make more definitive recommendations.

- *Stability balls and core activation:* Some studies show that stability training increases abdominal muscle activity, activating more motor units of the stabilizing muscles than traditional exercises and thus improving overall balance and core stability

(18, 30). In addition, stability balls stimulate parts of the cerebellum, vestibular system, and brain stem, which are responsible for posture, balance, and body control (30). Initial scientific support for stability ball training came from observations of greater activation of the rectus abdominis and external obliques during abdominal curl-ups on the stability ball compared with a stable surface (77). Research since has shown that use of a stability ball versus a stable surface leads to greater activation of the external obliques, transversus abdominis, internal obliques, erector spinae, and rectus abdominis as well as the abdominal stabilizers (8, 37, 52), suggesting that exercises intended to strengthen or increase the endurance of the core stabilizers should involve a destabilizing component. However, other studies do not show significant differences in abdominal muscle electromyography with the ball versus a stable surface (38, 71).

- *Stability balls and core training:* Training the core has become an area of emphasis in athletic strength and conditioning programs, health and fitness centers, and rehabilitation facilities (26). Prevailing beliefs hold that training the core is important for improving performance and reducing the risk of injuries and that core strengthening is vital for improving athletic performance (58). Use of stability balls is most associated with core training. Stability ball training has been used for many years in physical therapy settings to strengthen the musculature responsible for spinal stability (13), although little research has been performed to show it improves spine stabilization or helps decrease the risk of back pain (13).

However, stability ball exercises that require a neutral spine position may be appropriate for targeting the specific muscles that stabilize the spine during the early phase of training; they also may improve trunk endurance because of the sustained muscle activity needed to maintain a neutral position. Increasing back strength may provide some protection from low back pain when greater forces are required to perform a task (8, 26). Further, the spine may become unstable because of weak trunk stabilizer muscles, and a lack of back muscle endurance is strongly associated with low back pain.

■ *Other potential benefits:* Stability ball training offers several additional potential benefits:

- Improved balance, joint stability, proprioception, and neuromuscular control decrease the incidence of injury (28, 30).
- Acute increases are seen in heart rate and oxygen consumption (30).
- Strength, stability, balance, posture, proprioception, and flexibility in pregnant women increase. These adaptations result in stronger abdominal muscles, which help support the baby, decrease the incidence of back pain, and reduce the chances of accidental falls (45).

■ *Potential disadvantages:* Despite its advantages, stability ball training has possible drawbacks:

- Some studies have confirmed increased core stability with the use of stability balls, but this did not result in improved sport performance (17).
- Under unstable conditions, training at an intensity necessary to bring about increases in strength in trained individuals is not possible (35, 47, 69, 78).
- Sport performance might be better enhanced by free-weight exercises performed on a stable surface than exercises performed on a stability ball (80).

■ *Stability balls in sport performance training programs.* Few investigations have examined the effect of stability ball training on physical performance. Stability ball training enhanced core stability in swimmers, but this did not transfer to improved swim times (59). In runners, stability ball training significantly improved core stability but did not improve running performance (18, 69) or running posture (69). Thus, the anecdotal evidence supporting the use of stability ball training to enhance physical performance has not been scientifically substantiated (69), and there is no guarantee that improvements in core strength and power will transfer to improvements in sport performance (80).

■ *Importance of training specificity:* As with all training endeavors, the principle of specificity must be emphasized for optimal results (69, 80). Regarding the trunk, training in a supine or prone position on the stability ball may not transfer effectively to sports or activities performed predominately in upright positions. However, specificity also dictates that training activities should simulate the demands of a sport as closely as possible (80), and in some situations the use of a stability ball can increase the degree of specificity. Mogul skiing, shooting a puck in hockey, and surfing, for example, all involve generating forces under unstable conditions. Additionally, most sports involve a combination of stabilizing and force-producing functions (e.g., forehand in tennis, baseball pitcher windup), and resistance training under unstable conditions provides similar challenges to the neuromuscular system. Another important aspect of specificity is core stability requirements. Free-weight exercises performed on a stable surface might be more transferable to sport performance than exercises performed on a stability ball (80).

■ *Effect of unstable base on force output:* The value of unstable training for the limb musculature remains a matter of debate (35). A recognized limiting factor with resistance training under unstable conditions is reduced force-generating capabilities (35, 47, 69, 78). Isometric force output during unstable resistance exercise is significantly lower than during stable conditions (35). Similarly, in healthy subjects, the stimulus provided by stability ball training is insufficiently intense to increase muscular strength and thus does not appear to provide a training advantage (47). Squats and deadlifts performed under stable conditions at intensities as low as 50% of 1RM were shown to elicit greater muscle activation than stability ball exercises (47), which may suggest they are superior for increasing muscular strength and hypertrophy of the back extensors. The reduced force-generation capabilities elicited by unstable training have led to the suggestion that instability training devices should be used to augment traditional training methods (78). Nuzzo and colleagues (47), however, suggested that such training be excluded or limited because of the apparent lack of evidence that it improves strength, hypertrophy, or measures related to athletic performance.

Considering some of the disadvantages described previously, personal trainers might choose to incorporate instability into training programs via methods other than stability ball training. Two such methods are described here.

- *Emphasis on structural multijoint exercises:* Instead of emphasizing stability ball training, personal trainers should focus on structural multijoint exercises like squats and deadlifts because the intensity can be continually increased through changes in external loading (47). Additionally, because these are multijoint exercises that recruit multiple major muscle groups, they may be more time efficient than many stability ball exercises (47). However, because of its advantages, stability ball training should be viewed as an important supplement to more traditional methods of resistance training so that clients obtain the benefits of each training mode.

- *Instability with free-weight training:* Instability can be influenced not only by the base of support but also by the implements used. Free-weight training has been promoted as more beneficial than machines for training athletes partially because of the instability it offers (61). Free-weight training can provide a moderate degree of instability (80). Additionally, the use of unconventional methods, including accommodating resistance such as bands and chains, tires, and water-filled implements, has been shown to further create an unstable environment as compared with traditional training modalities (57). Another way to augment instability in free-weight training is to emphasize unilateral over bilateral dumbbell training (8). Many activities in daily life and in sport are unilateral. Unilateral exercises allow a higher degree of movement specificity than bilateral training and stimulate the trunk stabilizers more (8).

Safety and Correct Sizing

Because of their inherent instability, safety is a major concern with stability balls (30). Proper exercise technique must be emphasized to protect people from falling. It is important that people start off with basic, less complex exercises and increase the complexity over time. Jakubek (30) suggests using sandbags as stabilizing wedges. Further, people with long hair should tie it back so it does not get caught during movements. Finally, during stability ball training people need to use common sense; if an exercise causes pain, the personal trainer should modify the movement or the movement should be discontinued.

Another aspect of safety with the use of stability balls is making sure the ball is correctly sized. The individual should sit on the ball; the size is correct if the thighs are slightly above parallel to the floor.

Correct Positioning of the Stability Ball

An important but often overlooked aspect of maximizing the effectiveness of stability ball training is the positioning of the ball relative to the body. One investigation showed a significant increase in abdominal muscle activity when a crunch was performed on a stability ball in comparison to the same movement performed on the floor, but only when the ball was correctly placed (71). When the ball was placed high on the back, at the level of the inferior border of the scapula, abdominal muscle activity was significantly decreased as compared with either a lower ball position or a crunch performed on a stable surface. Placing the ball lower on the back requires elevation of a greater portion of the trunk during the crunch motion and requires greater trunk stabilization in the horizontal position because there is no support for the upper trunk from either the floor or the ball. Thus, performing the crunch using the lower ball placement requires more abdominal muscle activity than either performing using the higher ball placement or performing a traditional crunch (71).

Individuals with abdominal muscle weakness can use a high ball placement, allowing them to perform the crunch motion with less effort than would be needed on a stable bench or the floor. As their condition and fitness improve, the ball can gradually be positioned lower on the back to increase the training load and thus increase abdominal muscle activity (71).

GUIDELINES FOR STABILITY BALL TRAINING

As with any training method, it is important for the personal trainer to adhere to training guidelines to ensure that clients are maximizing their time and effort with the stability ball. Guidelines include the following:

- The stability ball should be fully inflated so that it is firm.

- The stability ball should be the correct size for the client. To determine the correct size, have the client sit on the ball with feet on the floor. In this position the thighs should be parallel or slightly above parallel to the floor. If the client has low back pain, the thighs should be slightly above parallel, with the knees lower than the hips.

- As with other modes of training, a warm-up session of 5 to 15 minutes should precede the actual workout. Activities such as brisk walking or jogging, walking up stairs, or calisthenic activities (e.g., jumping jacks, mountain climbers) can be used during the warm-up period. Warm-up activities performed on the stability ball have the advantage of training the stabilizing muscle groups, improving balance and coordination (75).

- Allow time for the client to become familiar with the ball. A client may be able to demonstrate superior strength in traditional types of exercises but still find stability ball exercises extremely challenging. This is especially true for clients who perform most of their training on machines. When an exercise is performed on a machine, the stabilizing muscles are not activated. Thus, when clients begin to use a stability ball, they may fatigue very rapidly, which leads to poorly performed repetitions.

- Emphasize correct technique. Attention to detail is critical when clients perform exercises on a stability ball. Many stability ball exercises look easy, but the slightest deviation from correct technique or position can have a negative effect on performance of the exercise. This is especially important to remember as the client becomes fatigued and it becomes more and more difficult to perform the exercise correctly.

- The number of sets and repetitions performed will depend on the fitness level of the client. Clients can perform the exercises in circuit training fashion or can perform the full number of sets on each exercise before advancing to the next exercise, depending on their fitness goals. As when beginning any exercise routine, clients should start with low volume and low intensity (e.g., 1 × 8) and gradually adjust the training variables as their fitness level improves (e.g., 3 × 15).

CONCLUSION

Personal trainers typically incorporate some form of stretching into their clients' programs, and it is important that they and their clients have a clear understanding of what flexibility is and how it relates to conditioning in general. Defined as the ROM of a joint or a series of joints, flexibility helps a joint to move freely through a full normal ROM and helps to improve performance and prevent injury. Many factors affect a client's flexibility, including joint structure, muscle and connective tissue, sex, temperature, and resistance training. Warm-up—which is not to be confused with stretching—is part of the foundation of an effective workout, increasing the client's body temperature and ROM.

In designing flexibility programs, the personal trainer should incorporate a combination of dynamic and static flexibility training. For some clients, it is appropriate to use a series or a combination of bodyweight, stability ball, manual resistance, and suspension training exercises.

Flexibility, Bodyweight, Suspension Training, Manual Resistance, and Stability Ball Exercises

▶ Video available within HK*Propel*

STATIC FLEXIBILITY EXERCISES

LOOK RIGHT AND LEFT

1. Stand or sit with the head and neck upright.
2. Turn the head to the right using a submaximal concentric muscle action.
3. Turn the head to the left using a submaximal concentric muscle action.

Primary Muscle Stretched

Sternocleidomastoid

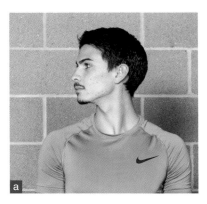 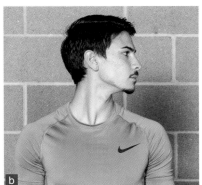

Common Errors

- Turning the torso as the head turns
- Not turning the head through the full comfortable range of motion

NECK FLEXION AND EXTENSION

1. Standing or sitting with head and neck upright, flex the neck by tucking the chin toward the chest.
2. If the chin touches the chest, try to touch the chin lower on the chest.
3. Extend the neck by trying to come as close as possible to touching the head to the back.

Primary Muscles Stretched

Sternocleidomastoid, suboccipitals, splenae

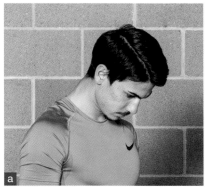 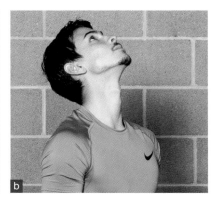

Common Errors

- Failing to go through a complete range of motion, either during flexion or extension
- Using a jerky, explosive type of action rather than pushing against, or resisting against, the force being applied to the head; all movements should be slow, continuous, and steady
- Using movements in the trunk, arms, or other parts of the body to assist in the movement at the neck; there should be no movement other than what is occurring at the neck

HANDS BEHIND BACK

1. Stand erect and reach behind the back with both arms.
2. Clasp the hands together and fully extend the elbows.
3. Slightly flex the knees and look straight ahead.
4. Raise the arms until a stretch is felt.

Common Errors

- Allowing the elbows to flex
- Flexing the torso forward or looking down at the floor

Primary Muscles Stretched

Anterior deltoid, pectoralis major

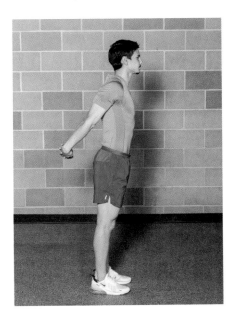

BEHIND-NECK STRETCH

1. Stand erect and raise the right arm to position it next to the right side of the head.
2. Flex the right elbow to allow the right hand to touch the back of the neck or upper back.
3. Raise the left arm to grasp the right elbow with the left hand.
4. Pull the right elbow toward (and behind) the head with the left hand (i.e., increase shoulder abduction) until a stretch is felt.
5. Repeat the stretch with the right hand grasping and pulling the left elbow.

Common Error

Flexing the torso forward or rounding the shoulders

Primary Muscles Stretched

Triceps brachii, latissimus dorsi

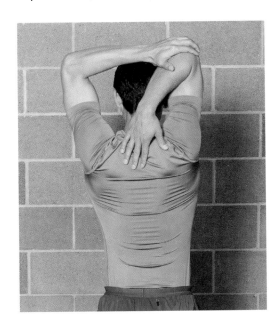

ASSISTED LAT STRETCH

1. Kneel on the floor facing a workout bench.
2. The elbows should be placed on top of the bench at a 90-degree angle.
3. Flex forward at the hips until the torso is parallel to the floor.
4. Continue to lean forward from the hips until the ears and upper arms align.

Common Errors

- Arching the back
- Cervical flexion

Primary Muscle Stretched

Latissimus dorsi

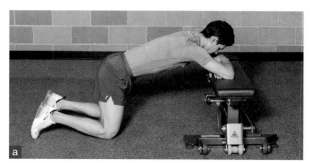

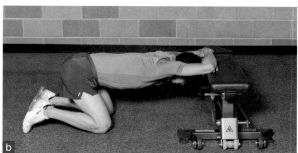

SIDE QUADRICEPS STRETCH

1. Lie on the right side of the body with both legs extended and the right elbow flexed at a 90-degree angle, positioned directly under the right shoulder.
2. Flex the left knee, pulling the left heel back toward the buttocks.
3. Grasp the front of the left ankle with the left hand, and pull the heel to touch the buttocks.
4. Repeat on the other side.

Common Errors

- Failing to maintain a neutral cervical spine
- Not keeping the elbow on the floor aligned with the shoulder

Primary Muscles Stretched

Iliopsoas, rectus femoris

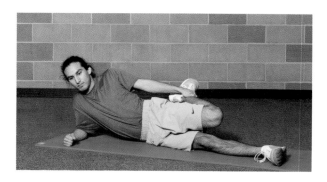

PRETZEL

1. Sit on the floor with the legs next to each other and extended away from the body.
2. With the torso upright, flex the right knee, cross it over the left leg, and place the right foot on the floor to the outside of the left knee.
3. Twist the torso to the right to position the back of the left elbow against the outside of the right knee.
4. Place the right palm on the floor 12 to 16 inches (30.5-40.6 cm) behind the hips.
5. Keeping the buttocks on the floor, use the right knee to hold the left elbow stationary while twisting the head and shoulders to the right until a stretch is felt.
6. Repeat the stretch with the left foot placed to the outside of the right knee and the right elbow against the outside of the left knee.

Primary Muscles Stretched
Internal and external obliques, piriformis, erector spinae

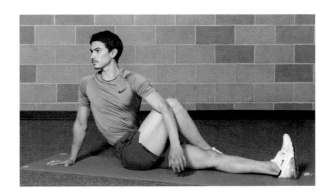

Common Errors

- Placing the elbow on the front of the thigh (rather than to the outside of the knee)
- Allowing the buttocks to rise off the floor

FORWARD LUNGE

1. From a standing position, take an exaggerated step forward with the right leg.
2. Flex the right knee until it is positioned over the right foot.
3. Keep the right foot on the floor, with both feet pointed straight ahead.
4. Keep the left leg almost fully extended (more than what is shown in the photo) with the heel lifted off the floor.
5. Allow the arms to hang at the sides or place the hands on the top of the right thigh or on the hips and look straight ahead.
6. With the torso fully upright, push the hips forward until a stretch is felt in the left hip flexors.
7. Repeat the stretch with the left leg positioned ahead of the body (i.e., lunge with the left leg).

Primary Muscles Stretched
Iliopsoas, rectus femoris, gluteus maximus, hamstrings

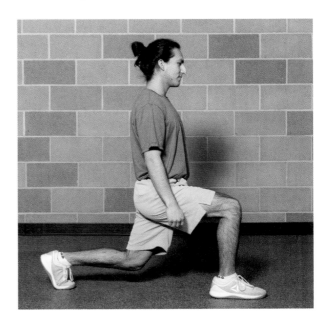

Common Errors

- Allowing the lead knee to flex too far beyond the toes of the lead foot
- Allowing the heel of the lead foot to lift off the floor
- Flexing the torso forward or looking down at the floor
- Allowing an anterior pelvic tilt (i.e., a forward pelvic tilt and increased low back arch)

LYING KNEE TO CHEST

1. Lie supine with the legs next to each other and extended away from the body.
2. Flex the right knee and hip to elevate the right thigh toward the chest.
3. Grasp the back of the right thigh (underneath the right knee).
4. Keep the left leg in the same starting position.
5. Use the arms to pull the right thigh farther toward the chest until a stretch is felt.
6. Repeat the stretch with the left knee pulled to the chest and the right leg extended away from the body.

Common Errors

- Grasping the front of the flexed knee (rather than the back of the thigh)
- Flexing the neck or arching the back
- Lifting the opposite leg off the floor

Primary Muscles Stretched

Gluteus maximus, hamstrings, erector spinae

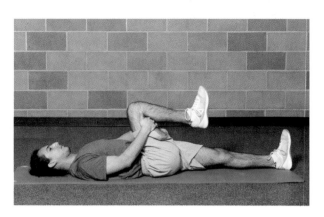

SEMISTRADDLE (MODIFIED HURDLER'S STRETCH)

1. Sit on the floor with the left leg extended away from the body and the sole of the right foot pressed against (or near to) the inside of the left knee.
2. The outside of the right leg will be touching or nearly touching the floor.
3. Keeping the back neutral, lean forward at the hips and grasp the toes of the left foot with the left hand.
4. Pull the toes of the left foot toward the upper body as the torso is flexed toward the left leg until a stretch is felt.
5. Repeat the stretch with the right leg extended away from the body and the sole of the left foot pressed against (or near to) the inside of the right knee.

Common Errors

- Allowing the extended thigh to externally rotate
- Rounding the shoulders or curling the torso toward the extended leg (rather than flexing the torso at the hips)
- Allowing the knee of the extended leg to flex

Primary Muscles Stretched

Hamstrings, erector spinae, gastrocnemius

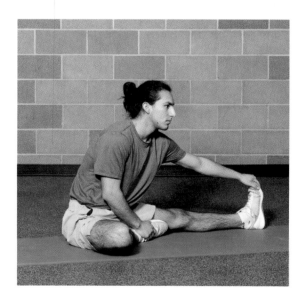

BUTTERFLY

1. Sit on the floor with the torso upright.
2. Flex the hips and knees and externally rotate the thighs to bring the soles of the feet together.
3. Lean forward at the hips and grasp the feet and move them toward the body.
4. Place the elbows on the inside of the legs.
5. Keeping the back neutral, slightly push the elbows down, pull the feet toward the upper body, and flex the torso forward until a stretch is felt.

Common Error

Rounding the shoulders or curling the torso toward the feet (rather than flexing the torso at the hips)

Primary Muscles Stretched

Hip adductors, gracilis

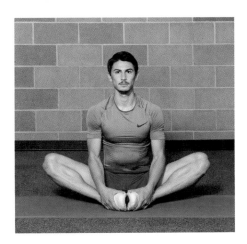

WALL STRETCH

1. Stand facing a wall with the feet shoulder-width apart and the toes about 12 inches (30.5 cm) from the wall.
2. Lean forward and place the hands on the wall.
3. Step back about 2 feet (61 cm) with the right leg and slightly flex the left knee.
4. Fully extend the right knee and keep the right heel on the floor.
5. Allow the elbows to flex to move the hips and torso closer to the wall until a stretch is felt.
6. Repeat the stretch with the left leg positioned behind the body (i.e., step back with the left leg).

Common Errors

- Moving the torso closer to the wall without also moving the hips forward
- Allowing the heel of the stepped-back foot to lift off the floor

Primary Muscles Stretched

Gastrocnemius, soleus (and Achilles' tendon)

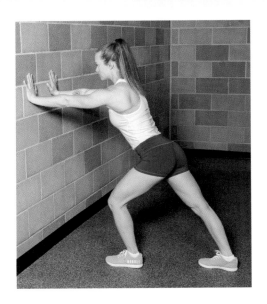

STEP STRETCH

1. Place one foot flat on top of a 3- to 4-inch (7.6-10.2 cm) step. Place the other foot on the edge of the step. To assist in maintaining balance, the client may use a dowel rod if necessary.
2. While keeping the legs extended, lower the heel of the foot on the edge of the step toward the floor as far as possible.
3. Repeat with the other leg.

Common Errors

- Losing balance
- Externally rotating the foot
- Excessively hyperextending the knee

Primary Muscles Stretched

Gastrocnemius, soleus (and Achilles' tendon)

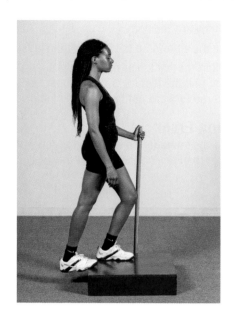

DYNAMIC FLEXIBILITY EXERCISES

ARM CIRCLE

1. Move the arms in wide circles, progressing from a position in which the arms are directly at the sides to a position in which the arms are directly overhead.
2. Allow movement to occur only at the shoulder joints (i.e., keep the elbows fully extended).
3. Perform the arm circles both forward and backward through a full comfortable ROM.

Common Error

Allowing the torso to flex and extend as the arms move in circles

Primary Muscles Stretched

Deltoids, latissimus dorsi, pectoralis major

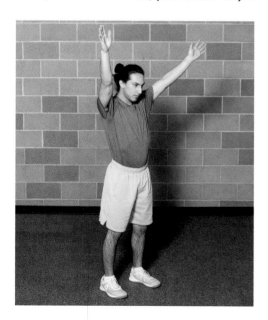

ARM SWING

1. Flex the arms at the shoulders to position the arms parallel to the floor in front of the body.
2. Swing the arms in unison to the right so the left arm is in front of the chest, the fingers of the left hand are pointing directly lateral to the right shoulder, and the right arm is behind the body.
3. Immediately reverse the movement direction to swing the arms in unison to the left.
4. Allow movement to occur only at the shoulder joints (i.e., keep the torso and head facing forward).
5. Alternate the arm swings to the right and left through a full comfortable ROM.

Common Error

Allowing the torso or neck to rotate in the direction of the arm swing

Primary Muscles Stretched

Latissimus dorsi, teres major, anterior and posterior deltoids, pectoralis major

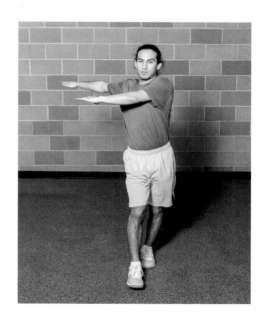

LUNGE WALK

1. Clasp the hands behind the head.
2. From a standing position, take an exaggerated step forward with the left leg.
3. Flex the left knee until it is positioned over the left foot.
4. Slightly flex the right knee to be just off the floor; both feet should be pointed straight ahead.
5. Keep the torso erect (or leaning back slightly), and look straight ahead.
6. Pause for a count in the bottom lunged position, stand up, and then repeat with the right leg, progressing forward with each step.

Common Errors

- Allowing the lead knee to flex too far beyond the toes of the lead foot
- Touching the knee of the trailing leg to the floor
- Flexing the torso forward or looking down at the floor

Primary Muscles Stretched

Iliopsoas, rectus femoris, gluteus maximus, hamstrings

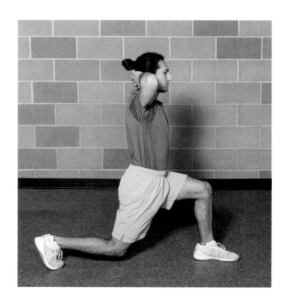

VARIATION: REVERSE LUNGE WALK

1. Clasp the hands behind the head.
2. From a standing position, take an exaggerated step backward with the right leg.
3. Flex the left knee until it is positioned over the left foot.
4. Slightly flex the right knee to be just off the floor; both feet should be pointed straight ahead.
5. Keep the torso erect (or leaning back slightly), and look straight ahead.
6. Pause for a count in the bottom lunged position, stand up, and then repeat with the left leg, progressing backward with each step.

Common Errors

- Allowing the lead knee to flex too far beyond the toes of the lead foot
- Touching the knee of the trailing leg to the floor
- Flexing the torso forward or looking down at the floor

Primary Muscles Stretched

Iliopsoas, rectus femoris, gluteus maximus, hamstrings

HOCKEY LUNGE WALK

1. Clasp the hands behind the head.
2. From a standing position, take an exaggerated step forward and diagonally to the right with the right leg.
3. Place the right foot on the floor 10 to 12 inches (25.4-30.5 cm) wider than the placement of the lead foot during the lunge walk exercise (page 295).
4. Keep the toes of both feet pointing straight ahead.
5. Flex the right knee until it is positioned over the right foot.
6. Slightly flex the left knee to be just off the floor.
7. Keep the torso erect (or leaning back slightly), and look straight ahead.
8. Pause for a count in the bottom lunged position, stand up, and then repeat with the left leg, progressing forward with each step.

Common Errors

- Allowing the lead knee to flex too far beyond the toes of the lead foot
- Touching the knee of the trailing leg to the floor
- Flexing the torso forward or looking down at the floor
- Stepping too laterally or pointing the feet medially or laterally

Primary Muscles Stretched

Iliopsoas, rectus femoris, gluteus maximus, hamstrings, hip adductors

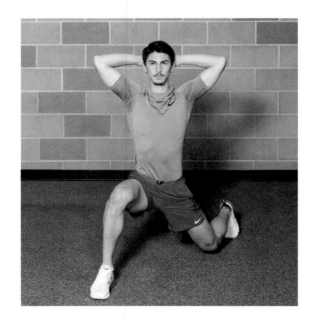

VARIATION: WALKING SIDE LUNGE

1. Clasp the hands behind the head.
2. Turn sideways, with the right shoulder pointing in the desired movement direction.
3. From a standing position, take an exaggerated lateral step to the right with the right foot.
4. Keeping the left knee extended, flex the right knee until it is positioned over the right foot and allow the hips to sink back and to the right.
5. Keep the torso erect (or leaning back slightly) and look straight ahead.
6. Pause for a count in the bottom lunged position, then stand back up, pivot on the right foot, and repeat with the left leg.

Common Errors

- Allowing the lead knee to flex too far beyond the toes of the lead foot
- Flexing the knee of the trailing leg
- Flexing the torso forward or looking down at the floor

Primary Muscles Stretched

Iliopsoas, rectus femoris, gluteus maximus, hamstrings, hip adductors

WALKING KNEE TUCK

1. From a standing position, step forward with the left leg and flex the right hip and knee to move the right thigh toward the chest.
2. Grasp the front of the right knee or upper shin.
3. Use the arms to pull the right knee farther up, and squeeze the right thigh against the chest.
4. Pause for a count in the knee tuck position, then step back down with the right leg, shift the body weight to the right leg, and repeat with the left leg, progressing forward with each step.
5. Try to pull the knee slightly higher with each repetition.

Common Error

Flexing the torso forward or looking down at the floor

Primary Muscles Stretched

Gluteus maximus, hamstrings

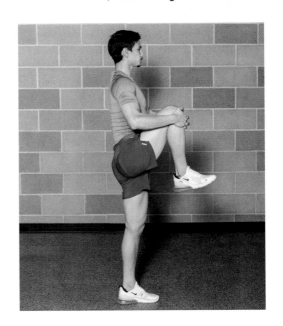

WALKING KNEE OVER HURDLE

1. Set up pair of staggered hurdles approximately 3 feet (1 m) tall, where the hurdles are on alternating sides of the body. (Alternatively, the stretch can be done with an imaginary hurdle as seen in the photo.) The first hurdle is to the right side; the second hurdle, which is a short distance beyond the first, is to the left side, and so on.

2. Walk forward and flex the right hip and knee and abduct the right thigh until it is parallel with the floor.

3. Lead the right knee over the first hurdle that is on the right.

4. Pause for a count in the highest thigh position, then step back down with the right leg, shift the body weight to the right leg, take one step, and repeat with the left leg, progressing forward with each step.

5. Try to lift the thigh slightly higher over the hurdle with each repetition.

Common Errors

- Leaning the torso too far away from the hurdle (rather than emphasizing hip abduction)
- Leading with the torso or the head over the hurdle (rather than with the lead knee)

Primary Muscles Stretched
Hip adductors

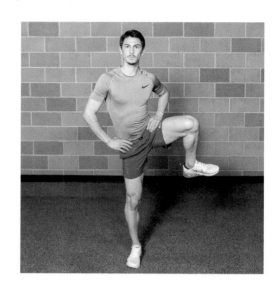

INVERTED HAMSTRING STRETCH

1. Assume a standing position.

2. While balancing on one foot, keep both knees nearly fully extended and flex forward at the hips so that the upper body (with neutral spine) and nonbalancing leg are approximately parallel to the floor.

3. Reach hands toward the floor, touching it if flexibility levels permit it.

4. Keep the hips squared to the floor throughout the duration of the stretch.

5. Return to the starting position, and perform this movement on the other leg.

Common Errors

- Rounding the back
- Not keeping the hips square to the floor

Primary Muscles Stretched
Hamstrings

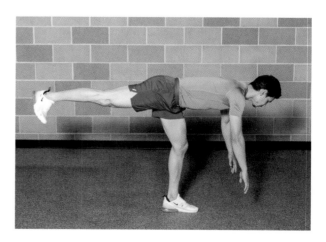

DYNAMIC PIGEON

1. Get on all fours with the hands positioned directly underneath the shoulders and the knees directly aligned under the hips.
2. Extend the right leg and cross it over the left leg behind the body at a 45-degree angle.
3. Keeping the right leg extended, shift the hips backward at a 45-degree angle toward the left. This movement will cause the left knee and hip to flex and rotate leaving the lower portion of the left leg resting on the floor in front of the body.
4. Without lifting the hands off the floor, hinge the torso over the left leg as low as possible, keeping the hips and shoulders parallel to the floor.

Primary Muscles Stretched

Iliopsoas, piriformis, gluteus maximus, hip adductors

5. Reverse the motion and return to the starting position by bringing the right knee back down underneath the right hip.
6. After bringing the right knee back, repeat the same action with the left leg.

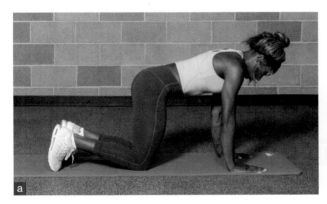 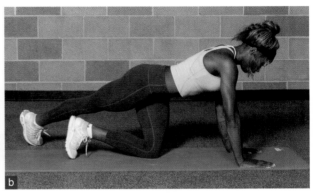

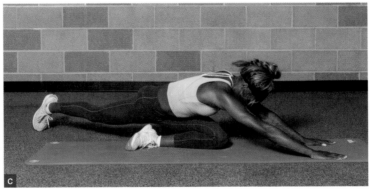

Common Errors

- Not keeping the shoulders parallel to the floor throughout the movement
- Allowing the hands to lift off the floor as the hips are shifted backward
- Not keeping the chest parallel to the floor throughout

HIGH KICK

1. Stand tall with the feet hip-width apart, with the arms positioned directly to the sides of the body.
2. Kick toward the sky using the right leg, and while keeping the knee slightly flexed, reach the left arm out at shoulder level in front of the torso.
3. Attempt to touch the foot of the kicking leg to the hand.
4. Continue this action, alternating arms and legs with each kick.

Common Errors

- Not keeping the torso upright throughout
- Not keeping the ankle dorsiflexed on each kick

Primary Muscles Stretched

Hamstrings, gluteus maximus

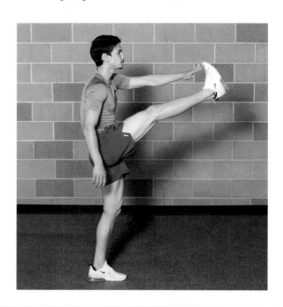

BODYWEIGHT EXERCISES

ABDOMINAL CRUNCH

1. Assume a supine position on the floor.
2. Flex the hips and knees and place the heels on a box.
3. Place the hands behind or at the sides of the head (to hold its weight only) or fold the arms across the chest or abdomen.
4. Curl the torso until the upper back is off the floor. Client should maintain a tucked or neutral head and neck position.
5. Keep the feet, buttocks, and lower back stationary at all times.
6. After completing the crunch, allow the torso to uncurl back down to the starting position.

Common Errors

- Raising the hips or feet
- Pulling the head with the hands
- Flexing the torso to a fully seated position

Primary Muscle Trained

Rectus abdominis

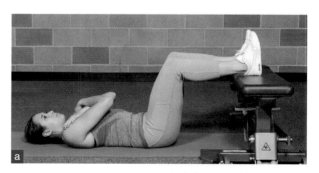

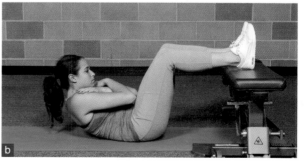

VARIATION: TWISTING CRUNCH

1. Assume a supine position on the floor.
2. Flex the hips and knees and place the heels on a box or bench.
3. Place the hands behind or at the sides of the head (to hold its weight only) or fold the arms across the chest or abdomen.
4. Twist (rotate) the torso to move the right shoulder toward the left thigh.
5. Continue flexing and twisting the torso until the upper back is off the floor.
6. Keep the feet, buttocks, and lower back stationary at all times.
7. After completing the crunch, allow the torso to uncurl and untwist back down to the starting position.
8. Alternate the direction of the twist with each repetition.

Common Errors

- Raising the hips or feet
- Pulling the head with the hands

Primary Muscles Trained

Rectus abdominis, internal and external obliques

BACK EXTENSION

1. Assume a prone position on the floor with the knees fully extended and the toes pointed down to the floor.
2. Clasp the hands behind the head.
3. Keeping the toes in contact with the floor, extend the torso (i.e., arch the back) to lift the chest off the floor.
4. After completing the extension, allow the chest to lower and return to the starting position.

Common Errors

- Flexing the knees or lifting the toes off the floor
- Rapidly rocking up and down on the hips (rather than performing the movement under control)

Primary Muscle Trained

Erector spinae

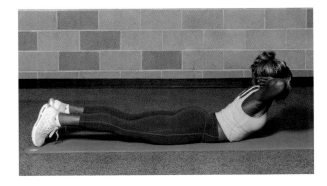

VARIATION: TWISTING BACK EXTENSION

1. Assume a prone position on the floor with the knees fully extended and the toes pointed down to the floor.
2. Clasp the hands behind the head.
3. Keep the toes in contact with the floor.
4. Extend and twist (rotate) the torso to move the right shoulder up and to the left.
5. Continue extending and twisting the torso until the chest is off the floor.
6. Keep the feet, buttocks, and lower back on the floor at all times.
7. After completing the extension, allow the chest to lower and untwist back down to the starting position.
8. Alternate the direction of the twist with each repetition.

Common Errors

- Flexing the knees or lifting the toes off the floor
- Rapidly rocking back and forth on the hips (rather than performing the movement under control)

PUSH-UP

1. Assume a prone position on the floor with the knees fully extended and the toes pointed down to the floor.
2. Place the hands on the floor, palms down, about 2 to 3 inches (5.1-7.6 cm) wider than shoulder-width apart, with the elbows pointed outward.
3. Keeping the body in a straight line and the toes in contact with the floor, push against the floor with the hands to fully extend the elbows.
4. After completing the push-up, lower the body by allowing the elbows to flex to a 90-degree angle. Alternatively, the personal trainer can place a soft object about the size of rolled-up socks or a foam half-roller on the floor beneath the client's chest and count the repetitions only when the client's chest touches the socks or roller.

Common Errors

- Allowing the hips to sag or rise (rather than keeping the body in a straight line)
- Performing the exercise through a reduced ROM

Primary Muscle Stretched

Erector spinae

Primary Muscles Trained

Pectoralis major, anterior deltoid, triceps brachii

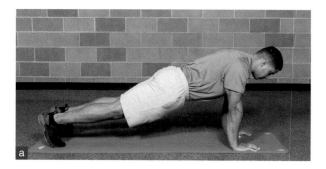

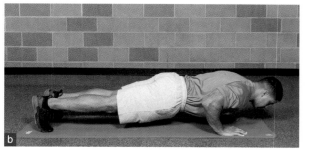

VARIATION: MODIFIED PUSH-UP

Modify the standard push-up technique by having the client assume a kneeling position, with the knees flexed to 90 degrees and the ankles crossed.

Common Errors

- Allowing the hips to sag or rise (rather than keeping the body in a straight line)
- Performing the exercise through a reduced ROM

<table>
<tr><td>Primary Muscles Trained</td></tr>
</table>

Pectoralis major, anterior deltoid, triceps brachii

HEEL RAISE

1. Stand on the floor or on the edge of a stair step, with one hand at the side or on the hip.
2. Place one hand on the wall or stair railing or use a dowel or pole to assist in balance.
3. The feet should be close together and flat on the floor. If on a stair step, place the balls of the feet on the edge of the step, with the rear portion of the feet extending off the step.
4. Elevate up onto the toes, then lower the heels through the full comfortable ROM.

Common Errors

- Using a ballistic movement to achieve a brief full range of motion contraction instead of slowly lifting and holding a full range of motion position
- Failing to achieve a true comfortable full range of motion position

<table>
<tr><td>Primary Muscles Trained</td></tr>
</table>

Gastrocnemius, soleus

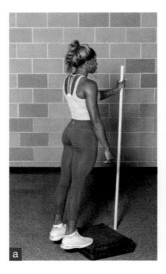
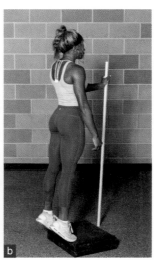

STEP-UP

1. Stand facing a chair, bench, or other sturdy object. The height of the object should be such that placing the foot on the object puts the knee at about hip height.
2. Place the entire left foot on the object.
3. Using the muscles of the left leg, bring the right foot up so that both feet are on top of the object.
4. Leaving the left foot on the object, step down with the right foot.
5. Repeat the stepping motion but with the right foot starting the movement.
6. Alternate the lead leg; a helpful strategy to is think or say, *left, right, right, left*; then *right, left, left, right*, and so on.

Common Errors

- Not placing the entire foot on the object, increasing the opportunity for the foot to slip off
- Pushing off with the foot on the floor to assist in the movement; rising up on the top of the object should occur as a result of muscular action originating from the leg placed on the object, not both legs

Primary Muscles Trained

Gluteus maximus, semimembranosus, semitendinosus, biceps femoris, vastus lateralis, vastus intermedius, vastus medialis, rectus femoris

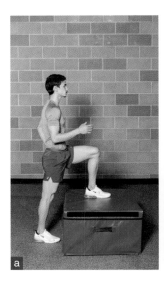
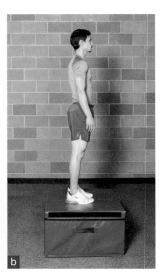

ZOMBIE SQUAT

1. Stand tall, with the feet shoulder-width apart and the toes turned slightly outward.
2. Extend the arms and position them at shoulder height.
3. While keeping the arms at shoulder height, squat and allow the ankles, knees, and hips to flex simultaneously during the eccentric phase.
4. Descend to where the thighs are parallel to the floor (or lower if possible) while keeping the trunk upright.
5. Return to the starting position, and repeat for the desired number of repetitions.

Common Errors

- As the squat is being performed, allowing the heels to come off the floor
- Allowing the knees to come together toward the midline of the body; the knees should track in the same direction as the toes

Primary Muscles Trained

Gluteus maximus, hamstrings, quadriceps

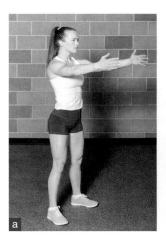
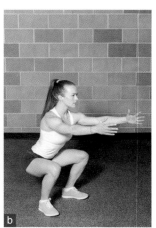

SHOULDER T (BENT-OVER REVERSE FLY)

1. Stand with the feet hip-width apart.
2. Keeping the knees slightly flexed, lean forward from the hips until the torso is approximately parallel to the floor.
3. Allow the arms to hang down toward the floor.
4. Keeping the elbows slightly flexed, raise the arms out to the sides of the torso, and point the thumbs upward toward the sky.
5. The arms should be at a 90-degree angle relative to the torso at the top of each repetition, thus forming a T shape with the torso.
6. Simultaneously retract the shoulder blades while depressing the scapulae.
7. Briefly pause at the top of each repetition.
8. Slowly lower the arms and return them to the starting position in front of the torso.

Common Errors

- Swinging the arms up by using the lower back or the legs
- Allowing the back to round
- Shrugging the shoulders and allowing the scapulae to elevate
- Using momentum to achieve the upward position

Primary Muscles Trained

Rhomboids, trapezius

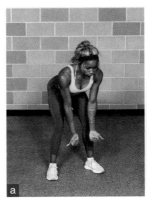
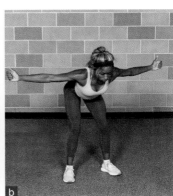

SINGLE-LEG HIP BRIDGE

1. Lie supine on the floor, with the knees flexed and heels on the floor.
2. Lift the left leg so the knee is directly above the hip.
3. While maintaining this position, drive the hips up as high as possible while keeping the torso in a neutral position. The right foot will be used to stabilize the lower body.
4. Pause at the top of this movement before slowly returning to the starting position.
5. Perform all repetitions for this side before switching legs.

Common Errors

- Failing to keep the non–weight-bearing leg static by allowing it to drop toward the floor
- Failing to maintain a neutral posture throughout the exercise movement
- Allowing the hips to rotate during the exercise movement

Primary Muscles Trained

Gluteus maximus, hamstrings

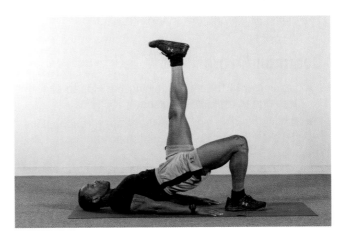

SUSPENSION TRAINING EXERCISES

SUSPENSION INVERTED ROW

1. Face the anchor point and hold the handles, with the palms either facing each other or upward.
2. Lean back while maintaining a neutral body posture, simultaneously allowing the arms to extend in front of the body until they are at or slightly above shoulder height.
3. Pull the torso toward the hands by flexing at the elbows and extending the shoulders.
4. Pull the elbows tight to the sides of the torso until the wrists are in line with the torso.
5. Pause at the top, then slowly return to the starting position.

Common Errors

- Leading with the hips or allowing the hips to sag when pulling the body upward
- Allowing the wrists to flex during the exercise movement

Primary Muscles Trained

Latissimus dorsi, rhomboids, biceps

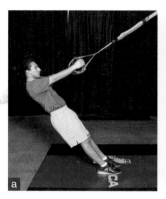 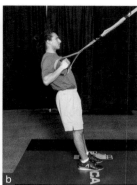

SUSPENSION Y-PULL

1. Face the anchor point and hold the handles, with the palms facing each other.
2. Lean back while maintaining a neutral body posture, simultaneously allowing the arms to extend in front of the body until they are at or slightly above shoulder height.
3. Without flexing the elbows, flex the shoulders and push the hands overhead and diagonally to form a Y with the arms and body.
4. Pause at the top, then slowly return to the starting position.

Common Errors

- Leading with the hips, allowing the hips to sag, or arching the back when pulling the body up
- Not maintaining tension on the straps throughout the full exercise movement (e.g., top position)

Primary Muscles Trained

Latissimus dorsi, rhomboids, trapezius, posterior deltoid

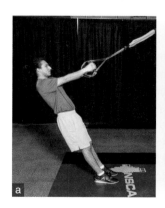 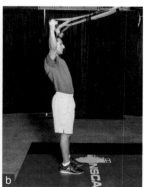

SUSPENSION AB FALLOUT

1. Facing away from the anchor point of a suspension trainer, grab the handles and lean the body forward in a push-up position, with the arms shoulder-width apart.

2. While maintaining a neutral torso position, and without flexing the elbows, continue to lean forward and extend the arms above the head as if diving into a pool.

3. Do not extend the arms past the point of being in line with the torso.

4. The range of motion should be limited to the client's ability to maintain a neutral torso position without losing the natural lumbar curvature or without pressure in the lower back.

5. From the end ROM, extend the shoulder joints and pull the handles back to return to the starting position. Be sure to maintain proper body alignment throughout the movement.

Primary Muscles Trained
Abdominals, erector spinae, latissimus dorsi

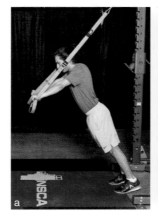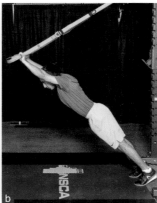

Common Errors

- Failing to maintain a neutral torso position for the duration of the exercise
- Allowing the elbows to flex

MANUAL RESISTANCE EXERCISES

MANUAL RESISTANCE LATERAL RAISE

1. Assume a standing position with the feet shoulder- to hip-width apart, knees slightly flexed, torso erect, shoulders back, and eyes focused straight ahead.

2. Position the hands to the side of the body so they are facing the thighs, and slightly flex the elbows.

3. At this point, the personal trainer, or partner, should stand behind the client with the hands on the client's forearms.

4. The client will raise the arms out to the sides; the elbows and upper arms should rise together and slightly higher than the forearms and hands.

5. As the client raises the arms, the personal trainer, or partner, applies resistance downward at an intensity that will allow the client to perform the target number of repetitions for the set.

6. During the eccentric phase, the client will attempt to resist against the personal trainer's attempt to push the client's arms down.

Primary Muscles Trained
Deltoids, trapezius

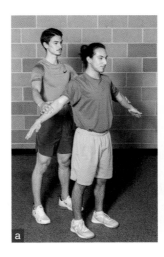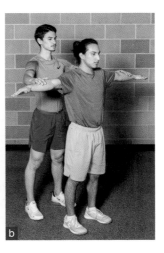

Common Errors

- Personal trainer, or partner, applying too much or too little resistance
- The client extending or flexing the elbows during the movement
- Flexing the torso forward on the descent
- Shrugging the shoulders, arching the back, and extending the knees on the ascent

MANUAL RESISTANCE SINGLE-ARM TOWEL ROW

1. Face the personal trainer, or partner, and assume a staggered stance position, with the right leg leading. (*Note:* More well-trained clients can stand with the feet shoulder-width apart rather than a staggered stance.)

2. Grab one end of a towel with the right hand while the personal trainer or partner grabs the other end of the towel with both hands.

3. While maintaining an upright torso and neutral posture, pull the towel toward the chest or upper abdominals.

4. Next, as the personal trainer pulls on the towel, resist

Primary Muscles Trained

Latissimus dorsi, teres major, rhomboids, posterior deltoid

against this force while slowly extending the elbows and returning to the starting position.

5. The personal trainer, or partner, provides resistance throughout the entire exercise movement by pulling the other end of the towel with both hands.

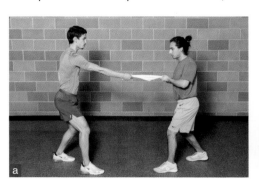

Common Errors

- Personal trainer, or partner, applying too much or too little resistance
- The client rotating the hips or torso during the movement

MANUAL RESISTANCE PUSH-UP

1. Assume a prone position on the floor, with the knees fully extended and the toes pointed down to the floor.

2. Place the hands on the floor, palms down, about 2 to 3 inches (5.1-7.6 cm) wider than shoulder-width apart, with the elbows pointed outward.

3. The personal trainer, or partner, straddles the client's torso, flexing forward at the hips while maintaining a neutral posture and applies a downward force onto the client's upper back.

4. Keeping the body in a straight line and the toes in contact with the floor, the client pushes against the floor (and against the personal trainer or partner) to fully extend the elbows.

5. During the eccentric phase, the client lowers the body by allowing the elbows to flex to a 90-degree angle while resisting the personal trainer's downward force onto the client's upper back.

Primary Muscles Trained

Pectoralis major, anterior deltoid, triceps brachii

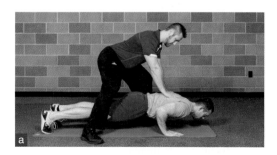

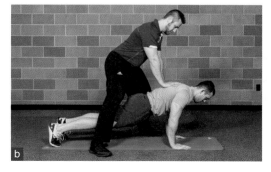

Common Errors

- Personal trainer, or partner, applying too much or too little resistance
- Allowing the hips to sag or rise (rather than keeping the body in a straight line)
- Performing the exercise through a reduced ROM

STABILITY BALL EXERCISES

EXTENDED ABDOMINAL CRUNCH

1. Lie supine on the stability ball with the lower-to-middle section of the back on the apex of the ball.
2. Place the feet flat on the floor about hip-width apart, with the thighs, hips, and lower abdomen approximately parallel to the floor.
3. Place the hands behind or at the sides of the head (to hold its weight only) or fold the arms across the chest or abdomen.
4. Curl the torso to raise it 30 to 40 degrees from the starting position.
5. Keep the feet on the floor and the thighs and hips stationary.
6. After completing the crunch, allow the torso to uncurl back down to the starting position.

Common Errors

- Raising the feet off the floor
- Allowing the hips to drop down off the side of the ball
- Pulling the head with the hands

Primary Muscle Trained

Rectus abdominis

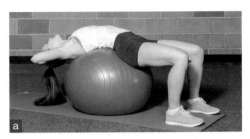

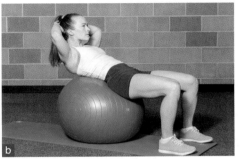

SUPINE LEG CURL

1. Lie supine on the floor, with the legs next to each other and extended away from the body.
2. Abduct the arms 90 degrees away from the torso, with the palms facing the floor.
3. Lift the hips off the floor to position the lower calves and back of the heels on the apex of the stability ball.
4. Begin the exercise with the ankles, knees, hips, and shoulders in a straight line.
5. Keeping the upper body in the same position, flex the knees (which will cause the ball to roll backward) to bring the heels toward the buttocks.
6. Continue flexing the knees to a 90-degree angle; the soles of the feet will finish near the apex of the ball.
7. Keep the knees, hips, and shoulders in a straight line.
8. After completing the leg curl, allow the knees to extend and the ball to roll forward to the starting position.

Common Error

Allowing the hips to flex or sag (rather than keeping them in line with the knees and shoulders)

Primary Muscles Trained

Hamstrings, gluteus maximus, erector spinae

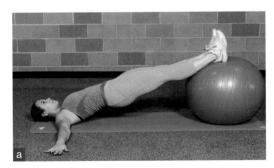

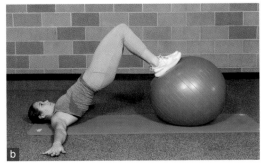

SUPINE HIP LIFT

1. Lie supine on the floor, with the legs next to each other and extended away from the body.
2. Abduct the arms 90 degrees away from the torso, with the palms facing the floor.
3. Keeping the hips on the floor, position the back of the heels on the apex of the stability ball.
4. Begin the exercise with the ankles, knees, and hips in a straight line.
5. Keeping the upper body in the same position, lift (extend) the hips until the feet, knees, hips, and shoulders are in a straight line.
6. After completing the hip lift, allow the hips to lower and return to the starting position.

Common Error

Allowing the knees to flex (rather than keeping them in line with the ankles and hips)

Primary Muscles Trained

Erector spinae, gluteus maximus, hamstrings

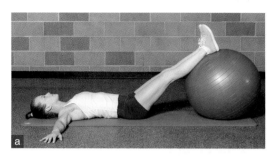

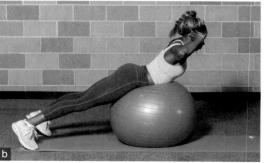

BACK HYPEREXTENSION

1. Lie prone on the stability ball, with the navel positioned on the apex of the ball.
2. Place the feet (toes) on the floor at least 12 inches (30.5 cm) apart, with the knees fully extended.
3. Clasp the hands behind the head.
4. Keeping the toes in contact with the floor, elevate the torso until it is fully extended (arched) and the chest is off the ball.
5. After completing the extension, allow the torso to lower and return to the starting position.

Common Errors

- Flexing the knees or lifting the toes off the floor
- Allowing the navel to move off the apex of the ball as the torso extends

Primary Muscle Trained

Rectus abdominis, internal and external obliques, quadratus lumborum, latissimus dorsi, teres major, erector spinae

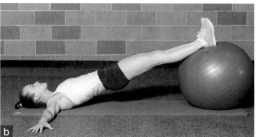

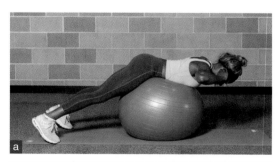

REVERSE BACK HYPEREXTENSION

1. Lie prone on the stability ball, with the navel positioned on the apex of the ball.
2. Place the hands (palms) on the floor at least 12 inches (30.5 cm) apart, with the elbows fully extended.
3. Begin the exercise with the knees extended and the toes in contact with the floor.
4. Keeping the hands in contact with the floor, elevate the legs with the knees held in extension until the hips are fully extended.
5. After completing the reverse extension, allow the legs to lower and return to the starting position.

Common Errors

- Flexing the knees or lifting the hands off the floor
- Allowing the navel to move off the apex of the ball as the legs are raised

Primary Muscles Trained

Gluteus maximus, erector spinae, hamstrings

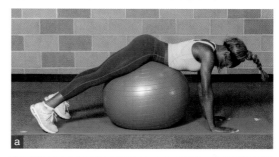

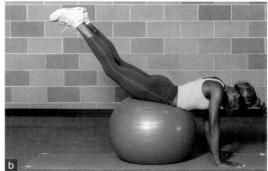

ELBOW BRIDGE

1. Kneel next to the stability ball and place the elbows and the back of the upper forearms on the ball.
2. While keeping the elbows and forearms on the ball, move the ball forward or reposition the kneeling location to create about a 90-degree angle at the elbows, shoulders, and knees.
3. Keeping the knees and toes on the floor and the elbows on the ball, begin the exercise by extending the knees to roll the ball forward until the elbows, shoulders, hips, and knees are nearly in a straight line and the back of the upper arms are on the ball.
4. After completing the elbow bridge, flex the knees to roll the ball backward to return to the starting position.

Common Errors

- Arching the back as the knees extend
- Raising the feet off the floor

Primary Muscles Trained

Rectus abdominis, internal and external obliques, quadratus lumborum, latissimus dorsi, teres major, erector spinae

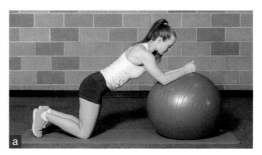

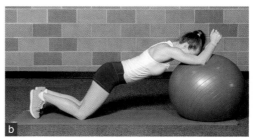

VARIATION: STRAIGHT ARM ROLL-OUT

1. Kneeling next to the stability ball, fully extend the elbows and place the hands on the stability ball.
2. While keeping the hands on the ball, roll the ball forward or reposition the kneeling location to create about a 90-degree angle at the shoulders and knees.
3. Keeping the knees and toes on the floor, begin the exercise by extending the knees to roll the ball forward until the hands, elbows, shoulders, hips, and knees are nearly in a straight line and the arms are across the ball.
4. After completing the roll-out, flex the knees to roll the ball backward to return to the starting position.

Common Errors

- Arching the back as the knees extend
- Raising the feet off the floor

Primary Muscles Trained
Rectus abdominis, internal and external obliques, quadratus lumborum, latissimus dorsi, teres major, erector spinae

STABILITY BALL PUSH-UP (FEET ON BALL)

1. Assume a push-up position with the shins and the instep of the feet on the stability ball and the elbows fully extended.
2. Position the feet, knees, hips, and shoulders in a straight line.
3. Allow the elbows to flex to lower the face to a position 1 to 2 inches (2.5-5.1 cm) from the floor while keeping the body in a straight line.
4. After reaching the lowest position, push with the arms to extend the elbows back to the starting position.

Common Errors

- Allowing the hips to sag or rise (rather than keeping the body in a straight line)
- Pushing slightly backward with the arms to move the body backward or roll the knees onto the ball

Primary Muscles Trained
Pectoralis major, anterior deltoid, triceps brachii

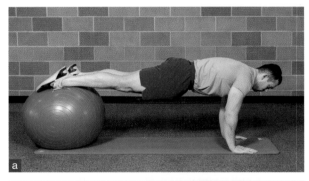

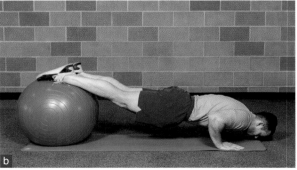

STABILITY BALL PUSH-UP (HANDS ON BALL)

1. Assume a prone position with the chest on the stability ball, feet on the floor, knees fully extended, toes pointed down to the floor, and hands placed on the sides of the ball facing one another.
2. Keeping the body in a straight line and the toes in contact with the floor, push against the stability ball with the hands to fully extend the elbows.
3. After completing the push-up, slowly lower the body by allowing the elbows to flex to a 90-degree angle.

Common Errors

- Arching the back as the knees extend
- Allowing excessive movement at the shoulder joint to maintain stability

Primary Muscles Trained

Pectoralis major, anterior deltoid, triceps brachii

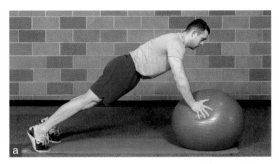

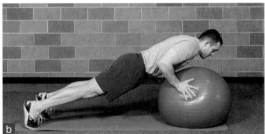

PIKE ROLL OUT AND IN

1. Assume a push-up position, with the instep of the feet on the stability ball and the elbows fully extended.
2. Position the feet, knees, hips, and shoulders in a straight line.
3. Keeping the knees and elbows fully extended, begin the exercise by flexing the hips to roll the ball forward until the toes are on top of the ball and the hips are nearly (ideally directly), over the shoulders.
4. After reaching the pike position, allow the hips to extend back to the starting position.

Common Errors

- Arching the back in the push-up position
- Hyperextending the neck in the pike position

Primary Muscles Trained

Rectus abdominis, internal and external obliques, quadratus lumborum, hip flexors

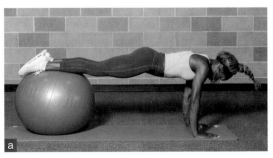

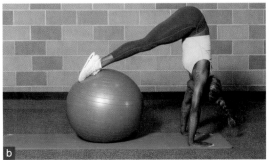

VARIATION: KNEE TO CHEST (JACKKNIFE)

1. Assume a push-up position, with the instep of the feet on the stability ball and the elbows fully extended.
2. Position the feet, knees, hips, and shoulders in a straight line.
3. Keeping the elbows fully extended, begin the exercise by raising the hips slightly and flexing the hips and knees to roll the ball forward until the hips and knees are fully flexed and the knees are near the torso.
4. After reaching the knee-to-chest position, allow the hips and knees to extend back to the starting position.

Common Errors

- Arching the back in the push-up position
- Allowing the elbows to flex in the knee-to-chest position

Primary Muscles Trained
Rectus abdominis, internal and external obliques, quadratus lumborum, hip flexors

STABILITY BALL SIDE CRUNCH

1. Lie on the left side of the body over a 22- to 26-inch (55.9-66 cm) stability ball so the navel is just above the top of the ball.
2. Without allowing the torso or hips to rotate, allow the torso to relax over the ball until a mild stretch is felt on the right side of the torso.
3. Anchor the feet in a staggered position against the base of a wall, with the right foot behind the left foot.
4. Cross the arms in front of the chest.
5. Without allowing the torso or hips to rotate, laterally flex the torso toward the wall until the upper body and the lower body are in a straight line.
6. Relax the torso to return to the starting position.
7. Repeat on the opposite side for the desired number of repetitions.

Common Errors

- Not stretching over the ball at the bottom of each rep
- Positioning the ball improperly underneath the torso (too high or too low)

Primary Muscles Trained
Internal and external obliques, abdominals

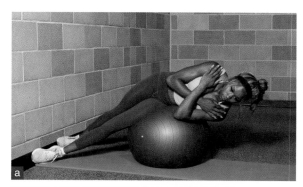

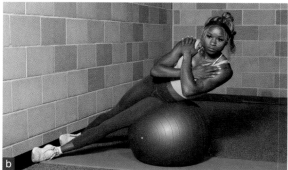

Study Questions

1. "The ability of a joint to move freely through the full normal range of motion (ROM)" defines which of the following?

   A. mobility

   B. flexibility

   C. dynamic flexibility

   D. static flexibility

2. Which of the following statements is *correct* regarding flexibility?

   A. Resistance training for flexibility should focus on antagonist muscles.

   B. Improper resistance training can impair flexibility.

   C. Resistance training reduces flexibility by making clients too muscular.

   D. Resistance training for flexibility should only use partial ranges of motion.

3. Which of the following is *incorrect* about warm-ups?

   A. Warming up is a part of the foundation of a successful practice session.

   B. Research shows that individuals who warmup before their main activity tend to be more mentally prepared.

   C. Often clients attempt to take shortcuts in the warm-up procedure.

   D. Warm-ups raise the total body temperature, but not that of the muscles themselves.

4. Which of the following is *true* about manual resistance training exercises?

   A. They are only used for partial, not full range of motion.

   B. They allow personal trainers to apply varying amounts of resistance during exercise.

   C. They are not beneficial practice to use for isometric muscle actions of the trunk.

   D. They require a lot of training equipment.

5. Guidelines for stability ball training include all of the following *except*

   A. Ensuring that the ball is inflated until firm.

   B. Correctly sizing the ball by ensuring that the client's knees are slightly below parallel when seated.

   C. Understanding that clients may fatigue easily when transitioning from machine exercises to those on a stability ball.

   D. Recognizing that it is beneficial to start with less complex exercises and build gradually.

CHAPTER 13

Resistance Exercise Technique

Ronald L. Snarr, PhD, and Alexis Batrakoulis, PhD

After completing this chapter, you will be able to

- comprehend the fundamental techniques for performing and instructing proper form for resistance training exercises,

- describe proper spotting techniques as well as situations in which they are needed,

- define appropriate training equipment and apparel, and

- recognize common resistance exercise technique errors.

One of the personal trainer's most important responsibilities to clients is to instruct and manage their exercise technique to ensure maximum benefit from resistance training in the safest possible environment. This chapter explains the benefits and physiological aspects of resistance training, safety, and resistance training technique. The chapter concludes with a detailed description of resistance training exercise techniques and spotting techniques.

COMMON TYPES OF RESISTANCE TRAINING EQUIPMENT

Although many variables must be taken into consideration when designing a resistance training program, choosing the proper equipment or machine is essential. The choice of modality should be based on several factors, including the client's training status (i.e., beginner, intermediate, or advanced), proficiency of the movement, anthropometrics (e.g., height, weight), and personal preference.

Resistance training equipment falls into three main categories:

- Constant resistance throughout a range of motion (ROM)
- Variable resistance throughout a ROM
- Constant speed of contraction during a given ROM

Each piece of equipment provides unique advantages; thus, common types of weight training machines, free weights, and alternative equipment will be described in this chapter.

Machines

Weight machines allow the individual to perform single or multijoint movements in a restricted and controlled plane of motion without a spotter, while increasing ease of use and stability for the client. Machines are particularly useful for special populations (e.g., elderly), inexperienced clients, and those

---

The authors would like to acknowledge the significant contributions of Thomas R. Baechle, Roger W. Earle, and John F. Graham to this chapter.

recovering from injury. However, all individuals, regardless of training status, can benefit from the addition of machine-based exercises within their resistance training regimen. Machines can also be adjusted to accommodate most individuals of varying heights and segment lengths; however, they may not be ideal for smaller or larger individuals depending on the machine's biomechanical design. Although machines have multiple advantages, they can be costly and can require large amounts of space; further, several units are often needed to target all the major muscle groups. This may particularly affect those who train in group settings, in one-on-one studios, or at home. Thus, personal trainers may opt for free weights or alternative resistance training equipment for a particular exercise if a machine is not feasible. The features of the most common types of resistance training machines are described next.

Selectorized

Selectorized machines use a series of cables and pulleys to lift a built-in vertical weight stack. These machines provide constant resistance and a preset movement pattern that theoretically helps reduce the risk of injury while ensuring proper exercise technique. Additionally, selectorized machines provide the client an easier and quicker way to change the weight selection as opposed to plate-loaded machines and free weights.

Plate Loaded

As compared with selectorized, **plate-loaded machines** require the use of external resistance via conventional free-weight plates. Since this involves manually loading the device with resistance, plate-loaded machines increase risk of injury to clients when loading and unloading weight. Plate-loaded machines are often capable of supporting more weight and offer a smoother movement pattern versus selectorized because of the diminished frictional resistance.

Cam

Cam-based machines offer a form of variable resistance that increases or decreases load assistance based on the strength curve; however, absolute load does not change throughout the ROM. These machines are based on joint kinetics and forces associated with the particular joint or joints used within the movement. For example, at the start of a chest press with the handles close to the body, a greater force production is required to push through the **sticking point** (the most difficult part of the exercise) as compared with the remainder of the movement. Thus, the cam allows for a greater load assistance earlier in the concentric phase and less assistance past the sticking point.

Rod or Linear Guided

Rod machines provide constant resistance during a given exercise and are usually plate loaded. These machines allow movement in a straight (linear) path only, thereby increasing stability. Additionally, most rod machines contain safety mechanisms that allow the use of heavier weights without a spotter; however, if applicable, a spotter is always recommended. The most common types of rod machines are the Smith machine, leg press, and hack squat.

Hydraulic

Hydraulic machines incorporate fluid-filled (oil or water) pistons and cylinders to achieve resistance as a client works through a given ROM. A major advantage of hydraulic machines is there are no external plates or weight stacks that may potentially cause an injury if a client loses his or her grip or is unable to complete the full ROM because of muscular failure. Additionally, the hydraulic resistance can be increased by either reducing the length of the lever or performing the movement quicker through a given ROM. Because pistons are used, the client can perform only the concentric portions of an exercise. For example, after performing a chest press–style movement by pushing the levers away from the body, the client must pull the handles back to the starting position. Thus, personal trainers must consider the implications of using concentric-only movements.

Air or Pneumatic

Air or **pneumatic machines** use compressed air cylinders rather than selectable weights or external plates to add resistance. Pneumatic machines allow individuals to perform high-velocity movements with a reduced risk of injury as compared with traditional resistance machines. Depending on the design of the machine, exercises can be performed in either one plane of motion or within a three-dimensional space. Each repetition is fully controlled via pressurized air, and resistance can be easily adjusted as needed. However, one of the major drawbacks is the need for an air compressor with each unit to supply the resistance. Additionally, pneumatic machines are costly, require different units to target all the major muscle groups, and require a large amount of space.

Isokinetic

Isokinetic machines, or accommodating variable-resistance machines, allow for the speed of contraction to be held constant throughout a given ROM. As an exercise is performed, the muscular effort from the client is matched with a proportional amount of resistance that maintains contraction speed. Unlike other resistance training machines, isokinetic machines are computer controlled and can be programmed to function through a specific ROM or provide concentric- or eccentric-only resistance. Because of their high cost and required knowledge of complex computer programming, isokinetic machines are typically found only in clinical, rehabilitation, and laboratory settings. Furthermore, they do not allow for exercises to be performed in multiple planes of motion or for certain multijoint movements (e.g., squat, bench press).

Free Weights

Unlike machine equipment, **free-weight equipment** such as barbells, dumbbells, and kettlebells allow unrestricted movement in all planes of motion, rather than a largely fixed movement path.

Barbells

One of the most common forms of free weights are **barbells**, which allow the client to perform multi- and single-joint movements in all planes of motion. Barbells are available in a variety of shapes, weights, and lengths. Thus, certain exercises may warrant proper fitting of the barbell to the client and exercise. For example, the bench press exercise is commonly performed with a longer straight bar, while the biceps curl often uses a shorter, bent EZ-curl bar to allow for a more natural position of the elbow and wrists.

A **standard barbell** is about 1 inch (2.5 cm) in diameter and weighs approximately 5 pounds per foot (about 7.5 kg per meter). Some standard barbells (there are also EZ-curl bar varieties) are fixed at a preset weight that cannot be adjusted but are typically available in 5- to 10-pound (2.5-5 kg) increments. An **Olympic barbell** is about 7 feet (2 m) long and weighs 45 pounds (20 kg), with the section where the weight plates are placed having a diameter of approximately 2 inches (5 cm).

Since barbells are free moving, the personal trainer should assess clients to determine if they possess the required coordination, stability, and increased knowledge of proper technique to safely perform a movement.

Dumbbells

Dumbbells allow for multi- and single-joint resistance training exercises to be performed within all planes of motion. Dumbbells vary in size and shape, ranging from 1 pound (0.5 kg) to over 100 pounds (45 kg), and are typically made from cast iron or rubber (with a steel handle). Equipment advantages include minimal space requirements, easily transportable, and the possibility of decreasing muscular imbalances through unilateral exercises. Although benefits include increased muscular strength and joint stability, an initial level of joint stability is required before a client can use free weights. Personal trainers should take this into account when working with specific populations.

Kettlebells

An alternative to dumbbells, **kettlebells** are a highly versatile modality and allow for a variety of exercises with minimal space and equipment. Where dumbbells have an equal weight distribution, kettlebells have an offset center of mass that allows for more momentum-based movements (e.g., swings). Kettlebells are typically made with cast iron, rubber, or hard plastics and have various sizes of hand grips (e.g., cast iron kettlebell handles increase in thickness as the weight increases), which may be a consideration for personal trainers working with special populations.

Alternative Equipment

The alternative category of equipment essentially includes all other types. By definition, most alternative equipment is like free-weight equipment because it permits motion in any movement plane; it is the relative uniqueness of this type of equipment compared with traditional resistance training equipment that labels it as alternative. Because of the somewhat higher skill level needed to use tires, weighted bags, ropes, instability devices, chains, medicine balls, slam balls, resistance bands, wooden clubs, and sleds, personal trainers should carefully consider if it is appropriate for a client to use one of these pieces of equipment and then provide clear instructions for its proper use.

Tires

Tire flipping is a form of training used to increase muscular strength and power while providing an increased level of instability as compared with traditional resistance equipment. Selecting the correct size tire for a client will depend on the weight, width, height, and tread of the tire. For instance, smaller, narrow tires may pose more difficulty for taller individuals, or worn treads may be difficult for those with poor grip strength. Before implementing tire flipping in a resistance training program, it is recommended that the client be able to perform a standard or sumo-style deadlift with proper technique. Additional considerations when performing tire flips are selecting an appropriate surface, providing a landing area clear from other equipment and individuals, ensuring the tire is in good shape (e.g., free from cuts, debris, or exposed metal), and proper spotting in case a client loses grip on the tire.

Weighted Bags

Weighted bags are a popular method of alternative resistance training because of their cost-effectiveness, portability, and unstable nature. Depending on the manufacturer, weighted bags can have various features, including handles or the ability to increase or decrease the weight. They are commonly filled with sand and provide a way for individuals to increase the intensity of a given exercise in environments not conducive to traditional free weights or gym equipment (e.g., outdoors). Weighted bags may also be incorporated in a program because of the constant unequal distributions of weight, which may transfer to the application of activities of daily living for clients or certain sports for athletes.

Ropes

Traditionally used within tactical populations, ropes have become an increasingly popular method of improving upper body strength and power, as well as muscular endurance and general conditioning depending on the specifics of the program (6, 12, 33). Ropes are often used for upper body pulling movements, climbing, and stationary movements, which allow the shoulder joint to be trained through various ranges of motions and planes. Exercises can involve creating undulating wavelike patterns, rope slams, rope climbs, and standing or seated rope pulls as well as partner-based training (collectively referred to as *battle rope training*). Before choosing rope training for a client, the personal trainer must consider the length, diameter, and weight of the rope because these variables affect the intensity of the exercise (12, 28). Additionally, manipulation of training variables, such as work-to-rest ratios, dual- versus single-arm movements, and movement speed, allows for a decrease or increase in a client's exercise intensity (26). Disadvantages of rope training include a large space requirement and a limitation in the range of motion that is trained during exercises with a high-speed component (e.g., battle rope slams).

Instability Devices

Instability devices allow for multi- or single-joint movements in an unstable environment. Theoretically, by either increasing the planes of motion or decreasing the amount of contact points with the floor, the individual must work harder to maintain balance and stability to complete the desired movement. Thus many exercises that use an instability device increase core strength and muscular endurance as well as balance and stability of either a specific joint or the entire body. Instability devices include stability balls, foam pads or mats, BOSU balls, suspension devices, and balance or wobble boards. Further information about the effectiveness and implementation of instability devices in a resistance training program is provided in chapter 12.

Chains

Chains are often used to increase external training load throughout a given range of motion. They are a form of variable resistance, meaning the external load increases as the weight is moved farther away from the floor (or the initial resting area or surface) of the chain. This style of training creates a greater resistance when the load passes the sticking point (figure 13.1*a*; 30a) and a reduced resistance during the lowering portion (i.e., eccentric phase) (figure 13.1*b*; 30a). The amount of resistance is affected by chain thickness, size, and manufacturing material. Table 13.1 displays the average amount of resistance as chain size increases in thickness (29).

Medicine Balls and Slam Balls

Medicine balls and slam balls are typically produced from various materials (e.g., leather, rubber, soft gel, air-filled) and available in 1- or 2-pound or 1- or 2-kilogram increments. Advantages of medicine ball training include the ability to perform traditional and power movements in a standing, seated, or supine position, as well the ability to throw or toss the ball at high speeds at a reduced risk of injury compared with traditional weights. Additionally, multiple clients can be trained at once because the ball can be transferred from person to person (e.g., a medicine ball pass) with minimal injury risk.

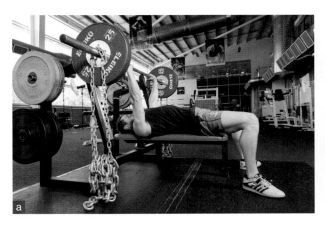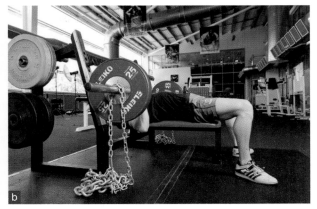

FIGURE 13.1   Bench press with added chain resistance. *(a)* In the starting position, the links of the chain are draped over each other (i.e., the chain is largely off the floor) so the client also has to handle the chain's weight. *(b)* As the client lowers the barbell to the chest, the resistance progressively decreases as the chain piles up on the floor.

TABLE 13.1   Mass, Length, and Diameter of Chains

Chain diameters	CHAIN LENGTHS				
	10 cm (3.9 in.)	50 cm (19.7 in.)	100 cm (39.4 in.)	150 cm (59.1 in.)	200 cm (78.7 in.)
6.4 mm (1/4 in.)	0.3 kg (0.7 lb)	1.3 kg (2.9 lb)	2.5 kg (5.5 lb)	3.8 kg (8.4 lb)	5.0 kg (11.0 lb)
9.5 mm (3/8 in.)	0.4 kg (0.9 lb)	1.9 kg (4.2 lb)	3.7 kg (8.2 lb)	5.6 kg (12.3 lb)	7.4 kg (16.3 lb)
12.7 mm (1/2 in.)	0.7 kg (1.5 lb)	3.7 kg (8.2 lb)	7.4 kg (16.3 lb)	11.1 kg (24.5 lb)	14.8 kg (32.6 lb)
19.1 mm (3/4 in.)	1.4 kg (3.1 lb)	7.0 kg (15.4 lb)	14.0 kg (30.9 lb)	21.0 kg (46.3 lb)	28.0 kg (61.7 lb)
22.2 mm (7/8 in.)	2.2 kg (4.9 lb)	10.8 kg (23.8 lb)	21.6 kg (47.6 lb)	32.4 kg (71.4 lb)	43.2 kg (95.0 lb)
25.4 mm (1 in.)	2.8 kg (6.2 lb)	14.0 kg (30.9 lb)	28.0 kg (61.7 lb)	42.0 kg (92.6 lb)	56.0 kg (123.5 lb)

Adapted by permission from D.T. McMaster (2009).

Resistance Bands

Resistance bands have become increasingly popular for their convenience, low cost, and versatility. Bands are frequently used within rehabilitation, personal training, and athletic settings and may supplement free-weight exercises. Often composed of thermoplastic or elastomer, bands range in shape and size. The tension provided by resistance bands is affected by several factors including the band stretch length, material, and thickness. Table 13.2 displays the most common length–tension relationships and tension predictive equations for resistance bands of varying widths (30). As bands increase in length, a greater tension is applied to the movement (variable resis-

tance), and there is a greater need for joint stability. For example, during the ascent phase of a barbell back squat, the bands provide the greatest amount of tension at the top of the movement (i.e., band is fully stretched). However, as the client begins the descent, the band will provide a gradual reduction in resistance.

Wooden Clubs

Wooden clubs resemble the shape of a baseball bat or bowling pin, with an offset center of mass. Originating in combat and martial arts settings, clubs have increased in popularity within personal training and strength and conditioning programs. Clubs typically range from 1 to 3 pounds (0.5-1.5 kg) and from 16 to 20

TABLE 13.2 Examples of Resistance Band Length–Tension Relationships

| Width (mm) | Color | Length–tension relationships | | | | | Tension prediction equation |
		110 cm (43.3 in.)	120 cm (47.2 in.)	130 cm (51.2 in.)	140 cm (55.1 in.)	150 cm (59.1 in.)	
14	Yellow	2.6 kg (5.7 lb)	5.7 kg (12.5 lb)	8.1 kg (17.8 lb)	9.8 kg (21.6 lb)	11.5 kg (25.3 lb)	$Y = -0.003x^2 + 0.98x -69.82$
22	Red	4.6 kg (10.1 lb)	9.6 kg (21.1 lb)	13.3 kg (29.3 lb)	16.6 kg (36.5 lb)	19.2 kg (42.2 lb)	$Y = -0.004x^2 + 1.38x - 99.49$
32	Blue	8.5 kg (18.7 lb)	14.8 kg (32.6 lb)	19.5 kg (42.9 lb)	23.9 kg (52.6 lb)	27.3 kg (60.1 lb)	$Y = -0.004x^2 + 1.60x - 114.86$
48	Green	6.8 kg (15.0 lb)	16.5 kg (36.3 lb)	24.0 kg (52.8 lb)	30.0 kg (66.0 lb)	49.3 kg (108.5 lb)	$Y = -0.007x^2 + 2.43x - 179.56$
67	Black	15.4 kg (33.9 lb)	29.1 kg (64.0 lb)	40.0 kg (88.0 lb)	49.3 kg (108.5 lb)	57.2 kg (125.8 lb)	$Y = -0.010x^2 + 3.73x - 269.21$

Adapted from McMaster et al. (30).

inches (40.6-50.8 cm) long but can be custom made up to 100 pounds (45.4 kg). Traditional exercises include various striking and swinging movements designed to increase shoulder joint stability, upper body and core muscular strength, and coordination. However, advanced technique and coordination are required, something personal trainers should consider when working with special populations.

Sleds

Resistance training sleds are used for exercises that require pulling, pushing, or dragging weights across a given surface. Exercises that use a sled are typically designed to increase muscular strength, power, or speed or a combination of those outcomes. Sleds range in weight from 10 pounds (4.5 kg) to 200 pounds (90.7 kg) and include the option to increase resistance using external loads, such as free-weight plates. Sleds allow exercises that target a specific muscle group (e.g., a seated sled pull for the back and biceps) or use the entire body (e.g., a walking sled push). However, certain exercises require advanced technique, balance, and stability, or have the client wearing a weight belt or harness to drag or pull (tow) the sled. Therefore, personal trainers should use caution when adding sled-based movements to a resistance training routine for individuals who do not possess proper balance, stability, or coordination.

> **Proper equipment selection is essential for creating an optimal resistance training program. Variables such as a client's training status, personal preference, familiarity, balance, coordination, strength, and knowledge of proper exercise technique should be taken into consideration.**

FUNDAMENTAL EXERCISE TECHNIQUE GUIDELINES

Several basic guidelines apply to performing nearly all resistance (weight) training exercises. The client must grasp some type of barbell, dumbbell, or handle, place his or her body in an optimal position, and follow a recommended movement and breathing pattern to promote safe and effective exercise technique.

Handgrip Types and Widths

The most frequently used handgrip positions in resistance training exercises are the **pronated grip**, with the palms down and the knuckles up (also called the **overhand grip**), and the **supinated grip**, with the palms up and the knuckles down (also called the

underhand grip) (figure 13.2, *a* and *b*; 30a). Examples of exercises that use these handgrips are the shoulder press, which uses a pronated grip, and the wrist curl, which uses a supinated grip. Some exercises, such as the dumbbell hammer curl and a version of the machine seated shoulder press, use a **neutral grip**. With this grip, the palms face in and the knuckles point out to the side, as in a handshake.

A grip that is often recommended for spotting the barbell (e.g., for the free-weight bench press exercise) is the **alternated grip**, in which one hand is pronated and the other is supinated (figure 13.2*c*; 30a). In the pronated, supinated, and alternated grips, the thumb is wrapped around the barbell so that the barbell is fully held by the hand. This thumb position creates a **closed grip**. When the thumb does not wrap around the bar-

bell but instead is placed next to the index finger, the position is called an **open** or **false grip** (figure 13.2*d*; 30a). When a client is preparing to perform a free-weight resistance training exercise using a barbell, it is also important for the personal trainer to instruct the client to place the hands a certain distance from each other. This placement is called the **grip width**. Figure 13.3 shows three grip widths: common (hands outside the legs near the width of the shoulders), wide, and narrow or close (inside the width of the shoulders). For most exercises, the hands are placed shoulder-width apart on the barbell. A client's body dimensions influence the decisions regarding actual hand placement, however. For all the grip widths, the hand position should result in an evenly balanced barbell.

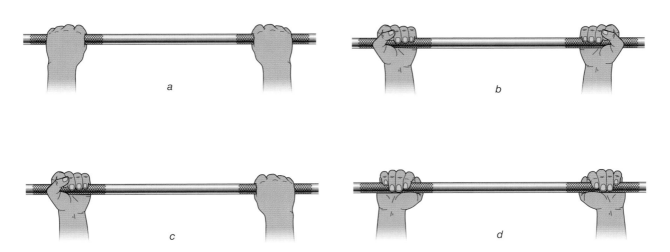

FIGURE 13.2 Bar grips: *(a)* pronated, *(b)* supinated, *(c)* alternated, and *(d)* false.

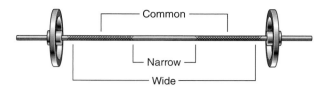

FIGURE 13.3 Grip widths.

Reprinted by permission from National Strength and Conditioning Association (2016, p. 352).

Starting Position

For all resistance training exercises, it is critical that the personal trainer instruct the client to assume, or get into, a correct initial body position. Demonstration of a new exercise given to a client should begin with how to establish a starting position. From this position, the client can maintain correct body alignment throughout the exercise, thereby placing the stress only on the targeted muscles. Standing exercises (e.g., back squat, barbell bent-over row, barbell upright row) typically require the client's feet to be at or between hip-width or shoulder-width apart, with the feet flat on the floor. Establishing a secure position in or on a machine typically requires the personal trainer to change the seat height, the position of all adjustable body and limb pads, or both the seat height and pad positions, to align the joint or joints involved in the exercise with the axis of the machine. For example, preparing a client to perform the leg (knee) extension exercise requires the personal trainer to adjust the position of the back pad forward or backward, the cam on the range limiter, and the ankle pad up or down to place the client's knee joints in line with the machine axis.

> Every demonstration of a new exercise given to a client should begin with establishing a stable starting position.

Five-Point Body Contact Position

Some free-weight and machine exercises are performed while the client is seated (e.g., leg press, machine chest press) or lying down on the back facing up (**supine**; e.g., dumbbell bench press, lying triceps extension, dumbbell fly). The exercises performed on a chair-like seat or a torso-length bench require the personal trainer to instruct the client to position his or her body in a **five-point body contact position** so that these body parts or segments contact the seat or bench and the floor or foot platform:

- Back of the head
- Upper back and rear shoulders
- Lower back and buttocks
- Right foot
- Left foot

For **prone** exercises, the client lies facedown (e.g., leg [knee] curl, back hyperextension); most of the front surface of the client's body is in contact with the floor or machine pads and handles. For example, the proper position for the leg (knee) curl exercise (i.e., the version where the client is lying fully flat on the pads) involves these five contact points:

- Chin (or one cheek if the head is turned to the side)
- Chest and abdomen
- Hips and front of the thighs
- Right hand
- Left hand

Breathing Considerations

The best recommendation personal trainers can give to clients about when and how to breathe during a resistance exercise is to exhale through the sticking point during the concentric phase and inhale during the easier part of the exercise (i.e., the eccentric phase). Typically, the sticking point occurs soon after the transition from the eccentric to the concentric phase. For example, since the sticking point of the barbell incline bench press exercise is reached when the barbell is about halfway up, the client should exhale through this portion of the movement. When lowering the barbell back down to the starting position, the client should inhale. This breathing strategy applies to nearly all resistance training exercises. A personal trainer can give the client these verbal directions: "Breathe out during the hardest part of the exercise and breathe in during the easier part of the exercise."

Valsalva Maneuver

Some exercises might require a variation of the typical breathing method for optimal performance. For these exercises, it may be helpful for the personal trainer to explain a different breathing pattern to certain clients. For example, clients who are resistance trained and will perform **structural exercises** (those that load the vertebral column; e.g., back squat, push press) or exercises that stress the lower back (e.g., bent-over row, deadlift, shoulder press) may benefit from temporarily holding their breath during the exercise.

This course of action produces what is referred to as the **Valsalva maneuver**. In this breathing practice, the **glottis** (the narrowest part of the larynx) is closed to keep air from escaping the lungs while the muscles of the abdomen and rib cage contract. This results in the individual trying to exhale against a closed throat. The outcome is that the diaphragm and deep muscles of the torso contract and generate intra-abdominal pressure against the **fluid ball,** which helps support the vertebral column internally, from the inside out, and significantly reduces the effort required of other muscles (e.g., the low back muscles during the back squat exercise) to perform the exercise (7). Thus, the client is better able to maintain correct posture and body alignment. The following are two breathing options, with sample verbal directions, that a personal trainer can give to advanced clients who are performing exercises that involve the Valsalva maneuver.

- *Option 1:* Inhale during the eccentric phase until just before starting the concentric phase; hold the breath through the sticking point; exhale. Verbal directions: "Take a breath in during the easiest part of the exercise; hold your breath until the hardest part of the exercise is completed, and then exhale."
- *Option 2:* Inhale before beginning a repetition; hold the breath through the sticking point of the concentric phase; exhale. Verbal directions: "Take a breath in before starting a repetition; hold your breath until the hardest part of the exercise is completed, and then exhale."

For an example of option 1, advanced clients attempting to lift heavy loads for the back squat exercise can take a breath in as they descend to the bottom or low position, perform the Valsalva maneuver, continue to hold the breath until right after the sticking point of the upward movement, and then exhale through the rest of the concentric phase back up to the starting or standing body position.

Despite its advantages, the Valsalva maneuver causes an increase in the pressure in the chest that can have the undesirable side effect of exerting compressive forces on the heart, making venous return more difficult. Also, the Valsalva maneuver can momentarily raise blood pressure to high levels that may cause dizziness, rapid-onset fatigue, blood vessel rupture, disorientation, and blackouts. Therefore, a personal trainer should not permit clients with any known or suspected cardiovascular, metabolic, or respiratory condition to hold their breath during resistance exercise. Personal trainers who conduct maximum or near-maximum muscular strength tests need to be aware of the advantages and disadvantages of encouraging or allowing their clients to use the Valsalva maneuver. Although it is important that the vertebral column be internally supported during these testing situations for safety and technique reasons, it is recommended that a client not overextend the time that the breath is held. Even resistance-trained and technique-experienced clients should be advised to hold their breath only momentarily (e.g., 1 to 2 seconds).

> **A personal trainer should not permit clients with any known or suspected cardiovascular, metabolic, or respiratory condition to hold their breath during resistance exercise.**

Weightlifting Belt Recommendations

Weight belts have been shown to increase intra-abdominal pressure during performance of a resistance training exercise (21, 24, 25). Therefore, the use of a weight belt can contribute by decreasing the compressive forces on the vertebral column, leading to a reduction in injury risk at near-maximal loads. Despite this benefit, if a client uses a weight belt for all resistance training exercises, the muscles of the lower back and abdomen may become unaccustomed to supporting the torso (21). Then, if the client performs an exercise without a weight belt, the weaker torso muscles may not be capable of generating enough intra-abdominal pressure to decrease the chance of injury. When determining whether a client should wear a weight belt during a resistance training exercise, the personal trainer should base the decision on the following guidelines:

- A weight belt is recommended for ground-based structural exercises that load the trunk and place stress on the lower back (e.g., back and front squat, standing shoulder press, deadlift) *and* involve lifting maximal or near-maximal loads. (Both conditions should exist; it is not necessary, for example, for the client to wear a weight belt when lifting lighter loads even when performing a structural exercise.)

- A weight belt is not needed for an exercise that does not directly load the trunk even if it might place a stress on the lower back (e.g., lat pulldown, bench press, biceps curl, leg extension).

> **A weight belt is recommended for ground-based structural exercises that involve lifting maximal or near-maximal loads.**

SPOTTING RESISTANCE TRAINING EXERCISES

When a client is performing a resistance training exercise, the personal trainer's primary responsibility is the client's safety. In addition to teaching and reinforcing proper exercise technique, the personal trainer may also serve as a **spotter** by physically assisting clients in completing the exercise to help protect them from injury. This need for a spotter is typically associated with free-weight exercises. Bars, dumbbells, and weight plates that are not restricted to a fixed movement path increase the possibility that a client will lose control and become injured. A spot can be given for a machine exercise, but it is not as necessary because clients are not exposed to the possibility that a bar, dumbbell, or weight plate could fall on them. This advantage does not imply that machine exercises do not require supervision or assistance, however (e.g., a client may need help with maintaining proper speed and range of motion).

A personal trainer may assist a client with **forced repetitions** (repetitions that are successfully performed with help from another person), but this type of assistance should not be confused with or substituted for spotting for safety.

Four free-weight exercise conditions require a spotter:

- Overhead (e.g., standing shoulder press)
- Over the face (e.g., bench press, lying triceps extension)

- With a bar on the upper back and shoulders (e.g., back squat)
- With a bar positioned on the front of the shoulders or clavicles (e.g., front squat)

Spotting Overhead or Over-the-Face Exercises

Many overhead and over-the-face resistance training exercises place the client in a sitting or standing position (e.g., shoulder press, overhead dumbbell triceps extension) or a supine position (e.g., bench press, dumbbell chest fly, lying triceps extension, dumbbell pullover). Because of the location of the barbell or dumbbell above the client's head or face, the potential for serious injury is greater during the performance of these exercises compared with most others. Also, to effectively provide enough assistance during an overhead exercise, the personal trainer must be at least as tall as the client. If this is not the case, then the personal trainer should modify the exercise so that the client is in a seated position. Some types of bench press and shoulder press benches have a small platform that places the spotter in a better position for spotting overhead or over-the-face exercises.

Barbell Exercises

When spotting over-the-face barbell exercises, the personal trainer should grasp the bar between the client's hands using an alternated grip (see figure 13.2c on page 232). This helps keep the bar from rolling out of the personal trainer's hands and onto the client's head, face, or neck. Also, the personal trainer should take a position as close to the client as possible—without creating a distraction—to be able to grab the bar quickly if necessary. Finally, to create a stable base of support, the personal trainer, if possible, should be in a neutral spine position rather than rounded-back position, with the feet flat on the floor in a staggered stance. With some bench frames there may not be enough room for the staggered stance, however.

Dumbbell Exercises

It is common to see people receiving spotting assistance at their upper arms or elbows while performing an overhead or over-the-face dumbbell exercise (figure 13.4a; 30a). This spotting technique may lead to injury if the individual's elbows quickly collapse while the spotter is lifting the upper arms or elbows. If that happens, the spotter probably will not be able to prevent

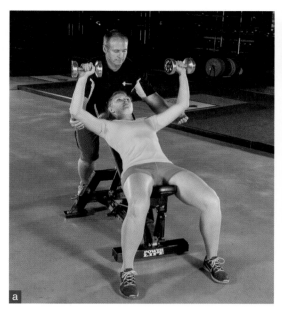 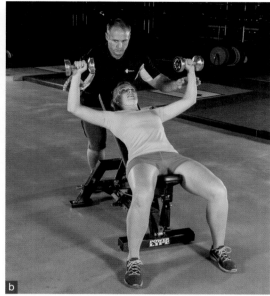

FIGURE 13.4   *(a)* Incorrect dumbbell spotting location. *(b)* Correct dumbbell spotting location.

the dumbbells from landing on the client's head, face, neck, or chest. The personal trainer should instead spot the client's wrists (figure 13.4b; 30a) very near to the dumbbell. For exercises that require the client to use two hands to hold one dumbbell (e.g., dumbbell pullover) or only one hand at a time to perform an exercise (e.g., overhead dumbbell triceps extension), the personal trainer should spot the lowest half of the dumbbell itself (i.e., the end closest to the floor).

> When a client is performing an overhead or over-the-face dumbbell exercise, the personal trainer should spot the client's wrists close to the dumbbell, not the upper arms or elbows.

Spotting Exercises With the Bar on the Back or Front Shoulders

Exercises that involve placing the bar across the shoulders at the base of the neck or the upper back (e.g., back squat, lunge, step-up) or on the front of the shoulders and across the clavicles (e.g., front squat) should also be spotted. As with the overhead or over-the-face exercises, to be an effective spotter, the personal trainer needs to be strong enough to handle the load lifted and needs to be at least as tall as the client. A variety of

methods can be used to spot these types of exercises. For example, the spotter can stand close behind the client (without impeding the execution of the exercise) and be prepared to "hug and lift" the client if he or she is not able to complete the set. To further guard against injury or accident, these types of exercises should be performed, if possible, inside a squat rack with the crossbars placed just below the lowest position the bar will reach during the downward movement phase.

Spotting Power Exercises

As a rule, explosive, or simply power, exercises (e.g., power clean, hang clean, push jerk, high pull, snatch) should not be spotted. Fast-moving bars are difficult for a personal trainer to spot and catch; trying to do so may result in injury to one or both parties. Because of this dynamic situation, power exercises should be performed in a segregated area or on a lifting platform in case the client "misses" (fails to complete a repetition) or loses control of the bar. Instead of physically catching the bar during a missed lift, the personal trainer should teach the client to push the bar away or simply drop it. Clients should be instructed that if the bar begins to fall behind the head, they should simultaneously let go of the bar and step or jump forward. It is also important to remove any equipment from the area in and around the space where power exercises are performed.

> ▶ **Power exercises should be performed in a segregated area or on a lifting platform without the use of a spotter.**

Number of Spotters

Once a personal trainer decides that a client requires a spot for an exercise, the next step is to determine how many spotters are necessary. If the load is beyond the personal trainer's ability to handle effectively, an additional spotter must be used. For example, it is common to use one spotter at each end of the bar during the front or back squat exercise. This technique requires spotters who are experienced because the spotters must perfectly synchronize when and how much they assist the client to keep the bar even and balanced. When excessively heavy loads are involved, three spotters may be appropriate.

Communication

Communication is the responsibility of both the client and the personal trainer. A client should be instructed to tell the personal trainer when he or she is ready to move the bar, dumbbells, or machine handles into the starting position (i.e., a **liftoff**). If the client needs help during the set, he or she should quickly ask or signal the personal trainer; and after the last repetition the personal trainer should help the client move the bar back onto the supports (i.e., **racking the bar**). Poor communication may cause the personal trainer to spot the client too soon, too late, or improperly. Therefore, the personal trainer should discuss all these issues with the client before the beginning of a set.

CONCLUSION

Personal trainers are responsible for teaching a client proper resistance training exercise technique to maximize the training effect of the exercises and create the safest training environment. This includes not only instructions on how to perform an exercise but also proper breathing guidelines and weight belt recommendations. The personal trainer must also know when and how to spot a client during a resistance training exercise and how to recognize and correct mistakes in a client's exercise technique.

A personal trainer should be familiar with all the exercises described in this chapter and should realize there has been no attempt to explain or provide photos of all possible technique and spotting variations. The exercise descriptions on the following pages offer the most accepted guidelines for resistance training exercise technique (5, 11, 22, 32). (Readers are encouraged to see references 1 through 4, 8 through 10, 13 through 20, 23, 27, 31, and 34 through 37 for additional guidelines.)

Resistance Training Exercises

▶ Video available within HK*Propel*

ABDOMEN AND CORE

CURL-UP

Starting Position

Assume a supine position on a floor mat.

Flex the knees to bring the heels near the buttocks.

Fold the arms across the chest or abdomen.

Upward Movement Phase

Flex the neck to tuck the chin toward the chest.

Keeping the feet, buttocks, and lower back stationary on the mat, with arms folded across the chest, curl the torso toward the thighs until the upper back is off the mat.

Downward Movement Phase

Allow the torso, then the neck, to uncurl and extend back to the starting position.

Keep the feet, buttocks, lower back, and arms in the same position.

Common Errors

- Raising the feet off the mat during the upward movement phase
- Raising the hips off the mat during the downward movement phase

Primary Muscle Trained
Rectus abdominis

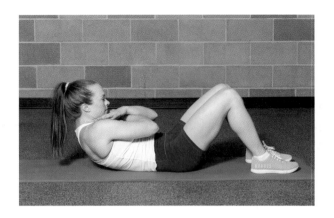

MACHINE ABDOMINAL CRUNCH

There are a variety of machine configurations for this exercise; the bullet points describe the machine shown in the photos.

Starting Position

Sit in the machine with the upper arms pressed against the arm pads, feet under the ankle roller pads, and hands grasping the handles with a closed grip.

Upward Movement Phase

Flex the hips up and the torso forward to curl the lower body and the upper body toward each other.

Keep the upper arms and ankles pressed against their respective pads during the movement.

Keep the buttocks and back pressed against the seat and back pad and keep a firm grip on the handles.

Downward Movement Phase

Allow the hips and torso to uncurl and extend back to the starting position while keeping the feet, legs, buttocks, and arms stationary.

Keep the buttocks and back pressed against the seat and back pad and keep a firm grip on the handles.

Common Errors

- Raising the buttocks off the seat during the movement
- Overemphasizing a pull with the legs or hands to help curl the torso

Primary Muscle Trained
Rectus abdominis

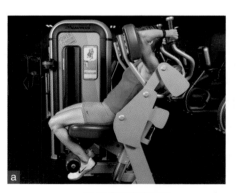

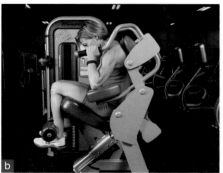

WOODCHOP

Starting Position

Stand beside the cable machine, with the feet positioned shoulder-width apart and the knees slightly flexed.

Grasp the cable handle with both hands above one shoulder, with the elbows fully extended.

Downward Movement Phase

Rotate the torso by pulling the handle down and across the body in a diagonal motion, passing the contralateral (opposite) thigh.

Elbows should remain fully extended.

Hips and knees can rotate slightly.

Upward Movement Phase

Return to the starting position in a slow and controlled manner by rotating the torso back to neutral.

After completing the set, repeat the same series of movements on the opposite side.

Common Errors

- Locking the knees and hips during the downward and upward movement phases

Primary Muscles Trained

Internal and external obliques, transversus abdominis, rectus abdominis

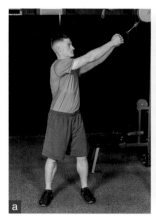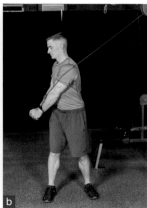

- Flexing the elbows while performing the exercise
- Using only the arms to complete the movement and not rotating the torso

ROMAN CHAIR BACK EXTENSION

Starting Position

Assume a prone position in the bench, with the upper thighs and lower hips in contact with the upper pad.

The top of the hips should lie slightly over the pad, while the back of the lower legs should be in contact with the lower pad.

The head, neck, and spine should remain in a neutral position throughout the movement.

Allow the upper body to be fully flexed over the upper pad; the result is approximately a 90-degree forward flexed position in the bottom position to start each repetition.

Upward Movement Phase

Contract the lower back, gluteal, and hamstring muscles to extend the torso until the body is in one line from the top of the head to the ankles.

Be sure to keep the spine and neck in a neutral position during the ascent.

Downward Movement Phase

Allow the hips to flex to slowly lower the upper body back to the starting position.

Keep the thighs and hips stationary and the spine and neck in a neutral position during the descent.

Common Errors

- Raising the thighs from the support pad during the upward movement phase
- Excessively arching the back at the end of the upward movement phase

Primary Muscles Trained

Erector spinae

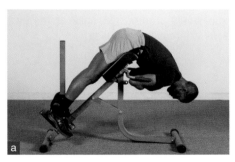

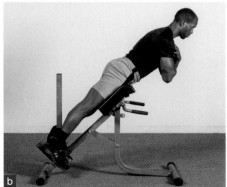

MACHINE BACK EXTENSION

Starting Position

Sit in the machine with the middle to upper back pressed against the back pad.

The torso should be in slight flexion and the hips aligned with the pivot point of the machine.

Place the feet on the machine frame or foot supports.

Grasp the handles with a firm, neutral, pronated grip or cross the arms across the chest.

Backward Movement Phase

Keeping the thighs and feet stationary, extend the torso by pushing back on the pad (lean backward).

Keep the back and neck in a neutral position throughout the movement and the back firmly pressed against the back pad.

If using handles, maintain a tight grip.

Forward Movement Phase

Allow the torso to flex (lean forward) and return to the starting position.

The upper back should remain firmly pressed against the back pad, with the thighs and feet stationary.

If using handles, maintain a tight grip.

Common Errors

- Pushing with the legs or buttocks rising from the seat during the backward movement phase
- Excessively arching the back at the end of the backward movement phase

Primary Muscles Trained

Erector spinae

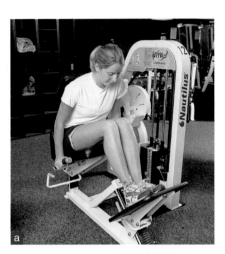

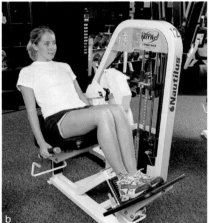

BACK

BENT-OVER ROW

Starting Position

Grasp the bar with a closed, pronated grip wider than shoulder width.

Feet should be shoulder-width apart, with a slight flex in the knee.

The neck and back should remain in a neutral, tightly packed position throughout the movement.

Lift the bar from the floor to a position at the front of the thighs using the first pull phase of the power clean exercise.

The torso should have a forward lean so that it is slightly above parallel to the floor.

Eyes should be focused a short distance ahead of the feet.

Allow the bar to hang, with the elbows in full extension.

Adjust the position of the knees, hips, and torso to suspend the weight plates off the floor.

Upward Movement Phase

Pull the bar up toward the upper abdomen (bottom of the rib cage).

Keep the elbows pointed away from the sides of the body, with the wrists straight.

The bar should touch the upper abdomen at the top of the movement.

At the highest bar position, the elbows should be slightly higher than the torso.

Downward Movement Phase

Allow the elbows to slowly extend back to the starting position.

The bar should follow a path close to the individual.

Keep the torso rigid, back neutral, and knees in the same flexed position.

After completing the set, perform the eccentric phase of a deadlift to return the bar to the floor.

Primary Muscles Trained

Latissimus dorsi, teres major, middle trapezius, rhomboids, posterior deltoid

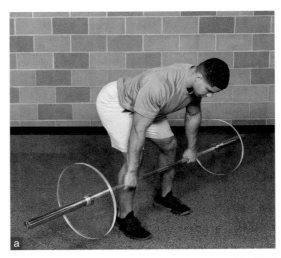

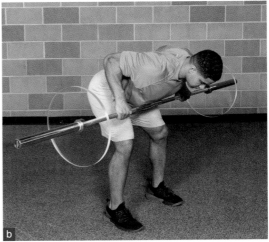

Common Errors

- Jerking the upper body, shrugging the shoulders, extending the torso, locking out the knees, curling the bar in the hands, or rising on the toes to help move the bar toward the upper abdomen.
- Allowing the upper back to round (losing the neutral spine position) during the movement.

ONE-ARM DUMBBELL ROW

Starting Position

Facing a bench, stand with the feet shoulder-width apart and knees slightly flexed.

Flex forward at the hips and place one hand, with the elbow fully extended for support, on top of a bench.

Pick up a dumbbell from the floor with a closed, neutral grip.

Adjust the upper body to assume a bent-over position with a neutral, rigid back that runs parallel to the floor.

The arm with the dumbbell should be fully extended.

Upward Movement Phase

Flex the elbow and extend the shoulder to lift the dumbbell up toward the body.

The upper arm should remain tight with the body, and the elbow should not flare at the top of the movement.

At the highest dumbbell position, the elbow should be in line with the torso.

The torso should remain flat and the body rigid throughout this phase.

Downward Movement Phase

Slowly extend the elbow back to the starting position while maintaining a neutral neck and spine.

After completing the set, switch sides and repeat again with the opposite arm.

Common Errors

- Jerking the upper body, rotating the torso, shrugging the shoulders, or only using the biceps to curl the dumbbell toward the body
- Allowing the upper back to round during the movement
- Flaring of the elbow
- Not fully extending the arm in the downward movement phase

Latissimus dorsi, teres major, middle trapezius, rhomboids, posterior deltoid

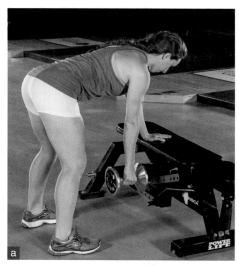

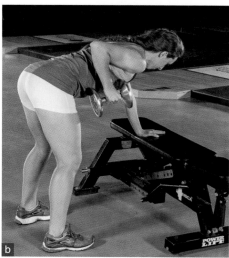

LAT PULLDOWN

Starting Position

Grasp the bar with a closed, pronated grip slightly wider than shoulder width.

Sit facing the machine stack, with the legs under the thigh pads and the feet flat on the floor.

Slightly lean the torso backward to create a path for the bar to pass by the face.

Allow the elbows to fully extend.

In this position, the weight to be lifted will be suspended above the rest of the stack.

Downward Movement Phase

Pull the bar down and toward the upper chest; the elbows should move down and back and the chest up and out as the bar is lowered.

Keep the feet, legs, and torso in the same position.

Touch the bar to the clavicles or upper chest.

Upward Movement Phase

Allow the elbows to slowly extend back to the starting position.

Keep the feet, legs, and torso in the same position.

After completing the set, stand up and return the weight to its resting position.

Common Errors

- Using an open grip on the bar
- Contracting the abdominal muscles and flexing the torso to assist in the downward movement phase
- Not fully extending the elbows during the upward movement phase
- Pulling the bar down behind the head to the back of the neck

Primary Muscles Trained

Latissimus dorsi, teres major, middle trapezius, rhomboids, posterior deltoid

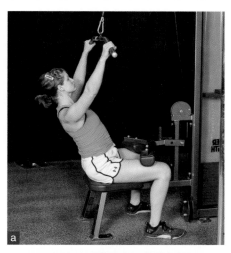

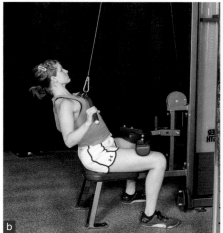

LOW PULLEY SEATED ROW

Starting Position

Facing the machine, sit on the floor (or on the long seat pad, if available).

Place the feet on the machine frame or foot supports.

Flex the knees and hips to reach forward and grasp the handle with a closed, pronated grip.

Get into an erect seated position with the torso perpendicular to the floor, knees slightly to moderately flexed, and the feet and legs parallel to each other.

Allow the elbows to fully extend, with the arms about parallel to the floor.

In this position, the weight to be lifted will be suspended above the rest of the stack.

Backward Movement Phase

Pull the handle toward the chest or upper abdomen.

Maintain an erect torso, with the knees in the same slightly or moderately flexed position.

Touch the handle to the sternum or upper abdomen.

Forward Movement Phase

Allow the elbows to slowly extend back to the starting position.

Maintain an erect torso, with the knees in the same slightly or moderately flexed position.

After completing the set, flex the knees and hips to reach forward, and return the weight to its resting position.

Common Errors

- Jerking the upper body or leaning back during the backward movement phase
- Curling the handle toward the torso during the backward movement phase
- Flexing the torso forward during the forward movement phase

Primary Muscles Trained

Latissimus dorsi, teres major, middle trapezius, rhomboids, posterior deltoid

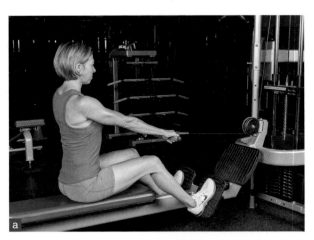

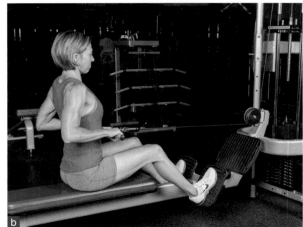

SEATED ROW (RESISTANCE BAND)

Starting Position

Grasp the handles of the resistance band with a closed, neutral grip.

Sit on the floor or mat with the knees slightly flexed, and evenly wrap the resistance band around the insteps of the feet.

Assume an erect position, with the torso perpendicular to the floor.

Hold on to the handles with the elbows fully extended, the arms about parallel to the floor, and the palms facing each other.

In this position, the resistance band should be nearly taut (not stretched); if it is not, take up the slack by wrapping the resistance band further around the feet.

Backward Movement Phase

Pull the handles toward the chest or upper abdomen.

Maintain an erect torso, with the knees in the same slightly flexed position.

Touch the hands to the sides of the torso.

Forward Movement Phase

Allow the elbows to slowly extend back to the starting position.

Maintain an erect torso, with the knees in the same slightly flexed position.

Common Errors

- Jerking the upper body or leaning back during the backward movement phase
- Curling the handles toward the torso during the backward movement phase
- Flexing the torso forward during the forward movement phase

Primary Muscles Trained

Latissimus dorsi, teres major, middle trapezius, rhomboids, posterior deltoid

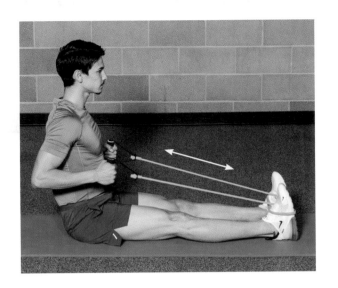

ARMS (BICEPS)

BICEPS CURL (BAR)

Starting Position

Grasp the bar with a closed, supinated grip at or slightly wider than shoulder width.

Stand erect with the feet shoulder-width apart and knees slightly flexed (slightly more than what is seen in the photos).

Position the bar in front of the thighs, with the elbows fully extended.

Position the upper arms against the sides of the torso and perpendicular to the floor.

Upward Movement Phase

Flex the elbows to move the bar in an upward arc toward the shoulders.

Keep the torso erect, the upper arms stationary, and the knees in the same slightly flexed position.

Flex the elbows until the bar is within 4 to 6 inches (10.2-15.2 cm) of the shoulders.

Downward Movement Phase

Allow the elbows to slowly extend back to the starting position.

Keep the torso, upper arms, and knees in the same position.

Common Errors

- Jerking the upper body, shrugging the shoulders, extending the torso, extending the knees, swinging the bar, or rising on the toes to help raise the bar
- Moving the elbows away from the sides of the torso (backward during the downward movement phase or forward during the upward movement phase)
- Keeping the elbows partially flexed at the end of the downward movement phase (a shortened range of motion)
- Bouncing the bar off the thighs to add momentum to help with the next repetition

Primary Muscles Trained

Biceps brachii, brachialis, brachioradialis

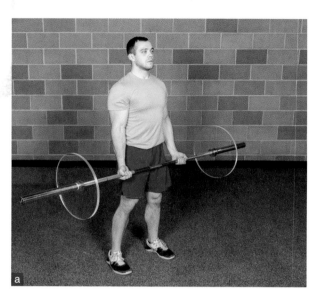

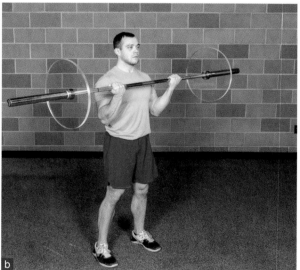

BICEPS CURL (EZ-CURL BAR)

Starting Position

Grasp the bar with a closed, supinated grip at or slightly wider than shoulder width.

The palms of the hands should be slightly tilted inward because of the shape of the EZ-curl bar.

Stand with an erect spine, feet shoulder-width apart and knees slightly flexed (slightly more than what is seen in the photos).

Position the bar in front of the thighs, with the elbows fully extended.

The upper arms should be tightly packed to the sides of the torso and perpendicular to the floor.

Upward Movement Phase

Flex the elbows to move the bar in an upward arc toward the shoulders.

The torso, knees, and upper arms should remain stable and stationary throughout the movement.

Flex the elbows until the bar is within 4 to 6 inches (10.2-15.2 cm) of the shoulders.

Downward Movement Phase

Allow the elbows to slowly extend back to the starting position.

Keep the torso, upper arms, and knees in the same position.

Common Errors

- Jerking the upper body, shrugging the shoulders, extending the torso, extending the knees, swinging the bar, or coming up on the toes to help raise the bar
- Moving the elbows backward during the downward movement phase or forward during the upward movement phase
- Shortening the range of motion by not putting the elbows into full extension
- Bouncing the bar off the thighs to add momentum to assist with the next repetition

Primary Muscles Trained

Biceps brachii, brachialis, brachioradialis

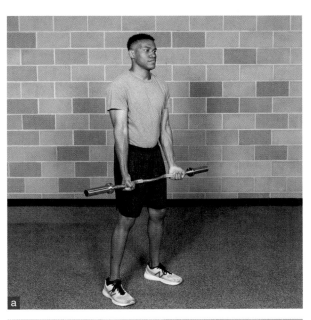

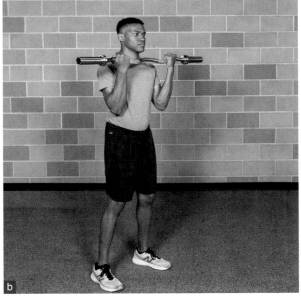

BICEPS CURL (RESISTANCE BAND)

Starting Position

Grasp the handles of the resistance band with a closed, supinated grip.

Position the feet shoulder-width apart, with the arches of both feet on top of a middle section of the resistance band.

Stand erect with the knees slightly flexed (slightly more than what is seen in the photos).

Position the handles outside of the thighs, with the arms at the sides and the palms facing forward.

In this position, the resistance band should be nearly taut (not stretched); if not, take up the slack by widening the stance or selecting a shorter band.

Upward Movement Phase

Flex the elbows to move the handles in an upward arc toward the shoulders.

Keep the torso erect, upper arms stationary, and knees in the same slightly flexed position.

Flex the elbows until the hands are within 4 to 6 inches (10.2-15.2 cm) of the shoulders.

Downward Movement Phase

Allow the elbows to slowly extend back to the starting position.

Keep the torso, upper arms, and knees in the same position.

Common Errors

- Shrugging the shoulders to help raise the handles upward
- Moving the elbows backward during the downward movement phase or forward during the upward movement phase
- Shortening the range of motion in the downward phase of the movement by not reaching full extension

Primary Muscles Trained

Biceps brachii, brachialis, brachioradialis

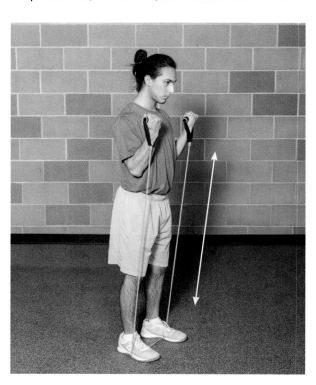

MACHINE (PREACHER) BICEPS CURL

Starting Position

Assume a seated position facing the chest pad of the machine.

Grasp the handles with a closed, supinated grip, with the elbows fully extended.

Position the upper arms on the angled upper arm pad(s), and align the elbows with the axis of the machine.

Place the feet on the machine frame, foot supports, or floor.

Sit erect and push the torso against the chest pad. If necessary, adjust the pad to position the torso perpendicular to the floor.

Upward Movement Phase

Keeping the torso, thighs, and feet stationary, flex the elbows to move the handles toward the face and shoulders.

Keep the torso and upper arms firmly pressed against their pads.

Flex the elbows until the handles are within 4 to 8 inches (10.2-20.3 cm) of the face and shoulders.

Downward Movement Phase

Allow the elbows to slowly extend back to the starting position.

Keep the torso and upper arms firmly pressed against their pads.

Common Errors

- Lifting the upper arms off the angled upper arm pad(s) during the upward movement phase
- Jerking the upper body or leaning back during the upward movement phase
- Rising off the seat during the downward movement phase
- Keeping the elbows partially flexed at the end of the downward movement phase, thereby shortening the range of motion

Primary Muscles Trained

Biceps brachii, brachialis, brachioradialis

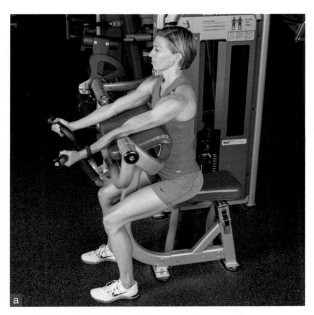

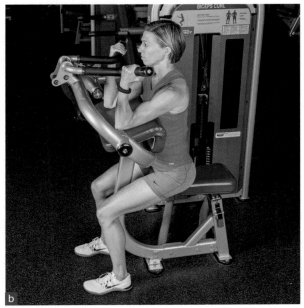

DUMBBELL ALTERNATING CURL

Starting Position

Grasp the dumbbells with a supinated grip.

Stand erect with the feet shoulder-width apart and knees slightly flexed.

A dumbbell should be in each hand and the elbows positioned just outside the torso along the sides of the body.

Upward Movement Phase

Flex one elbow to move the dumbbell in an upward arc toward the shoulders.

Flex the elbow until the dumbbell is within 4 to 6 inches (10.2-15.2 cm) of the shoulder.

Remain in an erect, stationary stance throughout the movement.

Downward Movement Phase

Allow the elbow to slowly return to full extension and resting along the side of the body.

After the dumbbell has returned to the starting position, begin the upward movement phase with the opposite arm.

Alternate arms until the set is completed. Keep the torso, upper arms, and knees in the same position.

Common Errors

- Jerking the upper body or leaning back during the upward movement phase
- Shortening the range of motion by keeping the elbows partially flexed at the end of the downward movement phase

Primary Muscles Trained

Biceps brachii, brachialis, brachioradialis

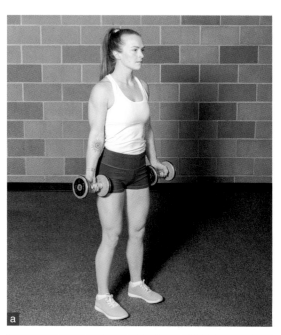

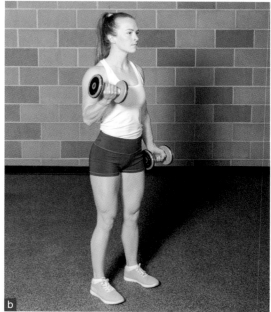

ARMS (TRICEPS)

TRICEPS EXTENSION (RESISTANCE BAND)

Starting Position

Grasp the handles of the resistance band with a closed, pronated grip.

Sit on the floor or mat with the buttocks on top of a middle section of the resistance band.

Assume an erect position, with the torso perpendicular to the floor and the legs crossed in front of the body.

Position the arms and handles behind the head and upper back with the elbows flexed, facing forward, and palms facing up.

In this position, the resistance band should be nearly taut (not stretched); if not, select a shorter band.

Upward Movement Phase

Keeping the wrist rigid, push one handle upward until the elbow is fully extended.

Maintain an erect torso, with the legs in the same position.

Downward Movement Phase

Allow the elbow to flex slowly by moving the handle down to the starting position.

Maintain an erect torso, with the legs in the same position.

After completing the set, repeat the movement with the other arm.

Common Errors

- Excessively arching the back during the upward movement phase
- Flexing the torso or tilting the head forward during the downward movement phase

Primary Muscle Trained

Triceps brachii

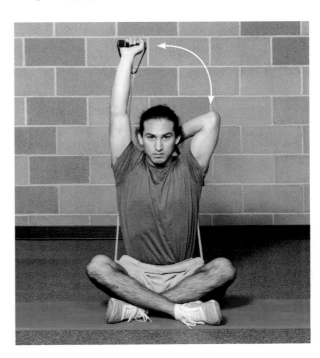

LYING TRICEPS EXTENSION

Client: Starting Position

Assume a supine position on a bench in the five-point body contact position.

On a signal, take the bar from the personal trainer.

Grasp the bar with a closed, pronated grip about 12 inches (30.5 cm) apart.

Position the bar over the chest, with the elbows fully extended and the arms parallel.

Point the elbows away from the face.

Personal Trainer: Starting Position

At the client's signal, grasp the bar with a closed, alternated grip (not where the client will grasp the bar, however) and lift it from the floor.

Stand erect and close to the head of the bench, but not so close as to distract the client.

Place the feet shoulder-width apart (even with each other or staggered), with the knees somewhat flexed.

At the client's signal, place the bar in the client's hands.

Guide the bar to a position over the client's chest.

Release the bar smoothly.

Client: Downward Movement Phase

Allow the elbows to slowly flex to lower the bar toward the nose, eyes, forehead, or the top of the head depending on the length of the arms.

Keep the wrists rigid and the elbows pointing away from the face.

Keep the upper arms parallel to each other and perpendicular to the floor.

Lower the bar to touch the top of the head or forehead.

Maintain the five-point body contact position.

Personal Trainer: Downward Movement Phase

Keep the hands in the alternated grip position close to—but not touching—the bar as it descends.

Slightly flex the knees, hips, and torso (if needed to stay close to the client) and keep the back neutral when following the bar.

Client: Upward Movement Phase

Push the bar upward until the elbows are fully extended.

Keep the wrists rigid and the elbows pointing away from the face.

Keep the upper arms parallel to each other and perpendicular to the floor.

Maintain the five-point body contact position.

After completing the set, signal the personal trainer to take the bar.

Personal Trainer: Upward Movement Phase

Keep the hands in the alternated grip position close to—but not touching—the bar as it ascends.

Slightly extend the knees, hips, and torso (if needed to stay close to the client) and keep the back neutral when following the bar.

At the client's signal, grasp the bar with an alternated grip, take it from the client, and return it to the floor.

Common Errors

- Allowing the elbows to flare to the sides during the movement
- Moving the upper arms away from their perpendicular position in relation to the floor
- Arching the back or raising the hips off the bench during the upward movement phase

Primary Muscle Trained

Triceps brachii

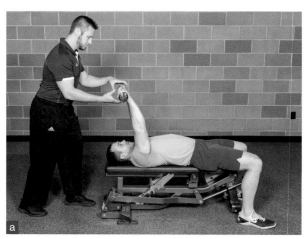

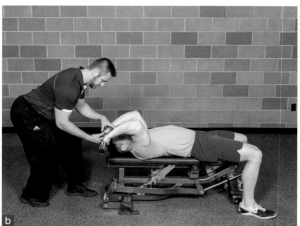

TRICEPS PUSHDOWN

Starting Position

Grasp the bar with a closed, pronated grip 6 to 12 inches (15.2-30.5 cm) apart. A minimum recommended grip width is close enough for the tips of the thumbs to touch each other when they are extended along the bar. A maximum grip width is one in which the forearms are parallel to each other.

Stand erect with the feet shoulder-width apart and knees slightly flexed.

Pull the bar down and position the upper arms against the sides of the torso, with the arms flexed.

Adjust the degree of elbow flexion to position the forearms approximately parallel to the floor.

Stand close enough to the machine to allow the cable to hang straight down when it is held in the starting position.

Keep the head in a neutral position, with the cable directly in front of the nose.

Keep the torso in position by holding the

- shoulders back,
- upper arms and elbows against the sides of the body, and
- abdominal muscles contracted throughout the exercise.

In this position, the weight to be lifted will be suspended above the rest of the stack.

Downward Movement Phase

Push the bar down until the elbows are fully extended.

Keep the torso and the upper arms stationary.

Upward Movement Phase

Allow the elbows to slowly flex back to the starting position.

Keep the torso, upper arms, and knees in the same position.

After completing the set, guide the bar upward to move the weight back to its resting position.

Common Errors

- Moving the elbows away from the sides of the torso (backward during the downward movement phase or forward during the upward movement phase)
- Flexing the torso during the downward movement phase
- Forcefully locking out the elbows during the downward movement phase
- Turning the head to the side during the movement

Primary Muscle Trained

Triceps brachii

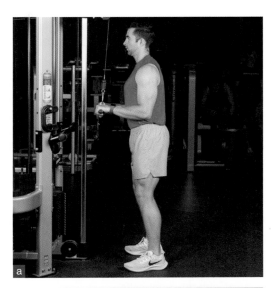

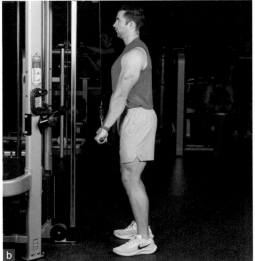

OVERHEAD TRICEPS EXTENSION

Starting Position

Sit on a bench with the upper body erect, the knees flexed, and the feet resting on the floor.

Grasp a dumbbell in each hand with a closed grip.

Position the arms and dumbbells over the head, with the elbows fully extended and palms facing each other.

Downward Movement Phase

Keeping the upper arms in line with the ears, flex the elbows to slowly lower the dumbbells behind the head. Continue lowering the weight until the forearms move below parallel to the floor.

Maintain an erect torso while keeping the upper arms in line with the ears during this phase.

Be sure to maintain control during the lowering phase to prevent contact of the head or neck with the dumbbells.

Upward Movement Phase

Extend the elbows to move the dumbbells back over the head until the starting position is reached.

Maintain control during this phase to prevent contact of the head with the dumbbells.

Common Errors

- Excessively arching the back
- Flexing the neck and trunk to clear the dumbbells over the head

Primary Muscle Trained

Triceps brachii

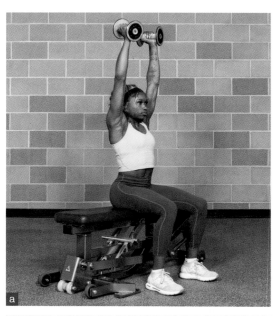

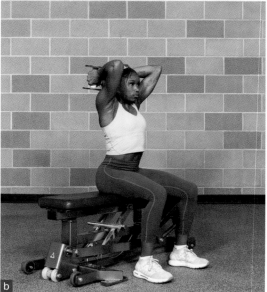

CALVES

MACHINE STANDING CALF (HEEL) RAISE

Starting Position

Facing the machine, place the balls of the feet on the nearest edge of the step, with the toes pointing straight ahead.

Move under the shoulder pads and stand erect, with the hips under the shoulders.

Position the feet and legs parallel to each other.

Slightly plantar flex the feet and ankles to lift the thigh pads to remove the supports. If there are none, then the position of the shoulder pads needs to be low enough that the exercise can be performed through a full range of motion.

Extend the knees fully, but not forcefully.

Allow the heels to drop down lower than the step in a comfortable, stretched position.

Upward Movement Phase

Fully plantar flex the feet and ankles.

Keep the torso erect, legs and feet parallel, and knees extended.

Downward Movement Phase

Allow the heels to slowly lower back to the starting position.

Maintain the same body position.

After completing the set, slightly flex the knees, replace the supports, and move out from under the shoulder pads.

Common Errors

- Allowing the ankles to invert or evert (i.e., rising on the big or little toes, respectively) during the upward movement phase
- Allowing the knees to flex during the downward movement phase or extend during the upward movement phase
- Bouncing the weight to add momentum to help with the next repetition

Primary Muscles Trained

Gastrocnemius, soleus

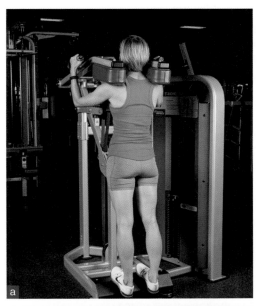

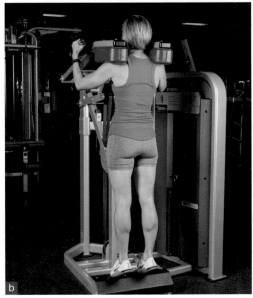

MACHINE SEATED CALF (HEEL) RAISE

Starting Position

Sit erect on the seat and place the knees and lower thighs under the pads, with the thighs parallel to the floor.

Place the balls of the feet on the nearest edge of the step, with the toes pointing straight ahead.

Position the feet and legs parallel to each other.

Slightly plantar flex the feet and ankles to lift the thigh pads to remove the supports.

Allow the heels to drop down lower than the step in a comfortable, stretched position.

Upward Movement Phase

Keeping the torso erect and the legs and feet parallel, fully plantar flex the feet and ankles.

Downward Movement Phase

Allow the heels to slowly lower back to the starting position.

Maintain the same body position.

After completing the set, replace the supports, and remove the feet.

Common Errors

- Allowing the ankles to invert or evert (i.e., rising on the big or little toes, respectively) during the upward movement phase
- Pulling with the hands or jerking the torso to help raise the weight
- Bouncing the weight to add momentum to help with the next repetition

Primary Muscles Trained

Soleus, gastrocnemius

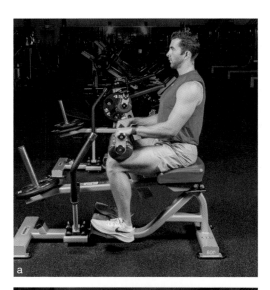

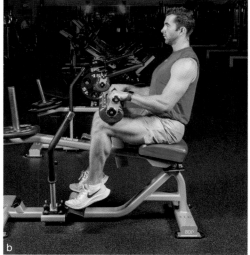

CHEST

FLAT BARBELL BENCH PRESS

Client: Starting Position

Assume a supine position on a bench in the five-point body contact position.

Place the body on the bench so that the eyes are below the bar.

Grasp the bar with a closed, pronated grip slightly wider than shoulder width.

Signal the personal trainer for a liftoff.

Guide the bar to a position over the chest, with the elbows fully extended.

Personal Trainer: Starting Position

Stand erect and very close to the head of the bench (but not so close as to distract the client).

Place the feet shoulder-width apart, in a staggered stance, with the knees slightly flexed.

Grasp the bar with a closed, alternated grip inside the client's hands.

At the client's signal, assist with moving the bar off the supports and to a height that allows the client's elbows to be fully extended.

Guide the bar to a position over the client's chest.

Release the bar smoothly.

Client: Downward Movement Phase

Allow the bar to lower to touch the chest at approximately nipple level.

Allow the elbows to move down past the torso and slightly away from the body.

Keep the wrists rigid and directly above the elbows.

Keep the forearms approximately perpendicular to the floor and parallel to each other.

Maintain the five-point body contact position.

Personal Trainer: Downward Movement Phase

Keep the hands in the alternated grip position close to—but not touching—the bar as it descends.

Slightly flex the knees, hips, and torso and keep the back neutral when following the bar.

Client: Upward Movement Phase

Push the bar upward and very slightly backward until the elbows are fully extended.

Keep the wrists rigid and directly above the elbows.

Maintain the five-point body contact position.

After completing the set, signal the personal trainer for assistance in racking the bar.

Keep a grip on the bar until it is racked.

Personal Trainer: Upward Movement Phase

Keep the hands in the alternated grip position close to—but not touching—the bar as it ascends.

Slightly extend the knees, hips, and torso and keep the back neutral when following the bar.

At the client's signal after the set is completed, grasp the bar with an alternated grip inside the client's hands and help to rack the bar.

Common Errors

- Bouncing the bar on the chest during the upward movement phase to help raise the bar past the sticking point
- Lifting the buttocks off the bench
- Raising the head off the bench during the movement

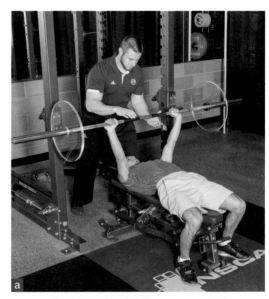

Primary Muscles Trained

Pectoralis major, anterior deltoid, triceps brachii

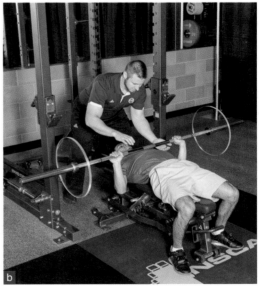

INCLINE DUMBBELL BENCH PRESS

This exercise can also be performed with a barbell using a closed, pronated grip slightly wider than shoulder width. When using a barbell, the spotter will assist by spotting the bar instead of the client's wrists.

Client: Starting Position

Grasp two dumbbells using a closed, pronated grip.

Lie in a supine position on an incline bench in the five-point body contact position.

Signal the personal trainer or spotter for assistance in moving the dumbbells into the starting position.

Press the dumbbells in unison to full elbow extension; arms should be parallel to each other above the head and face.

Personal Trainer: Starting Position

Stand erect and close to the head of the bench, but do not distract the client.

Place the feet shoulder-width apart, with the knees slightly flexed.

Grasp the client's forearms near the wrists.

At the client's signal, assist with moving the dumbbells to a position over the client's head and face.

Release the client's forearms smoothly.

Client: Downward Movement Phase

Lower the dumbbells in an arc motion, ending with the dumbbells slightly out and near the armpits, in line with the upper one-third area of the chest (between the clavicles and the nipples).

Keep the wrists stiff and directly above the elbows.

Maintain the five-point body contact position throughout the movement.

Do not arch the back or raise the chest to meet the dumbbells.

Personal Trainer: Downward Movement Phase

Keep the hands near—but not touching—the top of the client's forearms toward the wrists as the dumbbells descend.

Slightly flex the knees, hips, and torso and keep the back neutral when following the dumbbells.

Client: Upward Movement Phase

Push the dumbbells upward at the same rate in an arc motion.

Dumbbells should be slightly away from each other at the top of the movement.

Maintain stability in the arms by keeping the wrists stiff and directly above the elbows.

Maintain the five-point body contact position.

Personal Trainer: Upward Movement Phase

Keep the hands near—but not touching—the client's forearms near the wrists as the dumbbells ascend.

Slightly extend the knees, hips, and torso and keep the back neutral when following the dumbbells.

Pectoralis major, anterior deltoid, triceps brachii

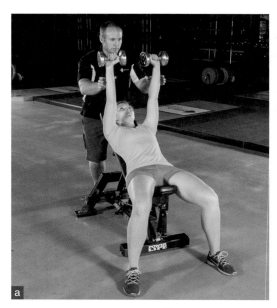

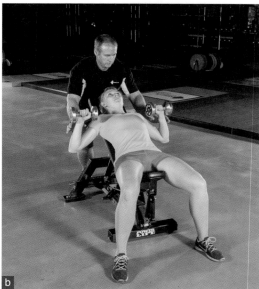

Common Errors

- Lifting the buttocks off the bench
- Excessively arching the back
- Raising the head off the bench during the movement

FLAT DUMBBELL FLY

Client: Starting Position

Assume a supine position on a bench in the five-point body contact position.

On a signal, take the dumbbells from the personal trainer (one at a time) and position them near or on the chest.

Rotate the dumbbells to a neutral grip position.

Signal the personal trainer for assistance to move the dumbbells into an extended elbow position over the chest, with the arms parallel to each other.

Slightly flex the elbows and point them out to the sides.

Personal Trainer: Starting Position

At the client's signal, lift the dumbbells from the floor into the client's hands (one at a time).

While the client adjusts the dumbbells, position one knee on the floor, with the foot of the other leg forward and flat on the floor (or kneel on both knees) very close to the head of the bench (but not so close as to distract the client).

Grasp the client's wrists.

At the client's signal, assist with moving the dumbbells to a position over the client's chest.

Release the client's wrists smoothly.

Client: Downward Movement Phase

Allow the dumbbells to lower at the same rate in a wide arc until they are level with the shoulders or chest.

Keep the dumbbell handles parallel to each other as the elbows move downward.

Keep the wrists rigid and the elbows held in a slightly flexed position.

Keep the dumbbells in line with the elbows and shoulders.

Maintain the five-point body contact position.

Personal Trainer: Downward Movement Phase

Keep the hands near—but not touching—the client's wrists as the dumbbells descend.

Client: Upward Movement Phase

Pull the dumbbells up toward each other in a wide arc back to the starting position; imagine the arc formed by the arms when hugging a very large tree trunk.

Keep the wrists rigid and the elbows held in a slightly flexed position.

Keep the dumbbells in line with the elbows and shoulders.

Maintain the five-point body contact position.

After completing the set, first slowly lower the dumbbells to the chest and armpit area, then signal the personal trainer to return them to the floor.

Primary Muscles Trained

Pectoralis major, anterior deltoid

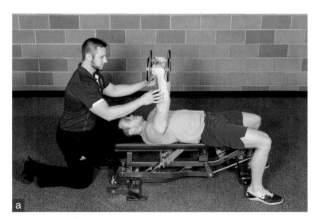

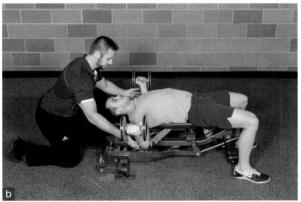

Personal Trainer: Upward Movement Phase

Keep the hands near—but not touching—the client's wrists as the dumbbells ascend.

At the client's signal, take the dumbbells from the client and return them to the floor.

Common Errors

- Allowing the elbows to flex and extend during the movement
- Lifting the buttocks off the bench
- Raising the head off the bench during the movement
- Lowering the dumbbells below chest level

PEC DECK (BUTTERFLY)

There are a variety of machine configurations for this exercise; the bullet points describe the machine shown in the photos. A common variation has forearm pads, elbow pads, or both. For that version, adjust the seat height before beginning the exercise to position the shoulders slightly above the bottom of the forearm pads (or in line with the elbow pads) with the elbows flexed to 90 degrees when the hands are holding on to the handles. During the movement, press the forearms and elbows against their respective pads to squeeze the handles together; do not pull the handles together using the hands.

Starting Position

Sit in the machine with the back, hips, and buttocks pressed against their pads.

If the seat is adjustable, move it up or down to

- position the feet flat on the floor in the seated position;
- position the shoulders in line with the handles; and
- position the upper arms approximately parallel to the floor when the hands are holding on to the handles.

Grasp the handles with a closed, neutral grip and the elbows in a slightly to moderately flexed position.

If the handles are too far back to be grasped from the seated position, push down on the foot pedal (if available), or request the assistance of a spotter.

Begin the exercise with the handles together in front of the chest.

Backward Movement Phase

Begin the exercise by allowing both handles to swing out and back slowly and under control.

Keep the wrists locked, the elbows held in the same slightly to moderately flexed position, and the upper arms approximately parallel to the floor.

Allow the handles to move back so they are level with the chest (a short distance farther than what is seen in the photo, if that is comfortable for the client's shoulders).

Forward Movement Phase

Move the handles out and then toward each other back to the starting position.

Keep the elbows held in the same slightly to moderately flexed position.

At the completion of the set, guide the handles backward to their resting position (one at a time, or with the assistance of a spotter).

Common Errors

- Positioning the seat too low or too high
- Swinging the handles back to add momentum to help with the next repetition

Primary Muscles Trained

Pectoralis major, anterior deltoid

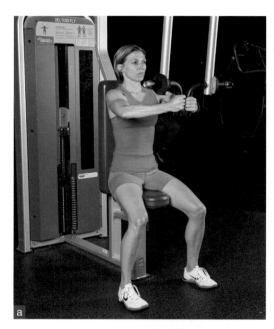

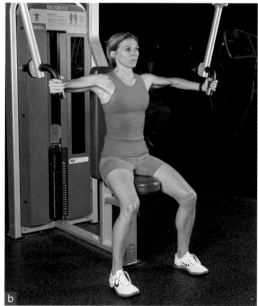

- Flexing the torso forward to help move the handles together

CHEST PRESS (RESISTANCE BAND)

Starting Position

Grasp the handles of the resistance band with a closed, pronated grip, and evenly wrap the band around the upper back at nipple height.

Stand erect with the feet shoulder-width apart and the knees slightly flexed (slightly more than what is seen in the photo).

Position the handles to the outside of the chest at or slightly above nipple height, with the palms facing down.

In this position, the resistance band should be nearly taut (not stretched); if not, select a shorter band.

Forward Movement Phase

Push the handles away from the chest until the elbows are fully extended.

Keep the arms parallel to the floor.

Maintain the erect standing position, with the heels on the floor and the knees slightly flexed.

Backward Movement Phase

Allow the handles to slowly move backward to the starting position.

Keep the arms parallel to the floor.

Maintain the erect standing position, with the heels on the floor and the knees slightly flexed.

Common Errors

- Forcefully locking out the elbows at the end of the forward movement phase
- Shortening the range of motion during the backward movement phase

Primary Muscles Trained

Pectoralis major, anterior deltoid, triceps brachii

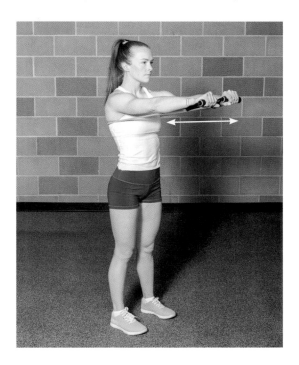

VERTICAL CHEST PRESS

Starting Position

Sit in the machine with the head, back, hips, and buttocks pressed against their pads.

If the seat is adjustable, move it up or down to

- position the thighs approximately parallel to the floor, with the feet flat in the starting seated position; and
- put the body in line with the handgrips (an imaginary line connecting both handgrips should cross the front of the chest at nipple height, although this may vary based on the machine's design).

Grasp the handles with a closed, pronated grip and move them forward so they begin at chest level. If the handles are too far back to be grasped from the seated position, push down on the foot pedal (if available), or request the assistance of a spotter to move the handles slightly forward.

Forward Movement Phase

Push the handles away from the chest until the elbows are fully extended.

Maintain the five-point body contact position.

Backward Movement Phase

Allow the handles to slowly move backward so they are level with the chest.

Maintain the five-point body contact position.

After completing the set, guide the handles backward to their resting position.

Common Errors

- Positioning the seat too low or too high
- Arching the back or pushing with the legs during the forward movement phase
- Flexing the torso forward to help move the handles forward
- Forcefully locking out the elbows at the end of the forward movement phase
- Shortening the range of motion during the backward movement phase

Primary Muscles Trained

Pectoralis major, anterior deltoid, triceps brachii

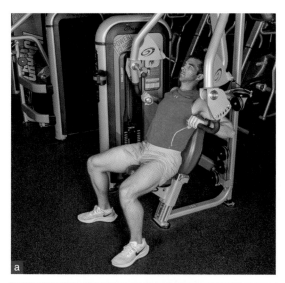

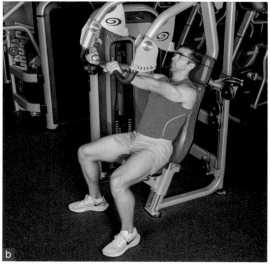

HIPS AND THIGHS

LEG PRESS

Starting Position

Sit in the machine with the back, hips, and buttocks pressed against their pads. (If the horizontal position of the foot platform or the seat is adjustable, move it forward or backward to allow the thighs to be parallel to the foot platform when seated in the starting position.)

Place the feet flat in the middle of the platform (or one foot on each pedal as seen in the photos) in a hip-width position, with the toes slightly pointed out.

Position the thighs and lower legs parallel to each other.

Grasp the handles or the sides of the seat.

Forward Movement Phase

Extend the hips and knees to push the platform or pedals forward (note that in some machines, the foot platform is fixed so the seat will move backward during this phase, or in machines with two pedals, the pedals will move independently).

Push to a fully extended position while maintaining the same upper body position and the heels in contact with the platform or pedals.

Backward Movement Phase

Allow the hips and knees to slowly flex to lower the weight.

Keep the hips and buttocks on the seat and the back pressed against the back pad.

Keep the legs parallel to each other.

Continue flexing the hips and knees to return to the starting position.

Common Errors

- Allowing the heels to lift off the platform or pedals, the buttocks to lose contact with the seat, or the hands to let go during the movement
- Allowing the knees to move in (via hip adduction) or out (via hip abduction) during the movement
- Locking the knees out at the end of the forward movement phase

Primary Muscles Trained

Gluteus maximus, semimembranosus, semitendinosus, biceps femoris, vastus lateralis, vastus intermedius, vastus medialis, rectus femoris

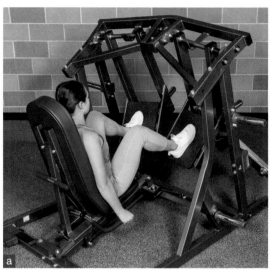

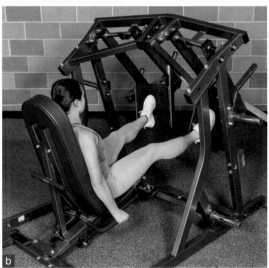

BACK SQUAT

Client: Starting Position

Step under the bar and position the feet parallel to each other.

Place the hands on the bar using the "high bar position" technique:

- Grasp the bar with a closed, pronated grip slightly wider than shoulder width.
- Dip the head under the bar and move the body to place the bar evenly above the posterior deltoids at the base of the neck.

Lift the elbows up to create a shelf for the bar to rest on.

Hold the chest up and out.

Pull the scapulae toward each other.

Tilt the head slightly up.

Once in position, signal the spotters for a liftoff.

Extend the hips and knees to lift the bar off the rack and take one or two steps backward (not as far as what is seen in the photos).

Position the feet shoulder-width or wider apart and even with each other, with the toes slightly pointed outward.

Keep the elbows lifted and backward to keep the bar on the shoulders.

Two Spotters: Starting Position

Stand erect at opposite ends of the bar, with the feet shoulder-width apart and the knees slightly flexed.

Grasp the end of the bar by cupping the hands together with the palms facing upward or forward.

At the client's signal, assist with lifting and balancing the bar (if needed) as it is moved out of the rack.

Release the bar smoothly in unison with the other spotter.

Hold the hands 2 to 3 inches (5.1-7.6 cm) below the ends of the bar.

Move sideways in unison with the client as the client moves backward.

Once the client is in position, assume a hip-width stance, with the knees slightly flexed and the torso erect.

Client: Downward Movement Phase

Allow the hips and knees to slowly flex while keeping a relatively constant angle between the torso and the floor.

Maintain a position with the back neutral, elbows high, and chest up and out.

Keep the heels on the floor and the knees aligned over the feet.

Continue allowing the hips and knees to flex until one of these three events first occurs (this determines the client's maximum range of motion; the lowest or "bottom" position):

- The thighs are parallel to the floor.

Primary Muscles Trained

Gluteus maximus, semimembranosus, semitendinosus, biceps femoris, vastus lateralis, vastus intermedius, vastus medialis, rectus femoris

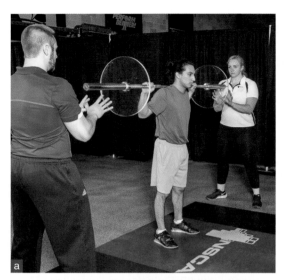

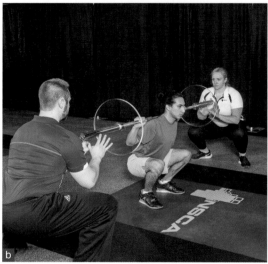

- The trunk begins to round or flex forward.
- The heels rise off the floor.

Two Spotters: Downward Movement Phase

Keep the hands close to—but not touching—the bar as it descends.

Slightly flex the knees, hips, and torso and keep the back neutral when following the bar.

Client: Upward Movement Phase

Extend the hips and knees at the same rate to keep a relatively constant angle between the torso and the floor.

Maintain a position with the back neutral, elbows high, and chest up and out.

Keep the heels on the floor and the knees aligned over the feet.

Continue extending the hips and knees to reach the starting position.

After completing the set, step forward and rack the bar.

Two Spotters: Upward Movement Phase

Keep the hands close to—but not touching—the bar as it ascends.

Slightly extend the knees, hips, and torso and keep the back neutral when following the bar.

After the set is completed, help the client rack the bar.

Common Errors

- Allowing the heels to lift off the floor, the torso to flex further forward, or the upper back to round during the upward movement phase
- Allowing the knees to move in (via hip adduction) or out (via hip abduction) during the movement
- Allowing the arms to relax or the elbows to drop down and forward

SQUAT (RESISTANCE BAND)

Starting Position

Grasp the handles of the resistance band with a closed, pronated grip.

Position the feet shoulder-width apart, with the toes slightly pointed outward and the arches of both feet on top of a middle section of the resistance band.

Position the handles to the outside and level with the top of the shoulders, palms facing forward.

Create a neutral spine position, with the chest held up and out and the shoulders back.

Flex the hips and knees to assume the lowest desired squat position.

In this position, the resistance band should be nearly taut (not stretched); if not, select a shorter band.

Upward Movement Phase

Extend the hips and knees at the same rate to keep a relatively constant angle between the torso and the floor.

Maintain the neutral spine position, with the chest held up and out.

Keep the heels on the floor and the knees aligned over the feet.

Continue extending the hips and knees to a fully standing position.

Downward Movement Phase

Allow the hips and knees to slowly flex while keeping a relatively constant angle between the torso and the floor.

Maintain the neutral spine position, with the chest held up and out.

Keep the heels on the floor and the knees aligned over the feet.

Continue allowing the hips and knees to flex until reaching the lowest desired squat position.

Primary Muscles Trained

Gluteus maximus, semimembranosus, semitendinosus, biceps femoris, vastus lateralis, vastus intermedius, vastus medialis, rectus femoris

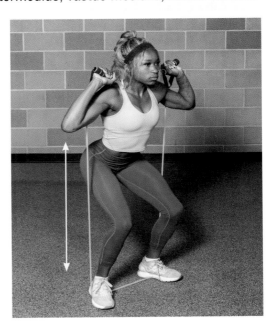

Common Errors

- Allowing the heels to lift off the floor, the torso to flex further forward, or the upper back to round during the upward movement phase
- Allowing the knees to move in (via hip adduction) or out (via hip abduction) during the movement

FRONT SQUAT

Client: Starting Position

Walk up to the bar and position the feet parallel to each other.

Place the hands on the bar using the "parallel arm position" technique:

- Grasp the bar with a closed, pronated grip slightly wider than shoulder width.
- Move the body to place the bar evenly on top of the anterior deltoids and clavicles.
- Fully flex the elbows and hyperextend the wrists to position the upper arms parallel to the floor. The back of the hands should be either on top of or just to the outside of the shoulders, right next to where the bar is resting on the deltoids.
- Hold the chest up and out.
- Pull the scapulae toward each other.
- Tilt the head slightly up.
- Once in position, signal the spotters for a liftoff.
- Extend the hips and knees to lift the bar off the rack and take one or two steps backward (not as far as what is seen in the photos).
- Position the feet shoulder-width or wider apart and even with each other, with the toes slightly pointed outward.
- Keep the elbows lifted and forward to keep the bar on the shoulders.

Two Spotters: Starting Position

Stand erect at opposite ends of the bar, with the feet shoulder-width apart and the knees slightly flexed.

Grasp the end of the bar by cupping the hands together, with the palms facing upward or forward.

At the client's signal, assist with lifting and balancing the bar (if needed) as it is moved out of the rack.

Release the bar smoothly in unison with the other spotter.

Hold the hands 2 to 3 inches (5.1-7.6 cm) below the ends of the bar.

Move sideways in unison with the client as the client moves backward.

Once the client is in position, assume a hip-width stance, with the knees slightly flexed and the torso erect.

Client: Downward Movement Phase

Allow the hips and knees to slowly flex while keeping a relatively constant angle between the torso and the floor.

Maintain a position with the back neutral, elbows high, and chest up and out.

Keep the heels on the floor and the knees aligned over the feet.

Continue allowing the hips and knees to flex until one of these three events first occurs (this determines the client's maximum range of motion; the lowest or "bottom" position):

Primary Muscles Trained

Gluteus maximus, semimembranosus, semitendinosus, biceps femoris, vastus lateralis, vastus intermedius, vastus medialis, rectus femoris

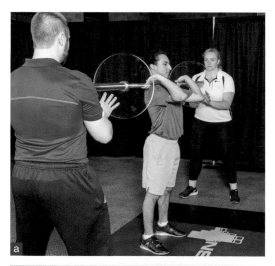

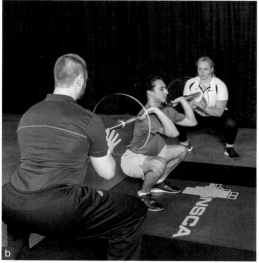

- The thighs are parallel to the floor.
- The trunk begins to round or flex forward.
- The heels rise off the floor.

Two Spotters: Downward Movement Phase

Keep the hands close to—but not touching—the bar as it descends.

Slightly flex the knees, hips, and torso and keep the back neutral when following the bar.

Client: Upward Movement Phase

Extend the hips and knees at the same rate to keep a relatively constant angle between the torso and the floor.

Maintain a position with the back neutral, elbows high, and chest up and out.

Keep the heels on the floor and the knees aligned over the feet.

Continue extending the hips and knees to reach the starting position.

After completing the set, step forward and rack the bar.

Two Spotters: Upward Movement Phase

Keep the hands close to—but not touching—the bar as it ascends.

Slightly extend the knees, hips, and torso and keep the back neutral when following the bar.

After the set is completed, help the client rack the bar.

BULGARIAN SQUAT

The Bulgarian (split) squat is not typically performed with a spotter. However, for clients who lack stability and balance, a railing, fixed stationary object, or spotter may be necessary. If using a barbell, then two spotters should be used, one on each side of the barbell.

Client: Starting Position

Place a barbell on the upper back and shoulders in either the high or low bar position with a closed, pronated grip.

For a dumbbell variation, hold a dumbbell in each hand with a closed, neutral grip and arms resting by the sides of the body.

Stand in front of a bench or box that is approximately knee height, with the feet approximately shoulder-width apart.

Facing away from the bench or box, take a moderate step forward with one leg and place the instep of the back foot on top of the bench or box.

Allow both knees to be slightly flexed, with the torso in a nearly erect position and tightly packed shoulders.

Two Spotters: Starting Position

The spotters should stand erect at opposite ends of the bar, with the feet hip-width apart and the knees slightly flexed.

Hold the hands 2 to 3 inches (5.1-7.6 cm) below the end of the bar.

If the dumbbell variation is performed, no spotter is needed.

Client: Downward Movement Phase

Flex the hip and knee of the forward leg simultaneously to lower the body in a vertical plane while keeping a relatively constant angle between the torso and the floor.

Keep the heel of the forward foot flat on the floor and the instep of the back foot on top of the bench or box.

Continue flexing the hip and knee until the front thigh is approximately parallel to the floor.

Common Errors

- Allowing the heels to lift off the floor, the torso to flex forward, or the upper back to round during the upward movement phase
- Allowing the knees to move in (via hip adduction) or out (via hip abduction) during the movement
- Allowing the arms to relax or the elbows to drop down and backward

Primary Muscles Trained

Gluteus maximus, semimembranosus, semitendinosus, biceps femoris, vastus lateralis, vastus intermedius, vastus medialis, rectus femoris

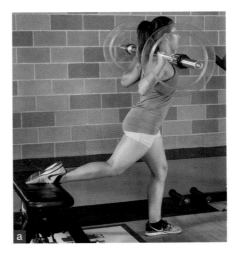

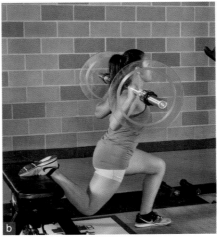

Two Spotters: Downward Movement Phase

Keep the cupped hands close to—but not touching—the bar as it descends.

Slightly flex the knees, hips, and torso and keep the back neutral when following the bar.

Client: Upward Movement Phase

Raise the bar under control by actively extending the forward hip and knee; extend the other hip and knee also to keep a relatively constant angle between the torso and the floor.

Maintain a neutral spine, and keep the torso upright.

Keep the forward knee aligned over the forward foot.

Do not flex the torso forward or round the spine.

Continue extending the hip and knee of the forward leg to reach the starting position.

Repeat for the desired number of repetitions, and then switch the forward leg.

FORWARD LUNGE

Client: Starting Position

Grasp the bar with a closed, pronated grip slightly wider than shoulder width.

Step under the bar and position the feet parallel to each other.

Place the bar evenly on the upper back and shoulders above the posterior deltoids at the base of the neck.

Lift the elbows up to create a shelf for the bar to rest on.

Hold the chest up and out.

Pull the scapulae toward each other.

Tilt the head slightly up.

Once in position, signal the spotter for a liftoff.

Extend the hips and knees to lift the bar off the rack and take two or three steps backward.

Place the feet hip-width apart, with the toes pointed ahead.

Personal Trainer: Starting Position

Stand erect and very close to the client (but not close enough to be a distraction).

Place the feet shoulder-width apart, with the knees slightly flexed.

At the client's signal, assist with lifting and balancing the bar as it is moved out of the rack (if needed).

Move in unison with the client as the client moves backward to the starting position.

Once the client is in position, assume a hip-width stance, with the knees slightly flexed and the torso erect.

Position the hands near the client's hips, waist, or torso.

Two Spotters: Upward Movement Phase

Keep cupped hands close to—but not touching—the bar as it ascends.

Slightly extend the knees, hips, and torso and keep the back neutral when following the bar.

Common Errors

- Allowing the lead knee to extend too far past the lead foot
- Allowing the torso to extremely flex forward during the downward movement phase
- Elevating the back foot too high
- Stepping too far forward with the front foot
- Not maintaining a neutral pelvis or spine

Primary Muscles Trained

Gluteus maximus, semimembranosus, semitendinosus, biceps femoris, vastus lateralis, vastus intermedius, vastus medialis, rectus femoris, iliopsoas (of the trailing leg), soleus and gastrocnemius (of the lead leg)

Client: Forward Movement Phase

Take one exaggerated step directly forward with one leg (the lead leg).

Keep the torso erect as the lead foot moves forward and contacts the floor.

Keep the trailing foot in the starting position but allow the trailing knee to slightly flex.

Plant the lead foot flat on the floor, pointing straight ahead or slightly inward. To help maintain balance, place this foot directly ahead from its initial position, with the lead ankle, knee, and hip in one vertical plane.

Allow the lead hip and knee to slowly flex. Once balance has shifted to be even on both feet, flex the lead knee to lower the trailing knee toward the floor. The trailing knee will flex somewhat further, but not to the same degree as the lead knee.

Keep the lead knee over the lead foot (which remains flat on the floor).

Lower the trailing knee—still slightly flexed—until it is 1 to 2 inches (2.5-5.1 cm) above the floor. At this point, the lead knee will be flexed to about 90 degrees, with the lower leg perpendicular to the floor.

Balance the weight evenly between the ball of the trailing foot and the entire lead foot.

Keep the torso perpendicular to the floor by "sitting back" on the trailing leg. Actual lunge depth, however, depends primarily on the client's hip joint flexibility.

Personal Trainer: Forward Movement Phase

Step forward with the same foot as the client.

Plant the lead foot 12 to 18 inches (30.5-45.7 cm) behind the client's foot.

Flex the lead knee as the client's lead knee flexes.

Keep the torso erect.

Keep the hands near the client's hips, waist, or torso.

Assist only when necessary to keep the client balanced.

Client: Backward Movement Phase

Shift the balance forward to the lead foot, and forcefully push off the floor by extending the lead hip and knee. As the lead foot moves back toward the trailing foot, balance will shift back to the trailing foot. This will cause the heel of the trailing foot to regain contact with the floor.

Maintain the same torso position.

Bring the lead foot back to a position next to the trailing foot.

Stand erect in the starting position, pause, and then alternate lead legs.

After completing the set, step forward and rack the bar.

Personal Trainer: Backward Movement Phase

Push backward with the lead leg in unison with the client.

Bring the lead foot back to a position next to the trailing foot.

Keep the hands near the client's hips, waist, or torso.

Stand erect in the starting position, pause to wait for the client, and alternate lead legs.

Assist only when necessary to keep the client balanced.

After the set is completed, help the client rack the bar.

Common Errors

- Stepping out too shallowly, causing the lead knee to extend too far past the lead foot
- Allowing the torso to flex forward during the forward movement phase
- Quickly jerking the torso backward during the backward movement phase
- Stutter-stepping backward during the backward movement phase
- Not maintaining a neutral pelvis or spine

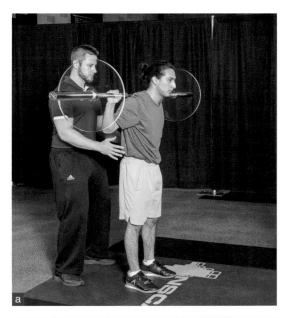

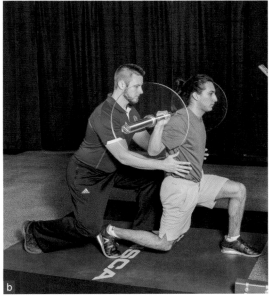

BARBELL HIP THRUST

Starting Position

Assume a seated position on the floor perpendicular to a flat bench, with the upper back firmly leaning against the long side of the bench. (Be sure that the bench is fixed and will not move during the exercise.)

Roll a loaded barbell over the legs, grasp the bar with a wide, pronated grip, and position the bar over the hips.

Flex the hips and knees to approximately 90 degrees and position the feet flat on the floor, shoulder-width apart.

Note: A pad may be placed on the bar to reduce any potential discomfort caused by the bar across the hips.

Upward Movement Phase

While keeping the feet flat on the floor, extend the hips to lift the bar from the floor. (The knees will extend also, but the muscular effort should be focused on the hip extensors.)

Use the upper back as a pivot point while firmly pressing against the bench.

Continue extending the hips until the torso and thighs are parallel to the floor.

Downward Movement Phase

Allow the hips and knees to slowly flex back to the starting position while using the upper back as a pivot point.

Continue to lower the bar until the buttocks are just above the floor, then perform the next repetition.

Keep the back neutral and the shoulder blades in contact with bench.

Common Errors

- Arching (hyperextending) the lower back during the upward movement phase
- Not extending the hips as far as needed at the top position (limited range of motion)
- Allowing the back to slide up and down the bench instead of being used as a pivot point

Primary Muscles Trained

Gluteus maximus, semimembranosus, semitendinosus, biceps femoris

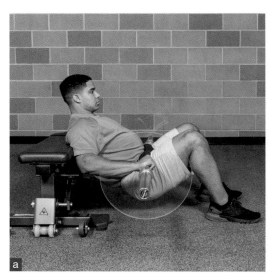

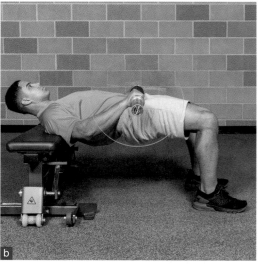

ROMANIAN DEADLIFT (RDL)

Starting Position

Grasp a barbell with a closed, pronated grip using either a clean (*a*) or snatch (*b*) grip. After performing the deadlift exercise to lift the bar off the floor, slightly to moderately flex the knees and keep them in this position throughout this exercise.

The barbell should be resting at midthigh height at the starting position.

Downward Movement Phase

Begin the exercise by flexing the hips and pushing them backward to perform a hip hinge.

Allow the torso to move forward, keeping the bar in contact with the thighs.

Keep the knees slightly flexed, and continue flexing the hips until the barbell has reached just below the knee.

Maintain a rigid torso and neutral spine, and keep the shoulders retracted.

Keep a normal lordotic position throughout the movement.

Upward Movement Phase

Slowly extend the hips while raising the torso back to the starting standing position.

Primary Muscles Trained

Gluteus maximus, semimembranosus, semitendinosus, biceps femoris, erector spinae

Keep the knees slightly flexed and the torso in a neutral spine position.

Make sure the barbell maintains contact with the thighs throughout the movement.

Do not hyperextend the back or flex the elbows.

Common Errors

- Arching (hyperextending) the lower back at the starting position
- Not keeping the bar close to the body throughout the movement
- Flexing forward instead of pushing the hips back throughout the downward movement
- Rounding the back throughout the movement

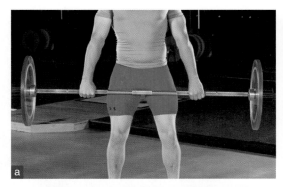

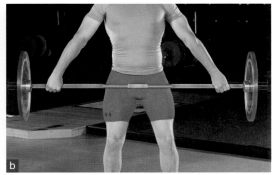

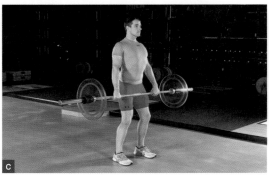

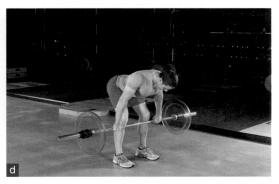

LEG (KNEE) EXTENSION

Starting Position

Sit in the machine with the thighs and back in the center of their pads (not to the left or right side) and the knees aligned with the axis of the machine. If the back pad is adjustable, move it forward or backward to align the knees with the axis of the machine, and position the buttocks and thighs so that the backs of the knees are touching the front end of the seat.

Hook the feet under the ankle pad or pads; if the pad is adjustable, position it so it is in contact with the instep of the foot.

Position the thighs, lower legs, and feet parallel to each other.

Grasp the handles or the sides of the seat.

Upward Movement Phase

Keeping the thighs, lower legs, and feet parallel to each other, extend the knees until they are straight.

Keep the torso erect and the back firmly pressed against the back pad.

Maintain a tight grip on the handles or the sides of the seat.

Downward Movement Phase

Allow the knees to slowly flex back to the starting position.

Keep the thighs, lower legs, and feet parallel to each other.

Keep the torso erect and the back firmly pressed against the back pad.

Maintain a tight grip on the handles or the sides of the seat.

Common Errors

- Allowing the hips or buttocks to lift off the seat during the upward movement phase
- Swinging the legs or jerking the torso backward to help raise the weight
- Forcefully locking out the knees at the end of the upward movement phase

Primary Muscles Trained

Vastus lateralis, vastus intermedius, vastus medialis, rectus femoris

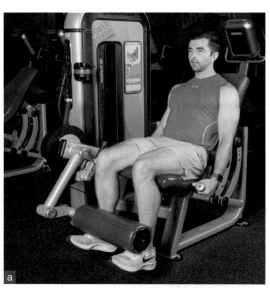

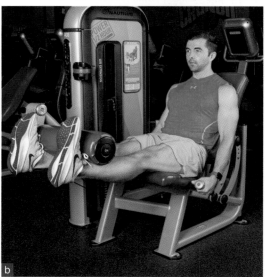

LYING LEG (KNEE) CURL

Starting Position

Assume a prone position on the machine, with the hips and torso in the center of their pads (not to the left or right side) and the knees aligned with the axis of the machine.

Hook the feet under the ankle pad or pads; if the pad is adjustable, position it so it is in contact with the back of the heel just above the top of the shoe.

Once in proper position, the knees should be hanging slightly off the bottom edge of the thigh pad.

Position the thighs, lower legs, and feet parallel to each other.

Grasp the handles or the sides of the chest pad.

Upward Movement Phase

Keeping the thighs, lower legs, and feet parallel to each other, flex the knees until the ankle pad touches (or nearly touches, depending on the machine) the buttocks.

Keep the torso stationary.

Maintain a tight grip on the handles or the sides of the chest pad.

Downward Movement Phase

Allow the knees to slowly extend back to the starting position.

Keep the thighs, lower legs, and feet parallel to each other.

Keep the torso stationary.

Maintain a tight grip on the handles or the sides of the chest pad.

Common Errors

- Allowing the hips to rise (using hip flexion) during the upward movement phase
- Swinging the legs backward to help raise the weight
- Locking out the knees at the end of the downward movement phase

Primary Muscles Trained

Semimembranosus, semitendinosus, biceps femoris

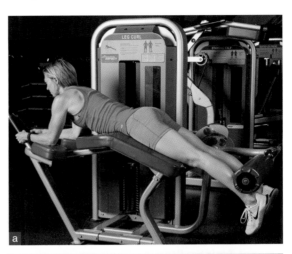

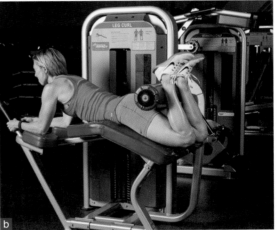

SHOULDERS

SHOULDER PRESS (BAR)

Client: Starting Position

Sit on a shoulder press bench and lean back to assume the five-point body contact position (if the back pad is long enough; if not, there will only be four points of contact). If the seat can be adjusted, modify its height to

- position the thighs parallel to the floor (with the feet flat) and
- allow the bar to move in and out of the rack without hitting the top of the head (the seat is too high) or having to half-stand up to reach the rack (the seat is too low).

Grasp the bar with a closed, pronated grip slightly wider than shoulder width.

Signal the personal trainer for a liftoff.

Press the bar over the head until the elbows are fully extended.

Personal Trainer: Starting Position

Stand erect on the step at the back of the bench or on the spotter's platform (if present) with the feet shoulder-width apart, if there is enough room, and the knees slightly flexed.

Grasp the bar with a closed, alternated grip inside the client's hands.

At the client's signal, assist with moving the bar off the rack.

Guide the bar to a position over the client's head.

Release the bar (or wrists) smoothly.

Client: Downward Movement Phase

Allow the elbows to slowly flex to lower the bar toward the head.

Keep the wrists rigid and directly above the elbows. The width of the grip will determine how parallel the forearms are to each other.

Extend the neck slightly to allow the bar to pass by the face as the bar is lowered to touch (or be at the level of) the clavicles and anterior deltoids.

Maintain the five-point body contact position.

Personal Trainer: Downward Movement Phase

Keep the hands in the alternated grip position close to—but not touching—the bar as it descends.

Slightly flex the knees, hips, and torso and keep the back neutral when following the bar.

Client: Upward Movement Phase

Push the bar upward until the elbows are fully extended.

Extend the neck slightly to allow the bar to pass by the face as it is raised.

Primary Muscles Trained

Anterior and medial deltoids, triceps brachii

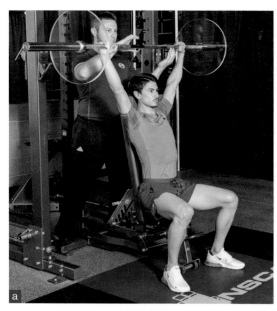

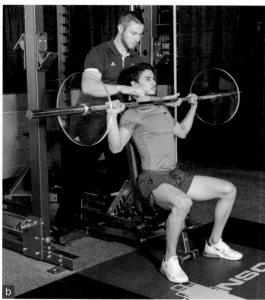

Keep the wrists rigid and directly above the elbows.

Maintain the five-point body contact position.

After completing the set, signal the personal trainer for assistance in racking the bar.

Keep a grip on the bar until it is racked.

Personal Trainer: Upward Movement Phase

Keep the hands in the alternated grip position close to—but not touching—the bar as it ascends.

Slightly extend the knees, hips, and torso and keep the back neutral when following the bar.

After the set is completed, help the client rack the bar.

Common Errors

- Pushing with the legs or rising off the seat to help raise the bar upward
- Excessively arching the back during the upward movement phase

MACHINE SHOULDER PRESS

Starting Position

Sit down and lean back to place the body in the five-point body contact position.

Grasp the handles with a closed, pronated grip.

Align the handles with the top of the shoulders by adjusting either the seat height or handle height (depending on the machine).

Upward Movement Phase

Push the handles upward until the elbows are fully extended.

Maintain the five-point body contact position.

Do not arch the lower back or forcefully lock out the elbows.

Downward Movement Phase

Allow the elbows to slowly flex to lower the handles to the starting position.

Maintain the five-point body contact position.

Common Errors

- Not executing the full range of motion
- Excessively arching the back during the upward movement phase

Primary Muscles Trained

Anterior and medial deltoids, triceps brachii

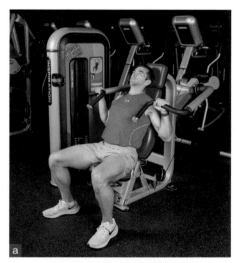

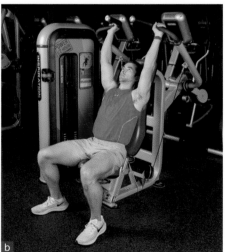

SHOULDER PRESS (RESISTANCE BAND)

Starting Position

Grasp the handles of the resistance band with a closed, pronated grip.

Sit on the floor or mat with the buttocks on top of a middle section of the resistance band.

Assume an erect position, with the torso perpendicular to the floor and the legs together and extended away from the body.

Slightly flex the hips and knees for balance.

Position the handles to the outside and level with the top of the shoulders, with the palms facing forward.

In this position, the resistance band should be nearly taut (not stretched); if not, select a shorter band.

Upward Movement Phase

Push the handles upward until the elbows are fully extended.

Keep the wrists rigid and directly above the elbows.

Maintain an erect torso, with the legs in the same position.

Downward Movement Phase

Allow the handles to slowly move backward to the starting position.

Maintain an erect torso, with the legs in the same position.

Common Errors

- Excessively arching the back during the upward movement phase
- Flexing the torso forward during the downward movement phase

Primary Muscles Trained

Anterior and medial deltoids, triceps brachii

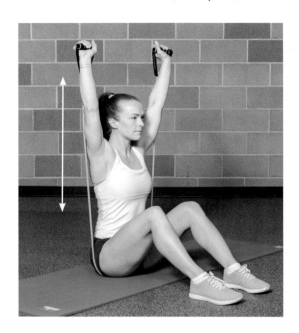

DUMBBELL LATERAL RAISE

Starting Position

Grasp two dumbbells with a closed, neutral grip.

Position the feet shoulder- or hip-width apart, knees slightly flexed, torso erect, shoulders back, and eyes focused ahead.

Move the dumbbells to the front of the thighs, positioning them with the palms facing each other.

Slightly flex the elbows and hold this flexed position throughout the exercise.

Upward Movement Phase

Raise the dumbbells up and out to the sides; the elbows and upper arms should rise together and ahead of (and slightly higher than) the forearms and hands/dumbbells. This movement is similar to pouring liquid out of a plastic jug.

Maintain an erect upper body position, with the knees slightly flexed and feet flat.

Continue raising the dumbbells until the arms are approximately parallel to the floor or nearly level with the shoulders. At the highest position, the elbows and upper arms will be slightly higher than the forearms and hands/dumbbells.

Downward Movement Phase

Allow the dumbbells to lower slowly back to the starting position.

Keep the knees slightly flexed, feet flat on the floor, and eyes focused ahead.

Common Errors

- Extending or flexing the elbows during the movement
- Shrugging the shoulders, arching the back, extending the knees, or rising on the toes to help raise the dumbbells upward
- Flexing the torso forward or allowing the body's weight to shift toward the toes during the downward movement phase

Primary Muscles Trained

Deltoids

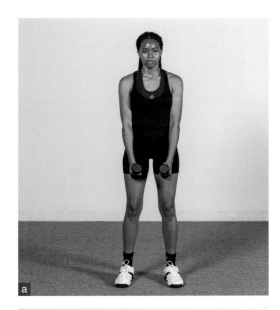

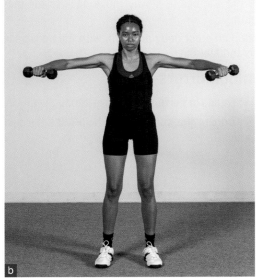

LATERAL RAISE (RESISTANCE BAND)

Starting Position

Grasp the handles of the resistance band with a closed, neutral grip.

Position the feet shoulder-width apart, with the arches of both feet on top of a middle section of the resistance band.

Stand erect with the knees slightly flexed.

Position the handles outside of the thighs, with the arms at the sides and the palms facing inward.

In this position, the resistance band should be nearly taut (not stretched); if not, take up the slack by widening the stance or selecting a shorter band.

Upward Movement Phase

Pull the handles up and out to the sides; the hands, forearms, elbows, and upper arms should rise together.

Maintain an erect body position, with the knees slightly flexed and feet flat.

Continue raising the handles until the arms are approximately parallel to the floor or nearly level with the shoulders.

Downward Movement Phase

Allow the handles to slowly move back to the starting position.

Maintain an erect body position, with the knees slightly flexed and feet flat.

Common Errors

- Extending or flexing the elbows during the movement
- Shrugging the shoulders to help raise the handles upward

Primary Muscles Trained

Deltoids

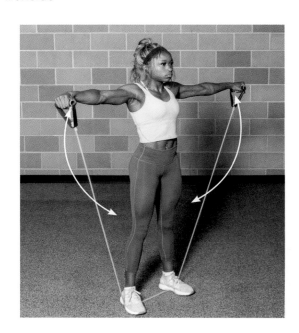

UPRIGHT ROW

Starting Position

Grasp the bar with a closed, pronated grip approximately shoulder-width apart or slightly wider.

Stand erect with feet shoulder-width apart, knees slightly flexed.

Rest the bar on the front of the thighs, with the elbows fully extended and pointing out to the sides.

Upward Movement Phase

Pull the bar up along the abdomen and chest toward the chin.

Keep the elbows pointed out to the sides as the bar brushes against the body.

Keep the torso and knees in the same position.

Do not rise on the toes or swing the bar upward.

At the highest bar position, the elbows should be level with or slightly higher than the shoulders and wrists.

Downward Movement Phase

Allow the bar to slowly descend back to the starting position.

Keep the torso and knees in the same position.

Common Errors

- Not maintaining an erect torso throughout the movement
- Not keeping the bar close to the body
- Lifting through the wrists and not the elbows

Primary Muscles Trained

Deltoids, upper trapezius

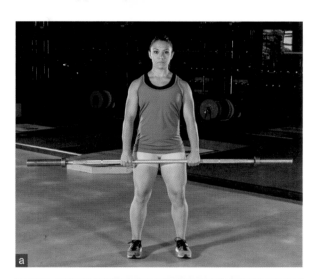

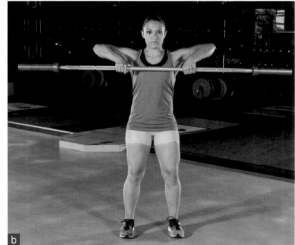

WHOLE BODY

POWER CLEAN

This exercise consists of four phases (first pull, scoop, second pull, and catch), but there is no pause between them; the bar is lifted (pulled up) from the floor to the front of the shoulders in one continuous movement.

Starting Position

Stand with the feet placed between hip- and shoulder-width apart, with the toes pointed slightly outward.

Squat down with the hips lower than the shoulders and grasp the bar with a closed, pronated grip.

Place the hands on the bar slightly wider than shoulder-width apart, outside of the knees, with the elbows fully extended.

Place the feet flat on the floor and position the bar approximately 1 inch (3 cm) in front of the shins and over the balls of the feet.

Position the body with the

- back neutral or slightly arched,
- trapezius relaxed and slightly stretched,
- chest held up and out,
- scapulae retracted,
- head in line with the spine or slightly hyperextended,
- shoulders over or slightly in front of the bar, and
- eyes focused straight ahead
- or slightly upward.

Upward Movement Phase: First Pull

Lift the bar off the floor by forcefully extending the hips and knees.

Keep a relatively constant angle between the torso and the floor.

Do not let the hips rise before the shoulders.

Maintain a neutral spine position.

Keep the elbows fully extended, the head neutral in relation to the spine, and the shoulders over or slightly ahead of the bar.

As the bar is raised, keep it as close to the shins as possible.

Upward Movement Phase: Scoop (Transition)

As the bar rises just above the knees, thrust the hips forward and slightly re-flex the knees to move the thighs against and the knees under the bar.

Keep the back neutral or slightly arched, the elbows fully extended and pointing out to the sides, and the head in line with the spine.

Upward Movement Phase: Second Pull

Forcefully and quickly extend the hips and knees and plantar flex the ankles.

Keep the bar near to or in contact with the front of the thighs.

Keep the bar as close to the body as possible.

Primary Muscles Trained

Gluteus maximus, semimembranosus, semitendinosus, biceps femoris, vastus lateralis, vastus intermedius, vastus medialis, rectus femoris, soleus, gastrocnemius, deltoids, trapezius

Keep the back neutral, the elbows pointing out to the sides, and the head in line with the spine.

Keep the shoulders over the bar and the elbows extended as long as possible.

When the lower body joints reach full extension, rapidly shrug the shoulders upward, but do not allow the elbows to flex yet.

As the shoulders reach their highest elevation, flex the elbows to begin pulling the body under the bar.

Because of the explosive nature of this phase, the torso will be erect or slightly hyperextended, the head will be tilted slightly back, and the feet may lose contact with the floor.

Upward Movement Phase: Catch

After the lower body has fully extended and the bar reaches near-maximal height, pull the body under the bar, and rotate the arms around and under the bar.

Simultaneously, the hips and knees flex into a quarter-squat position.

Once the arms are under the bar, lift the elbows to position the upper arms parallel to the floor.

Rack the bar across the front of the clavicles and anterior deltoids.

The bar should be caught at the anterior deltoids and clavicles with the

- head facing forward,
- neck neutral or slightly hyperextended,
- wrists hyperextended,
- elbows fully flexed,
- upper arms parallel to the floor,
- back neutral or slightly arched,
- knees and hips slightly flexed to absorb the impact of the weight,
- feet flat on the floor, and
- the body's weight over the middle of the feet.

Stand up by extending the hips and knees to a fully erect position.

Downward Movement Phase

Lower the bar to the thighs by gradually reducing the muscular tension of the arms to allow a controlled descent.

Simultaneously flex the hips and knees to cushion the impact of the bar on the thighs.

Squat down with the elbows fully extended until the bar touches the floor.

Common Errors

- Allowing the hips to rise before the shoulders during the first pull
- Allowing the upper back to round (i.e., losing the neutral spine position), especially during the first pull
- Extending the knees faster than the hips, before the hips, or both
- Allowing the bar to travel upward too far away from the body
- Using a "reverse curl" movement to move the bar into the catch position

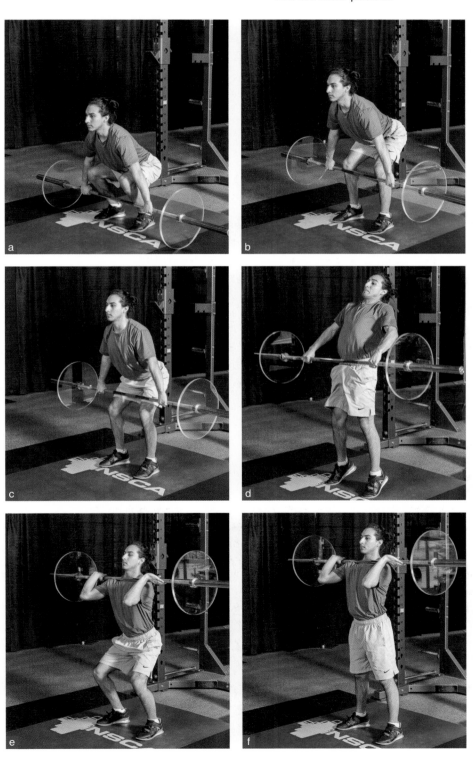

DUMBBELL SQUAT TO PRESS

Starting Position

Stand erect with the feet shoulder-width apart.

Grasp a dumbbell in each hand using a closed, neutral grip.

Position the dumbbells next to each shoulder, with the elbows flexed and palms facing forward (or each other, as shown in the photos).

The head and spine should be in a neutral, rigid position.

Downward Movement Phase

Maintaining a position with the back neutral and chest up, allow the hips and knees to flex to perform a squat.

Keep a relatively constant angle between the torso and the floor.

Keep the heels on the floor and the knees aligned over the feet.

Continue flexing the hips and knees until the tops of the thighs are parallel to the floor. (*Note:* More well-trained clients can squat lower than parallel.)

The dumbbells should remain next to the shoulders in a secure position during this phase.

Upward Movement Phase

Extend the hips and knees at the same rate to ascend out of the squat position toward the starting position.

As the body is rising, begin to press the dumbbells overhead until the elbows are fully extended.

Primary Muscles Trained

Gluteus maximus, semimembranosus, semitendinosus, biceps femoris, vastus lateralis, vastus intermedius, vastus medialis, rectus femoris, soleus, gastrocnemius, anterior and medial deltoids, trapezius, triceps brachii

Aim to achieve the ending position for both the squat and the press at the same time.

Keep the heels in contact with the floor and the knees aligned over the feet.

Keep the wrists stiff and above the elbows during the pressing motion.

Maintain a position with the back neutral and chest up throughout the ascent.

Common Errors

- Flexing the torso forward during the downward movement
- Not keeping the heels in contact with the floor
- Not maintaining the arms perpendicular to the floor at the top position
- Arching the lower back during the upward movement

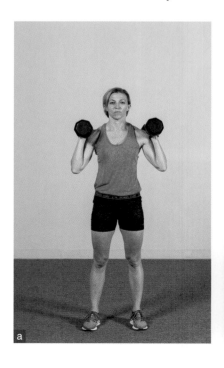 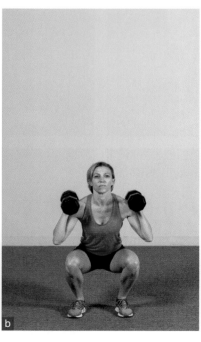 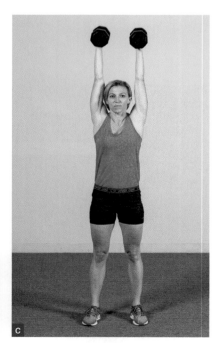

KETTLEBELL SWING

Starting Position

Stand straddling a kettlebell, with the feet flat and between hip- and shoulder-width apart, the toes pointed straight ahead.

Squat down with the hips lower than the shoulders and grasp the kettlebell with a closed, pronated grip.

Place the hands on the kettlebell, with index fingers touching or close together, inside of the legs, keeping the elbows fully extended.

Position the body with the

- back in a neutral spine position,
- shoulders retracted and depressed,
- feet flat on the floor, and
- eyes focused straight ahead or slightly upward.

Maintain a neutral spine or normal lordotic position while flexing the hips and knees to approximately a quarter-squat position, with the kettlebell hanging at arm's length between the thighs.

Backward Movement Phase

Begin the exercise by flexing at the hips to swing the kettlebell between the legs.

Keep the knees in a moderately flexed position, with the back neutral and the elbows extended.

Keep swinging the kettlebell backward until the torso is nearly parallel to the floor and the kettlebell is past the vertical line of the body.

Primary Muscles Trained

Gluteus maximus, semimembranosus, semitendinosus, biceps femoris, vastus lateralis, vastus intermedius, vastus medialis, rectus femoris

Forward and Upward Movement Phase

When the backward swing reaches its end point, reverse the movement by extending the hips and knees to move the kettlebell in an upward arc.

Allow momentum to raise the kettlebell to eye level, keeping the elbows extended and the back in a neutral spine position.

Downward and Backward Movement Phase

Allow the kettlebell to drop into the downswing.

Flex the hips and slightly flex the knees to absorb the weight by performing a hip hinge.

Keep the elbows fully extended and the back neutral.

Continue the downward-then-backward movement until the kettlebell passes under and then behind the body, then begin the upward movement phase for the next repetition.

Common Errors

- Allowing the back to round during the downward swing phase
- Performing a squat instead of a hip hinge on the swing phase
- Not keeping the head and neck in line with the spinal column

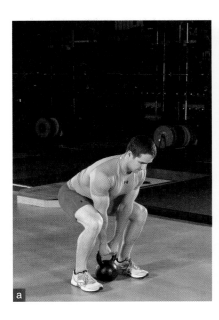
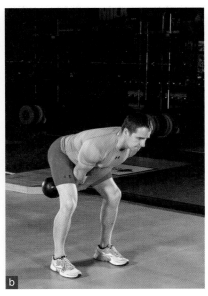
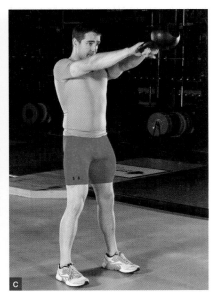

Study Questions

1. Which of the following is an advantage of machine-based training?

   A. enhanced ability to target specific muscle groups

   B. greater activation of stabilizer muscles

   C. improved muscle activation patterns in athletic movements

   D. stronger carryover to sport performance

2. What is the standard weight of an Olympic barbell?

   A. 25 lb (12 kg)

   B. 35 lb (16 kg)

   C. 45 lb (20 kg)

   D. 60 lb (28 kg)

3. Which of the following grips is used for the barbell shoulder press exercise?

   A. closed, pronated

   B. closed, supinated

   C. closed, neutral

   D. open, alternated

4. When spotting over-the-face barbell exercises, the personal trainer should grasp the bar with which type of grip?

   A. pronated grip, outside of the client's grip

   B. supinated, inside of the client's grip

   C. supinated grip, outside of the client's grip

   D. alternated grip, inside of the client's grip

5. Which of the following is *incorrect* regarding multiple spotters?

   A. More than two spotters are never necessary.

   B. It is common to use one spotter at each end of the bar during the front or back squat exercise.

   C. Multiple spotters must perfectly synchronize when and how much they assist the client.

   D. If the load is beyond the personal trainer's ability to handle effectively, an additional spotter must be used.

CHAPTER 14

Cardiovascular Exercise Technique

Benjamin H. Reuter, PhD, and Margaret T. Jones, PhD

After completing this chapter, you will be able to

■ provide recommendations relevant to cardiovascular activities;

■ provide advice in regard to proper exercise technique on treadmills, rowing machines, stair climbers, elliptical trainers, upper body ergometers, and stationary bicycles;

■ teach clients safe participation in group exercise classes; and

■ match clients with cardiovascular activities that are compatible with their preferences and physical capabilities.

The purpose of this chapter is to provide an overview of important considerations when one is prescribing cardiovascular exercise activities. These activities can be classified into machine (e.g., treadmill, stair climber, elliptical trainer, upper body ergometry) and nonmachine (e.g., walking, resistance, running, swimming) exercises. A single chapter cannot provide a complete description of these activities; but the most important aspects of proper cardiovascular exercise techniques are covered. Since personal trainers often work with various types of clients, some of whom may have special needs, it is helpful to know how to incorporate variety into training programs in order to achieve an array of training goals.

Warm-up and cooldown activities help the cardiovascular and musculoskeletal systems adjust to the selected exercise. Specific information about the design of warm-up and cooldown activities is included in chapters 12 and 16. Generally speaking, most clients are capable of performing a single exercise session continuously. However, it is recommended that personal trainers follow the general guidelines for frequency, intensity, and duration of cardiovascular exercise, discussed in chapter 16, when designing cardiovascular exercise programs. Finally, the general adaptations to the cardiovascular and pulmonary systems carry over well from one exercise modality to the next, but the stress placed on the musculoskeletal system will vary. Thus, personal trainers should pay careful attention to their clients as they adapt from one exercise modality to the next.

The authors would like to acknowledge the significant contributions of Travis W. Beck and J. Henry "Hank" Drought to this chapter.

CLOTHING AND FOOTWEAR

For safe and enjoyable participation in cardiovascular exercise, clients must wear appropriate clothing and footwear. Comfortable, loose-fitting clothing allows for ease of movement during aerobic activities. In hot and humid environments, the clothing should be as light as possible. In cold weather, clothing should be layered; much of the body's heat is lost through the head and extremities, so hats, gloves, and scarves are recommended to prevent excessive heat loss. Proper footwear is also important for weight-bearing activities like walking and running. Generally speaking, shoes should provide cushioning, stability, and comfort. The primary factor determining the quality of a running shoe is the compression capability, 50% of which is lost within 300 to 500 miles (~500-800 km) of use (12). Some running shoes are better than others; but in general, most running shoes should be replaced after 300 to 500 miles of use or every six months, whichever comes first. Runners with a high body weight or an unusual gait (e.g., over- or underpronation) may need to replace their shoes more often. Tables 14.1 and 14.2 provide recommendations for shoe selection based on the type of activity and footstrike characteristics, and figure 14.1 provides an illustration of **overpronation** and **underpronation**.

Running shoes are generally made with three different types of forms (also called **lasts**, or the mold a shoe is built on): straight, semicurved, or curved (figure 14.2). Overpronators may benefit from a motion-control shoe with a straight last. Underpronators may favor a shoe with a curved last that allows greater range of motion of the foot. Neutral footstrikers may benefit from shoes with a semicurved last and moderate direction- and foot-control features (10). A consultation with a podiatrist to analyze running biomechanics may be helpful for proper shoe selection.

> **Proper clothing and footwear selection should be a priority. Selections should match the specific activity as well as the environment in which the event will take place. For instance, light clothing allows for the dissipation of heat within hot and humid climates, while layered clothing protects heat loss in dry, colder environments.**

TRAINING ON CARDIOVASCULAR MACHINES

Common cardiovascular machines include treadmills, stair climbers, elliptical trainers, stationary bicycles, upper body ergometers (UBEs), and rowing machines. This section discusses the primary muscles used with each piece of equipment and the techniques that should be considered when using the equipment. Exercise

TABLE 14.1 Shoe Selection Based on Activity

| Activity | GENERAL SHOE CHARACTERISTICS | |
	Cushion	Lateral stability
Walking	Moderate	Moderate
Running	High	Low
Aerobics	Moderate to high	Moderate to high
Racket sports	Moderate	High
Cross-training	Moderate to high	Moderate to high

TABLE 14.2 Shoe Selection Based on Footstrike

Type of footstrike	Specific shoe characteristics
Neutral	Semicurved last; moderate motion control
Overpronators	Straight last; high motion control
Underpronators (supinators)	Curved last; high motion flexibility or straight

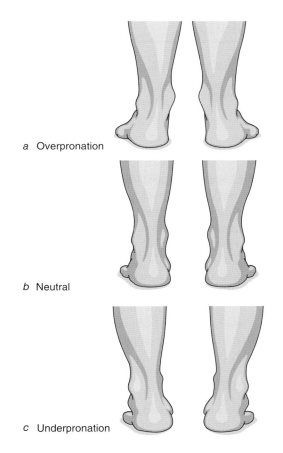

a Overpronation

b Neutral

c Underpronation

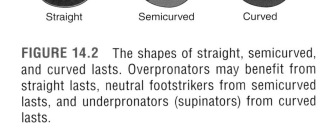

Straight   Semicurved   Curved

FIGURE 14.1 *(a)* Overpronation occurs when the foot collapses too far inward on the arch with each footstrike. *(b)* Neutral footstrike. *(c)* Underpronation (supination) occurs when footstrikes are too much on the outsides of the feet and have too little inward roll.

FIGURE 14.2 The shapes of straight, semicurved, and curved lasts. Overpronators may benefit from straight lasts, neutral footstrikers from semicurved lasts, and underpronators (supinators) from curved lasts.

technique for additional modalities (i.e., walking, race walking, running, swimming, and some popular group exercise classes) are also briefly discussed.

Treadmill

Primary Muscles Used

Quadriceps, hamstrings, gluteals, iliopsoas, tibialis anterior, gastrocnemius, soleus

Both walking and running can be performed on a treadmill. Important advantages of the treadmill include the conveniences of indoor exercise, handrail support, controlled speed and elevation, and a soft

landing surface to reduce the impact forces associated with footstrike.

Stepping on the Belt

Many clients will be familiar with a treadmill and how to step on the belt to begin exercising. However, elderly clients, those undergoing cardiac rehabilitation, and anyone who has not used a treadmill before may need assistance. Personal trainers can do the following to assist clients in need of help on a treadmill:

1. Instruct the client to hold on to the handrails while straddling the belt. Turn the treadmill on and set the speed to 1 mile (1.6 km) per hour. When the belt begins moving, instruct the client to step on the belt with one foot and then the other to begin

walking. Some clients may find it useful to "paw" the belt with one foot several times in order to become acclimated to the speed before stepping onto the moving belt with both feet.

2. Instruct clients to continue to hold the handrails if they feel unsure about their balance. Once they feel comfortable, however, they should let go of the handrails and swing their arms in a natural walking motion.

3. Instruct clients to try to remain at the front of the treadmill and in the center of the belt to reduce the risk of falling.

Treadmill Running

Clients accustomed to running outdoors will find it easier to run indoors on a treadmill, assuming the running speed is the same. This difference is caused by the lack of air resistance on a treadmill, so the body has only to keep up with the belt speed rather than propel itself forward. Thus, treadmill running at a given speed has a lower energy cost than running at the same speed outdoors. One can offset this difference by increasing the treadmill grade to approximately 1% (16).

> **When stepping on the treadmill to begin a workout, the client should place one foot on the belt at a time. The treadmill speed should be slow (e.g., 1 mile [1.6 km] per hour).**

Stair Climber

Primary Muscles Used

Quadriceps, hamstrings, gluteals, iliopsoas, tibialis anterior, gastrocnemius, soleus

The ground reaction forces at the knee during non-machine stair climbing can be three to six times body weight (8). Escalator-type stair climber machines help reduce these knee stresses because the downward stroke of the leg is assisted by the moving step. A disadvantage, however, is that these machines do not allow for variations in step height, which can make their use difficult for shorter clients. Pedal-based stair climbers allow for adjustment of stepping depth, and generally speaking, a greater stepping depth requires more muscle activation. A limitation of this exercise modality is that deconditioned clients may not be able to use a stair climber at even the lowest work levels (1).

Body Position

Stair climbers are designed to be used with the client facing and stepping forward onto the pedals. Thus, reversing the body position and facing out is not recommended as it can place excessive stress on the lower back, thereby increasing the risk for injury.

Hip movement during stair climbing is beneficial as long as it is in the sagittal plane. If there is excessive

REDUCING HANDRAIL USAGE

When possible, personal trainers should strive to reduce handrail usage by their clients for both the treadmill and stair climber. General procedures for achieving this include instructing the client to hold the handrails in the following progression.

1. Both hands lightly
2. The fingers of both hands
3. One hand, with the other arm swinging at the side
4. The fingers of one hand
5. Only one finger of one hand

It is recommended that clients progress through steps 1 to 5 in order, with the end goal being complete release of the handrails. For both the treadmill and stair climber, clients who use the handrails tend to support too much of their body weight, thereby reducing the workload demands. Excessive handrail usage can also compromise postural alignment, thereby increasing the risk for lower back injury.

side-to-side motion of the body, instruct the client to decrease the depth of the step or the step rate until this motion is minimized.

Range of Movement

Height and fitness level are the primary determinants of stair stepping depth. An appropriate range of movement is usually from 4 to 8 inches (10.2-20.3 cm). Excessive depth is usually indicated by side-to-side rocking of the hips, while a depth that is too shallow will not properly stress the target muscles, and, in turn, the cardiovascular system. Generally speaking, all clients should strive to achieve a stepping depth that promotes proper posture and works the muscles adequately.

Stepping Speed

Stepping speed generally ranges from 43 to 95 steps per minute (23a). A stepping speed that is too fast may cause either excessive hip movement (to keep up with the stepping depth) or short, fast steps (resulting in a stepping depth that is too shallow). Both of these extremes should be discouraged. It is important for the client to become comfortable with a stepping speed that elicits the appropriate metabolic demands yet encourages proper biomechanics.

> When clients are performing stair climbing or elliptical trainer exercise, the knee should not come forward in front of the toe when the leg is in the flexed position.

Elliptical Trainer

Primary Muscles Used

Quadriceps, hamstrings, gluteals, iliopsoas, tibialis anterior, gastrocnemius, soleus

Elliptical trainers combine the motions involved in stair climbing with those of walking or running. The advantage of elliptical trainers is that they are low impact, and most models allow the upper body to contribute to the movement. This is important from a practical standpoint because it increases the amount of muscle mass involved in the activity and therefore the total caloric expenditure.

Foot Placement and Handrail Usage

The whole foot should be in contact with the pedal surface at all times unless the machine requires lifting of the heel (e.g., figure 14.3). In addition, although many elliptical trainers do not have side handrails, the handrails on those that do should be used only for balancing purposes.

Body Position and Knee Placement

All clients who use the elliptical trainer should remain upright with the torso balanced over the hips. The hands should grip the handles, with the shoulders relaxed. In addition, the knees should not come in front of the toes since this position places additional strain on the joint that can lead to injury.

Cadence, Elevation, Resistance, and Direction of Movement

In general, movements with slow cadences resemble the walking motion, while those with fast cadences are closer to a running movement. Motions on medium-level inclines resemble walking and running up hills,

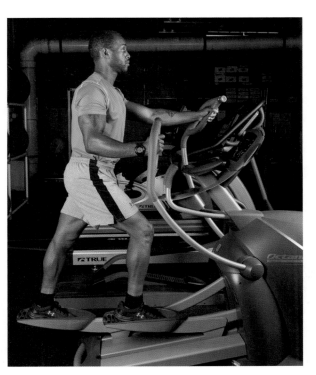

FIGURE 14.3 Proper elliptical trainer exercise technique: head up, looking straight ahead, and torso balanced over hips with no excessive forward lean.

while those on high inclines are similar to stair climbing. Another unique feature of elliptical trainers is that they allow pedaling in both the forward and backward directions, which allows the muscles to work in different ways. Therefore, changing the direction of movement may be a useful method for introducing variation into the exercise program.

> **Low-impact cardiovascular training machines (e.g., elliptical trainers, stationary bicycles), as well as swimming, can be used for clients who have orthopedic problems like arthritis and low back pain.**

Stationary Bicycle

Primary Muscles Used

Quadriceps, hamstrings, gluteals, tibialis anterior, iliopsoas, gastrocnemius, soleus

Stationary cycling is a non–weight-bearing, non-impact exercise. Thus, overweight clients and those with lower back and lower extremity orthopedic prob-

lems may benefit from the fact that their body weight is supported by the seat. A drawback, however, is that the exercise can be limited by local muscle fatigue, resulting in a suboptimal cardiovascular stimulus.

Seat Height

The seat height should allow for a slight bend in the knee joint at the bottom of the pedal stroke, which permits extension of the leg without locking of the joint, leaving the knee with about 25 to 30 degrees of flexion (figure 14.4). Clients can readjust the seat height if they feel the range of motion is too short or too long.

Handlebars and Body Positioning

Handlebar positioning should allow the back to be tilted forward from the hips, but not excessively rounded. Some stationary bicycles use "bullhorn," or drop, handlebars that allow for a variety of hand positions, including the following:

1. A pronated grip on the front of the handlebar, which requires a more upright posture
2. A neutral palms-facing-in grip on the sides of the handlebar, which uses more forward lean

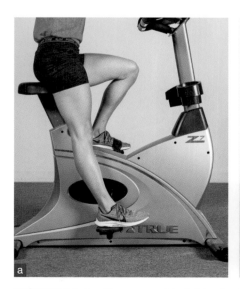 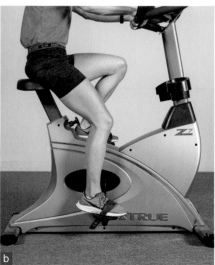 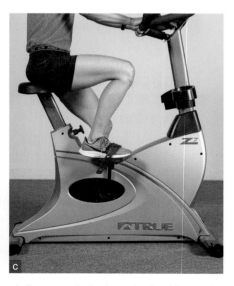

FIGURE 14.4 Proper seat height adjustment guideline options: *(a)* with the knee fully extended when the heel is on the pedal; *(b)* with the knee flexed about 25 to 30 degrees when the ball of the foot is on the pedal; or *(c)* with the pedal at 12 o'clock, the knee is approximately even with the hips and the thigh is approximately parallel with the floor. The result of these three options is that the knee will be slightly flexed (i.e., not locked out) as at the bottom of the pedal stroke.

3. A position in which the forearms rest on the sides of the handlebar, thereby supporting much of the upper body weight and encouraging forward lean

Many clients find it useful to adjust their hand positioning during longer rides, although some stationary bicycles do not allow for handlebar adjustments.

Cadence and Pedaling Action

In general, the most economical pedaling cadence ranges from 60 to 100 revolutions per minute (rpm), with beginners preferring lower pedaling rates and trained cyclists preferring higher cadences. Pedaling at too high a cadence, however, results in wasted energy due to added muscular work needed to stabilize the trunk (13, 17, 18, 24). Most clients are able to sense the pedaling cadence that allows for the greatest economy. In addition, most of the force production during cycling is applied in a forward and downward direction during the downstroke. For most clients, the upstroke contributes very little to the overall power output, and the quadriceps femoris and gluteal muscles generate nearly all of the power needed for the movement. In some cases, the calf muscles can aid in the downstroke, but they do not contribute significantly to the overall power output.

Semirecumbent Bike

Many training facilities have semirecumbent bikes that provide back support and a wider seat, which is particularly beneficial for overweight clients, those with low back pain, and pregnant women. Heart rate, oxygen consumption rate, and rating of perceived exertion on a semirecumbent bike are typically lower than on an upright bike (given the same workload). There are two primary reasons for this phenomenon: The back support of a semirecumbent bike reduces the workload placed on postural muscles, and the semirecumbent position prevents the heart from having to pump blood vertically against gravity (6). Figure 14.5 shows proper body positioning on a semirecumbent bike.

Group Indoor Cycling

Group indoor cycling generally provides a higher-intensity workout than does individual cycling. This form of cycling is usually performed with music in a class atmosphere, with instructors guiding the class on a simulated ride that lasts anywhere from 30 to 45 minutes. It is recommended that beginners develop a good baseline level of conditioning before starting a cycling class. They should do this on their own time; and when they feel they are ready, they should start

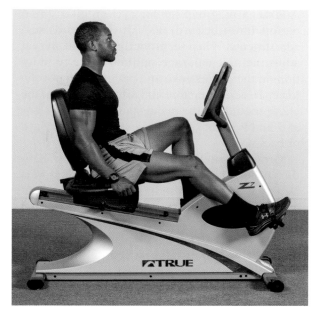

FIGURE 14.5 The upper body is supported in a seated position on a semirecumbent bike; the seat is adjusted to allow a slight bend at the knee (similar to the situation with a standard stationary bike).

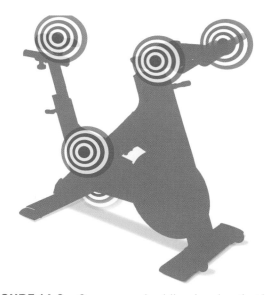

FIGURE 14.6 Group exercise bike showing that bike position is based on the five contact points of the body.
© BikeFit

with a beginning-level class and progress to more advanced classes.

Most bikes are highly adjustable, which allows for proper fit based on the five points of contact (i.e., feet on the pedals, hands on the handlebars, and ischial tuberosities on the seat (figure 14.6).

Additionally, group indoor cycling bikes often permit fore (forward) and aft (backward) seat adjustments. When set properly, fore and aft seat adjustments encourage optimal force production on the downstroke and better safety for the knee. To adjust the fore and aft seat position, the client should set the pedals parallel to the floor at 3 and 9 o'clock, then adjust the seat forward or backward.

Group indoor cycling bikes also allow handlebar height adjustments. Handlebar height is largely a function of individual preference, but a good starting point is to set the handlebar level with the tip of the saddle. Novices and clients with poor back flexibility may prefer the handlebar higher to allow a more upright sitting posture (figure 14.7a). Either way, the handlebar should be adjusted so that the arms are in a comfortable position, with the elbows slightly bent at a minimum of 15 degrees. The angle between the torso and the ground has been found to be most comfortable at about 55 degrees (21). Some bikes also include handlebar fore and aft positioning, which allows further adjustment to maximize comfort. A more forward-leaning upper body "racing" posture (figure 14.7b) is used more often during group indoor cycling than for standard stationary bicycling on electronic and generator-driven bikes.

Upper Body Ergometer

Primary Muscles Used

Pectoralis major, deltoids, latissimus dorsi, biceps brachii, triceps brachii

The upper body ergometer (UBE) is also known as the arm ergometer, arm crank ergometer, or arm cycle. The UBE has been used extensively in rehabilitation settings but can also provide an alternative cardiovascular conditioning workout for clients who have lower body extremity limitations or need a change of pace in their exercise programming.

This exercise modality requires a hand-pedaling action that involves the majority of the upper body musculature in the chest, back, shoulders, and arms. UBE exercise can be performed seated or standing, and the arm crank should be adjusted to the height of the shoulders. The length of the arm cranks should permit slight elbow flexion of the arm extended farthest from the body. The exercise intensity is raised by increasing pedal revolutions or resistance on the crank, or both. If the client is exercising from the seated position, the client's feet should be flat and remain in contact with the floor. Exercising from the standing position elicits a greater degree of lower body and core musculature involvement

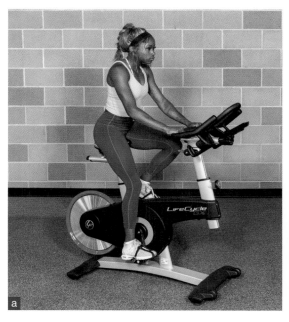
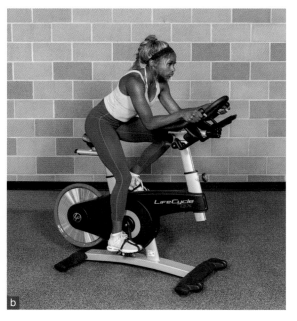

FIGURE 14.7 Proper body position on a group cycling bike *(a)* when not racing and *(b)* when racing.

because standing requires more global muscle activation than sitting to allow maintenance of a standing posture.

A point to consider when programming for UBE use is the difficulty of or unfamiliarity with upper body aerobic conditioning. Because of the smaller muscle mass involved in upper body exercise (as opposed to the lower body), clients may find it difficult to exercise at a high intensity for long periods. Therefore, it is recommended that the UBE first be introduced as a 5-minute warm-up or cooldown option. When incorporating it directly into the exercise session, start with interval training since the intermittent rest periods will permit more work to be accomplished by delaying the onset of muscular fatigue as compared to traditional steady-state training (11). When exercising with the UBE, it is recommended that pedaling occur in the forward and backward directions with both arms. Once a higher level of aerobic endurance is achieved, single-arm exercise can be incorporated into the workout.

Rowing Machine

Primary Muscles Used

Quadriceps, hamstrings, gluteals, tibialis anterior, gastrocnemius, soleus, biceps brachii, brachioradialis, brachialis, rectus abdominis, posterior and medial deltoids, trapezius, latissimus dorsi, teres major, erector spinae, flexor and extensor carpi ulnaris

Rowing is an excellent non–weight-bearing activity that stimulates both the upper and lower body. Since a large portion of the entire body's muscle mass is used to perform the rowing motion, the risk for local muscle fatigue is low. A disadvantage is that clients may be unfamiliar with the movement. As a result, beginners tend to perform the row using too much upper body movement. In addition, those with low back pain tend to round or flex the back too much. Thus, familiarization with proper body positioning is important when introducing rowing into an exercise program (figure 14.8).

Starting Position and the Drive

For the starting position, clients should be looking straight ahead, with an upright back and slight forward lean. The arms are straight in front of the body, and the hips and knees are flexed. From this position, they should perform the drive by extending the hips and legs forcefully while leaning the torso back slightly. After the hips and legs have been extended, the arms should be used to pull the handle to the abdomen.

The Finish, Recovery, and Catch

For the finish, the legs are fully extended, the torso leans backward slightly, the elbows are flexed, and the handle is pulled into the abdomen. The recovery, in turn, involves extension of the elbows followed by a forward lean of the torso at the hip joint. The catch resumes the starting position. Specifically, the torso leans forward slightly at the hips, the arms are straight, and the shins are vertical in preparation for the next stroke.

Resistance and Cadence

Although rowing machines have various designs, a common technique for altering resistance is to adjust the airflow. Specifically, an air vent controls the amount of air that reaches the flywheel. As more air is allowed through the vent, the resistance on the flywheel increases. However, the change in resistance is not linear on many air resistance rowing machines and can be affected by differences in machine design and elevation above sea level at which the machine is used.

It is important to remember that stroke rate has an effect on resistance. Regardless of the damper setting, the harder an individual pulls the greater the air resistance since more air is pulled across the flywheel. In addition, if the flywheel is allowed to slow during stroke recovery, bringing the flywheel speed back up can also increase the workout difficulty.

If the machine allows, clients may be able to change intensity based on the air drag on the flywheel. Thus, monitoring resistance and air drag will allow clients to maintain consistent resistance levels when they are not using the same rower for each workout. Beginners should start at a low resistance and stroke rate and increase the workload as their conditioning level improves. Most recreational rowers row at a moderate cadence of approximately 20 to 25 strokes per minute, and elite rowers generally row at a faster rate (e.g., 25-35 strokes per minute).

> The chosen cardiovascular training modality will depend partly on equipment availability, but it also must be comfortable for the client and able to help the client achieve his or her fitness goals. It is important to start the exercise program at a level that matches the client's fitness level and then follow a slow progression.

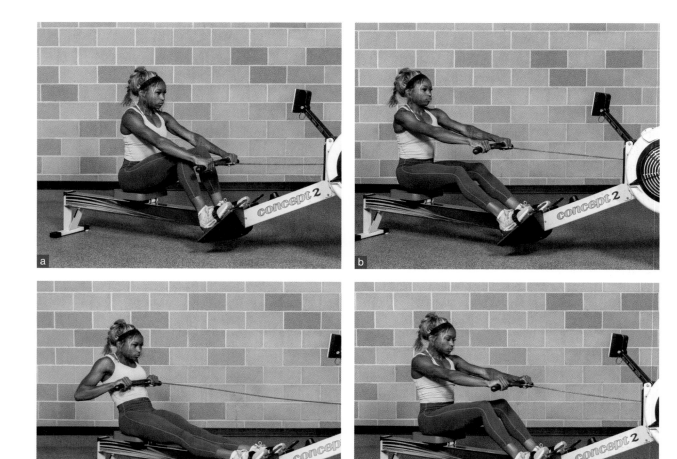

FIGURE 14.8 Proper body position on the rowing machine: *(a)* starting position (and the catch); *(b)* the drive; *(c)* the finish; *(d)* the recovery.

NONMACHINE CARDIOVASCULAR EXERCISE TECHNIQUES

Nonmachine exercises like walking and running are less expensive than machine activities and are often easy to fit into a client's schedule. This section deals with walking, running, swimming, group exercise classes, and aqua exercise.

Walking

Primary Muscles Used

Quadriceps, hamstrings, gluteals, iliopsoas, tibialis anterior, gastrocnemius, soleus

In general walking is an excellent exercise selection for beginners. However, as conditioning improves, clients should strive to achieve the proper body position, footstrike, hip action, and arm action.

Body Position

Proper posture is important during walking because it improves efficiency and decreases strain on the lower back and vertebral column. The personal trainer should educate clients that proper posture is characterized by "walking tall." A commonly used visual example is that of a string pulling the head upward and straightening the vertebral column. The shoulders should remain relaxed but not rounded, with the upper body positioned directly over the hips.

Footstrike

Footstrike during walking occurs when the heel strikes the ground and the body weight is transferred through the foot in a gentle rolling action from the heel to the ball of the foot. Abnormal footstrike patterns are usually characterized by excessive weight transfer to either the inside (pronation) or outside (supination) of the foot (see figure 14.1 on page 379), both of which can cause injury.

Hip Action

Light dynamic stretching before walking can improve hip mobility. Improved hip movement ensures adequate stride length. Gradually increasing stride frequency, stride length, or both is an excellent way to increase training intensity during walking.

Arm Action

Arm and leg action should be coordinated during walking, with the left arm swinging forward with the right leg, the right arm with the left leg. At fast walking speeds, the elbows should be flexed such that the joint angle is 90 degrees and the hands are brought upward to chest level. This swinging action from the hips to the chest and back helps propel the body forward. The arms should not swing across the body.

Race Walking

There is one primary difference between walking and race walking. In race walking, the leg must be fully extended from the time the foot lands until the body passes over the supporting leg. Competitive race walkers improve performance by maximizing stride length. This is accomplished by increasing hip rotation (i.e., the pelvic roll commonly used in race walking) (figure 14.9). The success of competitive race walkers is dictated by their ability to consistently produce stride lengths just a few inches longer than a normal stride length.

Running

Primary Muscles Used
Quadriceps, hamstrings, gluteals, iliopsoas, tibialis anterior, gastrocnemius, soleus

Running produces outstanding cardiovascular benefits and, like walking, is a low-cost exercise. It is time efficient for conditioned clients and sport spe-

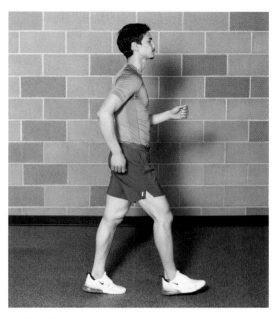

FIGURE 14.9 Proper race walking technique dictates that one foot must always be in contact with the ground, and the support leg must remain straight. Race walkers increase stride length with increased hip rotation.

cific for recreational athletes whose sport involves running. Many clients are unsure, however, when it is appropriate to incorporate running into their programs. Generally speaking, when clients can walk 3 to 4 miles (4.8-6.4 km) in an hour without becoming fatigued, they can start a walk/run program. These programs alternate periods of walking and running (e.g., a 1- to 2-minute run followed by a 3- to 5-minute walk), with this sequence repeated for the necessary duration. Progression is accomplished as the amount of running time is increased until running is continuous. Running is a high-impact activity; therefore, those who are overweight or have orthopedic problems may need lower-impact cardiovascular activities such as cycling or swimming.

The net energy cost of running is generally greater than for walking. For example, one study found that running 1,600 meters (about 1 mile) requires approximately 30% more total energy than walking for both men and women (14). Running requires specific techniques to conserve energy and reduce the risk of impact injury. Bouncing with each step should be avoided because it wastes energy through vertical displacement and increases shock. Footstrike abnormalities (e.g., overpronation, underpronation) have greater consequences during running than during walking because of the footstrike impact.

Body Position and Footstrike

Running is similar to walking in that clients should be told to "run tall" by keeping the head upright, the shoulders relaxed, and the torso balanced over the hips. Footstrike is achieved through a heel-to-ball rolling action. Specifically, the heel touches the ground first, and the body weight is spread through the foot with a gentle rolling action (figure 14.10). Thus, it is important for clients to concentrate on preventing the foot from slapping the ground as they run. Instead, running should be thought of as a gliding motion, with as little impact force as possible.

Arm Action

During long-distance running, the arms hang from relaxed shoulders and are bent at the elbows. Arm action occurs from the shoulders, but too much shoulder movement wastes energy. Much of the arm movement comes from the lower arm (forearm, wrist, and hand) by means of hinging at the elbow. In this way, the elbow is unlocked, and the angle at the elbow opens during the arm downswing and closes during the upswing. The forearms are carried between the waist and chest. If the arms are carried too high, the shoulders and upper back become fatigued. If the arms are carried too low, excessive forward lean may

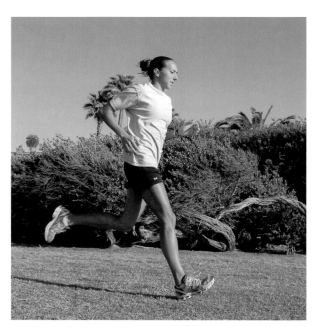

FIGURE 14.10 During long-distance or treadmill running, proper footstrike involves contact with the heel and then a gentle rolling action toward the ball of the foot for push-off.

© Human Kinetics; Photographer: Stacy Peterson.

occur. The hands are gently cupped (not clenched into fists), and the thumb softly touches the index finger. On the forward swing, the hands reach chest height. On the backward swing, the hands reach the hips at the side of the body. The arms and hands also move slightly inward, but the hands do not cross the midline of the body. The wrists should be relaxed but not held too loosely.

Stride Length

Running speed, like walking speed, is determined by stride length and stride frequency. To improve running performance, it is necessary to increase stride length, stride frequency, or both. Exact stride length depends on leg length, flexibility, strength, coordination, and level of fatigue. With each running step, the feet should land approximately under the hips. If the foot hits too far in front of the body's center of gravity, greater shock and a slight braking effect will occur. This is **overstriding,** or taking too long of a stride. Braking, as well as too much time spent in the air, makes overstriding inefficient. Many runners overreach with the front leg and foot in an effort to improve stride length. This is counterproductive and will likely cause braking. **Understriding** wastes energy since it prevents the body from advancing far enough with each stride. The best way to improve stride length is to increase rear leg drive by improving strength and to increase range of motion by improving flexibility.

Stride Frequency

Taking quicker, softer relaxed steps while keeping the feet low to the ground will increase stride frequency. People who are running for health benefits may not see the importance of improving stride frequency and stride length, since speed and racing are not the goal. However, a slow overstride usually results in a raised center of gravity and more time spent in the air, thereby leading to a harder landing and greater impact. In short, a slow overstride may cause not only loss of speed but also an increased risk of injury.

Swimming

Primary Muscles Used
Dependent on the stroke being used, but can be nearly a full-body activity

The four competitive swimming strokes are the front crawl, backstroke, breaststroke, and butterfly. All strokes can provide an excellent stimulus to the cardiovascular system and are low impact. It is recommended, however, that American Red Cross–certified water safety instructors be used to teach clients with no swimming experience before they begin a swim exercise program. A discussion of proper technique for all strokes is beyond the scope of this chapter; the following is a brief discussion of instruction on the front stroke.

The front crawl (also known as freestyle or front stroke) is the most popular and fastest stroke. Since this stroke uses both the upper and lower body, it is highly dependent on proper coordination, and it also provides an excellent stimulus to the cardiovascular system (3).

Body Position

With front crawl swimming, the body is prone and straight; the head should be held in a natural position, with the eyes looking at the bottom of the pool or slightly forward. Extraneous lateral or vertical movements should be avoided as much as possible since they reduce horizontal velocity. This straight and streamlined position also incorporates a body roll that is initiated by the hips and moves to the shoulders, legs, and feet. The head should be turned only to take a breath, and this turning should be an extension of the body roll, which involves four basic steps: rotation of the hips, lifting of the recovery arm, forward propulsion by the pulling arm, and leg kick that produces lateral force as the legs roll with the rest of the body. Body roll not only allows easier breathing and improves arm propulsion but also reduces drag forces and decreases shoulder stresses.

Arm Stroke

The arm stroke action in the front crawl provides as much as 80% to 90% of the propulsion force needed to move the body through the water. The arm stroke consists of three phases: the entry/catch phase, the power phase, and the recovery phase. Entry of the hand occurs in front of the shoulder and slightly lateral to the midline of the body. The elbow should be flexed slightly and held high, which allows the arm to enter the water cleanly and ensures an effective pulling position. The fingertips, hand, forearm, elbow, and shoulder all enter the water in the same location and in sequential order. The catch occurs just after entry and allows the hand and forearm to "catch" the water in front of the shoulder. The catch is important because it properly positions the hand and arm in order to pull effectively during the stroke. This action can be

thought of as "feeling" for the water, similar to the way a mountain climber grabs a piece of rock with an outstretched arm to pull the body upward.

The power phase is the primary propulsive phase of the arm stroke. The power phase pulls the body forward through the water by accelerating the hand and forearm backward with a pulling action. This action occurs in an S-shaped pattern in which the hand sweeps downward and slightly outward. The hand and arm then move slightly inward and backward toward the chest and middle of the body as the elbow is bent to roughly 90 degrees. The hand is then rotated to a neutral position with the palm facing backward, and the arm is extended outward, upward, and backward past the thigh. The last portion of the backward pull past the thigh is the most forceful portion of the power phase and is when the arm has maximum pulling capacity. In addition, this last part of the stroke should be coupled with the body roll to maximize propulsion. However, the S-shaped movements are very subtle and span a width of only 4 to 8 inches (10.2-20.3 cm) (figure 14.11; 18a). The fingers should be relaxed and slightly apart.

The final phase involves recovery and prepares the arm for another pull. First, the elbow is lifted high out of the water and the hand is turned inward toward the legs. The high elbow position allows the forearm to hang downward. Once the hand has cleared the water, it is brought forward and in position for the next power phase.

Leg Kick

The primary functions of the leg kick are to balance the body and help maintain a horizontal position. In most swimmers, the leg kick does not contribute meaningfully to forward propulsion (9, 15). During the front stroke, the leg kick is best described as a flutter kick that ranges in amplitude from 12 to 15 inches (30.5-38.1 cm). The downward thrust of the kick is the power portion, providing the most propulsion. The foot remains plantar flexed, with the kick originating from the hips and continuing with very slight knee extension and flexion. During the recovery portion of the kick (the upward thrust), the leg rises until the heel is just above the surface of the water.

Many swimmers use a two-beat kick, with the feet kicking two times for every arm cycle. However, with long-distance swimming the emphasis should be on kicking just fast enough to stay afloat to conserve energy. Elite swimmers usually try to maximize kicking propulsion. For example, high-level sprint

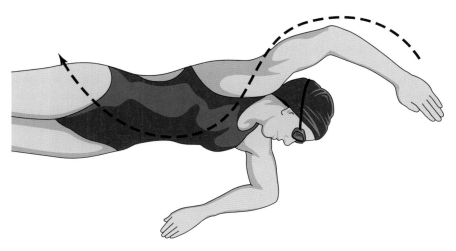

FIGURE 14.11 The subtle S-shaped hand pattern during the power phase of the front crawl arm stroke in swimming.
Adapted by permission from Maglischo (2003, p. 181).

swimmers primarily use a six-beat kick because they are not concerned with conserving energy.

Breathing

Breathing should occur when the head turns to the side as a natural part of the body rotation. The head stays level, with the forehead just higher than the chin. A breath can then be taken in the trough created by the head when it turns. Many beginners make the mistake of lifting the head, which causes the hips to sink. After the inhale, the head is turned back into the water with the body roll. At low intensities, it is possible to exhale through the nose only; but during maximal efforts, it is important to exhale forcefully through the mouth and nose to ensure complete exhalation.

Group Exercise Classes

Primary Muscles Used

Dependent on the exercises involved, but can be nearly a full-body activity

The traditional aerobics classes of the past have evolved to include many exercise modalities, such as kickboxing, step classes, group resistance training, aqua exercises, tai chi, and fitness yoga (2). These classes provide various cardiovascular activities that are choreographed with music. This section provides a brief discussion of aerobics, step classes, kickboxing, and aqua exercise. Safety is important during group exercise, particularly

good posture and body position. As with most exercises, the shoulders should be relaxed but not rounded, and the torso should be kept upright. In addition, during all activities that require knee flexion, the knee joint should not come in front of the toes.

> **Group exercise classes are an excellent way to improve cardiovascular fitness while allowing participants the opportunity to learn new movements or activities.**

Traditional Aerobics

Traditional aerobics classes generally range in duration from 45 to 75 minutes. Each session usually begins with a warm-up that includes dynamic preworkout stretching, followed by the aerobic activity, cooldown, and postworkout stretching. Each section has a different time requirement, based on the emphasis of the class session.

The aerobics portion of a class can be a combination of impact styles. In low-impact aerobics, one foot remains in constant contact with the floor. Ways of altering intensity include changing the amount of muscle mass used, lifting and lowering the center of gravity, and changing the range of motion and tempo, as well as side-to-side and forward and backward traveling. Low-impact aerobics is good for deconditioned, beginning, or obese clients as well as for senior clients and pregnant women, since the vertical impact forces are around 1 times body weight (25). With high-impact aerobics, both feet leave the floor during running, jumping, hopping, and leaping movements. This type of workout is vigorous and is appropriate only for well-conditioned clients. The vertical impact forces of high-impact aerobics have been measured at levels from 2.3 to over 2.7 times body weight (25).

Step Training

Step training uses a small platform ranging in height from 4 to 12 inches (10.2-30.5 cm). The participants step up and down to music while performing various movements and sequences using predominantly large muscle groups. Intensity can be increased by raising the step height, but this form of training is not appropriate for clients who have knee problems. Simply stepping up and down on a bench 6 to 8 inches (15.2-20.3 cm) high produces impact forces of approximately 1.4 to 1.5 times body weight, which is roughly the same as those for brisk walking. However, when the stepping speed is increased and propulsive moves are added, the impact forces may get as high as 2.5 times body weight (19, 23). Thus, propulsive moves should always be directed up onto the platform, and never down onto the floor. In addition, it is recommended that the step height for beginners produce a maximum of 60 degrees of knee flexion to reduce the risk for knee injury (7, 22).

Kickboxing

Kickboxing simulates martial arts training by using choreographed kicks and punching moves. These classes typically involve shadow boxing sessions rather than contact sparring against an opponent. They are usually 45 to 90 minutes in duration and require adequate time to warm up, cool down, and stretch.

The personal trainer should encourage beginners to learn the kickboxing moves correctly, since injuries often occur when clients try to do too much too soon. Beginners may also require at least one day of rest between classes to recover from workouts. More advanced clients can use punching combinations, speed kicking, and kicks above the waist after a proper warm-up. Some advanced clients will progress to heavy bags, speed bags, and other punching and kicking equipment.

Aquatic Exercise

Aquatic exercise is a safe training modality because the buoyancy of the water reduces the impact of landing on joints. This form of exercise is excellent for clients who are elderly, obese, deconditioned, or managing musculoskeletal conditions (5). Aqua exercise also has the advantage of not requiring swimming expertise. The exercises can be performed in shallow or deep water with an upright body position. Generally speaking, a body submerged to the waist bears 50% of its weight, one submerged to the chest bears 25% to 35%, and one submerged to the neck bears only 10% (5, 6). It is recommended to keep the arms submerged to maximize the water's resistance and optimize improvements to upper body musculature, balance, and coordination (4).

The basic aquatic movements include walking, jogging, kicking, jumping, and scissors (simultaneous arm and leg actions that are similar to those in cross-country skiing). Walking can be done with high knees, backward, sideways, and on the toes. Jogging can be performed either in place or with a traveling motion. Greater speed of movement results in higher intensity, and arm movements can be added to provide variety. Kicking movements with one leg can be forward, sideways, and backward; other kicking movements are knee lifts and leg curls. It is recommended that clients avoid hyperextension of the legs during all movements. Swimming flutter kicks can be performed when seated at the side of the pool or lying prone and holding on to the side of the pool. Larger-amplitude movements, like jumping and rebounding off the pool bottom, can increase workout intensity. Jumping activities can be performed on one or both feet, and variations include jumping jacks, traveling jumps, jumping with a twist, frog jumps, and leaps (4, 5, 20).

Before performing jumping movements, clients should learn proper landing technique—toes first, then onto the ball of the foot and finally the heel; the knees are "soft" (unlocked) and directly over the ankles to absorb bodyweight impact and reduce injury risk.

Other aquatic exercises include squats, lunges, leg extension and flexion, and forearm flexion and extension, just to name a few. Further, clients who are elite runners can use aquatic exercise or deep water running (or both) as a supplement to dryland running. This allows them to maintain both a high level of cardiovascular conditioning and running specificity. The feet can touch the bottom of the pool, or flotation devices can help the client stay afloat.

Clients often neglect to rehydrate after aquatic exercise because they may not have been sweating at high rates. However, respiration causes fluid loss, so clients should be instructed to drink plenty of fluids after workouts.

CONCLUSION

All cardiovascular activities should be performed with proper technique since poor technique can lead to injuries. The personal trainer is responsible for helping clients choose activities that are appropriate for their age and abilities. When possible, variety should be added to the program to decrease the chance for overuse injuries. Long-term adherence to the proper exercise program is an important key to maintaining a high level of physical fitness throughout one's life.

Study Questions

1. In cold conditions, much of the body's heat is lost through which of the following?

   I. head

   II. torso

   III. upper arms and legs

   IV. extremities

   A. I and II only

   B. II and III only

   C. III and IV only

   D. I and IV only

2. Which of the following is *incorrect* regarding stairclimber stepping speed?

   A. Stepping speed generally ranges from 43 to 95 steps per minute.

   B. Short, fast steps result in a stepping depth that is too shallow.

   C. The client should become comfortable with a stepping speed that elicits the appropriate metabolic demands and yet encourages proper biomechanics.

   D. The faster the stepping rate, the better.

3. During the finish phase of using the rowing machine, the handle should be pulled into which part of the client's body?

   A. hips

   B. abdomen

   C. chest

   D. shoulders

4. The arm stroke action in the front crawl provides as much as _____ of the propulsion force needed to move the body through the water.

   A. 20%-30%

   B. 40%-50%

   C. 60%-70%

   D. 80%-90%

5. When submerged under water up to the neck, the body bears what percentage of its dry land mass?

   A. 10%

   B. 20%

   C. 30%

   D. 40%

CHAPTER 15

Resistance Training Program Design

Brad J. Schoenfeld, PhD, and Ronald L. Snarr, PhD

After completing this chapter, you will be able to

- understand the application of specificity, overload, variation, progression, and sequencing;

- select exercises, determine training frequency, and arrange exercises in a specific sequence;

- determine how to estimate initial loads for clients;

- assign training loads, volumes, and rest period lengths based on client needs and appropriate sequential training methods;

- add variation between training sessions, training days, and training weeks; and

- determine when training loads need to be increased or varied.

Designing a safe and effective resistance training program is a multifaceted process in which the personal trainer must consider and manipulate specific training variables to achieve specific goals. Many personal trainers consider the resistance training program separate from the aerobic exercise or sprint interval program, but it is important to consider all elements when constructing the resistance training program. The best approach begins with an initial consultation to determine the client's goals, evaluate the client's health or medical history, and perform a fitness assessment (see chapters 9, 10, and 11). At this time, the personal trainer can find out the client's experience with resistance training and perform a cursory evaluation of his or her technical capabili-

ties. The information gathered will help the personal trainer develop the overall training program, which will include factors such as how often the client will train, types of exercises selected, training loads, repetition and set schemes, order of exercises, and rest intervals. To facilitate continued improvements, the personal trainer should consider a periodized training plan. Periodization may ensure that appropriate training variation and progression are used to minimize the potential for overtraining while maximizing improvements in the targeted training outcomes. Moreover, integrating variety into a training program can help with client motivation (6), which in turn may improve exercise adherence (61).

The authors would like to acknowledge the significant contributions of Roger W. Earle, Thomas R. Baechle, G. Gregory Haff, and Erin E. Haff to this chapter.

GENERAL TRAINING PRINCIPLES

Four principles should guide the development of effective resistance training programs: specificity, overload, variation, and progression. Any program that does not address each of these principles can result in a failure to meet client goals, poor adherence to the exercise plan, and potential litigation because of an increased risk of injury.

Specificity

The principle of **specificity** is a foundational aspect of every effective training program. Specificity of training refers to training a client in a specific way to produce a targeted change or result. The personal trainer can accomplish this by targeting specific muscle groups, energy systems, movement velocities, movement patterns, or muscle action types (18, 64, 67). For example, if a client wants to strengthen his or her leg muscles, the personal trainer will select exercises such as the back squat and leg press because of their emphasis on lower body development. This type of specificity is often referred to as **muscle group specificity** (18).

Another method of applying specificity to a client's training program is to target specific movement patterns. **Movement pattern specificity** is generally used with athletes or clients who wish to develop strength that translates to a specific activity or sport. For example, if the client is a volleyball player, the personal trainer considers the fact that volleyball involves repeated jumping movements. The personal trainer could target these movements by incorporating exercises such as back squats (or front squats), power cleans, and power snatches into the program because they mimic the jumping movements in volleyball. The more similar the resistance training exercise is to the movement pattern, the greater the likelihood of translation to the targeted activity (62). Exercises such as the Olympic lifts (i.e., cleans, snatches) appear to offer the most translation to sports because their movement patterns are similar to those performed in many sports and activities. See chapter 23 for further discussion of designing programs for clients with athletic aspirations.

Overload

Overload refers to a training stress or intensity that is greater than what a client is used to. If a program fails to adhere to the principle of overload, it will produce limited results. The most common methods of induc-

ing overload include increasing the weight lifted, having the client perform more repetitions or sets of a given exercise, shortening the rest interval between sets, and increasing the number of training sessions in a week. Although overload is an essential component of a resistance training program, the personal trainer should apply overload systematically and should adhere to the principles of progression and variation. Overload must be progressive to allow sufficient time for the client to adapt to the new training stimulus.

Variation

Variation refers to the manipulation of specific training variables (3, 67) such as volume, intensity, exercise selection, frequency of training, rest interval, and speed of movement (67). Appropriate training variation is essential when attempting to ensure long-term adaptation (41, 67). The best way to apply training variation is through the principles of **periodization** (67), which refers to the logical phasic manipulation of training factors to optimize specific training outcomes at specific time points (45). If appropriate training variation is not incorporated in the program, the rate of improvement will plateau (3, 67) or decrease, resulting in what is termed **monotonous program overtraining** (63).

The variation in the resistance training plan should not be haphazard, and the sequencing of training factors should be appropriate (67). For example, clients who want to maximize power and strength may undergo periods of training designed to target muscular strength followed by a period of power development. This type of sequencing has been shown to result in significantly greater improvements in performance compared with a program that lacks planned or sequenced variation (28). Additionally, varying exercises and modalities may increase client adherence and retention because it decreases training monotony. For example, clients who are not keen on resistance training routines may benefit from creative, nontraditional workouts as opposed to traditional strength training routines.

Progression

Regardless of how effective a training program is, it should not continue indefinitely without modification. As the client adapts to the training plan, the training stress or intensity must be altered to continue to induce positive adaptations. The process of altering training

SEQUENTIAL STEPS FOR DESIGNING A RESISTANCE TRAINING PROGRAM

To design an effective resistance training program, the personal trainer must make specific decisions about the manipulation of the **program design variables**, such as the training frequency, exercises used and how they are arranged, the structure of the program, the rest periods between sets, and the overall progression of the program. To facilitate the decision-making process, the personal trainer should consider a sequential approach. The culmination of this process is the establishment of a periodized training plan that increases the likelihood of the clients' achieving their predetermined training goals. The first step is to conduct an initial fitness consultation and evaluation, which serves as the foundation for the subsequent steps that are generally associated with the sequential approach.

1. Initial consultation and fitness evaluation
2. Determination of training frequency
3. Exercise selection
4. Arrangement of exercises (exercise order)
5. Training load: resistance and repetitions
6. Training volume: repetitions and sets
7. Rest periods
8. Training variation
9. Sequencing the training plan
10. Progression

stress as a client adapts is termed **progressive overload**. The stress is altered as the client becomes better trained (17), allowing him or her to continue advancing toward a specific training goal (3). Progression in resistance training must be applied systematically (3) and in proportion to the client's training status. Often, the effective application of progression in a program requires appropriate variation strategies and the use of periodized training models.

> **Successful resistance training programs must incorporate specificity, overload, variation, and progression. Ignoring any of these factors can limit the program's ability to stimulate the desired outcome, decrease adherence to the program, and increase the probability of injury and legal risk.**

INITIAL FITNESS CONSULTATION AND EVALUATION

Before any exercise program begins, it is essential that the personal trainer conduct an initial client consultation to assess compatibility, establish a client–trainer agreement, discuss the client's exercise goals, and determine the client's level of commitment (see chapter 9). After this discussion, the personal trainer needs to evaluate the client's exercise history and current level of fitness, identify strengths and weaknesses, identify areas of potential risk for injury, determine if contraindications to exercise exist, and refine the goals for the program (see chapters 9 and 10).

The initial consultation is an essential component of the resistance training program design process in that it gives the personal trainer valuable information about the client's training status. More specific information will be collected as the personal trainer assesses the client's initial resistance training status and resistance exercise technique experience, conducts a fitness evaluation and analyzes the results, and determines the client's primary goals.

Initial Resistance Training Status and Experience

The client's current training status and experience with resistance training will exert a significant impact on the training program to be developed. General information about the client's experience with resistance training can be gathered during the initial meeting (or soon afterward) when the client's exercise history is discussed.

The first step in determining the client's resistance training status is to have the client answer the general exercise history questions listed on the Health/Medical Questionnaire on page 166. The personal trainer then needs to obtain more specific information about the client's resistance training status and experience. A way to do this is to ask the client five basic questions (15):

1. Do you currently participate in a resistance training program?
2. How long have you been following a regular (one or more times per week) resistance training program?
3. How many times per week do you resistance train?
4. How intense (or difficult) are your resistance training workouts?

5. What types of resistance training exercises do you perform, and how many of them can you perform with proper technique?

These questions can be used to establish a basic understanding of the client's resistance training experience and as a tool for establishing a general classification of the training status. Table 15.1 offers one approach for classifying resistance training status on a continuum from beginner to advanced (60, 15). When the client's answers to the five questions match those shown in at least three of the five columns in one row, the estimated or predicted resistance training status is the one shown in the right-hand column. Although this basic classification system is useful, pigeonholing a client into a generalized training classification is difficult; at best, it helps establish a baseline starting point. The personal trainer must also make decisions about the client's responses based on professional knowledge and experience.

For example, if the client is not currently participating in a resistance training program but was following a regular training plan within the past four to six weeks, the answer to question 1 can be considered *yes*. In this case, the personal trainer would ask the client to answer questions 2 through 5 based on the recent training program. The decision to consider a recent

TABLE 15.1 A Method for Classifying Resistance Training Status

Question 1	Question 2	Question 3	Question 4	Question 5	
Do you currently participate in a resistance training program?[a]	How long have you been following a regular (one or more times per week) resistance training program?	How many times per week do you resistance train?	How intense (or difficult) are your resistance training workouts?	What types of resistance training exercises do you perform, and how many of them can you perform with proper technique?[b]	Estimated resistance training classification[c]
No	n/a	n/a	n/a	None	Beginner
Yes	≥2 months	1-2	Low intensity	3-5 machine exercises	
	4-6 months	2-3	Low to medium intensity	6-10 machine core and assistance exercises; 3-5 free-weight assistance exercises	
Yes	8-10 months	3	Medium intensity	11-15 machine core and assistance exercises; 6-10 free-weight assistance exercises; 3-5 free weight-core exercises	Intermediate
Yes	1 year	4	Medium to high intensity	>15 free-weight and machine core and assistance exercises	
Yes	1-1.5 years	4	High intensity	>15 free-weight and machine core and assistance exercises; 3-5 power/explosive exercises	Advanced
Yes	≥2 years	≥5	Very high intensity	>15 free-weight and machine core and assistance exercises; most power/explosive exercises	

Note: The personal trainer should realize that this method of classifying resistance training status will not apply to every client; the unique characteristics of each client need to be considered.

[a]If a client is not currently following a resistance training program but was participating in a regular resistance training plan in the past four to six weeks, the personal trainer could consider the answer to question 1 a *yes* and the client could answer questions 2 through 5 based on that recent program. The decision to equate participation in a recent program with participation in a current resistance training program is based entirely on the personal trainer's professional judgment regarding the particular client.

[b]As determined or evaluated by a qualified personal trainer; refer to section "Types of Resistance Training Exercises" on page 400 for a description of the various types of resistance training exercises.

[c]Classification of resistance training status is determined when the client's answers match the answers shown in at least three of the five columns in one row pertaining to resistance training exercise history and technique experience.

Adapted from Sheppard and Triplett (60) and Earle and Baechle (15).

resistance training program a current program is based solely on the personal trainer's professional judgment regarding the individual client's ability.

Fitness Evaluation

Typically the fitness evaluation involves an assessment of the client's resting heart rate and blood pressure, body composition, height, weight, girth, muscular strength, muscular endurance, aerobic fitness, and flexibility. In the context of this chapter, the fitness evaluation focuses on assessing or estimating the client's muscular strength and muscular endurance. Chapters 10 and 11 provide more information on fitness assessments.

After the fitness evaluation is completed, the personal trainer should compare the results with the normative or descriptive data presented in chapter 11. This comparison allows the personal trainer to determine the client's current level of fitness, establish a baseline for future comparisons as training status improves, and identify any strengths and weaknesses upon which to base goals. Additionally, the initial assessment may reveal contraindications to exercise that may require referring the client to a medical professional.

Primary Resistance Training Goal

Establishing the client's training goals is a very important part of the resistance training program design process. In keeping with the specificity principle, the client must train in specific ways to achieve desired results. Four primary resistance training goals include muscular endurance, hypertrophy (muscular size or tone), muscular strength, and muscular power.

Often the client's goals are not clearly identifiable. For example, it is uncommon for clients to say, "I want to follow a resistance training program for hypertrophy"; rather, they may say something more like "I want to have flatter abs." When the training goals are established during the initial consultation and fitness evaluation, the personal trainer will have to match the resistance training goals with the desires expressed by the client. Frequently during the consultation, the personal trainer needs to educate clients about the various goals that resistance training can address.

Muscular Endurance

A client may express a desire to improve muscular endurance with statements like "I want to have better endurance" or "I want to increase my stamina." Resistance training that targets **muscular endurance**, which is also termed *strength endurance training*, would address these goals by enhancing the ability of the targeted muscles to perform at a submaximal level for many repetitions or an extended period. The appropriate application of a resistance training program has great potential to improve muscular endurance (33, 66). Muscular endurance is commonly viewed as a part of aerobic exercise, as the muscle may contract thousands of times during a 20-minute activity such as running.

Hypertrophy

Statements like "I want my arms to be bigger, " "I want more size, " "I want to be more sculpted, " or "I want to change my body shape" suggest that the client wants to follow a program that will result in muscular hypertrophy or increased tone. **Hypertrophy** refers to an increase in muscle size, and hypertrophy training typically leads to an increase in fat free mass and a reduction in percent body fat.

Muscular Strength

Of the four resistance training goals, **muscular strength** is the easiest to establish. Clients often state this goal directly—"I want to get stronger." Although this is a common goal for athletes interested in a resistance training program designed to enhance their athletic performance (66), it may also be a goal for other clients. For example, older clients may say things like "I want to be able to carry my golf bag" or "I want to be able to get up and down the stairs better." Research suggests that older adults can improve their ability to engage in activities of daily living by increasing their muscular strength through performance of appropriate training programs (29, 35).

In comparison with resistance training programs that target muscular endurance or hypertrophy, a program that targets the development of muscular strength uses heavier training loads. Therefore, it is prudent for clients to develop proper form using relatively lighter loads before engaging in a program that targets muscular strength improvements.

Muscular Power

Traditionally, resistance training programs that target **muscular power** have been used only with athletes or clients who want to improve their sport performance abilities. Typically, statements like "I want to jump higher" or "I need to improve my speed and agility" suggest that the client would like to improve muscular power. Training programs that target muscular power have great potential to improve sport performance (4, 72). To maximize the benefits of these types of programs, it is prudent to sequence the client's training. For example, it has been shown that improvements in speed and jumping ability are greater when a program targeting muscular strength is performed before a program targeting muscular power (28).

Although power training has generally been used with athletes, research suggests it is also of benefit for older adult and nonathletic populations. Evidence indicates that older adults who engage in power-type training experience improvements in their ability to engage in activities of daily living (29) and in functional performance (31, 32).

DETERMINATION OF TRAINING FREQUENCY

Training **frequency** refers to the number of workouts a client will undertake for one week. Many factors contribute to the determination of the optimal frequency for an individual client. Factors such as the types of exercises used, the number of muscle groups trained per session, the structure of the program (volume and intensity), and the client's training status and overall fitness level dictate the training frequency (3). The client's work schedule, social schedule, and family obligations will also strongly influence how frequently the client can train.

Influential Factors

The primary factors the personal trainer should consider when determining training frequency is the client's training status, overall level of fitness, and time available for exercise. Lesser-trained clients usually require more rest between workouts, which lowers frequency, while highly trained clients are able to tolerate more frequency. However, the personal trainer may need to reduce the frequency of resistance training if the client's overall amount of physical or psychological stress is high because of other demands (e.g., work, social, or academic schedule; other forms of exercise; or some combination of all demands) (63). For example, if the client is a construction worker who performs repetitive lifting tasks at work, he or she may not want or be able to tolerate more than two or three days per week of resistance training. Moreover, daily schedules can potentially limit the availability to train, regardless of individual abilities. Taking all these considerations into account is paramount in determining optimal training frequency for a given client.

An influential factor that many personal trainers overlook is how the different components of the training program interact (36, 37, 45). Many personal trainers plan resistance, endurance, agility, and plyometric training without considering how each factor affects the overall workload. It is essential to examine how the various training activities interact and to take the client's overall workload into account. For example, if the client is running 30 minutes a day, five days per week, he or she may be able to tolerate only two days per week of resistance training.

Guidelines for Determining Training Frequency

When determining the training frequency, it is important to plan sufficient recovery into the program. A general rule that many personal trainers follow is to allow at least one day (but no more than three) between workouts that stress the same muscle group or groups (7, 43). More specific guidelines depend on a client's overall resistance training status (table 15.2; 48). Most novice (untrained beginner) and intermediate clients can experience the benefits of resistance training with as few as two or three days per week (3, 44, 50). It has been proposed that advanced clients generally can only maintain their strength gains and cannot increase strength levels when training just one or two days per week (3), but there is not enough research to draw strong conclusions on the topic. In general, the more frequent the sessions, the greater the strength gains, although it is not clear to what extent these increases are driven by associated higher training volumes (20).

Novice or Beginner Resistance Training Status

A general recommendation for the novice, or untrained beginner, to resistance training is to exercise two or three days per week when training the entire body (3, 12, 14, 34, 50). With this frequency, resistance training days should be nonconsecutive (i.e., Monday and Thursday; Tuesday, Thursday, and Saturday; or Monday, Wednesday, and Friday) to allow for appropriate recovery between sessions. Novice clients should have one to three days between resistance training session, but ideally no more than three, to facilitate recovery. If, for example, the client was to train on Monday and Wednesday, the amount of time between the Wednesday and the next Monday training session would be greater than three days and hypothetically result in a less effective training program. That said,

TABLE 15.2   General Guidelines for Resistance Training Frequency

Resistance training status	Recommended number of sessions per week
Novice or beginner	2-3
Intermediate	3 if using total body training
	4 if using a split routine
Advanced	3-6˙

˙Advanced resistance-trained clients may perform multiple sessions in one day.

Adapted from Ratamess et al. (48).

the significance of any difference in results remains questionable and at the very least would be specific to individual goals and abilities; ultimately, practical considerations regarding the client's availability would take precedence. As the client progresses from the novice to the intermediate level, a change in frequency is not always necessary (3). However, increasing the frequency to three or four days per week allows for greater program flexibility.

Intermediate Resistance Training Status

A general recommendation for the client who has achieved an intermediate training status is to increase the training frequency to three or four days per week (3). In the case of four weekly sessions, this means the client trains two or more days in a row. A common strategy is to use a **split body** (or just *split*) **routine**, which spreads four or more workouts evenly across the week. With this structure, the client has the option to train only one part of the body (e.g., upper body or lower body) (39), certain muscle areas (e.g., chest, back, or legs) (39), or certain movement patterns (i.e., push or pull) (67) during a given session. This structure allows for an increase in frequency while still providing sufficient time for recovery between sessions (43).

A common example of a four day per week split routine for the intermediate client includes upper body exercises on Monday and Thursday and lower body exercises on Tuesday and Friday (39). Even though the client is training two days in row, changing the targeted muscle groups ensures that individual muscles are provided with at least 48 hours' recovery between sessions. With this type of frequency split, the nonresistance training or rest days are consistently Wednesday, Saturday, and Sunday. More importantly, when training specific muscle groups or body parts, this split allows for optimization of results using higher volumes (50) or within-week variation (discussed later in this chapter).

Scheduling or financial concerns can affect the ability to increase training frequency. Some clients will simply not be willing or able to devote the time to train this often. Other clients may be willing and able to train more frequently but might not have the financial means to work with a personal trainer on the extra days. In the former case, availability will always dictate the ultimate number of days a client can train, and programming must be altered around his or her schedule. In the latter case, the personal trainer must work within the budgetary constraints, working directly with the client as frequently as finances allow and then providing an integrated routine to perform on alternate days.

Advanced Resistance Training Status

Depending on their goals, intermediate clients may need to increase their training frequency as they become more experienced and reclassified as advanced in status. A general recommendation is for advanced individuals to resistance train three to six days per week to allow for an increase in training stimulus (3). An option is to employ double split routines (27), performing two sessions on the same day, which increases the number of training sessions from 8 to 12 per week (3, 65). Some evidence supports a potential benefit to performing multiple short training sessions in one day for certain fitness outcomes (27, 65). However, such routines are not feasible from a scheduling standpoint for most clients.

Another method for increasing the frequency from five to six days is to use a split routine of three days on, one day off. With this structure, three distinct workouts target specific muscle groups, and the client completes one workout on three consecutive days and rests on the fourth day. A common strategy is to divide the program into upper body push exercises (i.e., chest, shoulders, triceps), lower body exercises, and upper body pull exercises (i.e., upper back, trapezius, and biceps). In this type of structure, the workouts are on unspecified days; that is, the rest day is not the same each week. As previously mentioned, scheduling and financial concerns will ultimately dictate a client's ability to increase frequency or work more frequently with a personal trainer. Such factors must be considered when making recommendations on the topic, as well as in creating customized programs.

EXERCISE SELECTION

The selection of exercises to be incorporated into the client's training program is influenced by the principle of specificity, the equipment available, the client's resistance training experience, the amount of time the client dedicates to training, and personal client preference. Once the personal trainer considers these issues, he or she can select exercises that maximize the training adaptations and increase the chances of achieving the client's specific training goals while maintaining motivation to exercise.

Influential Factors

When selecting exercises, the personal trainer should make decisions based on the specific needs of the client and the target goals established in the initial consultation with the client while considering individual preferences. Many factors will affect this decision-making process, including how much time a client dedicates to training. The time available can have a large impact on the number and complexity of exercises chosen for a given training session. For example, performing the back squat to target lower body development works a much greater portion of the body's musculature compared with performing leg curls and leg extensions, thereby potentially providing a more time-efficient option.

An additional factor is the equipment available to the client. Even if an exercise is effective, goal specific, and efficient, it cannot be a major part of a client's training plan if the required equipment is not available. To account for this, the personal trainer needs to gather an equipment inventory for the facility in which the client intends to train before planning the program. This important step can help avoid wasting time in constructing the training plan.

Another factor that will dictate the selection of exercises is whether the client can perform the exercise correctly. If the client is inexperienced in or unfamiliar with proper technique for an exercise, or if the extent of the client's experience is unknown, the personal trainer must provide a complete demonstration, explanation, and familiarization period in which to teach the client appropriate technique. This may require initially giving the client remedial exercises that can build a

foundation for more complex exercises in future programs. Inexperienced clients often are taught machine exercises and free-weight assistance exercises first because these require less skill than many of the core exercises (17, 64). (In this context, *core exercises* do not refer to exercises targeting the abdominal core. See the next section on types of resistance training exercises.) Following these recommendations can be effective in reducing the potential for litigation, decreasing injury risk, promoting adherence, and improving the overall effectiveness of the program.

Types of Resistance Training Exercises

There are a plethora of exercises from which to construct a resistance training program. These exercises can be classified as either core or assistance exercises based on the size of the muscles recruited, the complexity of the movement pattern, and the degree of contribution toward the client's training goals.

Core Exercises

Generally speaking, **core exercises** should form the bulk of a program because they are more effective than assistance exercises in helping clients achieve their specific training goals. However, the needs and abilities of the client will ultimately dictate the selection of exercises; there are no absolute rules in this regard. An exercise is classified as a core exercise if it

- involves two or more primary joints, which would make it a **multijoint exercise**, and
- engages large muscles while activating synergistic muscles.

One multijoint large muscle exercise has the potential to activate as many muscles or muscle groups as four to eight small muscle, single-joint assistance exercises (62, 64). A program that uses core exercises appropriately is more time-efficient than one that uses many small muscle exercises.

The personal trainer has many core exercises to choose from when constructing a program (see chapter 13). An example is the bench press, which involves movement at the shoulder and elbow joints while recruiting the pectoral muscles with synergistic help from the anterior deltoids and the triceps brachii.

If a core exercise loads the axial skeleton (places a load on the spine) (e.g., power clean, squat, front squat, shoulder press), it is further classified as a **structural exercise**. Structural exercises require the muscles of the torso to maintain an erect or near-erect position. For example, during the squat, the barbell loads the axial skeleton, and the musculature of the torso must maintain a near-erect position as the client descends and ascends. A structural exercise that is performed very quickly, such as the power clean or power snatch, is also classified as **power** or **explosive exercise** (e.g., push press, snatch or clean pull, high pull, push jerk). Although these types of exercises can be effective for developing muscular power, they are highly challenging to perform and thus tend to carry a greater risk of injury. Accordingly, personal trainers should weigh the costs and benefits when deciding whether such exercises are appropriate for a given client in accordance with his or her goals.

> **In the context of resistance training, core exercises refer to exercises that engage large muscles and multiple joints.**

Assistance Exercises

Assistance exercises are supplementary exercises performed to maintain muscular balance across a joint, help prevent injury, rehabilitate a previous injury, or isolate a specific muscle group or muscle. Exercises are classified as assistance exercises if they

- are **single-joint exercises**, engaging only one primary joint, and
- recruit a small amount of muscle mass (i.e., a small muscle group or area).

The extent of the inclusion of assistance exercises in program design will depend on the client's goals and abilities.

A popular assistance exercise is the barbell biceps curl. This exercise engages a small amount of muscle mass (biceps brachii, brachialis, and brachioradialis) and involves movement of only a single joint (the elbow). The pec deck and dumbbell fly are also classified as assistance exercises even though they engage the larger muscles of the chest. They involve movement only at the shoulder joint and place primary emphasis on the pectoral muscles.

Guidelines for Choosing Exercises

The exercises selected for a training program should meet the individual client's needs, whether the client is an elite athlete or a novice, is severely detrained, or has been recently injured.

For an untrained novice, the personal trainer should pay more attention to developing a training base, probably with assistance exercises or basic core exercises. In this situation, one may decide to target specific muscle groups or train each muscle group. This strategy involves choosing one exercise per muscle group: chest, shoulders, upper back, hips and thighs, biceps, triceps, abdominal muscles, and calves (43). As the client becomes better trained, the number of exercises per muscle group can be increased (43). Typically, this type of program uses small muscle or single-joint exercises, but programs should progressively incorporate more multijoint large muscle or core exercises.

Employing multijoint large muscle exercises can magnify the adaptive response and increase the overall metabolic cost of the training program. An example is the squat and press. This complex exercise engages a large amount of muscle mass, substantially increases the metabolic cost of training, and produces a substantial training effect. Other examples are power cleans, power snatches, and pulls. These all train the entire body and appear to be extremely effective training methods for athletes (62). With athletes, the more closely the exercise relates to the sporting movement pattern, the more likely the strength gains developed will translate to the sport (8, 17, 64, 67, 73). For example, when working with a volleyball or basketball player, the personal trainer should consider using exercises such as the power clean or power snatch since they involve a jumping movement, which is important in these sports. (See chapter 23 for guidelines on selecting exercises for a particular sport.)

In work with clients who have special needs, such as lower back problems or recent injuries, it is important to adapt the training program to address these issues. Accordingly, the personal trainer should work alongside, or seek guidance from, a medical professional for the proper selection of exercises. It is essential that a training program for these clients avoid exercises that are contraindicated or not recommended. For example, if a client was recently released from the care of a physical therapist for a shoulder impingement, the physical therapist may prescribe the dumbbell lateral raise in place of the overhead shoulder press to work the deltoid muscle group.

Finally, and importantly, client preference should be considered when deciding on exercise selection. Certain exercises are simply more enjoyable for a given individual. Matching personal preference with the client's goals and abilities will help build client motivation, which in turn can improve adherence.

> Client preference should be considered when choosing exercises so they match a client's goals and abilities in order to build client motivation and improve adherence.

EXERCISE ORDER

The **exercise order** or arrangement refers to the order in which the exercises are performed during the workout. The exercise order is dependent on many factors but is most strongly influenced by the type and characteristics of the exercises selected.

Influential Factors

Factors that influence the order of exercises include the goals of the client, fatigue-generating potential of the exercise, and type of exercise (core versus assistance).

One method for ordering exercises is to place them in a descending order of priority or application to the client's goals, activity, or, in the case of athletes, sport. With this type of structure, the client performs the exercises that target individual goals earlier in the workout when fatigue is lowest, performing less goal-specific exercises toward the end of the session.

A second method for arranging exercises is based on their type (core versus assistance). With this method, core exercises are performed first, and assistance exercises are performed later in the session. This arrangement allows the client to perform the more complex, multijoint core exercises under minimal levels of fatigue. In general, the personal trainer should attempt to maximize the client's ability to tolerate the training loads and complete all the exercises in one session by arranging the exercises to manage fatigue.

Guidelines for Arranging Exercises

There are many ways to arrange exercises in a training session (17). The ordering of exercises can be categorized into several primary methods, such as placing power and core exercises before assistance exercises, alternating push and pull exercises, and alternating upper and lower body exercises. There are also combination methods and secondary arrangement methods (tables 15.3 and 15.4).

Placing Power and Core Exercises Before Assistance Exercise

One of the most common guidelines is to order the exercises as follows:

> Power exercises → Core exercises → Assistance exercises

Conceptually, since power exercises and core exercises are often multijoint exercises and assistance exercises are typically single-joint exercises, the following is another possible order:

> Multijoint exercises → Single-joint exercises

Another way to think about exercise order is to consider the amount of muscle mass activated with the exercise. Large muscle exercises, which are generally core or multijoint exercises, should be performed before single-joint exercise:

> Large muscle exercises → Small muscle exercises

Regardless of the way one conceptualizes these exercise sequences, the basic structures noted here should be the most effective exercise sequencing methods for most clients.

These arrangements of exercises are effective because power or multijoint exercises require more effort, skill, and focus than single-joint assistance exercises and should be performed when the client is fresh (17). Historically it has been recommended that only athletes use power exercises, such as the Olympic lifts and their derivatives; but research suggests that all populations can use power-oriented exercises to achieve their training goals (11, 35). The caveat is that research investigating power training in the general population has focused on performing the concentric portion of traditional resistance training exercises at higher velocities (29), not with the use of Olympic lifts. The complexity of the Olympic lifts heightens their risk of injury, making their use questionable for the public. As previously mentioned, a cost–benefit analysis should be undertaken when deciding on the inclusion of specific exercises for a given individual.

Alternating Push and Pull Exercises

Another method of arranging exercises is to alternate push exercises (e.g., vertical chest press and triceps pushdown) with pull exercises (e.g., seated row and dumbbell biceps curl). It has been suggested that this system allows rest between exercises and ensures that the same muscle group is not used for two exercises

TABLE 15.3   Sample Exercise Order for Resistance Training Based on Exercise Type and Muscle Mass Activated

SAMPLE EXERCISE ORDER: POWER → CORE → ASSISTANCE				
Exercise order	**Exercise**	**Exercise classification**		
1	Power clean	Power exercises	Multijoint exercises	Large muscle exercises
2	Push press			
3	Front squat	Core exercises		
4	Bench press			
5	Triceps pushdown	Assistance exercises	Single-joint exercises	Small muscle exercises
6	Wrist curl			
7	Seated heel raise			

SAMPLE EXERCISE ORDER: MULTIJOINT → SINGLE JOINT				
Exercise order	**Exercise**	**Exercise classification**		
1	Squat + press	Core exercises	Multijoint exercises	Large muscle exercises
2	Back squat			
3	Incline bench press			
4	Leg curl	Assistance exercises	Single-joint exercises	Small muscle exercises
5	Three-way shoulder raise			

SAMPLE EXERCISE ORDER: LARGE MUSCLE → SMALL MUSCLE				
Exercise order	**Exercise**	**Exercise classification**		
1	Power snatch	Power exercises	Multijoint exercises	Large muscle exercises
2	Overhead squat	Core exercises		
3	Romanian deadlift			
4	Bent-over row	Assistance exercises	Single-joint exercises	Small muscle exercises
5	Lateral raise			
6	Abdominal crunch			

Note: These are simply examples of how exercises may be sequenced and do not represent complete resistance training workouts.

in a row (60). Although the push–pull system is commonly used, it is important to remember that core exercises can activate a vast array of muscles and that many will use the same muscle groups. For example, if a client performs the seated row (a pulling exercise) followed by the bench press (a pushing exercise), the sternal head of the pectoralis major will be activated in both exercises.

Alternating Upper and Lower Body Exercises

A traditional approach to ordering exercises requires the client to alternate between upper and lower body exercises (17). This type of ordering is typically used with a circuit weight training program and short rest intervals (e.g., ≤30 seconds). As with the push–pull system, this ordering may be best suited for machine-based training or when the predominant exercises selected are those classified as small muscle or assistance exercises.

Combination Arrangement Methods

It is possible to combine the most common methods of arranging exercises. Two or three of the previously mentioned methods can be combined: for example, core exercises and then assistance exercises that alternate push and pull. Often with a combination arrangement, a lower body exercise precedes an upper body exercise, although the opposite order appears to be equally as viable.

TABLE 15.4 Examples of Alternating Exercise Ordering Systems

SAMPLE EXERCISE ORDER: ALTERNATING PUSH AND PULL EXERCISES				
Exercise order	**Exercise**	**Exercise classification**		
1	Back squat	Push	Core	Multijoint
2	Leg curl	Pull	Assistance	Single joint
3	Standing heel raise	Push	Assistance	Single joint
4	Upright row	Pull	Assistance	Single joint
5	Incline bench press	Push	Core	Multijoint
6	Dumbbell biceps curl	Pull	Assistance	Single joint
7	Shoulder press	Push	Core	Multijoint
8	Lat pulldown	Pull	Assistance	Multijoint
SAMPLE EXERCISE ORDER: ALTERNATING UPPER AND LOWER BODY EXERCISES				
Exercise order	**Exercise**	**Exercise classification**		
1	Leg press	Lower body	Core	Multijoint
2	Bench press	Upper body	Core	Multijoint
3	Lunge	Lower body	Core	Multijoint
4	Shoulder shrug	Upper body	Assistance	Single joint
5	Leg extension	Lower body	Assistance	Single joint
6	Dumbbell shoulder press	Upper body	Core	Multijoint
7	Leg curl	Lower body	Assistance	Single joint
8	Triceps extension	Upper body	Assistance	Single joint

Note: These are simply examples of how exercises may be sequenced and do not represent complete resistance training workouts.

Secondary Arrangement Methods

Two popular secondary methods involve completing a set of two different exercises in succession without an intervening rest interval. If the two exercises coupled together train the same muscle group (e.g., incline bench press and incline dumbbell fly), the set is considered a **compound set** (60). Compound sets are often used by bodybuilders to induce muscular hypertrophy (17), although the efficacy of this strategy remains undetermined.

Another secondary arrangement, termed a **superset**, involves performing two exercises that activate opposing or antagonistic muscle groups (e.g., biceps curl and triceps press) with no rest between each exercise (17, 60, 64). Supersetting is popular among bodybuilders, individuals who are attempting to increase muscular endurance, and individuals with limited time for training (17). Whether supersets enhance results remains equivocal, but implementing this strategy can facilitate greater time-efficiency by increasing the training density of the exercise session.

TRAINING LOAD: RESISTANCE AND REPETITIONS

The training **load**, or the amount of weight to be used, is one of the most important factors to consider in the design of a training program. There are many ways to determine the training load. The assigned load will exert a large impact on the number of repetitions that can be performed and ultimately the types of physiological and performance adaptations stimulated (e.g., muscular strength versus muscular endurance). Ultimately, the interplay between the load and volume of training (repetitions × sets × resistance) is dictated by the type of training program established and the intended goals of the program.

Influential Factors

The load, number of repetitions, and targeted outcomes of a resistance training program are strongly related. For example, higher-intensity loads performed for fewer repetitions target the development of muscular strength. Lifting lighter loads for many repetitions enhances muscular endurance. In its most basic form, a client's training program would address specific goals and target them with selected repetition and load relationships. Additional factors to consider when assigning initial training loads are the differences in muscular demands between various modalities and the complexity of the exercise. For example, transitioning from bilateral to unilateral exercises (e.g., barbell bench press to dumbbell bench press) or exercises that require more stability and technique (e.g., machine-based chest press to barbell bench press) will alter the amount of weight than can be lifted by the individual. Furthermore, when progressing to exercises requiring more stability and skill, the focus of the personal training should be proper technique before establishing a training load. This, however, is a gross simplification of the training process.

Regardless of the client's goals, the training plan should include periods in which muscular endurance, strength, and potentially power are developed. Sequencing different repetition and loading schemes will magnify training adaptations and provide a greater chance of accomplishing the client's goals (28, 45, 67).

Another key consideration for the personal trainer when establishing training loads is the intensity of effort from the client. Reduced individual effort can greatly affect outcomes for any resistance training program. For example, if a prescribed range of 8 to 12 repetitions has been established, the client should not be able to perform more than 12 with a specific weight. If the client successfully performs the desired number of repetitions but could successfully perform a significant number of repetitions beyond the goal range (e.g., >3 repetitions), then benefits may not be maximized. Therefore, client effort should be monitored to ensure that the last few repetitions are challenging but do not compromise proper technique.

Determining Training Loads

Before assigning the training load and repetitions to be performed in each set, the personal trainer must determine the client's ability to properly perform an exercise as well as handle a specific load in a series of selected exercises. For example, the focus for any beginner or client who is unfamiliar with a movement is proper exercise technique before determining a training load. Thus, the initial sessions with a beginner may focus on assessing the individual's movement capabilities, strengths, and weaknesses. If a client

is unable to successfully perform an exercise, then regressions, assisted machines, or proper mechanics should be the priority. Once the client demonstrates proficiency with an exercise, the personal trainer can assign training loads.

The following are methods for accomplishing this directive:

- Repetition maximum testing (RM)
- Repetitions in reserve (RIR)
- Rating of perceived exertion (RPE)

Individual differences, variations in technical proficiency, and multiple equipment choices make it nearly impossible to calculate a testing load perfectly, so the personal trainer may rely on previous knowledge and personal expertise when determining an initial training load. One of the best approaches is to first establish a goal repetition range and then determine a maximal load for one or multiple sets of the respective exercise through trial and error, but erring on the side of caution for the initial load. For beginners and deconditioned clients, it may require several sessions to determine training loads as the client becomes more familiar with the exercises and proper technique.

Percentage of 1-Repetition Maximum Relationship

The repetition maximum (RM) is the maximal load the client can handle in a specific exercise for a specific number of repetitions. As the load becomes heavier, the number of repetitions the client can perform will decrease. Eventually the load will become so heavy that the client can perform only one repetition; this is the **1-repetition maximum (1RM)**. Conversely, the lighter the load, the more repetitions the client can perform. This association between 1RM and repetitions has been termed the **percentage of 1RM (%1RM)–repetition relationship**. Although this method is used for many load prescriptions, it is uncommon for the personal trainer to use 1RM testing. The biggest disadvantage of this method is that it is extremely time consuming, taking a half hour or more per exercise. This is generally not an efficient use of client training time. Additionally, clients who have been recently injured or are under medical supervision should abstain from 1RM testing. All things considered, 1RM testing should generally be reserved for more advanced clients and athletes who are primarily training with heavy loads. More information about this method of testing can be found in chapter 23.

Repetition Maximum

One of the most common methods for establishing training loads is to use an intensity that allows for performance of a specific number of repetitions, or what is known as a **repetition maximum (RM)** or **repetitions to failure**. In this method, clients lift the heaviest load they can for the selected repetition scheme (40). For example, clients performing 3 sets at a 12RM load would use the heaviest weight that would allow them to perform 3 sets with no less or more than 12 repetitions. A similar method, using what is called the **RM target zone** (also called the **repetition maximum zone**), is to assign a range, such as 10RM to 12RM (17). For a prescribed RM target zone, clients use the heaviest weight that allows them to perform the exercise for the number of repetitions within the range. Although this is probably not the best method for determining training loads, it can be used to assess core and assistance exercises. If RM testing is to be performed, the personal trainer should select a few key exercises, particularly core movements, to reduce the initial testing time for the client.

Higher RMs (i.e., 8 or more repetitions) can result in a large amount of accumulated fatigue during multiple trial sets, particularly for beginning or deconditioned clients (64). If RM testing is to be performed, the personal trainer should select a few key exercises, particularly core movements, to avoid a large amount of initial testing time for the client. Regardless of the client's training status, it is important for the personal trainer to monitor the client to prevent excessive fatigue that could result in an increased risk of injury; a general recommendation is to limit testing to 3 sets. Additionally, because of the stress placed on an iso-lated joint and tissues, the heaviest load for assistance exercises should be ~8RM (60).

The targeted RM and RM target zone methods for assigning initial training loads can be potentially problematic because in both instances the client is required to train to muscular failure. For clients who are beginners or deconditioned, RM training may lead to increased feelings of discomfort or increased levels of delayed-onset muscle soreness, which may reduce client retention, motivation, and adherence. Thus, this method of prescribing an initial training load may be more acceptable for intermediate and advanced populations. It is important to note that continually training to failure throughout each workout session can increase the time of recovery as well as the risk of overtraining (38). Therefore, incorporating load variation (described later in this chapter) into a resistance training routine may provide a more successful approach to training adaptations.

Rating of Perceived Exertion

A subjective method of determining an initial training intensity, based on the client's level of perceived effort or intensity, is known as the **rating of perceived exertion (RPE)**. The scale used most often within resistance training is the **OMNI-Resistance Exercise Scale** (figure 15.1; 51). Consisting of a 1 to 10 scale with visual aids, RPE can help personal trainers increase or decrease the exercise load based on client feedback (49). Each increment on the OMNI scale represents a 10% increase within the client's RM; the higher the rank (i.e., closer to 10), the greater the perceived intensity. By using a subjective rating, the personal trainer can gauge the intensity of a given

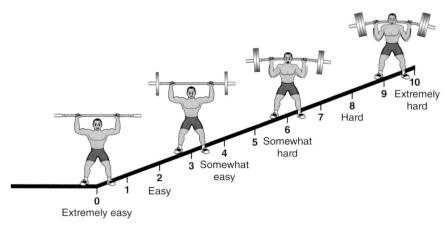

FIGURE 15.1 OMNI-Resistance Exercise Scale.

Reprinted by permission from Robertson (2004, p. 49).

set, exercise, or workout session from the viewpoint of the client. RPE also allows the personal trainer to monitor fatigue from session to session and adjust training loads accordingly. Therefore, the RPE scale has become crucial in assessing exercise intensity within special populations, such as clients who are elderly, are pregnant, or have other conditions that would contraindicate RM testing.

However, this method is not without limitations. Research suggests that familiarization with the scale plays a key role in gauging intensity (68). For example, individuals tend to report RPE scores that are less than maximal despite achieving the maximal repetition count for a given set load (30). Thus, depending on an individual's fitness level, a client's feedback is reliant on his or her understanding of the RPE scale. When implementing the RPE scale for novice clients, the personal trainer may combine it with other methods of determining an initial training load (e.g., repetitions in reserve) until the client gains a better understanding of the scale.

Repetitions in Reserve

An alternative method for prescribing training load is **repetitions in reserve (RIR)**, or **nonfailure training**. Unlike a repetition maximum, clients do not train to muscular failure within each set. Instead, a repetition value or range is selected based on the client's goal; however, the client is advised to stop a certain number of repetitions short of muscular failure. By using RIR and stopping short of failure, clients are less likely to experience higher levels of fatigue or muscle soreness, which potentially can increase client adherence and retention. Methods like %1RM and RM testing are based on a single day of testing and may not represent the day-to-day variation of a client's strength or fatigue due to previous workout sessions or physiological or psychological factors.

Furthermore, using %1RM or RM for loading prescription has inherent flaws because the number of repetitions achieved at a given percentage will vary substantially between individuals. For example, in one study the subjects completed an average of ~14 repetitions at 75% 1RM in the leg press; however, individual variance ranged from a low of 7 repetitions to a high of 24 repetitions (54). Thus, the RIR method allows for the adjustment of training load between sets within a given session and may provide a more accurate assessment of intensity within a given

repetition range (30). The RIR testing method is not accurate when sets are performed at low to moderate intensities, far from volitional fatigue; therefore it is best used when the resistance training program calls for sets to be performed a few repetitions shy of muscular failure (74).

However, a limitation of this approach is the training status of the client. Novice clients are less likely to accurately gauge the number of repetitions remaining in a set before fatigue (74). Therefore, personal trainers should not rely solely on RIR for initial training load prescriptions. A way to familiarize clients with this method is to prescribe a submaximal set with the instructions to stop 3 repetitions before muscular failure. Record the number of repetitions the client performs. After a rest period of 1 to 2 minutes, have the client perform another set of the same exercise, with the same load, to *failure* to determine if the client correctly estimated 3 RIR in the set (30).

Figure 15.2 can be used to improve the accuracy of the RIR method. Each value within the RPE 1 to 10 scale, modified by Zourdos and colleagues (74), corresponds to a categorical perceived effort (denoted as *RPE*) and a given number of RIR. For example, an RPE of 10 would be a maximal effort with no RIR, whereas an RPE of 8 or 9 would constitute a set performed with 1 or 2 RIR. Since the accuracy of the RIR diminishes as the number of remaining repetitions increases, RPE values of 1 to 4 correspond to *little to no effort* (i.e., an RPE of 1-2) and *light effort* (i.e., an RPE of 3-4). When incorporating the RIR method into a resistance training program, the personal trainer can use it in conjunction with other methods of initial load prescription. For instance, if a 10RM is known for a given exercise, the program may call for 2 sets of 10 repetitions with an RPE of 8 or 9, thereby informing the client to perform the set with 1 or 2 RIR.

Both the RPE and RIR methods are autoregulatory, meaning the client is subjectively making the decision of the exercise intensity. Therefore, to maximize benefits of the training program, the client must learn how to properly use these approaches before relying on them to establish an initial training load (74). However, any method used to determine the initial training load has room for error. For example, although an assessment may be designed to produce an intensity to be performed for 12 to 15 repetitions, it is possible that the client will perform less than 12 or more than 15 repetitions. Thus, the trial load will need to be adjusted to better target the client's goals. Table 15.5 (15, 60)

FIGURE 15.2 Resistance training–specific RPE.

Rating of Perceived Exertion (RPE)	Description of perceived exertion	Repetitions in reserve (RIR)
10	Maximum effort	0
9.5	No further repetitions but could increase load	0
9	1 repetition remaining	1
8.5	1 or 2 repetitions remaining	1 or 2
8	2 repetitions remaining	2
7.5	2 or 3 repetitions remaining	2 or 3
7	3 repetitions remaining	3
5-6	4-6 repetitions remaining	4 to 6
3-4	Light effort	--
1-2	Little to no effort	--

Reprinted by permission from Zourdos et al. (2016).

provides one possible method for making this adjustment by increasing the load if the client performs too many repetitions or reducing the load if the client performs too few. These adjustments are only guidelines and not without error (e.g., multijoint exercises may require larger load adjustments), but they provide a viable starting point for structuring the training plan. For example, if the client cannot complete 2 or more sets of 8 or 9 repetitions with a 105-pound (50 kg) load in the bench press, the load can be adjusted according to the information in table 15.5 to potentially achieve the desired number of repetitions. So if the client can perform only 6 repetitions with the 105-pound load, the load could be reduced by 5 pounds (2.5 kg).

Guidelines for Assigning Loads

When determining the loads to be used in a program, the personal trainer must consider the primary goals of the client (muscular endurance, hypertrophy, muscular strength, or muscular power). Different load and repetition schemes can have different training effects (table 15.6). It is recommended that various loading schemes be employed in a program (3, 67) to avoid overtraining, allow for progression, and maximize training adaptations. Results will also vary for exercises using upper versus lower body, multi- versus single-joint, and machine versus free weights. Thus, a better strategy is to program loading based on a given repetition range, as noted in table 15.6 (3, 15, 17, 44, 50, 67). During the initial stages of training, novice clients should simply focus on developing proper form across the spectrum of exercises that will be employed within the training program. It is generally best to employ a moderate- to higher-repetition scheme during this initial period, which allows for sufficient practice of movement patterns to enhance motor learning. Once technical competence is achieved in the chosen exercises, programming of load should shift to a more goal-focused approach.

Heavier loads (1RM-5RM) are required to optimize muscular strength (55). At least some training must be carried out in this loading zone on a regular basis for clients seeking maximal strength gains. Despite that, consistently training with very heavy loads may overstress joints and overtax the neuromuscular system, leading to neuroendocrine alterations that may bring about a nonfunctionally overreached state (18, 58). Thus strength-related goals can benefit from a periodized approach, whereby moderate and lighter loads are employed on a rotating basis. It should be noted that moderate- and light-load training do in fact increase dynamic strength, even in resistance-trained individuals (53, 57), just not to the same extent as heavy-load training. From a practical standpoint, unless a client's goal is to maximize strength, the spectrum of loading ranges will likely be sufficient to enhance force-producing capacity to carry out activities of daily living.

Muscular endurance benefits from the use of lighter loads with higher repetitions (>15RM) (10, 57). The longer time under tension associated with this loading zone enhances mitochondrial protein synthesis (9), which may in turn promote greater fatigue resistance

TABLE 15.5   Adjusting the Trial Load to Allow the Goal Number of Repetitions*

| Goal repetitions | REPETITIONS COMPLETED WITH THE TRIAL LOAD | | | | | | | | | |
	18	16-17	14-15	12-13	10-11	8-9	6-7	4-5	2-3	<2
14-15	+10	+5		−5	−10	−15	−15	−20	−25	−30
12-13	+15	+10	+5		−5	−10	−15	−15	−20	−25
10-11	+15	+15	+10	+5		−5	−10	−15	−15	−20
8-9	+20	+15	+15	+10	+5		−5	−10	−15	−15
6-7	+25	+20	+15	+15	+10	+5		−5	−10	−15
4-5	+30	+25	+20	+15	+15	+10	+5		−5	−10
2-3	+35	+30	+25	+20	+15	+15	+10	+5		−5

Load increase (+) or decrease (−) in pounds.

*Actual increases or decreases in load will be dependent on the specific exercise employed and individual genetic and lifestyle factors.

Adapted from Sheppard and Triplett (60) and Earle and Baechle (15).

TABLE 15.6   Training Load and Repetition Schemes for Targeted Goals

| Training emphasis | REPETITIONS | | | SETS | | |
	Novice	Intermediate	Advanced	Novice	Intermediate	Advanced
Muscular endurance	10RM-15RM	10RM-30+RM	15RM-30+RM	1-3	≥3	≥3
Hypertrophy	8RM-12RM	5RM-30+RM	5RM-30+RM	1-3	≥3	≥3
Muscular strength˙	≤6RM	≤3-6RM	≤1-6RM	1-3	≥3	≥3
Muscular power	n/a	3-6	1-6	n/a	1-3	3-6

˙These loads apply to core exercises; assistance exercises should use loads *lighter* than or equal to a 6RM.

Based on American College of Sports Medicine (3), Earle and Baechle (15), Fleck and Kraemer (17), Peterson et al. (44), Rhea et al. (50), and Stone et al. (67).

during repeated submaximal muscular work. It is also conceivable that the elevated metabolite accumulation from consistently training with lighter loads results in adaptations that improve muscle buffering capacity, although this hypothesis remains somewhat speculative.

Contrary to what many personal trainers believe, muscle hypertrophy can be achieved across a broad spectrum of loading ranges. Similar increases in muscle development are seen with loads as low as 30% of the 1RM compared with higher training intensities (>60% of the 1RM), provided training is carried out with a high degree of effort (55). Findings are consistent across populations and are observed in both untrained and resistance-trained individuals. This provides a wide range of options for customizing loading prescription to the client whose goal is to increase muscle mass. Those who have issues training with heavier loads (e.g., conditions such as osteoarthritis

or rehabilitation from injury) can achieve appreciable hypertrophy with lighter loads and thus decrease levels of stress on joints and soft tissues. However, evidence suggests that loads <30% of the 1RM may elicit suboptimal muscle growth compared with higher load intensities (42), indicating a minimum threshold for maximizing hypertrophic gains.

> **Although there are many ways to determine an initial training load, the initial focus of the personal trainer should be teaching proper exercise technique and movement proficiency. Once the client can properly perform the movement, a challenging load, based on the client's goal repetition range, can be incorporated.**

PROGRESSION

An essential component of any training program, **progression** is the process by which the client continues to move toward a predetermined goal, as opposed to **maintenance**, the point at which the goal has been achieved and the client is attempting to maintain that specific level of fitness. Progression should be considered a general training principle and is a function of training variation. It can be accomplished through increasing loads, volume, or frequency or making any number of alterations that modify the training stimulus. The most frequently used method for progressing clients is to change the load and volume lifted (i.e., additional sets or repetitions) for each exercise. Gradual and systematic changes in volume and load may also increase client behavioral changes, particularly for beginners, because seeing improvements toward their goals can increase motivation. As compared with moderate and advanced clients, beginners and deconditioned clients will make greater gains in strength during the initial weeks of a resistance training program; therefore, reassessment and training load adjustments may need to occur more frequently.

Progression is a systematic approach, and the intensity or challenge for resistance training sessions should ultimately increase over time. However, it is not required that each resistance training session be more challenging than the previous. As a client gains strength, personal trainers should progressively increase loads to maintain a given RIR within the target loading zone. A popular method for load progression is the **2-for-2 rule** (60), which is based on the achievement of goal repetitions for a training session. The rule states that if the client can complete 2 more repetitions than the repetition goal in the final set of an exercise for two consecutive training sessions, the load in all the sets for that exercise during subsequent training sessions can be increased. Generally speaking, loads should be increased by approximately 2.5% to 10%; the actual magnitude of increase will be specific to the client and the given exercise (table 15.7; 60). From a safety standpoint, it is best to be conser-

TABLE 15.7 Load Increases Based on Training Status, Body Area, and Exercise Type

Resistance training status	Body area	Type of exercise	APPROXIMATE LOAD INCREASE	
			Absolute increase (weight)	Relative increase (% of previous load)
Novice	Upper body	Core	2.5-5 lb	2.5%
			1-2 kg	
		Assistance	1.25-2.5 lb	1%-2%
			0.5-1 kg	
	Lower body	Core	10-15 lb	5%
			4-7 kg	
		Assistance	5-10 lb	2.5%-5%
			2-4 kg	
Intermediate or advanced	Upper body	Core	5-10+ lb	2.5%-5+%
			2-4+ kg	
		Assistance	5-10 lb	2.5%-5%
			2-4 kg	
	Lower body	Core	15-20+ lb	5%-10+%
			7-9+ kg	
		Assistance	10-15 lb	5%-10%
			4-7 kg	

Note: These load increases should be considered only guidelines and are best for programs with volumes of 3 sets of 5 to 10 repetitions.

Adapted from Sheppard and Triplett (60).

vative with the weight increase; loads can always be adjusted upward if needed. See table 15.8 (15) for an example of the 2-for-2 rule.

TRAINING VOLUME: REPETITIONS AND SETS

Volume in resistance training can be defined in several ways including the total number of sets, the total number of repetitions, or the amount of work performed (i.e., **volume load**), which is calculated as follows:

$$\text{Volume load} = \text{Total repetitions} \times \text{Load} \quad (15.1)$$

where *total repetitions* = sets × reps.

Although all these classifications are valid measures of volume, they each have inherent practical limitations. For example, using the number of repetitions as a marker of volume discounts the fact that a light-load/high-repetition set (e.g., 20RM) would have substantially more repetitions than a heavy-load/low-repetition set (e.g., 5RM). However, the neuromuscular stress of the initial repetitions in the light-load set would be much lower than that of the heavy-load set and thus would not necessarily receive equal weighting from an adaptive standpoint. Similarly, the volume load would be greater for the light- versus heavy-load set, but equating volume load between conditions would not necessarily be required to achieve a given fitness outcome as demonstrated by the superiority of heavy-load training on increasing strength despite a much lower total amount of work performed compared with light-load training (55).

As a general rule, **set volume** is arguably the best way to gauge training volume in personal training settings. Most meta-analyses on muscle strength and hypertrophy have used set volume to gauge outcomes. Moreover, evidence indicates that the total number of sets is a valid method for quantifying training volume with respect to muscle development for loading ranges between 6RM and 20+RM (5). That said, for training with very heavy loads (≤5RM), more sets would be required to achieve similar increases in hypertrophy, but not strength (53, 58).

Guidelines for Assigning Volume

Evidence indicates a dose–response relationship between set volume and muscle growth, with 10+ sets per muscle per week, spread across several different exercises, producing greater hypertrophic increases than lower volumes (56). Similarly, moderate- to

TABLE 15.8   Sample Load Increase Using the 2-for-2 Rule Notes and Observations

EXAMPLE: NOVICE CLIENT WHOSE REPETITION GOAL FOR THE BACK SQUAT EXERCISE IS 10				
Training session 1	**Set 1**	**Set 2**	**Set 3**	**Notes and Observations**
Weight	135 lb	135 lb	135 lb	
Repetitions completed	10	10	11	Exceeded goal by 1 repetition
Training session 2	**Set 1**	**Set 2**	**Set 3**	**Notes and Observations**
Weight	135 lb	135 lb	135 lb	
Repetitions completed	12	11	10	Did not exceed repetition goal
Training session 3	**Set 1**	**Set 2**	**Set 3**	**Notes and Observations**
Weight	135 lb	135 lb	135 lb	
Repetitions completed	12	12	12	Exceeded goal by 2 repetitions
Training session 4	**Set 1**	**Set 2**	**Set 3**	**Notes and Observations**
Weight	135 lb	135 lb	135 lb	
Repetitions completed	12	12	12	Exceeded goal by 2 repetitions in 2 consecutive training sessions
Next training session	**Set 1**	**Set 2**	**Set 3**	**Notes and Observations**
Weight	145 lb	145 lb	145 lb	10 lb added to all 3 sets
Repetition goal	10	10	10	

Adapted from Earle and Baechle (15).

high-volume resistance training programs produce greater strength increases compared with lower-volume programs (47). That said, substantial gains in both strength and hypertrophy can be made with lower-volume programs, particularly in the novice to intermediate phases of training. Thus, the need to use higher volume should be matched with a client's ultimate goals and take into account whether he or she seeks to maximize results or simply gain overall health and fitness. Moreover, time constraints also enter the equation. For clients with limited time availability (or finances) to train, relatively short workouts (~30 minutes) using lower training volumes can be both an effective and efficient strategy to meet these needs.

REST INTERVALS

The time between multiple sets, or the **rest interval**, can exert a strong impact on the physiological responses to a training session (60). The term *rest interval* can also refer to the time between exercises. Overall, the rest interval, whether between sets or exercises, is largely predicated on the goals of the client and the structure of the training plan.

Influential Factors

In general, there is a direct relationship between the load and the need for rest between sets; the heavier the load, the longer the rest needed between sets or exercises (17, 64). An additional consideration is the client's training status; untrained novice clients may require longer times between sets and exercises to achieve adequate recovery to maintain exercise technique.

Guidelines for Establishing Rest Intervals

The overall goals of the client play a large role in dictating assignment of the resistance training loads and volumes, both of which exert a large influence on the rest intervals chosen.

Resistance Training Status

Table 15.9 presents recommended rest interval lengths, but it is important to note that these are merely recommendations. Typically, they are not appropriate for untrained clients who are learning new exercises or attempting to master a technical exercise (3). With these clients it may be best to use a rest interval of 2 to 5 minutes to facilitate recovery between sets and exercises. As the client becomes more trained and has mastered the technical aspects of each lift, the recommendations presented in table 15.9 may become more appropriate (3, 17, 60, 64).

Resistance Training Goal

To tailor the training plan to the individual client's goals, the personal trainer must craft a program that allows enough rest between sets and exercises to permit the client to lift the selected loads for the assigned number of repetitions. The basic rest interval lengths for muscular endurance, hypertrophy, power, and strength, presented in table 15.9, are as follows:

- *Muscular endurance:* A relatively short rest interval, typically ≤30 seconds, is recommended for circuit-based training with exercises using dis-

TABLE 15.9 Rest Interval Recommendation Based on Training Goals

Training goal	Rest interval length
Muscular endurance	≤30 s
Muscular hypertrophy	≥2-3 min for multijoint exercises; 60-90 s for single-joint exercises
Muscular power	2-5 min
Muscular strength	2-5 min

Note: These rest intervals are only guidelines and should be interpreted with caution. Maintaining technique is of primary importance; if the rest interval length selected results in a reduction in technical proficiency, increase the rest interval duration. Also consider the rest interval length as a function of the total amount of work (volume load) encountered in a training set; the more work completed in a set, the longer the rest interval needs to be.

Based on American College of Sports Medicine (3), Fleck and Kraemer (17), Sheppard and Triplett (60), Stone and O'Bryant (64).

similar muscle groups (69), while up to 3 minutes' rest may be warranted between exercises using similar muscle groups (69).

- *Muscular hypertrophy:* A moderate to longer rest interval (≥2-3 minutes) is generally needed to maximize hypertrophy (19), because shorter rest intervals may compromise growth by impairing volume load. This recommendation seems particularly relevant to multijoint exercises, especially those involving free weights. Somewhat shorter rest intervals (60-90 seconds) may be appropriate for single-joint and machine-based exercise, as evidence indicates such movements are not substantially influenced by shorter recovery periods (59).

- *Muscular power:* Longer rest intervals of 2 to 5 minutes are warranted (64, 69) between maximal-effort sets.

- *Muscular strength:* Longer rest intervals are necessary for exercises targeting strength development (69). This is especially true for lower body or whole-body exercises (3, 71). The general recommendation is 2 to 5 minutes (43, 48).

VARIATION

Regardless of how effective or individualized a training program is, it will eventually need to be varied to ensure continued adaptation (3, 67). The concept of **variation** involves the appropriate alteration of training variables to produce adaptations over the long term (41, 67). One key component of variation is a purposeful sequencing of training factors (45, 67). If training is sequenced correctly, the adaptations stimulated by one period of training can exert a powerful effect on the next period of training, resulting in a summation of training effect (36, 37). If the resistance training plan includes appropriate and correctly sequenced variation, it will be incrementally more effective.

Much less training variation is needed with novice clients because any reasonable training plan generally will produce results (67). As clients become more trained, however, their progress may begin to slow if the plan does not include variation and progression. Maintenance of the same training plan without variation can induce what has been termed *monotonous overtraining* (63). If the training stimulus is unvaried for a long time (e.g., several months), even more experienced or trained clients can have an increased occurrence of overtraining symptoms (18a), potentially leading to impaired adaptations (25, 26, 28).

The best way to avoid stagnation is to include purposeful variation of the program design variables used to expose the client to training stimuli (13, 67). The many levels at which the personal trainer can alter the training stimulus include frequency, intensity, and volume of training, as well as the rest intervals between sets and exercises (13, 16, 43, 45, 67). Variation in the training plan can occur within a workout, during a week, or over a period of several weeks. Only a few of the possible methods for introducing variation into the training plan are presented here. (See chapter 23 for a detailed discussion of periodization, or a systematic method for inducing training variation.)

Within-Session Variation

During an individual training session, there are several ways to vary the training stimulus. One often employed method is to vary the intensity at which individual exercises are performed—some exercises are performed at higher intensities and others at lower intensities (67). For example, during a lower body workout, the personal trainer may employ a 5RM on the squat, a 10RM on the leg press, and a 15RM on the leg extension. A single session may employ some longer rest intervals and some shorter rest intervals. Typically, longer rest intervals are used with core exercises, and shorter rest intervals are used with assistance exercises (3, 52, 70).

Another way to vary the training stimulus during a session is to alter the set configuration (21, 22, 24). Traditionally sets are performed in a continuous fashion, with little or no rest between each repetition. Research suggests that one can modify the focus of a set by altering the inter-repetition rest interval to construct what has been termed a **cluster set** (24). A cluster set uses a rest interval of 5 to 45 seconds between each repetition (21). For example, if muscular endurance or conditioning is the focus, a shorter rest interval may be employed (~5 seconds). If power generation is the focus, rest intervals may be longer (~45 seconds). When employing cluster sets, the personal trainer can add an additional layer of variation by introducing changes to the loading used during each repetition of the set. There are three categories of cluster sets: the standard cluster set, in which the load is not altered across the set; the undulating cluster, in which the load is increased and then decreased within the set; and the ascending cluster, in which the load increases across the set (table 15.10; 22, 23, 24). Cluster sets offer another level of variation that can affect the focus of an individual training session.

TABLE 15.10 Sample Within-Cluster Set Structures

Type of cluster set	Sets	×	Repetitions	Inter-repetition rest interval (s)	Sample cluster set repetition loading structures									
Standard	1-3	×	10/1	5	80/1	80/1	80/1	80/1	80/1	80/1	80/1	80/1	80/1	80/1
	1-3	×	10/2	10	80/2	80/2	80/2	80/2	80/2					
	1-3	×	10/5	15	80/5	80/5								
Undulating	1-3	×	10/1	5	75/1	80/1	82.5/1	85/1	85/1	82.5/1	80/1	77.5/1	75/1	80/1
	1-3	×	10/2	10	77.5/1	80/1	85/1	80/1	77.5/1					
Ascending	1-3	×	10/1	5	55/1	60/1	65/1	70/1	75/1	85/1	90/1	95/1	100/1	105/1
	1-3	×	10/2	10	70/2	75/2	80/2	85/2	90/2					

Note: All weights based on a 1RM power clean of 100 kg (80 kg = 80% of the 1RM). Each set has an average intensity of 80 kg, or 80% of the 1RM. Rest interval lengths can be increased to 45 s depending on the goal of the training structure.

10/1 = 10 total repetitions broken into 10 clusters of 1; 10/2 = 10 total repetitions broken into 5 clusters of 2; 10/5 = 10 total repetitions broken into 2 clusters of 5.

Adapted from Haff et al. (22), Haff et al. (23), and Haff et al. (24).

Within-Week Variation

One of the best ways to incorporate variation into a training plan is to vary the intensity of exercises selected across the week (67). It may be difficult for clients to undertake high training loads across an entire week. As the week progresses, the client's cumulative stress (e.g., training, work, home, personal) is likely to increase steadily, and his or her ability to tolerate the training stress will decline (67); this increases the potential for overtraining (63). One strategy to combat this is to use light and heavy days of training; the light days allow the client to recover, thereby reducing the risk of overtraining (table 15.11).

There are a multitude of strategies for varying the training load, but one that is particularly easy to employ is varying the repetition range during the sessions across the week in an undulating fashion. This strategy, familiarly known as **daily undulating periodization**, involves structuring training sessions into heavy, moderate, and light training days. For example, a client who trains three days per week may have a target loading zone of 3RM to 5RM on Mondays, 8RM to 12RM on Wednesdays, and 15RM to 20RM on Fridays. This is an excellent programming method that can help maximize training adaptations while decreasing the risk of overtraining.

Between-Week Variation

The training program should vary between weeks, through alterations in volume, intensity, frequency, exercise selection, and training focus. For example, a four-week period of training may call for 3 sets of 10 repetitions (the top part of table 15.11). According to the principles of periodization, the average intensity could be increased for three weeks and then reduced during the fourth week, creating what is termed a 3:1 loading paradigm (the bottom part of table 15.11) (15, 90). There, the weekly volume load (e.g., week 1 = 79, 500 pounds; week 2 = 82, 650 pounds; week 3 = 85, 950 pounds; week 4 = 79, 950 pounds) and average training intensity (i.e., week 1 = 134 pounds; week 2 = 140 pounds; week 3 = 145 pounds; week 4 = 135 pounds) increase across the first three weeks. This type of loading is considered the most basic loading structure for resistance training, but there are other possibilities (e.g., a 2:1, 4:1, 3:2, or 4:2 structure). If these types of loading are coupled with daily variations as discussed previously, the client will be able to maximize training adaptations while minimizing the chances of overtraining.

Another way to incorporate variation between training weeks is to alter the training density. For example, week 1 may include four resistance training sessions, two high-intensity interval training sessions, and two aerobic training sessions. In this week, the focus is the resistance training. In the second week, the resistance training sessions could be reduced to three, the high-intensity interval training sessions increased to three, and the frequency of aerobic training maintained, thus changing the focus of the week to interval training. By manipulating the various training modes over the training week, the personal trainer can selectively target specific outcomes and manage

TABLE 15.11   Sample Daily and Weekly Variations (Upper Body–Lower Body Split Routine)

Day	Exercises	TARGET ZONE		INTENSITIES (LB)			
		Sets	Reps	Week 1	Week 2	Week 3	Week 4
Monday (heavy)	Back squat	3	10	200	210	220	205
	Single-leg squat	3	10	135	140	145	135
	Leg curl	3	10	120	125	130	120
	Leg extension	3	10	150	155	160	150
	Abdominal exercises	3	25	--	--	--	--
Tuesday (heavy)	Bench press	3	10	180	185	190	180
	Bent-over row	3	10	150	155	160	150
	Shoulder press	3	10	130	135	140	130
	Lat pulldown	3	10	140	145	150	140
	Triceps pushdown	3	10	100	105	110	100
	Biceps curl	3	10	95	100	105	95
Thursday (light)	Back squat	3	10	180	185	190	185
	Single-leg squat	3	10	120	125	130	125
	Leg curl	3	10	105	110	115	110
	Leg extension	3	10	135	140	145	130
	Abdominal exercises	3	25	--	--	--	--
Saturday (light)	Bench press	3	10	160	165	170	160
	Bent-over row	3	10	135	140	145	135
	Shoulder press	3	10	115	120	125	115
	Lat pulldown	3	10	125	130	140	125
	Triceps pushdown	3	10	90	95	100	90
	Biceps curl	3	10	85	90	95	85

	MONDAY			TUESDAY			THURSDAY			SATURDAY			WEEKLY		
Microcycle	Reps	VL	TI	Reps	VL	TI	Reps	VL	TI	Reps	VL	TI	Reps	VL	TI
1	120	18,150	151	180	23,850	133	120	16,200	135	180	21,300	118	600	79,500	134
2	120	18,900	158	180	24,750	138	120	16,800	140	180	22,200	123	600	82,650	140
3	120	19,650	164	180	25,650	143	120	17,400	145	180	23,250	129	600	85,950	145
4	120	18,300	153	180	23,850	133	120	16,500	138	180	21,300	118	600	79,950	135

Reps = repetitions; VL = volume load (reps × sets × pounds); TI = average training intensity (volume load ÷ total repetitions).

fatigue more efficiently, ultimately allowing the client to experience greater training adaptations. As previously noted, such programming decisions must be made in consideration with a client's availability or desire to train with higher frequencies.

SEQUENCING TRAINING

One of the classic mistakes made in the design of a resistance training program is not appropriately sequencing the training factors (28, 45, 67). Appropriately sequenced training programs result in superior

adaptations and performance gains (28). Conversely, an inappropriately sequenced training plan will blunt the physiological and performance adaptations that are expected from the training plan.

Generally, all clients should begin a resistance training program with a plan based on maximizing adherence and enjoyment. Although the client may have a specific end goal (e.g., muscular endurance or hypertrophy), these results will not be achieved if the client lacks consistency or dislikes the program, training methods, or personal trainer. With most clients purchasing sessions in small packages (e.g.,

6-12 sessions), it is difficult for the personal trainer to establish a long-term training program when the client may not renew the package. Therefore, the personal trainer should discuss the longevity of the training program with the client during the initial consultation as well as periodically thereafter. For example, it is not uncommon for a client to purchase a small package of sessions to learn the basics, after which the individual will train on his or her own. Thus, the personal trainer needs to maximize the time with the client to program a small number of sessions (e.g., six sessions over three weeks), promote adherence, and demonstrate the need for continued guidance from the personal trainer (i.e., renewal).

It appears that traditionally, personal trainers have targeted only the primary training goals (i.e., muscular endurance, hypertrophy, muscular strength, or muscular power) when designing a program. While at first glance this seems logical based on the principles of specificity, it has been hypothesized that there is an interdependence among the goals. For example, when maximal strength is the main desired training outcome, a period of training that targets hypertrophy should precede training that targets maximal strength.

> Training sequence targeting maximal strength
> = Hypertrophy training → Maximal strength training

By sequencing training in this fashion, greater levels of strength conceivably can be developed because of the underlying muscular adaptations stimulated by increasing muscle cross-sectional area.

Similarly, it is clear that if maximal power-generating capacity is the target outcome, the client needs to first develop overall strength levels.

> Training sequence targeting power development
> = Hypertrophy training → Maximal strength training → Muscular power training

The increases in muscle cross-sectional area would thus increase the ability to increase maximal strength, which would then contribute to maximizing muscular power development when the training focus shifts to power-based training.

These phases are important because they establish the training base, which lays the foundation for the development of other targeted goals (45, 64). Most clients can elicit benefits from several weeks of these phases of training as long as there are appropriate variations in volume and intensity. After an extended period of this type of training,

however, the client becomes less responsive to the stimulus and training adaptations will slow dramatically. This decrease in responsiveness, or reduction in received benefits, is also known as the **law of diminished returns**. At this time, the personal trainer should alter the training goals to obviate the problem by shifting the focus of the program toward the development of muscular strength, typically targeting strength development for two to five weeks. Most clients would then shift back to a muscular endurance or hypertrophy focus, but athletes would likely progress toward a muscular power–based plan. Regardless of the goals, the sequencing of training appears to result in a phase potentiation effect, whereby the attributes developed in one phase facilitate the physiological and performance adaptations seen in the subsequent phase (8, 36, 37, 64). When sequencing training, the personal trainer should consider the basic guidelines for the length of each phase presented in table 15.12 (64).

The client's overall training goals, as established early on by the personal trainer and client, will determine the sequence of the training plan. As noted previously, the goals will also help the personal trainer establish basic volume and loading parameters. However, no client can keep targeting the same goals indefinitely. Therefore, the program should vary the targeted goals by periodically altering the training target. For example, a client who is targeting muscular hypertrophy might perform a four-week period of hypertrophy training (e.g., 3 sets of 10) followed by three weeks of muscular strength work, then return to four weeks of hypertrophy training. Alternating between muscular strength and hypertrophy may produce greater increases in hypertrophy and strength (46). Three of many methods for sequencing training are shown in figure 15.3.

> Sequencing the training emphasis is critical for achieving specific training outcomes. A periodic shifting of targeted training goals in a sequential fashion prevents stagnation and overtraining while encouraging physiological and performance adaptations.

SAMPLE PROGRAMS FOR TARGETED TRAINING OUTCOMES

Numerous combinations of training programs can be constructed based on the sequential approach

TABLE 15.12   Training Factor Sequencing Guidelines

Phase of training	Length (weeks)	Ratio of heavy to light weeks (heavy/light)
Muscular endurance	2-4	2-3/1
Hypertrophy	2-4	2-3/1
Muscular strength	2-5	2-4/1
Muscular power	2-4	2-3/1

2-3/1 = 2 or 3 weeks with increasing loads followed by 1 unloading week. 2-4/1 = 2 to 4 weeks with increasing loads followed by 1 unloading week.

Adapted from Stone and O'Bryant (64).

to designing training plans. Remember that before focusing on strength or power development, the client should become proficient in exercise technique. Each program should be individualized to meet the client's needs and should meet all the general principles of training addressed at the beginning of this chapter. There are numerous possibilities; the programs presented in tables 15.13 through 15.15 on pages 419 to 424 are simply examples rather than definitive plans to apply to all clients.

Table 15.13 presents a plan that targets muscular endurance training for a novice client. The methods are primarily machine based, and the rest intervals are short (i.e., 30 s) to facilitate the development of muscular endurance. This program can be used for

a relatively brief period of time until a training base has been established; at this point the program should be modified so that training intensities can be based on a repetition maximum or an RPE prescribed load to maximize the client's adaptive responses. After completing this program, the client may opt to enter into a two- to four-week phase that targets muscular strength, depending on personal goals and abilities. Subsequently, the focus can be reoriented toward muscular endurance, and more advanced training techniques can be employed.

The program presented in table 15.14 is a four-week training block that targets muscular hypertrophy. This example is based on the client's stated goals of muscular hypertrophy. Training takes place four times per

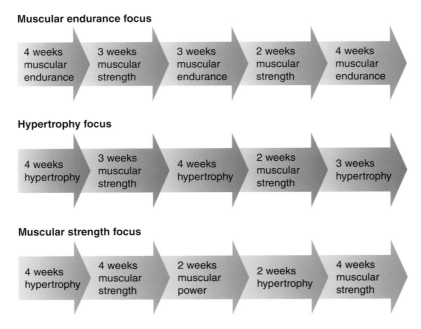

FIGURE 15.3   Sample 16-week program sequences.

week, employing a combination of exercise modalities. The program employs inter- and intra-intensity variation as indicated by the inclusion of heavy and light training days. The overall block exhibits a 3:1 loading paradigm: The load increases over the first three weeks, while the fourth week is an unloading week as indicated by the overall decrease in training intensity.

A sample training program that targets muscular strength is presented in table 15.15. This example includes a four-week block of training. The plan is for an advanced client who is targeting the maximization of muscular strength. Based on the client's level of development and experience, the plan calls for a frequency of four times per week (based on table 15.2). Most of the exercises are performed with free weights, with 3 sets of 5 repetitions for core exercises and 3 sets of 10 repetitions for assistance exercises. The initial training intensities are determined based on 5RM testing for the core exercises and 10RM testing for the assistance exercises. The program has a 3:1 loading structure, with heavy and light days to facilitate recovery and adaptation.

CONCLUSION

Designing a resistance training program requires the personal trainer to understand the concepts of specificity of training, overload, variation, progression, and sequencing. Many training factors can be altered to optimize outcomes, such as the exercises selected, frequency of training, overload, volume, intensity, rest interval, and sequence. Once the program is established, the personal trainer must vary and advance the plan to continue to help clients achieve their training goals in accordance with individual lifestyle-related factors.

Study Questions

1. Which of the following exercises has the *greatest* movement pattern specificity for a volleyball player?
   A. power clean
   B. bench press
   C. lateral raise
   D. curl-up

2. Which of the following is the recommended training frequency for a client with an intermediate resistance training status using a split training routine?
   A. 1
   B. 2
   C. 3
   D. 4

3. Which of the following is an example of the correct order of exercises, if the goal is to order exercises alternating between pushes and pulls?
   A. incline bench press, biceps curl, upright row, shoulder press
   B. upright row, incline bench press, shoulder press, biceps curl
   C. incline bench press, upright row, shoulder press, biceps curl
   D. incline bench press, shoulder press, upright row, biceps curl

4. For an *advanced* level client, with the goal of enhancing muscular endurance, which of the following would be an appropriate resistance exercise program design for the client's core exercises only?
   A. 10-15RM, 1-3 sets
   B. ≤6RM, >3 sets
   C. 8-12RM, 1-3 sets
   D. 15-30+RM, >3 sets

5. Which of the following levels of resistance training status would require the *least* variation to produce results from a client's training program?
   A. novice
   B. intermediate
   C. advanced
   D. highly advanced

TABLE 15.13 Sample Muscular Endurance Program: Alternating Upper and Lower Body Exercises

WORKOUT (TUESDAYS AND FRIDAYS)					
Exercise	Exercise type	Sets	Repetitions	Weight	Rest interval
Bench press	Free weights	2	15	50 lb	30 s
Leg press	Machine	2	15	150 lb	30 s
Seated row	Machine	2	15	30 lb	30 s
Leg (knee) curl	Machine	2	15	15RM	30 s
Shoulder press	Machine	2	15	20 lb	30 s
Leg (knee) extension	Machine	2	15	15RM	30 s
Biceps curl	Free weights	2	15	25 lb	30 s
Seated heel raise	Machine	2	15	15RM	30 s
Triceps pushdown	Machine	2	15	20 lb	30 s
Abdominal crunch	Body weight	2	25	N/A	30 s

EXPLANATION OF PROGRAM		
Initial consultation	Initial training status and experience based on table 15.1	Beginner
	Fitness evaluation	15RM testing
	Primary resistance training goal	Muscular endurance
Exercises	Exercise choices	Mixture of free weights, cam machine, and pivot machine exercise
	Core exercises	Bench press, leg press, seated row, and shoulder press
	Assistance exercises	Leg (knee) curl, leg (knee) extension, biceps curl, seated heel raise, triceps pushdown, abdominal crunch
	Number of exercises per muscle group	1 exercise per muscle group
Frequency	Frequency of training (table 15.2)	2 or 3 times per week spaced evenly throughout the week
Order	Primary methods	Complete the prescribed number of sets for each exercise, alternating between upper and lower body exercises
	Secondary methods	If circuit based, complete 1 set of each exercise, then repeat
Determining load[a]	Method	Based on client's 15RM

Exercise	Exercise type	Trial load	Number of repetitions completed
Bench press	Machine	50 lb	15
Leg press	Machine	140 lb	20
Seated row	Machine	25 lb	16
Shoulder press	Machine	35 lb	8
Biceps curl	Free weights	30 lb	12
Triceps pushdown	Machine	25 lb	13

(continued)

TABLE 15.13 *(continued)*

EXPLANATION OF PROGRAM	
Repetitions	Based on table 15.6 and the client's targeted goals.
	Repetition range is set based on client's classification: novice, 10-15RM reps; in this case, sets of 15 reps were chosen.
Sets	Based on table 15.6 and the client's classification: novice, one to three sets; in this case, two sets were chosen. The set structure presented is for the target sets and does not include warm-ups; two or three warm-up sets may be needed.
Rest periods	Rest periods are based on table 15.9. All sets and exercises have rest intervals of 30 s. If performing the exercises as a circuit, 30 s of rest between exercises is still recommended for novice clients.
Assigning load[b]	Assign the training load based on 15RM testing / Adjust the loads based on table 15.5.

		Exercise	Exercise type	Load adjustment	Equation	Assigned training load
		Bench press	Free weights	None needed	n/a	50 lb
		Leg press	Machine	+10	140 + 10 = 150	150 lb
		Seated row	Machine	+5 lb	25 + 5 = 30	30 lb
		Shoulder press	Machine	–15 lb	35 – 15 = 20	20 lb
		Biceps curl	Free weights	–5 lb	30 – 5 = 25	25 lb
		Triceps pushdown	Machine	–5 lb	25 – 5 = 20	20 lb

[a]15RM testing for these exercises should be conservative to avoid client fatigue; limit to three testing sets: leg (knee) curl, leg (knee) extension, and seated heel raise.

[b]Based on RM testing (note that the RM loads may have to be decreased because of the multiple assigned sets): Assign loads from 15RM testing for leg (knee) curl, leg (knee) extension, and seated heel raise.

TABLE 15.14   Sample Hypertrophy Program: Four Times Per Week Split Routine

Day	Exercise	Sets[a]	Repetitions	TRAINING LOADS (BASED ON AN RPE SCALE OF 1-10)			
				Week 1	Week 2	Week 3	Week 4
Monday	Back squat	3	10	7	8	9	6
	Leg extension	3	10	7	8	9	6
	Romanian deadlift	3	10	7	8	9	6
	Leg curl	3	10	7	8	9	6
	Standing heel raise + seated heel raise	3	10	7	8	9	6
	Hanging leg raise	3	25	--	--	--	--
Tuesday	Bench press	3	10	7	8	9	6
	Incline chest press	3	10	7	8	9	6
	Bent-over row	3	10	7	8	9	6
	Lat pulldown	3	10	7	8	9	6
	Shoulder press	3	10	7	8	9	6
	Biceps curl	3	10	7	8	9	6
	Triceps pushdown	3	10	7	8	9	6
Thursday	Leg press	3	10	6	7	8	6
	Lunge	3	10	6	7	8	6
	Hip thrust	3	10	6	7	8	6
	Glute-ham raise	3	10	6	7	8	6
	Standing heel raise + seated heel raise	3	10	6	7	8	6
	Abdominal crunch	3	25	--	--	--	--

Day	Exercise	Sets[a]	Repetitions	TRAINING LOADS (BASED ON AN RPE SCALE OF 1-10)			
				Week 1	Week 2	Week 3	Week 4
Saturday	Dumbbell chest press	3	10	6	7	8	6
	Incline fly	3	10	6	7	8	6
	Seated cable row	3	10	6	7	8	6
	Pull-up	3	10	6	7	8	6
	Lateral raise	3	10	6	7	8	6
	Hammer curl	3	10	6	7	8	6
	Overhead triceps extension	3	10	6	7	8	6

EXPLANATION OF PROGRAM

Initial consultation	Initial training status and experience based on table 15.1	Intermediate
	Fitness evaluation	10RM testing to determine initial training load
	Primary resistance training goal	Hypertrophy
Exercises	Exercise choices	Combination of free weights, machines, and cable exercises; based on client's abilities and proficiency of the movement
	Core exercises	Back squat, lunge, Romanian deadlift, bench press, shoulder press, bent-over row
	Assistance exercises	Biceps curl, triceps pushdown, leg curl, standing heel raise, seated heel raise, shoulder shrug
	Number of exercises per muscle group	1 or 2 exercises per muscle group
Frequency	Frequency of training (table 15.2)	3 or 4 times per week spaced evenly throughout the week
Order	Primary methods	Core exercise and then assistance exercises
		Exercises that train large muscle groups first and then exercises that train small muscle groups
		Multijoint exercises first, then single-joint exercises
	Secondary methods	Exercises performed in a superset: triceps pushdown, biceps curl
		Exercises performed in a compound set: heel raise, seated heel raise
Determining load	Method	Determine the training load based on 10RM testing; if needed, loads can be used to estimate a 1RM (protocol in chapter 11, but modified; see chapter 23 for conversion)

Exercise	Determine the training load using 10RM testing	Estimated 1RM
Bench press	165 lb	220 lb
Dumbbell incline press	40 lb (each hand)	55 lb (each hand)
Bent-over row	80 lb	110 lb
Shoulder press	90 lb	120 lb
Shoulder shrug	160 lb	215 lb
Biceps curl	90 lb	120 lb
Triceps extension	100 lb	135 lb
Back squat	225 lb	300 lb
Lunge	75 lb	100 lb
Romanian deadlift	150 lb	200 lb
Leg curl	120 lb	160 lb
Seated heel raise	110 lb	145 lb
Standing heel raise	120 lb	160 lb

(continued)

TABLE 15.14 *(continued)*

Repetitions	Based on table 15.6 and the client's targeted goals.
	Repetition range is set based on client's classification: intermediate, 5-30+ reps; in this case, sets of 10 reps were chosen.
Sets	Based on table 15.6 and the client's classification: intermediate, three or more sets; in this case, three sets were chosen. The set structure presented is for the target sets and does not include warm-ups; two or three or more warm-up sets may be needed.
Rest periods	Rest periods are based on table 15.9. All sets and exercises have rest intervals of 2-3 min. Only the superset of triceps pushdown and biceps curl and the compound set of standing and seated heel raise do not follow this recommendation.

Assigning load[a]	Assign the training load based on 10RM testing.	10RM testing is used to determine specific training zones with estimated RPE.

Exercise	10RM	RPE of 10	RPE of 9	RPE of 8	RPE of 7	RPE of 6
Bench press	165 lb	165-157 lb	157-149 lb	149-140 lb	140-132 lb	132-116 lb
Dumbbell incline press	40 lb (each hand)	40-38 lb	38-36 lb	36-34 lb	34-32 lb	32-30 lb
Bent-over row	80 lb	80-76 lb	76-72 lb	72-68 lb	68-64 lb	64-60 lb
Shoulder press	90 lb	90-86 lb	86-81 lb	81-77 lb	77-72 lb	72-68 lb
Shoulder shrug	160 lb	160-152 lb	152-144 lb	144-136 lb	136-128 lb	128-120 lb
Biceps curl	90 lb	90-86 lb	86-81 lb	81-77 lb	77-72 lb	72-68 lb
Triceps extension	100 lb	100-95 lb	95-90 lb	90-85 lb	85-80 lb	80-75 lb
Back squat	225 lb	225-214 lb	214-203 lb	203-191 lb	191-180 lb	180-169 lb
Lunge	75 lb	75-71 lb	71-68 lb	68-64 lb	64-60 lb	60-56 lb
Romanian deadlift	150 lb	150-143 lb	143-135 lb	135-128 lb	128-120 lb	120-113 lb
Leg curl	120 lb	120-114 lb	114-108 lb	108-102 lb	102-96 lb	96-90 lb
Seated heel raise	110 lb	110-105 lb	105-99 lb	99-94 lb	94-88 lb	88-83 lb
Standing heel raise	120 lb	120-114 lb	114-108 lb	108-102 lb	102-96 lb	96-90 lb

[a]Estimated 10RM values will be used to calculate the training zones for specific training sessions based on the RPE scale (figure 15.2).

TABLE 15.15 Sample Muscular Strength Program: Within- and Between-Week Variation

Day	Exercise	Sets[a]	Repetitions	Week 1	Week 2	Week 3	Week 4
				TRAINING LOADS (BASED ON AN RPE OF SCALE OF 1-10)			
Monday	Back squat	3	5	7	8	9	7
	Bench press	3	5	7	8	9	7
	Biceps curl	3	10	7	8	9	7
	Triceps pushdown	3	10	7	8	9	7
	Abdominal crunch	3	25	--	--	--	--
Tuesday	Deadlift	3	5	6	7	8	6
	Bent-over row	3	5	6	7	8	6
	Shoulder shrug	3	5	6	7	8	6
	Romanian deadlift	3	5	6	7	8	6
	Lat pulldown	3	10	6	7	8	6
	Abdominal crunch	3	25	--	--	--	--
Thursday	Back squat	3	5	6	7	8	6
	Bench press	3	5	6	7	8	6
	Biceps curl	3	10	6	7	8	6
	Triceps pushdown	3	10	6	7	8	6
	Abdominal crunch	3	25	--	--	--	--
Saturday	Deadlift	3	5	7	8	9	7
	Bent-over row	3	5	7	8	9	7
	Shoulder shrug	3	5	7	8	9	7
	Romanian deadlift	3	5	7	8	9	7
	Lat pulldown	3	10	7	8	9	7
	Abdominal crunch	3	25	--	--	--	--

EXPLANATION OF PROGRAM

Initial consultation	Initial training status and experience based on table 15.1	Advanced
	Fitness evaluation	5RM testing (core exercises) and 10RM testing (assistance exercises) to determine initial training load
	Primary resistance training goal	Muscular strength
Exercises	Exercise choices	Primarily free weights, but some machines for assistance exercises
	Core exercises	Back squat, bench press, deadlift, bent-over row, Romanian deadlift
	Assistance exercises	Biceps curl, triceps pushdown, shoulder shrug, lat pulldown
	Number of exercises per muscle group	1 or 2 exercises per muscle group
Frequency	Frequency of training (table 15.2)	3 or 4 times per week spaced evenly throughout the week
Order	Primary methods	Core exercise and then assistance exercises
		Exercises that train large muscle groups first and then exercises that train small muscle groups
		Multijoint exercises first, then single-joint exercises

TABLE 15.15 *(continued)*

Determining load	Method		Determine the training load based on 5RM and 10RM testing; if needed, loads can be used to estimate a 1RM (protocol in chapter 11, but modified; see chapter 23 for conversion)

5RM TEST RESULTS

Exercise	5RM	Estimated 1RM
Back squat	325 lb	375 lb
Bench press	260 lb	300 lb
Deadlift	285 lb	325 lb

10RM TEST RESULTS

Exercise	10RM	Estimated 5RM	Estimated 1RM
Bent-over row	140 lb	161 lb	185 lb
Lat pulldown	175 lb	300 lb	230 lb
Biceps curl	105 lb	122 lb	140 lb
Triceps pushdown	105 lb	122 lb	140 lb

Repetitions	Based on table 15.6 and the client's targeted goals.
	Repetition range is set based on client classification: advanced, six or fewer repetitions; in this case, sets of five reps were chosen.
Sets	Based on table 15.6 and the client's classification: advanced, three or more sets; in this case, three sets were chosen. The set structure presented is for the target sets and does not include warm-ups; two or three more warm-up sets may be needed.
Rest periods	Rest periods are based on table 15.9. All sets and exercises have rest intervals of 2-5 min.

Assigning load[a]

Assign the training load based on 5RM and 10RM testing.

5RM and 10RM testing are used to determine specific training zones with estimated RPE.

Exercise	5RM or 10RM	RPE of 10	RPE of 9	RPE of 8	RPE of 7	RPE of 6
Back squat	325 lb	325-310 lb	310-293 lb	293-277 lb	277-261 lb	261-245 lb
Bench press	260 lb	260-248 lb	248-235 lb	235-222 lb	222-209 lb	209-196 lb
Deadlift	285 lb	285-269 lb	269-255 lb	255-241 lb	241-226 lb	226-212 lb
Bent-over row	160 lb	160-153 lb	153-145 lb	145-137 lb	137-129 lb	129-121 lb
Shoulder shrug	195 lb	195-186 lb	186-176 lb	176-167 lb	167-157 lb	157-147 lb
Romanian deadlift	195 lb	195-186 lb	186-176 lb	176-167 lb	167-157 lb	157-147 lb

Exercise	10RM	RPE of 10	RPE of 9	RPE of 8	RPE of 7	RPE of 6
Lat pulldown	175 lb	175-166 lb	166-158	158-149 lb	149-140 lb	140-131 lb
Biceps curl	105 lb	105-100 lb	100-95 lb	95-89 lb	89-84 lb	84-79 lb
Triceps pushdown	105 lb	105-100 lb	100-95 lb	95-89 lb	89-84 lb	84-79 lb

[a]Estimated 5RM and 10RM values will be used to calculate the training zones for specific training sessions based on the RPE scale (figure 15.2).

CHAPTER 16

Aerobic Training Program Design

Mike Martino, PhD, and Nicole C. Dabbs, PhD

After completing this chapter, you will be able to

- design aerobic endurance training programs based on the principle of specificity and individual client goals;

- select the appropriate mode of aerobic exercise;

- determine aerobic endurance training intensity, frequency, and duration and understand their interactions and effects on the training outcome;

- determine training intensity using calculated target heart rate zones, rating of perceived exertion, or metabolic equivalents;

- design programs with proper warm-up, cooldown, and exercise progression; and

- apply long slow distance, pace/tempo, interval training, cross-training, arm exercise, and combination training in accord with client goals.

Aerobic endurance training is an essential component of any general exercise program. Health clubs and fitness centers dedicate large sections of their facilities to aerobic endurance training equipment, and the majority of athletic competitions for the general public are designed around aerobic endurance exercise (e.g., 10K and 5K runs, marathons, cycling tours, and sprint triathlons).

In 2018, the Department of Health and Human Services created the 2018 Physical Activity Guidelines Advisory Committee to analyze the scientific literature on physical activity and health. It was determined that the scientific findings on the relationship between exercise and health during the previous decade provide additional evidence for improved health benefits,

describe more diverse methods to achieve these health benefits, and suggest increased overall physical activity in Americans. The findings recommend 150 to 300 minutes per week of moderate-intensity physical activity and about 75 to 150 minutes of vigorous-intensity physical activity per week is considered within the target range. Physical activity can be categorized within the following four categories (90):

1. *Vigorous-intensity activity requiring ≥6.0 METs:* examples include walking very fast (4.5 to 5 mph [7-8 km/h]), running, carrying heavy groceries or other loads upstairs, shoveling snow by hand, mowing grass with a hand-push mower, or participating in an aerobics class. Adults generally spend less than 1% of waking time in vigorous activity.

The authors would like to acknowledge the significant contributions of Patrick Hagerman to this chapter.

2. *Moderate-intensity activity requiring 3.0 to <6.0 METs:* examples include walking briskly or with purpose (3 to 4 mph [5-6.5 km/h]), mopping or vacuuming, or raking a yard.

3. *Light-intensity activity requiring 1.6 to <3.0 METs:* examples include walking at a slow or leisurely pace (≤2 mph [≤3 km/h]), cooking, or standing while scanning groceries as a cashier.

4. *Physical activity requiring 1.0 to 1.5 METs:* referred to as sedentary activity.

Aerobic endurance training is often referred to as *aerobic exercise, cardiovascular exercise,* or *cardiorespiratory exercise.* These terms should be considered synonymous because they all refer to exercise that involves the cardiovascular and respiratory systems, including the heart, blood vessels, and lungs.

Designing an aerobic endurance training program necessitates an examination of the client's present level of fitness, exercise history, and fitness goals. One of the more common health-related goals among the general population is fat loss (often incorrectly referred to as "weight loss"), and a well-designed aerobic endurance training program should be a part of workouts for clients with this goal. Likewise, clients who wish to compete in a 10K race or complete a marathon will need specific training guidelines in order to meet their goals.

Previous chapters have dealt with determining fitness level and appropriate exercise levels. This chapter is devoted to properly designing aerobic exercise programs for a variety of clients.

SPECIFICITY OF AEROBIC ENDURANCE TRAINING

The same principle of specificity that applies to resistance training applies to aerobic endurance training. The **principle of specificity** states that the results of a training program will be directly related to the type of training performed (22). The results of a resistance training program will be specific to resistance training, and the results of an aerobic exercise program will be specific to aerobic endurance training. In other words, resistance training does not significantly improve maximal aerobic power ($\dot{V}O_2$max) (42, 45, 58). In addition, training that involves one mode of aerobic exercise will not guarantee equal improvement in a different aerobic exercise mode (9, 100). For instance, a person who has achieved a high level of aerobic conditioning through cycling will not nec-

essarily be able to produce the same aerobic performance, as measured by peak $\dot{V}O_2$ capability, during a running workout (73, 87, 99). The muscle activation patterns and oxygen requirements among exercise modes are not equal, so the responses and adaptations are not equal (11, 70, 100). Even though improvements in $\dot{V}O_2$ elicited from one exercise mode will help in other exercise modes, they will not do so to the same extent (10, 62, 92).

COMPONENTS OF AN AEROBIC ENDURANCE TRAINING PROGRAM

An aerobic endurance training program consists of several components that can be manipulated in a variety of ways to produce a number of particular outcomes. These components include the mode of exercise, intensity of training during each session, frequency of exercise sessions, and duration of each exercise session. A personal trainer needs to consider each component in relation to the client's personal goals, as well as in terms of how each component interacts with the other components.

Two hypothetical clients will serve throughout the remainder of this chapter to highlight some practical examples of integrating the components into an overall aerobic endurance training program. The first client, Becky, has a goal of completing a local 10K race in less than 50 minutes. The second client is Floyd, who wants to lose about 30 pounds (~14 kg) of body fat. Neither client has any musculoskeletal dysfunction, and each has received physician clearance for exercise. Client example 16.1 provides the initial status and goals of these two hypothetical clients.

Exercise Mode

The first step in designing aerobic endurance training programs is to decide on the mode of exercise. Exercise **mode** refers simply to what exercise or activity will be performed. As discussed in chapter 14, aerobic exercise modes include machine and nonmachine exercises. Athletes should choose the exercise mode that most closely mimics their specific sport or the movement they perform during competition. The same goes for a client who wishes to compete in an amateur event such as a 5K run or 25-mile (40.2 km) cycling tour. The decision about which exercise mode to use depends on several factors, including equipment

CLIENT EXAMPLE 16.1

Initial Client Status and Goals

Becky

Age: 30

Height: 5 feet 5 inches (165.1 cm)

Weight: 120 pounds (54.4 kg)

Goal: Complete 10K race in less than 50 minutes

Training status: Intermediate. Has run 3 to 5 miles (4.8-8 km) an average of two times a week for the past three years, at a pace and speed that is comfortable and not strenuous for her. Her 10K personal best is 53 minutes.

Other activities: Works as a receptionist, mostly sitting from 8 a.m. to 5 p.m. No other structured exercise or activities.

Floyd

Age: 52

Height: 6 feet 0 inches (182.9 cm)

Weight: 230 pounds (104.3 kg)

Goal: Lose about 30 pounds (~14 kg) of body fat

Training status: Beginner (untrained), former college baseball player. Has not been involved in a regular exercise program since college.

Other activities: Works long hours as a bank officer. Walks throughout the office during the day, but no more than 40 feet (12.2 m) at a time, and is usually sitting in his office. Teaches at the community college at night. No structured exercise or activity.

availability, personal preference, the client's ability to perform the exercise, and the client's goals.

The machine exercise modes use aerobic endurance training equipment and depend on what is available at the facility where the training will take place. Most fitness centers have a variety of aerobic endurance training equipment that typically includes treadmills, elliptical machines, stair climbers, stationary bikes, cross-country ski simulators, rowing ergometers, upper body ergometers, semirecumbent bikes, rotating climbing walls, and others.

If aerobic endurance training equipment is not available, nonmachine exercises can provide a variety of options as well. Nonmachine exercises comprise anything that allows the person to move freely and independently of equipment. This includes walking, jogging, running, swimming, water-resisted walking or running, skating, cycling, cardio kickboxing, and aerobic dance or step classes.

Machine exercise modes that appear similar to nonmachine exercise modes may not elicit the same cardiovascular response or provide the same ability to help clients reach their goals. For instance, running on a treadmill requires different motor patterns and muscle use than running on a track or trail. The propulsion is provided by the moving belt, so running on the treadmill does not require use of the muscles of the leg and hip to push the client forward. Likewise, riding a stationary bike uses the same muscles to turn the crank as a regular bike but does not require the muscles to provide balance; nor is there a headwind or friction between the ground and tires on a stationary bike. The mode of exercise used should match the needs and goals of the client, especially if the client is training for a running or cycling event.

Clients' personal preferences on exercise mode have a great influence on how well they will adhere to the program (72, 76). Selecting activities or exercises that clients enjoy will help them complete the training program as it was designed, rather than cutting corners to shorten the exercise session or decrease the intensity.

The mode of exercise must also be matched to the client's physical abilities. Clients with lower body orthopedic concerns may be limited in their ability to perform certain exercises because of impact strain on the foot, knee, or hip. These clients would be better served by a nonimpact form of exercise. Clients who have limitations in joint range of motion need an exercise that works within their capacity. For instance, a client with diagnosed shoulder impingement may not be able to use an upper body ergometer (arm bike).

The initial exercise mode must also be within the client's current $\dot{V}O_2$ capacity. In many cases clients have not had a graded exercise test to determine their $\dot{V}O_2$max. Without data to help determine what a client is capable of, it is always prudent to begin with an enjoyable exercise mode. A client who used to walk or ride a bike might begin a new exercise program by resuming those activities. This method will prevent situations in which clients are instructed to perform an activity that is inappropriate for them. For instance, if a running program is assigned to a client who does not have the fitness capacity to complete a brisk walk, he or she will not be able to participate in an exercise session of sufficient duration to elicit any improvement. A different, less demanding exercise mode is needed instead.

Finally, exercise mode should match the client's ultimate goals for specificity of training. For instance, Becky, who wishes to complete a 10K race, will spend a good deal of time running on an outdoor track or trail, or indoors using a treadmill during inclement weather. In a different approach, Floyd, who is interested in losing body fat, will need to purposely expend calories, which does not necessitate any particular piece of equipment or mode of exercise; he can use several different modes of exercise to provide variety in his workouts.

> **The decision about which exercise mode to use depends on several factors, including equipment availability, personal preference, the client's ability to perform the exercise, and the client's goals.**

Exercise Intensity

The intensity of exercise sessions is the main determinant of both exercise frequency and training duration. The intensity level required to reach the client's goal must be ascertained before the frequency and duration of exercise sessions are determined.

Regulating and monitoring exercise intensity are key to prescribing the correct aerobic endurance training program and preventing over- or undertraining. A certain threshold of $\dot{V}O_2$ or **heart rate reserve (HRR)**, which is the difference between a client's maximal heart rate and resting heart rate, must be attained during an aerobic exercise session before improvements in the cardiovascular system are seen (39, 49, 55, 69, 80, 97). Oxygen uptake reserve ($\dot{V}O_2R$ = difference between $\dot{V}O_2$max and resting $\dot{V}O_2$) has been shown to equate fairly evenly to the HRR. Since it is not common to have laboratory-assessed $\dot{V}O_2$max or $\dot{V}O_2R$ data for a personal training client, using HRR to determine exercise intensity is acceptable (46, 55, 66, 85).

Ultimately, the necessary aerobic exercise threshold depends on a client's initial fitness level, but for the apparently healthy adult, moderate to vigorous intensity is 40% to 89% of HRR (2, 84, 85). Extremely deconditioned clients may need to begin at an intensity of 30% to 39% of HRR (2). Depending on their fitness level, some may find 50% of HRR strenuous, while more advanced clients may find 85% of HRR insufficient to elicit cardiovascular system improvements. If the exercise intensity is too high, overtraining and injury may result. If the intensity is too low, the physiological stimulus to improve will be insufficient, and it will take longer to reach the goals that have been set. The key to knowing where to begin lies in examining the client's exercise and medical history and in the results of any recent exercise testing. It is always smart to begin conservatively and increase the intensity as needed, rather than beginning too high and risk overtraining and poor adherence.

Target Heart Rate

Heart rate and oxygen consumption ($\dot{V}O_2$) are closely related. During exercise, heart rate increases with increases in workload, and an increase in workload necessitates an increase in oxygen consumption. Therefore, as heart rate nears a client's maximal heart rate (MHR), a greater percentage of $\dot{V}O_2$max is being used. Table 16.1 illustrates a range of percent $\dot{V}O_2$max and the related percent HRR and percent of maximal heart rate (%MHR). This relationship has been shown to be consistent across age, sex, coronary artery disease status, fitness level, training status, muscle groups exercised, and testing mode (29, 81, 82, 98). Because of this relationship, heart rate is often used as a quick and easy way to measure exercise intensity.

The only way to determine a client's true MHR is to perform a graded exercise test that takes the client to the point where the heart rate does not increase with an increase in workload. At this point the heart has reached its maximal beat per minute (beat/min) capacity. For safety's sake, it may be recommended that a physician be present during a maximal graded exercise test on a client (68). Refer to chapter 9 for discussion on the conditions warranting the presence of a physician during exercise testing. Instead of performing a maximal graded exercise test, the personal trainer can use an estimate of a client's MHR in most cases, determined through a variety of methods. Table 16.2 provides the most common ways MHR is calculated.

A commonly used **age-predicted maximal heart rate (APMHR)** equation is as follows:

$$\text{APMHR} = 220 - \text{Age} \qquad (16.1)$$

This is only an estimate, with an error range of ±10 to 15 beats/min (43, 94). This error range is important to note when calculating target heart rate training zones. For example, a 20-year-old client with an APMHR of 200 may actually have an estimated MHR as low as 185 (200 − 15) or as high as 215 (200 + 15) when the error range is taken into account. The APMHR will therefore actually be maximal for some, unattainable for others, and submaximal for the rest (56). However, a client should never reach MHR during the course of submaximal aerobic endurance training, so the age-predicted estimate provides a close approximation that is acceptable for designing aerobic exercise programs (94). Using APMHR is not advisable for clients taking medications such as βblockers that blunt the heart rate response to exercise. In these clients, the medication prevents heart rate from rising above a certain point independent of the exercise intensity or workload. Before using APMHR to prescribe exercise intensity, the personal trainer must determine that the client is not taking any heart rate–altering medications; if the client is doing so, an alternative prescription for intensity not based on heart rate is necessary. Refer to chapter 20 for discussion of heart rate–altering medications.

If APMHR has been calculated, an appropriate exercise intensity training zone, or **target heart rate range (THRR)**, can be determined through one of two different calculations.

Percent of Age-Predicted Maximal Heart Rate

Once the APMHR is known, a range of exercise intensities based on known relationships between percentages of the APMHR and $\dot{V}O_2$max can be determined. For the apparently healthy adult, 46% to 90% of $\dot{V}O_2$max approximates to 64% to 95% of the APMHR, which provides the moderate to vigorous stimulus to improve aerobic function (2). Other ranges may be calculated depending on the client's medical history, any complications present, and physician recommendations. Because initial fitness level greatly affects the minimal threshold for cardiovascular improvement, for clients who are very deconditioned, a lower range of 57% to 63% of APMHR may be more appropriate (26, 50, 59, 77).

To determine the intensity training zone using a percentage of APMHR for an apparently healthy adult (called the **percent of APMHR method**), multiply the client's APMHR by 57% [the bottom of the light-intensity classification (2)] or 64% [the bottom of the moderate-intensity classification (2)] and 95% [the top

TABLE 16.1 Relationship Between $\dot{V}O_2$max, HRR, and MHR

%$\dot{V}O_2$max	%HRR	%MHR
37	30	57
45	39	63
46	40	64
63	59	76
64	60	70
90	89	95
91	90	96
100	100	100

%$\dot{V}O_2$max = percent of maximal oxygen uptake; %HRR = percent of heart rate reserve; %MHR = percent of maximal heart rate.

TABLE 16.2 Alternative Formulas for Estimating Maximal Heart Rate

Author	Equation	Population
Åstrand (5)	HRmax = 220 − age	Men and women aged 4-34 years
Fox et al. (23)	HRmax = 216.6 − (0.84 × age)	Small group of men and women
Gulati et al. (30)	HRmax = 206 − (0.88 × age)	Asymptomatic middle-aged women
Tanaka et al. (86)	HRmax = 208 − (0.7 × age)	Healthy men and women

HRmax = maximal heart rate.

of the vigorous-intensity classification (2)]. The results provide the lower and upper limits of exercise heart rate needed for improving cardiovascular function (table 16.3, using 64% and 95% of APMHR).

$$\text{Target heart rate (THR)} = \text{APMHR} \times \text{Exercise intensity} \quad (16.2)$$

Percent of Heart Rate Reserve: The Karvonen Formula The **Karvonen formula** is related to the percent of APMHR formula but allows for differences in resting heart rate (RHR) (48, 49). To use this formula, the personal trainer will need to obtain the client's RHR. The best time to measure RHR is first thing in the morning upon waking but before getting out of bed. Clients should be taught how to take their resting heart rate using a radial pulse palpation (index and forefinger over the radial pulse) for 1 minute. To obtain the HRR, subtract the RHR from the APMHR:

$$\text{HRR} = \text{APMHR} - \text{RHR} \quad (16.3)$$

The HRR is the available increase in heart rate over the RHR, up to the APMHR. In other words, the HRR is the number of beats per minute that the heart rate can increase from resting up to maximal. For instance, a 40-year-old client has an APMHR of 180; if he or she has an RHR of 70, then his or her HRR is 110 beats/min (an APMHR of 180 minus an RHR of 70).

As mentioned earlier, 40% to 89% of HRR is needed to improve cardiovascular function. To determine the target training zone, multiply the HRR by 40% and 89%, and then add the RHR back to each answer to obtain the lower and upper heart rate limits. Failure to add the RHR back to the answer will result in an underestimated training zone that will not provide the desired improvements. In the case of this client, his or her HRR of 110 beats/min × 0.40 = 44 and × 0.89 = 98. When we add the RHR of 70 to these values, we get a THRR of 114 to 168.

$$\text{Low end of THR} = (\text{HRR} \times \text{Lower exercise intensity value}) + \text{RHR} \quad (16.4)$$

$$\text{High end of THR} = (\text{HRR} \times \text{Higher exercise intensity value}) + \text{RHR}$$

The benefit to using HRR is that it is specific to the client because it is based on that client's baseline RHR. As a client becomes more fit and the RHR decreases, the HRR will increase; this represents a greater reserve to draw from.

As shown in table 16.3, in most situations, using the Karvonen formula provides slightly larger training ranges than the percent of APMHR formula (28, 66). To calculate exercise heart rate range, use 64% to 95% of APMHR or 40% to 89% of HRR. Both will

TABLE 16.3 Aerobic Endurance Training Exercise Heart Rates

Age	APMHR (beats/min)	PERCENT OF APMHR METHOD		KARVONEN FORMULA METHOD*	
		64%	95%	40%	89%
80	140	90	133	98	132
75	145	93	138	100	137
70	150	96	143	102	141
65	155	99	146	104	146
60	160	102	152	106	150
55	165	106	157	108	155
50	170	109	162	110	159
45	175	112	166	112	163
40	180	115	171	114	168
35	185	118	176	116	172
30	190	122	181	118	177
25	195	125	185	120	181
20	200	128	190	122	186
15	205	131	195	124	190

APMHR = Age-predicted maximal heart rate.
*Assumes a resting heart rate of 70 beats/min.

provide a heart rate range that produces an appropriate exercise stimulus to improve cardiovascular fitness (2, 49, 54). Note that untrained or beginning clients probably should begin with a THR based on the lower half of the APMHR intensity range (e.g., 57% to 63% of APMHR), and more trained clients typically can tolerate intensities in the upper half of the HRR range (e.g., 60% to 89% of HRR). See "Exercise Intensity Calculations Using Heart Rate" for exercise intensity formulas and sample calculations for both methods.

> **To calculate exercise heart rate range, assign an exercise intensity of 64% to 95% of APMHR or 40% to 89% of HRR.**

Wearable Technology

Properly determining exercise intensity is a primary concern when implementing an aerobic training program. Wearable technology can help the personal trainer monitor a client's physical activity, and recent progress has made it more affordable and accessible. One main feature of several wearable technology devices is heart rate monitoring, allowing individu-

als to track heart rate during activities of daily living and exercise. Wearable technology comes in a variety of forms but most often as heart rate straps, smart watches, finger sensors, and compression clothing with built-in technology; additional features may estimate daily steps, daily calories expended, daily minutes of activity, GPS tracking, or exercise intensity. These devices can be useful for tracking a client's progress and goals not only within a particular session but also over time since they often include smartphone apps that save individual data. Additionally, if worn outside of the exercise session, wearable technology allows the personal trainer to gain a deeper insight into a client's daily physical activity and provide appropriate programming based on HR, calories expended throughout the day or week, step counts, and multiple other physiological or psychological variables.

Percent of Functional Capacity

If a client's **functional capacity** (measured as $\dot{V}O_2max$) has been determined through a physician-supervised graded exercise test, the true MHR will be known. In this situation, it is best to use the measured MHR rather than an estimate. Either the Karvonen formula or the percent of APMHR formula (using the

---

EXERCISE INTENSITY CALCULATIONS USING HEART RATE

Percent of APMHR Method

Formula

Age-predicted maximal heart rate (APMHR) = 220 − age

Target heart rate (THR) = (APMHR × exercise intensity)

Do this calculation twice for the lower and upper limits to determine the target heart rate range (THRR).

Example: 30-year-old client; 70% to 85% of APMHR

APMHR = 220 − 30 = 190 beats/min

THR (70%) = 190 × 0.70 = 133 beats/min

THR (85%) = 190 × 0.85 = 162 beats/min

THRR = 133 to 162 beats/min

Karvonen Method

Formula

Age-predicted maximal heart rate (APMHR) = 220 − age

HRR = APMHR − RHR

Target heart rate (THR) = (HRR × exercise intensity) + RHR

Do this calculation twice for the lower and upper limits to determine the target heart rate range (THRR).

Example: 30-year-old client; 40% to 89% of HRR; RHR = 70 beats/min

APMHR = 220 − 30 = 190 beats/min

HRR = 190 − 70 = 120 beats/min

THR (40%) = (120 × 0.40) + 70 = 118 beats/min

THR (89%) = (120 × 0.89) + 70 = 177 beats/min

THRR = 118 to 177 beats/min

actual MHR in place of the APMHR) can be used to determine the aerobic exercise training zone.

Ratings of Perceived Exertion

An additional method, to be used along with heart rate calculation methods, is a **rating of perceived exertion (RPE)** scale. An RPE scale helps clients monitor their exercise intensities using a rating system that accounts for all of the body's responses to a particular exercise intensity. A client must be taught to quantify the stress of the exercise session in terms of both physiological and psychological factors, based on the mode of exercise; environment (e.g., temperature, humidity); intensity of the effort; and extent of strain, discomfort, or fatigue (27, 57, 75). An RPE is meant to measure not just how fast the heart is beating but also exertion, respiration, and emotional responses to exercise.

Often during graded exercise testing, clients are asked to give an RPE during each successive workload. These RPEs are paired with the $\dot{V}O_2$ of that workload so that when the test is completed, any given workload and $\dot{V}O_2$ has a known RPE. Because the personal trainer now knows what exertion rating corresponds to a given workload, he or she can use the RPE to determine approximate $\dot{V}O_2$ during exercise without the need to directly measure $\dot{V}O_2$. For example, if it is known that a particular $\dot{V}O_2$ elicited an RPE of 7 on a 1 to 10 scale during the YMCA cycle ergometer test (see chapter 11), during the next exercise session the personal trainer can approximate that same $\dot{V}O_2$ intensity with a different exercise mode by simply adjusting the intensity of the exercise to the point where the client rates the exercise at an RPE of 7. Figure 16.1 shows an example of an RPE scale.

The numerical ratings on the RPE scale are associated with adjectives that describe the effort needed to maintain the given exercise level. These ratings range from "Nothing at all" to "Maximum effort." Teaching a client to differentiate between exertion levels may take some time. The lowest level of each scale can be compared with lying still and not exerting any effort at all, while the highest level of each scale is the maximal amount of effort the client is capable of producing. The difficulty in using RPE is that very few clients will have ever actually reached the upper levels of effort and therefore cannot perceive what a 10 actually feels like. The RPE will have a greater degree of subjectivity in clients who have not completed a maximal stress test. To untrained, deconditioned clients, an exercise level that produces a heart rate of 60% HRR may seem maximal because they are unaccustomed to exercise and do not really know what a maximal effort is. Only through training and changes in exercise intensities will such clients learn the true meaning of the rating adjectives and how to accurately report their RPE.

A downside to using RPEs is that they vary between clients and between exercise modes for any given heart rate (64). Rating of perceived exertion scales should be used along with heart rate measurements so that over time, a pattern of exercise intensity for a given client can be established. Combining THHR and RPE in an exercise prescription will allow the personal trainer to determine the different effects a mode of exercise has on the client. For instance, while riding a stationary bike, a client may be working at 80% of THR and report an RPE of 7, whereas the same client running on a treadmill at 80% of THR may report an RPE of 9. Differences in mode of exercise will often include different amounts of muscle use and energy expenditure, which will change %THR, RPE, or both. Therefore, the personal trainer should avoid general exercise prescriptions based simply on an RPE, as they do not take individual differences into account.

The strength of RPE scales is that they allow for more than just a measurement of heart rate. These scales can be used when traditional heart rate intensity prescriptions are inaccurate because of the influence of medications or illness. When combined with heart rate, RPE allows assessments of whether the exercise intensity is providing enough of a stimulus for a particular client. For instance, if an advanced client is exercising at 80% of HRR and indicates an RPE of 4 on a 1 to 10 scale, an increase in exercise intensity is appropriate. In contrast, if a new client indicates

FIGURE 16.1 Sample rating of perceived exertion (RPE) scale.

Rating	Description
1	Nothing at all (lying down)
2	Extremely little
3	Very easy
4	Easy (could do this all day)
5	Moderate
6	Somewhat hard (starting to feel it)
7	Hard
8	Very hard (making an effort to keep up)
9	Very, very hard
10	Maximum effort (can't go any further)

a rating of 9 but has an actual exercise heart rate equal to 70% of HRR, the personal trainer should reduce exercise intensity until the client becomes better trained. The personal trainer must remember that an RPE is an indicator of overall effort, not just heart rate, so the client may be including feelings of fatigue, respiratory effort, pain, and mental effort or stress among other factors.

Metabolic Equivalents

Exercise intensity can also be prescribed in terms of **metabolic equivalents (METs)**. One MET is equal to 3.5 ml · kg^{-1} · min^{-1} of oxygen consumption and is considered the amount of oxygen required by the body to function when at rest (60). Therefore, any given MET level is an indication of how much harder than rest a particular activity is. For example, an activity that has a 4 MET rating is four times harder than rest, meaning it requires the body to work four times harder than at rest. In order to accurately prescribe an exercise intensity based on METs, the personal

trainer or physician must perform a maximal graded exercise test on a client to obtain the maximal MET level possible for that client (i.e., $\dot{V}O_2$max divided by 3.5). Without this information, assigning a percentage of maximal METs is not possible.

There are published MET approximations as shown in table 16.4 (1, 2). These approximations can be used to prescribe a variety of activities for the client's total exercise program and to compare the energy requirements of one activity with another. Client example 16.2 provides updated information for the hypothetical clients with sample intensity prescriptions based on various methods.

Training Frequency

Training **frequency** refers to how often the workouts are performed (e.g., the number of training sessions per week). The frequency of training sessions depends on the client's goals, current fitness level, duration, intensity, and recovery time required for the exercise.

CLIENT EXAMPLE 16.2

Exercise Intensity

A variety of intensities are provided for each client. The personal trainer should choose one based on the mode of exercise and the intensity monitoring tools that are available (e.g., heart rate monitor or RPE). (Refer to chapter 11 for illustrations and instructions on how to measure a client's heart rate manually.)

Becky

Age: 30

RHR: 65

APMHR: 190 beats/min

70% to 85% HRR: 153 to 171 beats/min

RPE: 5 to 6

METs: 12.5 (8 min/mile pace)

Because Becky is somewhat trained, her THRR can be set at 70% to 85% of her HRR. Her current 10K personal best time is 53 minutes, which is about 8.5 minutes per mile. Although Becky's workouts may vary from day to day, to reach her goal time of under 50 minutes she needs to increase her average training pace to 8 minutes per mile. Her personal trainer can monitor her ability to tolerate this increase in exercise intensity by either an RPE or heart rate.

Floyd

Age: 52

RHR: 74

APMHR: 168 beats/min

70% to 80% APMHR: 118 to 134 beats/min

RPE: 3 to 4

METs: 3 to 3.8 (walking at 2.5-3.5 mph [4-5.5 km/h]); 5.5 (stationary cycling at 100 watts; refer to chapter 11 to convert watts to an exercise work rate)

Because Floyd is untrained, his THRR can be set at 70%-80% of his APMHR. The MET intensities chosen for Floyd will allow him to exercise at a pace he can sustain as a beginner for weight-bearing exercises, and a little harder (5.5 METs) for non–weight-bearing exercises. Until Floyd becomes accustomed to exercise and can give accurate RPEs, his personal trainer should monitor his exercise intensity by regularly measuring his heart rate during the exercise session.

TABLE 16.4 Estimated Metabolic Equivalents for Various Activities

METs	Activity
1.0	Lying or sitting quietly, doing nothing, lying in bed awake, listening to music, watching a movie
2.0	Walking, <2 mph (<3.2 kph), level surface
2.5	Stretching, hatha yoga
2.8	Walking, 2 mph (3.2 kph) slow pace, level surface
3.0	Walking, 3.0 mph (4 kph), level, firm surface
3.0	Pilates, general
3.5	Resistance training (weight) training, multiple exercises, 8-15 reps at varied resistance
3.5	Stationary cycling, 30-50 watts, very light to light effort
3.5	Calisthenics, home exercise, light or moderate effort, going up and down from the floor
3.5	Golf, using a power cart
3.5	Rowing machine, 50 watts, light effort
4.3	Walking, 3.5 mph (5.6 kph), level, firm surface
4.3	Golf, walking and carrying clubs
4.5	Tennis, doubles
4.5	Basketball, shooting around
5.0	Aerobic dance, low impact
5.0	Walking, 4 mph (6.4 kph), level surface, very brisk pace
5.0	Resistance training, squats, slow or explosive effort
5.5	Water aerobics, water calisthenics
5.5	Badminton, social singles and doubles
5.5	Step aerobics (with a 4 in. [10.2 cm] step height)
5.8	Swimming laps, freestyle, slow, moderate or light effort
6.0	Outdoor cycling, 10-12 mph (16.1-19.2 kph), leisure, slow, light effort
6.0	Resistance training (free weights, Nautilus or Universal machine), powerlifting or bodybuilding, vigorous effort
6.0	Basketball, nongame
6.3	Walking, 4.5 mph, level surface, very, very brisk pace
6.8	Cross-country skiing, 2.5 mph (4 kph), slow or light effort, ski walking
6.8	Stationary cycling, 90-100 watts, moderate or vigorous effort
7.0	Walking, 4.5 mph (7.2 kph), level, firm surface, very, very brisk
7.0	Badminton, competitive
7.0	Rowing machine, 100 watts, moderate effort
7.3	Aerobic dance, high impact
7.5	Step aerobics (with a 6-8 in. [15.2-20.3 cm] step height)
8.0	Basketball, game
8.0	Calisthenics (e.g., push-ups, sit-ups, pull-ups, jumping jacks), vigorous effort
8.0	Circuit training (kettlebells, some aerobic movements), with minimal rest, vigorous intensity
8.0	Outdoor cycling, 12-14 mph (19.3-22.4 kph), moderate effort
8.0	Tennis, singles

METs	Activity
8.3	Walking, 5 mph (8 kph), level, firm surface
8.5	Rowing machine, 150 watts, vigorous effort
8.5	Step aerobics (with a 6-8 in. [15.2-20.3 cm] step)
8.8	Stationary cycling, 101-160 watts, vigorous effort
9.0	Cross-country skiing, 4-4.9 mph (6.4-7.9 kph), moderate speed and effort
9.5	Step aerobics (with a 10-12 in. [25.4-30.5 cm] step height)
9.8	Swimming laps, freestyle, fast, moderate/hard effort
10.0	Running, 6 mph (9.7 kph) (10 min mile)
10.0	Outdoor cycling, 14-16 mph (22.5-25.6 kph), racing or leisure, fast, vigorous effort
10.5	Running, 6.7 mph (10.8 kph) (9 min mile)
11.0	Stationary cycling, 161-200 watts, vigorous effort
11.5	Running, 7 mph (11.3 kph) (8.5 min mile)
12.0	Outdoor cycling, 16-19 mph (25.7-30.6 kph), very fast, racing
12.0	Rowing machine, 200 watts, very vigorous effort
12.3	In-line skating, 13-13.6 mph (20.9-21.9 kph), fast pace, exercise training
12.3	Running, 8.6 mph (13.7 kph) (7 min mile)
12.5	Cross-country skiing, 5-7.9 mph (8-12.7 kph), brisk speed, vigorous effort
12.8	Running, 9 mph (14.5 kph) (6 min, 40 s mile)
14.0	Stationary cycling, 201-270 watts, very vigorous effort
14.5	Running, 10 mph (16.1 kph) (6 min mile)
15.0	Cross-country skiing, >8 mph (>12.9 kph), racing
15.8	Outdoor cycling, >20 mph (>32.2 kph), not drafting
16.0	Running, 11 mph (17.7 kph) (5.5 min mile)

MET = metabolic equivalent.

Adapted from Ainsworth et al. (1) (consult this reference for a comprehensive list of the MET level for 821 specific activities) and ACSM (2).

As noted earlier, the 2018 Physical Activity Guidelines Advisory Committee has recommended that all individuals accumulate 150 to 300 minutes per week of moderate-intensity physical activity or about 75 to 150 minutes of vigorous-intensity physical activity per week as a valid option (90). The committee also stated that exercise bouts of any length contribute to the health benefits associated with the accumulated volume of physical activity (90). The American College of Sports Medicine (ACSM) recommends that most adults engage in moderate-intensity cardiovascular exercise training for ≥30 minutes per day on five days of the week for a total of 150 minutes per week,

vigorous-intensity cardiovascular exercise training for ≥20 minutes per day on three days of the week (≥75 minutes per week), or a combination of moderate- and vigorous-intensity exercise to achieve a total energy expenditure of ≥500 to 1,000 MET-minutes per week (2, 26). While the distribution of activity across the week may be less important, the ACSM recommends that aerobic physical activity is spread throughout the week, preferably across three or more days, which may also help to reduce the risk of injury and prevent excessive fatigue (2).

Beginning clients (e.g., no participation in a regular aerobic exercise program for the past six months) should start with the minimum number of sessions per week, spaced out evenly (table 16.5). As fitness levels improve, the frequency of training can increase. As the number of exercise sessions per week increases, the frequency should not exceed the frequency that a client is willing to adopt and maintain (46). For example, despite the common examples shown, some clients may have only the weekdays (or just the weekends) to exercise, so the personal trainer will need to design an exercise schedule around when the client is available. Most desirably, however, the client's rest days should be placed in between exercise days to space them evenly throughout the week.

In the case of Becky, because she is already running twice a week, her exercise prescription can begin at three or four days per week. Floyd, on the other hand, as a non-exerciser, will begin with two days per week, although he has the flexibility and desire to exercise in the morning before work and during his lunch hour.

Ultimately, the frequency of exercise must be balanced with the duration and intensity of exercise. In general, exercise sessions of longer duration or higher intensity require more recovery time and are therefore performed less frequently, whereas exercise sessions of shorter duration or less intensity do not require as much recovery time and can be performed more often (68).

> **Exercise sessions of long duration and high intensity require longer recovery times and therefore cannot be performed very often; short-duration exercise at low intensity does not require as much recovery time and can be performed more frequently.**

Exercise Duration

Exercise **duration** is a measure of how long an exercise session lasts. Along with training frequency, exercise duration depends on the client's goals, current fitness levels, and the intensity of the exercise. The greater the intensity of an aerobic exercise session, the greater the $\dot{V}O_2$ requirement and the less time a client will be able to spend exercising at that level (78).

The 2018 Physical Activity Guidelines Advisory Committee stated that the duration of aerobic endurance training should range from a minimum of 30 minutes up to 60 minutes (90). In addition, the committee noted that the total exercise duration could be achieved in smaller 10-minute bouts to accumulate the total aggregate time (90). The American Heart Association recommends between 30 and 60 minutes for the purposes of health promotion and cardiovascular disease prevention (3). The ACSM recommends at least 150 to 300 minutes per week of moderate intensity, or 75 to 150 minutes a week of vigorous intensity aerobic physical activity, or an equivalent combination of moderate and vigorous physical activity (2).

If time constraints prevent a client from dedicating a block of time large enough to meet exercise duration needs, or if the client is very deconditioned, shorter **intermittent exercise** bouts can be substituted. If the intensity is moderate to high, intermittent exercise bouts of at least 10 minutes each can improve the aerobic fitness of all but the most advanced clients (18, 34, 65). Intermittent bouts have also been shown to improve adherence to exercise in people who are unaccustomed to physical activity (54). For clients who are severely deconditioned and unable to complete even a 10-minute exercise bout, several shorter bouts

TABLE 16.5 Sample Exercise Frequency Options

	BEGINNER		INTERMEDIATE		ADVANCED
	5 days of rest	4 days of rest	3 days of rest	2 days of rest	1 day of rest
Day	2 days of exercise	3 days of exercise	4 days of exercise	5 days of exercise	6 days of exercise
Sunday	Rest	Rest	Rest	Rest	Exercise
Monday	Exercise	Exercise	Exercise	Exercise	Exercise
Tuesday	Rest	Rest	Exercise	Exercise	Exercise
Wednesday	Rest	Exercise	Rest	Rest	Rest
Thursday	Exercise	Rest	Exercise	Exercise	Exercise
Friday	Rest	Exercise	Exercise	Exercise	Exercise
Saturday	Rest	Rest	Rest	Exercise	Exercise

of exercise with rest periods in between will allow them to build up to a continuous bout.

Beyond the recommended minimum of 30 minutes, the human body is capable of withstanding hours of aerobic endurance exercise, as is evident in athletes who complete iron-distance triathlons, 24-hour ultramarathons, or cycling races of 100 miles (160 km) or more. The total duration of a given client's program is ultimately determined by that client's personal goals, the intensity level of a given workout, and the client's ability to fit the training session into his or her schedule. In the case of Becky, she has been running 3 to 5 miles (4.8-8 km) at about an 8.5 min/mile pace for an exercise duration of 25 to 42 minutes. Since her goal of completing a 10K in less than 50 minutes requires a continuous exercise bout, intermittent training throughout the day will not offer her sufficient training specificity; therefore, she must adjust her schedule (e.g., exercise before or after work) to allow for longer exercise sessions. In contrast, Floyd's goal of weight loss does not require sustained bouts of exercise; and although he will be able to eventually sustain a longer exercise bout, he may begin with two 10- to 15-minute sessions each exercise day.

> **Exercise duration is inversely related to exercise intensity.**

Progression

One of the keys to designing a proper aerobic endurance training program is exercise **progression**. For purposes of training the general population, aerobic endurance training programs can be divided into two distinct types: **improvement** and **maintenance**. The type of program the personal trainer designs for a client depends on the client's initial fitness level and training background. The untrained beginner will always start with an improvement program; a client who has been exercising but wants to improve will also use an improvement program; and a client who just wishes to maintain his or her current level of aerobic endurance will use a maintenance program.

Improvement in aerobic endurance training can be measured as an increase in $\dot{V}O_2$ capacity, or an increased tolerance for longer durations or higher intensities. Following an improvement program requires making periodic, progressive increases in exercise frequency, duration, or intensity. As a general rule, weekly increases in frequency, intensity, or duration should be no more than 10%, and increases should be made only after the body has adjusted to the new program. Constraints on a client's available training time, along with the fact that there are only seven days in a week, often mean that exercise frequency and duration reach their upper limits before exercise intensity does, after which improvements in aerobic capacity will have to result from increases in intensity. In other words, the client will have only so much time available to exercise, but he or she can continually (albeit gradually) increase exercise intensity. Client example 16.3 updates the information on the sample clients and illustrates options for progression of their workouts.

The maintenance program is reserved for clients who want to maintain their current level of fitness or who have progressed through the improvement program and have reached the upper limits of how intensely they wish to train. Maintenance of aerobic capacity requires significantly less effort than trying to improve it. Over the long term, clients can maintain improvements from an aerobic endurance training program if they reduce the frequency of training to no fewer than two sessions per week but maintain the duration and (especially) the intensity during the exercise sessions they do perform (39, 40, 41). Additionally, to keep a client motivated during a maintenance program and to facilitate continued adherence, the personal trainer can design the program to use a variety of exercise modes (33). Another use of a maintenance program is for a client who wishes to take some time off from training (or needs to because of a business trip or vacation); this person can decrease the total volume of aerobic exercise for a few weeks by as much as 70% without negatively affecting $\dot{V}O_2$max (61).

> **As a general rule, weekly increases in frequency, intensity, or duration should be limited to no more than 10%.**

Warm-Up and Cooldown

Regardless of which program a client is using, appropriate warm-up and cooldown procedures should be integrated into the exercise sessions. The purpose of a warm-up is to increase blood flow to the muscles that will be used during the workout, slowly increase heart rate so that oxygen debt is minimized, prepare the nervous system for action, and increase muscle core temperature to cause more complete unloading of oxygen from the blood to the muscles (31, 79, 91). Proper warm-up involves a slow progression from small, simple movements to the larger, more complicated movements that mimic those used during the exercise session (21, 51). For instance, if a client will be running, a proper warm-up will include progression from normal walking with the arms at the sides, to slow jogging with a swinging of slightly bent arms, to running with full pumping of the arms at a 90 degrees bend in the elbows. The client should allow enough time in each activity for the heart rate to increase to meet metabolic demands before progressing further.

The cooldown uses the same progression in reverse. The client progresses from running to jogging to walking, allowing the heart rate to decrease and reach a lower steady state before slowing down. Clients can do additional flexibility exercises after the cooldown. See chapter 12 for more information on warm-up, cooldown, and flexibility exercises.

CLIENT EXAMPLE 16.3

Six-Week Progression

Becky

Becky indicated that she can work out only three days a week. Since she has been running 3 to 5 miles (4.8-8 km) at about an 8.5 min/mile pace (25-42 minutes) twice a week, her six-week program will concentrate on gradually increasing the distance she runs while maintaining the faster training pace (8 min/mile) needed to prepare her for running a 10K in her goal time.

Week 1: Three days (Mon, Wed, Fri): running 3 miles (4.8 km) in 24 minutes

Week 2: Three days (Sun, Tue, Thu): running 4 miles (6.4 km) in 32 minutes

Week 3: Three days (Mon, Wed, Fri): running 4.5 miles (7.2 km) in 36 minutes

Week 4: Three days (Sun, Tue, Thu): running 5 miles (8 km) in 40 minutes

Week 5: Three days (Mon, Wed, Fri): running 5.5 miles (8.9 km) in 44 minutes

Week 6: Three days (Sun, Tue, Thu): running 6 miles (9.7 km) in 48 minutes

Floyd

Floyd indicated he can begin with working out two days a week (although he has each weekday available), in two 15-minute sessions each exercise day. His six-week program will concentrate on increasing the number of days and the duration of exercise while keeping him within his APMHR training zone of 118 to 134 beats/min.

Week 1: Two days (Mon, Thu), two times each day (in the morning before work and during the lunch hour)—walking on a treadmill at 2.5 to 3.5 miles (4-5.6 km) per hour for 10 to 15 minutes

Week 2: Three days (Tue, Thu, Sat), two times each day: in the morning before work—riding the stationary bike at 100 watts for 10 to 15 minutes; during the lunch hour—walking on a treadmill at 2.5 to 3.5 miles (4-5.6 km) per hour for 10 to 15 minutes

Week 3: Four days (Mon, Tue, Thu, Fri), once each day—riding the stationary bike at 100 watts for 20 to 25 minutes

Week 4: Four days (Mon, Tue, Thu, Fri), once each day—walking on a treadmill at 2.5 to 3.5 miles (4-5.6 km) per hour for 15 to 20 minutes

Week 5: Five days (Mon, Tue, Wed, Thu, Fri), once each day (Floyd can decide when)—three times a week (Mon, Wed, Fri), walking on a treadmill at 2.5 to 3.5 miles (4-5.6 km) per hour for 20 to 25 minutes; two times a week (Tue, Thu)—riding the stationary bike at 100 watts for 25 to 30 minutes

Week 6: Five days (Mon, Tue, Wed, Thu, Fri), once each day (Floyd can decide when)—walking on a treadmill at 2.5 to 3.5 miles (4-5.6 km) per hour for 25 to 30 minutes

TYPES OF AEROBIC ENDURANCE TRAINING PROGRAMS

There are many ways to design aerobic endurance training programs, but all will contain the components previously discussed. As mentioned earlier, the first step is deciding which mode or modes of exercise to use. Sometimes choosing more than one mode is appropriate. For instance, outdoor running, cycling, and swimming are all dependent on the weather. Combining machine and nonmachine exercises that mimic each other can provide a continued training stimulus when the environment is not conducive to outdoor workouts. Running outside or on a treadmill, cycling or riding a stationary bike, and swimming in a lake or in a pool can all provide the stimulus needed for improvement if adjustments for duration and intensity are made. The exercise mode must be one that the client will enjoy and can perform without any problems or pain, and one that provides enough of a challenge to stimulate improvement.

After exercise modes have been selected, the frequency, duration, and intensity can be combined in a number of ways, each of which will produce a different effect. The final program may take the form of long slow distance training, pace/tempo training, interval training, circuit training, or cross-training. The most important determinant of how to combine these components is the goal of the client.

Long Slow Distance Training

In **long slow distance (LSD) training**, exercise sessions should be performed at an intensity less than that normally used so that the duration of the workout can be longer. For example, during LSD, a client capable of running at a 6 min/mile pace may exercise at an 8 min/mile pace for a longer distance. A client who normally rides a stationary bike for 30 minutes at 150 watts may ride for 1 hour at 100 watts. The basic premise of LSD is to increase exercise duration at a lower intensity than normal. A good indicator of proper intensity other than percent of HRR is whether the client can carry on a conversation during the exercise session. The idea is not to speak at length, but to be able to talk without becoming short of breath. Typical training sessions last between 30 minutes and 2 hours and, to prevent overtraining, should not take place more than twice a week (17, 93).

Once target intensity is achieved, the exercise can continue as long as the client is able to maintain a heart rate within the prescribed zone and as long as energy is available. When heart rate increases beyond the training zone, the anaerobic systems begin to provide energy at the expense of carbohydrate and glycogen stores, and volitional fatigue will quickly follow. Once the client's heart rate begins to increase without an increase in workload, the exercise session is complete. For the beginning exerciser, this may occur after only a brief period of time (10 to 15 minutes). With subsequent exercise sessions, the client can increase the duration of exercise as cardiovascular system improvements allow for greater perfusion of oxygenated blood, delivery of energy substrates, and removal of waste products.

Personal trainers should note that not all clients will initially be able to achieve the 40% to 89% HRR training zone or be able to continue the exercise for more than a short time. Seriously deconditioned clients will require a lower starting point and a slower increase in both intensity and duration.

Pace/Tempo Training

For clients who wish to improve their cardiovascular endurance and who are capable of working at the highest percentages of their heart rate range, **pace/tempo training** can help improve $\dot{V}O_2max$. This type of training allows clients to train for short periods at their goal pace, which will be higher than their current pace. Pace/tempo training sessions typically last between 20 and 30 minutes and require clients to exercise at their lactate threshold (15, 17). The workout can be performed either intermittently or steadily. **Intermittent pace/tempo training** involves work bouts of 3 to 5 minutes with rest periods of 30 to 90 seconds, repeated until the desired pace cannot be maintained. During the rest period, clients may engage in very light (slow) walking to prevent any blood pooling in the legs. Intermittent pace/tempo training is best suited for clients who typically do not tolerate an intensity at their lactate threshold for very long. Over time, these clients will increase their tolerance and can progress to steady pace/tempo training. **Steady pace/tempo training** involves one bout of exercise lasting 20 to 30 minutes, sustained at the desired pace. Because pace/tempo training requires that a higher intensity be achieved during a workout session, the duration of the workout is reduced. Pace/tempo training should be performed only one or two times a week. Client example 16.4 provides a sample intermittent pace/tempo workout.

CLIENT EXAMPLE 16.4

Sample Intermittent Pace/Tempo Workout for Becky

Overall Parameters

Intervals: 3 to 6 minutes

Intensity: 80% to 89% $\dot{V}O_2$max or 8 METs

Rest between intervals: 60 seconds

Mode: Elliptical machine with 1 to 10 levels

Total time completed at goal pace/intensity: 30 minutes

Elliptical Machine

Warm-up

Three minutes at level 8, 60 seconds rest

Four minutes at level 8, 60 seconds rest

Five minutes at level 8, 60 seconds rest

Six minutes at level 8, 60 seconds rest

Five minutes at level 8, 60 seconds rest

Four minutes at level 8, 60 seconds rest

Three minutes at level 8

Cooldown

CLIENT EXAMPLE 16.5

Sample Training Programs With Long Slow Distance, Interval, and Pace/Tempo

Because LSD, interval, and pace/tempo programs require a firm aerobic base, these sample programs should be viewed as a progression to be used after some tolerance for exercise has been established through consistent and regular aerobic endurance training.

BECKY (REST DAYS: TUESDAY, THURSDAY, FRIDAY, SUNDAY)			
	Monday	**Wednesday**	**Saturday**
Type of training	Long slow distance	Interval	Pace/tempo
Activity	Outdoor running	Treadmill	Outdoor running
Distance or duration	15K-20K (9.3-12.4 miles)	60 min	30 min steady
Pace or intensity	9-10 min/mile pace	5 min work period at a 6 min/mile pace (10 mph [16 km/h]) alternated with a 5 min rest period at a 12 min/mile pace (5 mph [8 km/h])	8 min/mile pace

FLOYD (REST DAYS: SATURDAY, SUNDAY)			
	Monday and Thursday	**Tuesday and Friday**	**Wednesday**
Type of training	Interval	Long slow distance	Pace/tempo
Activity	Stationary cycle	Treadmill	Stationary cycle
Distance or duration	30 min	60 min	20 min intermittent
Pace or intensity	5 min work period at 150 watts alternated with a 5 min rest period at 75 watts	3 miles [4.8 km] per hour	Four 5 min work periods at 80% to 89% $\dot{V}O_2$max alternated with a 1 min rest period

Interval Training

Interval training programs get their name from the alternating periods of high- and low-intensity exercise performed over a given session. Interval training can involve short periods of exercise at intensities at or above the lactate threshold and $\dot{V}O_2$max, alternated with longer periods of lesser intensities. Interval training can also involve high-intensity exercise ($\geq 90\%$ $\dot{V}O_2$max) with periods of rest in between, also known as **high-intensity interval training (HIIT)**.

The benefit of interval training is that with the correct spacing of work and rest, clients can accomplish a greater amount of work at higher intensities that are normally not possible with a continuous, steady-state aerobic program. Exercising at such a high intensity ($\geq 90\%$ $\dot{V}O_2$max) requires a large contribution from both the anaerobic and aerobic energy systems, thereby quickly inducing fatigue. With interval training, the length of time spent exercising is kept relatively short, and the rest periods are lengthened to allow for more complete recovery between exercise intervals. Thus, complete fatigue is delayed. Alternatively, if a client attempted a continuous training session (i.e., non-interval based) at an intensity $\geq 90\%$ $\dot{V}O_2$max for as long as possible, fatigue would set in within a few minutes and the exercise intensity would need to be lowered. However, during the course of an interval program, a client may train at the high intensity for several short periods, with rest in between, allowing for a greater total amount of time spent at the highest intensity.

For instance, clients who want to increase their maximal running or cycling speeds may use intervals of all-out sprinting or cycling efforts, alternated with rest periods in which they continue moving at a lower-intensity recovery pace. Refer to chapter 11 on how to estimate $\dot{V}O_2$max to maximize high-intensity interval training. Additionally, clients who wish to burn the maximum number of calories in a set amount of time could employ interval training. In this case, alternating high and low intensities, instead of using one set intensity, allows the client to burn a greater number of calories, in a time-efficient manner, during a workout (4, 6, 12).

Properly adjusting the work-to-rest ratio is essential to allow the client to complete the prescribed exercise session. For instance, the duration of each interval performed at a high intensity ($\geq 90\%$ $\dot{V}O_2$max) can range from 5 seconds to 8 minutes (depending on the intensity, goal, number of intervals, and work-to-rest ratio). Thus, the entire HIIT session can last from ~5

to 30 minutes, with work-to-rest ratios varying from 1:1 to 1:8 depending on the ability of the client to perform successive high-intensity intervals. As the client fatigues, the rest interval can be lengthened to allow for greater recovery between work bouts. Extending the rest interval beyond 1:8 reduces the amount of time that can be spent doing high-intensity work in a fixed-length exercise session and thus reduces the total amount of work done and improvement made. The 1:1 to 1:8 work-to-rest ratios cause beneficial adaptations in cardiovascular endurance by increasing the lactate threshold (i.e., right shift), the number of mitochondria, and the body's ability to buffer metabolic by-products (e.g., H^+) from the muscles and bloodstream (19, 93).

Clients should use interval training and HIIT only after they have established a firm aerobic base and are able to maintain the prescribed exercise intensity for a period roughly equal to the total time that will be spent on interval training (52). As an example, a client who is able to maintain a steady-state HRR training zone for 60 minutes could perform interval training for up to 60 minutes (exercise and rest time combined).

Almost any aerobic endurance exercise can be selected for an interval training workout. If the intensity can be adjusted quickly and easily, aerobic endurance training machines can be used in the same way that outdoor exercises are used for interval training. For variety, interval bouts can be done on one aerobic modality and the rest bouts performed on another. For example, an interval training program could involve using the stair climber for the work period and the treadmill for the rest period. However, with shorter work-to-rest ratios (e.g., 1:1), this method may not be feasible because of the limited time to switch modalities. Client example 16.5 provides a sample training program with LSD, interval, and pace/tempo routines.

> **Research supports the development of an aerobic foundation before integrating advanced metabolic conditioning training modalities like high-intensity interval training (HIIT), advanced resistance training circuits, or boot camp–style programming.**

Circuit Training

Circuit training can involve resistance training only or can combine resistance training with aerobic endurance training, where the client performs short intervals of aerobic endurance training between resis-

CLIENT EXAMPLE 16.6

Sample Hybrid Cardiovascular Circuits

Hybrid cardiovascular circuits and boot camp–style workouts incorporate a variety of exercises, including popular training implements, in an interval-type workout. These circuits can include multiple stations (lasting approximately 10 to 60 seconds), without rest or with rest (10 to 30 seconds) in between stations. Personal trainers can effectively use these circuits to increase heart rate in a fun and creative way to enhance exercise adherence over time.

Circuit Example 1

Station 1: Standing double arm waves with battle ropes

Station 2: Core stability station (side bridge)

Station 3: Outer circle waves with battle ropes

Station 4: Walking lunge with 6- to 12-pound (3-6 kg) medicine ball trunk rotations

Station 5: Core stability station (plank)

Station 6: Standing overhand power wave with battle ropes

Station 7: 15 to 25 jumping jacks

Station 8: Core stability station (side bridge)

Station 9: Overhead mace swings with battle ropes

Station 10: Half-kneeling wood chops with resistance band

Station 11: Inner circles with battle ropes

Station 12: Overhead counterclockwise mace swings with battle ropes

Circuit Example 2

Station 1: Standing power wave with battle ropes

Station 2: Active recovery station (jogging, 200 to 400 yards or meters)

Station 3: Kettlebell hip swings

Station 4: Active recovery station (jogging, 200 to 400 yards or meters)

Station 5: Standing double arm wave with battle ropes

Station 6: Active recovery station (jogging, 200 to 400 yards or meters)

Station 7: Standing S wave with battle ropes

Station 8: Active recovery station (jogging, 200 to 400 yards or meters)

Station 9: Sandbag alternation rotational lunge

Station 10: Active recovery station (jogging, 200 to 400 yards or meters)

tance training sets. The goal is to increase heart rate to the training zone and keep it there for the duration of the exercise session, thus inducing improvement in cardiovascular endurance and muscular endurance at the same time. Unfortunately, most investigations on variations of circuit training have shown that although strength increased, $\dot{V}O_2$max did not significantly improve compared with values for participants in an aerobic exercise–only program or a combined circuit training and aerobic program (32, 63, 89). Those research studies that did show small improvements in $\dot{V}O_2$max due to circuit training required the subjects to train at heart rates close to 90% HRR (16).

However, although circuit training has not been shown to significantly increase $\dot{V}O_2$ in many cases, there is no evidence that $\dot{V}O_2$ decreases during a circuit training program. Therefore, it may be a useful tool in a maintenance program. Circuit training can also be used with beginning clients as a means of introducing them to both resistance and aerobic endurance training

Sample Cross-Training Workouts

Cross-training workouts should be designed around the total volume or duration of exercise the client is capable of. The following examples are progressions to be used after some tolerance for exercise duration has been established through consistent and regular aerobic endurance training.

Becky

> *Monday:* 60 minutes on the treadmill
>
> *Wednesday:* 60 minutes on the stationary bike
>
> *Friday:* 30 minutes on the stair climber

Floyd

> *Monday:* 10 minutes on the treadmill, 10 minutes on the stationary bike, 10 minutes on the stair climber
>
> *Tuesday:* 10 minutes on the rowing machine, 10 minutes on the elliptical trainer, 10 minutes on the treadmill
>
> *Thursday:* 30 minutes on the stationary bike
>
> *Saturday:* 20 minutes walking outdoors, 15 minutes on the rowing machine

when their available time for training is short. Client example 16.6 provides some sample hybrid cardiovascular circuit workouts.

Cross-Training

Cross-training is a method of combining several exercise modes for aerobic endurance training. In order for cross-training to be effective in maintaining or improving $\dot{V}O_2$max, the intensity and duration of each exercise must be of sufficient quantity with respect to the client's fitness level (95, 96). For clients who wish to do cross-training, the personal trainer must prescribe the intensity and duration of each mode of exercise individually while keeping the combined volume of exercise within the client's capabilities. The benefit of cross-training is that it distributes the physical stress of training to different muscle groups during the different activities and increases the adaptations of the cardiovascular and musculoskeletal systems (51, 67, 101).

The result of cross-training is that it overcomes the limitations of specificity of training. That is, when a client has a goal that cannot be met with use of one particular exercise, competing in a triathlon for instance, cross-training is a way of obtaining that goal.

Aerobic endurance cross-training can be accomplished by two different means: using different modes of exercise each training period, rotating through two or more modes within a week; or using several different exercise modes within the same workout. With the first option, a client may train on the treadmill one day, cycle outdoors the next, and then finish the week on a rowing machine. The second option entails setting up a series of exercise modes that can be completed back to back. For example, instead of doing 30 minutes on the treadmill, the client may complete 10 minutes each on the treadmill, elliptical trainer, and arm ergometer.

The key to making cross-training effective is ensuring that clients work within their prescribed training zone with each exercise mode. Different exercises may elicit different heart rates for a given workload or speed, so individualization of the program for each mode is necessary. Client example 16.7 provides some sample cross-training workouts.

Arm Exercise

Many aerobic endurance activities primarily involve the major muscles of the lower body. However, arm exercises are becoming more popular, are often part of cardiac rehabilitation programs, and are a contributing source of power for swimming. To prescribe a THRR based on a percent of APMHR, the personal trainer must make a downward adjustment of 10 to 13 beats/min when calculating the APMHR because heart rate is higher during arm exercise than during leg exercise for any given workload (20, 24, 25, 47, 88). Additionally, the $\dot{V}O_2$max for arm exercise is significantly lower

SAMPLE COMBINED AEROBIC AND RESISTANCE TRAINING PROGRAMS

Goal: Increased Muscular Strength, Maintenance of Aerobic Endurance

1. Perform initial aerobic endurance training for 8 to 10 weeks: three or four days a week, 40% to 89% HRR, 30 to 60 minutes.
2. Reduce aerobic endurance training to two days per week, 40% to 89% HRR, 30 minutes, and begin resistance training.

Goal: Increased Aerobic Endurance, Maintenance of Muscular Strength

1. Perform 8 to 10 weeks of initial resistance training.
2. Reduce resistance training to two days per week and begin aerobic endurance training three or four days per week, 40% to 89% HRR, 30 to 60 minutes.

than that for leg exercise (20, 47). The result is that the lactate threshold is reached at lower intensities than during leg exercise (71).

Upper body ergometers (UBEs or arm bikes) are the most common type of arm-specific equipment found in fitness centers. Many stationary bicycles, elliptical trainers, and stair climbers have an attachment that allows the arms to work in a push–pull motion and may be used in an arms-only mode for upper body aerobic endurance exercise. Likewise, the arm portion of a rowing machine may be isolated if the feet are placed on the floor so that the body does not slide back and forth.

Arm exercise is probably the most underused type of aerobic endurance exercise. To increase variety, arm work can be added to programs that mainly use lower body exercises. Arm exercise is especially helpful in providing some aerobic endurance exercise to clients who have orthopedic problems in the lower body, such as an injury to the foot, knee, or hip.

Combined Aerobic and Resistance Training

Quite often, clients undertake aerobic endurance and resistance training programs simultaneously. Although the benefits of both are clear and there is no doubt that both should be part of a complete training program, there is a downside to combining these two types of training. Research has shown that when properly designed resistance training and aerobic endurance training programs are combined, the increase in strength gains will be blunted while $\dot{V}O_2$ increases normally. Clients will see increases in aerobic endurance similar to those they would have seen if they had done only aerobic endurance train-

ing, but the increases in strength from the resistance training portion of their program will be smaller than if they had done only resistance training (7, 14, 35, 36, 44). Along with reduced maximum strength gains, combined programs result in reductions in the amount of muscle girth gains and in specific speed- and power-related performances (16, 36, 53). On the other hand, the addition of anaerobic resistance training to an aerobic endurance training program seems to improve low-intensity aerobic endurance (37, 42, 83).

A relatively sedentary client who is just beginning to exercise will show improvements from both aerobic and resistance training when using both programs within a total workout. However, for more advanced clients who are reaching plateaus in improvement, it is doubtful they will obtain the full benefits of both programs at the same time because there will be little to no recovery time (days off to rest).

To remedy this problem, the personal trainer can design a program to allow the client to complete the aerobic endurance training program before beginning the resistance training program. For instance, a client could perform eight weeks of aerobic endurance training only, followed by eight weeks of resistance training with only the minimal amount of aerobic endurance training needed for maintenance. This would allow the client to increase $\dot{V}O_2$max and establish an aerobic base first, then work on increasing muscular fitness (e.g., strength) while maintaining the improved $\dot{V}O_2$ (8, 13, 38). After the initial 16 weeks, the client could begin alternating periods of aerobic endurance training and minimal resistance training for maintenance of strength with periods of resistance training and minimal aerobic endurance training for maintenance of aerobic endurance (39). This style of program provides continued increases in both aerobic endurance and muscular strength, although at a reduced rate in comparison with training only for one or the other, but also allows for changes in program variables such as mode and intensity to enhance variety. See the "Sample Combined Aerobic and Resistance Training Programs" for combined training programs based on differing training goals.

CONCLUSION

Designing aerobic endurance training programs that meet clients' goals and improve the working capacity of the cardiovascular and respiratory systems requires careful thought and accurate calculations. Because of individual differences in exercise preference, long-term goals, and current training status, the personal trainer must take care when manipulating the components of intensity, duration, and frequency. When program components are properly aligned, improvements in $\dot{V}O_2$max for an individual are limited only by genetics. Incorporation of different training methods such as long slow distance, pace/tempo training, interval training, circuit training, cross-training, arm exercises, and the combination of aerobic and resistance training will allow clients to continue making improvements in aerobic capacity and overall fitness.

Study Questions

1. Which of the following represent the recommend amount of physical activity per week for Americans?

   I. 150-300 minutes moderate intensity

   II. 60-120 minutes moderate intensity

   III. 30-60 minutes vigorous activity

   IV. 75-150 minutes vigorous activity

   A. I only

   B. III only

   C. I and IV only

   D. II and III only

2. The personal trainer is designing an aerobic exercise program for a 43-year-old client who has a resting heart rate of 75 beats/min. Using the Karvonen method, which of the following is the target heart rate range if the personal trainer assigns an intensity of 60% to 70% of the client's HRR?

   A. 106 to 123 beats/min

   B. 136 to 146 beats/min

   C. 123 to 137 beats/min

   D. 154 to 165 beats/min

3. As a general rule, weekly increases in frequency, intensity, or duration should be no more than which of the following?

   A. 5%

   B. 10%

   C. 15%

   D. 20%

4. Circuit training can increase strength and $\dot{V}O_2$max concurrently, with $\dot{V}O_2$max improving to the same extent as compared to an aerobic-exercise only program.

   A. true

   B. false

5. Which of the following is *incorrect* regarding combining aerobic and resistance exercise?

   A. Both aerobic and resistance exercise should be part of a complete training program.

   B. The increase in strength gains will be blunted compared to strength training alone.

   C. $\dot{V}O_2$ improvements will be blunted compared to aerobic training alone.

   D. Muscle girth gains will be blunted compared to strength training alone.

CHAPTER 17

Plyometric and Speed Training Program Design and Technique

Jason C. Casey, PhD, and Chris A. Bailey, PhD

After completing this chapter, you will be able to

- explain the mechanics and physiology of plyometric and speed-enhancing exercises,
- identify the phases of the stretch–shortening cycle,
- understand the different roles of plyometric and speed training,
- recommend proper equipment for use during plyometric exercise performance,
- design safe and effective plyometric and speed training programs, and
- provide instruction in correct plyometric and speed training technique and recognize common errors.

In an effort to improve sport performance, athletes at all levels want an advantage that allows them to outplay their opponent. Athletes are looking for ways to become quicker and more explosive, for ways to jump higher and sprint faster. Plyometric and speed training are two training techniques that allow athletes of all ages and abilities to accomplish these goals. Although not typically emphasized in the design of programs for personal training clients, plyometric and speed training are important components of a well-balanced plan to improve not only sport performance but also job performance and activities of daily living. Exercises designed to train clients to jump higher and run faster are arguably essential program components. Further, because so many injuries occur as the result of an inability to control decelerative forces, the use of both plyometric and speed training, with their emphasis on the efficient production and use of ground reaction forces, should be considered an integral part of any program whose goal is injury prevention. Another benefit of note is increased bone mass (57), of particular importance for those at risk of osteoporosis. Moreover, plyometric training has been demonstrated to be a potentially valuable tool in combating aging-related issues (40, 85). Additional benefits of incorporating plyometric and speed training components include overall enhanced coordination, increased agility, and improved anaerobic and general conditioning (55).

A plyometric movement is a quick, powerful movement consisting of an eccentric muscle action, also known as a countermovement or prestretch, followed by an immediate powerful concentric muscle

The authors would like to acknowledge the significant contributions of Vanessa van den Heuvel Yang, Kevin Messey, Stacy Peterson, Robert Mamula, and David H. Potach to this chapter.

action (90). Speed is simply the ability to achieve high velocity. Both plyometrics and speed rely heavily on the stretch–shortening cycle (SSC) to elicit the desired outcome. Since all functional activities are composed of a series of repetitive SSCs, it is essential to incorporate exercises that strengthen clients in these areas (21). The purpose of plyometric exercise is to use the stretch reflex and natural elastic components of both muscle and tendon to increase the power of subsequent movements and strengthen the muscles and tendons functionally (14, 21, 55, 61, 93). Speed training exercises are designed to use these same mechanical and neurophysiologic components, in concert with technique and muscular strength, to produce larger ground forces, thereby allowing clients to run faster. This chapter describes how to use plyometric and speed training exercise effectively as part of an overall training program.

PLYOMETRIC MECHANICS AND PHYSIOLOGY

Successful, goal-directed movements—athletic, job related, and functional—depend on all active musculotendinous structures working in concert at appropriate velocities. The term used to define this force–speed relationship is *power* (see chapter 4 for a detailed definition of power). When used correctly, plyometric training has consistently demonstrated the ability to improve the production of muscle force and power (45, 82). This increased production of muscular power is best explained by two proposed models as discussed in this section—mechanical and neurophysiological (90). The function of each model is then summarized by a description of the SSC.

Mechanical Model of Plyometric Exercise

In the **mechanical model**, elastic energy is stored after a rapid stretch and then released during a subsequent concentric muscle action, thereby increasing the total force production (1, 11, 46). A common model presents the function of the musculotendinous unit as a relationship between three mechanical components: the series and parallel elastic components and the contractile component (CC) (figure 17.1, row 2). The **series elastic component (SEC)** is a primary contributor to force production during plyometric exercises. Although the SEC includes some muscu-

lar components (actin and myosin), it is composed mainly of tendon (14). When the musculotendinous unit is stretched, as during an eccentric muscle action, the SEC acts as a spring and is lengthened, storing elastic energy. If the muscle then immediately begins a concentric muscle action, the stored energy is released, contributing to the total force production by naturally returning the muscles and tendons to their resting configuration. If a concentric muscle action does not occur immediately following the eccentric action, or if the eccentric phase is too long or requires too great a motion about the given joint, the stored energy dissipates and is lost as heat. Consequently, no plyometric effect will occur (14, 61).

Neurophysiological Model of Plyometric Exercise

The **neurophysiological model** involves a change in the force–velocity characteristics of the muscle's contractile components caused by stretch (31); concentric muscle force is increased with the use of the stretch reflex (figure 17.1, row 3) (6-8). The **stretch reflex** is the body's involuntary response to an external stimulus that causes a rapid stretching of the muscle. In response to this rapid stretch, a signal is sent to the spinal cord, which in turn sends a message back, resulting in a concentric contraction of the same overstretched muscle (61). The stretch reflex responds to the rate at which the muscle is stretched (17, 44, 58). An example of the stretch reflex in action is the quick knee jerk reaction that occurs when the patellar tendon is hit by an external stimulus such as a reflex hammer. A quick stretch of the patellar tendon occurs when the reflex hammer contacts with the tendon. The quadriceps muscle then senses this stretch and responds with an involuntary concentric contraction, resulting in the knee jerk as seen by the observer (17, 58).

This reflexive component of plyometric exercise is composed primarily of muscle spindle activity. Muscle spindles are sensory receptors located within the muscle near the musculotendinous junction. They are sensitive to the rate and magnitude of a stretch; when a quick stretch is detected, muscular activity reflexively increases (44, 58, 61). This reflexive response increases the activity in the agonist muscle, thereby increasing the force the muscle produces (6-8, 52). Although response time of the reflex does not really change with training, the strength of the response in terms of the muscle contraction elicited does increase with training, resulting in power gains. The faster a muscle is stretched, the greater the concentric force after the stretch, eliciting increased power output (17). As with the mechanical model, if a concentric muscle action does not immediately follow a stretch (e.g., due to an excessive delay between the stretch and concentric action or with a movement occurring over too large a range), the **potentiation**, or enhancement, of the stretch reflex is negated (14, 61).

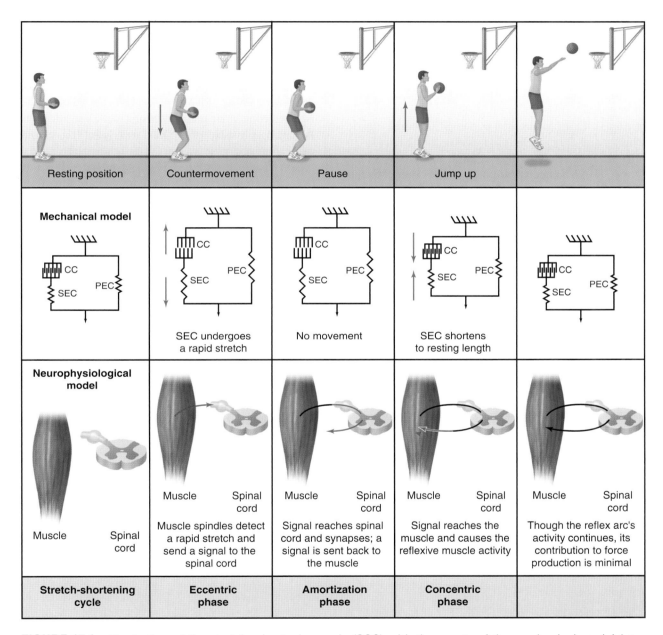

FIGURE 17.1   Illustration of the stretch–shortening cycle (SSC) with the events of the mechanical model (row 2) and neurophysiological model (row 3) that occur during each of its three phases (row 4). For example, during the eccentric phase of the SSC (column 2)—that is, the client's countermovement—the series elastic component (SEC) undergoes a rapid stretch that the muscle spindles detect, which then send a signal to the spinal cord.

Reprinted by permission from Albert (1995).

Stretch–Shortening Cycle

The **stretch–shortening cycle (SSC)** is a model explaining the energy-storing capabilities of the SEC and stimulation of the stretch reflex that facilitate a maximal increase in muscle recruitment over a minimal amount of time. The SSC involves three distinct phases (table 17.1). Although these phases outline the individual mechanical and neurophysiological events of the SCC, all the events listed do not necessarily occur within the given phase, as some events may last longer or require less time than the given phase allows. The **eccentric phase**—the deceleration phase—involves preloading the agonist muscle group(s). During this phase, the SEC stores elastic energy and the muscle spindles are stimulated (4). To visualize the eccentric phase, think about a basketball jump shot. The eccentric phase is the countermovement, beginning at the initiation of the half-squat motion and continuing until the bottom of the movement (figure 17.1, column 2).

The **amortization phase**, or transition phase, is the time between the eccentric and concentric phases—the time from the end of the eccentric phase to the initiation of the concentric muscle action. This is the turnaround time from landing to takeoff and is the most important part of the plyometric exercise because it is critical for power development (61). There is a delay between the eccentric and concentric muscle actions during which the spinal cord begins to transmit signals to the agonist—stretched—muscle group. For a period of milliseconds, an isometric contraction occurs as the body prepares to change direction. This phase must be kept short. If the amortization phase lasts too long, the energy stored during the eccentric phase will be dissipated as heat, and the stretch reflex will not increase muscle activity during the concentric phase (61). Consider again the basketball jump shot. Once the person's downward half squat has stopped, the amortization phase has begun. As soon as upward movement begins, the amortization phase has ended (figure 17.1, column 3).

The **concentric phase** is the body's response to the events occurring during the eccentric and amortization phases. During this final phase of the SSC, the energy stored in the SEC during the eccentric phase is either used to increase the force of the subsequent movement or is dissipated as heat. Use of the stored elastic energy increases the force produced during the concentric phase movement to a level above that of an isolated concentric muscle action (10, 82). In addition, the agonist muscle group performs a reflexive concentric muscle action as a result of the stretch reflex. Again visualize the jump shot. After the half squat, as soon as movement begins in an upward direction, the concentric phase of the SSC has begun and the amortization phase has ended (figure 17.1, column 4). In this example, one of the agonist muscles is the quadriceps femoris. During the countermovement, the quadriceps femoris undergoes a rapid stretch (eccentric phase); there is a delay in movement (amortization phase); then the muscle acts concentrically to extend the knee, allowing the person to push off the floor or ground (concentric phase) (figure 17.1, columns 2, 3, and 4, respectively).

> The stretch–shortening cycle describes the stretch reflex and stored elastic energy–induced increases in concentric force production that follow a rapid eccentric muscle action.

TABLE 17.1 Stretch–Shortening Cycle

Phase	Action	Physiological event
I—Eccentric	Stretch of the agonist muscle	• Elastic energy is stored. • Muscle spindles are stimulated. • Signal is sent to spinal cord.
II—Amortization	Pause between phases I and III	• Nerves synapse (meet) in spinal cord. • Signal is sent to stretched muscle.
III—Concentric	Shortening of agonist muscle fibers	• Elastic energy is released from the SEC. • Stretched muscle is stimulated by the nerve.

SEC = series elastic component.

WHEN TO USE PLYOMETRIC EXERCISE

It should seem obvious that plyometric training offers significant benefits to athletic clients in that most sporting movements rely on quick, powerful movements to be successful (2, 61). Which other populations may benefit from use of these types of movements is less clear. This bias has allowed plyometric exercise to become an ignored training modality for the general population. Many non-athletic clients, however, may benefit from the increases in muscular power production that plyometric training provides. The ability of the personal trainer to identify non-athletic clients who may benefit from plyometrics, as well as those for whom plyometrics are not necessary or perhaps contraindicated, is an essential skill for designing individualized exercise programs.

Training and Sport Performance

When training clients whose goals include becoming more explosive in their sport, components of the training regimen must include exercises that mimic the movements occurring in that sport. Being able to train clients to produce greater muscular force (power) at a faster speed will provide them the edge in performance they are looking for. Increased production of muscular power is an established outcome of participation in a plyometric training program (1, 11, 45, 46, 61, 73, 82, 91). The ability to produce more muscular power has been associated with improved sport performance (including increased jump performance, decreased sprint times, and increased strength) (3, 25, 60, 81). Plyometric training, then, is an ideal exercise mode when the goal is to improve muscular power production (60, 61, 73). In addition, plyometric training prepares athletes for the deceleration–acceleration and change-of-direction requirements in most sports by improving their ability to perform these types of tasks. An additional benefit of moderate plyometric training in average-distance runners is an improved **running economy** (the distance run per amount of oxygen consumed) (83).

Training and Work Performance

In addition to sport performance, participation in a plyometric training program has the potential to improve performance in certain jobs involving physical work (54). Though this has not been sufficiently examined in the literature, an analysis of some job requirements indicates that the production of muscular power is a key to movement efficiency and may improve job output. For example, police officers, firefighters, or clients preparing for military training must be able to run quickly, change direction effectively, and jump onto or over objects (e.g., fences) in preparation for their occupational demands.

Exercise and Injury Prevention

Decreasing the incidence of injury, especially in populations who are at a greater risk of injury than others, is an important consideration when designing an exercise training program. There is great interest in the effectiveness of plyometric training for decreasing risk of injury. Studies have shown that athletic injury rates decrease following participation in a plyometric training program (5, 13, 45, 94). Research has also shown that proper plyometric training improves bone mineral content, muscle recruitment, strength, body control, and balance (14, 65, 93). The increased bone mineral content development could lead to a decreased risk of osteoporosis later in life.

Since plyometric training teaches the neuromuscular system to quickly perform an SSC while also focusing on proper technique and biomechanics, the client develops the ability to control all joints in the kinetic chain. This results in an improved stability of the entire body (94). These results suggest that the plyometric program should focus on proper jumping and landing mechanics, which will carry over into the client's athletic or work activity. When the client engages in activities in either work or play that incorporate jumping and landing components, he or she will do so correctly, which will decrease the risk of injury. Plyometric training improves dynamic joint stability (14) and the ability to control the body during activities (e.g., controlled knee positioning during landing). This can help decrease the chances of knee issues like patellofemoral pain syndrome and anterior cruciate ligament injuries (14, 65, 79). Also, the increased ability to control the body has the potential to reduce the risk of falls that could result in fractures (85, 93).

It is difficult, however, to extrapolate the results of these studies to different populations. A component of plyometric training is eccentric control of movement, which research has shown may decrease the risk of injury (76). Eccentric training may therefore be a compromise for clients who wish to engage in injury prevention activities but for whom plyometric training is not appropriate. Eccentric training can consist of normal weight training with a focus on the eccentric phase of the lift. The personal trainer can guide clients to perform a lift with both the concentric and eccentric phases but to perform the eccentric phase more slowly. Even more effective is having clients perform the eccentric phase on their own and the personal trainer assist with the concentric phase. This technique allows clients to resist more weight than they would without assistance.

> Although plyometric training is primarily thought to enhance athletic performance, other populations may benefit as well. Along with increases in power, properly applied plyometric training programs have been shown to decrease injury rates and improve bone mineral content, muscle recruitment, strength, body control, and balance.

PLYOMETRIC SAFETY CONSIDERATIONS

There has been no research to delineate populations for whom plyometric training is contraindicated, though analysis of a client's age, experience, and current training level may help identify clients who are and are not ready for plyometric training. To reduce the risk of injury and to improve the performance of plyometric exercises, the client must understand proper plyometric technique and possess a sufficient base of strength, speed, and balance. In addition, the client must be sufficiently mature both physically and psychologically to participate in a plyometric training program.

Plyometric exercise is not inherently dangerous; however, as with all modes of exercise, there is a risk of injury. Injuries may be caused by an accident, but they more typically occur when training procedures are violated. Improper program design, inadequate instruction and supervision, or an inappropriate training environment can contribute to increased injury risk. Often these injuries occur when the muscles are fatigued, since fatigue affects the body's proprioceptive ability. Ankle and knee sprains are the most common injuries that occur with plyometrics because of breaks in form resulting from muscular fatigue (17). In addition, whenever the client adds more difficult exercises or movements or trains at an increased intensity level, there is an increased risk of injury until the client becomes proficient at the exercise (55). Personal trainers must understand and address these and other risk factors to improve client safety. The following factors must be considered when prescribing plyometric exercise.

Age and Maturity

Plyometric training places great stress on the body, so it is important to consider all factors to ensure that the client's health is not compromised. Plyometrics at certain intensities are safe for the majority of populations; however, modifications to intensity and volume must also be made based on age.

Research shows that plyometrics are safe and beneficial for youth (32). Guidelines indicate that as soon as the client is mature enough to accept and follow directions, plyometrics can be safely integrated into the training program (32, 33). In fact, this is an ideal time to implement plyometrics within a comprehensive training program, including resistance and flexibility training, because a youth's body is very moldable and adept at learning these motor skills (33, 53). In addition to improving running velocity and vertical jump, plyometrics can help improve bone strength, balance, and coordination and decrease sport injury rate in young clients (32, 53, 92). However, the addition of high-intensity lower body plyometrics could place young clients at an increased risk for bone injury because the epiphyseal plates (growth plates) of the bones of prepubescent children have yet to close (51, 56). Therefore, it is important that plyometric programs follow the recommended guidelines.

When developing a plyometric program for youth, personal trainers should focus on teaching the proper technique, especially jumping and landing techniques, described later in the chapter (32, 33, 42, 53). Young clients should not focus on competing with or outperforming others, but rather on improving their own performance and mastering the skill. The exercises should be low-intensity plyometrics performed at the beginning of a session, before the client is fatigued (55). This ensures that the client has proper neuromuscular and postural control to perform the exercises correctly. Increased errors and injuries are likely to occur if the client is tired. Incorporating plyometric exercises into a dynamic warm-up is ideal. The exercises should take the form of fun and creative activities that resemble structured play and games so that the actual training goal is not apparent to the child (72, 75). Examples include having the child react to balls, run obstacle courses, perform jumping jacks, play hopscotch, or mimic being chased (32, 33, 72).

For adolescent clients, it is appropriate to incorporate low-intensity plyometric exercise into the training regimen as long as the client has met all the safety conditions outlined later (75, 77, 93). The personal trainer should emphasize proper technique as well, since adolescents are still developing neuromuscular control. It is safe to perform low-intensity plyometrics at small volumes, incorporating them into warm-up activities. Once these low-intensity exercises have been mastered, the client may perform moderate-intensity exercises (17, 79).

The other population of concern is older clients. Because of decreasing bone strength as one ages as well as the possibility of degenerative joint conditions, the aging population may need to avoid high-intensity plyometrics. However, it is very beneficial for older people to continue training the SSC (75) by integrating low- to moderate-intensity plyometrics into their training program. The older client should begin with low-intensity exercises and progress to moderate-intensity plyometrics only when the personal trainer has ensured the client is able to safely and correctly perform the exercises (63). Properly performed high-intensity resistance training can have positive results for people older than 60 (26). This outcome suggests that the addition of plyometrics may be beneficial, as long as the client is medically cleared and has met all the safety conditions.

For all ages, physical maturity should not be the sole determinant of plyometric preparedness. Psychological maturity and acuity are necessary before someone begins plyometric training. The client must respond positively to the personal trainer's instructions to proceed with plyometric training. If he or she does not, plyometric training should be postponed. Injury, overtraining, or undertraining may result if the client is inattentive to instructions.

Posture, Flexibility, and Stability

Many lower body plyometric drills require the client to move in nontraditional patterns (e.g., double-leg zigzag hops and backward skips) or on a single leg (e.g., single-leg tuck jump and single-leg hops). These types of drills necessitate a solid base of support on which the client can safely and correctly perform the exercises. Even lower-intensity drills performed by clients just beginning a plyometric program require sufficient balance to prevent injury. As a result, it is essential that the personal trainer assess whether the client can safely meet the demands of plyometric training. The fundamental position that all lower body plyometric exercises originate from and end in is the partial (half) squat. Therefore, it is essential that the personal trainer begin by assessing the client's ability to hold this position (79) in order to determine his or her potential to land properly with each exercise.

For both the partial-squat position and the squat movement itself, the client's feet should be flat on the floor or ground and approximately shoulder-width apart, with the knees directly over or slightly posterior to the toes. The chin should be tucked in slightly, the scapulae should be slightly retracted, and the trunk should be parallel to the tibias. The client's body weight should be centered over a stable base of support (79), and the client must maintain this position in proper form.

Once the client can hold this position, he or she should perform a bodyweight squat. The personal trainer should have the client stand with feet approximately shoulder-width apart. To initiate the squat movement, the client should anteriorly rotate the pelvis, then flex at the ankles, knees, and hips while keeping the trunk parallel to the tibias throughout the entire range of motion. Also, the knees should remain either posterior to the toes or directly over them, and the feet should remain flat on the floor or ground, avoiding liftoff of the heels if possible. Common errors include rounded shoulders, a forward head, a flexed thoracic spine, a posterior pelvic tilt, and a heel liftoff (79).

Once clients can both hold a proper double-leg squat position and perform a proper bodyweight squat, they may begin low-intensity plyometric exercises. When performing low-intensity plyometrics, they must learn to maintain the proper alignment, providing a strong base for dynamic action (79). Errors in alignment will increase the chance of injury and also increase contact time during the amortization phase, resulting in less than optimal concentric force (79, 94).

Before the personal trainer increases the level of exercises, the client should be able to hold a single-leg squat position (i.e., standing, quarter squat, or half squat) as shown in table 17.2. These are divided into level of difficulty; each test position must be held for 30 seconds (86). For example, a client doing plyometric training with double-leg drills for the first time must be able to balance on one leg for 30 seconds without falling. This indicates that the client has enough balance and leg strength to do double-leg drills. An experienced client beginning an advanced plyometric training program involving single-leg drills should be able to maintain a single-leg half squat for 30 seconds without falling. The added dimension of the half squat indicates the client has enough strength on the leg to do single-leg plyometric exercises. Note that the surface on which the balance testing is performed must be the same as that for the plyometric drills.

Strength

Before adding plyometrics to a client's workout program, the personal trainer must also take the client's level of strength into consideration. Clients who have never participated in a resistance training program should be precluded from taking part in a plyometric training program. Plyometric training requires significant strength and muscle control, especially during the eccentric phase. For this reason, clients should be encouraged to perform a resistance training program that includes standard exercises (e.g., squat, bench press, deadlift) before beginning a plyometric training program.

If the client does not possess sufficient muscular strength, plyometrics should be delayed until certain standards—originally intended for athletes—are met. Because research has yet to define a prerequisite level of strength, the following are the only published recommendations available for personal trainers to use when determining a client's readiness to participate in a plyometric training program:

- For lower body plyometrics, the client's 1RM squat should be at least 1.5 times his or her body weight (47, 55, 69, 88).

- Clients weighing more than 220 pounds (99.8 kg) should exercise caution when considering plyometric exercise choices (see the "Physical Characteristics and Proficiency" section for additional details). Increased body mass results in increased compressive forces, so avoiding high-volume and high-intensity plyometric exercises may be beneficial (47, 69, 88).

- An alternative measure of prerequisite upper body strength is the ability to perform five clap push-ups in a row (69, 88).

Although these guidelines provide a good rule of thumb, it is not necessary for clients to possess this level of strength to engage in low to moderate levels of plyometric activity, like simple jumps in place, as long as they can tolerate moderate loading during a resistance program and have proper landing technique (14, 61). When moving a client to more advanced levels of plyometric exercises, such as depth jumps, it is recommended that the personal trainer follow the strength guidelines listed (75). However, personal

TABLE 17.2 Balance and Strength Prerequisite Tests

Level[a]	Position[b]	Drill variation[c]
Beginning	Standing	Double leg
		Single leg
Intermediate	Quarter squat	Double leg
		Single leg
Advanced	Half squat	Double leg
		Single leg

[a]Each of these levels corresponds with a drill's intensity level (e.g., beginning-level balance corresponds with low-intensity plyometric drills).

[b]The client is required to maintain each position within each variation for 30 s before attempting plyometric exercises of the same intensity and the more difficult balance test.

[c]The type of prerequisite test (i.e., how many legs are used) needs to match the intended type of plyometric drill (e.g., the beginning client has to pass the standing single-leg balance test to qualify to perform single-leg plyometric drills).

trainers should recognize that it is possible to modify even high-intensity plyometric exercises to make them appropriate for a client's strength level so that he or she can perform them safely and still achieve similar gains.

Another aspect of strength that is very important to assess is core strength (61, 75). **Core strength** is the body's ability to control its center of mass in response to forces on the trunk generated by other parts of the body, including upper and lower extremities (66, 75, 94). In other words, the core is responsible for maintaining balance and postural stability during all activities (66, 75). Core strength directly affects all other aspects of strength. A strong core provides a solid base for all other muscles and joints to work from, thereby allowing them to function in an optimal manner. A weak core will negatively affect the manner in which muscles and joints function since the base of support is weak and therefore unstable. A direct effect of a weak core is a longer amortization phase, which will compromise the plyometric effect (61). Overall, proper form will be compromised, performance will be hindered, and the chance of injury will increase with poor core strength (94).

Speed

Perhaps a more specific requirement for plyometric training participants is speed of movement. Because plyometric exercise relies on quick movements, the ability to move rapidly is essential before a client begins a plyometric program. In the absence of research specifying the level of speed necessary for plyometric exercise, personal trainers can use the following guidelines. For lower body plyometrics, the client should be able to perform 5 repetitions of a squat with 60% body weight in 5 seconds or less (69, 88). To satisfy the speed requirement for upper body plyometrics, the client should be able to perform 5 repetitions of the bench press with 60% body weight in 5 seconds or less. Like the strength guidelines presented previously, these speed requirements were originally intended for athletic populations. Should a client lack the speed of movement described here, he or she may begin a plyometric training program that starts with lower-intensity drills that do not rely as heavily on speed (e.g., two-foot ankle hop, standing long jump, double-leg vertical jump).

Landing Position

For lower body plyometrics, proper landing technique is essential to maximize the effectiveness of the exercise and minimize the risk of injury. This is especially true for depth jumps. If the center of gravity is offset from the base of support, performance will be hindered and injury may occur (79). If the earlier squat assessment reveals proper posture, flexibility, and stability, the personal trainer should begin assessing and training landing technique.

During the landing, the shoulders should be over the knees; the knees should be over or slightly posterior to the toes, with the ankles, knees, and hips flexed and the feet approximately shoulder-width apart (figure 17.2). Clients should reduce forces gradually upon landing and maintain a dorsiflexed position of the ankle, with the feet in full contact with the floor or ground. Clients should also keep their weight more on the ball of the foot and not on the heel. This position allows a quick turnaround on the landings so that the client spends as little time as possible on the floor or ground, achieving maximum power output (17). Instilling a proper landing technique will also teach the client to control the body's center of gravity within the base of support (79).

Landings can be taught during several exercises, including a vertical jump followed by a freeze in the landing position to allow proper analysis of the landing position, a forward or backward jump followed by a freeze in the landing position, or even a lateral jump followed by a freeze in the landing position. It is important that the personal trainer provide constant feedback during and after each drill or exercise in order to instill proper technique.

For plyometric jumps, hops, leaps, bounds, skips, and quick foot drills, clients should concentrate on keeping their knees and their thumbs up. This will help with balance by keeping the workload centered around the hips and legs. Normally, when the knees are brought up quickly, as is the case with these exercises, the tendency is for the shoulders to drop forward. To prevent this, clients should focus on holding their hands in a position in which the thumbs are pointing up toward the sky, which forces the torso to remain in a more upright position. This also helps with maintaining balance (75). Also, the arms should be brought behind the midline of the body so they

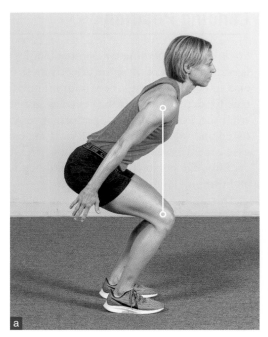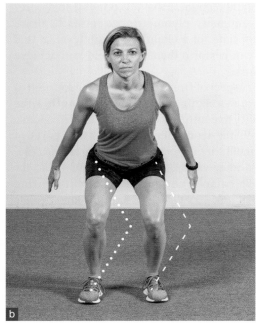

FIGURE 17.2 Proper plyometric landing position. *(a)* The shoulders are in line with the knees, which helps place the center of gravity over the body's base of support. *(b)* The knees are in line with the feet. There is no valgus (dotted line) or varus (dashed line) deviation.

can move forward and up rapidly to help increase the strength of the muscle action (17, 75).

Medical History

As with other forms of exercise, joint structure, posture, body type, and previous orthopedic injuries must be examined and reviewed before the start of a plyometric training program. Previous injuries or abnormalities of the spine, lower extremities, or upper extremities may increase a client's risk of injury during plyometric exercise. Specifically, clients with a history of muscle strains, pathological joint laxity, or spinal dysfunction (including vertebral disc dysfunction or compression injuries) (38, 39) should exercise caution when beginning plyometric training (47). Clients with a history of such conditions should receive medical clearance from a licensed physician before beginning plyometric activity. Any preexisting injury may require modifications to plyometric activity. For example, a client with patellofemoral pain may not be able to squat without pain and thus should not be doing high-intensity plyometric exercises like depth jumps. Before beginning any plyometric training,

the client should be able to tolerate activities of daily living without pain or joint swelling (14).

Medical conditions, such as certain illnesses, osteoporosis, arthritis, or diabetes, may not respond well to plyometric activities. Therefore, personal trainers should require formal medical clearance before starting a client on plyometric activities. They should be well informed of the client's medical history and should ensure that the client has had a recent physical examination from a licensed physician (79).

MINIMUM REQUIREMENTS FOR PARTICIPATION IN A PLYOMETRIC TRAINING PROGRAM

- Proper technique for each drill
- At least three months of resistance training experience
- Sufficient strength, speed, and balance for the level of drill used
- No current injuries to involved body segments

Physical Characteristics and Proficiency

A specific characteristic warranting caution is client size because greater body weight increases joint compressive forces. Guidelines exist (69, 79, 88) for clients who weigh more than 220 pounds (99.8 kg); they may be at increased risk of injuring lower extremity joints when performing plyometric exercises or, more specifically, depth jumps from heights greater than 18 inches (45.7 cm). Note that these guidelines may incorrectly imply that a client who weighs 219 pounds (99.3 kg) can perform plyometric exercises without limitations but a client who weighs 221 pounds (100.2 kg) is contraindicated. Moreover, client size does not adequately reflect all aspects of morphology (e.g., there are 250-pound [113.4 kg] American football players who can do backflips). Thus, personal trainers need to take individual client factors into account when designing a plyometric training program.

It is also important to make progressions in plyometric exercise selection that are appropriate for the skill level of the specific client. For example, a client should gain proficiency in exercises involving double-leg takeoffs before progressing to single-leg takeoffs.

Equipment and Facilities

In addition to the participant's level of fitness and health, the area where the client performs plyometric drills and the equipment used may significantly affect safety.

Landing Surface

To prevent injuries, the landing surface used for lower body plyometrics must have adequate shock-absorbing properties but not be so soft that it significantly increases the transition between the eccentric and concentric phases. A grass field, field turf, a suspended floor, and rubber mats are good surface choices (17, 47, 61, 79). Clients may progress to harder surfaces that encourage higher rates of energy return (50). Surfaces such as concrete, tile, and hardwood are not recommended because they are not sufficiently shock absorbent (47, 61). Performing exercises on these surfaces can lead to a variety of lower extremity injuries. Mini-trampolines and excessively thick exercise mats (≥6 inches [15.2 cm]) and may extend the amortization phase, thus preventing efficient use of the stretch reflex.

Training Area

The amount of space needed depends on the drill. Most bounding and running drills require at least 33 yards (or 30 m) of straightaway, though some drills may require a straightaway of 109 yards (or 100 m). For most standing, box, and depth jumps, only a minimal surface area is needed; but adequate height—9.8 to 13.2 feet (3-4 m)—is required.

Equipment

Boxes used for box jumps and depth jumps must be sturdy, should have a nonslip top, and should be closed on all sides. Boxes should also have few, if any, sharp or abrupt edges. Box heights should range from 6 to 42 inches (15.2-106.7 cm) (2, 17) with landing surfaces of at least 18 inches by 24 inches (45.7 cm by 61 cm) (17). The box should be constructed of sturdy wood (e.g., 3/4-inch [1.9 cm] plywood) or heavy-gauge metal. To further reduce injury risk, ways to make the landing surface nonslip are to add nonslip treads, mix sand into the paint used on the box, or affix rubberized flooring to the top of the box (17).

Plastic cones of varying heights (from 8 inches up to 24 inches [20.3-61 cm]) can be used as items to jump over during plyometric exercises. Since the cones are flexible, they are less likely to cause injuries if the client lands on them (17). Stairways, bleachers, and stadium steps also provide a viable plyometric training area. One must make sure they are safe for jumping on before the client begins the activities. Concrete steps are not a preferred surface since the concrete is unyielding (17). Medicine balls can be used for upper extremity plyometric exercises as well as in conjunction with some lower body exercises. They should be easy to grip, durable, and of varying weights (17).

Proper Footwear

Plyometrics require footwear with good ankle and arch support, good lateral stability, and a wide, nonslip sole (69, 88). Shoes with a narrow sole and poor upper support (e.g., running shoes) may invite ankle problems, especially with excessive lateral movements.

Supervision

In addition to the safety considerations already mentioned, clients must be closely monitored to ensure proper technique. Plyometric exercise is not intrinsically dangerous when performed correctly; but as with other forms of training, poor technique may unnecessarily predispose a client to injury. It is especially important for personal trainers to monitor client jumping and landing technique for lower extremity drills. In particular, personal trainers must instruct clients to avoid extremes of lateral knee motion (i.e., valgus and varus movements; see figure 17.2 on page 456) and to minimize time spent on the floor or ground. Knees should line up with the second and third toes while not passing ahead of them (anteriorly), and the amortization phase should be kept as short as possible. If the client deviates from these norms, drill intensity should be lowered to allow successful completion of each drill. Common technique errors are provided for each drill at the end of this chapter.

PLYOMETRIC PROGRAM DESIGN

Plyometric exercise prescription is similar to resistance and aerobic exercise prescriptions (36). After an evaluation of the client's needs, the mode, intensity, frequency, duration, recovery, progression, and a warm-up period must all be included in the design of a sound program. Unfortunately, there is little research demarcating optimal program variables for the design of plyometric exercise programs. Therefore, in addition to the available research, personal trainers must rely on the methodology used during the design of resistance and aerobic endurance training programs and on practical experience when prescribing plyometric exercise. When in doubt about volume, frequency, or intensity, it is best to err on the side of caution (50). The guidelines that follow are based in part on Chu's work (16, 17) and the NSCA's position statement (69).

Needs Analysis

As with other training modalities, when incorporating plyometric exercise into a training program the personal trainer must perform a needs analysis to evaluate a client's current abilities. Specifically, the personal trainer determines the client's needs and the requirements of the client's activities and lifestyle. A combination of the following factors helps in the analysis of a client's needs:

- *Age:* Does the client's age predispose the client to injury and therefore preclude plyometric training?
- *Training experience and current training level:* Has the client been resistance training? If so, what types of exercises has he or she been performing?

Has he or she participated in a plyometric training program? If so, when?

- *Injury history:* Is the client currently injured? Has he or she experienced an injury that might affect his or her ability to participate in a plyometric training program?
- *Physical testing results:* What are the client's abilities as they relate to muscular power production (e.g., vertical and standing long jump results)?
- *Training goals:* What does the client want to improve? A specific movement (e.g., throwing)? A particular skill (e.g., volleyball hitting)? An on-the-job activity (e.g., loading a truck)?
- *Incidence of injury in a client's job or chosen activity:* What is the risk of injury in the client's chosen activity? Is the activity relatively sedentary (e.g., student or office worker)? Does the activity require constant change of direction (e.g., racquetball player or construction worker)? If the activity is dynamic, is the client prepared for it physically?

Client example 17.1 illustrates one form of the plyometric needs analysis. Near the end of this discussion of program design are sample programs for each of these six clients, illustrating the "how" of program design.

Mode

The **mode** of plyometric training is determined by the general part or parts of the body that are performing the given exercise. For example, a depth jump is a lower body plyometric exercise, whereas a medicine ball chest pass is an upper body exercise.

Lower Body Plyometrics

Lower body plyometrics are appropriate for clients involved in virtually any sport—including soccer, volleyball, basketball, and baseball—as well as in nonathletic activities or occupations that require muscular power production or quick changes of direction. These types of activities require participants to produce a maximal amount of force in a minimal amount of time. Soccer and basketball require quick, powerful movements and changes of direction from competitors. A client who plays basketball is an example of one who would benefit greatly from a plyometric training program because basketball players must jump repeatedly for rebounds.

Needs Analysis for Plyometric Exercise

Sport Client A

A healthy 30-year-old male has been fairly active all of his life and has joined a YMCA basketball league. He is currently in a resistance training program and performed plyometrics two years ago. He is 6 feet (182.9 cm) tall, weighs 200 pounds (90.7 kg), and has a 16-inch (40.6 cm) vertical jump and a 180-pound (81.6 kg) 1RM squat. He wants to

1. increase his vertical jump to improve his ability to rebound the basketball and
2. run up and down the court faster as well as change directions quickly.

Sport Client B

A healthy, 28-year-old female fast-pitch softball player has played first base for the past five years but is transitioning to an outfield position. She trains with weights one or two times a week with a circuit weight training program for both the upper and lower body. She is 5 feet, 3 inches (160 cm) tall and weighs 125 pounds (56.7 kg). Her testing session reveals a 60-pound (27.2 kg) 1RM bench press and an 11-inch (27.9 cm) vertical jump. She requests help in improving her

1. ability to cover right field and
2. arm strength to help throw the ball to the infield.

Work Client A

A 35-year-old firefighter participates in a resistance training program five days a week with both upper and lower body exercises. He was in a plyometric training program six months ago. He is 6 feet, 2 inches (188 cm) tall and weighs 225 pounds (102.1 kg). He has a 5.3-second 40-yard (36.6 m) dash time, 225-pound (102.1 kg) squat, and 20-inch (50.8 cm) vertical jump. In addition to the necessary cardiovascular training, he has requested help in improving his

1. lifting ability and
2. speed while carrying the hose.

Work Client B

A 40-year-old female warehouse worker has had difficulty the past two months lifting boxes up and onto shelves at or above shoulder level. She has no complaints of pain and has been cleared by the company physician of any musculoskeletal dysfunction. She is 5 feet, 10 inches (177.8 cm) tall and weighs 150 pounds (68 kg). Her estimated 1RM bench press is 70 pounds (31.8 kg); estimated 1RM squat is 135 pounds (61.2 kg); and vertical jump is 13 inches (33 cm). She has never participated in a resistance training program. She has come to a personal trainer in the hope of improving her

1. arm strength, especially when pushing boxes onto a shelf, and
2. leg strength to assist her in lifting the heavier boxes.

Injury Prevention Client A

A healthy 14-year-old female soccer player is preparing to try out for her high school soccer team. She is 5 feet, 7 inches (170.2 cm) tall and weighs 110 pounds (49.9 kg). She has not performed 1RM testing, but her vertical jump is 12 inches (30.5 cm). Her parents are concerned she will get hurt because she is playing with much older girls. She has been involved in a general resistance training program for the past six months but has never participated in a plyometric training program. The parents have requested help for their daughter to

1. reduce her risk of injury and
2. "get in shape."

(continued)

CLIENT EXAMPLE 17.1 *(continued)*

Injury Prevention Client B

A 55-year-old female masters-level tennis player is returning to play following a yearlong layoff and is concerned about "losing a step" and injuring herself. She has not had any serious injuries. She is 5 feet, 6 inches (167.6 cm) tall and weighs 150 pounds (68 kg). Physical testing reveals an estimated 1RM squat of 140 pounds (63.5 kg), vertical jump of 10 inches (25.4 cm), and 40-yard (36.6 m) dash of 7.0 seconds. She has been resistance training for the past four months. She would like to

1. improve her speed when coming to the net and
2. reduce her risk of injury.

Lower body plyometric training allows the client's muscles to produce more force in a shorter amount of time, thereby allowing the person to jump higher. There are a wide variety of lower body plyometric drills with various intensity levels and directional movements. Descriptions of lower body plyometric drills are provided in table 17.3 and in general are listed from lower to higher intensities.

Upper Body Plyometrics

Rapid, powerful upper body movements are requisites of several sports and activities, including golf, baseball, softball, and tennis. As an example, a baseball pitcher routinely throws a baseball at 80 to 100 mph (129-161 km/h). To reach velocities of this magnitude, the pitcher's shoulder joint must move at over 6,000 degrees per second (28, 34, 37, 70). Plyometric

training of the shoulder joint would not only increase pitching velocity but may also prevent injury to the shoulder and elbow joints, although further research is needed to substantiate the role of plyometrics in injury prevention.

Plyometric drills for the upper body are not used as often as those for the lower body and have been studied less thoroughly. Nonetheless, they are essential for athletes requiring upper body power (68) and may help clients who need greater levels of upper body strength. Plyometrics for the upper body include medicine ball throws, catches, and push-up variations. With plyometric throws, the initial countermovement requires the individual to "cock" the arms, torso, or both—that is, move the arms slightly backward or rotate the torso away from the direction of the throw *before* the actual throw.

TABLE 17.3 Lower Body Plyometric Drills

Type of jump	Definition	Examples
Jump in place	Jumping and landing in the same spot, performed repeatedly, without rest between jumps	Squat jump, double-leg tuck jump, split squat jump
Standing jump	• Maximal-effort jumps involving either vertical or horizontal components • Recovery between repetitions required	Double-leg vertical jump, standing long jump, front barrier hop
Multiple hops and jumps	• Drills involving repeated movements • Commonly viewed as a combination of jumps in place and standing jumps	Double-leg hop, front barrier hop
Bounds	• Drills that involve exaggerated movements with greater horizontal speed than other drills • Volume for bounding typically measured by distance; normally greater than 98 ft (29.9 m)	Skip, alternate-leg bound—double arm, lateral bound
Box drill	• Multiple hops and jumps using a box to jump on or off • Height of the box dependent on the size of the client, the landing surface, and goals of the program	Jump to box, drop freeze
Depth jump	Drills in which the client assumes a position on a box, steps off, lands, and immediately jumps vertically, horizontally, or to another box	Depth jump, depth jump with standing long jump

Intensity

Plyometric **intensity** refers to the amount of effort exerted by the muscles, connective tissues, and joints during performance of an exercise and is controlled both by the type of drill and by the distance covered (e.g., height of a jump) (table 17.4) (14, 17, 33). The intensity of plyometric drills ranges from low-level skipping that places less stress on the joints to high-level depth jumps that apply significant stress to the agonist muscles and joints (table 17.4). Intensity should be determined by both the ability of the body to handle the load and the ability of the client to maintain proper technique while performing the exercise (14). If technique suffers, the personal trainer should drop the intensity until the client can perform the exercise while maintaining the proper technique.

Intensity should be kept at a low level for those just beginning a plyometric program. Double-leg jumps in place, double-leg standing jumps, and simple skips are appropriate for such clients. Youth and adolescent clients should begin with 1 or 2 sets of 6 to 8 repetitions to ensure quality repetitions in each set (32, 33). When in doubt, it is better to underestimate the physical ability of youth clients and have them do fewer repetitions. Rather than concentrating on advancing intensity, the personal trainer should focus on ensuring proper technique to prevent injury when the client is ready for more advanced drills. Intensity can be increased by raising the platform height for box jumps or depth jumps, increasing the distance of bounds, and incorporating more advanced exercises like those involving single-leg takeoffs—and for the very advanced client, adding light weights or weighted vests (table 17.5). If intensity is too high because of excessive loading during the eccentric phase, an increase in the amortization phase may result, negating the plyometric benefit of the exercise (14, 61).

Frequency

Frequency is the number of plyometric training sessions per week and depends on the client's age, ability, and goals (17). Often frequency and intensity are inversely proportional (14). Frequency increases as intensity decreases and vice versa. A low number of repetitions of low-intensity plyometric exercises can be performed multiple times per week. As for moderate-intensity plyometric training, research shows that training two times per week is best and results in improved jumping ability, jump contact times, maximal concentric and isometric strength, and 22-yard (20.1 m) sprint time at the greatest training efficiency (14, 25). For youth and adolescent clients, plyometric training may be performed up to two times per week on nonconsecutive days.

Recovery

Rather than concentrating on the frequency, many personal trainers rely more on the **recovery time** (the time between repetitions, sets, and workouts) of plyometric training sessions (17). Since plyometric drills often involve maximal efforts to improve anaerobic power, adequate recovery is required (14, 69, 88). The time between sets is determined by a proper work-to-rest ratio (i.e., a range of 1:5 to 1:10) (17, 30, 79) and is specific to the volume and type of drill being performed. That is, the higher the intensity of a drill, the more rest the client requires. For example, rest between sets of a plyometric skip will be shorter than the rest between sets of a depth jump (17). Recovery for depth jumps may range from 5 to 10 seconds of rest between single repetitions to 2 to 3 minutes between sets.

TABLE 17.4 Plyometric Exercises Listed by Intensity

Low intensity	Medium intensity	High intensity
Ankle flip	Double-leg hop	Cycled split squat jump
Skip	Alternate-leg bound—double arm	Single-leg vertical jump
Squat jump	Split squat jump	Single-leg hop
Standing long jump	Double-leg tuck jump	Depth jump
Double-leg vertical jump	Front barrier hop	Depth jump with standing long jump
Jump to box	Drop freeze	Lateral bound
Chest pass	Depth push-up	
Overhead throw	45-degree sit-up	
Side-to-side throw		

TABLE 17.5 Factors Affecting the Intensity of Lower Body Plyometric Drills

Factor	Effect
Points of contact	The ground reaction force is greater in single-leg lower body plyometric drills than during double-leg drills. More stress will be placed on the extremity's muscles, connective tissues, and joints when switching from double-leg to single-leg drills.
Speed	Increases in speed will increase the drill's intensity.
Height of the drill	Increases in the height of the body's center of gravity will increase the force upon landing.
Participant's weight	Athletes with higher body weight will experience more stress placed on muscles, connective tissues, and joints. Adding external weights (in the form of weight vests, ankle weights, and wrist weights) will increase the drill's intensity.

Shorter recovery periods between sets do not allow for maximum recovery and will thus attenuate the potential benefits as well as potentially heighten the risk of injury from compromised form. Plyometrics is an anaerobic activity designed specifically to improve neuromuscular reactions, explosiveness, quickness, and the ability to generate forces in certain directions (17, 74). Each plyometric repetition requires a maximal effort in order to be effective (79). Generally speaking, rest times of 60 to 120 seconds between drills should allow for full or nearly full recovery (75), and 48 to 72 hours between plyometric sessions is typically recommended (17, 79). Additionally, athletes or clients should not perform drills for a given body area on subsequent days (69). This is especially applicable to beginners, who should have at least 48 hours of rest time (17). Using these typical recovery times, most clients should perform one to three plyometric sessions per week.

Volume

Plyometric **volume** is the total work performed during a single workout session (14, 17) and is typically expressed as the number of repetitions and sets performed. Often plyometric volume is expressed as the number of contacts (each time a foot, the feet together, or a hand contacts the surface) per workout (14, 17), but it may also be expressed as distance, as with plyometric bounding. For example, a client beginning a plyometric training program may start with a double-arm bound for 33 yards (or 30 m) per repetition but advance to 109 yards (or 100 m) per repetition for the same drill (17). Lower body plyometric volumes vary for clients of different needs (i.e., client age and goals; resistance training and plyometric experience); suggested volumes are provided in table 17.6. Upper body plyometric volume is typically expressed as the number of throws or catches per workout. As for the

number of repetitions, it is suggested that sets be kept to 8 to 12 repetitions each, with fewer repetitions for exercises that are more intense and more repetitions for exercises that are less intense (75).

The entire plyometric exercise session for beginners should never exceed 30 minutes. Adequate warm-up and cooldown should be included. Advanced clients may do longer workouts that may require a longer recovery (17). The effectiveness of the plyometric workout should not be determined by the level of fatigue the client feels. Using fatigue as a guideline often results in overtraining, pain, and overuse injuries. It is the quality of the exercise, not the quantity, that produces the most increases in power (17, 79). The volume of the plyometric session must relate inversely to the intensity of the drill. If the level of the plyometrics is considered low to moderate, the total number of foot contacts can be higher. Volume should increase only if technique is maintained without any adverse effects such as pain (14).

Exercise Order

If plyometric exercises are being incorporated into a workout, they should be performed before any other exercise. In order to get maximum benefits, they must be done accurately. The client will benefit only from the number of reps performed well (17, 75). Also, previously fatigued muscles and tendons can become overstressed by the high demands placed on them during a plyometric workout if it is performed after other activities. This can lead to overtraining and injury (75).

The guidelines of mode, intensity, frequency, and volume can now be applied to the sample clients introduced in client example 17.1. See client example 17.2 for sample plyometric programs designed for these clients on page 465.

TABLE 17.6 General Plyometric Volume Guidelines Based on Age and Experience

Age	No resistance training experience	More than 3 months general resistance training experience	More than 3 months resistance training experience, including power exercises	More than 1 year general resistance training experience	More than 1 year resistance training experience, including power exercises	Resistance training but no plyometric training experience	Resistance training and plyometric training more than 1 year ago	Resistance training and plyometric training within past year
≤13	Nr	Nr	Nr	Nr	Nr	Nr	Nr	Nr
14-17	Nr	40-60	40-60	60-80	80-100	40-60	60-80	80-100
18-30	Nr	60-80	60-80	80-100	100-120	80-100	100-120	120-140
31-40	Nr	40-60	60-80	60-80	80-100	60-80	80-100	100-120
41-60	Nr	40-60	40-60	60-80	60-80	40-60	60-80	80-100

Volume is expressed as number of foot contacts (lower body plyometrics) or throws and catches (upper body plyometrics). The volumes included in this table should be modified according to individual client goals and abilities.

Nr = not recommended (i.e., no plyometric training for a client in this situation).

Progression

Plyometric exercise is a form of resistance training and thus must follow the principles of **progressive overload**—a systematic increase in training frequency, volume, and intensity through the use of various combinations. Plyometric progression should take place systematically, with learning and demonstrating proper landing position as the beginning point. Once proper landing technique is established, the personal trainer can advance clients by adding horizontal or vertical components and gradually move through the intensity levels (in an appropriate manner according to the client's training status and experience) with a vigilant focus on form. For example, clients should first begin with a low-intensity plyometric program, which could include such drills as skips, squat jumps, and standing long jump (17, 75). A client who is considered to be at an intermediate level, including high school clients who have been exposed to weight training, can perform moderately intense plyometric exercises such as split squat jumps or bounding. Once the client has matured, become proficient at moderately intense plyometric exercises, and has a strong resistance training background, high-intensity plyometrics including cycled split squat jumps, depth jumps, and exercises with external resistance and vertical or horizontal components may be incorporated into the training program

(17). Across the various types of drills, clients should start with double leg versions of lower body exercises and progress to single leg drills only after becoming fully adjusted to the stress of plyometric training.

Warm-Up

As with any training program, the plyometric exercise session must begin with general and specific warm-ups (refer to chapter 12 for discussion of warm-up). The general warm-up may consist of light jogging or using a stationary bicycle at low intensity, while a specific warm-up for plyometric training should consist of low-intensity dynamic movements similar in style to those performed during plyometric exercises. Refer to table 17.7 on page 464 for a description of dynamic warm-up drills that are generally appropriate for most clients.

> **Plyometric programs must include the many elements essential to effective training program design. After a needs analysis, the variables to be included in the program design are mode, intensity, frequency, recovery, volume, program length, progression, and warm-up.**

TABLE 17.7 Plyometric Warm-Up Drills

Dynamic warm-up drill	Description
Lunging	Performed to improve the client's readiness to move into a variety of positions
	May be performed in a variety of directions (e.g., forward, diagonal, backward)
Toe jogging	Jogging while not allowing the heels to touch the floor or ground
Straight-leg jogging	Jogging while maintaining an extended (or nearly extended) knee
Butt kicker	Jogging and allowing the heels to touch the buttocks through knee flexion
Skipping	Exaggerated mode of reciprocal upper and lower body movements
Footwork	A variety of drills that require changes in direction (e.g., shuffling, sliding, carioca, backward running)

Starting Levels for Plyometric Exercises

If the client is deemed ready for plyometric exercises, several tests can be performed to help determine the level at which the client should complete vertical jumps, depth jumps, box jumps, and the medicine ball toss (74, 75).

A vertical jump is performed with the client standing next to a wall with both feet flat on the floor or ground. The client fully reaches and touches the wall, the point that will be used as the baseline measurement. The client should jump off both feet and touch the wall at the highest point of the jump. The distance between the initial reach mark and the mark made at the highest point of the jump is the client's vertical jump height. The client should perform five trials, taking the best three jumps (74, 75). The result will be used in evaluating the height of the box used for the depth jump.

To perform a depth jump, the client steps off boxes of varying heights onto a firm or grass surface. Clients should begin with a 12-inch (30.5 cm) box. After stepping off the box and landing, the client immediately jumps up in an attempt to reach or surpass the mark placed on the wall during the vertical jump test. The height of the box should increase by 6 inches (15.2 cm) until the client can no longer jump to the vertical jump height. Rest between each jump should be about 1 to 2 minutes. The box height at which the max vertical jump height was attained is the height the client should train at for this exercise. If a client cannot reach the vertical jump height from the 12-inch box, either the height of the box should be decreased or the client should avoid depth jumps until he or she gets strong enough (17, 74, 75).

The personal trainer can use a box jump test to determine the maximum height of the box for box jump plyometric training. The client stands flat-footed directly in front of a box, about arm's length away. The client jumps up on the box and lands cleanly and softly. After each successful attempt, the height may be increased until the client finds it very difficult to jump onto the box. The greatest height at which the client can land successfully should be the height at which the client trains box jumps. Mats should be placed around the box, and trained spotters should be present to catch the client in an unsuccessful attempt (74).

To determine the weight of the medicine ball to use for chest passes, the personal trainer should have the client sit in a straight-back chair strapped in with a belt. The client performs a chest pass with a weighted medicine ball with as much force as possible. If the ball travels more than 12 feet (3.7 m), the client should try again with a heavier ball. If the ball travels less than 10 feet (3 m), the client should use a lighter medicine ball for medicine ball chest passes (74).

SPEED TRAINING MECHANICS AND PHYSIOLOGY

Most sports depend on the speed of execution; for example, regardless of whether a client is a sprinter, cross country runner, or swimmer, success depends on the ability to perform a given task in the shortest time possible. Speed training has been classically considered a modality for improving sport function. Indeed, many of the concepts discussed in this section are difficult to incorporate into personal training programs for those uninvolved in sport. For example, the appropriateness of training to improve speed in soccer and base running in baseball should seem obvious. Training to improve speed in a work setting is more challenging to envision and difficult to defend as an appropriate exercise mode for the personal trainer to choose. The paragraphs that follow, then, use primarily athletic settings and situations as examples. Some nonsporting applications, however, are provided as appropriate.

CLIENT EXAMPLE 17.2

Sample Plyometric Programs for Client Examples

Client	Mode	Intensity[a]	Frequency (sessions per week)[a]	Volume[a]	Activity-specific drills[b]
Sport client A	Lower body	Medium	2	100 contacts	Double-leg tuck jump Standing long jump Double-leg vertical jump Double-leg hop Jump to box Drop freeze
Sport client B	Lower and upper body	Low	1	60 contacts 20 throws for UB	Standing long jump Double-leg hop Skip Jump to box Chest pass
Work client A	Lower and upper body	Medium-high	2	100 contacts for LB 20 throws for UB	Split squat jump Standing long jump Double-leg vertical jump Single-leg jump Jump to box Chest pass Depth push-up
Work client B	Although this client would benefit from plyometrics eventually, because she has not previously participated in a resistance training program she must begin there and can progress to plyometric training after 3 months.				
Injury prevention client A	Lower body	Low	1	40 contacts	Split squat jump Double-leg vertical jump Skip
Injury prevention client B	Lower and upper body	Low to medium	1	40 contacts	Split squat jump Standing long jump Single-leg jump Lateral bound

[a]The values for these variables represent beginning levels; each will be advanced according to client tolerance and performance. (See client example 17.1 for descriptions of these clients.)

[b]The drills provided for each client are examples of exercises that are appropriate based on the client's background, goals, and experience. *Note:* The client is not expected to include all of the listed drills in the program.

Speed Training Definitions

The basis of **speed training**, accomplished in a variety of ways, is the application of maximal force in a minimal amount of time. This simply means that if clients are to move more quickly, they must *explode* when their feet are on the ground. **Speed-strength** is this application of maximum force at high velocities (84). People improve speed-strength in essentially the same way they improve muscular power production, by performing rapid movements both with and without resistance. Examples include weightlifting-type movements (e.g., power clean, hang clean, snatch) and plyometric exercise; each of these exercise modes is performed quickly to potentiate muscle force through the release of stored elastic energy and the stretch reflex. Therefore, to improve speed-strength, the exercise prescription should rely on powerful exercises and avoid those requiring slow movement (80).

Speed-endurance is the ability to maintain running speed over an extended duration (typically longer than 6 seconds) (29). The development of speed-endurance helps prevent a client from slowing down during a maximal-speed effort. Consider a soccer player caught from behind on a breakaway or a police officer on foot who is unable to keep up with a fleeing suspect. Each of these illustrates poor speed-endurance; that is, each person either slowed down or was unable to accelerate because of fatigue.

Sprinting Technique

Technique evaluation is an important tool to use when assessing movement efficiency and, ultimately, in training to improve speed. The basic techniques of running are presented in chapter 14; running for speed, or sprinting, although similar, is a considerably different form of training. Like running, sprinting is a somewhat natural activity, although it may be performed in a variety of ways. Because of this relative normalcy, technique training should initially focus on optimizing form and correcting faults (15); developing completely new movement patterns is typically unnecessary. The form and faults that characteristically need correction center on posture and action of the legs and arms. Maximizing sprinting speed, therefore, depends on a combination of optimal body posture, leg action, and arm action (figure 17.3, *a* and *b*) (27, 41, 49, 72, 78).

Posture

During the acceleration phase, the body should lean forward approximately 45 degrees for 13 to 16 yards (or 12 to 15 m). When one is looking at a client who is accelerating, the angle between the lower leg and the foot will be much greater than when he or she is running at maximum speed. After the 13 to 16 yards of acceleration, the client should quickly move upright to a less than 5-degree lean during maximal speed (with the lean coming from the ground up, not the waist up). With the body maintained in a relaxed, upright position, the head, torso, and legs should be aligned at all times. Although commonly viewed as a controlled fall (9), sprinting may be more accurately described as a series of ballistic strides in which the body becomes a projectile as it is propelled forward repeatedly. The head should be relaxed and show minimal movement, and eyes should be focused straight ahead.

Leg Action

Two main phases of the sprint technique are outlined in the literature: the driving phase and the recovery phase (19). During the **driving phase**, or support phase, the lead foot, driven by the hip extensors

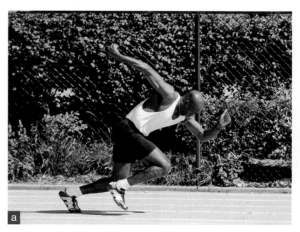
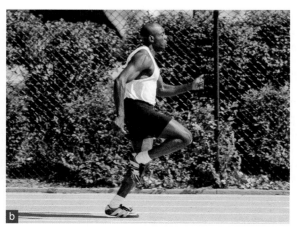

FIGURE 17.3   Proper sprinting technique. *(a)* At initial acceleration, the body should be leaning forward approximately 45 degrees and *(b)* should then quickly move upright to a less than 5-degree lean.

(gluteals), lands on the lateral aspect of the forefoot, just in front of the client's center of gravity. At footstrike, the quadriceps muscles must contract to prevent excessive knee flexion resulting in the loss of elastic energy. The ankle should remain dorsiflexed and the great toe extended. The gluteals and hamstrings should then contract so the client pulls himself or herself forward. The client should begin plantar flexing the foot once the hip crosses over the foot until the completion of toe-off. Ground contact time should be minimal while allowing explosive leg movement.

The **recovery phase** begins the moment the client's foot completely leaves the ground. As soon as the client enters the recovery phase of the sprint, he or she must immediately dorsiflex the ankle and extend the great toe. This places the leg in proper position so that, upon contact with the ground, the ground can push back against the body. The client can then use the ground's reactive force to propel forward. Leaving the foot on the ground too long causes the foot to absorb too much of the ground's force that would otherwise be used to help the client move more efficiently and effectively (71). He or she must also flex the knee, driving the foot directly toward the buttocks. This helps shorten the lever, which allows the leg to swing forward more quickly (19, 71). As the heel moves toward the buttocks, the leg swings forward as if the client is attempting to step over the opposite knee. The knee then extends to approximately a 90-degree position and then becomes nearly straight as the foot moves down and forward, driven toward the ground by the hip extensors. Increasing sprinting speed should increase the height the foot moves toward the buttocks (the heel kick).

Running heel-to-toe instead of landing on the lateral aspect of the forefoot is a common error. This causes balance issues as well as improper absorption of ground forces by the lower extremity structures, leading to hamstring injuries over time (19). Also, clients with poor flexibility may have trouble bringing the heel toward the buttocks.

Arm Action

Remaining relaxed, each elbow should be flexed to approximately 90 degrees (19, 71). Movement must be an aggressive front-to-back action originating from the shoulder with minimal frontal plane motion. The arm movement must be an aggressive backward hammering or punching motion and occur opposite to the leg motion in order to assist in balance and provide

momentum for the legs (19, 71). Also, if the client is aggressive with driving the arms back, the stretch reflex at the shoulder will activate and automatically force the arms forward. Hands should rise to shoulder level during the anterior arm swing and should pass the buttocks when moving posteriorly.

Common errors for arm swing include locking the upper arm into place and moving only the lower arm rather than having the action created at the shoulder; allowing the arm to cross the midline of the body; improper arm swing distance; and emphasizing a forward motion of the arm swing rather than a backward motion (19, 71). If a client allows the arm to cross the body's midline, upper body rotation will occur, slowing him or her down. As for the arm swing distance, clients tend to either bring the hand past the shoulders or not bring the hand back far enough, stopping short of their hips.

Acceleration

In general, it will take the client approximately 13 to 16 yards (12-15 m) of acceleration to achieve the proper technique (18). During these first yards, the client focuses on increasing both velocity and stride length. Initially, footstrike will occur behind the body, rather than in front of the center of gravity, but this changes quickly over the 13 to 16 yards. Also, the client will have increased body lean and be focused more on the driving phase and less on the recovery phase of the sprint technique (18, 19). This increased body lean positions the client so he or she can place stronger emphasis on front-side running mechanics (i.e., high knee punch, dorsiflexion) and minimal emphasis on back-side mechanics (i.e., plantar flexion, heel-to-hip contact).

> During a sprint, support time should be kept brief while braking forces at ground contact are minimized and the backward velocity of the lower leg and foot at touchdown is maximized. Maximizing sprinting speed depends on a combination of optimal body posture, leg action, and arm action.

Speed Training Program Design

As with plyometric exercise prescription, research on program design for speed training is sparse and therefore practical experience must be the guide. Speed training exercise prescription uses typical program design variables to provide a safe and effective plan to improve a client's speed.

Mode

The mode of speed training is determined by the speed characteristics that the given drill is designed to improve. Speed training focuses on three areas: form, stride frequency, and stride length. Improving sprinting technique may be accomplished in a number of ways, including sprint performance, stride analysis, and specific form drills. Drills designed to improve form are provided at the end of this chapter. Since form drills are performed at a slower speed, they should not substitute for actual sprint training. Form drills are great to include in the warm-up (19).

Within an analysis of running speed, stride frequency and stride length have an intimate relationship. In general, as both the **stride frequency** (the number of strides performed in a given amount of time) and **stride length** (the distance covered in one stride) increase, running speed improves. During the start, speed is highly dependent on stride length. Stride length drills help improve the rhythm of the sprinter's stride (20, 22). The personal trainer should first measure the client's leg length from the greater trochanter to the floor, then multiply this measurement 2.3 to 2.5 times for females and 2.5 to 2.7 times for males. This is the client's optimal stride length range. For example, if a male client has a leg length of 36 inches (91.4 cm), the client's optimal stride length range is 90 to 97.2 inches (228.6 to 246.9 cm). Drills should be performed anywhere from 60% to 105% of optimal stride length, but the personal trainer should mark the distances of the optimal stride length so the client has a foot placement target during the drill (20, 22). Using the 90-inch optimal stride length, 60% of 90 is 54 inches (137.2 cm), and 105% of 90 inches is 94.5 inches (240 cm). Therefore, stride length drills should use between 54 and 94.5 inches per stride.

As sprinting speed increases, frequency becomes the more important variable (62, 79, 92). Of the two components, stride frequency is likely the more trainable because stride length is highly dependent on body height and leg length (62, 64). Stride frequency is typically increased through the use of fast leg drills, **sprint-assisted training** (running at speeds greater than a client is able to independently achieve [(23)]), and resisted sprinting (20). With sprint-assisted training, the supramaximal speed forces clients to take more steps than they are accustomed to taking

during a typical sprint. Assuming that stride length remains the same as during normal sprinting, increasing the frequency of strides will help them run faster. Methods used to accomplish sprint-assisted training include downgrade sprinting (3-7 degrees), high-speed towing, and use of a high-speed treadmill. Regardless of the method used, sprint-assisted training should not increase speed by more than 10% of the client's maximal speed.

Sprint-assisted training is an advanced technique that requires careful instruction and demonstration on the part of the personal trainer and clear understanding on the part of the client. Sprint-assisted training may cause clients to alter their technique, which will affect running without assistance. Further, a proper warm-up to each session should be considered mandatory.

Resisted sprinting is used to help a client increase stride length, as well as speed-strength, by increasing the client's ground force production during the support phase (24, 27, 31, 41, 49), which is arguably the most important determinant of speed (80). Again, while maintaining proper form, clients may use uphill sprinting; running in sand or in water; or sprinting while being resisted by a sled, elastic tubing, a partner, or a parachute (20, 63). Resisted sprinting is used especially to improve the acceleration of the sprint (24). Resisted towing and uphill running are two exercises that work well to improve the acceleration of the sprint because they increase trunk lean, stance duration, and horizontal force production during the propulsive phase of the stance (24, 43). Resisted sprinting should not increase external resistance by more than 10% (48, 59). The personal trainer should use heavier resistance when the goal is to improve the acceleration phase and lighter resistance when the goal is to improve maximum velocity (24). Too much external resistance may negatively alter running mechanics (i.e., increase ground contact time, decrease stride length, or decrease hip extension), thereby compromising performance outcomes (20). Another measure for gauging the amount of resistance is to use an external load that is equal to or less than 15% of the client's body mass. The resistance level can also be assessed by looking at performance. If performance decreases by more than 10%, the load being used is too heavy and will have detrimental effects on sprinting technique. Resisted sprinting should be performed over relatively short distances, anywhere from 11 to 33 yards (or 10-30 m) (67).

As with most other speed training techniques, resisted sprinting targets clients who aspire to improve speed-strength. Adding resistance to a non-athletic client's gait, however, may also improve function. For example, attaching elastic tubing to provide resistance to a 70-year-old client during walking may improve his or her ability to walk up hills or may increase confidence during walking, thereby reducing the risk of injury from a possible fall. Providing resistance to a construction worker by having the individual push a weighted implement or sled may improve his or her ability to push a wheelbarrow filled with cement.

Although nearly all clients may perform form drills, sprint-assisted and -resisted training may be too advanced for some. A more general mode of speed training that most clients can easily perform is interval sprinting. The client sprints (or runs or walks, depending on abilities) as fast as possible over a given distance or for a predetermined amount of time, then rests. After the rest period, the client repeats the bout. In performing interval training, clients are able to maintain higher-intensity work periods (i.e., sprint/run/walk) by interspersing them with times of rest (35).

> When properly employed, assisted and resisted sprints may improve sprinting performance. Assisted sprints may be used if the goal of training is to increase stride frequency, whereas resisted sprints may be used when the goal is to increase stride length.

Intensity

Speed training intensity refers to the physical effort required during execution of a given drill and is controlled both by the type of drill performed and by the distance covered. The intensity of speed training ranges from low-level form drills to sprint-assisted and -resisted sprinting drills that apply significant stress to the body. Sprinting should be performed at close to maximum speed to ensure proper sprinting mechanics, stride length, and stride frequency (20). Distance is determined according to the goals of the client. Training acceleration requires covering short distances (less than 20 yards or meters), whereas training maximum velocity requires covering longer distances (greater than 20 yards or meters) (20).

Frequency

Frequency, the number of speed training sessions per week, depends on the client's goals. As with other program variables, research is limited on the optimal frequency for speed training sessions; again, personal trainers must rely on practical experience when determining the appropriate frequency. For clients who are athletes participating in a sport, two to four speed sessions per week is common; non-athletic clients may benefit from one or two speed sessions per week.

Recovery

Because speed training drills involve maximal efforts to improve speed and anaerobic power, adequate recovery (the time between repetitions and sets) is required to ensure maximal effort with each repetition (69, 88). The time between repetitions is determined by a proper work-to-rest ratio (i.e., a range of 1:5 to 1:10) and is specific to the volume and type of drill. That is, the higher the intensity of a drill, the more rest a client requires. Recovery for form training may be minimal, whereas rest between repetitions of downgrade running may last 2 to 3 minutes. Although near-full recovery is optimal for ensuring maximal effort with each repetition, having clients work on speed drills when they are less than 100% recovered may actually be beneficial as well, because it may be more specific to the type of tasks they will have to accomplish. However, consistently training for speed in a fatigued state will not yield optimal results (87). In fact, consistently training in a fatigued state may slow the client down, as this is teaching the client's body to run at slower speeds. It also interferes with body coordination, which results in training poor speed technique (19, 20). Recovery from sessions should last 24 to 48 hours depending on the intensity of the previous sprint training session.

Volume

Speed training volume typically refers to the number of repetitions and sets performed during a session and is normally expressed as the distance covered. For example, a client beginning a speed training program may start with a 33-yard (or 30 m) sprint but advance to 109 yards (or 100 m) per repetition for the same drill. As with intensity, speed training volume should vary according to the client's goals.

Progression

Speed training must follow the principles of progressive overload—a systematic increase in training frequency, volume, and intensity through various combinations. Typically, as intensity increases, volume decreases. The program's intensity should progress from

1. low to high volume of low-intensity speed drills (e.g., stationary arm swing) to
2. low to high volumes of moderate intensity (e.g., front barrier hop) to
3. low to high volumes of moderate to high intensity (e.g., downhill sprinting).

Warm-Up

As with any training program, the speed training session must begin with both general and specific warm-ups (refer to chapter 12 for a discussion of warm-up). The specific warm-up for speed training should consist of low-intensity dynamic movements. Once mastered, many of the form drills provided at the end of this chapter may be incorporated into warm-up drills.

SPEED TRAINING SAFETY CONSIDERATIONS

Although not inherently dangerous, speed training—like all modes of exercise—places the client at risk of injury. Injuries during speed training commonly occur because of insufficient strength or flexibility, inadequate instruction or supervision, or an inappropriate training environment.

Pretraining Evaluation

To reduce the risk of injury during participation in a speed training program, the client must understand proper technique and possess a sufficient base of strength and flexibility. In addition, the client must be sufficiently prepared to participate in a speed training program. The following evaluative elements will help determine whether a client meets these conditions.

Physical Characteristics

As with other forms of exercise, it is necessary to examine and review joint structure, posture, body type, and previous injuries before a client begins a speed training program. Previous injuries or abnormalities of the spine, lower extremities, and upper extremities may increase a client's risk of injury

during a speed training program. An area of concern is hamstring flexibility and strength; as the swing leg—the leg not on the training surface—transitions from an eccentric muscle action to concentric, the hamstring must be prepared to undergo extreme amounts of stretch (during the eccentric phase of the movement) followed by nearly instantaneous concentric muscle action. If this muscle is not prepared (through both strength and flexibility training), injury risk increases.

Technique and Supervision

When a client will be performing speed training drills, it is essential that the personal trainer demonstrate and monitor proper movement patterns and sprint technique—as previously described—to maximize the drill's effectiveness and to minimize the risk of injury. Proper technique will ensure efficient and faster running, whereas poor technique will not only slow the client down but also predispose him or her to injuries due to overloading of tissues (19). Posture and proper arm and leg actions are especially important characteristics for the personal trainer to watch. Should the client not demonstrate correct technique, intensity must be lowered to allow successful completion of each drill. Common technique errors are listed for each drill at the end of this chapter.

Exercise Surface and Footwear

In addition to proper participant fitness, health, and technique, the area where the client performs speed training drills may affect safety. To prevent injuries, the landing surface used for speed training drills must possess adequate shock-absorbing properties but must not be so absorbent as to significantly increase the transition between the eccentric and concentric phases of the SSC. Grass fields, suspended floors, and rubber mats are good surface choices (47). Avoid excessively thick exercise mats (6 inches [15.2 cm] or more) because they may lengthen the amortization phase, thus not allowing efficient use of the stretch reflex. In addition, footwear with good ankle and arch support and a wide, nonslip sole is required (69, 88).

COMBINING PLYOMETRICS AND SPEED TRAINING WITH OTHER FORMS OF EXERCISE

Plyometrics and speed training are just parts of a client's overall training program. Many sports and activities use multiple energy systems or require other forms of exercise to properly prepare athletes for their competitions or to help them reach their goals. A well-designed training program must address each energy system and training need.

Resistance, Plyometric, and Speed Training

Combining plyometric and speed training with resistance training requires careful consideration to optimize recovery while maximizing performance. The following list and table 17.8 provide appropriate guidelines for developing a program that combines these different, but complementary, modes of training:

- In general, clients should perform *either* lower body plyometric training, speed training, *or* lower body resistance training on a given day, but not more than one of these types of training on the same day.
- It is appropriate to combine lower body resistance training with upper body plyometrics, and upper body resistance training with lower body plyometrics.
- Performing heavy resistance training and plyometrics on the same day is not usually recommended (36). However, some athletes may benefit from **complex training**—a combination of resistance and plyometric training—by performing plyometrics followed by high-intensity resistance training. If an individual is engaging in this type of training, adequate recovery between the plyometrics and other high-intensity lower body training, including speed training, is essential.
- Traditional resistance training exercises may be combined with plyometric movements to further

enhance gains in muscular power (91). For example, performing a squat jump with approximately 30% of one's 1RM squat as an external resistance further increases performance (91). This is an advanced form of complex training that should be performed only by clients with previous participation in high-intensity plyometric training programs.

Plyometric and Aerobic Exercise

Many sports and activities require both a power and an aerobic component. It is necessary to combine multiple types of training to best prepare clients for these types of sports. Because aerobic exercise may have a negative effect on power production during a given training session (12), it is advisable to perform plyometric exercise before the longer, aerobic endurance–type training. The design variables do not change and should complement each other to most effectively train the athlete for competition or help a client meet his or her goals. Studies actually indicate that plyometrics may improve long-distance running performance and decrease incidence of injury (21, 81, 89); therefore adding low-intensity bounding-type drills to nonrunning days may improve long-distance running performance.

> Plyometric exercise should be incorporated into an overall training program, including both strength and aerobic exercise. Speed training may be combined with plyometric and resistance training, but this requires careful planning to optimize recovery while maximizing performance.

TABLE 17.8　Sample Schedule for Resistance, Plyometric, and Speed Training

Day	Resistance training	Plyometric training	Speed training
Monday	Upper body	Lower body	Rest
Tuesday	Lower body	Upper body	Rest
Wednesday	Rest	Rest	Technique and sprint-assisted drills
Thursday	Upper body	Lower body	Rest
Friday	Lower body	Upper body	Rest
Saturday	Rest	Rest	Technique and sprint-resisted drills
Sunday	Rest	Rest	Rest

CONCLUSION

The ability to apply force quickly and provide an overload to the agonist muscles is the major goal of plyometric training, a benefit to most sporting activities and many occupations. Further, because the ability to move rapidly is needed in sport, speed training may be another important component to include for clients active in competitive and recreational sports. The performance of each of these forms of exercise requires the proper application of force to the floor or ground in a minimal amount of time. If the force used is insufficient or takes too long to generate, the ability to effectively accelerate, change direction, or overtake an opponent is lost.

In addition to improving the potential to succeed in sport, speed and especially plyometric training may improve function on the job or may reduce the risk of injury. Many occupations require employees to lift or move large objects, move quickly, or otherwise perform explosive movements. Using the plyometric and speed training principles outlined is an ideal way to improve the speed-strength quality important to so many activities. In addition, the ability to decelerate efficiently and under control is indispensable to any attempt to reduce a client's risk of injury. Proper performance of plyometric drills helps clients learn how to decelerate when landing from a jump or when changing directions.

Plyometric training and speed training should not be considered ends unto themselves but rather as components of an overall program (in addition to resistance, flexibility, and aerobic endurance training and proper nutrition). Clients possessing adequate levels of strength perform plyometric and speed training drills more successfully. Further, combining these modes of exercise with others allows clients to optimize performance, regardless of sport or activity requirements.

Study Questions

1. Which of the following is *not* a component of the mechanical model of plyometric exercise?

    A. series elastic

    B. parallel

    C. contractile

    D. mechanical

2. Clients should be able to perform a 1-repetition maximum squat at 1.5 times their body weight before participating in any form of plyometric training.

    A. true

    B. false

3. Which of the following modifications *increases* the intensity of a plyometric drill?

    A. *decrease* the height of the drill

    B. *increase* the client's weight

    C. *increase* the client's points of contact with the ground

    D. *decrease* the speed of the drill

4. During the start, speed is most dependent on _____. At top speed, speed is most dependent on _____.

    A. stride length; stride length

    B. stride frequency; stride length

    C. stride length; stride frequency

    D. stride frequency; stride frequency

5. Which of the following is *incorrect* regarding combining plyometric exercise and aerobic exercise?

    A. Aerobic exercise may have a negative effect on power production.

    B. Plyometric training should be performed *after* aerobic training.

    C. Adding low-intensity bounding-type drills to non-running days may improve long-distance running performance.

    D. Many sports and activities require both a power and an aerobic component.

Plyometric and Speed Drills

LOWER BODY PLYOMETRIC DRILLS

ANKLE FLIP

Intensity level: Low

Direction of jump: Vertical

Beginning position: Stand with feet shoulder-width apart. Body should be upright.

Arm action: None

Preparatory movement: None

Upward movement: Pushing off using only ankles, hop up in place, plantar flexing ankles fully with each jump.

Downward movement: Land in starting position. Repeat the motion.

Common Errors

- Clients add a countermovement.
- Clients do not fully plantar flex ankles.
- Clients jump and land asynchronously; that is, feet neither leave nor contact the floor or ground at the same time.

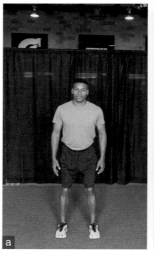
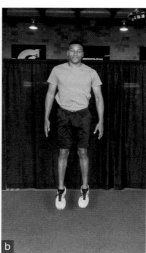

SQUAT JUMP

Intensity level: Low

Direction of jump: Vertical

Beginning position: Descend into a squatting position (thighs are slightly above parallel with the floor or ground), with feet shoulder-width apart. Hands should be placed behind the head, with fingers interlocked.

Arm action: None

Preparatory movement: None

Upward movement: Jump upward explosively to a maximal height.

Downward movement: Land in the squat position and immediately repeat the jump.

Common Error

Clients descend slightly before the upward movement. There should be no countermovement after getting set in the squat position.

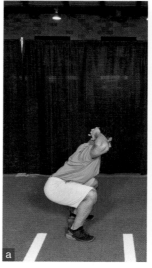
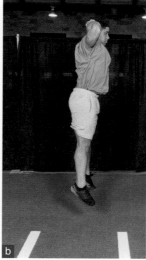

STANDING LONG JUMP

Intensity level: Low

Direction of jump: Horizontal

Beginning position: Assume a comfortable upright stance, with feet shoulder-width apart.

Arm action: Double arm

Preparatory movement: Begin with a countermovement.

Upward movement: Explosively jump forward and up, using arms to assist with jumping to a maximal horizontal distance.

Downward movement: Land in the starting position and repeat jump. Allow complete rest between repetitions.

Advanced variation: Progress to multiple jumps without a pause between jumps. Immediately, upon landing, jump forward again. Keep landing time short. Use quick double-arm swings when performing repetitions. This changes the intensity to medium.

Common Error

Clients jump and land asynchronously; that is, feet neither leave nor contact the floor or ground at the same time.

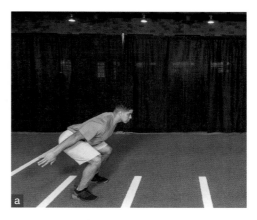

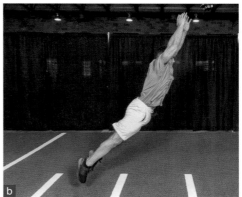

DOUBLE-LEG VERTICAL JUMP

Intensity level: Low

Direction of jump: Vertical

Beginning position: Assume a comfortable upright stance, with feet shoulder-width apart.

Arm action: Double arm

Preparatory movement: Begin with a countermovement.

Upward movement: Explosively jump up with both legs, using both arms to assist and reach for a target.

Downward movement: Land in the starting position and repeat the jump. Allow complete recovery between jumps.

Advanced variation: Increase the intensity of the double-leg vertical jump by performing it without a rest between jumps. Immediately upon landing, begin the jump again. Ground contact time between jumps should be minimal. This changes the intensity to medium. One can further progress the jump using one leg only. This changes the drill's intensity to high.

Common Errors

- Clients do not jump and land in the same place.
- Countermovement is too deep.
- Countermovement is too shallow.

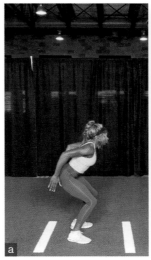

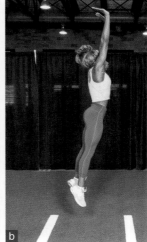

DOUBLE-LEG HOP

Intensity level: Medium

Direction of jump: Horizontal and vertical

Beginning position: Assume a comfortable upright stance, with feet shoulder-width apart, knees slightly bent, and arms at side.

Arm action: Double arm

Preparatory movement: Begin with a countermovement.

Upward movement: Jump as far forward as possible.

Downward movement: Land in the beginning position and immediately repeat the hop.

Advanced variation: Progress to perform the hop with one leg only. This changes the drill's intensity from medium to high.

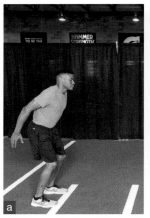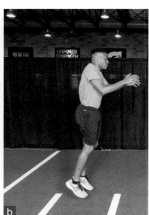

Common Errors

- Amortization phase (i.e., time on the floor or ground) between hops is too long.
- Clients do not maintain proper posture.

SPLIT SQUAT JUMP

Intensity level: Medium

Direction of jump: Vertical

Beginning position: Assume a lunge position with one leg forward (hip and knee joints in approximately 90 degrees of flexion, with knee directly over foot) and the other behind the midline of the body.

Arm action: Double or none

Preparatory movement: Begin with a countermovement.

Upward movement: Explosively jump up, using the arms to assist as needed. Maximum height and power should be emphasized.

Downward movement: When landing, maintain the lunge position (same leg forward) and immediately repeat the jump. After completing a set, rest and switch front legs.

Advanced variation: While off the floor or ground, switch the position of the legs so the front leg is in the back and the back leg is in the front. When landing, maintain the lunge position (opposite leg forward) and immediately repeat the jump. This changes the drill's intensity from medium to high.

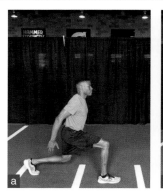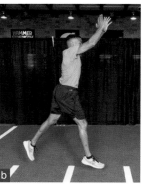

Common Errors

- The lunge position is too shallow.
- Amortization phase (i.e., time on the floor or ground) is too long.
- Clients do not jump and land in the same place; lateral and anterior or posterior movement are excessive.
- Clients' shoulders do not remain back and in line with the hips, leading to decreased stability.

DOUBLE-LEG TUCK JUMP

Intensity level: Medium

Direction of jump: Vertical

Beginning position: Assume a comfortable upright stance, with feet shoulder-width apart.

Arm action: Double arm

Preparatory movement: Begin with a quick counter-movement.

Upward movement: Explosively jump up, driving the knees to the chest. Pull the knees to the chest and quickly grasp the knees with both hands and release before landing.

Downward movement: Land in the starting position and immediately repeat the jump. Ground contact time between jumps should be minimal.

Advanced variation: Progress from pausing in between each jump to multiple jumps without a pause in between jumps to jumps with one leg only (high intensity).

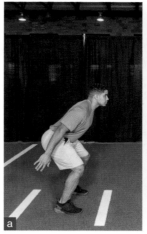
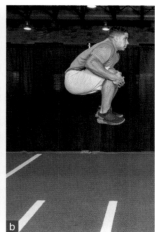

Common Errors

- Amortization phase (i.e., time on the floor or ground) is too long.
- Clients do not jump and land in the same place; there is excessive lateral and anterior or posterior movement.

CYCLED SPLIT SQUAT JUMP

Intensity level: High

Direction of jump: Vertical

Beginning position: Step forward with one leg into a lunge position (hip and knee joints flexed to approximately 90 degrees) and the other leg behind the midline of the body.

Arm action: Double arm or none

Preparatory movement: Begin with a countermovement.

Upward movement: Jump upward explosively, assisting with the arms as needed, emphasizing maximal height and power. Switch leg positions while in the air.

Downward movement: Maintain the lunge position upon landing, but the legs should have switched positions. Immediately repeat the jump.

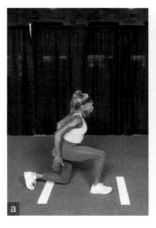
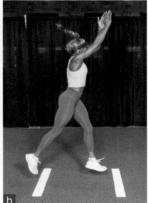

Common Error

Clients lunge too deeply. The stretch-shortening cycle may not effectively contribute to subsequent jumps.

SINGLE-LEG VERTICAL JUMP

Intensity level: High

Direction of jump: Vertical

Beginning position: Assume a comfortable upright stance while standing on one foot. Hold the nonjumping leg in a stationary position, with the knee flexed.

Arm action: Double arm

Preparatory movement: Begin with a countermovement.

Upward movement: Jump upward explosively, assisting with the arms as needed, emphasizing maximum height while reaching for a target.

Downward movement: Land in the beginning position and repeat jumps using the same leg. Allow for recovery between jumps. Repeat with the opposite leg after a short rest.

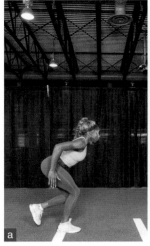 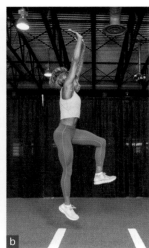

Common Errors

- Clients do not jump and land in the same place.
- Countermovement is too shallow.

SINGLE-LEG HOP

Intensity level: High

Direction of jump: Horizontal and vertical

Beginning position: Assume a comfortable upright stance while standing on one foot. Hold the nonjumping leg in a stationary position, with the knee flexed.

Arm action: Double arm

Preparatory movement: Begin with a countermovement.

Upward movement: Jump forward explosively, assisting with the arms as needed.

Downward movement: Land in the beginning position and repeat jumps using the same leg. Repeat with the opposite leg after a short rest.

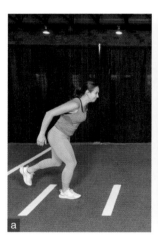 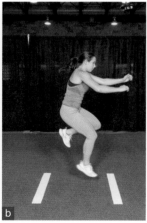

Common Errors

- Clients do not jump and land in the same place.
- Amortization phase (i.e., time on the floor or ground) between hops is too long.
- Clients do not maintain proper posture.

SKIP

Intensity level: Low

Direction of jump: Horizontal and vertical

Beginning position: One leg is lifted to 90 degrees of hip and knee flexion.

Arm action: Reciprocal (as one leg is lifted, the opposite arm is lifted)

Preparatory movement: Begin with a countermovement.

Upward movement: Jump up and forward on one leg. The opposite leg should remain in the starting position until landing. Drive the toes of the lead leg up, knee forward and up, and keep the heel under the hips.

Downward movement: Land in the starting position with the same leg. Repeat the motion with the opposite leg.

Advanced variation: This drill may also be performed backward. Jump up and backward on one leg. Land in the starting position with the same leg. Repeat the motion with the opposite leg.

Common Error

Movements are not coordinated (i.e., clients have difficulty coordinating the transition from one leg to the other).

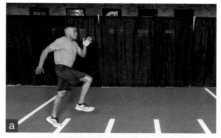
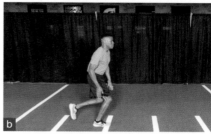
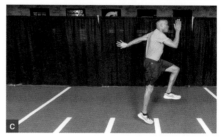

ALTERNATE-LEG BOUND—DOUBLE ARM

Intensity level: Medium

Direction of jump: Horizontal and vertical

Beginning position: Assume a comfortable upright stance, with feet shoulder-width apart.

Arm action: Double arm

Preparatory movement: Jog at a comfortable pace; begin the drill with the right foot forward.

Upward movement: Push off with the right foot as it contacts the floor or ground. During push-off, bring the left leg forward by flexing the thigh to a position parallel with the floor or ground and the knee at 90 degrees. During the flight phase of the drill, the arms will reach forward then move back in preparation for the left foot to contact the floor or ground.

Downward movement: Land on the left leg and immediately repeat the sequence with the opposite leg upon landing. A bound is an exaggeration of the running gait; the goal is to cover as great a distance as possible during each stride.

Alternate variation: Instead of reaching forward with both arms during the flight phase, reach with a single arm while the opposite leg is in the flight phase.

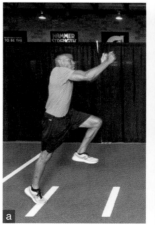
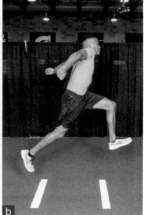

Common Error

Clients do not have appropriate balance between the horizontal and vertical components of the bound.

LATERAL BOUND

Intensity level: High

Direction of jump: Lateral

Beginning position: Stand on one leg (this becomes the stance leg).

Arm action: Double arm

Preparatory movement: Begin with a countermovement.

Upward movement: Begin by driving the nonstance leg and upper extremities toward the stance leg. Then, push off the stance leg and drive the upper extremities to laterally jump as far as possible away from the beginning position of the stance leg in the frontal plane.

Downward movement: Land on the foot of the nonstance leg (now that leg becomes the stance leg). Immediately upon landing, jump back in the opposite direction to land on the foot of the original stance leg. Repeat, with minimal rest time between bounds.

Common Errors

- Amortization phase (i.e., time on the floor or ground) is too long.
- Clients jump ahead or behind the frontal plane.
- Landing is unbalanced.

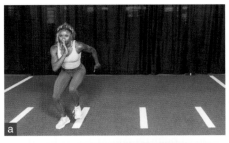

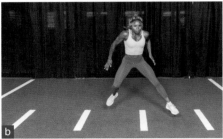

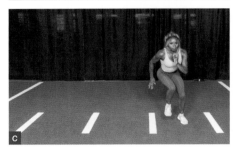

JUMP TO BOX

Intensity level: Low

Equipment: Plyometric box, 6 to 42 inches (15.2-106.7 cm) high

Direction of jump: Vertical and slightly horizontal

Beginning position: Facing the plyometric box, assume a comfortable upright stance, with feet shoulder-width apart.

Arm action: Double arm

Preparatory movement: Begin with a countermovement.

Upward movement: Jump onto the top of the box using both feet.

Downward movement: Land on both feet in a semi-squat position; step down from the box and repeat.

Advanced variation: Increase the intensity of this jump by clasping the hands behind the head or increasing the box height (initial height should be set at 6 inches [15.2 cm]).

Common Errors

- Clients' knees and feet separate in an effort to clear the front edge of the box.
- Countermovement is too deep.
- Box is too tall for client's height or abilities.

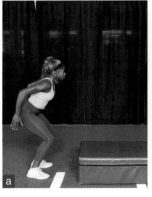

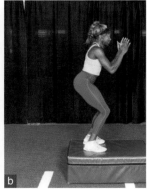

FRONT BARRIER HOP

Intensity level: Medium

Direction of jump: Horizontal and vertical

Equipment: Two or more barriers such as cones or hurdles (a second barrier ahead of the client is not seen in the photos)

Beginning position: Assume a comfortable upright stance facing the first barrier, with feet shoulder-width apart.

Arm action: Double arm

Preparatory movement: Begin with a countermovement.

Upward movement: Jump over the first barrier with both legs, using primarily hip and knee flexion to clear the barrier. Keep the knees and feet together without lateral deviation.

Downward movement: Land in the starting position and immediately repeat the jump over the next barrier.

Alternate variation: This drill may also be performed laterally. Stand to either side of the barrier; jump over the barrier with both legs. Land in the starting position and immediately repeat the jump to the starting side.

Advanced variation: To increase the intensity of barrier hops, progressively increase the height of the barrier

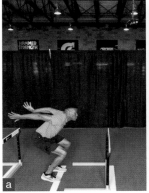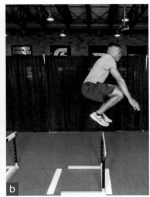

(e.g., from a cone to a hurdle) or perform the hops with one leg only. This changes the drill's intensity from medium to high.

Common Errors

- Amortization phase (i.e., time on the floor or ground) between hops is too long.
- Clients' knees and feet separate in an effort to clear the barrier.

DROP FREEZE

Intensity level: Medium

Equipment: Plyometric box, 12 to 42 inches (30.5-106.7 cm) high

Direction of jump: Vertical

Beginning position: Assume a comfortable upright stance, with feet shoulder-width apart on the box.

Arm action: None

Preparatory movement: Step from box.

Downward movement: Land on the floor or ground in a partially-squatted position, with both legs quickly absorbing the impact upon touchdown.

Common Errors

- Clients land asynchronously; that is, feet do not contact the floor or ground at the same time.
- Box is too tall for client's height or abilities.
- Clients jump off the box instead of stepping off the edge of the box.

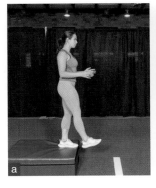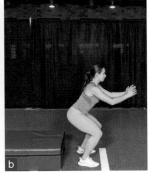

DEPTH JUMP

Intensity level: High (vary the intensity by increasing the height of the box)

Equipment: Plyometric box, 12 to 42 inches (30.5-106.7 cm) high

Direction of jump: Vertical

Beginning position: Assume a comfortable upright stance, with feet shoulder-width apart on the box; toes should be near the edge of the box.

Arm action: Double arm

Preparatory movement: Step from box. When stepping from the box, step straight out. Do not first jump up or lower your center of gravity while stepping down because these adjustments will change the initial height from which the exercise is performed.

Downward movement: Land on the floor or ground with both feet.

Upward movement: Upon landing, immediately jump up as high as possible, emphasizing a vertical jump with minimal horizontal movement.

Common Errors

- Amortization phase (i.e., time on the floor or ground) is too long.
- Clients do not jump and land in the same place; there is excessive lateral and anterior–posterior movement after landing.
- Box is too tall for client's height or abilities.

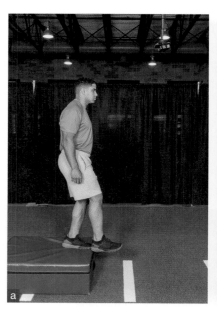
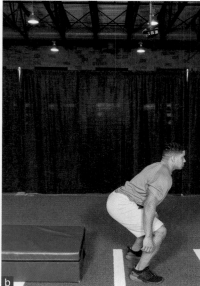
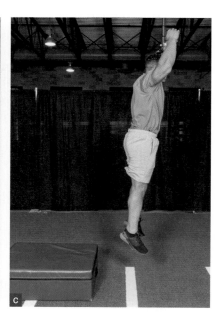

DEPTH JUMP WITH STANDING LONG JUMP

Intensity level: High (vary the intensity by increasing the height of the box)

Equipment: Plyometric box, 12 to 42 inches (30.5-106.7 cm) high

Direction: Vertical and horizontal

Beginning position: Assume a comfortable upright stance, with feet shoulder-width apart on the box; toes should be near the edge of the box.

Arm action: Double arm

Preparatory movement: Step from box.

Downward movement: Land on the floor or ground both feet. Time on the floor or ground should be kept to a minimum.

Upward movement: Upon landing, immediately jump forward as far as possible.

Common Errors

- Clients jump up slightly when stepping off the box, thus changing the height from which the exercise is performed.
- Clients lower their center of gravity before stepping off the box, thus changing the height from which the exercise is performed.

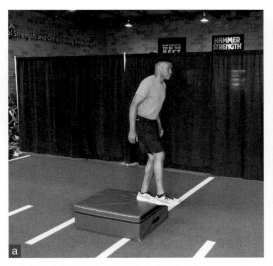
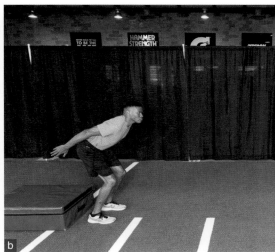
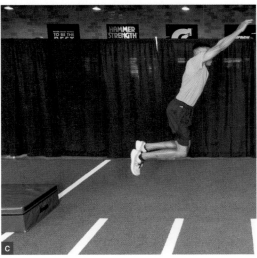
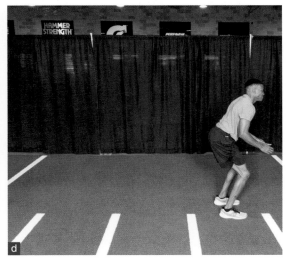

UPPER BODY PLYOMETRIC DRILLS

CHEST PASS

Intensity level: Low (begin with a relatively light medicine ball, and increase intensity by increasing the weight of the ball)

Equipment: Medicine or plyometric ball; partner

Direction of throw: Forward

Beginning position: Assume a comfortable upright stance, with feet shoulder-width apart; face the personal trainer or a partner approximately 10 feet (3 m) away. Raise the ball to chest level with elbows flexed.

Preparatory movement: Begin with a countermovement.

Arm action: Using both arms, throw (or push) the ball to the partner by extending the elbows. When the partner returns the ball, catch it, return to the beginning position, and immediately repeat the movement.

Common Errors

- Amortization phase (i.e., time ball is in hands) is too long.
- Ball is too heavy.

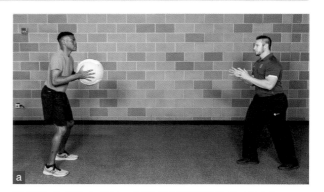

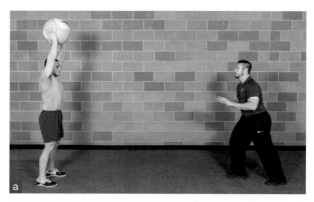

OVERHEAD THROW

Intensity level: Low (begin with a relatively light medicine ball, and increase intensity by increasing the weight of the ball)

Equipment: Medicine or plyometric ball; rebounder or partner

Direction of movement: Forward and down

Beginning position: Assume a comfortable upright stance, with feet shoulder-width apart, facing a rebounder or partner approximately 10 feet (3 m) away. Raise the ball overhead with both arms.

Preparatory movement: Begin with a countermovement.

Arm action: Using both arms, throw the ball toward the rebounder or partner, extending the elbows. When the rebounder or partner returns the ball, catch it over-head and immediately proceed to the next throw. For a downward movement, partners can bounce the ball on the surface between them and catch it on the rebound.

Common Errors

- Amortization phase (i.e., time ball is in hands) is too long.
- Ball is too heavy.

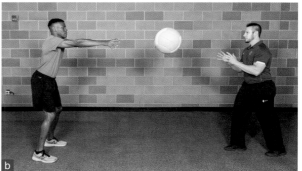

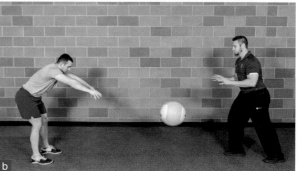

SIDE-TO-SIDE THROW

Intensity level: Low (begin with a relatively light medicine ball, and increase intensity by increasing the weight of the ball)

Equipment: Medicine or plyometric ball; rebounder or partner

Direction of movement: Forward (after rotation)

Beginning position: Assume a comfortable upright stance, with feet shoulder-width apart and knees moderately flexed, facing a rebounder or partner approximately 10 feet (3 m) away. Hold the ball in front of the torso, with both arms flexing at the elbows.

Preparatory movement: Begin with a countermovement.

Arm action: Using both arms, throw the ball toward the rebounder or partner, extending the elbows. When the rebounder or partner returns the ball, catch it and immediately proceed to the next throw.

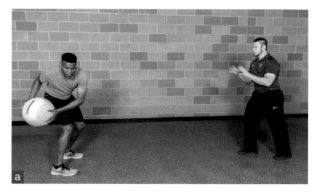

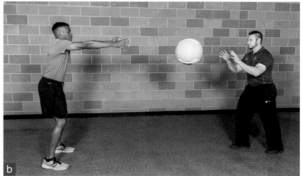

Common Errors

- Amortization phase (i.e., time ball is in hands) is too long.
- Ball is too heavy.

DEPTH PUSH-UP

Intensity level: Medium (increase intensity by increasing the size [diameter] of the medicine ball)

Equipment: Medicine ball 6 to 12 inches (15.2-30.5 cm) in diameter. The medicine ball should be selected based on its height and the size of the client. Initially, the ball height should be selected so that the client's chest nearly contacts the ball in the fully descended position.

Direction of movement: Vertical

Beginning position: Lie in a push-up position, with the hands on the medicine ball and elbows extended.

Preparatory movement: None

Downward movement: Quickly remove the hands from the medicine ball and drop down. Contact the floor or ground with the hands slightly more than shoulder-width apart and the elbows slightly flexed. Allow the chest to almost touch the medicine ball.

Upward movement: Immediately and explosively push up by extending the elbows to full extension. When the upper body is at maximal height during the upward movement, the hands should be higher than the medicine ball (not shown). Quickly place the palms on the medicine ball and repeat the exercise.

Advanced variation: To increase the intensity of this drill, perform it as described with the feet placed on an elevated surface (e.g., a plyometric box).

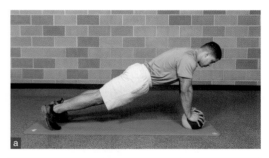

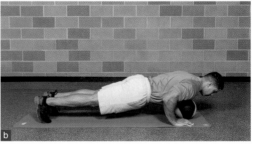

Common Errors

- Amortization phase (i.e., time hands are on the floor or ground) is too long.
- Ball is too big, increasing the distance from the beginning position to the bottom of the downward movement.

45-DEGREE SIT-UP

Intensity level: Medium (begin with a relatively light medicine ball, and increase the intensity by increasing the weight of the ball)

Equipment: Medicine or plyometric ball; partner

Beginning position: Sit with the trunk at approximately a 45-degree angle to the floor or ground. The personal trainer or partner should be standing in front with the medicine ball.

Preparatory movement: The partner throws the ball to outstretched hands.

Downward action: Once the partner throws the ball, catch it using both hands, allow some trunk extension (not seen in photo b), and immediately return the ball to the partner. The force used to return the ball to the partner should be predominantly derived from the abdominal muscles.

Common Errors

- Eccentric phase (i.e., amount of trunk extension) is too long.
- Ball is too heavy.

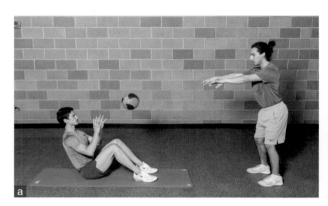
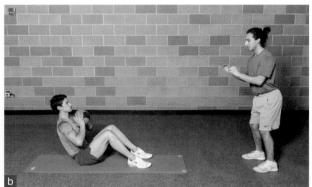
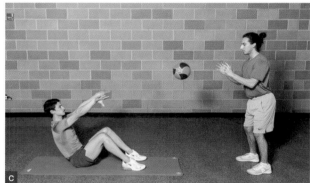

STRIDE FREQUENCY SPEED DRILLS

STATIONARY ARM SWING

Intensity level: Low

Purpose: Teaches proper arm swing technique and upper body control

Beginning position: Initial position is seated, progressing to kneeling, standing (as seen in the photo), walking, and finally jogging. Elbows should be at about 90 degrees of flexion, with the left hand next to the left hip and the right hand in front of the right shoulder. (Note that the client's left elbow in the photo should be flexed closer to 90 degrees.)

Movement: Maintaining the elbows at approximately 90 degrees and keeping the hands relaxed, drive the arms forward and back at the shoulder in a sprinting-type motion. The hands' arc of motion should be from shoulder level anteriorly to just past the hips posteriorly.

Advanced variation: Progression moves from seated to kneeling to standing to walking and finally to jogging. Each progression appropriately challenges the ability to stabilize the core and control the body, which leads to good form when jogging.

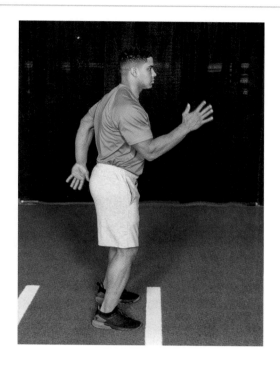

Common Errors

- Arms cross the line of the body; arm swing should be maintained in the sagittal plane.
- Arm motion does not originate from the shoulder.
- Arm swing either goes too high past the shoulder or not back far enough to the hips.
- Arm swing is often not forceful enough; be sure to maintain an aggressive hammering or punching motion.

ANKLING

Intensity level: Low

Purpose: Teaches how to lift the feet off the ground and how to properly place them back on the ground during sprinting. Proper position of the foot will minimize the amount of time spent on the ground, minimize power lost into the ground, and minimize injuries due to the additional stress absorbed by the body with the increased ground time.

Beginning position: Start in a neutral, upright position, with feet hip-width apart. Focus on one leg at a time. Keep the legs stiff.

Movement: Move forward until the hips have passed over the feet. As soon as the right heel begins to lift off the ground, dorsiflex the ankle approximately 90 degrees and extend the great toe, picking the foot up off the ground. The leg should move forward slightly (approximately one-quarter the length of the foot), with this movement initiated from the hips. As this is occurring, quickly plantar flex the right foot and make contact with the ground with the lateral forefoot and ball of the foot, pulling the body over the foot. Immediately repeat this action. Make sure the legs remain stiff throughout the drill. Focus on the movement at the ankle as well as getting the foot off the ground as quickly as possible. Repeat this dorsiflexion–plantar flexion action with just the right foot over the course of 30 feet (9.1 m), making as many foot contacts with the ground as possible. Steps should be no greater than one-quarter of foot length. Switch legs.

Advanced variations: Alternating feet while walking; straight-leg bounding while ankling, focusing on one leg at a time; straight-leg bounding while ankling, alternating legs; running while ankling, alternating legs.

Common Errors

- Clients have difficulty getting to 90-degree dorsiflexion with great toe extension and maintaining that position until foot contact.
- Clients are running on the toes rather than landing on the forefoot and having the foot pull the body's center of gravity.
- Legs are not staying stiff.
- Steps are greater than one-quarter the length of the foot.
- Ball of foot is spending too much time on the ground between each contact.

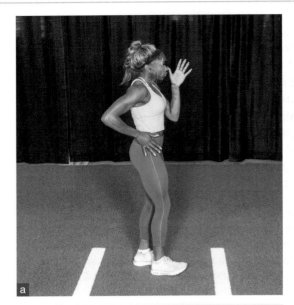

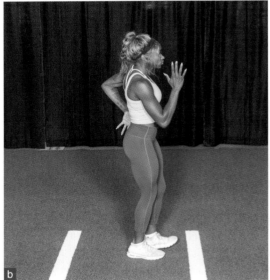

BUTT KICKER

Intensity level: Low

Purpose: Builds on the ankling drill. Teaches to bring the heel to the buttocks immediately after plantar flexion of the ankle during the sprinting motion.

Beginning position: Assume a comfortable, upright stance, with feet shoulder-width apart. Begin to jog.

Movement: Pull the heel toward the buttocks, contracting the hamstrings to swing the lower leg back. Allow the heel to "bounce" off the buttocks.

Advanced variation: Imagine a wall right behind you. Perform a butt kicker, but instead of having the heel drive posterior to the hips, bring the heel up along the imaginary wall to reach the buttocks, forcing the heel of the recovery leg to stay anterior to the buttocks. This variation improves knee lift during the flight phase of sprinting. This shortens the lever so the mass of the leg is closer to the axis of rotation, allowing the leg to be cycled forward more quickly during sprinting.

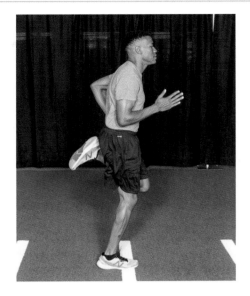

Common Errors

- Clients are forcing the heel toward the buttocks instead of allowing the heel to elevate toward the buttocks.

- There is excessive thigh motion; the thigh should not move too much—concentrate on moving at the knee versus the hip joint.

HIGH KNEE DRILL

Intensity level: Low to moderate

Purpose: Trains hip flexors and reinforces foot positioning taught during ankling drill; reinforces front-side mechanics while reinforcing dorsiflexion and conditioning the hip flexors.

Beginning position: Assume a comfortable, upright stance, with feet shoulder-width apart. Begin to walk, focusing on one leg at a time.

Movement: Plantar flex the right ankle as the hips move over the right foot. As soon as the right heel lifts off the ground, immediately dorsiflex the right ankle and extend the great toe of the right foot as in the ankling drill. At the same time, flex the right hip and knee until the right thigh is parallel to the ground. Then, keeping the ankle dorsiflexed and toe extended, drive the right foot back into the ground by extending the right hip and knee, placing the lateral aspect of the right forefoot slightly in front of the hips.

Advanced variations: Walking, focusing on one leg at a time, no arm swing; repeat, adding arm swing; walking, alternating legs, no arm swing; repeat, adding arm swing; skipping, focusing on one leg, no arm swing; repeat, adding arm swing; skipping, alternating legs, no arm swing; repeat, adding arm swing; running, alternating legs, no arm swing; repeat, adding arm swing

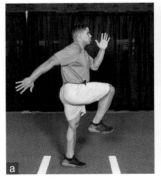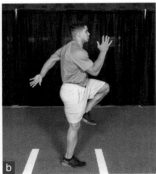

Common Errors

- Inability to stand tall during this drill because of weak hip flexors and core; trunk will flex as the hip flexes.
- Inability to keep the ankle dorsiflexed and great toe extended when flexing the hip.

FAST LEG DRILL

Intensity level: High

Purpose: Move lower extremities at a faster speed than during normal running

Beginning position: Perform at a walk, beginning with the right foot.

Movement: After the third step, perform a fast sequence of the following motions: bring the heel to the hip with the ankle dorsiflexed and great toe extended as in the butt kicker; bring the right knee forward as if stepping over the opposite foot; flex the hip so that the thigh is parallel to the ground (more than what is seen in the middle photo), then unfold the leg and drive the foot to the ground as in the high knee drill. Repeat every third step.

Advanced variations: Ankling for three steps, then fast leg motion for one step, focusing on one leg at a time; ankling for three steps, then fast leg motion for one step, alternating legs; ankling for two steps, then fast leg motion for one step, alternating legs; straight-leg bounding for three steps, then fast leg for one step, focusing on one leg at a time; straight-leg bounding for two steps, then fast leg for one step, alternating legs; straight-leg bounding for one step, then fast leg for one step, focusing on one leg at a time; continuous fast leg for distance.

Common Errors

- Ankles are not dorsiflexed enough.
- Hips are not flexed enough; thigh does not become parallel to the ground, and the movement is cut short.

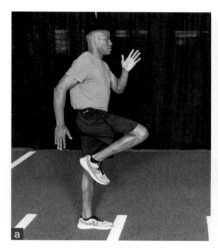 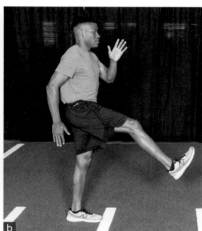 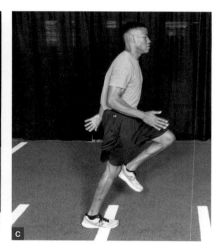

UPHILL SPRINT

Intensity level: High

Equipment: A 3- to 7-degree uphill sprinting surface

Beginning position: At the bottom of the downhill area, assume a comfortable, upright stance, with feet shoulder-width apart.

Movement: Maintaining correct posture and technique, sprint 33 to 55 yards (30.2-50.3 m) uphill.

Common Errors

- Sprinting speed slows more than 10%; do not exceed a 7-degree slope, and decrease the slope if slowdown continues.
- Clients do not maintain proper form; decrease the slope until proper technique returns.

PARTNER-RESISTED SPRINTING

Intensity level: High

Equipment: 10 to 20 yards (9.1-18.3 m) of rubber tubing or band (actual length depends on available space); partner

Purpose: Works on increasing stride length, achieving full hip extension, and spending minimal time in contact with the ground.

Beginning position: With the client in front (the person on the right in the photo), the personal trainer or a partner attaches one end of the tubing or band to the client, then holds the other end. The client moves approximately 5 yards (4.6 m) ahead while the partner maintains the beginning position.

Movement: With the beginning distance maintained, the client begins sprinting while the partner resists. The partner should resist only enough for the client to slow speed by 10%. The client should sprint for a distance of only 10 to 15 yards (or meters).

Common Errors

- Sprinting speed slows more than 10%; decrease resistance until proper technique returns.
- Clients do not maintain proper form; decrease distance until proper technique returns.

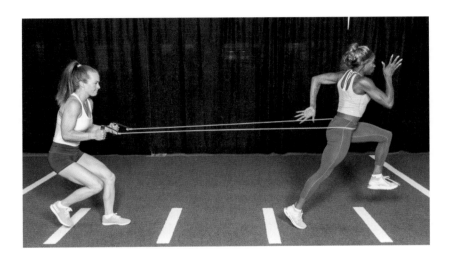

STRIDE LENGTH SPEED DRILLS

DOWNHILL SPRINT

Intensity level: High

Equipment: A 3- to 7-degree downhill angled sprinting surface

Purpose: Running at a greater velocity than one is normally capable of. This allows the body to learn how to run at greater stride frequencies, which will then transfer to nonresisted running or flat sprinting.

Beginning position: At the top of the downhill area, assume a comfortable, upright stance, with feet shoulder-width apart.

Movement: Maintaining correct posture and technique, sprint 30 to 50 yards (or meters) downhill. Do not run at speeds greater than 106% to 110% of maximum speed.

Common Errors

- There is excessive braking or deceleration; do not exceed a 7-degree slope, and decrease the slope if braking continues.
- Clients do not maintain proper form; decrease the slope until proper technique returns.

PARTNER-ASSISTED TOWING

Intensity level: High

Equipment: 10 to 20 yards (9.1-18.3 m) of rubber tubing or bungee (actual length depends on available space); partner

Purpose: Running at a greater velocity than one is normally capable of. This allows the body to learn how to run at greater stride frequencies, which will then transfer to nonresisted running or flat sprinting.

Beginning position: The tubing or bungee is attached to both the client (the person on the left in the photo) and the personal trainer or a partner, with the partner in front. The partner moves approximately 5 yards (4.6 m) ahead while the client maintains the beginning position.

Movement: The partner initiates the running, with the client beginning almost immediately after. The client should run with a slight lean in an upright position, focus-

ing on stepping up and over the other knee, dorsiflexing the feet when in the air, making contact with the ground on the ball of the foot, and maintaining a good powerful arm drive.

Common Errors

- There is insufficient assistance; the partner must be at least as fast as the client.
- Clients do not maintain proper form with increased speed. The client begins to brake to slow down, which results in his or her leaning back and making contact with the heel instead of the ball of the foot. In turn, the client spends too much time in contact with the ground, decreasing the stride length, getting slowed down, and over time predisposing himself or herself to overuse injuries. The partner should decrease the sprinting speed until proper technique returns.

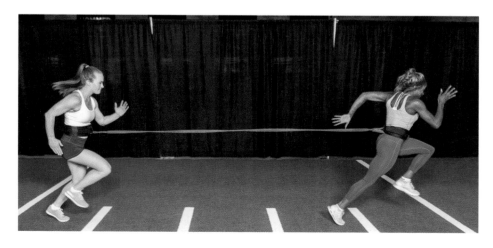

CHAPTER 18

Clients Who Are Preadolescent, Older, or Pregnant

Wayne L. Westcott, PhD, and Avery D. Faigenbaum, EdD

After completing this chapter, you will be able to

- describe developmentally appropriate physical activity programs for preadolescents that demonstrate an understanding of age-related needs and concerns,

- explain the health benefits of senior exercise and outline exercise guidelines for older adults, and

- discuss exercise recommendations and precautions for pregnant women.

The purpose of this chapter is to present general training considerations and specific exercise guidelines for three groups of people who typically need modified workouts to maximize their conditioning benefits and minimize their injury risk. Preadolescent youth, older adults, and pregnant women can safely perform aerobic endurance exercise for improved cardiovascular fitness, as well as resistance training for increased musculoskeletal fitness. However, because each of these special populations has particular characteristics, personal trainers must incorporate a number of recommendations into exercise programs for them.

PREADOLESCENT YOUTH

Preadolescence refers to a period of time before the development of secondary sex characteristics (e.g., pubic hair and reproductive organs) and corresponds roughly to ages 6 to 11 years in girls and 6 to 13 years in boys. Preadolescent youth (also referred to as *children* in this chapter) should be encouraged to participate regularly in a variety of physical activities that enhance aerobic endurance, strength, flexibility,

and skill-related fitness abilities (i.e., agility, balance, coordination, reaction time, speed, and power). Regular participation in physical activity programs can improve health- and skill-related components of physical fitness and have been found to enhance psychosocial well-being in school-age youth (40, 42, 43). Furthermore, increasing opportunities for regular moderate to vigorous physical activity (MVPA) may support academic achievement and favorably influence brain structure and function in youth (14, 57). Health and fitness organizations support and encourage children's participation in daily MVPA that is consistent with the needs and abilities of the participants (51, 56, 60).

The promotion of physical activity among youth has become a major public health concern because the number of children who are overweight and obese continues to increase worldwide, and the physical activity level of most boys and girls is down (3, 48). The percentage of overweight boys and girls in the United States has more than tripled since the 1980s (2), and many children who are overweight have one or more risk factors for cardiovascular disease (59). The amount of time children spend with electronic media (e.g., television, video games, and computers) has grown considerably, and active travel to school (e.g., walking and cycling) continues to decline (44, 61).

The negative health consequences of childhood obesity and physical inactivity include the appearance of coronary fatty streaks and type 2 diabetes in children and teenagers (1, 35). The increasing incidence of type 2 diabetes in youth is particularly troubling because conditions related to uncontrolled diabetes such as kidney failure, blindness, and limb amputation will occur earlier in life. Notably, the loss of glycemic control in youth with uncontrolled type 2 diabetes is rapid and may follow an aggressive disease course (39). In addition to premature morbidity and mortality, the increasing burden of physical inactivity on the economy and health care costs is staggering (12). Without concerted efforts to increase participation in MVPA throughout the day, it seems these trends will continue.

Since physical activity behaviors established during childhood tend to carry over into adulthood (54), the key is to value the importance of daily physical activity early in life and help children develop healthy habits as an ongoing lifestyle choice. Personal trainers who model and support participation in developmentally appropriate fitness activities that are safe, fun, and supported by cultural norms can have a powerful influence on a child's health and activity habits. Well-organized personal training sessions that give boys and girls the opportunity to experience the mere enjoyment of physical activity can have long-lasting effects on their health and well-being. Thus, the goal of youth fitness programs is not only to engage boys and girls in a variety of age-appropriate games and activities but also to make youth aware of the intrinsic value and benefits of physical activity so they become adults who participate regularly in exercise and sport. Regular physical activity is recognized as one of the most important steps youth can take to improve their health and fitness (56).

Youth Physical Activity

Because youth have different needs than adults and are active in different ways, adult exercise guidelines and training philosophies should not be imposed on children. Watching boys and girls on a playground supports the contention that the natural activity pattern of children is characterized by sporadic bursts of moderate- to vigorous-intensity activity with brief periods of low-intensity activity or rest as needed. While adults often exercise within a predetermined target heart rate zone, children are intermittently active and often choose to exercise in a spurt-like pattern characterized by haphazard increases and decreases in exercise intensity (46). Thus, personal trainers should not expect preadolescents to exercise in the same manner as adults. The assumption that children are inactive simply because they do not perform continuous physical activity is inaccurate.

This does not mean that exercising continuously for 30 minutes or more within a predetermined target heart rate range (e.g., 70% to 85% predicted maximal heart rate) is not beneficial for children. Rather, it means this is not the most appropriate method for training preadolescents because most children prefer not to perform prolonged periods of continuous aerobic endurance training. Furthermore, cardiorespiratory adaptations such as increased aerobic capacity may be less noticeable in children compared with older adults (4). **High-intensity interval training (HIIT)**, characterized by short bouts of vigorous-intensity exercise (i.e., workloads $\geq$90% $\dot{V}O_2$peak interspersed with brief rest periods), is more similar to children's habitual activity pattern. HIIT is a feasible and time-efficient method for improving cardiometabolic health outcomes in children (15). Since physical activity intensity appears to have a significant impact on cardiometabolic health in youth (53), personal trainers can integrate vigorous bouts of physical activity into youth fitness programs with small-sided games and fitness circuits.

Personal trainers also need to be aware of physiological differences between children and adults. Children have a higher breathing frequency and a lower tidal volume than adults at all exercise intensities (45). Thus, it is normal for healthy children to breathe rapidly during a fitness workout. Children also exhibit a lower stroke volume and higher heart rate at all exercise intensities (45). Maximal heart rates do not change much during childhood, and it is not uncommon for a child's heart rate to exceed 200 beats/min during a vigorous fitness workout. Moreover, maximal heart rate prediction equations developed for adults may have limited accuracy in children (8). Years ago clinicians observed that children tend to be "metabolic nonspecialists" with regard to fitness performance (5), and more recent observations suggest the interplay between anaerobic and aerobic exercise metabolism is indeed different in children than in older populations (19). Unlike what is seen in adults who tend to specialize in sports such as weightlifting or long-distance running, the strongest child in class is likely to be the best at aerobic endurance events too. Personal trainers should appreciate the lack of metabolic specialization in children and should expose boys and girls to a variety of sports and activities during this developmental period (31).

Although the absolute level of physical activity required to achieve and maintain fitness in youth has not yet been determined, over the past few years several organizations and committees have developed youth physical activity guidelines (56, 60). It has been recommended that children participate daily in 60 minutes or more of MVPA that is developmentally appropriate, is enjoyable, and involves a variety of activities (56). In addition to participation in structured programs such as physical education classes, personal training sessions, and team sports, lifestyle physical activities including playground games, walking or biking to and from school, and physical chores around the home (e.g., yard work) can contribute to the amount of time children engage in physical activity. Reducing the amount of time children spend watching television, playing video games, or surfing the Internet can considerably increase the time they have available for physical activity.

Most children can remain physically active for 30 minutes or more provided the exercise intensity varies throughout the session and they are given the opportunity to take short breaks when needed. Even sedentary children can perform relatively large volumes of physical activity by alternating moderate to vigorous physical activity with brief periods of rest and recovery. Instead of a 30-minute jogging workout, the personal trainer can create a circuit of 8 to 12 stations that includes bodyweight movements (e.g., jumping jacks, push-ups, and squats), fitness rope exercises, medicine ball activities, balancing drills, and shuttle runs. As fitness levels improve, it becomes possible to decrease the rest period between stations and make the activities at each station more challenging. With qualified instruction, enthusiastic leadership, and adherence to safety issues, children can safely enhance their muscular strength and fundamental movement abilities and be better prepared for successful and enjoyable participation in recreational activities and sport.

> **Youth should be encouraged to participate daily in 60 minutes or more of moderate to vigorous physical activity as part of active play, outdoor games, recreational sports, active transportation, and school activities.**

Resistance Training for Youth

A compelling body of evidence indicates that resistance training can be a safe, effective, and worthwhile method of conditioning for preadolescents provided appropriate guidelines are followed (6, 9, 20). Despite the traditional belief that resistance training was inappropriate or unsafe for children, the qualified acceptance of youth resistance training by medical and fitness organizations is widespread (17, 32, 52). Public health recommendations encourage children to participate in muscle strengthening and bone strengthening activities, and resistance training is now recognized as foundational for long-term athletic development (31, 56).

The traditional concern that resistance training could damage the epiphyseal plates of children or impede the statural growth of young weight trainers caused some people to recommend that children not participate in resistance training. Current observations indicate no evidence of decrease in stature in preadolescent boys and girls who resistance train in supervised programs, and epiphyseal plate fractures have not been reported in any prospective youth resistance training study published to date (20, 32). There is no scientific evidence that the risks associated with competently supervised and well-designed youth resistance training programs are greater than those of other recreational activities that children regularly participate in (20, 32). However, children should not resistance train on their own without guidance from a qualified professional because the inappropriate use of exercise equipment and unsafe behavior can result in injury (38). These findings underscore the importance of providing close supervision, safe training equipment, and ongoing instruction for all youth resistance training programs.

Muscle Strength Gains and Other Benefits

Many studies have convincingly shown that children can increase muscular strength above and beyond that accompanying growth and maturation by participating in a well-designed resistance training program (6, 18, 30). Strength gains of roughly 30% to 40% have been observed in children following short-term (8-12 weeks) programs. Various combinations of sets and repetitions and different training modalities—including child-size weight machines, free weights (barbells and dumbbells), medicine balls, elastic bands, and bodyweight exercises—have proven to be safe and effective methods of conditioning for healthy children (23, 33).

Since children lack sufficient levels of circulating androgens to stimulate increases in muscle hypertrophy, it appears that neural adaptations are primarily responsible for training-induced strength gains in preadolescents (29). Intrinsic muscle adaptations (i.e., changes in excitation–contraction coupling, myofibrillar packing density, and muscle fiber composition), as well as improvements in motor skill performance and the coordination of the involved muscle groups, could also contribute to gains in strength. Longer training periods and more precise measuring techniques (e.g., computerized imaging) may uncover the potential for training-induced muscle hypertrophy in preadolescent youth.

In addition to increasing muscle strength, regular participation in strength-building activities can positively influence several measurable indexes of health and fitness. Reports indicate that regular participation in youth resistance training programs may increase bone mineral density, develop motor performance skills (e.g., vertical jump and sprint speed), facilitate weight control, improve cardiometabolic health, and support participation in MVPA (9, 24, 49, 50). Others have noted significant improvements in the mental health of youth who participated in resistance training interventions (10).

It has also been reported that overweight youth can benefit from participation in exercise programs that include resistance training (11, 26). Overweight youth seem to enjoy resistance training because it is characterized by short periods of physical activity interspersed with brief rest periods between sets. Although resistance training may not result in a high caloric expenditure, this type of training has proven to be an important component of weight management programs for overweight youth, who often lack the motor skills and confidence to be physically active (25, 47). Clearly, an important first step in encouraging overweight youth to exercise is to increase their confidence in their ability to be physically active, which in turn may lead to an increase in physical activity and potentially an improvement in body composition

and metabolic health. This is particularly important because overweight youth typically have limited experience participating in structured exercise programs.

Reducing Sport-Related Injuries

Since many sports have a significant strength or power component, stronger and more powerful children will be better prepared for the demands of sports practice and competition (6, 18, 28). Young athletes who participate in conditioning programs that include resistance training are more likely to experience success and are less likely to drop out of sport because of frustration, embarrassment, failure, or injury than those who do not (7, 55, 58). A long-term athletic development model that emphasizes resistance training right from the start is needed to maximize physical development and minimize injury risk (31).

A growing number of aspiring young athletes are not prepared for the demands of sport practice and competition (22, 37). Epidemiological reports show a decline in field measures of muscular fitness in school-age youth in a majority of countries (22). To better prepare boys and girls for sport training and competition, children who have been physically inactive for two to three months (e.g., no regular participation in recreational physical activities or sport) should be encouraged to participate in a supervised integrative conditioning program (two or three times per week) that includes strength-building activities and drills that enhance agility, balance, coordination, and power (36, 41). In some cases, youth may need to spend less time practicing sport-specific skills and more time enhancing fundamental fitness abilities in order to establish a sound fitness base prior to sport training. As children enhance their physical literacy and begin to gain confidence and competence in their physical abilities, they may be more likely to participate in exercise and sport as an ongoing lifestyle choice (21).

Comprehensive conditioning programs that include resistance training have proven to be an effective strategy for reducing sport-related injuries in adolescent athletes, and it is possible that similar effects would be observed in children (27, 41, 55). Although the total elimination of youth sport injuries is an unrealistic goal, acute and overuse injuries associated with youth sport could be significantly reduced if more emphasis were placed on the development of muscular strength and fundamental fitness abilities than on sport-specific skills (27, 36, 58). This may be particularly important for young female athletes, who appear to be more susceptible to knee injuries

(41). Although additional clinical trials are needed to determine the best method for reducing sport-related injuries in children, it seems prudent for personal trainers to encourage inactive youth to participate in at least six to eight weeks of integrative fitness conditioning that includes resistance training before sport participation. Ideally, young athletes should participate in year-round strength and conditioning in a systematic manner to optimize training adaptations and athletic performance (33).

Guidelines for Youth Resistance Training

The belief that resistance training is unsafe or inappropriate for children is not consistent with its documented benefits or with the needs of modern-day youth (18, 32, 50). There is no minimum age for participation in a youth resistance training program, but all participants should have the emotional maturity to accept and follow directions and should understand the benefits and risks associated with this type of training. While five- and six-year-olds may enjoy strength-building animal-like movements such as crocodile planks, gecko lunges, and bunny hops, seven- and eight-year-olds may be ready for more structured resistance training using their own body weight or external loads (16, 17). Although a medical examination before participation in a resistance training program is not mandatory for apparently healthy children, it is recommended for youth with signs or symptoms suggestive of disease and for youth with known disease (52).

Since resistance training is a learned skill, it is important for youth to begin at a level commensurate with their physical abilities to optimize skill competency and program adherence. If the volume and intensity of training exceed a child's capabilities and if the prescribed exercises are too demanding, the enjoyment of the resistance training experience may begin to wane and the risk of injury may increase. When introducing preadolescents to resistance training activities, it is always better to underestimate their abilities than to overestimate them and risk an injury. A light to moderate weight (≤60% of an estimated 1RM) that can be lifted for 1 or 2 sets of 8 to 12 repetitions appears to be a safe and effective training resistance for children beginning an introductory resistance training program. As resistance training skill competency increases, additional sets with heavier loads (60% to 80% of an estimated 1RM) and more complex exercises can be incorporated into the training program. Young athletes with

a high resistance training skill competency may use heavier loads (≥85% of an estimated 1RM) to optimize training-induced adaptations and performance (18, 30, 32). Importantly, the intensity and volume of resistance training need to be systematically varied over time because prolonged exposure to high-intensity or high-volume training may increase the risk of overtraining or overuse injuries (33).

The following are generally accepted guidelines for youth resistance training:

- Qualified adults should provide supervision and instruction.
- The training environment should be safe and free of hazards.
- Resistance training should be preceded by a 5- to 10-minute dynamic warm-up.
- Begin with 1 or 2 sets of 8 to 12 repetitions of a variety of exercises.
- Include exercises for the upper body, lower body, and midsection.
- Increase resistance gradually (e.g., about 5% to 10%) as resistance training skill competency improves.
- Resistance train two or three nonconsecutive days per week.
- Children should cool down with less intense calisthenics and static stretching.
- Vary the resistance training program over time to optimize gains and prevent boredom.

Personal trainers working with a group of children should individually prescribe workloads and ask children to do the best they can within the allotted time period instead of setting one workload for all children in the group (e.g., 10 push-ups or 20 pounds [9.1 kg] on the chest press exercise). Personal trainers and children should work together to determine the workload that is most appropriate for each child's needs and abilities. Although some children may want to see how much weight they can lift during the first workout, their energy and enthusiasm should be redirected toward developing proper form and technique on a variety of exercises. In addition, basic education on fitness room etiquette, realistic outcomes, and safety concerns including appropriate spotting and proper storage of equipment should be part of all youth resistance training programs (23).

No matter how big or strong a child is, adult resistance training guidelines and training philosophies should not be imposed on young resistance training clients. Parents, teachers, coaches, and personal trainers who work with children should not overlook the importance of having fun and developing a more positive attitude toward resistance training and all types of physical activity. The importance of creating an enjoyable exercise experience for all participants should not be overlooked, since enjoyment has been shown to mediate the effects of youth exercise and sports programs (13, 34). Long-term adherence to any type of exercise program is more probable when children are internally driven to do their best and when they feel good about their performances. If qualified supervision is present and if age-related training guidelines are followed, resistance training can be a safe, effective, and enjoyable method of conditioning for preadolescent boys and girls.

Teaching Preadolescent Youth

Although boys and girls should be aware of the potential health- and fitness-related benefits associated with regular physical activity, enthusiastic leadership, creative programming, and age-related teaching strategies are more likely to get youth "turned on" to physical activity (19). Personal trainers need to respect children's feelings while appreciating the fact that they think differently than adults. Personal trainers should not forget about the importance of play, which is one of the ways children learn (62). If personal trainers display physical vitality, relate to children in a positive manner, understand how children think, and participate in activities with children, their efforts are likely to be worthwhile and long lasting. The sidebar provides general recommendations for personal trainers who work with children.

Of note, getting children ready for a fitness workout is not just about low-intensity aerobic exercise and static stretching. A well-designed warm-up can set the tone for the training session and establish a desired tempo for the upcoming activities. If a warm-up is slow and monotonous, then performance during the main physical activities that follow may be less than expected. However, if the warm-up is up-tempo and exciting and contains variety, performance during the fitness lessons will likely meet or exceed expectations. Moreover, dynamic warm-up activities that are active, engaging, and challenging and that provide an opportunity for children to gain confidence in their abilities to perform fundamental movement skills are more enjoyable than traditional "stretch and hold" activities. A reasonable suggestion is to perform dynamic activities during the warm-up and static stretching during the cooldown.

Since a major objective of youth fitness programs is for physical activity to become a habitual part of children's lives, personal trainers must strive to increase each participant's self-efficacy or self-confidence regarding physical abilities. To achieve this objective, personal trainers should provide clear instructions and demonstrations so that participants can learn new exercises, experience success, make friends, and develop a sense of mastery of specific skills. Thus, the focus of personal training sessions should be on positive experiences instead of stressful competitions. It is unlikely that children will continue in a fitness program if they do not understand the instructions or are unable to perform the exercises. The development of successful youth programs requires preparation, coordination, and an awareness of individual differences in stress tolerance.

> **When children have fun, make friends, and experience success, they are more likely to engage in physical activities as a lifestyle choice.**

RECOMMENDATIONS FOR PERSONAL TRAINERS WHO TRAIN CHILDREN

- Provide close supervision, and listen to each child's concerns.
- Speak to children using words they understand.
- Greet each child by name on arrival.
- Praise children for doing a good job.
- Realize that children are active in different ways than adults.
- Design activities that ensure equal participation and enjoyment.
- Gradually progress the fitness program.
- Play down competition and focus on skill improvement, personal successes, and having fun.
- Remind children that it takes time to learn a new skill and get in shape.
- Offer a variety of activities and avoid regimentation.
- Emphasize the importance of healthy food choices.
- Inform parents about the benefits of regular physical activity.

OLDER ADULTS

Older adults experience a variety of health issues associated with aging, including sarcopenia, osteopenia, obesity, diabetes, cardiovascular disease, and musculoskeletal problems such as arthritis and low back pain (86). However, the underlying causes of these and many other age-related health issues may be overlooked by both patients and physicians.

Muscular Fitness

A largely unrecognized aspect of the aging process is the progressive loss of muscle (**sarcopenia**) that occurs at a relatively rapid rate in adults who do not perform regular resistance exercise (19, 32). Older adults who do not resistance train experience a 5% to 10% reduction in muscle mass every decade (58, 62). This muscle loss is responsible for about 90% of the strength loss experienced with aging (81) and is largely due to the lower proportion of type II muscle fibers in older adults (53). One study reported that adults in the 60 to 80 age range have approximately half as many type II motor units as adults in the 20 to 40 age range (26). Sarcopenia is associated with **osteopenia** (reductions in bone mineral density), and older adults who do not resistance train also experience a 10% to 30% reduction in bone mineral density every decade (46, 62). In addition to a weaker musculoskeletal system, muscle loss is accompanied by an average resting metabolic rate reduction of 3% per decade, which facilitates fat gain (65).

Unfortunately, many men and women are unaware of these age-associated physiological changes. Inactive adults typically experience more fat gain than muscle loss, resulting in a higher body weight. Consequently, they may not realize their muscle mass is decreasing. As illustrated in figure 18.1 (83b), an average 50-year-old female may weigh 30 pounds (13.6 kg) more than she did at age 20 but may have 15 pounds (6.8 kg) less muscle and 45 pounds (20.4 kg) more fat, for a 60-pound (27.2 kg) change in her body composition (23% fat vs. 47% fat). Similarly, because fewer than 2.5% of older adults perform sufficient physical activity to meet the minimum recommendations for weekly exercise (83), most older men and women are unaware that their muscle strength is decreasing at the rate of 10% to 20% per decade (75) and that their muscle power is decreasing at the rate of 30% to 40% per decade (75).

Health Benefits of Resistance Exercise

The insidious declines in muscle mass, muscle strength, and muscle power have important implications for both the quantity of life and the quality of life in aging adults. With respect to the quantity of life, being stronger appears to be associated with a longer life span. Although a correlation should not be confused with causation, research has shown that older adults who have a higher level of muscular fitness have a lower risk of premature death from cancers, cardiovascular disease (CVD), and all-cause mortality (56). A 2019 study with more than 12,500 participants concluded that, independent of aerobic activity, "low-to-moderate frequency and amount of resistance exercise are associated with reduced risk of nonfatal CVD events, total CVD events, and all-cause mortality" (57, p. 506). With respect to the quality of life, research reveals a wide variety of health benefits associated with regular resistance exercise, including the following physiological adaptations (65, 86).

Increased Muscle Mass

Several resistance training studies with older adults have shown significant increases in muscle mass that are similar to those attained by younger adults who perform resistance exercise (15, 42, 67, 88). On average, resistance exercise enables older adults to increase muscle mass by about 1 pound (0.5 kg) per month over the first few months of resistance training (15, 42, 67, 88), which effectively reduces (or reverses) the muscle loss (sarcopenia) associated with inactivity (32).

Increased Bone Mineral Density

Resistance training protocols that incorporate relatively heavy loads (approximately 80% of the 1RM) provide effective stimuli for both muscular development and bone development (83a). Multiple studies with older men and women have shown significant increases in bone mineral density after several months of regular resistance exercise (47, 62). However, the rate of bone development is considerably lower than the rate of muscle development. On average, resistance training enables older adults to increase bone mineral density by about 1% per year (47, 62), which effectively reduces (or reverses) the bone loss (osteopenia) experienced by older adults who do not perform this type of exercise (90).

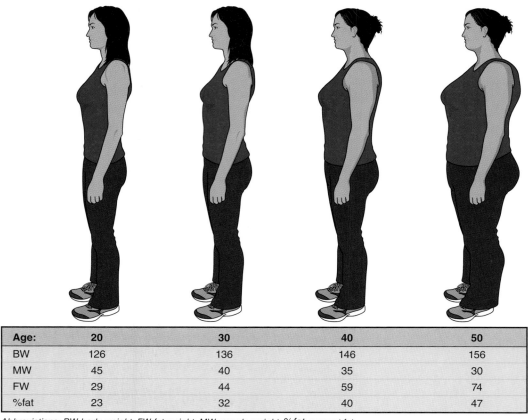

Age:	20	30	40	50
BW	126	136	146	156
MW	45	40	35	30
FW	29	44	59	74
%fat	23	32	40	47

Abbreviations: BW, body weight; FW, fat weight; MW, muscle weight; %fat, percent fat.

FIGURE 18.1 Bodyweight and body composition change throughout the life of an adult.

Reprinted by permission from Westcott (2003, p. 9).

Increased Energy Expenditure

Resistance training is a vigorous physical activity that uses calories during both the exercise performance and during the postexercise recovery period. Resistance training causes microtrauma in the exercised muscle, which requires protein for tissue building and energy from stored carbohydrates and fats for remodeling processes. Heden (39) reported a 5% increase in resting energy expenditure for three days after a low-volume resistance workout (10 exercises, 1 set each), while Hackney (38) reported a 9% increase in resting energy expenditure for three days after a high-volume resistance workout (8 exercises, 8 sets each). On average, older adults who perform regular resistance exercise elevate their resting energy expenditure by about 7% (15, 42, 67), equivalent to approximately 100 additional calories used every day at rest. Therefore, older adults who begin resistance training may experience a reduction in body fat due to the increased energy expenditure during and after this metabolically demanding activity.

Reduced Body Fat

Resistance exercise uses calories during training sessions because of the relatively high muscular effort and between training sessions because of the associated elevations in resting energy expenditure for recovery and repair. For example, a 25-minute circuit resistance training session may use about 200 calories for exercise performance. Three weekly workouts would therefore total about 2,400 calories per month. Assuming a 7% increase in resting energy expenditure of approximately 100 calories per day, this would burn another 3,000 calories per month. The sum of these resistance training and muscle remodeling energy expenditures is, therefore, about 5,400 calories per month, which is equivalent to approximately 1.5 pounds (0.7 kg) of fat. Several resistance training studies with older adults have found a monthly muscle gain of about 1 pound (0.5 kg) and a monthly fat loss of about 1.5 pounds (0.7 kg) during the first few months of regular resistance exercise (15, 67, 85).

Research has also shown significant intra-abdominal fat reduction in older adults (82) after standard resistance training programs. Causal factors may include increased metabolic rate, improved insulin sensitivity, and enhanced sympathetic activity associated with resistance exercise (43). After reviewing the studies related to resistance exercise and fat reduction, Strasser and Schobersberger (76) concluded that resistance training is recommended in the management of obesity and metabolic disorders. It is also noted that bodyweight change does not necessarily reflect the fat loss benefits of resistance exercise because of the concurrent gain in muscle mass and fluid volume.

Reduced Risk of Diabetes

An association exists between overweight or obesity and type 2 diabetes, which is predicted to affect more than 30% of American adults by the middle of this century (11). A major literature review (29), a comprehensive meta-analysis (77), and the American Diabetes Association (73) all recommend resistance training for the prevention and management of type 2 diabetes. In addition to reducing overall body weight and body fat (15, 67, 85, 88), resistance exercise decreases intra-abdominal fat (82), which appears to be associated with reduced insulin resistance in older adults (50). Numerous studies have shown that resistance training improves insulin response and glycemic control (18), and there is evidence that this may be the most effective physical activity for lowering blood sugar (HbA1c) levels (14).

Reduced Risk of Cardiovascular Disease

Well-designed resistance training programs enhance both muscular fitness and cardiovascular health. In fact, a comprehensive research review by Strasser and Schobersberger (76, p. 6) concluded that "resistance training is at least as effective as aerobic endurance training in reducing some major cardiovascular disease risk factors." Resistance training has been shown to improve four key factors associated with cardiovascular disease risk.

First, regular resistance exercise reduces body fat and intra-abdominal fat (15, 42, 67, 82, 88). Because of its positive impact on resting metabolism, resistance exercise may have a greater effect on fat loss than aerobic activity (15, 38, 42, 65, 67). Fat reduction has been shown to reduce other cardiovascular disease risk factors, including elevated plasma cholesterol, elevated plasma glucose, and elevated resting blood pressure (77).

Second, properly performed resistance training lowers resting blood pressure. Several studies have demonstrated significant reductions in systolic and diastolic blood pressures from as little as 10 weeks of resistance exercise (24, 88). A meta-analysis by Cornelissen and Fagard (24) found average resting blood pressure reductions of approximately 6 mmHg systolic and 5 mmHg diastolic associated with standard resistance training programs.

Third, many researchers have reported significant improvements in blood lipid profiles after resistance training (45). Evidence indicates that resistance exercise can increase HDL (good) cholesterol levels between 8% and 21%, decrease LDL (bad) cholesterol levels between 13% and 23%, and reduce triglyceride levels between 11% and 18% (1). Even elderly individuals (70 to 87 years) who performed resistance exercise attained significant and desirable changes in HDL cholesterol, LDL cholesterol, and triglyceride panels (27).

Fourth, there is evidence that resistance exercise can improve vascular condition, which facilitates circulation and arterial blood flow (4). Although more research on this resistance training adaptation is warranted, the enhanced endothelial function and arterial conductance associated with resistance training represent important cardiovascular benefits.

Based on these beneficial physiological responses to resistance exercise, it would appear that resistance training can reduce the risk of cardiovascular disease by favorably addressing the predisposing factors of metabolic syndrome (43, 76, 77). Research indicates that postcoronary patients experience similar health-related benefits from appropriate resistance exercise protocols (28) and should be encouraged to participate in medically approved resistance training programs.

> **Research reveals that older adults can significantly improve their cardiovascular health by performing regular resistance exercise.**

Reduced Risk of Certain Cancers and Treatment Side Effects

The speed at which food moves through the gastrointestinal system may be associated with colon cancer risk, and moving food more quickly through the gut may lessen the probability of this disease. Research has demonstrated a nearly 60% increase in gastrointestinal transit speed in older men after three months of resistance exercise (49). Resistance training may, therefore, be an effective means for addressing age-related gastrointestinal health issues, as well as for reducing the risk of colon cancer.

Specific prostate cancer treatments may also influence overall health and fitness levels because side effects include reduced muscle strength and mass, reduced bone mass, and increased fat mass. However, after five months of twice weekly resistance training, older prostate cancer patients receiving androgen-deprivation therapy experienced significant increases in muscle strength, quadriceps muscle thickness, functional performance, and balance, while preserving body composition and bone mineral density (33).

Reduced Musculoskeletal Discomfort

There are many causes and symptoms of musculoskeletal discomfort, including infirmities such as low back pain, arthritis, and fibromyalgia. Studies have shown that resistance exercise is an effective intervention for reducing low back pain (36, 69) because there appears to be a positive association between weak lumbar spine muscles and low back discomfort (36). Strong lumbar spine muscles provide greater musculoskeletal function, support, control, and force absorption, thereby reducing the risk of low back injury and structural degeneration (36).

Resistance training appears to be effective for easing the pain of osteoarthritis (52). Research has demonstrated that even individuals with advanced knee osteoarthritis can perform progressive resistance exercise and attain substantial strength gains in the muscles of the knee joint (48).

Adults with fibromyalgia have responded favorably to appropriate programs of resistance exercise (9). As a result, the Ottawa Panel has produced evidence-based clinical and practical resistance training guidelines for the management of fibromyalgia (13). It should be noted that physician approval may be warranted when working with these and other special populations.

Enhanced Mental and Emotional Health

Resistance training interventions have shown significant increases in cognitive abilities of older adults (17). For example, a training program consisting of both resistance and aerobic exercise significantly enhanced cognitive processes in older adults as compared with aerobic activity alone (23). In addition to improvements in memory and cognition, twice weekly resistance training has demonstrated increases in brain white matter volume (8). Resistance training is not limited to physiological adaptations—research has demonstrated significant improvements in physical self-concept, total mood disturbance, fatigue, positive engagement, revitalization, tranquility, and tension in older women who performed resistance training and aerobic activities (3). A classic study found that more than 80% of the depressed elderly participants showed no signs of clinical depression after 10 weeks of a standard resistance training routine (74); thus, resistance exercise may be an effective intervention for reducing depression symptoms in people with diagnosed depression (74).

Improved Physical Abilities

Aging is accompanied by a reduction in physical abilities that decreases functionality for performing activities of daily living. Resistance exercise can reverse some of the physical dysfunction experienced by older adults through increased muscle strength and power (6). In one study, elderly nursing home residents (mean age 89 years) significantly improved their functional independence measures for performing activities of daily living after 14 weeks of brief resistance training sessions (85). Research has also demonstrated improved movement control (6), balance (40), physical performance (40), and walking speed (70) in older adults, each of which may reduce the risk of falls and related injuries.

Improved Mitochondrial Function

A major factor in functional abilities is mitochondrial activity. Mitochondria control several cell functions and serve as the power source of each muscle cell. Aging is associated with genetic changes that cause varying degrees of mitochondrial impairment with respect to energy production and muscle performance. Research has shown that short-rest circuit resistance training (performing 1 set of 10 to 15 different exercises with minimum transition time between exercises) can increase mitochondrial content and oxidative capacity in the exercised muscle tissue (65). One study found that six months of progressive resistance exercise reversed mitochondrial dysfunction in older adults (59). The participants in this study (mean age 68 years) experienced desirable changes in 179 genes associated with age and exercise, resulting in mitochondrial characteristics similar to those of moderately active young adults (mean age 24 years). Beneficial modifications in mitochondrial gene expression are another impressive reason for older adults to perform resistance exercise.

Summary of Resistance Training Health Benefits

The main purpose of performing resistance exercise is to increase muscular strength, mass, and endurance. However, there are numerous health-related benefits associated with regular resistance training, many of which are particularly important for older adults. As presented in this section, these include increased muscle mass, increased bone mineral density, increased resting metabolism, reduced body fat, reduced risk of diabetes, reduced risk of cardiovascular disease, reduced risk of colon cancer, reduced musculoskeletal discomfort, enhanced mental and emotional health, improved physical function, and improved mitochondrial function.

> Resistance training has been shown to reduce the risk of several degenerative problems that are common to older adults, including sarcopenia, osteopenia, high blood pressure, unfavorable blood lipid profiles, insulin insensitivity, delayed gastrointestinal transit, low back pain, and metabolic syndrome.

Cardiovascular Fitness

Cardiovascular fitness plays an equally important role in reducing the risk of prevalent health issues, such as type 2 diabetes (73), coronary heart disease (66), and stroke (34). Properly performed aerobic endurance exercise (frequently called *aerobic activity* or *cardio training*) is associated with impressive physiological changes and health benefits that positively affect both quantity and quality of life.

Health Benefits of Aerobic Activity

Consider the following physiological adaptations within the heart, circulatory system, and blood that result from appropriate aerobic activity (30).

- *Heart:* Appropriately performed aerobic endurance exercise stimulates the heart to become a more effective and efficient blood pump. The physiological adaptations include increased stroke volume, enabling the heart to pump more blood with each contraction, for enhanced cardiac output; and decreased resting heart rate, giving the heart muscles more time to rest between contractions, allowing the heart chambers more time to fill with blood between contractions, and giving the heart tissue more time to receive its own blood supply between contractions.

- *Circulatory system:* Appropriately performed aerobic activity stimulates the circulatory system to become a more effective and efficient blood delivery network. The physiological adaptations include increased size of blood vessels, enabling greater blood carrying capacity; increased number of blood vessels, enabling greater blood distribution; and increased tone of blood vessels, enabling better blood flow control.

- *Blood:* Appropriately performed cardio training stimulates the blood to become a more effective and efficient transporter. The physiological adaptations include increased blood volume, enabling greater transport capacity, and increased number and mass of red blood cells, enabling greater oxygen and carbon dioxide carrying capacity.

These beneficial changes within the cardiovascular system can increase older adults' aerobic capacity ($\dot{V}O_2$max) up to 25% depending on training factors (72). Higher cardiovascular fitness levels reduce the risk of premature demise. In a study with more than 10,000 middle-aged men, those in the least fit quintile (20%) had 3.4 times greater relative risk of death than those in the most fit quintile (10). Another study of almost 3,000 public safety officers found that among those with elevated blood pressure, officers with low fitness had more than 5 times greater risk of heart attack than those with high fitness (64). Similarly, among those with elevated blood cholesterol, officers with low fitness had more than 4 times greater risk of heart attack than those with high fitness (64).

Higher levels of cardiovascular fitness are associated with lower resting blood pressure (63), better blood lipid profiles (80), reduced abdominal fat (37), enhanced insulin sensitivity (44), improved mitochondrial function, (12) and increased brain volume of white and gray matter (22).

Summary of Aerobic Training Health Benefits

The American College of Sports Medicine has summarized numerous evidence-based health benefits of aerobic endurance exercise, including reduced risk of obesity, osteoporosis, osteoarthritis, chronic obstructive pulmonary disease, type 2 diabetes, congestive heart failure, coronary heart disease, peripheral vascular disease, stroke, depression, dementia, constipation, and sleep disorders (21). Additionally, research has demonstrated that aerobic fitness is a better predictor of all-cause mortality than is body fat (78).

Exercise Recommendations for Older Adults

Resistance exercise and aerobic activity are associated with reduced risk of mortality (55) and increased longevity (54), which are important considerations for older adults. With respect to physical, mental, and emotional health, the information in the preceding sections clearly demonstrates that resistance exercise and aerobic activity are effective means for improving these quality of life components. It is therefore recommended that older adults perform a regular and appropriate physical activity program that includes both strength and aerobic endurance training (87).

Resistance Training Guidelines

Older adults are encouraged to perform basic single-joint and multijoint exercises using equipment that enables progressive increases in the training resistance, such as weight stack machines, air pressure machines, free weights, and elastic bands. The following resistance training guidelines are recommended for older men and women.

Exercise Selection

A well-designed resistance training program for older adults should include exercises that cumulatively address all the major muscle groups. The 2019 NSCA Position Statement on Resistance Training for Older Adults (31) recommends that older men and women emphasize multijoint resistance exercises that concurrently work two or more muscle groups. For example, the following four standard multijoint exercises using free weights or resistance machines effectively work nine of the major muscle groups:

1. *Squat or leg press:* Quadriceps, hamstrings, gluteus maximus

2. *Bench press or chest press:* Pectoralis major, deltoids, triceps

3. *Bent-over row or lat pulldown:* Latissimus dorsi, deltoids, biceps

4. *Free weight or machine shoulder press:* Deltoids, triceps, upper trapezius

The NSCA Position Statement (31) also suggests that older adults perform single-joint exercises that better isolate specific muscle groups, including the following:

1. *Leg extension:* Quadriceps
2. *Leg curl:* Hamstrings
3. *Triceps extension:* Triceps
4. *Biceps curl:* Biceps
5. *Low back extension:* Erector spinae
6. *Abdominal curl:* Rectus abdominis

If feasible, older adults should perform both multijoint and single-joint resistance exercises because not all muscles involved in a given exercise are worked equally during multijoint movements (20). When training in this manner, it is recommended that multijoint exercises (which typically require more muscle mass and heavier resistance) be performed before single-joint exercises (which typically require less muscle mass and lighter resistance). For example, the chest press exercise would typically be performed before the triceps extension exercise, and the back row exercise would typically be performed before the biceps curl exercise. Exercises that load the hips and spine, such as properly performed squats and deadlifts, may be particularly relevant for older adults with respect to bone loss.

Exercise Repetitions and Resistance

There is an inverse relationship between the amount of resistance used and the number of repetitions that can be completed, generally based on the heaviest resistance that can be performed for 1 repetition (i.e., the 1RM). The 1RM is typically estimated in older adults by means of multirepetition or repetitions in reserve assessment protocols. See chapter 15 for further information regarding the repetition maximum and the repetitions in reserve methods for establishing training loads. A standard resistance training recommendation is to use a resistance that permits 8 to 12 properly performed repetitions. Most people can perform 8 repetitions with about 80% of their estimated 1RM and 12 repetitions with about 70% of their estimated 1RM. The majority of productive resistance training studies in older adults used an 8- to 12-repetition range (15, 49, 62, 67, 85, 88). However, other studies have reported similar results when using sets of 12 to 16 repetitions (60% to 70% of an estimated 1RM), as well as sets of 4 to 8 repetitions (80% to 90% of an estimated 1RM) (7, 79). As shown in figure 18.2

(87a), an acceptable resistance range may extend from 60% to 90% of the 1RM.

Although studies have demonstrated significant strength gains when training with weight loads less than 60% of the 1RM (71), it is recommended that most older adults begin training with resistances that can be performed for 10 to 15 repetitions (31). Once they have strengthened their muscles and connective tissues, they may progress to weight loads that can be performed for 8 to 12 repetitions (31). Well-conditioned older adults who prefer to train with relatively heavy resistance may then advance to weight loads that can be performed for approximately 4 to 8 repetitions (5). The 2019 NSCA Position Statement on Resistance Training for Older Adults (31) recommends that older men and women progress to exercise resistances up to 85% of the 1RM, which can generally be performed for 4 to 6 repetitions depending on the number of sets completed.

Exercise Sets

For older adults, the number of exercise sets to be performed within a resistance training session is largely dictated by training status. The 2019 NSCA Position Statement on Resistance Training for Older Adults (31) recommends that previously untrained older men and women initially perform a single set of each resistance exercise. For beginning participants, particularly older adults, single-set training can be as effective as multiple-set, higher-volume regimens during the initial phases of an exercise program (16). For instance, several studies have demonstrated similar increases in muscle mass (approximately 1 pound

[0.5 kg] per month) between single- and multiple-set training when using sets between 8 and 12 repetitions (15, 42, 67, 88). Additionally, higher-volume training (i.e., 12, 14, and 22 sets vs. 10 sets) did not appear to influence muscle gains in novice older adults (15, 42, 67, 88). However, as these individuals begin to increase muscular strength, muscular endurance, and exercise enthusiasm, they may progress to 2 to 4 sets of each exercise (31, 87). With the incorporation of multiple-set training, a dose–response relationship indicates that maximal benefits are observed at 3 or 4 sets per exercise, with no additional benefits and potential decreases in benefits beyond 4 sets (51, 68). It is advisable for older adults to rest 2 to 3 minutes between successive training sets to facilitate tissue recovery and energy replenishment in the exercised muscles (60).

Exercise Progression

The most effective stimulus for increasing muscle mass and strength is a systematic increase in the exercise resistance. Progressive resistance exercise is productive within the previously recommended repetition ranges and may be performed safely by means of a double progressive training protocol, which alternately increases the exercise repetitions and the exercise resistance (87). A standard recommendation, known as the **two-for-two rule**, is to train with a given resistance until the target number of repetitions is exceeded by 2 reps for 2 consecutive workouts. For example, a person using an 8- to 12-repetition protocol would raise the resistance when 14 repetitions are completed (on the last set) for two consecutive training sessions.

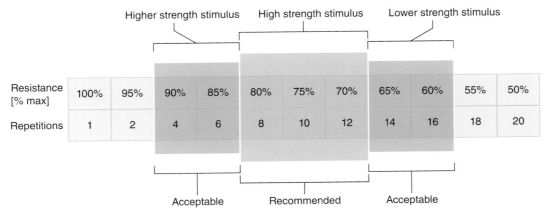

FIGURE 18.2 Resistance and repetition relationships for recommended resistance training protocols for older adults.

Reprinted by permission from Westcott and Baechle (2010, p. 22).

When this is achieved, the resistance is increased by approximately 5% for the next workout, which typically reduces the number of repetitions that can be performed, and the process is repeated.

Exercise Frequency

Most older adults train all the major muscle groups during each exercise session. Research using total body workouts has produced varying results with respect to training frequency. Hunter and associates (41) found no significant differences in strength development when training one, two, or three nonconsecutive days per week. DeMichele and colleagues (25) reported similar strength gains when training two days or three days per week that were significantly greater than training one day per week. A similar study with more than 1,600 participants found identical increases in lean mass when training two days or three days per week that were significantly greater than training one day per week (88). It is therefore recommended that older adults perform resistance training workouts two or three nonconsecutive days each week for significant improvements in muscle strength and muscle mass. For those who prefer to train more frequently, a sample split-routine workout protocol is to perform upper body resistance exercises on Mondays and Thursdays and to perform lower body resistance exercises on Wednesdays and Saturdays.

Exercise Range

It would appear that specificity of training applies to the range through which the target muscles are exercised. Maximum strength gains are experienced in the trained movement range, with (progressively) less strength increases outside the trained movement range (36). For this reason, as well as for enhanced joint flexibility, it is recommended that older adults perform each resistance exercise throughout the largest movement range that does not cause joint discomfort. Training only through the pain-free range of movement is an important guideline for older adults, especially for those who have some form of arthritis or other joint conditions.

Exercise Speed

Research indicates that muscle strength may be best increased by training with moderate to heavy resistance at moderate movement speeds (61). Conversely, muscle power may be best increased by training with moderate resistance at fast movement speeds (89). Heavy resistance is generally considered to be greater than 80% of the client's estimated 1RM, whereas moderate resistance is generally considered to be 60% to 80% of an estimated 1RM. Moderate movement speeds are generally considered to be 2 seconds or longer for concentric muscle actions (and the same for eccentric muscle actions). Fast movement speeds are generally considered to be 1 second or shorter for concentric muscle actions (with 2 seconds or longer for eccentric muscle actions). It is advisable for older adults to begin their training program with a strength emphasis, using exercise resistance that can be performed for 10 to 15 controlled repetitions (60% to 70% of the 1RM), then progress to 6 to 12 controlled repetitions (70% to 85% of the 1RM) (31).

After increasing muscle and connective tissue strength, older adults should add power training to their exercise program, performing faster concentric muscle actions with lower resistance. According to the 2019 NSCA Position Statement on Resistance Training for Older Adults, older adults should include some high-speed concentric muscle actions using 40% to 60% of their estimated 1RM to promote muscle power development (31). Because of the higher muscle force requirements for overcoming inertia, it is essential for older adults to use biomechanically correct exercise technique when performing faster-speed free-weight movements. An alternative power training mode that essentially eliminates the issues of inertia and momentum is air pressure (pneumatic) equipment. Another option for older adults training power is medicine balls, which are relatively light and can be moved very quickly. Because medicine balls offer minimal inertia and can be released at the end of the concentric muscle action, they facilitate fast movement speeds with low injury risk (5).

Exercise Breathing

For older adults, the recommendation to breathe naturally during exercise performance is inadequate. Older adults must be careful to avoid breath holding, known as the **Valsalva maneuver**, because doing so can increase internal chest pressure to levels that impede blood flow, elevate blood pressure, and even cause light-headedness or blackouts (35). Consequently, the personal trainer should advise older adults to breathe continuously throughout every concentric and eccentric muscle action. More specifically, older adults should be trained to exhale throughout each concentric muscle action and to inhale throughout each eccentric muscle action, because this procedure facilitates smaller increases in internal chest pressure.

Aerobic Training Guidelines

Older adults are advised to perform 20 to 60 minutes of aerobic activity three to five days a week, depending on the exercise intensity (2). Training intensity may be estimated by the type of exercise performed, by heart rate response during the exercise session, or by perceived physical exertion using a 10-point scale. For most practical purposes, there is an inverse relationship between training intensity and training duration. For example, a 20-minute running session would be typically performed at a higher heart rate and perceived physical exertion, whereas a 60-minute walking session would typically be performed at a lower heart rate and perceived physical exertion. This section presents aerobic training recommendations for exercise selection, intensity, duration, and frequency for older adults.

Exercise Selection

Physical activities that involve rhythmic, large muscle movements are recommended for improving cardiovascular health and aerobic fitness. Weight-bearing activities such as walking, jogging, running, stair climbing, stepping, skating, cross-county skiing, elliptical training, and dancing are excellent forms of aerobic exercise. Older adults who have difficulty doing ambulatory activities may attain similar cardiovascular benefits by performing weight-supported aerobic exercises, such as recumbent cycling, upright cycling, rowing, water aerobics, and swimming. These activities may be interchanged without altering the aerobic adaptations. For example, an older adult may choose to cross-train during a given exercise session (e.g., treadmill walking and recumbent cycling) or do different aerobic activities on different days of the week. Regardless of the aerobic endurance exercises selected, the following performance factors are closely associated with the conditioning effects.

Exercise Intensity

Cardiovascular health benefits may be realized from performing moderate-intensity aerobic activity, such as walking, which increases exercise heart rate, on average, to approximately 65% to 75% of maximum heart rate (2). Cardiovascular health benefits and physical fitness benefits may be attained from performing vigorous-intensity aerobic activity, such as jogging or running, which increases exercise heart rate to approximately 75% to 95% of maximum heart rate (2). Because older adults may have relatively large variations in maximum heart rate and may take medications that affect heart rate response to exercise, other means of assessing training intensity have been recommended. One way is the 10-point scale of perceived physical exertion or exercise effort (2). Using the 0 to 10 scale of physical exertion, moderate-intensity aerobic activity generally corresponds to an exercise effort level of 5 or 6, whereas vigorous-intensity aerobic activity generally corresponds to an exercise effort level of 7 or 8. Another means for assessing training intensity is the talk test. Moderate-intensity aerobic activity can be performed while talking in regular sentences, whereas vigorous-intensity aerobic activity limits speaking to brief phrases or short questions and answers. A general guideline for older adults is to begin aerobic training with moderate-intensity aerobic activity and gradually progress to vigorous-intensity aerobic activity, assuming no health issues or physical limitations.

Exercise Duration

The recommendations for older adults for aerobic endurance exercise duration calls for 30 to 60 minutes a day of moderate-intensity aerobic activity or 20 to 30 minutes a day of vigorous-intensity aerobic activity (2). Although longer-duration aerobic endurance exercise sessions may be more beneficial, minimum-duration aerobic workouts should be both effective and manageable for most older adults. On a weekly basis, it is recommended to accumulate 150 or more minutes of moderate-intensity aerobic activity, or to accumulate 75 or more minutes of vigorous-intensity aerobic activity, or a combination of both intensity levels (2).

Exercise Frequency

The recommended exercise frequency for moderate-intensity aerobic activity is five or more days each week (2). The recommended exercise frequency for vigorous-intensity aerobic activity is three or more days each week (2). An older adult who chooses to perform both moderate-intensity aerobic activity and vigorous-intensity aerobic activity could do 40 minutes of walking on Mondays and Thursdays and 20 minutes of jogging on Wednesdays and Saturdays, for a combined exercise total of 120 minutes per week.

Older Adult Training Considerations

It is undoubtedly a greater health risk to continue a sedentary lifestyle than to begin a sensible exercise program. However, because of a variety of physical issues that may require specific training modifications, it is recommended that older adults check with their physician before beginning a physical conditioning program. Table 18.1 lists some of these conditions and adjustments that clients or personal trainers can make to promote a safe exercise experience.

Once approved for physical activity, older adults should emphasize resistance training for the musculoskeletal system and aerobic endurance exercise for the cardiovascular system, incorporating the training recommendations in this chapter. If they perform both activities during the same workout, the order of strength and aerobic endurance exercise is essentially a matter of personal preference (84). They should begin each training session with some warm-up activity (e.g., easy cycling or treadmill walking) and end each training session with similar cooldown activity that includes some flexibility exercise. Stretching may be performed most safely and effectively after physical activity when the muscles are warm and relaxed. It is also advisable for older adults to keep accurate records of their training sessions to document progress as well as to note any issues that may require activity alterations. If possible, older adults should have periodic body composition assessments to determine changes in lean mass and fat mass that cannot be ascertained by bodyweight measures.

TABLE 18.1 Conditions Common to Older Adults and Suggested Adaptations

Condition	Adaptations
Dry skin	Clients can apply lotion to elbows, knees, and contact points before exercising.
Poor balance	Clients should begin with weight-supporting machine exercises before progressing to weight-bearing free-weight exercises and functional training.
	Clients should begin with weight-supporting aerobic endurance exercise such as stationary cycling before progressing to weight-bearing alternatives such as treadmill walking and stair climbing.
	Clients should avoid hard-to-control exercises such as lunges or step-ups.
	Clients can perform exercises in a seated or lying position instead of standing.
Propensity for injuries	Clients should train only in uncluttered facilities.
	Clients should use controlled movement speeds.
	Clients should emphasize proper posture and exercise positioning.
Susceptibility to colds and flu	Clients should drink plenty of fluids.
	Clients should obtain ample rest and sleep (at least 8 h a night).
	Clients should shower or wash face and hands after exercise session.
Reduced flexibility	Clients should warm up for 5-10 min prior to exercise.
	Clients should perform appropriate stretching exercises at end of training session.
	Clients should avoid exercises that require extreme movement ranges such as lunges.
Reduced tolerance to heat and humidity	Clients should train in climate-controlled facilities whenever possible.
	Clients should schedule training sessions earlier in the day.
	Clients should drink plenty of fluids, especially water.
	Clients should wear lightweight and light-colored exercise attire.
Difficulties seeing, hearing, or both	Personal trainers should speak clearly and concisely with sufficient volume.
	Personal trainers should use large-print materials and workout cards.
	Personal trainers should give precise exercise demonstrations and manual assistance when necessary.
	Personal trainers should frequently ask clients if they understand instructions and exercise performance procedures.

Fall Prevention in Older Adults

The most prevalent cause of injury (both fatal and non-fatal) in older adults is falling. A predisposing factor in older adults' higher risk of falling is muscular weakness. Unfortunately, many older adults do not address this problem by performing muscle strengthening exercises, but instead choose to reduce their physical activities. Of course, this results in accelerated rates of muscle loss (sarcopenia), bone loss (osteopenia), and functional abilities, thereby increasing the risk and severity of falls. The American College of Sports Medicine (2) recommends balance training for older adults who are subject to falls or have mobility issues. Generally, balance training programs include progressions from more stable postures to less stable postures (e.g., double-leg stand to single-leg stand), less to more challenging locomotor movements (e.g., straight walking to circle walking), and higher to lower sensory input (e.g., standing with both eyes open to standing with both eyes closed).

In addition to balance training and home safety precautions (e.g., better lighting, nonslip surfaces, reduced clutter, glasses on when not in bed), older adults should perform appropriate resistance exercises to attain and maintain higher levels of muscular strength. As presented in the "Improved Physical Abilities" section, resistance training can significantly enhance an older adult's balance (4), movement control (6), walking speed (70), physical performance (40), and functional independence (85), all of which may reduce the risk of falling and associated injuries. It is therefore recommended that older adults perform regular resistance exercise, along with other appropriate practices, to lessen the likelihood of both falling and serious musculoskeletal injury in case of a fall.

PREGNANT WOMEN

Women who are pregnant may seek out exercise programs for a number of reasons. They may feel self-conscious about their changing bodies, be concerned about having a healthy baby, want to stay in shape throughout their pregnancies, want to be able to handle the physical rigors of labor and delivery, or need additional social interactions and support during this new phase in their lives. Healthy pregnant women without complications who exercise regularly may continue participating in appropriately adjusted sessions of physical activity, thereby maintaining cardiovascular and muscular fitness throughout pregnancy and the postpartum period (1, 3, 12).

Since most pregnant women do not achieve the minimum recommendation of weekly physical activity (9), personal trainers should address perceived barriers, such as lack of time, and raise awareness about the potential physical and mental benefits of exercise during pregnancy (16). Previously inactive women may also benefit from regular exercise during pregnancy, although a program consistent with their physical capabilities should involve professional guidance, motivation, and a gradual increase in physical activity (12, 13). For pregnant women not currently active, short bouts of walking can be sensibly integrated into a pregnancy lifestyle to overcome perceived barriers and improve health outcomes (3, 7). Of note, some pregnant women prefer to start exercising during the second trimester after the nausea, vomiting, and fatigue from the first trimester subside (10). In any case, pregnant women should consult with a health care provider before initiating an exercise program or modifying a current program. Likewise, elite female athletes who wish to become pregnant should discuss specific issues regarding their health and training program with their medical team (5). In the presence of obstetric or medical complications, it may be necessary to alter the exercise program or training regimen as determined by the client's obstetrician.

Benefits of Exercise During Pregnancy

Most pregnant women who follow physician recommendations can attain maternal health and fitness benefits while subjecting the developing fetus to minimal risk (4, 12, 13). According to the 2020 report of the American College of Obstetricians and Gynecologists Committee on Obstetric Practice, "Women with uncomplicated pregnancies should be encouraged to engage in aerobic and strength-conditioning exercises before, during, and after pregnancy" (1, p. e178). Other organizations also suggest combining aerobic exercise and resistance training during pregnancy instead of performing aerobic exercise alone to improve health outcomes (3, 12). The following are some of the benefits for pregnant women who engage in properly designed prenatal exercise programs (1, 3, 14, 17):

- Improved aerobic and muscular fitness
- Faster return to prepregnancy weight, strength, and flexibility levels
- More energy reserve

- Shorter active phase of labor and less pain
- Less maternal weight gain
- Improved mood, self-concept, and psychologic well-being
- Reduced feelings of stress, anxiety, and depression
- Increased likelihood of adopting permanent healthy lifestyle habits
- Decreased risk of gestational diabetes mellitus
- Decreased risk of cesarean and operative vaginal delivery
- Reduced risk of preeclampsia
- Fewer obstetric interventions
- Facilitated recovery from labor
- Reduced postpartum belly

Participation in an exercise program may also reduce the risk of developing conditions associated with pregnancy including **preeclampsia** (pregnancy-induced hypertension) and **gestational diabetes mellitus** (a form of diabetes first diagnosed during pregnancy) (1, 12, 14). It appears that the physiological and psychological benefits associated with regular physical activity may play a role in reducing the risk of preeclampsia (1,12, 14). Moreover, the favorable effects of regular physical activity on insulin secretion, insulin sensitivity, and glucose metabolism may improve glucose tolerance and thereby reduce a woman's risk of developing gestational diabetes mellitus (15). Exercise training may also be beneficial in preventing or treating other conditions including low back pain, pelvic floor muscle dysfunction, pregnancy-related urinary incontinence, and chronic musculoskeletal conditions (1, 12, 14). In the absence of either medical or obstetric complications, pregnant women should accumulate at least 150 minutes of moderate intensity exercise each week to achieve health benefits and reductions in pregnancy complications (3, 12).

> ▶ **Healthy pregnant women should be encouraged to participate in daily physical activity throughout pregnancy.**

Fetal Response to Exercise

Some research has revealed reduced birth weight in babies whose mothers performed a higher volume of moderate- to vigorous-intensity exercise throughout their pregnancies (6). The lower birth weight apparently resulted from a decreased amount of subcutaneous fat in the newborn. Moderate-intensity exercise accumulated over a minimum of three days per week may therefore be advisable for active pregnant women (12).

Maternal exercise during pregnancy is associated with a 10 to 30 beat/min increase in fetal heart rate, but there are no documented adverse fetal effects related to exercise-induced fetal heart rate changes (1). With respect to preterm labor, the American College of Obstetricians and Gynecologists states that in the majority of healthy pregnant women without additional risk factors for preterm labor, exercise does not increase either baseline uterine activity or the incidence of preterm labor or delivery (1).

Accommodating Mechanical and Physiological Changes During Pregnancy

Medical and fitness organizations provide the following recommendations for accommodating the cardiovascular, respiratory, mechanical, metabolic, and thermoregulatory changes experienced during normal pregnancy (1, 3, 12).

Cardiovascular Response

Because pregnancy alters the relationship between heart rate and oxygen consumption, personal trainers can use the RPE scale or the "talk test" to prescribe aerobic exercise intensity (3). Generally, an RPE rating on the original 6 to 20 scale between 13 and 14 (1) seems appropriate for moderate-intensity aerobic conditioning during pregnancy. At this intensity, pregnant women should be able to keep up a conversation while walking, swimming, or stationary cycling. Pregnant women who exercise at this intensity for 30 minutes at least five days per week will accumulate the recommended 150 minutes of moderate-intensity physical activity weekly (3). Since women who were highly active before pregnancy may exercise at a higher RPE (e.g., 14 to 17 on the 6 to 20 scale), exercise programs need to be individually prescribed, and women may need to adjust the exercise intensity, duration, or both on any given day depending on how they feel.

After the first trimester of pregnancy, the back-lying (supine) position results in restricted venous return of blood to the heart because of the increasingly larger uterus. This position reduces venous return and subsequent cardiac output and may cause supine hypotension (1, 3). Consequently, exercises performed on the back should be phased out of the client's training program before the start of the second trimester. These include abdominal curl-ups or sit-ups, bench presses, supine exercises on the stability ball, and stretching exercises with the back on the floor.

As an alternative, women can perform core exercises in the quadruped (on hands and knees) or side-lying position (see figures 18.3 and 18.4) and upper and lower body resistance training exercises in the seated position. For example, instead of performing the barbell bench press exercise to enhance upper body strength, pregnant women can use the vertical chest press machine or perform wall push-ups or a resistance band exercise in the seated position to strengthen the same muscle groups.

Because of changes in the center of gravity later in pregnancy, it also may be advisable for some pregnant women to use weight machines, which provide more stability and support than the corresponding free-weight exercises (e.g., machine biceps curl rather than standing dumbbell curl). This recommendation may be particularly important for previously sedentary women who want to resistance train.

Respiratory Response

Pregnant women may increase their minute ventilation by almost 50%, resulting in 10% to 20% more oxygen use at rest (1). Consequently, less oxygen is available for aerobic activity. Additionally, as the pregnancy progresses, the enlarging uterus interferes with diaphragm movement, increasing the effort of breathing and decreasing both subjective workload and maximum exercise performance. Personal trainers should adjust exercise programs accordingly so that pregnant women do not train at high levels of fatigue or reach physical exhaustion.

Pregnant women should be cautioned to avoid the Valsalva maneuver because breath holding during exertion places excessive pressure on the abdominal contents and pelvic floor. A general resistance training recommendation is to exhale on exertion or through the concentric phase of a repetition. (See chapter 13 for additional breathing guidelines.)

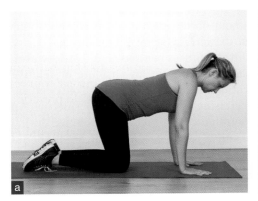 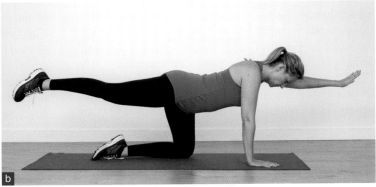

FIGURE 18.3   Core exercise performed in the quadruped position: *(a)* beginning position and *(b)* final position.

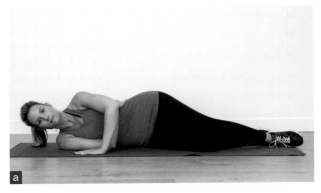 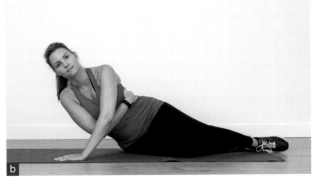

FIGURE 18.4   Core exercise performed in side-lying position: *(a)* beginning position and *(b)* final position.

Mechanical Response

As the uterus and breasts become larger during pregnancy, a woman's center of mass changes. This may adversely affect her balance, body control, and movement mechanics in some physical activities. Consequently, exercises requiring balance and agility should be carefully prescribed, with special attention to activity selection during the third trimester of pregnancy.

Although any activity that presents the potential for falling or even mild abdominal trauma should be avoided, some activities designed to enhance physical balance may be beneficial for pregnant women. For example, personal trainers may include gentle stretching and dynamic flexibility activities that may help women achieve physical balance during pregnancy and help them become more aware of body movements during exercise (3, 12). Because of joint laxity during pregnancy, exercises should be performed slowly and in a controlled manner to avoid damage to the joints. Furthermore, pregnant women should avoid participating in activities that present a high risk of falling or abdominal trauma. They should also avoid scuba diving because of the risk of decompression sickness to the fetus (1, 3).

Although it is important to strengthen all the major muscle groups, personal trainers should include pelvic floor muscle training because these muscles provide the basis for postural support and reduce the risk of urinary incontinence during and after pregnancy (3, 5, 12). Pelvic floor muscle training (e.g., **Kegel** exercises) involve tightening and relaxing muscle groups in the pelvic floor. With proper instruction, a woman can learn not only how to contract these muscles but also how to relax them so that the baby can be delivered more easily. Specific guidelines for performing Kegel exercises are beyond the scope of this chapter but are available in most books on pregnancy.

Metabolic Response

The need for more oxygen during pregnancy is paralleled by the need for more energy substrate. Pregnant women typically use an extra 300 kilocalories per day to meet the increased metabolic requirements for homeostasis of their expanded life functions. The obvious indication is for pregnant clients to attain an adequate intake of nutrient-dense foods and stay well hydrated through a balanced diet in accordance with dietary recommendations for the general population (11). Of note, pregnant women should be sure to take sufficient quantities of calcium, vitamin B_{12}, vitamin D, iron, and folic acid to achieve a healthy pregnancy outcome (11). Since the negative effects of poor mater-nal nutrition can be devastating, all pregnant women should receive nutrition counseling from a qualified professional to develop healthy habits that can be continued postpartum.

Thermoregulatory Response

Pregnancy elevates a woman's basal metabolic rate and heat production, which may be further increased by exercise. Exercise-associated rises in body temperature may be most likely in the first trimester of pregnancy. During this period, pregnant clients should facilitate heat dissipation through adequate hydration, appropriate clothing, and optimal environmental surroundings. If a client feels overheated or fatigued during an exercise session, the personal trainer should decrease the exercise intensity and begin the cooldown. Severe headaches, dizziness, and disorientation are indications of potential serious conditions that require referral to a client's health care provider. Pregnant women should be made aware of safe exercise guidelines and should know when to reduce the exercise intensity or stop exercising.

Contraindications for Exercise

Women without obstetric or medical complications can continue to exercise during pregnancy and derive related health and fitness benefits (1, 3, 12). However, certain conditions present an absolute or relative contraindication for exercise (see the "Contraindications for Exercising During Pregnancy" sidebar). An absolute contraindication precludes exercise during pregnancy and a relative contraindication should be evaluated by a physician before a pregnant client participates in exercise.

Additionally, any of the following warning signs is a reason to discontinue exercise and seek medical advice during pregnancy:

- Vaginal bleeding
- Abdominal pain
- Regular painful contractions
- Amniotic fluid leakage
- Dyspnea before exertion
- Dizziness
- Headache
- Chest pain
- Muscle weakness affecting balance
- Calf pain or swelling

Source: American College of Obstetricians and Gynecologists (1).

Exercise Guidelines

Although additional clinical trials are needed to further examine the effects of different types, frequencies, and intensities of exercise on the mother and baby, the following exercise guidelines apply to healthy pregnant women without exercise contraindications (1, 3, 12):

- Check with your health care provider before you begin exercising.
- Include a warm-up and cooldown period in any exercise program.
- Resistance training for the major muscle groups can be performed provided that a resistance permitting multiple repetitions (e.g., 12-15) is used. Isometric contractions and motionless standing should be avoided.
- Include pelvic floor muscle training such as Kegel exercises.
- Begin with short sessions and gradually increase to at least 20-30 minutes per day on most or all days of the week to accumulate at least 150 minutes of moderate-intensity aerobic exercise a week.
- Physical activities such as walking, swimming, or group exercise are favored for reducing injury risk and continuing the exercise program throughout pregnancy.

CONTRAINDICATIONS FOR EXERCISING DURING PREGNANCY

Absolute Contraindications

- Hemodynamically significant heart disease
- Incompetent cervix, cervical insufficiency, or cerclage
- Intrauterine growth restriction[a]
- Multiple gestation at risk for premature labor[b]
- Persistent second or third trimester bleeding
- Placenta previa after 26-28 wk of gestation
- Preeclampsia or pregnancy-induced hypertension[c]
- Premature labor during the current pregnancy
- Restrictive lung disease
- Ruptured membranes
- Severe anemia
- Uncontrolled or poorly controlled hypertension[d]
- Uncontrolled thyroid disease[e]
- Uncontrolled type 1 diabetes
- Unexplained persistent vaginal bleeding, such as in second or third trimester
- Other serious cardiovascular, respiratory, or systemic disorder

Relative Contraindications

- Anemia or symptomatic anemia
- Cervical dilation
- Chronic bronchitis, mild/moderate respiratory disease, or other respiratory disorders
- Eating disorder
- Extreme morbid obesity
- Heavy smoker
- History of extremely sedentary lifestyle
- History of spontaneous preterm birth, premature labor, miscarriage, or fetal growth restriction
- Malnutrition or extreme underweight
- Mild/moderate cardiovascular disease
- Orthopedic limitations
- Poorly controlled seizure disorder
- Poorly controlled type 1 diabetes
- Recurrent pregnancy loss
- Unevaluated maternal cardiac dysrhythmia
- Other significant medical conditions

[a]The American College of Obstetricians and Gynecologists (ACOG) guideline specifies intrauterine growth restriction in current pregnancy as a relative contraindication (2a).

[b]The Canadian guideline specifies triplets and higher as an absolute contraindication and a twin pregnancy after the 28th wk as a relative contraindication (12).

[c]The Canadian guideline specifies gestational hypertension as a relative contraindication (12).

[d]The ACOG guideline specifies poorly controlled hypertension as a relative contraindication (2a).

[e]The ACOG guideline specifies poorly controlled hyperthyroidism as a relative contraindication (2a).

Reprinted by permission from American College of Sports Medicine (2022, p. 187).

- Exercise should not continue past the point of fatigue and should never reach exhaustive levels but should be performed at a comfortable level at which you can maintain a conversation.

- Avoid straining or stretching to the point of discomfort.

- Exercise in the supine position should be avoided after the first trimester.

- Large increases in body temperature should be minimized through adequate hydration, appropriate clothing, and optimal environmental surroundings during exercise. Hot yoga and hot Pilates should be avoided.

- Stay well hydrated, and avoid exercising in hot, humid conditions.

- Wear proper footwear and loose-fitting clothing.

- Use equipment in good condition.

- Sports and activities that present the potential for even mild abdominal trauma or loss of balance should be avoided. Examples of sports and activities to avoid include soccer, basketball, horseback riding, scuba diving, in-line skating, outdoor cycling, and plyometric training.

- Do not exercise if you have a fever.

- See your health care provider if you experience bleeding, a large amount of discharge, or swelling in your face and hands.

- Because many of the physiological and morphological changes of pregnancy persist for several weeks postpartum, gradual exercise may begin approximately 4 to 6 weeks after a normal vaginal delivery or about 8 to 10 weeks (with medical clearance) after a cesarean delivery.

Postpartum Care

The weeks after pregnancy can be referred to as the "fourth trimester" since this critical period can influence the health and well-being of both the woman and infant (2). During the postpartum period, women are recovering from childbirth, caring for a newborn, and managing additional challenges that may include lack of sleep, pain, fatigue, urinary incontinence, or mental health disorders. Thus, comprehensive medical care during this time should include a full assessment of physical, social, and psychological well-being in order to address immediate needs and set the stage for long-

term health. Additionally, care during this period may include management of pregnancy-induced conditions such as diabetes or hypertension, other obesity-related disorders, or large accumulations of adipose tissue (2).

Since optimal postpartum care should promote the overall health and well-being of women, the importance of physical activity should not be overlooked. In addition to the cardiometabolic benefits of regular physical activity, strong evidence demonstrates that moderate-intensity physical activity, such as brisk walking, can reduce the symptoms of postpartum depression (8). By selecting enjoyable physical activities, socializing with family and friends, and setting realistic goals, women can improve a variety of physiological and psychological factors during the postpartum period through regular exercise.

In the absence of medical complications, physical activity can be resumed after pregnancy but should be done so gradually (3). Healthy women should be encouraged to be physically active and attain a healthy weight. Women who habitually engaged in moderate to vigorous physical activity before and during pregnancy may be able to resume aerobic and resistance exercise sooner provided they discuss their exercise plans with their primary maternal care provider (1, 3). In addition to exercises that enhance cardiovascular and musculoskeletal fitness, pelvic floor exercises should be incorporated into the postpartum exercise program. Performing Kegel exercises, or pelvic floor muscle training, postpartum can enhance the function of the pelvic floor musculature and reduce the onset of urinary incontinence (18).

CONCLUSION

Regular participation in physical activity can offer observable health and fitness benefits to preadolescent youth, older adults, and pregnant women. However, because each of these special populations has particular characteristics, personal trainers should be cognizant of exercise recommendations that address individual needs and abilities. In many cases, exercise modifications will be needed to enhance the safety, efficacy, and enjoyment of exercise programs for clients with special needs. Due to the health risks associated with physical inactivity throughout the life course, concerted efforts are needed to prescribe the appropriate volume of exercise in order to promote adherence, optimize adaptations, and enhance overall well-being.

Study Questions

1. What is the recommended amount of time youth should be encouraged to participate daily in moderate to vigorous physical activity?

   A. 15 minutes

   B. 30 minutes

   C. 45 minutes

   D. 60 minutes

2. On average, resistance exercise enables older adults to increase muscle mass by how much over a few months of resistance training?

   A. 1 lb (0.5 kg)

   B. 3 lb (1.4 kg)

   C. 5 lb (2.3 kg)

   D. 8 lb (3.6 kg)

3. The NSCA recommends that older adults begin resistance training with loads that can be lifted for approximately how many repetitions?

   A. 2-4

   B. 4-8

   C. 10-15

   D. 20-25

4. Which of the following is *not* a benefit of exercise during pregnancy?

   A. shorter active phase of labor and less pain

   B. fewer obstetric interventions

   C. increased possibility of preeclampsia

   D. reduced postpartum belly

5. Which of the following is *correct* regarding postpartum care and exercise?

   A. In the absence of medical complications, physical activity should resume gradually.

   B. Sedentary women are at no disadvantage beginning exercise following childbirth than women who engaged in regular exercise throughout pregnancy.

   C. Pelvic floor muscle training postpartum can reduce the onset of urinary incontinence.

   D. Moderate-intensity physical activity can reduce the symptoms of postpartum depression.

CHAPTER 19

Clients With Nutritional or Metabolic Concerns

Abbie Smith-Ryan, PhD, and Cassandra Forsythe, PhD, RD

After completing this chapter, you will be able to

- delineate the scope of practice of the personal trainer working with people who have nutritional or metabolic concerns;

- discuss the appropriate exercise prescription and program design for individuals who are obese or overweight, who have hyperlipidemia or diabetes, or who have an eating disorder;

- describe general nutritional guidelines for individuals with these nutritional or metabolic concerns; and

- discuss lifestyle change strategies (diet, exercise, and behavior changes) that will improve the health status of people with these nutritional or metabolic concerns.

Advances in technology, industrialization, and automation have reduced the demand for vigorous job-related tasks, increased sedentary time, and greatly increased food availability. Along with other factors, these societal changes have led to an increased prevalence of obesity, hyperlipidemia, and diabetes, as well as a trend toward disordered eating and eating disorders. Personal trainers are likely to encounter clients with one or more of these conditions and should therefore perform screening as described in chapter 9, obtaining medical clearance when needed (34).

SCOPE OF PRACTICE

Clients with the conditions discussed in this chapter should be referred to their physicians for medical care and to a registered dietitian (RD) for medical nutrition therapy; a personal trainer's role is limited to exercise program design and execution, along with lifestyle change support. Personal trainers should not diagnose or prescribe care for their clients nor accept or train clients who have medical conditions that may exceed their level of knowledge and experience. Instead, such clients should be referred to the appropriate health care professionals (34).

To explain further, personal trainers should always stay within their scope of practice and not engage in any modalities they are not trained in (such as skeletal manipulations, interpreting blood work, or prescribing a therapeutic diet). A personal trainer not only can harm a client because of lack of knowledge of these treatments but also may cause

The authors would like to acknowledge the significant contributions of Douglas B. Smith, Ryan Fiddler, Christine L. Vega, and Carlos E. Jiménez to this chapter.

permanent complications that could result in legal trouble. The first rule of any personal trainer is do no harm, so it is very important that personal trainers focus on what they are trained to do, which is to prescribe exercise programs based on clients' needs and desires and to monitor clients for correct exercise execution. They may give general nutrition advice based on the current Dietary Guidelines for Americans (27) to assist with weight loss and healthy eating patterns, but they should not try to prescribe a therapeutic diet, or create a rehabilitation plan for a client, or tell a client how or when to take medications based on their blood work. The personal trainer should always respect the top of the medical team—the medical doctor—and work respectfully with any other health care providers a client interacts with, becoming part of an effective team the client will remember positively.

> **Personal trainers must not diagnose or prescribe care, nor should they train clients with medical conditions outside of their knowledge and experience; instead, they should always refer the client to an appropriate health care professional and stay within their scope of practice as a personal trainer.**

OVERWEIGHT AND OBESITY

Worldwide, obesity tripled between 1960 and 2014, affecting more than 1.9 billion adults (38). According to 2017-2018 data from the U.S. National Health and Nutrition Examination Survey (NHANES), between 1999-2000 and 2017-2018, the prevalence of obesity (body mass index ≥30) in American adults (age 20+) increased from 30.5% to 42.4%, and the prevalence of severe obesity (body mass index ≥40) increased from 4.7% to 9.2% (45a). For men, 40.3% of those aged 20 to 39, 46.4% of those aged 40 to 59, and 42.2% of those aged 60 and over were classified as obese. For women, the figures are 39.7% of those aged 20 to 39, 43.3% of those aged 40 to 59, and 43.3% of those aged 60 and over (45a).

These figures may increase even more in the future: National surveys in the United States have shown that the prevalence of obesity in childhood and adolescence has more than quadrupled among children ages 6 to 11 years and more than tripled among adolescents ages 12 to 19 years (53); these increases have been associated with reduced activity levels (71, 78, 84, 88). The Office of the Surgeon General (82, 83) has reported several important findings:

- Risk factors for heart disease, such as high cholesterol and high blood pressure, occur with increased frequency in overweight children and adolescents compared with those of a healthy weight.
- Type 2 diabetes, previously considered an adult disease, has increased dramatically in children and adolescents.
- Overweight adolescents have a 70% chance of becoming overweight or obese adults, and this increases to 80% if one or more parent is overweight or obese.
- The most immediate consequence of overweight, as perceived by children themselves, is social discrimination.

Overweight and obesity are a significant public health problem. The condition of being overweight or obese raises the risk of morbidity from hypertension, hyperlipidemia, type 2 diabetes, cardiovascular disease, stroke, gallbladder disease, osteoarthritis, sleep apnea and respiratory problems, and endometrial, breast, prostrate, and colon cancers (58). Further, higher body weights and body fat percentages are associated with increases in all-cause mortality. Overweight and obesity have been designated as the second leading cause of preventable death in the United States (62, 63).

Definitions of Overweight and Obesity and Important Differences

A person whose weight is higher than what is considered a normal weight, when adjusted for height, is classified as being overweight or obese. **Overweight** is defined as a body mass index (BMI) of 25 to 29.9 kg/m^2 and **obesity** as a BMI of ≥30 kg/m^2 (62). The BMI describes relative weight for height and significantly correlates with total body fat content. BMI has limitations for individuals who are muscular (overestimates overweight and obesity) and for persons such as those of advanced age who have lost muscle mass (underestimates BMI) (63). The BMI should be used to assess overweight and obesity in addition to monitoring changes in body composition, if available (62, 63).

See "Body Mass Index" on pages page 247 in chapter 11 for the BMI formulas in pounds and inches or kilograms and meters. Table 11.4 on page 245 provides the National Heart, Lung, and Blood Institute (NHLBI) BMI classifications (62, 63, 64). See "Calculating BMI" on page 206 for examples of how to calculate BMI using nonmetric and metric units.

To select appropriate prevention strategies and design effective exercise programs, the personal trainer must understand the complex and important differences between overweight and obesity (13):

- People who are obese have a significantly greater excess of weight, particularly adipose tissue mass, than those who are overweight. Additionally, obese individuals have a higher percentage of fat mass as opposed to muscle mass.

- In general, persons who are obese are more likely to have had a larger positive energy balance over a longer time than those who are overweight. This positive energy balance is caused not only by a decrease in physical activity but also by an increase in food consumption (18). A neutral energy balance occurs when an individual is consuming as many calories as he or she expends, resulting in no change of body weight. A positive energy balance, or consuming more calories than are expended, will result in an increase in body weight; a negative energy balance, or the consumption of fewer calories than are expended, will result in a decrease in body weight.

- On average, a person who is obese has a higher resting metabolic rate and expends more energy on activities than those who are overweight or normal weight. The reason is that moving a heavy mass around requires more energy (18).

> Clients who are overweight may benefit simply by increasing physical activity along with some minor changes in their diets. Those who are obese should concentrate on both reducing caloric intake and increasing physical activity.

Causes and Correlates of Overweight and Obesity

No one theory completely answers the question of how and why obesity occurs. Although a positive energy balance—due to the increased availability of calorie-rich food coupled with a sedentary lifestyle—is a major factor in the worldwide increase in obesity, there are other factors to consider (87). The Surgeon General's *Overweight and Obesity: Health Consequences* reported that body weight is a combination of genetic, metabolic, behavioral, environmental, cultural, and socioeconomic influences and that behavioral and environmental factors contribute largely to overweight and obesity (83). These two factors may also provide the greatest opportunity for actions and interventions designed for prevention and treatment (83).

Environmental factors can include food availability, socioeconomic status, and lack of access to exercise facilities such as a gym or a track. Behavioral factors include eating patterns determined by individual preferences and ethnic backgrounds, including overeating or binge eating, and activity patterns (19). Genetic and metabolic factors can include differences in resting metabolic rate, levels of lipoprotein lipase and other enzymes, sympathetic nervous system activity, and dietary-induced thermogenesis. Some of these variables serve as true predictors of body fat gain, allowing them to be considered risk factors. In other cases, researchers do not know whether the relationship is causal or whether the correlate is secondary to being obese. In most cases, the associations are in fact secondary and are a result of obesity (18).

Decreasing sedentary behavior is a key factor for disease prevention, particularly in those who are overweight or obese (75). There is a significant linear relationship between hours of daily sedentary behavior and metabolic syndrome (41). Replacing sedentary time with exercise has been shown to significantly reduce cardiovascular disease, BMI, and cholesterol (47), supporting a key role personal trainers play in improving their clients' health.

Fat Distribution

It is important not only to note whether a client falls into the overweight or obese category but also to discern the pattern of fat distribution. There are two types of fat distribution: android obesity and gynoid obesity. **Gynoid obesity** (pear-shaped body) denotes the condition in which high amounts of body fat have been deposited in the hip and thigh areas. Alternatively, **android obesity** (apple-shaped body) is characterized by high amounts of body fat in the trunk and abdominal areas. This presence of excess fat in the abdomen, out of proportion to total body fat, acts as an independent predictor of disease risk for type 2 diabetes, hypertension, and CVD (62, 63).

Measuring Abdominal Fat

Researchers have suggested that central obesity poses a more significant CVD risk than does total obesity, and that waist circumference and waist/hip ratio may be better predictors of atherosclerosis and CVD risk than BMI (31, 58). Furthermore, there is a positive correlation between abdominal fat content and the waist circumference measurement (58, 63). The personal trainer can use waist circumference as a clinically acceptable measurement to assess the client's abdominal fat content before and during a weight loss program (58, 63). Proper measurement of the waist circumference is explained in chapter 11, page 211. For adult clients with BMIs between 25 and 34.9 kg/m², men whose waist circumference exceeds 40 inches (or 102 cm), and women whose waist circumference exceeds 35 inches (or 88 cm) have an increased risk of developing type 2 diabetes, dyslipidemia, hypertension, and CVD (58, 63). Note that these waist circumference limits are not useful in terms of incremental risk prediction in clients with a BMI ≥35 kg/m², as these individuals will automatically exceed the cutoff points because of their higher weight. The sidebar, "Assessing Abdominal Fat in Clients Who Are Overweight or Obese," contains practical recommendations for conducting measurements of abdominal fat in clients who are overweight or obese.

Skinfold measurement of persons who are obese can be difficult; correctly placing the calipers requires a good deal of experience. Additionally, the process can be demeaning to a client who is obese because of the size of the skinfold. Because BMI and waist circumference are easy to measure, personal trainers are encouraged to use these measurements for both initial and follow-up assessments. In fact, demonstrating the loss of inches can have a strong impact on a client, potentially improving adherence. Circumference measurements can also be taken of other parts of the body (e.g., the hips, arms, and thighs) to track progress in terms of weight loss.

If available, measurement of fat mass and fat free mass can be very helpful for tracking changes. A number of methods are available, with varied cost and portability (see chapter 11). Newer technology that may be useful incudes portable ultrasound (A-mode ultrasound) and 3D body imaging.

Controlling Cardiovascular Risk Factors Associated With Obesity

Table 11.4 on page 245 in chapter 11 adds the disease risk of increased abdominal fat to the disease risk of BMI (58, 63). As is evident, the increased abdominal fat distribution moves an individual in the overweight or the class I obesity category to an even higher disease risk category. The categories in the table indicate relative risk, not absolute risk (58, 63). In other words, the comparison of risk is being made relative to a normal weight. This is in contrast to the calculation of absolute risk for disease, which is determined by a summation of risk factors (62, 63).

Cardiovascular disease (CVD) is the leading cause of death for people of most racial and ethnic groups in the United States, including African Americans, Hispanics, and Caucasians (16). Risk factors for CVD include nonmodifiable factors, such as older age and family history. **Modifiable risk factors**—those that

ASSESSING ABDOMINAL FAT IN CLIENTS WHO ARE OVERWEIGHT OR OBESE

- Use waist circumference and BMI measurements in lieu of skinfold measurements.
- Conduct the assessment in a private setting and assure the client that no one else will see the results.
- Conduct the assessment in a matter-of-fact yet sensitive manner. Avoid uncomfortable humor.
- If the client is too embarrassed for someone to measure his or her waist, allow the client to conduct the measurement after having received instruction.
- Tell the client beforehand to wear thin clothing, and allow him or her to keep all clothes on during the measurement if he or she is uncomfortable about removing clothing. Although the measurement will not be as accurate, it will provide a starting point and avoid embarrassment.
- Retesting wearing the same clothing will keep the clothing's thickness a constant factor.
- The following cutoffs indicate an increased risk for type 2 diabetes, dyslipidemia, hypertension, and CVD in individuals with a BMI between 25 and 34.9 kg/m² (17, 18):

  Men: >40 inches (>102 cm)

  Women: >35 inches (>88 cm)

can be changed with lifestyle and behavior changes—include high blood pressure (hypertension), high total and LDL cholesterol levels (hyperlipidemia), diabetes, and obesity (particularly central obesity). These risk factors are often a result of lifestyle choices such as lack of physical activity, poor dietary habits, smoking, and excessive alcohol use.

Personal trainers can make a significant impact on risk for CVD by helping clients adopt a consistent physically active lifestyle that involves varied physical activities (biking, swimming, dancing) and a structured, supervised exercise regimen. Along with these positive changes in activity, the personal trainer can help clients adopt good eating habits, find a smoking cessation specialist if needed, and share resources that can help them reduce their alcohol intake if necessary. In clients who are overweight or obese, these consistent lifestyle changes should help them reduce their body weight to a more ideal number, which, according to the American Heart Association is a sustained loss of 3% to 5% of body weight (51). However, be mindful that weight loss should not be the only goal. In other words, the client must understand that an increase in physical activity, along with the cessation of smoking and the consumption of a heart-healthy diet, with or without weight loss, will still significantly improve health status. This allows personal trainers to measure the success of their interactions with a client not only in weight loss but also in positive lifestyle changes.

Benefits of Exercise in a Weight Reduction Program for Obesity

Including physical activity in a weight reduction program provides physiological and psychological benefits. The exact mechanism by which physical activity affects weight loss, and the degree to which it does so, is not yet completely understood; regardless, exercise should be included in a weight loss program to ensure a better chance of success. A review of the literature showed that adults with obesity who participated in physical activity realized modest weight loss and a lowering of the risk factors for CVD (82). Importantly, physical activity appears to confer cardioprotective benefits irrespective of whether or not weight is lost (57a).

It seems that some of the physiological benefits of exercise may not translate to weight loss as much as previously thought. For example, a person with obesity who has low aerobic fitness is often unable to perform exercise of sufficient duration or intensity

to expend enough calories to meet the targeted daily caloric deficit. Hence, although the exercise session is important, a decrease in calories consumed would have an even greater effect on weight loss. Still, an exercise program is important for its positive effect of lowering the risk factors for CVD, along with other general physiological and psychological benefits (see "Benefits of Exercise in a Weight Loss Program").

The psychological and emotional benefits of exercise deserve further research, but the existing studies and experiential data indicate such benefits do occur. An exercise program that improves motivation and commitment also leads to the possible psychological outcomes of increased well-being and mood, improved body image, improved self-esteem and self-efficacy, and improved coping abilities (13). For example, the enhanced well-being and self-esteem produced by physical activity may generalize to other areas of life and lead to improved dietary adherence. In other words, the client feels more productive and more in control of his or her life and is therefore better able and more willing to make the proper choices of food and portion sizes. Figure 19.1 (13) provides an overview of the proposed mechanism and potential pathways that link exercise to success in weight control.

BENEFITS OF EXERCISE IN A WEIGHT LOSS PROGRAM

- Increases energy expenditure
- Reduces the risk of heart disease more than weight loss alone
- May help reduce body fat and prevent the decrease in muscle mass that often occurs during weight loss
- May decrease abdominal fat
- Decreases insulin resistance
- May contribute to better dietary compliance, including reduced caloric intake
- May not prevent the decline in resting metabolic rate associated with a low-calorie diet, but may minimize the decrease
- Improves mood and general well-being
- Improves body image
- Increases self-esteem and self-efficacy
- Serves as a coping strategy

Based on NIH and NHLBI (63); Baker and Brownell (13).

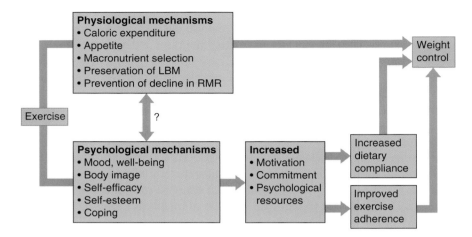

FIGURE 19.1 Proposed mechanisms linking exercise and weight control.

LBM = lean body mass; RMR = resting metabolic rate.

Reprinted by permission from Baker and Brownwell (2000, pp. 311-328).

Although the results of research on the benefits of physical activity for weight loss are mixed, strong evidence indicates physical activity is necessary for long-term weight maintenance (81). Regular physical activity not only improves weight loss and physical fitness during the weight loss phase of a weight management program but also ensures that clients maintain their target weight over time. One of the main goals of the personal trainer should be to help clients establish the habit of consistent exercise.

> Although physical activity may or may not help a client lose weight, it reduces many obesity-related risk factors and is critical for long-term weight maintenance.

Successful Weight Management Programs for Obesity

In general, the most successful weight management programs consist of a combination of diet modification, increased physical activity, and lifestyle change (62, 63). Personal trainers work with their clients not only to increase physical activity levels but also to provide support for lifestyle change, which includes finding ways to be more physically active at work (walking up a floor to the restroom, taking the stairs rather than the elevator) or at home (gardening, pushing a lawnmower, raking leaves, shoveling); finding a community of people who enjoy eating healthy more often than not and exercising regularly while being social (like being part of group fitness classes); and reducing unhealthy lifestyle habits such as smoking or excessive drinking.

Dietary Modification

The majority of clients who are overweight or obese need to adjust their diets in order to achieve a caloric deficit resulting in weight loss. Personal trainers should refer these clients to a registered dietitian. The RD will most likely evaluate the client's diet, design an appropriate calorie-reduced yet nutrient-dense diet, offer follow-up, answer questions and address concerns, and solve any problems. Referral to an RD is highly recommended for clients who are obese and who have hyperlipidemia, and it is necessary for clients with diabetes. (Diabetes is managed by a physician, normally in conjunction with an RD.)

To be effective, the diet must be designed in accordance with the client's cultural and ethnic background, should include the client's food preferences, should take into account the availability and cost of the food in the diet, should contain a selection of foods that will decrease the risk of other nutritionally related cardiovascular risk factors such as hyperlipidemia and high blood pressure, and should fit into the client's particular lifestyle (63). To help meet these goals, the diet should follow the latest Dietary Guidelines for Americans (27) and meet the Dietary Reference Intakes (DRIs) for all nutrients. Once the diet is individualized to the client's needs and preferences, the personal trainer can be of great help in supporting and motivating the client to adhere to the diet.

Most weight loss in persons who are obese occurs primarily because of decreased caloric intake. The NHLBI guidelines recommend that a diet be individually planned to create a deficit of 500 to 1,000 kcal per day to facilitate a weight loss of 1 to 2 pounds (0.5-0.9 kg) per week. This moderate reduction in calories is recommended to achieve a slow yet progressive weight loss. Excess weight will gradually decrease with this level of caloric intake. (The target amount also depends on the amount of exercise the client performs on a daily basis; in other words, if the client expends 250 kcal a day in an exercise session, the diet may have to be reduced by only 250 to 750 kcal per day, which may make it easier to adhere to.)

The exact calorie load for each individual is determined with the calorie calculation formulas on page 110 of chapter 7 and trial-and-error adjustments. It is recommended that caloric intake be reduced only to the level required to maintain weight at a desired level.

As a general guideline, women should consume diets containing no fewer than 1,200 to 1,500 kilocalories (kcal)/day, and men should consume a diet no lower than 1,500 to 1,800 kcal/day (63). Intakes of 1,200 to 1,600 kcal/day may also be appropriate for women who weigh 165 pounds (74.8 kg) or more, or for women who exercise regularly (63). If a client consumes a 1,600 kcal/day diet and does not lose weight, it may be advisable to try the 1,200 kcal/day diet. On the other hand, if a client gets hungry on the lower-calorie diet or is without sufficient energy to make it through the day or to engage in physical activity, he or she may need to consume an additional 100 to 200 kcal/day (63).

Very-low-calorie diets (VLCDs) of less than 800 kcal/day are sometimes used when needed for weight loss in obese individuals (BMI >30 kg/m²). VLCDs should be prescribed only by physicians with specialized training and experience. These diets require special monitoring and supplementation and should be used only in limited circumstances (65).

Overall, a variety of dietary approaches can produce weight loss in overweight and obese adults (60, 61b). The sidebar, "Scientifically Supported Dietary Approaches for Weight Loss," lists dietary approaches to weight loss that are supported by strong scientific evidence if reduction in dietary energy intake is achieved (61b).

Although it is outside the scope of practice for personal trainers to offer dietary prescription and counseling to their clients, personal trainers can support their clients' efforts by offering nutrition education or orientation. Topics may include low-calorie food choices, low-fat food preparation techniques, food label reading, holiday eating strategies, the importance of adequate hydration, ways to include more fruits and vegetables in the diet, and so on.

> **Dietary prescription or counseling is beyond the personal trainer's scope of practice; instead, the personal trainer can offer nutrition education and discuss the concept of fueling around workouts. Clients can follow many dietary approaches to achieve weight loss.**

Weight Loss Guidelines

An initial and reasonable goal of a weight loss program is about 10% reduction in body weight. A reasonable time to achieve this goal is six months (63). After six months, the personal trainer along with the dietitian and physician can set new goals. Even if the client only reaches this initial 10% reduction and maintains it, he or she has accomplished a significant decrease in the severity of the obesity-associated risk factors (62, 63). In fact, the literature indicates that a reduction of only 3% to 5% of body weight is sufficient to achieve a reduction in health risk (4).

Many clients find it difficult to lose weight after the first six months because of a decrease in their resting metabolic rate as well as in their motivation to continually follow a diet and exercise regimen. Additionally, their energy requirements decrease as their weight decreases (less mass to move around means less workload). Thus, an even larger increase in the dietary goals (further decrease in calories) and physical activity goals (further increase in activity levels) is needed to create an energy deficit at the lower weight (63).

After the initial goal of a 7% to 10% reduction in body weight has been achieved, the personal trainer and client can set new goals for weight loss, if appropriate. The benefits of achieving a moderate weight loss over a long period of time far outweigh the benefits of losing a great deal of weight quickly only to gain most of it back. This situation of weight regain, especially when repeated a number of times, undermines the benefits of participating in a weight loss program in terms of time spent, financial costs, and possible decreases in self-esteem (63).

SCIENTIFICALLY SUPPORTED DIETARY APPROACHES FOR WEIGHT LOSS

- The European Association for the Study of Diabetes guidelines, which focus on targeting food groups rather than formal prescribed energy restriction while still achieving an energy deficit. The diet recommends six or more servings of whole-grain breads and cereals, three or more servings of vegetables and two of fruit, two or more servings of low-fat milk, and one or more servings of lean meat, dried beans, or lentils. The guidelines advise reducing dietary fat, salt, and sugar intakes.

- Higher-protein diet (25% of total calories from protein, 30% of total calories from fat, and 45% of total calories from carbohydrate), with provision of foods that realize an energy deficit.

- Higher-protein Zone-type diet (five meals per day, each with 40% of total calories from carbohydrate, 30% of total calories from protein, and 30% of total calories from fat) without formal prescribed energy restriction but with a realized energy deficit.

- Lacto-ovo-vegetarian diet (no meat, fish or poultry; only dairy and eggs) with prescribed energy restriction.

- Low-calorie diet with prescribed energy restriction.

- Low-carbohydrate diet (initially <20 g/day carbohydrate) without formal prescribed energy restriction but with a realized energy deficit.

- Low-fat vegan-style (no animal foods at all) diet (10% to 25% of total calories from fat) without formal prescribed energy restriction but with a realized energy deficit.

- Low-fat diet (20% of total calories from fat) without formal prescribed energy restriction but with a realized energy deficit.

- Low-glycemic-load diet, either with formal prescribed energy restriction or without formal prescribed energy restriction, but with realized energy deficit.

- Lower-fat (≤30% fat), high-dairy (four servings per day) diets with or without increased fiber or low-glycemic-load foods with prescribed energy restriction.

- Macronutrient-targeted diets (15% or 25% of total calories from protein; 20% or 40% of total calories from fat; 35%, 45%, 55%, or 65% of total calories from carbohydrate) with prescribed energy restriction.

- Mediterranean-style diet with prescribed energy restriction.

- Moderate-protein diet (12% of total calories from protein, 58% of total calories from carbohydrate, and 30% of total calories from fat) with provision of foods that realize an energy deficit.

- High-glycemic-load or low-glycemic load meals with prescribed energy restriction.

Reprinted from National Heart, Lung, and Blood Institute (61b).

> **Reducing body weight by 7% to 10% over six months is an appropriate initial goal; at that time, new goals can be set. It is much better to lose a moderate amount of weight relatively slowly than to lose a large amount quickly and then regain most of it. Many dietary approaches and exercise regimens can be used to achieve sustainable weight loss.**

Physical Activity

Moderate levels of physical activity for at least 30 minutes, most days of the week, are recommended for clients who are overweight or obese and who are beginning an exercise program (62, 63). A moderate level of physical activity is defined as the amount of activity that uses approximately 150 kcal/day, with a total of approximately 1,000 kcal/week (2). In fact, the Centers for Disease Control and Prevention, the American College of Sports Medicine (ACSM), the

Surgeon General, and the National Institutes of Health (NIH)/NHLBI make the following recommendation as expressed in the NHLBI *Practical Guide*: "All adults should set a long term goal to accumulate at least 30 minutes or more of moderate-intensity physical activity on most, and preferably all, days of the week" (63, p. 3). A review of the most current literature on this subject reinforces these guidelines. The ACSM recommends a minimum of 150 to 300 minutes per week of moderate-intensity (40%-59% $\dot{V}O_2R$ or heart rate reserve [HRR]) or 75 minutes of vigorous-intensity (≥60% $\dot{V}O_2R$ or HRR) physical activity to effectively prevent weight gain for individuals who are overweight or obese (2). Furthermore, the guidelines suggest that overweight and obese clients progress to a level of physical activity of at least 250 minutes per week or 50 minutes per day five days a week to enhance long-term weight loss maintenance (2). For the purposes of weight loss, some individuals may need to progress to 60 to 90 minutes per day of moderate- to vigorous-intensity physical activity. Examples of moderate amounts of physical activity are shown in table 19.1 (63).

It is important to consider the concept of progression when designing a physical activity program for a client. Many clients who are obese may not be able to start with a moderate-level activity program. For these clients, the initial activities may have to be low in intensity or even simply a matter of focusing on increasing the tasks of daily living. For example, clients might

- take a walk after lunch,
- walk to a coworker's desk or office instead of using the phone,
- use stairs instead of an elevator or escalator,
- walk to pick up lunch instead of ordering a delivery,
- get off the bus or subway at least one stop early and walk the remainder of the way,
- park in a space at the mall that is farther from the entrance and requires more walking,
- walk to the neighborhood mini-mart to pick up milk instead of driving the block or two,
- walk the dog,
- do yard work, or
- play actively with children or grandchildren.

A well-designed progressive program reduces injury risk in addition to making the beginning exercise sessions comfortable and tolerable. Many people with obesity, because of their sedentary lifestyles, have very low functional capacities. What may seem like a moderate intensity or a moderate amount of physical activity to a personal trainer may actually be a great

TABLE 19.1 Examples of Moderate Amounts of Physical Activity

Common chores	Sporting activities	Less vigorous, more time*
Washing or waxing a car for 45-60 min	Playing volleyball for 45-60 min	↑
Washing windows or floors for 45-60 min	Playing touch football for 45 min	
Gardening for 30-45 min	Walking 1.75 miles (2.8 km) in 35 min	
Wheeling self in wheelchair for 30-40 min	Basketball (shooting baskets) for 30 min	
Pushing a stroller 1.5 miles (2.4 km) in 30 min	Bicycling 5 miles (8 km) in 30 min	
Raking leaves for 30 min	Dancing fast (social) for 30 min	
Walking 2 miles (3.2 km) in 30 min	Water aerobics for 30 min	
Shoveling snow for 15 min	Swimming laps for 20 min	
Stair climbing for 15 min	Basketball (playing a game) for 15-20 min	
	Jumping rope for 15 min	↓
	Running 1.5 miles (2.4 km) in 15 min	More vigorous, less time

Note: A moderate amount of physical activity is roughly equivalent to physical activity that uses approximately 150 kcal of energy per day, or 1,000 kcal per week.

*Some activities can be performed at various intensities; the suggested durations correspond to expected intensity of effort.

Adapted from NIH and NHLBI (63).

challenge to an obese individual. An exercise program that is too demanding may lead to soreness to which clients are unaccustomed. These uncomfortable sensations may lead to a loss of motivation, discouraging a client from continuing with the program.

As clients lose weight and increase their functional capacity, exercise of increased intensity and increased duration can be programmed. Although longer sessions of moderate-intensity activities (such as fitness walking) can involve the same amount of activity and caloric expenditure as shorter sessions of higher-intensity exercises (such as running), it is best to go with the longer-duration, lower-intensity exercise (at least at the start of the program) in order to prevent injury and promote adherence to the program. Examples of appropriate exercises include fitness walking, fitness swimming, aqua fitness classes, indoor and outdoor cycling, rowing, hiking, square dancing, and aerobic dance in addition to resistance and flexibility training.

An additional 100 to 200 kcal/day expended doing common chores and recreational activities will promote an even larger caloric deficit with a concomitant increase in fat loss, functional capacity, and lean body mass (63). All this increased activity along with programmed exercise sessions will add up and contribute to the caloric deficit needed to ensure weight loss and subsequent weight maintenance.

> **Individuals who are obese may need to start with low-intensity activities to increase their physical activity each day. Keep progression in mind, and slowly move them to more moderate-intensity exercises as their capacity increases. Their long-term goal is to accumulate 30 minutes or more of moderate-intensity physical activity on most, and preferably all, days of the week.**

Lifestyle Change Support for Obesity

Lifestyle change support consists of various strategies that can help clients adhere to their physical activity and diet programs. Lifestyle change support helps clients identify the obstacles that are keeping them from following the program and then uses a problem-solving approach to design and implement strategies to overcome these obstacles. It is not easy for anyone to change well-established behaviors and to overcome the obstacles to those changes. Specifically, the techniques of self-monitoring, rewards, goal setting, stimulus

control, and dietary behavior changes may help clients see how continuing with their current weight loss or weight maintenance program and will allow them to make realistic long-term lifestyle changes (67).

Self-Monitoring of Lifestyle Changes

The practice of clients' taking note of their activity and diet behaviors and recording them is referred to as **self-monitoring**. Recording food and calorie intake, bouts of exercise and physical activity, moods when eating, where a food was eaten, weight lost or gained, and so forth can provide valuable information for both the personal trainer and the client. Further, in some cases, just self-monitoring a behavior can bring about positive changes as clients become keenly aware of what they are doing and can make immediate changes (63). Self-monitoring can help the client and personal trainer

- identify behaviors that put the success of the program at risk,
- identify obstacles to engaging in physical activity or eating healthfully, and
- chart progress to both motivate the client and serve as a basis for the reward system.

As an example of identifying risky behaviors, a diet history form that notes the food consumed, time of food consumption, site of food consumption, and even the mood of the client at the time may reveal that the client tends to eat high-calorie snacks, in relatively large amounts, when sitting in front of the television. The client could be advised to prepare a bowl of cut fresh vegetables or a controlled amount of unbuttered popcorn to consume during a show. Or clients may detect on the form that upon arrival home from work they make a trip directly to the refrigerator to eat whatever is available. They could solve this problem by eating a piece of fruit on the way home and then waiting until the planned dinner is prepared and on the table.

Self-monitoring of exercise behaviors also helps identify obstacles to engaging in the prescribed amount of physical activity. For example, the client and personal trainer may have agreed that they would meet twice a week for a resistance training session and that the client would engage in a 30- to 45-minute walk on alternate days. Inspection of the exercise self-monitoring form may reveal that the client exercised on the days when an early morning walk before work was scheduled. Conversely, when the client planned to walk in the afternoon, he or she never got around to it because of work constraints and finally was too tired to exercise upon arrival at home. This client would need to plan future exercise sessions in the morning.

Rewards for Lifestyle Accomplishments and Changes

Rewards can be used to encourage and acknowledge attainment of the client's behavioral goals or specific outcomes. An effective reward is something that is desirable to the client, awarded on a timely basis, and contingent upon meeting the goal (63).

Rewards can be big or small, tangible or intangible, awarded by the client's family or by the client, or awarded to the client by the personal trainer. Tangible rewards include items like a new blouse, an exercise outfit, or a book. Intangible rewards usually include some pleasant use of time such as a fishing excursion, an afternoon at the mall, quiet time to read a book, or a weekend getaway to a country inn. Usually, small rewards are given for attainment of steps within the goal or a short-term goal, while bigger awards are granted for attaining a long-term goal, such as the target 10% reduction of body weight within a six-month period. Ideally rewards should not revolve around food.

Goal Setting for Weight Loss and Lifestyle Change

Goal setting is covered in chapter 8. When a personal trainer is working with clients who are overweight or obese, it is especially important to set goals that are realistic and to set short-term goals within long-term goals. For example, a client may have the goal of losing 20 pounds (9.1 kg) over a six-month period. Breaking this down to 3 to 4 pounds (1.4-1.8 kg) per month enables the client to celebrate the attainment of each goal. Fortunately, if the client does not achieve the whole weight goal in the first six months but has achieved some of the smaller goals, he or she will most likely still feel motivated to continue the program (85).

However, focusing only on weight loss goals as opposed to behavior change can set clients up for failure. Using behavior change goals in addition to weight loss goals will help clients see the value in continuing the program, even when they experience plateaus in weight loss. For example, a goal may be to walk 40 minutes at least four times per week. If the client meets this goal, he or she is successful, regardless of the amount of weight lost.

Goal setting is to be used in conjunction with self-monitoring and rewards. Additionally, the client can commit to a self-contract. In a self-contract, the client usually outlines a desired goal or behavior (e.g., to lose half a pound [0.2 kg] per week for a total of 2 pounds [0.9 kg] per month; to walk 30 minutes at least four times per week). The client will also decide on the reward for achievement of the goal. The "Activity and Exercise Contract" on page 528 is an example of a self-contract.

Stimulus Control for Weight Loss

Stimulus control consists of identifying the social or environmental cues that seem to trigger undesired eating patterns or nonparticipation in physical activity and then modifying those cues (4). Sometimes the term *environmental trigger* is used in place of *stimulus*, because triggering is exactly what happens. Something in the environment sets off an undesirable behavior, and the client starts engaging in unwanted eating patterns. For example, a client may always eat popcorn and drink a soda at a movie despite not being hungry, overeat at a buffet, overeat while working at his or her desk, or tend to have rich desserts when out with a particular friend.

Using the self-monitoring strategy, reflection, or both, the client may be able to identify these cues in the environment and problem solve ways to manage the situation. For example, clients who eat popcorn at the movies even when they are not hungry could eat either a smaller meal or a salad before leaving home and then enjoy popcorn while watching the movie. If a client eats large amounts at a buffet, a solution could be to go only to restaurants where food is served from a menu. Clients who unwittingly overeat while working at their desks may be advised to make a rule to snack only away from the desk. Clients who tend to overeat or overdrink when they go out with a particular friend may need to decide to meet the friend for a nonfood activity like shopping or going for a walk. The problem-solving step either seeks to eliminate the cue or to manage it in a way that prevents overeating.

Food Consumption Behavior Changes

Food consumption behavior changes may also help the client eat less without feeling deprived (63). Some clients should be encouraged to slow the rate of eating. Eating too fast does not allow the body time to identify the satiety signals that develop before the end of a meal. Clients can also use smaller plates to make portion sizes appear bigger. The use of smaller plates is also recommended at buffets to prevent taking large amounts of food. Some clients do best by eating only three meals a day in order to avoid eating too many snacks, while others do better with four to six small meals because they tend to overeat at a meal when they eat only three times per day. Clients who tend to skip or delay meals and overeat later because they are overly hungry must consider tightly scheduling their meals to avoid this problem. Because every client is different, there is no recipe for eating patterns that will work best for each. Through trial and error, the personal trainer and client will find what works best.

ACTIVITY AND EXERCISE CONTRACT

I, _____ , will incorporate the following activity or exercise into my daily/weekly schedule for the week of _____ .

Extra physical activities* I will incorporate into my daily routine:

Activity	Where	When	Number of times performed	Duration

Formal exercise sessions** in which I will participate:

Name of exercise or program	Where	When	Duration	Time per week

*Examples include taking the stairs at work and taking a 10-minute walk at lunch.

**Examples include a session with a personal trainer, a 30-minute walk, an aerobics class, or lap swimming.

If I fulfill this one-week contract, I will reward myself by:

_____

_____

_____

Signature: _____ Date: _____

From *NSCA's Essentials of Personal Training*, 3rd ed., edited for the National Strength and Conditioning Association by B. Schoenfeld and R. Snarr (Champaign, IL: Human Kinetics, 2022).

Exercise Concerns of Clients Who Are Overweight or Obese

There are a number of physiological and biomechanical concerns to consider when working with individuals who are overweight or obese. The following concerns may affect the exercise program design, exercise selection, and instruction of the client (79): heat intolerance, movement restriction and limited mobility, weight-bearing stress, posture problems and low back pain, balance concerns, and hyperpnea and dyspnea.

Heat Intolerance

Heat intolerance is a result of the added insulation of excess fat. Compared with persons of average body composition, it is harder for individuals with obesity to thermoregulate, especially under hot and humid conditions (4). The personal trainer should encourage clients to wear loose-fitting clothes when working out in moderate and hot temperatures. On particularly hot or humid days, any of the following modifications should be considered: lowering the intensity of the workout to avoid discomfort and a possible heat emergency; training in a temperature-controlled environment; swimming or performing aqua exercise for the cardiovascular training component of the workout; conducting the resistance training in the pool; and water walking and jogging in the pool. Personal trainers must ensure that the client stays hydrated (see chapter 7 for recommendations).

Movement Restriction and Limited Mobility

In people who are obese, movement restriction or limited mobility due to the excess fat mass may require the modification of various exercises (4). For example, excess fat on the thigh and calf may make it difficult for a client to perform a quadriceps stretch with the leg held behind and the foot pressed into the buttock. For a more suitable quadriceps stretch, the client could lower the back knee and press the hips forward from a calf stretch. Alternatively, the client could perform an active stretch of the quadriceps by using the hamstring muscles to bend the knee as far back as the fat mass allows while performing a pelvic tilt to put the hip into extension. Although these modifications might not allow a full stretch of the quadriceps, they would provide some flexibility training benefit.

As another example, a client may be unable to reach his or her leg (because of the restriction imposed by the abdominal fat mass) in order to move it toward the chest during a back-lying hamstring stretch. In this case, the client could wrap a towel around the back of the thigh to perform the assisted passive stretch, or simply perform an active stretch of the hamstrings by using the hip flexors to put the leg into the stretch position. The personal trainer needs to observe the client performing various stretches and exercises in order to make the modifications specific to the client's limitations.

Weight-Bearing Stress

Weight-bearing stress on the joints is a concern for people who are overweight or obese, especially those who have osteoarthritis or musculoskeletal injuries (72). Low-impact activities, not necessarily low in intensity, will prevent some of this stress. For example, fitness walking causes less stress to the joints than jogging or running. Other low-impact activities include indoor and outdoor cycling; swimming; aqua aerobics; shallow-water walking, jogging, and aerobics; deep-water running; hiking; and rowing (not advised if the client has a movement restriction due to the fat mass). Activities that require sustained single-limb support (standing on one leg for an extended period of time while performing exercises with the other leg) can also impose an excessive weight-bearing stress on the involved joints, especially the hips. Many traditional aerobics classes and balance activities include such standing legwork. A way to avoid this situation is to alternate the supporting leg frequently when performing these exercises.

Posture Problems and Low Back Pain

Because of the stress of the abdominal fat mass on the spine and often inadequate strength of the muscles of the abdominal wall, posture problems and low back pain are not uncommon in persons who are obese. This situation may cause lordosis of the lower spine, with or without an accommodating kyphosis of the upper spine, along with other possible postural changes. Further, the hip flexors in persons with obesity can be quite strong owing to the repeated load of moving a large mass around; this further contributes to the muscular imbalance caused by weaker abdominal muscles. Therefore, the personal trainer must prescribe a variety of exercises to strengthen the abdominal muscles along with flexibility exercises for the hip flexors (e.g., iliopsoas). Because of the larger fat mass and weaker abdominal muscles, some abdominal exercises may have to be modified. Further, attention must be given to exercises to strengthen the muscles of the upper back and increase the flexibility of the chest muscles. Clients with significant or chronic low back pain should be referred to an orthopedist for an evaluation. The physician may refer the client to a physical therapist for a back education and rehabilitation program in addition to the personal training sessions.

Balance Concerns

Clients who are obese may have little experience in movement and sport and may not have had the chance to develop good balance. Unfortunately, when clients do start to fall because of lack of balance in a movement, the excess weight, lack of experience in proprioceptive adjustments, and lack of adequate strength can contribute to a greater difficulty in righting themselves. Therefore, the personal trainer should include balance training, but on a progressive basis, and needs to observe, correct, and spot the client during the various exercises that require good balance.

Hyperpnea and Dyspnea

Hyperpnea (increased respiratory rate) and dyspnea (labored or difficult breathing) during exercise can be both uncomfortable and a source of anxiety to clients who are obese (72). Although some hyperpnea or dyspnea is expected during an exercise session, persons with obesity may experience more because of their low functional capacity. This condition can be disquieting and uncomfortable enough to cause them to give up on the exercise training due to fear. The personal trainer can avoid problems in this area by ensuring that clients are working at the appropriate exercise intensity by using a rating of perceived exertion scale (see chapter 16). The use of interval training, especially at the beginning of an exercise program, is highly recommended because the rest intervals (active or inactive) will allow clients to bring their breathing into better control. With time, the work intervals can be increased, and the rest intervals can be decreased.

Exercise Prescription and Program Design for Clients Who Are Overweight or Obese

The components of a well-rounded exercise program for those who are obese or overweight include aerobic conditioning, resistance training, and flexibility training (table 19.2; 2). The personal trainer and client must first come to an agreement regarding how many days a week they will schedule and the content of the workout sessions. For example, they could decide that the personal training sessions will consist of all three of the components or only a warm-up followed by a resistance and flexibility training program. This would mean the client would perform aerobic conditioning on days alternate to the personal training session days, before the personal training sessions, or both. The initial sessions should contain the aerobic conditioning phase so that the personal trainer can supervise, instruct, motivate, and ensure that the client is working both correctly and efficiently on the cardiovascular training program. If the client has any difficulty complying with the cardiovascular program, this component should remain within the personal training session.

Aerobic Conditioning

A typical exercise prescription for a person who is overweight or obese calls for five days of participation in an aerobic conditioning program to ensure that the client expends the maximal calories possible during the week and establishes a regular physical activity habit. Some clients may not be able to start with the full cardiovascular component of the exercise program. In this case the beginning sessions need to be low in intensity, and the client would also be asked to work at increasing daily living activities as described earlier. Even when clients do achieve a full workout, it is important to encourage meeting their daily activity levels so they expend more calories, thereby enhancing weight loss.

Some individuals will have a very low fitness level, making it difficult to walk one lap of a track without stopping to rest. In such a situation, the personal trainer should consider a circuit training program. For example, the client would walk one-half of the track, stop to do a bodyweight calisthenic or exercise with a band, walk another half lap, stop to perform another exercise for 10 to 20 repetitions, and so on until he or she has walked a mile. With time, the client would increase the length of the walk intervals until he or she can walk half a mile before stopping to do half of the resistance exercises, and then complete the next half-mile before performing the last half of the resistance exercises. Eventually the client will be able to walk a mile or two without stopping before doing the exercises.

TABLE 19.2   Exercise Prescription for Clients Who Are Obese

Mode	Frequency, intensity, duration	Guidelines and concerns
Aerobic conditioning	• Minimum recommendation = 30 min most days of the week (150 min/week) • ≥5 days/week to maximize caloric expenditure • Eventual goal = 300 min/week • Moderate intensity (40%-59% $\dot{V}O_2R$ or HRR) to vigorous intensity (≥60% $\dot{V}O_2R$ or HRR)	• Use low-impact activities. • Take appropriate precautions because of increased risk of orthopedic injury, cardiovascular disease, and hyperthermia. • Initially emphasize increasing duration rather than increasing intensity to optimize caloric expenditure. • Modify equipment as necessary (e.g., wide seats on cycle ergometers and rowers). • Intermittent exercise of at least 10 min in duration is an effective alternative to continuous exercise.
Resistance training	• 2 or 3 days/week on nonconsecutive days • 1 or more sets initially progressing to 2-4 sets of 8-12 reps per set • Initial loads of 60-70% 1RM • Training for each major muscle group (chest, shoulders, upper and lower back, abdomen, hips, and legs) • Gradual load increases	• Can begin with bodyweight exercises. • Can intersperse with aerobic exercise. • Modify equipment as necessary (e.g., larger-framed machines). • Can complement aerobic conditioning (i.e., to maintain or gain lean body weight).
Flexibility training	• 2 or 3 days/week • Hold static stretches for 10-30 s, 2-4 repetitions of each exercise.	• Perform stretches for all the major muscle groups. • Stretch to the point of feeling tightness or slight discomfort.

Adapted from ACSM (2).

Resistance Training

A position stand by the ACSM (4, p. 466) states that "although the effects of resistance training on body weight and composition may be modest, resistance training has been associated with improvements in CVD risk factors in the absence of significant weight loss." Furthermore, the position stand cited research supporting the following benefits of resistance training: improvements in high-density lipoprotein cholesterol (HDL-C) (52), low-density lipoprotein cholesterol (LDL-C) (42, 47), and triglyceride levels (70); improvements in insulin sensitivity (28, 30, 48, 52); reductions in glucose-stimulated plasma insulin concentrations; and reductions in systolic and diastolic blood pressures (50, 66). The design of the resistance training program will depend on the available equipment along with the abilities and limitations of the client. It is recommended that the personal trainer check with the client for any orthopedic problems such as hip, back, or knee injuries and modify the program and specific exercises accordingly. Clients can start with bodyweight exercises and move on to machines or light free weights. The personal trainer must keep in mind that the client has a built-in workload with the excess body weight.

People who are obese are often quite strong in the lower body because of adaptations from carrying excess body weight. Hence, upper body strength should be well addressed in a training session. Still, since the major goals of the resistance training session are to expend calories and increase muscle mass, emphasis should be on the largest muscle groups and core exercises; the client should not spend a great deal of time on the smaller muscle groups. In general, one should follow the guidelines for resistance training presented in chapters 13 and 15.

Flexibility Training

Although stretching exercises typically do not result in large expenditures of energy, they are important for preventing injury and maintaining range of motion around the joints. Light stretching can be included in the warm-up, while more intense stretches would be included at the end of an exercise session or after resistance training exercises in order to develop flexibility. This timing ensures that the muscles are well warmed and thus more pliable. Stretches should be performed for all the major muscle groups.

Stretches must be modified in accordance with the client's structural and physiological limitations. The personal trainer must be cognizant of the limited range of motion of clients who are overweight or obese. For instance, in a sitting toe touch, the client may only be able to reach just below the knees. In this case, the goal would not be to reach the toes but to stretch until light tension is felt.

Obesity Paradox

Despite the negative consequences of obesity, it should be noted that many obese individuals are still healthy (53). In fact, obese individuals with moderate aerobic fitness have a lower health risk than their leaner counterparts with low aerobic fitness (53). The personal trainer should understand that obesity is not the primary factor when creating a program for a client. Baseline fitness should be the primary consideration as opposed to weight when establishing where to start with a client.

HYPERLIPIDEMIA

Blood lipid disorders, including hyperlipidemia and dyslipidemia, are risk factors for CVD. **Hyperlipidemia** is a general term for elevated concentrations of any or all of the lipids (fats) in the blood, such as cholesterol, triglycerides (TGs), and lipoproteins. Called *high cholesterol* by the general population, hyperlipidemia usually indicates high levels of low-density lipoprotein (LDL) cholesterol with or without high TGs (43, 44). The term **dyslipidemia** refers to abnormal lipid (fat) levels in the blood, lipoprotein composition, or both. Hyperlipidemia-associated lipid disorders are considered the cause of **atherosclerotic cardiovascular disease** (hardening of the arteries, which can lead to heart attack and stroke); thus, treatment of hyperlipidemia plays a crucial role in the management of patients with CVD or those at increased risk of CVD. Moreover, increased LDL cholesterol levels are found to be positively correlated with increased CVD risk and are often the focus of physicians (14). Because LDL cholesterol contributes to fatty buildups and narrowing of the arteries (**atherosclerosis**), it is often called the "bad" cholesterol. High LDL cholesterol at any age can cumulatively increase the risk for heart disease and stroke.

In 2013, the American College of Cardiology (ACC) and the American Heart Association (AHA) released guidelines for treatment of high blood cholesterol to update the previous Adult Treatment Panel III (ATP III) report of the National Cholesterol Education Program (64). In 2018, these guidelines were updated (45) to reflect a paradigm shift in the treatment of high blood cholesterol. Under the 2018 guidelines, there is no ideal target blood level for LDL cholesterol, but in principle, "lower is better" and an optimal total cholesterol level is about 150 mg/dL, with LDL cholesterol at or below 100 mg/dL. The new guidelines also deemphasize the importance of high-density lipoprotein (HDL) cholesterol, terming it "seemingly non-atherogenic," whereas previously, high HDL cholesterol was thought to be protective. Experts believe that HDL acts as a scavenger, carrying LDL (bad) cholesterol away from the arteries and back to the liver, where the LDL is broken down and passed from the body. But HDL cholesterol does not completely eliminate LDL cholesterol. Only one-third to one-fourth of blood cholesterol is carried by HDL. However, a healthy HDL cholesterol level may protect against heart attack and stroke, while low levels of HDL cholesterol increase risk. HDL cholesterol levels can be improved with diet and exercise.

If a client has diagnosed high cholesterol, it is important for the personal trainer to communicate with the client's physician. The physician will be the one to monitor levels and suggest pharmacological treatment if changes in the client's lifestyle do not improve blood lipid concentrations.

Possible Causes of Hyperlipidemia

Table 19.3 offers a review of the possible causes and treatment of unfavorable LDL, HDL, and triglyceride levels (10, 45).

High LDL cholesterol levels are related to family history, genetic disorders, overweight and obesity, sedentary lifestyle, smoking, poor (atherogenic) diet, prediabetes (insulin resistance, glucose intolerance), diabetes, and other diseases as well as certain drugs (e.g., βblockers, anabolic steroids, progestational agents) (10, 45). The personal trainer can help clients increase their physical activity levels, assist them with weight reduction, and suggest improved dietary choices based on the Dietary Guidelines for Americans (27), all of which can play a role in reducing LDL cholesterol levels (12).

The possible causes of low HDL levels, which are also correlated to insulin resistance, include elevated triglycerides, overweight and obesity, physical inactivity, and type 2 diabetes. Other causes include cigarette smoking, high carbohydrate intake (especially simple sugars), and certain drugs.

TABLE 19.3 Possible Causes of and Treatment Strategies for Unfavorable Lipid Levels

Lipid	Possible etiology (possible causes)	Possible treatment strategies[a]
High LDL levels	• Abdominal obesity • Sedentary lifestyle • Overweight and obesity • Poor diet[b] • Insulin resistance • Glucose intolerance • Genetic predisposition • Genetic disorders • Other diseases, such as hypothyroidism, obstructive liver disease, chronic renal failure • Certain drugs (e.g., progestins, anabolic steroids, corticosteroids)	• Weight reduction • Improved dietary choices • Reduced calorie consumption where appropriate • Increased physical activity • Drug therapy • Control of other risk factors (such as smoking, hypertension)
Low HDL levels	• Overweight and obesity • Sedentary lifestyle • Elevated triglycerides • Insulin resistance • Type 2 diabetes • Cigarette smoking • High carbohydrate intake (>60% of kilocalories) • Certain drugs (e.g., βblockers, anabolic steroids, progestational agents)	• Control of LDL level • Weight reduction • Physical activity • Smoking cessation • Improved diet, including control of caloric and carbohydrate intake • Drug therapy
Triglycerides	• Overweight and obesity • Sedentary lifestyle • Cigarette smoking • Excessive alcohol intake • High carbohydrate intake (>60% of kilocalories) • Insulin resistance • Other diseases, such as type 2 diabetes, chronic renal failure, nephritic syndrome • Certain drugs (e.g., corticosteroids, estrogens, retinoids, higher doses of βblockers) • Genetic disorders	• Control of LDL level • Physical activity • Weight reduction • Improved diet including control of caloric and carbohydrate intake • Restriction of excessive alcohol intake • Drug therapy

[a]The client's physician will decide on each client's specific treatment strategy in accordance with that person's specific condition and its severity.

[b]A poor diet is high in saturated fats, high in trans fatty acids, high in calories, high in simple sugars, low in fruits and vegetables, or any combination of these.

Adapted from Grundy et al. (45) and Arnett et al. (10).

Factors that can raise triglycerides to higher than normal levels in the general population include obesity and being overweight, lack of physical activity, cigarette smoking, excess alcohol intake, and high-carbohydrate diets, as well as several diseases (type 2 diabetes, chronic renal failure, and nephritic syndrome) and genetic disorders and some medications.

Lifestyle Treatment for Hyperlipidemia

The ACC/AHA recognizes that the foundation for managing risk factors for CVD is adoption of a healthy lifestyle (10, 45). This includes achieving a healthy body weight, increasing physical activity, and stabilizing blood sugar levels through healthier dietary patterns. These changes will improve the lipid profile and provide other benefits for the cardiovascular system, muscular system, and overall mental health (7). People with hyperlipidemia should consume a diet that emphasizes intake of vegetables, fruits, whole grains (oats, rice), legumes (black beans, kidney beans, edamame), lean protein sources, and nontropical vegetable oils (olive oil, canola oil), while limiting intake of sweets, sugar-sweetened beverages, and red meats (10). These recommendations should be adjusted based on appropriate calorie requirements, personal and cultural food preferences, and nutritional therapy for other medical conditions, including diabetes. Caloric intake should be adjusted to prevent weight gain, or in overweight or obese patients, to promote weight loss. The dietary pattern for lowering blood cholesterol levels is commonly known as a heart-healthy diet, especially when combined with physical activity and weight loss, if needed. It is best to work with an RD to help clients achieve these dietary goals; the personal trainer should focus on helping clients exercise effectively and achieve an ideal body composition.

Physical activity and changes to other lifestyle factors can improve hyperlipidemia. In general, adult clients should engage in at least 150 minutes per week of accumulated moderate-intensity or 75 minutes per week of vigorous-intensity aerobic physical activity (or an equivalent combination of moderate and vigorous activity) (10). If they are unable to meet these goals, engaging in at least some moderate- or vigorous-intensity physical activity, even if less than the recommended amount, can be beneficial. They also should be encouraged to discontinue smoking, reduce alcohol intake, and manage stress levels through exercise and other healthy behaviors.

Dietary Fat Modification

The ACC/AHA urge people to eat a healthy diet and decrease consumption of saturated fats and trans fats (10, 45). Saturated fats are found mostly in animal products such as red meat, milk, cheese, butter and cream, and tropical oils (i.e., palm oil and coconut oil). They are usually solid at room temperature. Trans fatty acids are formed when a liquid fat is converted to solid fat through a process called hydrogenation. Many manufacturers use hydrogenated fats and oils (which contain trans fatty acids) in their ingredients because it increases the shelf life and improves texture and consistency. There are currently no safe levels of trans fat to consume each day, so clients should keep their daily intake as low as possible.

To keep trans-fat intake low, clients should avoid foods that contain partially hydrogenated oils (most processed foods like cookies, crackers, fried snacks, and baked goods). These will contain some level of trans fat, even if the label states "trans-fat free." Avoid using shortening, an example of trans fat in its purest form. Finally, many fast foods and fried foods are currently high in trans fatty acids. Some restaurant chains now use nonhydrogenated or trans-fat free oils to fry their foods. Overall, look for foods that are labeled "trans-fat free" or those that use liquid vegetable oils instead of hydrogenated oils in the ingredient list.

To encourage healthy fat intake, clients should choose foods rich in monounsaturated and polyunsaturated fats from olive and canola oils, nuts, seeds, avocados, olives, flaxseed, soy, and fatty fish such as salmon.

Omega-3 is one type of essential polyunsaturated fat that has additional protective benefits against cardiovascular disease, including lowering triglycerides, protecting against irregular heartbeat, decreasing the risk of a heart attack, and lowering blood pressure. Fish are good food sources of omega-3, especially cold-water fish like mackerel, salmon, herring, and sardines. Smaller amounts of this protective fat can be found in flaxseeds, chia seeds (salvia), walnuts, soybeans, and canola oils. To reap the protective benefits of omega-3 fatty acids and other beneficial nutrients in these foods, clients should incorporate fish into at least two meals per week and add plant-based sources of omega-3 fats, such as algae (from supplements). Plant omega-3 sources (walnuts and flaxseeds) have other benefits for cardiovascular health beyond just the essential omega-3 fats and should be included in the diet regularly.

For dietary cholesterol, recommendations were updated in 2015 by the American Heart Association and the Dietary Guidelines for Americans (27). Doctors and RDs previously advised a limit of dietary cholesterol of 300 mg per day, with 200 mg recommended if a person had active heart disease. Now, through substantial research and observation, the limits on dietary cholesterol have been lifted. Research has shown that dietary cholesterol itself is not harmful and does not significantly increase the body's blood cholesterol levels and thus CVD risk (20). Cholesterol is a natural substance produced in the body and is found in animal-based foods. It's a precursor for most hormones (testosterone, estrogen, progesterone) and is necessary to support healthy levels of vitamin D in the blood. We need cholesterol in our bodies and our diets (in reasonable amounts) for optimal health. The body produces most of the cholesterol it needs in the liver and intestines from fats, sugars, and proteins, and any excess in the diet is balanced by a change in the body's internal production.

Problems arise when individuals consume too many saturated and trans fats in their diets, not necessarily dietary cholesterol. These fats cause the liver to produce too much LDL ("bad") cholesterol, which winds up in artery-clogging deposits. For this reason, experts generally recommend avoiding trans fats altogether and limiting saturated fats through smart food choices. However, replacing saturated and trans fats with carbohydrates (versus unsaturated fats) is not the answer; a diet high in carbohydrates and very low in fats does not reduce LDL cholesterol; rather, it decreases HDL ("good") cholesterol, increases triglycerides, and is hard for most people to follow (74). Unhealthy fats should be replaced with mono- and polyunsaturated fatty acids.

Limiting Sugar From Beverages and Foods for Heart Health

The American Heart Association (AHA) recommends limiting the amount of added sugars people consume to no more than half of their daily discretionary calorie allowance because of the relationship between increased sugar intake, particularly sugar-sweetened beverages, and decreased cardiometabolic health (49). For most American women, that is no more than 100 kcal per day, or about six teaspoons of sugar (30 g). For men, it is 150 kcal per day, or about nine teaspoons (45 g). The AHA recommendations focus on all added sugars, without singling out any particular types, such as high-fructose corn syrup. The Dietary Guidelines for Americans (27) also puts a limit on sugar to 10% of calories per day from added sugars for optimal health and ideal body weight, which equates to 200 kcal (50 g of sugar). Overall, limiting sugar in the diet is a recommendation all people can benefit from.

Sugar-sweetened beverages (SSBs) are the largest source of added sugar in the diet. They include carbonated and noncarbonated soft drinks, fruit drinks, and sports drinks that contain added caloric sweeteners and are low in nutritional quality. A large body of evidence supports a strong link between intake of SSBs and weight gain and risk of type 2 diabetes, which is the basis of many dietary guidelines and policies targeting SSBs (49). Consumption of sweetened beverages is also a significant risk factor for cardiovascular diseases and related issues.

The personal trainer can encourage clients to meet their hydration needs with water or other nonsweetened beverages rather than sports drinks. Clients who use sugar in their coffee or tea can be encouraged to use as little as possible. If water is not their preferred beverage because of taste, a good substitute is filtered water, or a squeeze of lemon might improve the taste. Another option is nonsweetened sparkling water, which in a study conducted and published in the *American Journal of Clinical Nutrition* was found to be just as hydrating as plain water (56).

Exercise Prescription and Program Design for Clients With Hyperlipidemia

Regular physical activity is one of the lifestyle therapies advocated by the ACC/AHA for prevention and treatment of high blood cholesterol levels and CVD. These guidelines are derived from the 2018 Physical Activity Guidelines for Americans (69). Regular physical activity lowers CVD risk by improving blood lipid levels, reducing blood pressure, reducing insulin resistance (improving blood sugar levels), and improving cardiovascular function.

A significant change since the 2008 Physical Activity Guidelines for Americans in the 2018 recommendations (69) is that previously, aerobic physical activity for adults had to be accumulated in bouts, or sessions, that lasted at least 10 minutes to count toward meeting the key guidelines. Evidence shows that the total volume of moderate to vigorous physical activity is related to many health benefits; bouts of a prescribed duration are not essential. Sufficient physical activity for cardiovascular health and reducing blood cholesterol is defined as

- at least 150 minutes of moderate-intensity physical activity (e.g., 30 minutes, five days a week), or
- at least 75 minutes of vigorous-intensity physical activity (e.g., 25 minutes, three days a week), or
- a combination of moderate- and vigorous-intensity aerobic activity, and
- at least two days of moderate- to high-intensity muscle strengthening activities (such as resistance training) for additional health benefits.

A resistance training program is recommended (24) and should follow the guidelines provided in chapter 15. In light of these benefits, it is prudent for the personal trainer to provide clients with a well-rounded exercise program that includes aerobic, resistance, and flexibility training components.

Any activity is better than nothing, so if clients cannot make it to the gym to work out five days a week, they can engage in lifetime physical activities—those they can do alone or with a group of people, such as bicycling, hiking, kayaking, or dancing, and that they can do throughout their lifetimes. The personal trainer can even organize a group hike for clients to encourage them to try new activities and promote regular daily physical activity.

METABOLIC SYNDROME

Metabolic syndrome (MetS) is a progressive (develops slowly over time) pathophysiological state that puts a person at increased risk for developing metabolic disease (such as type 2 diabetes) and atherosclerotic cardiovascular disease (77). The components of MetS include abdominal obesity, atherogenic dyslipidemia (hyperlipidemia, or low HDL cholesterol, or both), elevated blood pressure (hypertension), and insulin resistance with or without glucose intolerance (elevated blood glucose concentrations). This syndrome has also been referred to as *syndrome X*, *cardiometabolic syndrome*, *dyslipidemic hypertension*, and *insulin resistance syndrome*, but *MetS* is the term most used by health care professionals. The *Third Report of the Expert Panel on Detection, Evaluation, and Treatment of High Blood Cholesterol in Adults (Adult Treatment Panel III) Executive Summary* from 2001 (64) offers the most accepted clinical definition of this syndrome.

Persons having three or more of the following criteria are defined as having MetS (37, 64):

1. Abdominal obesity: waist circumference >40 inches (>102 cm) in men and >35 inches (>88 cm) in women
2. Hypertriglyceridemia: ≥150 mg/dl (1.69 mmol/L)
3. Reduced HDL-cholesterol: <40 mg/dl (1.04 mmol/L) in men and <50 mg/dl (1.29 mmol/L) in women
4. Elevated blood pressure: ≥130/85 mmHg
5. Elevated fasting glucose: ≥100 mg/dl (≥5.5 mmol/L)

Disease risk and risk of adverse health outcomes rise exponentially with an increased number of MetS elements, and there are other elements of MetS not typically measured in a clinical setting or as widely appreciated such as high apolipoprotein B, small LDL particle size, endothelial dysfunction, and prothrombotic and proinflammatory states. A disadvantage of these criteria is that they do not fully encompass the pathophysiological complexity of the syndrome; recognize predisposition to different types of end-organ damage; or account for health disparities according to race, sex, or socioeconomic status (SES) in screening or treatment (77). For example, Malay women with MetS had different factor patterns with greater importance of hypertension, insulin resistance, and triglycerides when compared with other South Asian women (9). This and other findings (26) emphasize

the variability of race, sex, and SES that is not well captured by standard MetS paradigms. Thus, personal trainers must be mindful of the diversity of their clients, both in their interest and desire to exercise and their potential ability to screen for disease risk factors.

In U.S. adults, the prevalence of the MetS is 35% in men and 33% in women and increases dramatically with increasing obesity (41). In fact, its increase in prevalence parallels the rise in obesity and type 2 diabetes (6). Because it is forecasted that over half of the U.S. population will be obese by the year 2030, rates of MetS will almost certainly rise over the next decade.

People with MetS often have apple-shaped, or android, body types, characterized by high amounts of fat in the trunk and abdomen. Researchers have found that abdominal fat cells deposit high amounts of triglycerides into the bloodstream. The nearby liver uptakes this fat and produces VLDL (very-low-density lipoprotein) molecules, which transport triglycerides to the cells of the body. Upon releasing triglycerides, VLDLs convert into LDLs. It is these LDL molecules that carry large amounts of cholesterol and deposit it around the body. Therefore, high levels of LDL cholesterol molecules in the bloodstream are associated with an increased risk of coronary heart disease and stroke due to the progression of atherosclerosis. The elevation in triglycerides is also believed to disrupt blood glucose regulation. The resulting rise in insulin levels may, in turn, stimulate sympathetic nervous system regulation, which increases blood pressure.

The MetS has both a genetic and a behavioral component. Family history increases one's risk for developing this syndrome, in addition to cigarette smoking, a sedentary lifestyle, alcohol consumption, a poor diet, and stress. Early intervention that includes weight loss through dietary modification and enhanced physical activity can significantly delay or prevent the development of this syndrome (40, 46).

Exercise and Dietary Modification for MetS

Exercise and proper nutrition are the first line of treatment for MetS because they influence all components of this disorder. These lifestyle choices are modifiable risk factors that can prevent and reverse MetS and its consequences.

Regular physical activity helps reduce excess body fat. Exercise also improves the sensitivity of the cells to insulin, thus normalizing blood insulin levels and decreasing blood glucose levels. It helps decrease blood pressure and can increase HDL cholesterol levels. Ross and Despres (73) reported that leading health organizations promote the use of physical activity as a therapeutic strategy for management of MetS (73); even in the presence of MetS, increased physical activity is associated with a substantially reduced risk of atherosclerotic CVD (20).

Nutritional modification for MetS should focus on dietary patterns (food groups and food choices) rather than specific macronutrients, given inconclusive evidence to date for a positive independent effect of macronutrient composition on reduced disease risk (63) and long-term adherence rates. Balanced dietary patterns that stress whole foods and limit sugar, saturated and trans fats, and processed foods, such as the Mediterranean diet, have been shown to reduce blood pressure, improve lipids, reduce inflammation, and optimize body weight (35, 36). Healthy dietary patterns for reducing MetS criteria include foods that have a high content of vitamins, minerals, antioxidants, fiber, and unsaturated and omega-3 fatty acids (36).

Personal trainers should work in conjunction with the client's physician and an RD to ensure the client's success in dealing with the various conditions of MetS (1). They can encourage their clients to follow the Dietary Guidelines for Americans (27) and promote a balanced, whole food approach.

> ▶ **Early intervention that effects weight loss through dietary changes and increased physical activity can significantly delay or prevent the onset of metabolic syndrome.**

DIABETES MELLITUS

Diabetes mellitus is a group of metabolic diseases characterized by an excessively high (or uncontrolled) blood glucose level. Some of the signs and symptoms of diabetes include

- increased frequency of urination,
- increased thirst,
- increased appetite, and
- general weakness.

The diagnosis of diabetes mellitus is based on two separate fasting glucose levels of 126 mg/dl or higher. Other options for diagnosis include two 2-hour postprandial (i.e., after a meal) plasma glucose measurements of 200 mg/dl or higher after a glucose load of 75 g or two casual glucose readings of 200 mg/dl. Chronic uncontrolled diabetes is associated with long-term damage to various body organs including the eyes, kidneys, nerves, heart, and blood vessels. Diabetes is the leading cause of blindness, renal failure, and lower extremity amputations.

Types of Diabetes

The major types of diabetes mellitus are type 1, type 2, and gestational diabetes. **Type 1 diabetes mellitus**, formerly known *as insulin-dependent diabetes mellitus (IDDM)* or *juvenile diabetes*, is associated with pancreatic beta cell destruction by an autoimmune process, usually leading to absolute insulin deficiency. Approximately 10% of patients with diabetes have type 1, and most of these people develop the disease before the age of 25. Exogenous insulin by either injection or pump is required for survival. People with uncontrolled or newly diagnosed type 1 diabetes are prone to developing diabetic ketoacidosis. Diabetic ketoacidosis is a metabolic acidosis caused by the accumulation of **ketones** (a fuel the body will make from fat when it cannot use glucose because of insulin insensitivity) owing to severely depressed insulin levels. The initial symptoms are frequent urination, nausea, vomiting, abdominal pain, and lethargy. If left untreated, the condition may progress to coma.

Type 2 diabetes mellitus, formerly referred to as *non–insulin-dependent diabetes mellitus (NIDDM)*, is characterized by insulin resistance in peripheral tissues and an insulin secretory deficit of the pancreatic beta cells. This is the most common form of diabetes mellitus (about 90% of cases) and is highly associated with a family history of diabetes, older age, obesity, poor dietary choices, and lack of exercise. The treatment for type 2 diabetes usually includes diet modification, weight control, regular exercise, and oral hypoglycemic agents.

Gestational diabetes mellitus is a condition during pregnancy in which glucose levels are elevated and other diabetic symptoms appear during pregnancy in women who have not previously been diagnosed with diabetes. Gestational diabetes is not caused by a lack of insulin but by **insulin resistance**. Insulin resistance is an impaired response of the body's cells to insulin, therefore reducing the ability to clear glucose from the bloodstream and resulting in elevated blood glucose levels. All diabetic symptoms usually disappear after delivery, but affected mothers are at increased risk of developing type 2 diabetes mellitus later in life. Approximately 6% of all pregnant women in the United States are diagnosed with gestational diabetes (54). Treatment for gestational diabetes typically includes dietary modification and exercise, but when those methods do not work, doctors may prescribe medications or insulin.

Exercise Prescription and Program Design for Clients With Diabetes Mellitus

Exercise is an essential component of diabetic management. In both types of diabetes mellitus, exercise can increase insulin sensitivity and glucose use, thus lowering blood glucose levels and medication requirements (28). In addition, regular physical activity reduces other risk factors related to CVD such as hypertension, dyslipidemia, and obesity. Although exercise is highly beneficial for clients with diabetes, there are some potential complications, such as **hypoglycemia** (a low blood glucose level of 65 mg/dl or lower), that the personal trainer needs to keep in mind when designing and supervising an exercise program (22, 23).

Before beginning an exercise program, clients with diabetes should have a medical evaluation to assess their glycemic control and to screen for any complications that may be exacerbated by exercise. Cardiac stress testing performed by a medical professional is also generally recommended for all clients with diabetes who are planning to engage in moderate-intensity exercise and are considered at risk for heart disease. This group includes clients who are older than 35 years, those with type 2 diabetes of more than 10 years' duration, those with type 1 diabetes of more than 15 years' duration, and those with evidence of microvascular disease (retinopathy or nephropathy) (22, 23).

Clients exhibiting organ damage from long-standing diabetes need to be careful and must abstain from certain exacerbating physical activities. For example, individuals with peripheral neuropathy are at an increased risk of ulceration and infection of the feet because of lack of sensation and decreased healing reaction. Therefore, in this condition, low-impact exercises, such as swimming and biking, may be preferable to walking and jogging. Also proper footwear—shoes that are comfortable and well fitted—is essential to prevent blisters and other foot injuries. Any dizziness, weakness, or shortness of breath should alert the per-

sonal trainer to the possibility of cardiac disease and the need for a medical evaluation. Contraindications to exercise for persons with diabetes are listed in the following sidebar.

Glycemic Control and Exercise

The principal risk of exercise among those who have diabetes is hypoglycemia (blood glucose level of 65 mg/dl or lower). This is of greater concern for patients who have type 1 diabetes than for those with type 2 (33).

Factors that predispose to hypoglycemia during exercise include

- increased exercise intensity,
- longer exercise time,
- inadequate caloric intake before exercise,
- excessive insulin dose,
- insulin injection into exercising muscle, and
- colder environmental temperatures.

The mechanism for exercise-induced hypoglycemia is related to the fact that exercise enhances the absorption of exogenous insulin, increases the muscle uptake of glucose, and impairs the mobilization of glucose in blood. Signs of hypoglycemia include apparent loss of concentration, shaking or shivering, sweating, tachycardia, and loss of consciousness. See the sidebar

CONTRAINDICATIONS TO EXERCISE FOR CLIENTS WITH DIABETES

- Blood glucose >250 mg/dl and ketones in urine for type 1 diabetes (5)
- Blood glucose >300 mg/dl without ketones for type 1 diabetes (5)
- Client is not feeling well or is dehydrated
- Proliferative retinopathy—clients with this condition should avoid strenuous high-intensity activities
- Severe kidney disease
- Loss of protective sensation in the feet (peripheral neuropathy)—clients with this condition should avoid outdoor walking and jogging (swimming or biking is recommended)
- Acute illness, infection, or fever
- Evidence of underlying CVD that has not been medically evaluated

HYPOGLYCEMIA

Signs and Symptoms of Hypoglycemia

- Sweating
- Hunger
- Palpitations
- Headache
- Tachycardia
- Anxiety
- Tremor
- Dizziness
- Blurred vision
- Confusion
- Convulsion
- Syncope
- Coma

Responding to a Client Who Has Hypoglycemia

1. Consider dialing 911 (or a similar emergency number).
2. Measure blood glucose level with glucose monitoring device (if available).
3. If the blood glucose level is below 70 mg/dl or the client is known to have diabetes and is having signs or symptoms of hypoglycemia, provide 15 g of carbohydrate, which is equivalent to any of the following:
   - About three or four glucose tablets
   - 1/2 cup (~120 ml) of regular soft drink or fruit juice
   - About six saltine crackers
   - 1 tablespoon (~15 g) of sugar or honey
4. Wait about 15 minutes and remeasure glucose level. If the level remains under 70 mg/dl, provide another 15 g of carbohydrate. Repeat testing and giving food or tablets until blood glucose level rises above 70 mg/dl.

for a comprehensive list of the signs and symptoms of hypoglycemia and a recommended response to hypoglycemia. Personal trainers working with clients who have diabetes should know how to recognize the signs of hypoglycemia and be able to manage hypoglycemia cases with glucose or fructose foods and drinks when affected individuals are unable to treat themselves. Clients with diabetes should always wear a medical alert identification bracelet where it can be easily seen in case of a hypoglycemic reaction.

Blood glucose measurements using portable glucose monitors are an essential part of the exercise prescription. Clients should monitor their blood sugar before and after exercise and also every 30 minutes during prolonged exercise. According to the American Diabetes Association, people with type 1 diabetes should not exercise if their glucose level is greater than 300 mg/dl or greater than 250 mg/dl with urinary ketones (6). The ACSM has recommended that individuals with type 2 diabetes can participate in exercise as long as they feel well and are adequately hydrated, although they should use caution if their blood glucose levels exceed 300 mg/dl without ketones (5). Exercising at these levels can worsen the hyperglycemia and promote ketosis and acidosis. On the other hand, individuals with pre-exercise glucose levels below 100 mg/dl are

at risk of developing hypoglycemia during or after exercise; therefore, they should ingest a carbohydrate-rich snack before exercise.

Adjustment of medication dosage, either insulin or oral hypoglycemic drugs, as well as proper timing of meals, is the key for maintaining good glycemic control during physical activity. Exercise should generally be scheduled 1 to 2 hours after a meal, or when the hypoglycemic medication is not at its peak activity. After exercise, carbohydrate stores should be replenished according to the duration and intensity of the activity. The client's physician will direct the patient's insulin use. This is normally done in conjunction with a dietitian to ensure that a hypoglycemic event does not occur. The personal trainer should never advise a client about the use of insulin or the timing of meals. Should a client experience regular episodes of lack of blood glucose control, the client should be sent back to his or her physician for care.

Finally, each client with diabetes has a unique metabolic response to exercise. No general guideline can take the place of intelligent self-observation and regular glucose monitoring in developing an individualized plan to facilitate safe, enjoyable exercise. Guidelines for aerobic conditioning and resistance exercise are shown in table 19.4 (2, 5, 23).

TABLE 19.4 Exercise Prescription for Clients With Diabetes

Mode	Intensity, frequency, duration	Guidelines and concerns
Aerobic conditioning	• 3-7 days/week with no more than 2 consecutive days without exercise • At least 150 min/week at moderate to vigorous intensity for most adults with diabetes (for adults able to run steadily at 6 mph (10 km/h) for 25 min, 75 min/week of vigorous activity may provide similar cardioprotective and metabolic benefits) • 60%-89% $\dot{V}O_2R$ or HRR (corresponding RPE of 14-17 on a 6-20 scale)	• A snack may be needed before exercise. • Monitor blood glucose before and after exercise. • Include a 5- to 10-min warm-up and cooldown period. • Monitor intensity via RPE, especially if the client is taking a heart rate–altering medication. • Both HIIT and continuous exercise training are appropriate activities for most individuals with diabetes.
Resistance training	• A minimum of 2 nonconsecutive days/week, but preferably 3 days • Moderate (50-69% 1RM) to vigorous (70-85% 1RM) loads • 1-3 sets of ~10-15 reps to near fatigue per set on every exercise early in training. • At least 8-10 multijoint exercises for all major muscle groups in the same session (whole body) or sessions split into selected muscle groups	• Can begin with bodyweight exercises and progress to free weights, resistance bands, or resistance machines. • Clients with well-controlled diabetes can progress to strength training (i.e., higher loads, fewer repetitions). • Beginning training intensity should be moderate, involving ~10-15 reps per set, with increases in weight or resistance undertaken with a lower number of reps (~8-10) only after the target number of reps per set can consistently be exceeded.
Flexibility and balance training	• ≥2 or 3 days/week flexibility, 2-4 reps of each exercise per muscle group • ≥2 or 3 days/week for balance, for any duration of light to moderate intensity • Hold static stretches for 10-30 seconds	• Stretching: Perform static, dynamic, and other types; yoga. • Balance (for older adults): Practice standing on one leg, exercises using balance equipment, lower body and core resistance exercises, tai chi. • Continue to work on flexibility and balance, increasing duration or frequency over time.

Adapted from American College of Sports Medicine (2), American College of Sports Medicine and American Diabetes Association (5), and Colberg et al. (23).

Aerobic Conditioning

Exercise prescription for clients with diabetes mellitus should include aerobic physical activity with a frequency of three to seven days a week, for 20 to 60 minutes per day at moderate to vigorous intensities, based primarily on subjective experience of "moderate" to "very hard" (2). People who are unconditioned can perform exercise at a lower intensity level for a longer duration, at least until they achieve a higher level of fitness. Exercise sessions should begin with a low-intensity warm-up and stretching of the muscle to be exercised and should conclude with a cooldown period. These activities ease the cardiovascular transition between rest and exercise and help prevent muscle and joint injuries. Balducci and colleagues (11) reported the effects of regular aerobic exercise on patients with type 2 diabetes; regular aerobic

exercise improved glycemic control, lipoprotein and lipid control, and bodyweight control and increased insulin sensitivity. The authors also reported that exercising at a vigorous level may have a higher benefit than exercising at low to moderate levels. Given the important of cardiorespiratory fitness, ACSM guidelines indicate that a greater emphasis should eventually be placed on vigorous intensity aerobic exercise if not contra-indicated by diabetes-related complications, However, clients should be instructed to work to voluntary fatigue, not to exhaustion.

Resistance Training

The recommendation for resistance training for individuals with diabetes is two or three days a week, with sessions including at least 1 set of each of 8 to 10 different exercises using the major muscle groups. Each set should consist of about 10 to 15 repetitions, with the amount of weight increased (and number of repetitions reduced) only after the target number of repetitions per set can consistently be exceeded. For clients with diabetes who are 50 years of age and older or who have other health conditions such as hypertension, more repetitions (~12 to 15+) at a lower weight may be more suitable (2, 68). Balducci and colleagues (11) reported that participation in a regular resistance training program offers the same benefits (improved glycemic control, increased insulin sensitivity, increased lean body mass, and increased overall functionality) as participating in a regular aerobic exercise program. Furthermore, participation in a mixed aerobic training and resistance training program may offer the optimal benefit for improvement of glycemic index control compared with either one alone.

Flexibility, Balance, and Other Training

Flexibility exercise for each of the major muscle–tendon groups performed on two or more days a week maintains joint range of movement. Although flexibility training may benefit individuals with all types of diabetes, it should not substitute for other recommended activities (i.e., aerobic and resistance training) because flexibility training has minimal effects on glucose control, body composition, and insulin action. Clients with diabetes who are 50 years and older should perform exercises that maintain or improve balance two or three times a week since balance and flexibility are reduced with age, particularly if these individuals have peripheral neuropathy. Many exercises for the lower body (e.g., single-leg Romanian deadlift) and core (e.g., standing alternating knee lifts) also improve balance and can be included in programming. Yoga and tai chi can be added based on individual preferences to increase flexibility, strength, and balance.

EATING DISORDERS

Eating disorders (EDs) are considered a mental illness; they include a wide range of conditions that involve an unhealthy focus on food, body weight, and appearance. The obsession with these factors can become so strong that it disrupts an individual's health, job performance, social and family relationships, and daily activities. Although an exact incidence cannot be calculated, it is estimated by the National Eating Disorders Association that about 30 million men and

women will experience an ED in their lifetime in the United States (61a). In 2017, Harvard's Strategic Training Initiative for the Prevention of Eating Disorders (STRIPED) asked the Centers for Disease Control and Prevention (CDC) to monitor eating disorders as part of national disease surveillance efforts because the exact prevalence is not known (53a), and eating disorders can affect all systems of the body, potentially resulting in death. This request from Harvard has been supported by the U.S. Congress, and the initiative is moving forward.

There are many forms of eating disorders described in the *Diagnostic and Statistical Manual of Mental Disorders* (*DSM*) and *International Classification of Diseases and Related Health Problems* (*ICD*). *DSM* has the most widely used classification. In *DSM-5*, the best characterized EDs are anorexia nervosa (AN), bulimia nervosa (BN), and binge eating disorder (BED), referred to as the three typical EDs (21). Other EDs are referred to as atypical and are classified as other specified feeding or eating disorders (OSFEDs); this new term of *OSFED* replaced the previously used terminology, eating disorder not otherwise specified (EDNOS) (39). An OSFED is defined as a feeding and eating disorder that causes clinically significant distress or impairment in social life but does not meet the full criteria for typical EDs; this includes atypical AN, atypical BN, atypical BED, purging, and night eating syndrome (39).

Personal trainers have a responsibility to educate clients about the risks of disordered eating, but they also must be sure not to promote unnecessary or risky behaviors to lose weight or to let their clients set unrealistic goals. Although a personal trainer would not be the sole cause of a client's eating disorder (the client would have to be already susceptible), an inappropriate comment or goal can trigger someone to engage in disordered eating practices, which in turn could possibly lead to an ED. Overall, personal trainers need to be sure they help each client set a bodyweight goal that is realistic and in accordance with the client's genetic makeup, which has a significant effect on both the client's metabolism and body type.

> It is the responsibility of the personal trainer to avoid promoting risky weight loss behaviors or setting unrealistic goals.

COMMON SYMPTOMS OF AN EATING DISORDER

Emotional and Behavioral

- General behaviors and attitudes indicating that weight loss, dieting, and control of food are becoming all consuming
- Preoccupation with weight, food, calories, carbohydrates, fat grams, and dieting
- Appearing uncomfortable eating around others
- Food rituals (e.g., eats only a particular food or food group [e.g., condiments], excessive chewing, does not allow foods to touch)
- Skipping meals or taking small portions of food at regular meals
- Any new practices with food or fad diets, including cutting out certain foods or entire food groups (no sugar, no carbohydrates, no dairy, vegetarianism or veganism)
- Withdrawal from usual friends and activities
- Frequent dieting
- Extreme concern about body size and shape
- Frequent checking in the mirror for perceived flaws in appearance
- Extreme mood swings

Physical

- Noticeable fluctuations in weight, both up and down
- Stomach cramps; other nonspecific gastrointestinal complaints (e.g., constipation, acid reflux)
- Menstrual irregularities—missing periods or having a period only while on hormonal contraceptives (this is not considered a true period)
- Difficulties concentrating
- Abnormal laboratory findings (anemia, low thyroid and hormone levels, low potassium, low white and red blood cell counts)
- Dizziness, especially upon standing
- Fainting
- Feeling cold all the time
- Sleep problems
- Cuts and calluses across the top of the finger joints (a result of inducing vomiting)
- Dental problems, such as enamel erosion, cavities, discoloration of teeth, and tooth sensitivity
- Dry skin and hair; brittle nails
- Swelling around area of salivary glands
- Fine hair on body (lanugo)
- Muscle weakness
- Yellow skin (in the context of eating large amounts of carrots)
- Cold, mottled hands and feet or swelling of feet
- Poor wound healing
- Impaired immune functioning

Adapted from National Eating Disorders Association (61a).

Disordered Eating and Restrictive Dieting

The development of an eating disorder sometimes passes through the stages of dieting for weight loss, disordered eating or restrictive dieting, and then possibly a clinically diagnosable ED. Clients may start out by dieting to lose weight and become frustrated when the weight loss does not seem fast enough or significant. This frustration, even desperation, causes them to restrict their diet even further. When this does not work from their viewpoint, they may start to experiment with even more dangerous restrictive dieting practices such as the use of **diuretics** (a medication that increases the rate of urination, hence increasing water loss), diet pills, self-induced vomiting, food **faddism** (eating only one or a few specific foods or following fad diets), fasting, using saunas to sweat weight off, spitting out food that has been chewed, and using laxatives or even enemas. Unfortunately, these practices do not work. Although there may be a loss of weight according to the scale, the lost poundage can often be attributed to water loss or lean tissue (muscle) as opposed to body fat.

The exact cause of EDs is not fully understood but may start with disordered eating or restrictive dieting sitting on a foundation of genetic, biological, behavioral, psychological, and social factors that raise a person's risk. There is a wide range in the frequency of restrictive eating practices. Some people may engage infrequently in one of the techniques mentioned, while others may do so several times a day. For individuals who are genetically predisposed to eating disorders, dieting can be the catalyst for heightened obsessions about weight and food. Dieting also intensifies feelings of guilt and shame around food, which may ultimately contribute to a cycle of restricting, purging, bingeing, or excessive exercise.

Personal trainers can reduce their clients' risk of developing an eating disorder by helping them appreciate the functionality of their bodies, setting achievable physical activity goals they can be proud of, and encouraging them to reinforce intuitive eating habits and follow the Dietary Guidelines for Americans (27). Maintaining a regular and enjoyable physical activity routine can help clients feel better about their bodies and improve their outlook on life, which can serve as protective factors against the development of an ED. It is not the job of a personal trainer to scold a client for disordered eating habits but instead to help clients feel more positive about themselves and their abilities. If the personal trainer offers sound exercise education, appropriate goal setting, and support, the client will be less likely to develop restrictive eating habits that develop into an eating disorder.

Anorexia Nervosa

The definition of **anorexia nervosa (AN)** was revised in *DSM-5*. Anorexia nervosa is characterized by

- "restriction of energy intake relative to requirements, leading to a significant low body weight (in context of what is minimally expected for age, sex, developmental trajectory, and physical health);
- intense fear of gaining weight or becoming fat or persistent behavior that interferes with weight gain (even though significantly low weight); and

- disturbance in the way one's body weight or shape is experienced, undue influence of body shape and weight on self-evaluation, or persistent lack of recognition of the seriousness of the current low body weight (distorted body image)" (21, p. 533).

Weight loss is usually facilitated through the restriction of food intake in conjunction with excessive exercise and may include the aforementioned disordered eating practices. The psychological and emotional problems associated with anorexia may include low self-esteem and compulsive behavior, among others. Further, the condition of any extremely malnourished person may lead to symptoms of apathy, confusion, social isolation, and nonresponsiveness (39).

The two subtypes of AN are the **restricting type** and the **binge eating and purging type** (39). An individual with the restricting type of anorexia does not regularly engage in binge eating or purging behaviors, although he or she does severely restrict food intake

SELECT WARNING SIGNS FOR ANOREXIA

- Dramatic loss of weight
- Denial; feelings of being fat even when thin; obsession with weight, diet, and appearance
- Use of food rituals or avoidance of social situations involving food
- Obsession with exercise; hyperactivity
- Sensitivity to cold
- Use of layers of baggy clothing to disguise weight loss
- Fatigue (in later stages)
- Decline in work, school, or athletic performance
- Growth of baby-fine hair over face and body (lanugo)
- Yellow tint to skin, palms, and soles of feet (from high levels of carotene)
- Hair loss, dry hair, dry skin, brittle nails
- Loss of muscle mass and tone
- Slow pulse at rest; light-headedness on standing up quickly
- Frequent constipation, abdominal pain, cold intolerance, lethargy or excess energy

Adapted from National Eating Disorders Association (61a).

in terms of the type and amount of food consumed over a period of at least three months (39); this is the most common type of anorexia. Restriction may take many forms (e.g., maintaining a very low calorie count, restricting types of food eaten, eating only one meal a day) and may follow obsessive and rigid rules (e.g., eating only food of one color). Alternatively, individuals with the binge eating and purging type of AN regularly engage in binge eating followed by purging behaviors (39).

If a personal trainer notes the signs listed in "Select Warning Signs for Anorexia" in a client, it becomes important to refer the client to a physician for a comprehensive treatment plan, which usually includes medical, dietary, and psychological or spiritual counseling from a team of professionals (physician, dietitian, psychologist, or religious or spiritual counselor). It may be hard for individuals with anorexia to acknowledge they have a problem. Therefore, the personal trainer should share this list with the client in the hopes of getting the person to seek help.

Bulimia Nervosa

Bulimia Nervosa (BN) is a serious psychiatric disorder that consists of recurring episodes of **binge eating** (the consumption of abnormally large amounts of food in a short period of time) followed by **purging behaviors** (self-induced vomiting or the misuse of laxatives, diuretics, or enemas) (39). An episode of binge eating is characterized by both of the following:

- Eating, in a discrete period of time (e.g., within any 2-hour period), an amount of food that is considerably larger than most people would eat during a similar period of time and under similar circumstances.
- A sense of lack of control over eating during the episode (e.g., a feeling that one cannot stop eating or control what or how much one is eating).

Whereas an individual with anorexia exhibits strict control of food intake, the individual with bulimia is experiencing a loss of control (39).

Bulimia nervosa often starts with weight loss dieting. The resulting food deprivation and inadequate nutrition can trigger what is, in effect, a starvation reaction—an overriding urge to eat. Once the person gives in to this urge, the desire to eat is uncontrollable, leading to a substantial binge on whatever food is available (often foods with high fat and sugar content),

followed by compensatory behaviors. A repeat of weight loss dieting often follows, leading to a cycle of bingeing, purging, and exercising that becomes more compulsive and uncontrollable over time. The goal of the personal trainer is to discourage restrictive eating patterns for weight loss.

The diagnosis of BN comes when the binge eating and purging behaviors occur on an average of at least once a week for at least three months. Even if these behaviors occur less frequently, steps should be taken to break the cycle. Early detection and intervention can prevent further or permanent damage to the body, mind, and spirit.

It is not easy to recognize bulimia. In fact, it often goes undetected. Individuals with bulimia often try

SELECT WARNING SIGNS FOR BULIMIA

- Difficulties with activities that involve food
- Deceptive behaviors related to food
- Self-induced vomiting
- Laxative, diuretics, or enema use
- Excessive exercise
- Overconcern with body shape
- Weight fluctuations of more than 10 pounds (4.5 kg)
- Traces of odor of vomit on the breath
- Scabs or scars on knuckles
- Swollen, persistently puffy face and cheeks
- Broken blood vessels in the face and eyes
- Sore throat and dental problems
- Abdominal symptoms
- Rapid weight changes of 2 to 5 pounds (0.9-2.3 kg) overnight
- Erratic performance in work, sport, and academics
- Lacerations of the oral cavity
- Diarrhea
- Constipation
- Fatigue
- Anxiety or depression

Adapted from National Eating Disorders Association (61a).

to hide the condition from their family and friends. People with bulimia can be of normal weight or slightly overweight, come from diverse backgrounds, and practice many types of eating behaviors. They frequently have weight fluctuations greater than 10 pounds (4.5 kg) because of alternate binges and fasts (39). It is important for personal trainers to be familiar with the signs, effects, and behaviors associated with bulimia so they may be able to identify the condition in a client and refer him or her for help (see "Select Warning Signs for Bulimia").

Binge Eating Disorder

Binge eating disorder (BED) is an illness characterized by frequently eating excessive amounts of food, often when not hungry (57). According to the *DSM-5* criteria, to be diagnosed as having BED a person must display (15, p. 2) the following:

- "Recurrent episodes of binge eating (as described in the section on bulimia).
- The binge eating episodes are associated with three or more of the following:
  - Eating much more rapidly than normal
  - Eating until feeling uncomfortably full
  - Eating large amounts of food when not feeling physically hungry
  - Eating alone because of feeling embarrassed by how much one is eating
  - Feeling disgusted with oneself, depressed, or very guilty afterward
- Marked distress regarding binge eating is present.
- Binge eating occurs, on average, at least once a week for three months.
- Binge eating is not associated with the recurrent use of inappropriate compensatory behaviors as in BN and does not occur exclusively during the course of BN or AN."

Binge eating disorder is associated with more subjective distress regarding the eating behavior and commonly other co-occurring psychological problems. Binge eating disorder can affect anybody, regardless of age, sex, or ethnicity. In fact, research suggests equal percentages of males and females experience BED. It is also the most common of eating disorders.

SELECT WARNING SIGNS FOR BINGE EATING DISORDER

- Evidence of binge eating
- Does not appear comfortable eating around others
- Shows extreme concern with body weight and shape
- Eating more rapidly than normal
- Periods of uncontrolled, impulsive, or continuous eating
- Eating in secret
- Avoiding social situations, particularly those involving food
- Eating normal quantities in social settings and bingeing when alone
- Low self-esteem and embarrassment over physical appearance
- Feeling extremely distressed, upset, and anxious during and after a binge episode
- Fluctuations in weight
- Low self-esteem

Adapted from National Eating Disorders Association (61a).

Other Specified Feeding or Eating Disorders (OSFEDs)

The **other specified feeding or eating disorder (OSFED)** classification was previously known as "eating disorder not otherwise specified" (EDNOS). Despite being considered a catch-all classification that was sometimes denied insurance coverage for treatment because it was seen as less serious, OSFEDs are serious, life-threatening, and treatable eating disorders. The category was developed to encompass those individuals who did not meet strict diagnostic criteria for AN or BN but still had a significant eating disorder.

According to the *DSM-5* criteria (21), to be diagnosed as having an OSFED a person must present with feeding or eating behaviors that cause clinically significant distress and impairment in areas of functioning but do not meet the full criteria for any of the other feeding and eating disorders. Because of changes to all eating disorder criteria, this catch-all category is no longer quite as expansive.

The *DMS-5* currently lists the following five clinical examples of OSFED (21):

1. Atypical anorexia nervosa (all criteria for anorexia nervosa are met; despite significant weight loss, the individual's weight is within or above the normal range)
2. Bulimia nervosa of low frequency or limited duration
3. Binge eating disorder of low frequency or limited duration
4. Purging disorder
5. Night eating syndrome

Prevalence of Eating Disorders in Women and Men

Eating disorders are higher among women than men but are significant in both sexes. In fact, the prevalence of EDs in males is on the rise (55, 76); based on population survey data (76), it is estimated that one in four people affected by an ED is male. *DSM-5* removed **amenorrhea** (lack of menstrual cycles) (8) as a criterion for AN partly to refute the stereotype that AN affects only females. However, more males than females will underreport eating disorders, and as such, the actual prevalence is hard to determine.

Binge eating disorder is most common in males compared with AN or BN. Indeed, some researchers report that males account for 40% of all BED cases (86). In males with BN, purging often manifests as compulsive exercise; self-induced vomiting or the use of laxatives is less common (86). AN is least frequently seen in men, possibly because men are less likely to be interested in the emaciated look of AN. However, a male's desire for leanness or a "ripped" appearance can drive AN symptomology. Male bodybuilders have high rates of both EDs and muscle **dysmorphia** (body dissatisfaction), which drives their quests in the gym (32, 61).

The Female Athlete Triad and Relative Energy Deficiency in Sport

Eating disorders and any dissatisfaction with body image, or pressure to achieve a certain body composition in sports, may push athletes of both sexes to restrict their energy intake, which could lead to a reduction in sport performance and compromised bone and metabolic health. In females, scientists have discovered an interplay between hormones, energy intake, and bone health, termed the **female athlete triad**. The triad consists of (25) the following:

- Low energy availability with or without disordered eating
- Menstrual dysfunction
- Low bone density

The label includes the word *athlete* because this condition was first discovered in young female athletes. In actuality, it affects a wide range of women of any age with different levels of activity, not just athletes (3). It is not the participation in exercise or sport that causes the triad, but the misguided goal of girls and women to become unrealistically lean, consequent to their thinking that this will improve sport performance or appearance. Activities that are at highest risk are those that focus on leanness and aesthetics (such as gymnastics, volleyball, and figure skating) and aerobic endurance (such as cross country running because a lighter body weight may make a female faster).

Low energy availability in a female means she is not consuming enough calories to meet her energy requirements. This could be from restrictive eating or lack of knowledge of proper calorie intake. When a woman experiences menstrual dysfunction, her menstrual cycles are altered: They may be longer than normal, or she may miss a period entirely. This can lead to loss of bone mineral density, which increases the risk of stress fractures. Any woman who experiences a stress fracture should be referred to a physical therapist for evaluation.

Scientists who discovered and named the female athlete triad also saw the same pattern in males: low energy availability (with or without disordered eating), hypogonadotropic hypogonadism (low testosterone and androgenic hormones), and low bone mineral density (29, 80). Consequently, male athletes may be predisposed to developing bone stress injuries, and these injuries can be the first presenting feature of associated triad conditions.

The concept of relative energy deficiency in sport (RED-S) has been proposed as a replacement for the female athlete triad and has been adopted by the International Olympic Committee (59). This model includes both sexes and focuses on **low energy availability**

(LEA) as the basis for all metabolic irregularities that can occur. LEA is described as a mismatch between an athlete's energy intake (diet) and the energy expended in exercise, leaving inadequate energy to support normal bodily functions required to maintain optimal health and exercise performance. An inadequate energy intake relative to energy expenditure affects all metabolic systems of the body including endocrinological (hormonal), skeletal, gastrointestinal, immunological, and psychological. Personal trainers should be alert to low food intake in their clients, especially those who compete in aesthetic sports, and emphasize the importance of a balanced, nutritious, and adequate food intake to help them look, feel, and function better. When appropriate, clients should be referred to health care professionals (such as an RD) for evaluation and follow-up.

> Low energy availability is a mismatch between food intake and energy expenditure such that essential metabolic functions are compromised. Personal trainers should always encourage diets of adequate caloric consumption and that follow the Dietary Guidelines for Americans.

Exercise Prescription and Program Design for Clients Recovering From an Eating Disorder

Clients with a diagnosed eating disorder should receive clearance from their physician before returning to an exercise program. An exercise program can be beneficial, both physically and emotionally, but the program must be designed so that it is safe and does not prompt a return to the use of exercise as a purging technique. The physician must determine whether and when it is medically safe for the client to start exercising.

When resuming a client's exercise program, the personal trainer needs to reassess the client. Clients who have experienced complications from the eating disorder (abnormal electrolytes, an irregular heartbeat, having passed out at any time) will not be able to exercise until the problem is corrected or alleviated. Once a client with a resolving eating disorder returns to exercise, it may be important to monitor heart rate and blood pressure.

An exercise program should deemphasize weight loss and emphasize exercise with a low energy demand, such as moderate resistance training instead

PROGRAM DESIGN FOR CLIENTS RECOVERING FROM AN EATING DISORDER

- Require the client recovering from an eating disorder to see a physician for a complete medical exam before returning to or continuing an exercise program.
- Do not prescribe a vigorous exercise program.
- Help the client engage in a well-rounded program of aerobic conditioning, resistance training, and flexibility exercise.
- Ensure adequate hydration and rehydration.
- Encourage the client to ingest an adequate dietary intake.
- Encourage the client to consume 200 to 400 kcal of complex carbohydrates during the first 30 to 90 minutes after an exercise session.
- Schedule exercise sessions so that the client does not exercise every day and takes two or three days off a week.
- Check the client's blood pressure and pulse.
- Do not allow high-impact exercises (like jumps) if the client has a stress fracture.
- Maintain regular communication with the client's physician, RD, and other health care professionals.
- If a client experiences any of the following signs or symptoms, he or she should seek medical clearance before continuing the exercise program: light-headedness, irregular heartbeat, nausea, injuries, abnormal blood pressure levels or pulse.

of vigorous, or moderate aerobic activity instead of high intensity (2). A return to high-energy expenditure exercise should be delayed until the client is cleared by a physician. Moderate resistance exercise will help preserve lean body mass, although its effectiveness will be severely compromised if the client does not consume adequate calories and nutrients.

The personal trainer may encounter an individual who has a significant eating disorder but refuses to see a physician. Although it may be tempting to continue to train the client, the personal trainer (as one of very few people who may be in touch with the client) should require a medical release before continuing. Should the client refuse to see a physician, the personal trainer should discontinue the training sessions, especially if the client experiences light-headedness, irregular heartbeat, nausea, injuries, or abnormal pulse or blood pressure levels during exercise.

CONCLUSION

Personal trainers play a valuable role in helping clients with obesity, hyperlipidemia, diabetes, and eating disorders achieve fitness and health goals through adherence to a healthy diet and a well-designed exercise program. Personal trainers should strongly consider the value of working in conjunction with the client's physician and with an RD in order to ensure the client's complete success. In so doing, they can play a significant role in the client's health care team.

Study Questions

1. Which of the following is *incorrect* regarding the scope of practice of professionals involved in nutritional or metabolic concerns?

    A. Clients should be referred to physicians for medical care.

    B. Clients should be referred to registered dietitians for medical nutrition therapy.

    C. Personal trainers may help in diagnosing or prescribing care.

    D. Personal trainers should not accept or train clients who have medical conditions that may exceed their level of knowledge and experience.

2. The NHLBI guidelines recommend that a diet be individually planned to create a deficit of _____ kcal per day to facilitate a weight loss of _____ per week.

    A. 500-1000; 3-4 lb (1.3-1.8 kg)

    B. 1000-2000; 3-4 lb (1.3-1.8 kg)

    C. 500-1000; 1-2 lb (0.5-0.9 kg)

    D. 1000-2000; 1-2 lb (0.5-0.9 kg)

3. Which of the following can occur in obese individuals during exercise?

    A. hyperpnea

    B. dyspnea

    C. both hyperpnea and dyspnea

    D. neither hyperpnea nor dyspnea

4. It is recommended that individuals with diabetes should go no more than how many consecutive days *without* exercise?

    A. 1

    B. 2

    C. 3

    D. 4

5. Which of the following is *incorrect* regarding how a personal trainer should approach a client recovering from an eating disorder?

    A. Require the client recovering from an eating disorder to see a physician for a complete medical exam.

    B. Prescribe a vigorous exercise program.

    C. Ensure adequate hydration and rehydration.

    D. Do not allow high-impact exercises (like jumps) if the client has a stress fracture.

CHAPTER 20

Clients With Cardiovascular or Respiratory Conditions

Cindy M. Kugler, MS, Steven M. Laslovich, PhD, and Paul Sorace, MS

After completing this chapter, you will be able to

- understand the pathophysiology and risk factors for hypertension, myocardial infarction, cerebrovascular accident, peripheral vascular disease, asthma, chronic obstructive pulmonary disease (COPD), and exercise-induced bronchoconstriction;

- understand the stages of the various diseases and how exercise can be used to enhance the client's quality of life; and

- know when it is appropriate to refer a client to a medical professional.

Cardiovascular and respiratory diseases present a challenge not only to the traditional health care provider but also to the personal trainer. Although deaths related to diseases of the heart have continued to decline since the late 1990s, cardiovascular disease remains the leading cause of death in the United States (figure 20.1; 47, 60).

Hypertension is a major risk factor for cardiovascular disease, with myocardial infarctions (heart attacks) and cerebrovascular accidents (strokes) being the most common cardiovascular events that personal trainers may encounter. In addition to providing information about these common conditions, this chapter includes information about training clients with peripheral arterial disease, because such clients can benefit a great deal from aerobic conditioning.

Respiratory disease in general is a topic well beyond the scope of this chapter. However, this chapter addresses three common airway problems: chronic obstructive pulmonary disease (COPD), asthma, and exercise-induced bronchoconstriction. Asthma and exercise-induced bronchoconstriction are conditions often seen in personal training clients, and exercise programming should be guided by the client's health care provider. In contrast, the primary pulmonary rehabilitation and training programs of individuals with COPD will need to be directly overseen by specialized respiratory medical personnel (whose level of training is beyond that of a personal trainer). However, in the client with COPD, the personal trainer may be part of the team involved in the long-term maintenance of the individual's medically prescribed aerobic and musculoskeletal fitness programs.

To properly guide, educate, and train cardiovascular and respiratory patients, the personal trainer must understand the pathophysiology of the disease and be able to recognize the early signs of inadequate blood circulation and labored breathing during

The authors would like to acknowledge the significant contributions of Moh Malek and Robert Watine to this chapter.

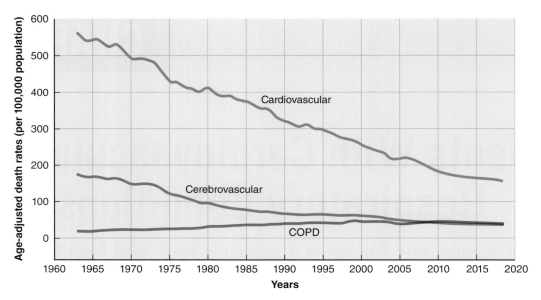

FIGURE 20.1   The three primary categories of the causes of death in the United States (age-adjusted): Cardiovascular disease, cerebrovascular disease, and chronic obstructive pulmonary disease (COPD).

Based on data from U.S. National Center for Health Statistics (47, 60).

training. This said, personal trainers can have a dramatic positive impact on the quality of life for their clients as long as they pay careful attention to the signs. Additionally, it is important for the personal trainer to approach the exercise regimen as part of a team with the physician as the leader. Any client who has a medical condition or disease should receive clearance from his or her physician. Of course, liability waivers should be signed by all parties to provide as much protection as possible should issues of liability ever arise (see chapter 25 for more information).

HYPERTENSION

Hypertension, or high blood pressure, is a disease not just of the old but of the young as well (56, 57, 58). Hypertension is largely an idiopathic disease, meaning it occurs without a known cause; 95% of cases are idiopathic. The other 5% are typically caused by multiple secondary factors (e.g., diet, sedentary lifestyle) (22). This small percentage of cases may be curable, but most cases are treated and managed via prescription medications and lifestyle interventions. Although hypertension is highly prevalent, a large portion of individuals may not display any signs or symptoms of the disorder until a cardiac event occurs. Thus, no person, not even a doctor, can look at 10 people in a room and pick out who has the disease and who does

not. This is why hypertension is considered one of the "silent killers." Although a blood pressure reading of 120/80 mmHg is often considered average, the American Heart Association and American College of Cardiologists announced new guidelines in 2017, now classifying this reading (i.e., 120/80 mmHg) as *elevated* blood pressure (62).

Elevated blood pressure puts an individual at risk for a stroke or heart attack or both. People cannot determine how high their blood pressure is based on how they feel. If a person truly were to perceive his or her blood pressure to be high, it would most likely be in the range of a hypertensive crisis with associated chest pains, visual blurring, neurological deficits, or some combination of these.

Blood pressure risk stratification is shown in table 20.1. The stages are stratified into normal, elevated, and stage 1 and stage 2 hypertension. These stratifications are based on the presence of major risk factors (e.g., smoking, dyslipidemia, diabetes mellitus, age greater than 60, postmenopause, and family history), as well as being male, having target organ damage (TOD), and having clinical cardiovascular disease (CCD). Any clients with stage 1 or greater readings should not begin an exercise program until their pressure is controlled and a physician has cleared them for exercise (12, 16).

Target organ damage includes cardiac, brain, kidney, peripheral vascular, and retinal disease.

TABLE 20.1   Categories of Blood Pressure in Adults

BP category	SBP		DBP
Normal	<120 mmHg	And	<80 mmHg
Elevated	120-129 mmHg	And	<80 mmHg
Hypertension: Stage 1	130-139 mm Hg	Or	80-89 mmHg
Hypertension: Stage 2	≥140 mm Hg	Or	≥90 mmHg

Note: Individuals with systolic blood pressure (SBP) and diastolic blood pressure (DBP) in two different categories should be designated to the higher BP category. Elevated blood pressure, or hypertension, is based on an average of more than two readings obtained on more than two occasions by a physician (62).

Target organ cardiac disease refers to left ventricular thickening or hypertrophy due to untreated or inadequately treated hypertension, history of exertional chest pain or angina, previous heart attack, having had reperfusion surgery (e.g., coronary bypass, stenting, or balloon angioplasty), and overall cardiac dysfunction (e.g., heart failure, cardiomyopathy). Stroke and peripheral vascular disease have pathophysiology similar to that of coronary artery disease. Kidney disease results in glomerular dysfunction, leading to the kidneys' inability to cleanse the blood, as well as affecting blood flow to and from the kidney, which can lead to hypertension as well. Retinal disease is a function of hemorrhages from high blood pressure, thereby affecting eyesight with the potential for the development of blindness.

A client with elevated readings and no major risk factors is potentially treated with lifestyle modification (e.g., proper nutrition, exercise). A client with stage 1 or stage 2 hypertension requires physician intervention for treatment and clearance before working with a personal trainer (62).

> A blood pressure reading of 120/80 mmHg is considered *elevated* blood pressure, not normal blood pressure. When systolic and diastolic pressures fall into different categories, use the higher category to classify a client.

Management of Hypertension

Lifestyle modification for clients with hypertension includes nonpharmacologic interventions (e.g., proper exercise, weight loss, and dietary changes). General lifestyle changes include an adequate amount of sleep, reduction in daily sodium intake, adequate potassium intake, weight loss if needed, limiting alcohol intake, performing aerobic activity for 90 to 150 minutes per week, eating a diet rich in fruits and vegetables and low in fat, and the cessation of smoking (62).

The **Dietary Approaches to Stop Hypertension (DASH)** diet has received a great deal of favorable publicity for lowering blood pressure. It entails reducing saturated fats, cholesterol, and total fat intake. Emphasis is on more fruits, vegetables, low-fat dairy products, whole-grain products, fish, poultry, and nuts; reductions in red meat, sweets, and sugar-containing beverages; and an increase in foods rich in magnesium, potassium, calcium, protein, and fiber.

Clients with hypertension may be taking one or more medications to control their blood pressure. The classes of medications include β-blockers, calcium channel blockers, ACE (angiotensin converting enzyme) inhibitors, ARBs (angiotensin receptor blockers), diuretics, and α-blockers. The exact mechanisms of action of these medications are beyond the scope of this chapter except for the fact that they all lower blood pressure. Diuretics cause blood volume depletion. However, the personal trainer should never restrict clients' use of fluids or worry about their use of electrolyte solutions. Calcium channel blockers, α-blockers, and β-blockers cause vasodilation, with the potential for blood pooling. Angiotensin-converting enzyme inhibitors and ARBs exert their effects on the kidneys' vasculature. These medications can cause blood pooling, which necessitates a longer period for cooldown, especially after treadmill walking, jogging, running, and resistance training. Additionally, β-blockers not only slow the heart rate but also prevent it from elevating as a normal response to exercise. This makes it difficult to use heart rate as a measure of intensity and necessitates use of the rating of perceived exertion (RPE) scale (e.g., figure 11.4 on page 204).

Safety Considerations for Clients With Hypertension

What is most promising for the client and exciting for the personal trainer is that the client with controlled hypertension can exercise with limited restrictions. A few simple precautions allow for the application of all modalities. There are numerous benefits, but exercise may be especially beneficial to clients with hypertension. Several studies have shown significant reductions in resting blood pressure after long-term exercise. A review of the literature, by meta-analysis, revealed approximate decreases in systolic and diastolic pressures of 4.5/3.8 mmHg and 4.7/3.1 mmHg, respectively, from long-term resistance and aerobic training (17, 23, 30, 31, 32, 33, 36, 37, 40, 44). A systolic pressure of 220 mmHg or diastolic pressure of 105 mmHg is considered grounds for exercise termination (5).

Generally, progression should be gradual, avoiding any large increases in the components of the exercise prescription, especially intensity (5). An extended cooldown is also recommended. Vigorous intensity is not contraindicated, but moderate intensity will optimize the risk-to-benefit ratio (5). Taking blood pressures before exercise, during peak exercise, and again after cooldown will ensure client safety and help with adjustment of the exercise prescription.

> **Clients with controlled hypertension can exercise with limited restrictions.**

Contraindications

As for which exercises are contraindicated, these include any type of activity that would increase intrathoracic pressure, thereby decreasing blood flow return to the heart, with a corresponding decrease in cardiac output. Essentially this means any exercise with an associated prolonged Valsalva maneuver (greater than 2 seconds). The burden is on the personal trainer to be certain not only that clients are performing exercises in a technically correct manner but also that they are breathing properly. Individuals whose blood pressure is not controlled should consult their physician before exercising.

Safe Exercises

Clients with controlled hypertension may participate in many types of training including, but not limited to, the use of free weights, weight machines, body weight, or elastic bands; aerobic exercise (walking, jogging, swimming); and circuit weight training. Essentially all exercises are permissible (6). If a client with hypertension has a comorbid condition, however, the choice of exercise may be altered or restricted (59).

Comorbid conditions include the following:

- *Musculoskeletal conditions or diseases:* degenerative joint diseases, rheumatologic diseases
- *Neurological disorders:* stroke, myasthenia gravis, muscular dystrophy
- *Vascular diseases:* carotid artery disease, cardiac conditions, aneurysms

Exercise Guidelines for Clients With Hypertension

The individual with hypertension will benefit from progressing and increasing total weekly exercise energy expenditure because greater volume can lead to greater improvements in blood pressure. Benefits can also be magnified if weight loss occurs during the training program, if needed. For maximized benefits, progressing to accumulate more than the minimum recommendation of 150 minutes per week is advisable (4). In individuals with other chronic diseases or disabilities, starting at a self-selected intensity and duration and progressing slowly to meet the recommended guidelines may be appropriate (4). Aerobic exercise should be performed five to seven days per week for a minimum of 30 minutes (may be accumulated in 10-minute bouts) at a moderate intensity of 40% to 59% of $\dot{V}O_2$ or heart rate reserve or an RPE of 12 to 13 (5).

As with the cardiovascular exercise, resistance training should be gradual, avoiding large increases in intensity. The Valsalva maneuver (breath holding) can result in high blood pressure; thus, this practice should be avoided during resistance training (5). The rest interval should initially be 2 to 3 minutes (or longer) to allow the client to fully recover between sets. This will allow for physiological compensation from the exercise, which is especially necessary because of the potential use of prescription medications for hypertension control (45). Resistance training should be performed on two or three days per week, performing 2 to 4 sets of 8 to 12 repetitions of each of the major muscle groups per session to total ≥20 minutes per session. Intensity should be moderate, starting at 60% to 70% of the 1RM; older adults and novice exercisers should begin with 40% to 50% of the 1RM (5).

EXERCISE GOALS FOR CLIENTS WITH HYPERTENSION

- Increase $\dot{V}O_2$max and ventilatory threshold.
- Increase maximal work and aerobic endurance.
- Increase caloric expenditure.
- Control blood pressure.
- Increase muscular strength and endurance.

MYOCARDIAL INFARCTION, STROKE, AND PERIPHERAL ARTERY DISEASE

Myocardial infarction (MI), stroke, and peripheral artery disease (PAD) are major health and economic burdens. Heart disease and stroke continue to be in the top 10 causes of death in the United States (14). According to the Centers for Disease Control and Prevention, peripheral artery disease affects approximately 8.5 million adults in the United States over the age of 40 (20). Beyond the physiological effects, there are true psychological problems, whether the client realizes them consciously or not. These can manifest themselves in many ways, from a fear of exercise (e.g., fear of the precipitation of another acute event) to the other end of the spectrum of fearlessness on the part of the client. The attitude of "I'll show you; I can beat this thing, I'll just push through the barriers" must be watched for when working with these clients. Thus, the personal trainer must actively listen to clients and pay attention to the messages being relayed via nonverbal cues and innuendo. The personal trainer needs to be knowledgeable in the pathophysiology of these conditions as well as the probable comorbidities, secondary conditions, and psychological effects (49, 54).

Pathophysiology

The pathophysiology is essentially the same for all three diseases, resulting in occlusive disease of the heart, brain, or peripheral cardiovascular system (26). An atheromatous (lipid-cholesterol) plaque forms within the lumen (the open space within a blood vessel), resulting in **atherosclerosis**. Focal inflammation around the area of the plaque occurs, leading to its instability. Over time, a collagen cap develops to stabilize the area, with a subsequent overlaying by smooth muscle cells (the normal inside lining of the blood vessel) (figure 20.2; 26). Depending on the timeline, the outcomes can be very different.

If the collagen cap and smooth muscle cells grow to a point of stability, the diameter of the blood vessel is dramatically reduced. This results in decreased blood flow, with the potential for turbulent flow to develop, as well as sludging of the circulation and the development of a thrombus (blood clot) that can either

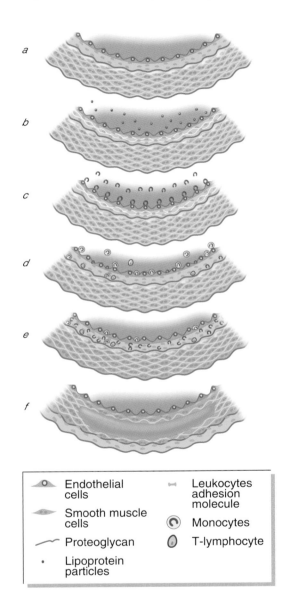

Symbol		Symbol	
	Endothelial cells		Leukocytes adhesion molecule
	Smooth muscle cells		Monocytes
	Proteoglycan		T-lymphocyte
•	Lipoprotein particles		

FIGURE 20.2 Development of a collagen cap. A normal artery *(a)* with the innermost layer of endothelial cells. As plaque (lipoprotein molecules) accumulates *(b-e)*, a cap or layer of collagen is eventually created and covered by a layer of smooth muscle cells (fibers) *(f)*.

Reprinted by permission from Fauci et al. (1998, pp. 1345-1352)

occlude the lumen or break off and flow downstream to occlude a more distal site. While the collagen cap is still soft and unstable, it can rupture (figure 20.3; 26) and release all the material within to flow downstream and cause sudden occlusive disease. A mature collagen cap does not rupture as easily and thus is more stable, allowing the body to dissolve the thrombus and thereby prevent it from reaching critical mass. A homeostatic mechanism with antithrombin III provides this protection. The collagen cap rupture is more dangerous, since the sudden release of the intracap material sent flowing distally can cause an acute MI or a cerebrovascular accident (CVA). The problems associated with the stable collagen cap typically affect peripheral circulation but can also be seen in the coronary arteries, as in **angina** (chest pain due to insufficient blood flow to the heart).

Risk Factors

Risk factors for atherosclerosis include diabetes, high blood cholesterol, high blood pressure, obesity, tobacco use, family history, and lifestyle (e.g., nutrition and dietary choices; reduced exercise and physical activity). High blood pressure increases the systemic vascular resistance, which increases the intracardiac pressure within the left ventricle to allow for systole to occur. During systole there is a compression of the cardiac vessels that feed the heart. When the pressure exceeds a certain threshold, there is a decrease in or a lack of flow to the interior of the heart, and thus chest pain occurs. Of course, with corresponding high cholesterol and cap formation, a rupture can occur, causing the same end result. This can also take place in the coronary arteries.

Diabetes exerts an acceleration effect on the process of vascular disease and thus has an independent effect on the pathophysiology of heart attacks. Nicotine (e.g., via smoking or vaping) increases systemic vascular resistance and thus there is an increase in blood pressure, causing an effect similar to that described in the previous section. People who are obese require more blood vessels to feed the adipose tissue. This effectively increases the cardiac workload, affecting the circulatory efficiency of the heart's pumping action. Over time, this can lead to the development of one of the various types of cardiomyopathy and heart failure. As for family history, anyone who has a first-degree relative (parent or sibling) with known cardiac disease diagnosed before the age of 55 (male relative) or 65 (female relative) has an increased risk (5).

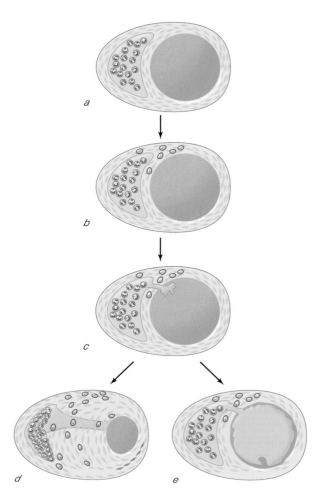

FIGURE 20.3 Rupture of an immature collagen cap. If a normal artery *(a)* begins to develop a collagen cap *(b)* that ruptures *(c)*, the artery can become partially *(d)* or fully *(e)* occluded.

Reprinted by permission from Fauci et al. (1998, pp. 1345-1352).

Myocardial Infarction

When a heart attack, or **myocardial infarction (MI)**, occurs, cardiac muscle potentially dies. Medical professionals intervene to try to salvage some of the damaged tissue or even reverse the entire process altogether. The extent of debilitation depends on the amount and location of the heart muscle that is damaged as well as on the timing of revascularization to restore blood flow (through an intervention such as percutaneous transluminal coronary angioplasty) and salvage tissue. The personal trainer, however, will be working with a client who has had a heart attack, has gone through cardiac rehabilitation, and has been discharged from the physician to continue with an exercise program. This places the personal trainer in a most opportune position to get the most recent test data on the new client—exercise stress test results, echocardiogram results, and a letter of clearance and recommendations from the cardiologist.

These reports give the personal trainer the needed information regarding where the doctor left off and thus where the personal trainer can begin (i.e., intensity level, among other parameters). The stress test provides the maximal oxygen uptake that enables one to determine the intensity level. It also becomes important to recognize that a subpopulation of clients have underlying coronary artery disease without associated chest pain during activity. These individuals are at risk for sudden death if they exercise to the point of coronary artery spasm, which can lead to an acute heart attack and possibly even sudden cardiac death, with a sudden stoppage of beating of the heart. Again, the stress test can reveal whether an individual is in this subclass. The personal trainer should not train these clients because they should exercise in a medically monitored setting.

> Initial exercise training post-MI should be performed in a cardiac rehabilitation setting under the supervision of a physician. Medical recommendations and guidelines can then be relayed to the personal trainer to allow for proper program prescription postrehabilitation.

Exercise Guidelines for Post-MI Clients

Post-MI clients are not to be trained until they have received clearance from their cardiologist, cardiovascular surgeon, or both (25). At that point, the medical professional must be able to provide an intensity level and training range for the personal trainer to work with. The medical professional should provide a metabolic equivalent of task (MET) level or $\dot{V}O_2$peak or $\dot{V}O_2$max for the personal trainer to use as a baseline for design of a program. The program should also be sent to the doctor for approval, or at the very least be placed in the client's medical file.

What is most important is for the personal trainer to be cognizant of, and monitor for, abnormal signs and symptoms. Some of these signs and symptoms are chest pain, palpitations, shortness of breath, diaphoresis, nausea, neck pain, arm pain (left or right), back pain, and a sense of impending doom.

One caveat is that many post-MI clients have comorbid diseases, such as diabetes and PAD. Peripheral arterial disease is discussed later in this chapter, and programming for clients with diabetes is addressed in chapter 19.

Exercise Program Components for Post-MI Clients

The personal trainer will need to obtain clearance and any recommendations from the client's cardiologist before working with this population. Ideally, the personal trainer should obtain any available stress test results and the last exercise prescription from cardiac rehabilitation to aid in the continuation, effectiveness, and safety of the ongoing exercise programming (4). Exercise considerations for the post-MI client include performing an extended warm-up and cooldown, including both upper and lower body aerobic modalities, and avoiding breath holding during resistance exercise and when doing static stretching. Additionally, monitoring signs and symptoms such as chest pain, dizziness, shortness of breath, and blood pressure is necessary before, during, and after each session (5). The recommendation for aerobic conditioning is three to five days per week of 20- to 60-minute sessions at an intensity of 40% to 80% of $\dot{V}O_2$ or heart rate reserve or an RPE of 12 to 16 (5). This may vary with some clients, and the personal trainer may opt to start the client at a lower intensity and slowly progress. Resistance training should be performed two or three days per week, 10 to 15 repetitions of 8 to 10 exercises total, working all major muscle groups. Intensity should be moderate (e.g., 60%-80% of an estimated 1RM or an RPE of 11-13) (5).

> Exercise programming for the post-MI client should include monitoring signs and symptoms for an arising cardiac issue, such as shortness of breath, chest pain, arm pain, diaphoresis, and heart palpitations.

Cerebrovascular Accident

Stroke, or **cerebrovascular accident (CVA)**, is a brain injury caused when blood flow to an area of the brain is cut off by either a blood clot or bleed due to a ruptured blood vessel. A stroke can affect the way you

GOALS FOR CLIENTS WHO HAVE HAD A MYOCARDIAL INFARCTION

- Increase aerobic capacity.
- Decrease blood pressure.
- Reduce risk of coronary artery disease.
- Increase ability to perform leisure, occupational, and daily living activities.
- Increase muscular strength and endurance.

move, feel, communicate, think, and act. Effects and changes are based on the severity and location of the stroke. Physical activity and exercise can positively influence many of the physical, psychosocial, and risk factors poststroke. For example, exercise can positively affect fatigue, depression, cognitive function, and emotional well-being. Physical improvements can be made in activities such as walking ability, mobility, joint stiffness, strength, and balance (63).

Exercise Guidelines for Post-CVA Clients

The post-CVA client faces many challenges, all depending on which area of the brain has been affected. For instance, many individuals after CVA have difficulty with simple daily tasks because of a loss of motor function, often in the arm, leg, face, or mouth. Others have trouble hearing, speaking, or understanding spatial arrangements—or they may even ignore one side of their bodies. A left-brain CVA will affect the right side of the body, resulting in motor deficits of the right arm, leg, or both. A right-brain CVA will affect the left side of the body.

A properly instituted exercise program can significantly improve the life of people who have had a CVA. The program, however, must begin where the post-CVA rehabilitation left off. Therefore, the personal trainer needs to have close contact with the rehabilitation team in order to establish goals and the direction of postrehabilitation training.

> **Exercise can significantly improve the quality of life of an individual who has had a stroke. Personal trainers may train post-CVA clients who have no neurological deficit and are released by a physician to exercise in a fitness setting.**

Exercise Program Components for Post-CVA Clients

Before the start of the initial program, the personal trainer needs to obtain clearance from the stroke client's primary medical provider along with recommendations, limitations, and current exercise information from the rehabilitation professionals. The physical and occupational therapy program is typically followed for three to six months after a stroke. Once the individual is able to work with a personal trainer, the program should focus on maintaining an active lifestyle, preventing another stroke or cardiovascular event, and improving physical function. To aid in exercise prescription, it is recommended that poststroke clients undergo a stress test under the supervision of a physician or other medically trained personnel (15). Personal trainers may also need to closely supervise stroke clients because of possible balance and stability issues or medication side effects (e.g., dizziness, postural hypertension, fatigue, and heat intolerance) (55). Thus, machine-based and supported exercises may be warranted initially when working with these individuals.

After a stroke, peak exercise capacity is typically diminished and the energy costs of physical activity are increased; therefore, lower intensities are needed for exercise prescription. Aerobic exercise recommendations call for three to five days per week of 20- to 60-minute sessions (or multiple 10-minute sessions throughout the day) at an intensity of 40% to 70% of $\dot{V}O_2$ or heart rate reserve or an RPE of 11 to 14. Resistance exercise should be performed two days per week on non-consecutive days for 1 to 3 sets of 8 to 15 repetitions at 50% to 70% of the 1RM, for a total of 8 to 10 exercises addressing all major muscle groups. Intensity should be an RPE of 11 to 14 on a 6 to 20 scale (15). Slow and judicious evaluation of the client for starting loads is a responsibility of the personal trainer. Stroke clients should avoid excessive blood pressure and the use of the Valsalva maneuver. Although some stroke patients may experience limited use of a limb or one side of the body, resistance training for the healthy limb will have a crossover effect on the compromised limb. Thus, the affected side may experience gains in strength despite not actively being worked.

Flexibility and stretching are also important considerations when training the poststroke patient. Too often the post-CVA patient experiences **joint contractures** as a result of the lack of motion around the joint. Over time, bone remodeling by osteoclasts and osteoblasts will occur until the joint becomes calcified, essentially rendering the joint frozen. Early range of motion training may prevent this from happening. Range of motion exercises should be performed before and after each training session (for as little as 5 minutes) as well as on non-training days.

Static, dynamic, or proprioceptive neuromuscular facilitation (PNF) stretching is recommended two or three days per week of 2 to 4 repetitions, holding for 10 to 30 seconds (15). Also recommended for the post-stroke client are neuromuscular exercises, which can help develop new neurological pathways to the affected limbs via the recruitment of dormant channels. Balance and coordination exercises can help decrease the fear of falling and improve safety during activities of daily living. Coordination and balance activities should be included two or three days per week and may include tai chi, yoga, hand–eye challenges, and active video or computer games (15). The personal trainer should be attentive for possible mood issues such as frustration, decreased motivation, and anxiety because these changes are common in CVA patients.

Peripheral Arterial Disease

Peripheral arterial disease (PAD) is a systemic vascular disorder in which there is atherosclerotic narrowing of peripheral arteries, arterial stiffness, and impairments of regulatory mechanisms governing peripheral artery blood flow. Although PAD is a common disease of older adults, the majority of individuals may be undiagnosed (11). The combination of atherosclerotic changes, arterial stiffness, and regulation of blood flow with PAD can result in mismatches between oxygen supply and demand in exercising lower limb muscles. Many people with PAD have no symptoms, but some experience various degrees of **claudication**. Claudication is described as aching, or cramping, in one or more of the calves, thighs, or buttocks during activity such as walking or climbing stairs. These symptoms are characterized as intermittent claudication (IC) because they typically resolve fairly quickly upon resting. The stages of PAD (table 20.2; 48) can range from no symptoms to debilitating leg muscle pain, lower limb ulcerations or infections, markedly limited ability to walk longer distances, and decreased overall quality of life. The four major stages of the Fontaine classification scale of PAD are based on clinical symptoms, while the seven Rutherford stages include clinical symptoms along with associating objective findings observed in PAD-related lower limb ulcerations.

Importantly, PAD is a strong risk factor for adverse cardiovascular events including myocardial infarction and stroke (46). Individuals with PAD may therefore also present with ischemic heart disease and cerebrovascular disease. Because of this, pharmacological management of PAD typically involves various combinations of lipid-lowering antihypertensive and antithrombotic or vasodilator drugs.

TABLE 20.2   Classification of Peripheral Arterial Disease

FONTAINE SCALE		RUTHERFORD SCALE		
Stage	Description	Grade	Category	Description
I	Asymptomatic	0	0	Asymptomatic
IIa	Mild claudication (after 200 meters)	I	1	Mild claudication
IIb	Moderate to severe claudication (before 200 meters)	I	2	Moderate claudication
		I	3	Severe claudication
III	Ischemic rest pain, mostly in the feet	II	4	Ischemic rest pain
IV	Lower limb or foot ulcerations, gangrene, or necrosis	III	5	Minor tissue loss
		III	6	Major tissue loss

Adapted from Norgren et al. (36a).

Exercise Guidelines for Clients With Peripheral Arterial Disease

Since the pathophysiology of PAD is present throughout the body, the personal trainer must be aware that exercise in a client with PAD may cause a cardiac event. Therefore, it is preferable for the client with PAD to be cleared from a cardiac viewpoint by an exercise stress test before embarking on a training program (5). For the same reasons as in cardiac and stroke patients, aggressive lifestyle changes must occur along with hyperlipidemia management.

Generally, as the patient begins to exercise there is an increased demand for oxygen in the working muscle. Therefore, the patient's rating of pain may increase; however, it should be noted that each patient may respond differently depending on their level of pain tolerance. Nevertheless, the personal trainer needs to work in accordance with the patient's physician.

Since PAD is a systemic cardiovascular disease, the personal trainer must be aware that clients with PAD require the same exercise programming and monitoring considerations as those with cardiovascular disease and hypertension. Depending on the severity of their leg symptoms, individuals with IC may be able to walk continuously for only a limited time (e.g., 1 to 5 minutes) before having to stop because of claudication pain. The client will not say it hurts or aches a little; it will hurt or ache a lot. Clients will not be able to "walk through" the pain; rather they will need to stop, sit down, and rest. However, although PAD is a vascular disease, clients with PAD presenting with claudication symptoms have the potential to make substantial gains in lower limb exercise, walking, and stair negotiation capacities.

Treadmill-based supervised exercise training (SET) three times per week, spanning 12 to 26 weeks, is an effective and safe therapy for improving walking capacity in those with and without IC (27). Mechanisms for the increases in walking capacity from SET may be related to a combination of improved blood flow regulation, skeletal muscle metabolic function, and walking biomechanics (29). The goal with treadmill-based exercise training is to lengthen the walking time and shorten the rest interval until the exercise becomes one long continuous activity.

Because of increased risk for adverse cardiovascular events, individualized treadmill-based SET programs in those with claudication symptoms are performed in hospital or cardiac rehab settings by qualified personnel and involve close cardiovascular monitoring.

FIGURE 20.4 Claudication pain rating scale.

Rating	Description
1	No pain or discomfort
2	Onset of claudication
3	Mild pain or discomfort
4	Moderate pain or discomfort
5	Severe pain or discomfort

> It is recommended that a client with PAD be cleared from a cardiac viewpoint by an exercise stress test before embarking on any exercise training programs, and all exercise programming should be in accordance with the client's physician.

Treadmill-based SET programs typically involve intermittent bouts of walking exercise to the point of mild (claudication pain scale = 3) to moderate (claudication pain scale = 4) lower limb claudication discomfort followed by a short rest period until symptoms completely resolve (usually 2-5 minutes but variable among individuals) (29) (see figure 20.4 for the scale). The bouts of exercise and rest are repeated and typically slowly progressed over time so that sessions last from 10 to 30 minutes, eventually up to 60 minutes (29).

Other forms of exercise that can benefit the health of an individual with PAD, with or without claudication symptoms, include home-based walking programs, resistance training, and flexibility exercise using the same general **FITT principles** (frequency, intensity, timing, type) for other forms of cardiovascular disease. All of these can be modified to the individual's capacities and capabilities. Six to eight resistance exercises targeting all major muscle groups, but focusing more on large lower limb musculature if time is limited, performed twice per week on nonconsecutive days with intensities of 60% to 80% of the 1RM are recommended (5). A reasonable goal is to have the client perform these resistance exercises in 2 or 3 sets of 8 to 12 repetitions (5).

CHRONIC OBSTRUCTIVE PULMONARY DISEASE

The term **chronic obstructive pulmonary disease (COPD)** refers to a group of chronic inflammatory lower respiratory lung diseases (emphysema, chronic bronchitis, and in some cases severe asthma) that result in persistent respiratory symptoms and obstructed airflow. Symptoms include constant cough, chronic mucus production, shortness of breath, inability to take a deep breath, and wheezing. Primarily caused by smoking but also by respiratory infections and exposures to environmental air pollutants, COPD is the third leading cause of death in the United States according to the American Lung Association (8). There are 15 million individuals in the United States diagnosed with COPD, and this number is projected to continue rising (38).

Of note for personal trainers, many individuals with COPD experience exercise intolerance not only because of pulmonary dysfunction but also from associated skeletal muscle wasting, weakness, and alterations in muscle fiber composition (50, 52, 64). The combination of these factors in the individual with COPD results in earlier onset of muscle fatigue and decreased physical activity levels (contributing to disuse atrophy), and it can have a negative influence on the individual's health-related quality of life (65).

Exercise is considered the best available means for improving muscle function and exercise tolerance in patients with COPD (35, 53). Traditionally, individuals with COPD are assigned to multidisciplinary outpatient center–based pulmonary rehabilitation programs that include aerobic exercise and inspiratory muscle training as centerpieces of the program. Studies demonstrate that resistance training is a beneficial component of pulmonary rehabilitation, leading to meaningful improvements in skeletal muscle strength and lung function for individuals with COPD (43). Furthermore, home-based exercise programs with minimal clinical supervision encompassing combined aerobic and resistance training have been shown to strengthen both skeletal and respiratory muscles (24, 34).

> ▶ **Individuals with COPD should begin exercise in a formal pulmonary and respiratory rehabilitation facility. After COPD patients complete formal pulmonary rehabilitation and obtain physician clearance, the personal trainer can then become involved, encouraging long-term maintenance of a prescribed home exercise program, smoking cessation, and continuation of a medical plan.**

ASTHMA AND EXERCISE-INDUCED BRONCHOCONSTRICTION

Asthma is a chronic airway disease affecting people of all ages (1 in 7 children and 1 in 15 adults in the United States) (2). Asthma is characterized as a hypersensitivity or hyperreactivity to various types of stimuli resulting in reversible narrowing of the lower airways (**bronchoconstriction**) (3). The triggers (stimuli) associated with asthma appear to be remarkably diverse, ranging from lower air temperatures, viral respiratory infection, stress, tobacco smoke, respiratory allergens, and exercise (10). The combination of airway narrowing, swelling, and mucus production can trigger periods of mild to severe coughing, wheezing, shortness of breath, and chest tightness. Although there are different clinical forms of asthma, the vast majority of clients with previously diagnosed asthma (~60%-90%) will experience symptoms of acute bronchoconstriction after the initiation of physical activity or exercise (1). Thus exercise itself can be one of the triggers for acute bronchial narrowing, independent of other triggers or mechanisms related to airway narrowing in asthma.

The acute but reversible airway narrowing associated with exercise is termed **exercise-induced bronchoconstriction (EIB)** (previously called *exercise-induced asthma*) (39). EIB, in general, appears to depend on the type and intensity of exercise as well as the environmental conditions where exercise or physical activity occurs. EIB can also develop in otherwise healthy individuals (children, adults, and athletes) without a clinical asthma diagnosis. Although it is not fully understood whether the pathogenesis of EIB is the same across both nonasthmatic and asthmatic individuals, many of the common symptoms of asthma (**dyspnea** [difficult or labored breathing], coughing, wheezing, shortness of breath, excessive mucus production, and chest tightness or pain) are also seen in the nonasthmatic with EIB.

It is thought that the normal hyperventilation that occurs during exercise causes a loss of heat and a drying of the airways. These changes along with other factors can trigger acute (early phase) bronchoconstriction. EIB varies but usually occurs between 2 and 5 minutes after the initiation of exercise, peaks after approximately 10 minutes, and typically resolves in about an hour after exercise stops (28). Individuals with asthma or EIB can also experience bronchoconstriction 1 to 6 hours after exercise (late phase) due to airway edema (28). The actual onset, peak, and postexercise duration of EIB depend on the presence and severity of clinical asthma, the environmental conditions, or both.

Pharmacological Asthma Management

In general, asthma medications are prescribed to help control and manage asthma, usually characterized as being either bronchodilators or anti-inflammatory in nature. Their effects may be short acting, used for quick therapeutic relief of asthma symptoms, or long acting, aimed at long-term asthma maintenance and prophylaxis. The proper use of medications is often a key influence on the ability to consistently exercise and be physically active. Importantly, those with poorly controlled or severe asthma are more likely to present with EIB than patients with well-controlled or milder disease (61). Questions or concerns regarding the use of asthma medications with exercise should be addressed directly with the prescribing physician.

Asthma Action Plans

For the personal trainer, careful monitoring of current and past asthma symptoms, severity, and exposures to triggering mechanisms (e.g., temperature, humidity, and allergens) can guide the exercise prescription process. Although athletes and asthmatic individuals can successfully manage many aspects of their asthma condition, it is extremely unwise for individuals with asthma or EIB to independently self-manage their asthma when exercising without proper and ongoing medical advice and guidance. As recommended by the American Lung Association and CDC all individuals with asthma should have and stick to an **asthma action plan** (AAP). An AAP is a written individualized worksheet that identifies the processes and actions that will help prevent worsening of asthma symptoms; it also provides guidance for when to directly contact a health care provider or when to seek emergency care (13).

Those working with and developing physical activity and exercise training programs for people with asthma should review their medically directed AAPs. If a client does not have an AAP, the personal trainer should encourage the individual's health care provider to develop one. The basic format of an AAP seen in table 20.3 (42) should include emergency contact information, contact information of the individual's health care provider, asthma classification (intermittent, mild, moderate, severe), current medications and their individualized uses, and identified triggers of asthma.

Exercise Guidelines for Individuals With Asthma

Individuals with asthma often demonstrate lower tolerances for exercise owing to a combination of factors including overall decreased lung function, EIB, muscular deconditioning, and decreased aerobic fitness (9). The personal trainer must realize that bronchoconstriction can be a significant factor in a client's exercise tolerance and performance. Since those demonstrating EIB are especially sensitive to air temperature and humidity, postpone exercise sessions when conditions of temperature and humidity are more extreme in order to lower the risk and severity of EIB (41).

Large muscle aerobic activity helps improve cardiovascular fitness, but it is essential to slowly build up the client's level of aerobic exercise in order to reduce the risk and severity of acute EIB. This includes providing shorter periods of activity and longer rest periods than with otherwise healthy individuals. Personal trainers working with individuals with asthma should consider using a **dyspnea scale** (i.e., a 0-10 scale that rates the level of shortness of breath, not perceived exertion; see figure 20.5 for an example) early on and throughout their exercise programming. Although aerobic exercise programing to improve cardiovascular fitness should be specifically tailored to the individual, having the client stay within the 3 to 4 range on the dyspnea scale can be a means of controlling the intensity of the exercise.

Individuals with asthma must be properly instructed to consistently perform a minimum 10- to 15-minute variable-intensity aerobic warm-up (e.g., combinations of flexibility exercises, walking, and jogging) to reduce the risk for developing EIB during the performance of higher-level exercise activities. To reduce the likelihood of an acute EIB response after the formal exercise period has ended, the personal trainer should prescribe a cooldown exercise to allow airway temperature to return to normal more gradually. Additionally, careful monitoring of postexercise responses related to acute bronchoconstriction should be a standard practice with all asthmatic individuals engaging in exercise programs.

> In the client with asthma, exercise intensity can be monitored using the dyspnea scale. Many clients with asthma may not be able to achieve standard training heart rates but will still gain meaningful physiological improvements.

TABLE 20.3   Asthma Action Plan

Zone	Peak flow rate (if used)	Associated conditions or symptoms	Exercise considerations
Green	80%-100% of previously best spirometer-measured peak flow rate (PFR) *Peak flow rate at this level suggests asthma is under reasonably good control* Follow the prescribed action plan for management	Currently breathing well Currently no coughing or wheezing Sleeping well at night	Status quo; no specific modifications to currently prescribed training Use adequate warm-up and cooldown to help prevent or control postexercise bronchoconstriction
Yellow	50%-79% of previous best spirometer-measured PFR *PFR at this level signals caution: Airways are beginning to constrict* Follow the prescribed action plan for management	Complaining of some problems breathing Experiencing cough, wheezing, or chest tightness Awakening at night because of asthma symptoms	*Caution:* Consider adequate trial with proper warm-up. Recheck PFR (if being used by the client) Remove from any suspected external asthma triggers Resume training when PFR returns to green zone Use adequate cooldown to help prevent or control postexercise bronchoconstriction
Red	<50% of previously best spirometer-measured PFR *PFR at this level signals a medical alert* Severe airway narrowing may be occurring; follow action plan and seek medical care	Demonstrating considerable difficulty breathing Breathing getting worse instead of better Medications not effectively reducing symptoms	*No exercise:* seek medical attention as described in the action plan Return to training when directed by medical provider and PFR returns to green zone

Note: An AAP is a written plan that uses three stoplight color zones (green, yellow, red) to guide medical treatment toward maintaining asthma control. Personal trainers should be aware of their clients' AAPs as they relate to current exercise programming.

Adapted from Laslovich and Laslovich (31a); based on data from American Lung Association (5) and Centers for Disease Control and Prevention (13).

FIGURE 20.5   Sample dyspnea scale.

Rating	Degree of breathlessness
0	None
0.5	Very, very minor
1	Very minor
2	Minor
3	Modest
4	Approaching serious
5	Serious
6	
7	Very serious
8	
9	Very, very serious
10	Absolute

Most individuals with asthma can safely perform resistance training to improve muscular fitness with lower risk of provoking EIB when incorporating low-resistance, high-repetition exercises. The benefits of a well-designed resistance training program (two or three days per week) for increasing strength, muscular endurance, and neuromuscular coordination are similar for clients with asthma as for those who are otherwise healthy. Specific to untrained asthmatic individuals, exercises using lower resistance (e.g., an RPE of 11-13) and higher repetitions (2-4 sets of 10-15 repetitions per set) and focusing on major muscle groups with extended rest intervals (3-4 minutes between sets) may be more easily tolerated initially with lowered risk of provoking EIB (51). However, although specific exercise training guidelines for individuals with asthma have yet to be firmly established, general FITT recommendations pertaining to aerobic, resistance, and flexibility training can be modified to each individual's capacities and capabilities (5). As with aerobic training, resistance and musculoskeletal flexibility training should include an extended warm-up and cooldown activities to reduce the risk for developing EIB.

The personal trainer should be aware that individuals with asthma may report various levels of anxiety and fear about exercising with asthma. It is helpful to address openly with all clients their concerns regarding their abilities to exercise. Both asthmatic individuals and those with nonasthmatic EIB present challenges for the personal trainer but can significantly benefit from a well-monitored exercise program to improve fitness, performance, and overall activity.

CONCLUSION

Working with clients who have cardiovascular and respiratory conditions poses unique challenges. The guidelines in this chapter have been presented with the idea of simplifying topics that can be very complex. It is common with these populations to present with more than one of these diseases or conditions. The personal trainer should have information on the client's clinical status including health history, current symptoms, medications, and any absolute or relative contraindications to exercise before implementing an exercise program. Beginning with an exercise prescription for the condition of highest risk or greatest limitation helps the personal trainer prescribe exercise appropriately, progress exercise safely, and have a positive impact on their clients' health. The personal trainer and client should set goals that are easy to attain, because reaching goals will help clients psychologically want to continue to train while limiting the risk of adverse effects.

Study Questions

1. Which of the following is *incorrect* regarding hypertension?
    A. refers to high blood pressure
    B. largely occurs without a known cause
    C. only impacts the older population
    D. most cases are treated and managed via prescription medications and lifestyle interventions

2. Activities that increase intrathoracic pressure are contraindicated because this can _____ blood flow return to the heart, with a corresponding _____ in cardiac output.
    A. increase; increase
    B. increase; decrease
    C. decrease; increase
    D. decrease; decrease

3. Which of the following risk factors for myocardial infarction, stroke, and peripheral artery disease increases systemic vascular resistance, ultimately leading to chest pain?
    I. smoking
    II. obesity
    III. diabetes
    IV. high blood pressure
    A. I only
    B. IV only
    C. II and III only
    D. I and IV only

4. A 63-year-old client with peripheral arterial disease describes significant pain when walking for 5 minutes or more. Which of the following programs would best help her increase the amount of time she is able to walk pain free?
    A. Have the client walk through the pain for 2 minutes after the pain begins.
    B. Decrease the duration to 2 minutes at the same intensity.
    C. Have the client take a short rest break once the pain begins, and then continue walking until the pain returns.
    D. Discontinue walking as a form of exercise since it is too painful.

5. What is the recommended range for a client to exercise in when using the dyspnea scale?
    A. 1 to 2
    B. 3 to 4
    C. 5 to 6
    D. 7 to 8

CHAPTER 21

Clients With Orthopedic, Injury, or Rehabilitation Concerns

Morey J. Kolber, PhD, PT, Dean Robert Somerset, BSc, and Michael G. Miller, PhD

After completing this chapter, you will be able to

- recognize common types of injury and orthopedic concerns;

- understand the impact of injury on physical function;

- describe the goals of each phase of tissue healing; and

- describe the personal trainer's role in relation to specific orthopedic, injury, and rehabilitation concerns.

The increased acceptance of the personal training profession and the limitations of health insurance coverage have created a unique practice opportunity for personal trainers with individuals recovering from an orthopedic injury. In many situations, the time needed for full restoration of function and movement and return to activity goals of the client after an orthopedic injury exceeds the reimbursement limits of the health care provider. Thus, people frequently rely on the expertise of a personal trainer to design individualized, safe, and effective programs to support a full recovery and facilitate a return to activity. To successfully manage the needs of this clientele population, a personal trainer must understand the types of orthopedic injury, the timeline for tissue healing, general psychophysiological factors that contribute to injury recovery, and how injury may affect movement and function. Failure to recognize the framework

of the healing process will unnecessarily slow the healing timeline, interfere with the full restoration of client function, and potentially cause more discomfort within the recovery than needed.

This chapter is not intended to provide detailed rehabilitation protocols for specific injuries, nor is it designed to take the place of medical advice given by qualified health care professionals. Rather, the intent is to provide a general framework to guide the delivery of personal training services to meet the unique needs of clients with orthopedic injuries or impairments. The information contained in this chapter should ultimately be augmented by collaborative communication and input from health care professionals to maximize client function and outcomes and should not be considered as diagnostic- or treatment-based guidelines.

Of note, personal trainers are not qualified to provide medical treatments of any kind, including making

The authors would like to acknowledge the significant contributions of Kyle T. Ebersole, David T. Beine, David H. Potach, and Todd Ellenbecker to this chapter.

diagnoses, applying manual therapies, administering medications, or prescribing specific dietary plans. To provide these services, personal trainers must attain relevant board-recognized designations or state licensure in the specific areas of expertise and have liability or malpractice insurance. Therefore, personal trainers need to review their respective state or local practice acts in order to become familiar with their scope of duty.

INJURY CLASSIFICATION

Musculoskeletal injuries are characterized and classified based on a variety of factors including onset and type of tissue damaged. Macrotrauma and microtrauma are mechanism-based terms used to classify injury onset. **Macrotrauma** refers to an injury with a sudden and obvious episode of tissue overload and subsequent damage. The acuteness of a macrotrauma differs from the insidious onset and frequently chronic nature of microtraumatic injuries (67). The lack of overt trauma suggests that **microtrauma** results from the accumulation of tissue damage across time. Although microtrauma is often referred to as an "overuse injury," this type of injury is not always caused by repeated physical activity (30). Thus, not all microtrauma injuries will recover from rest alone. For example, microtrauma may be due to training errors (e.g., poor program design, progressing too early, inadequate rest or recovery), suboptimal training surfaces (e.g., too hard or uneven), faulty biomechanics or technique during performance, insufficient motor control, decreased flexibility, or skeletal malalignment (29).

The type of injury (e.g., strain, sprain, fracture) is determined by the tissue involved (e.g., muscle, tendon, joint, bone). An understanding of common orthopedic injury classifications will provide an appreciation for the tissue healing timeline and inform decisions relative to exercise program design and progression. Table 21.1 describes common musculoskeletal injuries.

IMPACT OF INJURY ON FUNCTION

Injury often results in several physical impairments, including limitations to range of motion (ROM), strength, balance, and coordinated functional movement patterns. Additionally, it is important to recognize the possible psychological effects of injury on an individual and the subsequent recovery process and timeline.

Range of motion can be especially affected since injury creates changes in all tissues. After trauma, **exudate** (i.e., injury by-products) and **collagen cross-links** (i.e., scar tissue) are deposited. **Ground substance** (gel-like material) decreases, resulting in **fibrosis** (a condition in which tissue becomes less supple and more dense, hard, and contracted), which limits the flexibility of connective tissue. Limitations in ROM can be even further complicated should a period of immobilization follow the onset of injury or if circulation is impaired because of age or a medical condition.

The progression of ROM or stretching exercises can depend on the type of tissue, severity of injury, stage of healing, and the person's motivation. If the injury is not too severe and motion is allowed shortly after the onset, active ROM is primarily used (and preferred because it does not require outside assistance). If there is a period of reduced activity or immobilization after the injury, then collagen cross-linkage formation can be more significant and may require repeated lengthy stretches to regain as well as maintain ROM, even after full motion has been achieved. If the deposited collagen is new, it still should be supple and will respond reasonably well to active or passive short-term stretches. If it is several months after the injury, the tissue may be less pliable and will require prolonged stretches if the ROM is still deficient.

The magnitude of the effect of injury on the expression of strength will depend on the extent of the injury, the area or type of tissue injured, the amount of time the person has been immobilized or disabled by the injury, or some combination of these. There can be damage to the muscle itself, or pain and swelling can contribute to the inhibition of a muscle or group of muscles (43, 47). After injury, the rate of muscle loss is greater than the rate of gain; thus, building strength is an important component of a rehabilitation program (49, 56, 67).

Injury-related deficits in neuromuscular control and **proprioception** (an awareness of the body's position and movement) are due to microscopic nerve damage in soft tissue, called **deafferentation**, and disruption in the sensory feedback pathways used for joint stabilization and neuromuscular coordination (67, 68, 90). More simply, this can affect the person's ability to normally interpret peripheral sensations and respond with the appropriate coordinated muscle action to protect the injured area. Thus, the injured tissue and associated structures (i.e., joint) are more prone to reinjury as well as to developing incorrect substitution patterns.

TABLE 21.1   Common Musculoskeletal Injuries

Injury	Description
Muscle **contusion**	Commonly referred to as a bruise and occurs from a sudden and forceful blow to the body. The result is formation of a **hematoma** (blood tumor) in tissues surrounding the injured muscle. Speed of healing depends on extent of damage and internal bleeding. Contusions may severely limit movement of the injured muscle.
Muscle **strain**	Often the result of an abnormal muscle action leading to a stretching or tearing of the muscle fibers. Strains are assigned a grade or degree (first, second, third) to indicate severity of injury. A first- or second-degree strain is a partial tear, whereas third degree reflects a complete tearing of the muscle tissue. Pain, strength limitations, and motion restrictions may increase with an increase in the grade; however, complete ruptures may present with reduced pain from the muscle itself.
Tendinopathy	A more recently accepted term to describe the collective effects of tendinitis and tendinosis.
Tendinitis	Inflammation of a tendon. This microtrauma injury is frequently associated with obvious swelling and pain around the injured tendon. If left uncorrected or if the tissue is not allowed to fully heal, may lead to tendinosis.
Tendinosis	Represents a histological definition of tendinopathy and involves further breakdown and structural degeneration of the injured tendon. In advanced stages, tendon tears may occur.
Ligament **sprain**	Trauma to the tissues that connect bones and contribute to joint stability. Ligament sprains occur when an excessive force (i.e., due to a change in movement direction) moves the joint beyond its anatomical limits and stretches the ligament. Ligament sprains are assigned grades (1, 2, 3) to indicate severity of injury. An increase in the grade may be associated with greater pain and tenderness, swelling, joint instability, and loss of function. A grade 3 sprain, also referred to as a **rupture**, may present considerable instability although reduced pain.
Joint **dislocation**	A joint dislocation occurs when a synovial joint moves beyond its normal anatomical limits (i.e., a complete separation of joint surfaces). If there is only a partial loss of articular contact, it is a **subluxation**.
Osteochondrosis	Osteochondrosis refers to degenerative changes in the epiphyses of bones, particularly during periods of significant growth in children. The exact causes of osteochondrosis is not fully understood. Terms commonly used to describe variations of osteochondrosis are *osteochondritis dissecans* and *apophysitis*.
Osteoarthritis	Condition characterized by a loss of (degeneration) of articular cartilage and abnormal bony outgrowths (**osteophytes**) in a joint. Can occur in any joint but is most common in weight-bearing joints such as the hip, knee, and ankle.
Bursitis	**Bursae** are small fluid-filled synovial membrane sacs designed to reduce friction between tissues such as tendon and bone. When irritated, the bursa becomes inflamed, resulting in bursitis. Bursitis commonly occurs in the hip, knee, elbow, and shoulder and is usually accompanied by swelling, pain, and partial loss of function.
Bone **fracture**	A partial or complete disruption of a bone due to direct trauma.
Bone **stress fracture**	A microtraumatic injury that may result from an abnormal muscle action, fatigue-related failure in the stress distribution across the bone, dramatic change in exercise or training ground surface (e.g., wood to grass), excessive training volume, or a combination of these factors.

Much like the deficits in neuromuscular control after injury are the related compromises in balance and postural control. Although balance can be perceived to be a simple task, muscular weakness, proprioceptive deficits, and ROM deficits can alter the person's ability to appropriately sense and react to maintain balance (67). Injury causes damage to soft tissue and its neural tissue, resulting in impairments in adequate neural feedback in an injured extremity and contributing to decreased proprioceptive mechanisms to maintain balance (3, 25, 32).

Although injury is often associated with physiological impairments, the psychological effects must not be overlooked. The psychological reactions and adaptations can depend on the extent of the injury and rehabilitation (67). Short-term injuries and rehabilitation can be a mild inconvenience for the person, who may exhibit responses of impatience and even optimism to return to activity; but longer-term injuries and rehabilitation can create reactions of anger, frustration, fear, and even isolation, to name a few. The resultant effects may include loss of vigor, alienation, irrational thoughts, apprehension, and dependence on the therapist. All of these are influenced by an individual's personal coping skills, social support, experience with previous injury, and personality traits.

That said, each person does not respond similarly or equally to an injury, and any recovery or training programs should be managed individually (72). Additionally, establishing a good rapport with the person and forming an authentic relationship can serve as a catalyst for optimal recovery (86).

TISSUE HEALING AFTER INJURY

Despite the significant volume of literature and information available, there remain many unanswered questions concerning the specific aspects of the tissue healing process. It is generally agreed, however, that all tissues follow a pattern of healing that includes three phases: inflammation, repair or proliferation, and remodeling. Although each phase is associated with known outcomes, tissue healing occurs across a continuum of considerable overlap, with no definitive beginning or end. It is imperative that the personal trainer understand the tissue healing process because introducing a task or exercise before the injured tissues' readiness to tolerate the load or stress can ultimately impede full healing or cause additional injury (or both). Figure 21.1 summarizes and depicts the overlapping nature of the healing phases.

Inflammatory Phase

Inflammation is the body's initial reaction to injury and is necessary for normal healing to occur. During the **inflammatory phase**, several events contribute to both tissue healing and an initial decrease in function. After tissues are damaged, chemical mediators, including histamine and bradykinin, are released. These substances increase blood flow and capillary permeability, causing **edema** (the escape of fluid into the surrounding tissues), which inhibits contractile tissue function and significantly limits the injured client's activity level. In addition, the inflammatory substances may noxiously stimulate sensory nerve fibers, causing pain that may contribute to decreased function. An important attribute of the inflammatory phase is the influx of platelets, which release growth factors to stimulate healing, fibroblasts for structural support, and signaling molecules that help establish blood supply to injured areas. After an acute injury, this phase typically lasts two or three days but may be as long as five to seven days in the presence of a compromised blood supply and more severe structural damage, as well as after surgery (67). Although the inflammatory phase is critical for tissue healing, if it does not end within a reasonable amount of time, further healing may not occur, thereby delaying the rehabilitation process.

The goal during the inflammatory phase is to prepare for the new tissue formation that occurs during the subsequent phases of tissue healing (66). A healthy environment for new tissue regeneration and formation is essential to prevent prolonged inflammation and disruption of the production of new blood vessels and collagen. To achieve these goals, active rest and passive modalities, including ice, compression, and elevation, are the primary treatment options; however, treatment options will change as the client progresses into the subacute phase. Although a rapid return to preinjury activity is important, the damaged tissue requires rest for protection from additional injury. Therefore, active treatment to the injured area, including exercise, is not recommended during the early acute phase. For more information on acute and chronic injury treatment options, please refer to *NSCA's Essentials of Training Special Populations*.

> **Rest maximizes the natural physiological processes of the inflammatory phase and supports appropriate tissue healing.**

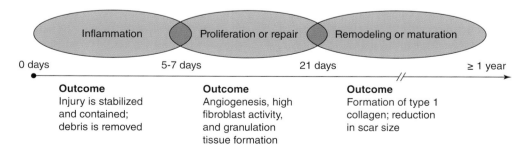

FIGURE 21.1 Healing phases with physiological outcomes.

Repair Phase

Although the inflammatory phase may continue, tissue repair begins within three to five days after injury, or potentially up to seven days in severe cases, and may last anywhere from a few weeks to two months. There is no definitive ending of the inflammatory phase or definitive beginning of the repair phase; rather it is a transitional flow. The **repair phase** of healing allows for the replacement of tissues that are not viable after injury or surgery (67). In an attempt to improve tissue integrity, the damaged tissue is regenerated (i.e., scar tissue is formed). New capillaries and connective tissue form in the area, and collagen fibers (the structural component of the new tissue) are randomly laid down to serve as the framework on which the repair takes place (27). Collagen fibers are strongest when they are parallel and lie longitudinally to the primary line of stress, yet many of the new fibers are laid down transversely. This random alignment does not allow optimal strength of the new tissue and therefore limits its ability to transmit and accept force.

The goals during the repair phase are to prevent excessive muscle atrophy and joint degeneration of the injured area, promote collagen synthesis, and avoid disruption of the newly formed collagen fibers (67). These cautions must be balanced with the gradual introduction of low-load stresses to promote increased collagen synthesis and prevent loss of joint motion. To protect the new, relatively weak collagen fibers, resistive exercises affecting the damaged tissue should be avoided. Specific exercises should be used during the repair phase only after consultation with the client's physician, athletic trainer, physical therapist, or more than one of these. Submaximal isometric exercise may be performed, provided it is pain-free and otherwise indicated. Submaximal isometric exercise can promote strength, but at intensities low enough that newly formed collagen fibers are not disrupted.

Remodeling Phase

The weakened tissue produced during repair is strengthened during the **remodeling phase** of healing. Much like the previous transition from inflammation to repair, the change from repair to remodeling is gradual. In the remodeling phase, production of collagen fibers has decreased significantly, allowing the newly formed tissue the opportunity to improve its structure, strength, and function. With increased loading, the collagen fibers of the newly formed scar tissue begin to hypertrophy (undergo enlargement or growth) and align themselves along the lines of stress, increasing the strength of the newly formed tissue and allowing for the injured client's return to function. Although strength of the collagen fibers improves significantly, the new tissue will likely never be as strong as the tissue it has replaced (1, 14, 27). Tissue remodeling can last up to two to four months or even beyond one year after injury depending on severity, type and location of tissue involved, previous injury, surgery performed, complications, age of client, and so on (48).

Optimizing tissue function is the primary goal during this final phase of healing. Clients improve function by continuing the exercises performed during the repair phase and by adding more advanced, activity-specific exercises that allow progressive stresses to be applied to the injured tissue. Progressive tissue loading allows improved collagen fiber alignment and fiber hypertrophy, optimizing the scar's tensile strength. Ultimately, rehabilitation and reconditioning exercises must be functional to facilitate a return to activity. Strengthening should transition from general exercises to activity-specific exercises designed to replicate movements common in given sports and activities.

> **Full restoration of tissue function after injury can be optimized through careful alignment of activities with the physiological phase of tissue healing.**

ORTHOPEDIC CONCERNS AND THE PERSONAL TRAINER

It is not uncommon for a personal trainer to have a client with an injury history. Therefore, personal trainers should have a basic familiarity with common injuries and orthopedic conditions. However, it is important for personal trainers to understand their limitations and scope of practice—it is not the personal trainer's responsibility to determine movement or exercise restrictions. Rather, personal trainers should be able to determine appropriate exercise strategies based on any movement restrictions or limitations commonly associated with an injury or established in consultation with the client's health care team, including the physician, athletic trainer, or physical therapist. In many situations, a client's health care team may be augmented with additional professionals such as a licensed nutritionist or sport psychologist. A personal trainer should establish effective communication across the entire health care team and frequently consult with team members before making significant advancements in the exercise activities of a client with an orthopedic injury.

It can be somewhat difficult to determine the appropriate exercises and progression for a client with an injury concern. Selection of exercises and activities for an individual recovering from injury should be informed by the injury timeline as well as observation of the client for signs and symptoms suggestive of ongoing injury complications. The most easily observable cardinal signs are pain (*dalor*), swelling, warmth (*calor*) and redness (*erythema* or *rubor*), loss of ROM and flexibility, and decreased strength and function. The presence of any of these classic signs and symptoms may be an indication of inappropriate exercise or of advancing the individual too quickly. It is good practice to increase only one exercise parameter at a time to make it easy to determine what may have triggered the negative response, should one occur. Table 21.2 should give readers an appreciation for using the physiology of healing to guide the selection of exercises.

The underlying pathophysiology for each type of orthopedic injury, surgical procedure, or disease process will be associated with specific exercise and movement guidelines based on indications, contraindications, and precautions. An **indication** is an activity that will benefit the injured client (66). For example, a client who recently had a knee replacement must maintain upper extremity function, so the personal trainer may design a program that allows the client to continue performing upper extremity resistance training exercises during rehabilitation of the knee. A **contraindication** is an activity or practice that is inadvisable or prohibited because of the given injury (66). For example, during rehabilitation from reconstruction of the knee's anterior cruciate ligament, a client must protect the anterior cruciate ligament graft, meaning that closed chain activities are more favored and open chain activities are contraindicated within a certain healing timeline. Therefore, the final 30 degrees of the leg extension exercise is contraindicated because it can place the graft in a compromised position. This is also an excellent example of a situation in which communication with the client's physician, athletic trainer, or physical therapist is essential to the outcome of the injury. A **precaution** is an activity that may be performed under supervision of a qualified personal trainer and according to client limitations and symptom reproduction (66). For example, although this is typically not advised, clients with anterior shoulder instability may perform the bench press provided they avoid excessive shoulder horizontal abduction (i.e., the upper arms stay above parallel to the body).

Because of the many different surgical procedures currently used, designing exercise programs for clients after surgery can be challenging. Typically these clients have undergone some form of formal rehabilitation or have been instructed in a home exercise program after the surgical procedure. Unfortunately, rehabilitation exercise programs often fail to allow the client's return to full function, whether because of limitations of insurance coverage or a lack of client compliance. These place the personal trainer in an ideal position to improve function through both traditional and nontraditional exercise programs. Before designing these programs, however, it is important that the personal trainer not only generally understand the surgical procedure but also understand and abide by the contraindications and precautions brought about by the surgery.

TABLE 21.2 Integration of Rehabilitation Goals Across Healing Timeline

Rehabilitation goals	Inflammatory phase	Repair/proliferation phase	Remodeling phase
Control pain and inflammation (PRICE: protection, rest, ice, compression, elevation)	X		
ROM, flexibility		X	Maintain
Balance, proprioception, neuromuscular control		X	X
Strengthening		X	X
Functional strengthening			X
Return to preinjury activity			X

It is beyond the scope of this chapter to give an in-depth description of every injury, surgical procedure, or disease process. Likewise, it is difficult to provide all the possible injury-specific exercise and movement guidelines. The sections that follow offer general descriptions for common orthopedic injuries and conditions, as well as guidelines to use when designing exercise programs for these clients. This information should not be considered a substitute for injury or postsurgical protocols. Nor should it replace the guidance of other health care providers. Rather, this brief discussion of select injuries and orthopedic conditions is intended to augment the personal trainer's base of knowledge, thereby improving communication with health care providers and ultimately supporting recovery of the client's function in a safe, efficient manner. It is imperative that the personal trainer contact the client's physician, athletic trainer, or physical therapist for a description of the injury or surgery and obtain a list of acceptable movement and exercise guidelines before beginning an exercise program.

> An appreciation for the physiology of healing will allow for appropriate selection of exercises and support of a client's full recovery.

LOW BACK

As one of the leading causes of pain and disability (5), low back pain has become a significant concern not only for health care providers but also for personal trainers hired by clients with this diagnosis. *Low back pain* is a catch-all term involving several different diagnoses including, but not limited to, disc dysfunction, muscle strain, lumbar **spinal stenosis** (i.e., a narrowing of the spaces in the spine, resulting in nerve compression), spondylolysis, and spondylolisthesis. Each of these diagnoses presents differently and requires a different treatment approach; yet each can be logically treated through promotion and reinforcement of pain-reducing postures and movements (also referred to as an individual's **directional preference**), as well as avoidance of any movement that causes the back pain to increase or to radiate or spread over a larger area. For example, if a person has pain with bending forward, it would be recommended that he or she avoid this movement and maybe even perform extension exercises provided these do not produce pain. Persons with disc herniation typically respond

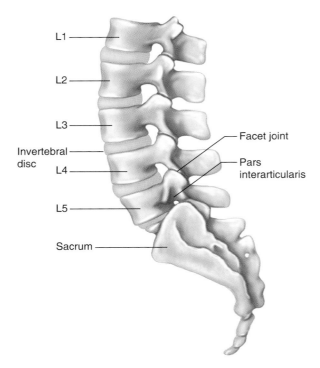

FIGURE 21.2   Lumbar spine anatomy.

best to exercises involving lumbosacral extension, while those diagnosed with lumbar spinal stenosis tend to favor flexion (64). The aim of this section, then, is to apprise the personal trainer of appropriate and inappropriate movements and exercises for clients with given diagnoses. Figure 21.2 shows the basic anatomy of the lumbosacral spine and is referred to throughout this section.

Low Back Pain

Low back pain can be acute, subacute, or chronic and can be caused by a strain, a sprain, disc herniation, osteoarthritis, tight muscles or trigger points, hypomobility, hypermobility, or sacroiliac dysfunction, to name a few. In any case, there are often similar contributing factors associated with low back pain. Low back pain can cause a vicious cycle of pain, decreased function, and loss of muscular support that, if not properly regained, can reappear frequently. Pain in the low back causes muscular inhibition, particularly in the multifidus, lumbar erector spinae, psoas, and transversus abdominis, all normally under automatic control and critical for providing segmental control and stabilization of the spine (71). Once inhibition occurs, the muscles become weak and function improperly. If the pain decreases, these muscles may still be weak because their return to normal function is not automatic once pain ceases; this may lead to future and repeated episodes of low back pain and dysfunction (39).

Movement and Exercise Guidelines

The low back and trunk have a functional muscular anatomy, frequently referred to as the **core**, that is important for performance. Likewise, nearby musculature can have a strong influence on proper low back function. Thus, it is not uncommon to have hypomobility in one segment and hypermobility in an adjacent segment of the low back. For example, the hamstrings, even though they may be considered a lower extremity muscle group, can cause excessive forward flexion of the lumbar area due to the posterior pull on the pelvis, especially during movement, which can result in low back pain. Here, the recommendation may be as simple as stretches or exercises directed at increasing hamstring length.

Low back pain responds well to spinal stabilization exercises, posture corrections, and flexibility exercises. Proper assessment for either tightness or weakness of contributing musculature is essential, and common culprits are located in the hip: hip flexors, hip lateral rotators (gluteals), and hamstrings (67). The extensors of the low back and the abdominal muscles are essential for stability and support; thus strengthening these areas is necessary. Additionally, people without low back injury tend to stabilize or fulcrum about the ankle. Those with low back pain, however, tend to stabilize or fulcrum about the hips and low back to maintain an upright posture in balance tasks, thus increasing or making them more prone to difficulties in controlling postural sway and balance (60). Therefore, people with low back pain, especially those with hypermobility or instability problems, should have balance work incorporated into their programs (62).

In general, a proper assessment of flexibility or ROM and the contributing deficits should be conducted. Flexibility exercises to improve areas deficient in ROM may be done frequently. They should not create pain and may even need to be performed in the opposite direction of painful motions. Establishing pain-free low back and pelvic neutral stabilization exercises and body mechanics should be a primary strengthening goal before progressing to trunk strengthening exercises and eventually more advanced stability and dynamic exercises (67). Should the client have a considerable history of low back pain or a low back injury or experience an increase of symptoms, or if the personal trainer

is unclear about the condition or status, a consultation with the medical providers (e.g., athletic trainer, physical therapist, or physician) is warranted.

Lumbar Disc Injury

In all sections of the vertebral column, the bodies of each vertebra are connected to each other by **intervertebral discs** (figure 21.3). These discs absorb shock and stabilize the vertebral column by preventing excessive shear. Each disc has two layers; the **annulus fibrosus** is the tough outer layer that surrounds the **nucleus pulposus**, the gelatinous inner layer (65). In the lumbar region of the back, the annulus fibrosus is reinforced anteriorly by the strong anterior longitudinal ligament; because the posterior longitudinal ligament narrows in the lumbar region, the support it is able to provide to the posterior aspects of the intervertebral discs is limited. This limited posterior support is one cause of posterolateral disc herniations, the most common type of disc herniation.

When an intervertebral disc herniates, part of the nucleus pulposus makes its way through the outer annulus fibrosus, resulting in tissue damage that causes inflammation; this inflammation, coupled with the potential for the herniation to compress the nerve or other sensitive tissues, may be responsible for low back pain and the potential for referred pain into the lower extremity (73). The irritation can manifest itself in several ways. The client may feel pain in the back; or changes may occur in the lower extremities, including pain, abnormal sensation, and weakness. In

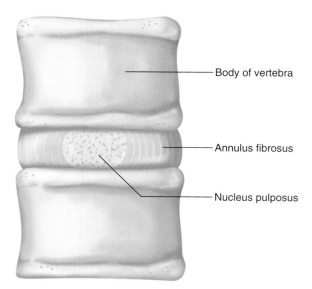

FIGURE 21.3 The components of the intervertebral disc.

addition to the weak posterior mechanical restraints to disc herniation, position is a significant contributor to lumbar disc dysfunction and injury. Excessive flexion (i.e., forward bending) tends to push the disc's nuclear material posteriorly, encouraging it to move beyond its normal confines toward the spinal canal and nerve roots. Clients who have a herniated disc should seek treatment from a qualified medical professional, whose treatment plan may include therapeutic exercise.

Movement and Exercise Guidelines

For the reasons just outlined, clients with herniated lumbar discs are generally encouraged to avoid lumbar flexion in favor of extension to prevent the posterior protrusion of the disc material (89). Therefore, they should avoid exercises involving significant lumbar flexion and should perform strengthening and stabilization activities in a natural lordosis. Resistance training contraindications may include full sit-ups, while precautions may include the squat, all rowing movements (e.g., seated row, bent-over row), and the deadlift. Aerobic exercise precautions may include bicycle riding (because of possible increased flexion with forward lean), using a rowing ergometer, and performing flexion-based movements in aerobic dance. Flexibility is important with a client who has a herniated disc, but stretching exercises involving flexion should be prescribed with caution; contraindicated flexibility exercises include hamstring stretches emphasizing lumbar flexion (e.g., standing toe touch) and other stretches requiring similar movements in the lumbar spine. Precautions may include gluteal, hip adductor, and upper back stretches.

Muscle Strain

As previously discussed, muscle strains are tears to muscle fibers. Strains to the muscles of the lumbosacral spine may have a variety of causes, including direct trauma and overuse. Traumatic muscle strains require completion of the various phases of tissue healing, with guidance from the client's health care practitioner. An overuse injury, on the other hand, requires the client to correct any improper posture and movement patterns. Retraining muscles to function in their intended manner will enable them to work more efficiently, thereby decreasing the abnormal stresses on the affected muscle or muscles.

Movement and Exercise Guidelines

Movement and exercise restriction after muscle strain is highly dependent on the muscle that has been strained. Once the medical provider has determined which muscle or muscles have been strained, exercises and movements that rely on that muscle should be avoided. For example, if the erector spinae muscles have been strained, resisted lumbar extension exercises (e.g., Roman chair back extension) and exercises requiring static maintenance of the normal lumbar lordosis (e.g., bent-over row) should be avoided during the early phases of tissue healing; these and similar exercises may be included in exercise programming during the remodeling phase once the pain subsides in the injured muscle's primary actions.

Spondylolysis and Spondylolisthesis

Spondylolysis is a defect, or fracture, of the pars interarticularis region of a lumbar vertebra (an arched area of the vertebra that connects the superior and inferior facet joints—see figure 21.4) (37, 40). **Spondylolisthesis** is the possible progression of spondylolysis, a forward slippage of one vertebral body on another (46, 80). Although causes vary, spondylolysis and spondylolisthesis commonly occur after lumbar extension injuries or in persons participating in activities requiring lumbar extension (e.g., divers and football linemen). Clients with spondylolysis and spondylolisthesis typically describe low back pain and possible lower extremity radicular pain, paresthesia (tingling), or muscle weakness. Complaints most often increase with lumbar extension and improve with flexion.

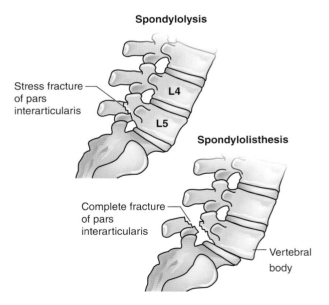

FIGURE 21.4 Spondylolysis and spondylolisthesis.

Movement and Exercise Guidelines

Like clients with lumbar spinal stenosis, clients with spondylolysis or spondylolisthesis should focus on strengthening the muscles surrounding the spine and should avoid exercises involving lumbar extension. Most abdominal exercises are appropriate, especially crunches and exercises for the obliques and transversus abdominis, as are stabilization-type exercises such as those performed on stability balls (provided that lumbar extension is not involved). In contrast to the situation with lumbar spinal stenosis, walking and other forms of standing cardiovascular exercise should not be considered contraindications for clients with spondylolysis or spondylolisthesis. Rather, it is a good idea to encourage these modes of exercise, although they may require modification to adapt to each client's needs. For example, if a client is unable to perform on a stair stepper for more than 10 minutes because of increased low back pain, exercise duration should be kept under that level and then gradually increased as tolerated. Additionally, rapid increases or changes in activity parameters (e.g., frequency, intensity, length of time, type of activity, surface) can produce symptoms, even in seemingly trained athletes. Table 21.3 provides a movement guide for clients with low back pain.

> Effective assessment for posture and movement impairments is essential for establishing appropriate pain-free low back and pelvic stabilization and flexibility exercises.

SHOULDER

Because of the inherent mobility of the shoulder joint and the need for dynamic muscular stability for proper function, the shoulder is an area where specific exercises after injury and surgery can have a tremendous influence on the client's overall function. The anatomy of the shoulder allows for great mobility of the joint, but this can also make it more susceptible to injury, whether acute, traumatic, atraumatic, chronic, or overuse. In the shoulder, it is necessary to consider posture, muscular balance, scapulothoracic control, ROM, and even the relationship to the trunk and hip for the joint to perform as a highly synchronous and balanced complex.

The trunk and hips are vital to shoulder function. The legs and trunk provide 51% to 55% of the total kinetic energy and total force for overhead activities (44). Consequently, a program for the shoulder should include strengthening exercises for the hip rotators, hip abductors, and hip extensors, as well as the abdominal and low back stabilizing muscles.

Another aspect that is essential to shoulder function is correct posture, and any person performing shoulder exercises or with a history of injury should have a posture assessment. A head-forward posture or rounded shoulders (**kyphotic posture**) are common faults and cause medial rotation of the humerus and protraction of the shoulder, as well as weakness of the posterior aspect (scapular retractors and lateral rotators) and tightness of the anterior aspect (pectoralis minor musculature) (67). This can prevent full elevation motion of the humerus and contribute

TABLE 21.3 Low Back Pain Movement and Exercise Guidelines

Diagnosis	Movement contraindications	Exercise contraindications	Exercise indications
Disc injury	• Lumbar flexion • Lumbar rotation	• Sit-up • Knee-to-chest stretch • Spinal twist • Exercises that increase or produce lower extremity symptoms (pain, tingling, burning)	• Passive lumbar extension stretches • Isometric abdominal and extensor strengthening, progressing to lumbar stabilization program while maintaining natural lordosis
Muscle strain	• Passive lumbar flexion (during inflammatory phase) • Active lumbar extension (during inflammatory phase)	Knee-to-chest stretch	None during inflammatory phase, progressing to gentle flexion stretching, followed by extension strengthening
Spondylolysis and acute or subacute spondylolisthesis	• Lumbar extension	• Squat • Shoulder press • Push press	• Knee-to-chest stretch • Abdominal crunch • Pelvic neutral stabilizations • Isometric gluteal strengthening

to subacromial impingement as well as rotator cuff tendinopathy and tears.

Muscle imbalance can contribute to shoulder injuries by affecting the force couples within the joint. In the glenohumeral joint, the external rotators form a force couple with the internal rotators, and the rotator cuff with the deltoid. This muscle balance is particularly important since the rotator cuff assists not only in producing shoulder motion but also in compressing the humeral head into the glenoid fossa, promoting stability and proper joint movement. Individuals who have greater muscle imbalances are more likely to experience subacromial impingement syndrome and shoulder pain (44c). In the scapulothoracic region, the upper trapezius and levator scapulae elevate the scapula; the middle trapezius and rhomboids adduct the scapula; the lower trapezius adducts and depresses the scapula; the serratus anterior abducts and upwardly rotates the scapula; and the pectoralis minor depresses the scapula and restricts upward rotation. The glenohumeral and scapulothoracic muscles act collectively to provide a synchronous and consistent relationship to produce shoulder movement (66). Common muscle imbalances include a decreased external to internal rotation ratio in strength, as well as increased activity of the upper trapezius and deltoid, decreased activity of the lower trapezius and rhomboids, and serratus anterior inhibition (67, 76).

When considering these issues, note that rotator cuff strengthening should be done with lower resistance loads or by choosing exercises that preferentially activate the rotator cuff as opposed to the deltoids (e.g., side-lying external rotation). Increased loads or more advanced exercises activate the deltoid, which can be counterproductive to rotator cuff strengthening and create unwanted superior translation of the humeral head, thus counteracting the rotator cuff exercises and making the area more susceptible to impingement (12). Additionally, fatigue of the scapular muscles can affect shoulder performance; thus endurance activities, especially those in the closed chain that promote enhanced scapular stability, should be included (67). Again, should there be any uncertainty regarding the appropriate exercises and progressions, consultation with the medical care team should occur.

The following sections present an overview of each shoulder injury or surgical procedure, followed by specific exercise indications and contraindications. Included are estimates of the general time frames during which exercise can be most appropriately used. As with all of the conditions described in this chapter, the personal trainer should consult with the client's health care team including the physician, athletic trainer, or physical therapist before advising the client on any exercises.

Subacromial Impingement Syndrome

Subacromial impingement syndrome is a pinching of the supraspinatus, the long head of the biceps tendon, or the subacromial bursa under the acromial arch (figure 21.5). Subacromial impingement syndrome occurs concurrently with rotator cuff tendinopathy, and thus the discussion for impingement applies to rotator cuff pathology (44c). Impingement has many contributory factors; some are changeable with conservative treatment, and others require surgical intervention (e.g., subacromial decompression). Causative factors that may necessitate surgery include anatomic or bony abnormalities (e.g., "hooked" acromion that compresses the subacromial structures). Factors that may be altered include muscle imbalances, poor posture and scapular control, and improper exercise technique or overuse of the shoulder, typically overhead (e.g., baseball pitchers, swimmers).

Many athletic trainers and physical therapists, after reducing inflammation, focus on exercises to improve muscular imbalance and endurance, ROM (if limited), scapular control, and posture. Once formal rehabilitation has ended, a personal trainer has the important responsibility of continuing the exercises performed during rehabilitation. After rotator cuff

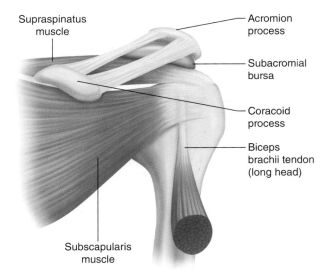

FIGURE 21.5   Anterior aspect of the shoulder.

strength and scapular stability have returned, often as the client notes significantly decreased or absent shoulder pain, personal trainers gradually add typical resistance training exercises.

The rotator cuff muscles position the humeral head in the shallow glenoid, thereby resisting the upward migration of the humeral head into the acromion. Further, muscles attaching to the scapula—primarily the upper and lower trapezius, serratus anterior, and levator scapulae—rotate the scapula during overhead movements. When any of these muscles become weak or fail to function properly, subacromial impingement may occur.

Movement and Exercise Guidelines

Figures 21.6 through 21.10 depict a series of rotator cuff exercises that elicit high levels of rotator cuff activation while minimizing compensation from other muscle groups (6, 67). These exercises are a staple of nonoperative and postoperative shoulder rehabilitation programs (18) and are indicated in postrehabilitation training programs to continue rotator cuff strengthening and maintain proper muscular balance. Because the rotator cuff muscles function primarily in an endurance role, these exercises are typically performed with light weights (seldom more than 4 pounds [1.8 kg]) and high repetitions (sets of 15-20 repetitions). The exercises are chosen for their muscle activation characteristics and because the shoulder is placed in safe, neutral environments below 90 degrees of elevation and with the arm in a forward position relative to the body (anterior to the frontal plane). These positions minimize rotator cuff impingement and allow for pain-free exercise in most individuals.

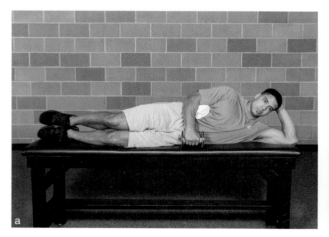 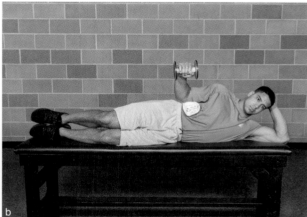

FIGURE 21.6   Side-lying external rotation: *(a)* beginning position; *(b)* end position.

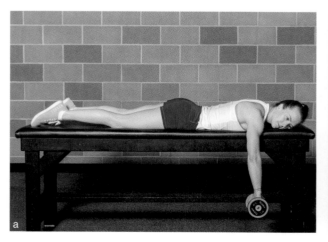 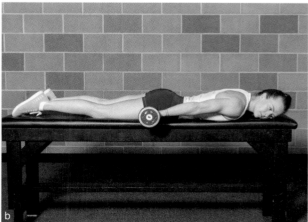

FIGURE 21.7   Prone shoulder extension: *(a)* beginning position; *(b)* end position.

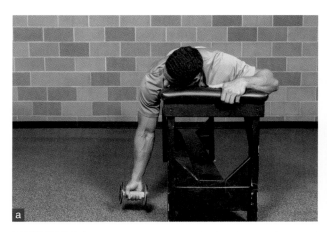
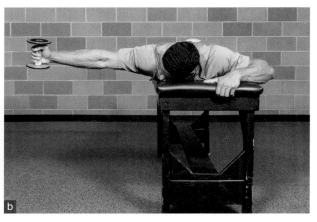

FIGURE 21.8   Prone horizontal abduction: *(a)* beginning position; *(b)* end position. (*Note:* Perform with the palm facing down if anterior instability is present.)

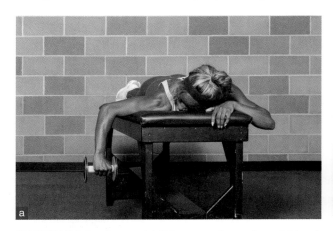
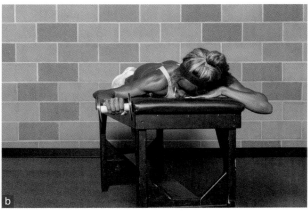

FIGURE 21.9   Prone 90/90 external rotation: *(a)* beginning position; *(b)* end position.

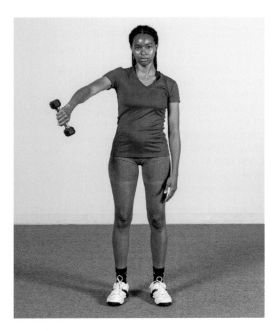

FIGURE 21.10   Standing empty can raise.

Clients who have had subacromial impingement syndrome should concentrate on continued rotator cuff and scapular exercises. Multiple types of rowing exercises targeting the rhomboids and middle and lower trapezius, focusing on scapular retraction and depression, are recommended. Overhead pressing exercises (e.g., shoulder press) and all forms of the bench press exercise should be prescribed cautiously; the decline bench press stresses this area the least and may therefore be an appropriate exercise choice in reintroduction of the bench press. The upright row should also be prescribed with caution, as rowing too high (elbows up too high relative to shoulder height) may aggravate impingement-type pain (44c). It is safe to prescribe exercises such as the lat pulldown by having the client pull the bar in front to the chest, rather than behind the neck, and focusing on activating the latissimus dorsi to depress the humeral head. Further to these exercises, evidence suggests that eccentric overload exercises for the rotator cuff reduce pain and increase function among individuals with subacromial impingement syndrome (11a).

Some cardiovascular exercises may also pose problems for the client recovering from shoulder impingement syndrome. For example, a VersaClimber should be considered a precaution because it places the shoulder in prime position for impingement (i.e., overhead) if strength of the rotator cuff muscles and scapular stabilizers has yet to return. Caution must also be used with overhead sports (tennis, baseball, volleyball, swimming) because the compulsory overhead component of these activities may increase the likelihood of impinging structures within the shoulder.

Glenohumeral Joint Anterior Instability

In anterior shoulder (glenohumeral joint) instability, the head of the humerus moves too far forward, resulting in possible injury, subluxation, or dislocation (31). Management of individuals with this condition is one of the greatest challenges facing medical professionals in orthopedic sports medicine. Because posterior instability occurs less frequently, the discussion here is limited to management of anterior instability, but guidelines for all directions of instability are listed in table 21.4.

TABLE 21.4 Shoulder Movement and Exercise Guidelines

Diagnosis	Movement contraindications[a]	Exercise contraindications[a]	Exercise indications
Subacromial impingement syndrome	Overhead or painful motions	• Shoulder press • Lateral dumbbell raise with internally rotated shoulder • Upright row above shoulder level • Incline bench press	• Rotator cuff strengthening exercises • Pain-free exercises • Posterior shoulder stretches
Instability	• Anterior: combined external rotation with >90-degree abduction; horizontal abduction posterior to plane of torso • Posterior: combined internal rotation, horizontal adduction, and flexion • Inferior or multidirectional: full elevation, dependent arm	• Bench press[b] • Pec deck[b] • Push-up[b] • Behind-the-neck lat pull-down and shoulder press • Pectoral stretches using externally rotated shoulder positions	• Rotator cuff strengthening exercises • Scapular strengthening • Stabilization: static to dynamic
Rotator cuff pathology	Resisted overhead movements	• Painful exercises • Similar contraindications to subacromial impingement syndrome	• Rotator cuff strengthening exercises • Eccentric loading exercises

[a]Consult with a medical professional to determine when or if these movements are no longer contraindicated for a specific client.

[b]Use a close-grip hand position (bench press), with hands no wider than shoulder width (push-up), and avoid the last 10 to 20 degrees of shoulder extension or horizontal abduction past the torso (pec deck).

Research has shown that after an anterior dislocation of the shoulder, recurrent dislocations can occur in as many as 90% of young, active individuals while only 30% to 50% of middle-aged individuals redislocate their shoulders. Tremendous advances have been made in rehabilitative and surgical methodology to treat people with shoulder instability. Surgical management of shoulder instability has progressed to include procedures using primarily arthroscopy, as well as high-tech instruments that literally shrink the joint capsule (thermal capsulorrhaphy) to assist in stabilizing the humeral head within the glenoid.

Movement and Exercise Guidelines

Exercise indications for instability (i.e., rotator cuff and scapular strengthening) are similar to those for impingement, since ultimately the rotator cuff is the primary dynamic stabilizer of the glenohumeral joint. Figures 21.6 through 21.10, as well as the contraindications listed in table 21.4, provide guidelines for performing exercises in a safe manner (44b). Movements that involve greater than 90 degrees of elevation while placing the hands and arms behind the plane of the shoulder (i.e., extension past the frontal plane or the 90/90 high five position) are dangerous because they may place the shoulder in an unstable position (44b). These criteria for shoulder exercises have led to a safe zone that restricts movement to below 90 degrees of elevation of the shoulder and anterior to the frontal plane of the body (figure 21.11) (19).

Clients with unstable shoulders may choose either a conservative, exercise-based approach or surgery as a remedy for instability. Individuals with unstable shoulders—both conservatively and surgically treated—frequently wish to return to traditional resistance training or aerobic conditioning activities or both. It is imperative that exercise modifications be incorporated to protect the structures that were repaired during the surgical procedures. Following these exercise modifications may prove to be a permanent part of the individual's lifting program to ensure that shoulder stability is not compromised (figure 21.12) (31).

Once a client has completed treatment for an unstable shoulder, most aerobic training activities are generally safe to perform, with the exception of some aerobic dance steps, swimming (specifically the freestyle, backstroke, and butterfly), and racket sports. Flexibility exercises that place the shoulder in a position outside the aforementioned safe zone are contraindicated (e.g., the hands-behind-back stretch and the behind-neck stretch, p. 289) because of the adverse stresses placed across an already unstable shoulder joint. One common stretch that should be avoided is the pectoral stretch, which places the shoulder joint in 90 degrees of elevation with 90 degrees of external rotation, also referred to as the 90/90 or high-five position (44b). Table 21.4 provides a movement guide for clients experiencing shoulder dysfunction.

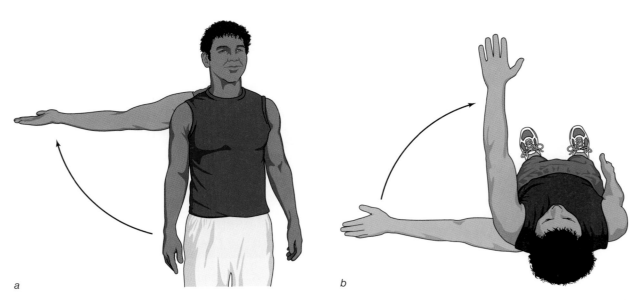

a   *b*

FIGURE 21.11　Safe zone exercise positions. Arm should be *(a)* below shoulder level and *(b)* in front of the body's frontal plane.

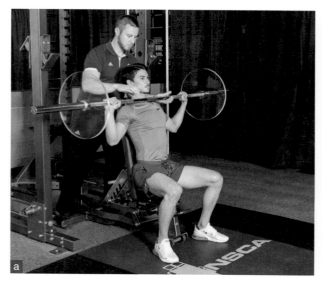
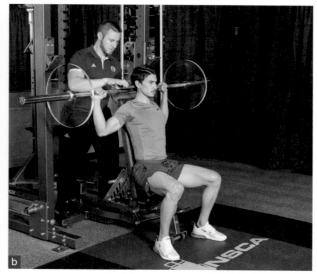
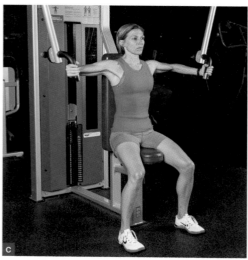
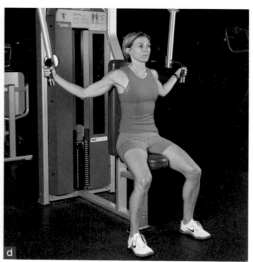
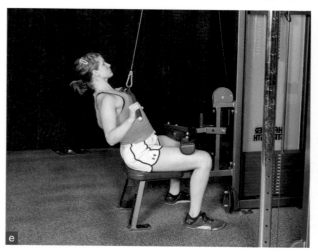
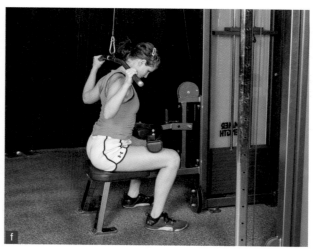

FIGURE 21.12 Exercise modification and anterior capsule stress. The photos in the left-hand column show exercises being performed correctly so as to not stress the anterior capsule. Harmful anterior capsule stress results when these exercises are performed incorrectly, as shown in the right-hand column. *(a)* Correct technique: front-of-face shoulder press. *(b)* Incorrect technique: behind-the-neck shoulder press. *(c)* Correct technique: pec deck. *(d)* Incorrect technique: excessive horizontal abduction and external shoulder rotation with pec deck. *(e)* Correct technique: front-of-face lat pulldown. *(f)* Incorrect technique: behind-the-neck lat pulldown.

Rotator Cuff Repair

A rotator cuff repair is typically carried out when damage to the rotator cuff tendons—most often the tendon of the supraspinatus muscle—includes a tear that is "full thickness," meaning the rotator cuff is not merely frayed but has a tear that goes through its entirety. These tears cause significantly altered joint mechanics (63) and are traditionally repaired using either sutures or suture anchors (fasteners that help reattach the torn tendon to its insertion), most often with an arthroscopic technique unless the repair involves multiple tendons, which may require an open incision.

Surgical repair of the rotator cuff requires periods of immobilization in a sling after surgery, with movements limited to passive range of motion. The exact amount of time spent in a sling without active movement (often up to six weeks) is determined by the surgeon and is dictated by factors such as the individual's age, tissue quality, and presence of additional injuries found at the time of surgery. Although most clients undergo formal physical therapy during their time in the sling, movements are limited to passive ROM and maintenance of elbow, wrist, and hand function.

Movement and Exercise Guidelines

Overzealous client activity and inappropriate exercise introduction can lead to failure of the rotator cuff repair and disastrous results (9). Exercises for the scapular muscles and rotator cuff (figures 21.6 through 21.10) are also used with these clients, but often not until 8 to 12 weeks postsurgery. Discharge from formal rehabilitation is usually three to four months after the rotator cuff repair. The exercises in figures 21.6 through 21.10 should be emphasized during the postrehabilitation programming to ensure continued activation of the rotator cuff musculature.

Contraindicated or precautionary exercises for these clients are also listed in table 21.4. Overhead lifting and exercises such as push-ups and bench presses place the shoulder in a position of stress and can result in overload to the rotator cuff. Aerobic endurance activities that cause discomfort or pain (e.g., swimming, VersaClimber) should be limited. Typically, aerobic endurance training using lower body exercises such as walking, running, and stair stepping is well tolerated and safe for inclusion during shoulder rehabilitation. Additionally, one complication of rotator cuff surgery is loss of ROM, the extent dependent on the amount of immobilization after the surgery. The ROM loss usually includes the patterns of external rotation, internal rotation, and abduction. This finding further complicates the performance of traditional exercises, such as those that place the shoulder and arm posterior to (behind) the head.

Several of the shoulder conditions discussed in this section preclude performance of standard upper extremity resistance training exercises. Responsible intervention by a personal trainer should include screening of individuals who may be at risk when performing these exercises. Table 21.5 describes appropriate modifications that can be made to common exercises and movements to reduce unwanted stress on the shoulder joint. Including rotator cuff and scapular exercises as a core aspect of any upper extremity training program is recommended because of the important role these muscles play in providing movement and stabilization of the shoulder complex.

> **Shoulder exercises should be anchored using an approach that ensures stability of the joint during functional activities through engagement of the scapular and rotator cuff muscles.**

TABLE 21.5   Shoulder Exercise Modifications

Exercise	Modification
Shoulder press	Clients should lower the barbell in front of the head in order to minimize anterior shoulder stress.
Bench press	When lowering the bar, clients with shoulder dysfunction should not allow the bar to touch the chest at its lowest point in order to minimize anterior shoulder stress. A towel roll or bar pad may be used to limit depth.
	Clients should keep the upper arms near the body to limit horizontal abduction and decrease shoulder stress.
Pec deck or chest fly exercises	During the eccentric phase, clients with shoulder dysfunction should not allow the pads to pass behind the body at their most posterior position in order to minimize anterior shoulder stress.
Lat pulldown	Clients should pull the bar down in front of the head in order to minimize anterior shoulder stress.

CONDITIONS REQUIRING SHOULDER EXERCISE MODIFICATION

Exercise for clients with the following conditions is not contraindicated. Each condition, however, requires specific modifications to allow exercise participation.

- Subacromial impingement syndrome
- Rotator cuff repair
- Rotator cuff tendinitis
- Glenohumeral joint instability (prior dislocation or subluxation)
- Acromioclavicular joint injury (separation)
- Glenohumeral joint osteoarthritis

ANKLE

The ankle sprain is one of the most common sport-related injuries, accounting for 10% to 28% of all athletic injuries (41, 74, 75). Ankle sprains are often linked to sports requiring sudden stops, changes of direction, and jumping such as soccer and basketball. An inversion sprain resulting in damage to the lateral ligaments is the most frequently reported type of ankle sprain. The lateral aspect of the ankle is primarily stabilized by three ligaments: anterior talofibular, posterior talofibular, and calcaneofibular (figure 21.13) (41, 74, 75). Most lateral ankle sprains primarily involve the anterior talofibular ligament because of its relative weakness and inability to withstand the force placed on the ankle in an inverted, plantar flexed, and internally rotated position. Although the posterior talofibular and calcaneofibular ligaments are likely to be damaged, it is generally believed that higher levels of inversion force are needed to sprain these ligaments. Thus, a sprain involving the posterior talofibular or calcaneofibular ligaments will likely be quite severe.

Perhaps because of the prevalence of the lateral ankle sprain, many individuals choose to self-treat. Thus, the personal trainer may work with a client who sustained a mild lateral ankle sprain or has been recently discharged from formal rehabilitation after a more severe sprain. An inappropriately managed lateral ankle sprain, however, can lead to chronic ankle instability. To minimize the potential for chronic problems with the ankle, it is important for the personal trainer to encourage the client to seek an evaluation by a physician or clinician before establishing an exercise plan.

Movement and Exercise Guidelines

Vigorous exercise is generally discouraged in the initial phase of ankle rehabilitation. The primary focus should be on controlling the pain and inflammation and protecting the joint to allow for ligament healing (43). The degree of weight bearing will depend on

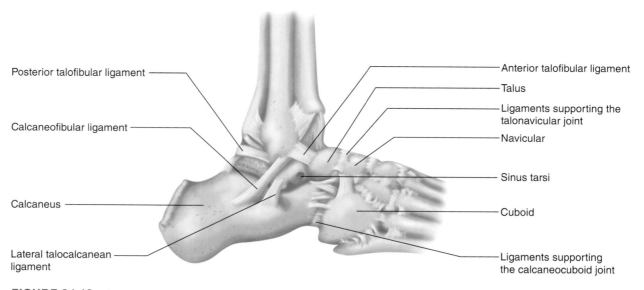

Posterior talofibular ligament

Calcaneofibular ligament

Calcaneus

Lateral talocalcanean ligament

Anterior talofibular ligament

Talus

Ligaments supporting the talonavicular joint

Navicular

Sinus tarsi

Cuboid

Ligaments supporting the calcaneocuboid joint

FIGURE 21.13   Lateral ligaments of the ankle.

the severity of the injury. In general, early ambulation, even if minimal, is encouraged because a small amount of stress promotes more complete tissue healing. During this early phase of recovery, the client may experience lower leg muscle atrophy and loss of balance and postural control. As is the case with other musculoskeletal injuries, the magnitude of the functional deficits will depend on the severity of the injury. Once swelling and pain have subsided, exercises and activities can become more aggressive. In addition to maintaining aerobic fitness (e.g., stationary bike), emphasis should be placed on restoring ROM, strength, and proprioception and should progress to more functional (both simple and complex) tasks (43, 82).

Evidence suggests that a balanced training program can reduce the risk of ankle sprains (52, 84). Balance programs, like other training paradigms, should be progressive in design and gradually incorporate a variety of more difficult and complex tasks. For athletes, the balance program should eventually transition to an in-season phase reflecting a lesser volume and frequency (84). Many of the balance and postural control tasks used as part of exercise protocols for other lower extremity injuries and conditions apply to the ankle as well. For example, a single-leg balance on a stable surface, advancing to an unstable surface (e.g., foam pad, BOSU ball), with and without eyes open; plyometric jumping and agility tasks; and running progressions (e.g., advancing from straight-line running to change-in-direction cuts) can be effective in restoring function to an injured ankle (13, 43, 69, 73, 74, 82). Table 21.6 provides movement guidelines for a lateral ankle sprain.

> Gradually progressing an injured ankle from non–weight-bearing to weight-bearing activities and subsequently incorporating strength, ROM, and balance or proprioception exercises will properly prepare the joint for more functional activities. Supportive devices, such as tape or braces, may help support the ankle joint during rehabilitation and for light to moderate activities.

KNEE

As with the shoulder, the knee is susceptible to a variety of injuries. Here we discuss three common conditions of the knee: anterior knee pain, anterior cruciate ligament injury, and total knee arthroplasty. Again, we do not give detailed descriptions of injury pathophysiology and surgical procedures. Rather we provide an overview of these procedures, discuss general rehabilitation, and outline exercise considerations (indications and contraindications) after discharge from formal rehabilitation. Figure 21.14 illustrates the ligaments of the knee.

Anterior Knee Pain

The term *anterior knee pain* is at times used interchangeably with *runner's knee*, but it is referred to clinically as **patellofemoral pain syndrome (PFPS)**

TABLE 21.6   Ankle Movement and Exercise Guidelines

Diagnosis	Movement contraindications	Exercise contraindications	Exercise indications
Inversion ankle sprain	Inversion with weight bearing	Activities requiring loaded or full weight bearing based on pain and mobility tolerance	• Open chain ROM exercises and strength activities until weight bearing is permitted • Functional progression and neuromuscular activities (balance and proprioception) per tolerance

Note: This information is based on an acute inversion ankle sprain and emphasizes early phases of recovery. Severity of the sprain will determine the level of allowable activity. Once full weight bearing is allowed, closed chain and more functional activities can be incorporated.

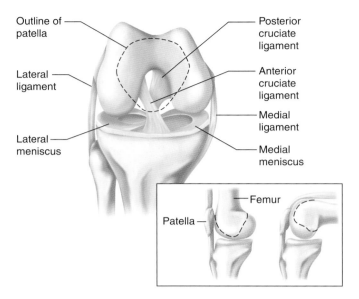

FIGURE 21.14 Ligaments of the knee joint. Anterior aspect of the right knee, flexed at 90 degrees, with patella removed to show the intracapsular cruciate ligaments and the femoral condyles slightly raised to show the menisci. The collateral ligaments are located at the center of the joint but lie outside the joint cavity.

and is a common clinical diagnosis in young adults, associated with general anterior or retropatellar knee pain in the absence of other apparent pathology (17, 67, 88). Patellofemoral pain syndrome is a multifactorial condition with suggested etiologies associated with intrinsic factors such as malalignment of the lower extremity, quadriceps weakness, or neuromuscular inefficiencies of the thigh musculature (or some combination of these) (17, 42, 88). A common malady among personal training clients, anterior knee pain can be associated with a variety of diagnoses (e.g., chondromalacia, iliotibial band friction syndrome, irritated plica, patellar tendinitis). Clients commonly describe pain with prolonged sitting and when walking up and down stairs. Consensus, however, is lacking regarding its cause and treatment. This lack of consensus is likely related to the multifactorial etiological nature of this condition, with proposed causes including overuse (particularly with running), overload, biomechanical faults, and muscular imbalance. Although the diagnosis of anterior knee pain is common, treatment demands an individualized approach based on the underlying precipitating factors and coexisting injuries that are specific to the client. That said, all diagnoses have several treatment commonalities, and rehabilitation frequently focuses on reducing pain and inflammation, correcting biomechanical faults, and optimizing tissue function.

Movement and Exercise Guidelines

Anterior knee pain has been referred to as the "miserable alignment syndrome," and the cause has been described as a combination of factors including femoral anteversion, patellar malalignment, increased quadriceps angle (Q-angle), and tibial external rotation (17). Overuse and training on unsuitable surfaces are common contributors to anterior knee pain and often occur with running, jumping, and bicycling activities. Collectively, these factors alter the tracking of the patella in the trochlear groove, resulting from tightness of surrounding tissues (e.g., lateral retinaculum, iliotibial band), imbalance in the forces acting on the patella, and possibly a change in foot biomechanics (e.g., excessive or improper pronation or supination) (17, 51). Thus, education on proper running surfaces (concrete vs. asphalt vs. treadmill), appropriate footwear, and the benefits of cross-training is quite important in addressing overuse.

Muscular imbalances surrounding anterior knee pain commonly relate to the relationship between the vastus lateralis and a portion of the vastus medialis, the vastus medialis obliquus (VMO). The common belief is that the vastus lateralis overpowers the VMO and pulls excessively on the patella, causing the patella to move laterally when the quadriceps muscles are active. Although it is possible that such an imbalance exists, its treatment is rather controversial. It would seem logical to strengthen the VMO to improve this balance, but research has yet to demonstrate that preferential VMO recruitment is possible. Other research has suggested that in addition to the strength and function of the quadriceps, proximal muscle weakness (e.g., gluteus medius) may be a contributing factor to anterior knee pain. Specifically, weakness in the gluteus medius will allow the contralateral pelvis to drop, thereby forcing the stance limb into a position of internal femoral and tibial rotation (17, 42). This change in the alignment of the pelvis, femur, and tibia may also facilitate hyperpronation of the foot and exacerbate the already poor alignment pattern (17).

Because the quadriceps muscles help clients walk up stairs and assist deceleration of the body during walking on level surfaces and down steps, general quadriceps strengthening does improve patellofemoral function and reduce anterior knee pain. However, weakness in the gluteal muscles will decrease an individual's general ability to stabilize the lower extremity, particularly during dynamic movements. Thus, specific exercises emphasizing unilateral balance tasks

and targeting hip strength are an essential component of treatment and prevention of anterior knee pain. Care must be taken, however, to use exercises that do not adversely stress the patellofemoral joint.

No exercises are explicitly contraindicated for clients experiencing anterior knee pain, but some exercises require caution. Additionally, most open kinetic chain exercises, such as knee extension, increase patellofemoral joint load in the last 30 degrees and should be avoided. High-impact aerobic dance or step aerobics, as well as aerobic endurance training that places the knee in positions such as deep lunging or squatting, would be contraindicated. Typically, cycling (provided seat height is appropriate) and water-based aerobic training activities are recommended to minimize impact and trauma to the knee joint and maintain an individual's aerobic condition during training. It is also common for clients with anterior knee pain to use a form of taping (e.g., McConnell), bracing, or orthotics to assist with stabilization of the patella and support proper mechanical alignment. Table 21.7 provides movement guidelines for anterior knee pain and other knee problems.

TABLE 21.7   Knee Movement and Exercise Guidelines

Diagnosis	Movement contraindications	Exercise contraindications	Exercise indications
Anterior knee pain*	• Closed chain knee movements with >90 degrees of knee flexion • Open chain knee movements 0 to 30 degrees of knee flexion	• Full squat; full lunge • End range of leg (knee) extension • Stair stepper with large steps	• 1/4 to 1/2 squat and leg press • Partial lunge and leg (knee) curl • Stair stepper with short, choppy steps • Hip abductor, gluteus maximus, and gluteus medius strengthening • Spinning or cycling • Single-leg balance
Anterior cruciate ligament reconstruction	Open chain knee movements <45 degrees of knee flexion	End range of leg (knee) extension	• 3/4 squat and leg press • Step-up • Leg (knee) curl • Stiff-leg deadlift • Elliptical trainer
Total knee arthroplasty	High-impact activity	• Full squat • Full lunge	• 1/4 to 1/2 squat and leg press • Partial lunge • Leg (knee) extension and leg (knee) curl • Stationary bicycle • Aquatics, swimming

*Although these movement and exercise contraindications are commonly used, it should be remembered that individual clients react to anterior knee pain differently; therefore, for clients with this general diagnosis, the ranges of motion and exercises provided should be considered relative. Exercises and movements that cause anterior knee pain become absolute contraindications and should be eliminated from the client's exercise program.

Anterior Cruciate Ligament Reconstruction

The **anterior cruciate ligament (ACL)** is a major stabilizing structure of the knee. Injury to the ACL can lead to joint instability during landing and pivoting tasks (7, 16, 50). The ACL primarily limits anterior tibial translation and rotation relative to the femur (7, 16, 50). Because of these important functions, reconstruction is a common treatment choice for joint laxity and possible functional instability, especially for active, competitive people and those with high-demand occupations (e.g., firefighting, construction).

Advances in surgical technique and more aggressive and accelerated postoperative rehabilitation programs have allowed individuals to return to functional activities sooner and with fewer complications than in the past (78). Anterior cruciate ligament reconstruction techniques commonly use either the central third of the patellar tendon as the graft source or a muscle graft from the semitendinosus or gracilis. There is conflicting evidence as to the relative strength of each graft (2, 4, 24), and each has its own set of advantages and disadvantages. In any case, exercises after ACL reconstruction are an extremely important part of a person's return to function and prevention of ACL reinjury, under close guidance from the supervising physician.

Movement and Exercise Guidelines

For the most part, rehabilitation and postrehabilitation contraindications and precautions are the same for the two types of grafts (tendon vs. muscle). The primary difference is that semitendinosus and gracilis grafts preclude postoperative active or resistive knee flexion exercise until approximately four to six weeks after surgery. For both the patellar tendon and muscle grafts, discharge from formal rehabilitation can be as early as three to four months after surgery. Ideally, upon discharge individuals should have reestablished full ROM, lower extremity strength (particularly the musculature around the hip and knee), and static and dynamic balance (38).

During rehabilitation, both open and closed kinetic chain exercises are important parts of the overall program. In **open kinetic chain exercises**, the distal aspect of the extremity can move freely in space (13, 20). Examples of open kinetic chain exercises include the straight-leg raise; leg (knee) extension (figure 21.15); leg (knee) curl; and hip flexion, extension, abduction, and adduction. The open kinetic chain leg extension exercise should be prescribed with caution; research has shown that the greatest amount of anterior tibial translation—hence the greatest stress on the ACL graft—occurs in the final 30 degrees of leg extension in an open kinetic chain (87). Therefore, the ROM of open kinetic chain leg extension exercises should extend from 90 degrees of knee flexion to only 45 degrees of knee extension to decrease stresses placed on the ACL graft. Clients should adhere to this important modification, at a minimum, for the first six months to one year after surgery to protect the maturing graft and minimize damaging stress application.

Closed kinetic chain exercises (figure 21.16) are performed with the distal part of the extremity fixed to an object that is either stationary or moving (13, 20). Examples include the leg press, squat, lunge, step-up, and unilateral stance activities. Translation of the tibia relative to the femur is minimized because of the weight bearing and muscular cocontraction (quadriceps and hamstring muscles) during closed kinetic chain exercises; further, these exercises allow multiple joints and muscle groups to be trained simultaneously. Research (58) has shown that people with ACL reconstruction who perform bilateral closed kinetic chain exercise shield the injured limb from weight bearing for up to a year after surgery, placing a greater percent-

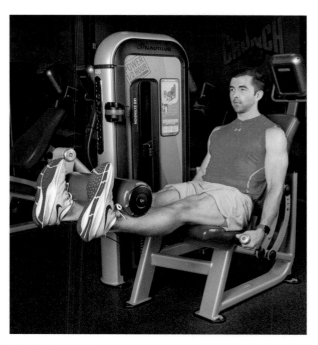

FIGURE 21.15 Example of an open kinetic chain exercise for the quadriceps.

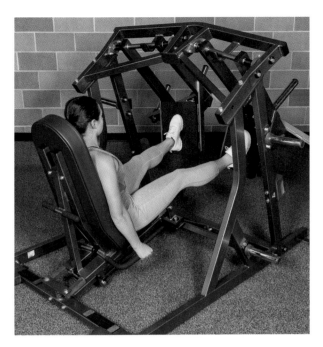

FIGURE 21.16 Example of a closed kinetic chain exercise for the quadriceps, hamstrings, and gluteal muscles.

age of weight bearing on the uninjured limb. They do this subconsciously and without volition. Therefore, reliance on only bilateral closed kinetic chain exercise activities for individuals after ACL reconstruction may result in inadequate training stimulus to the injured limb and suboptimal loading paradigms. Use of unilateral stance and exercise patterns such as single-leg squats and step-ups help ensure that this training compensation does not occur (13).

Incorporating plyometric training is generally acceptable because explosive power and the ability to rapidly change direction are necessary skills for most athletes recovering from ACL surgery (38, 69, 70). However, it is important that the personal trainer understand and establish proper landing mechanics before initiating or advancing a client to plyometric exercises.

The personal trainer should consider a dynamic warm-up to prepare these clients for an exercise session (70). A dynamic warm-up will promote posture, balance, stability, and flexibility across multiple planes of movement (70), all of which are essential to support the needs of a postsurgical ACL client. The warm-up can be tailored to meet the individual abilities and fitness levels of the client but should include activities that emphasize full ROM across all major joints and require general and sport-specific motor skills.

For example, Gambetta (28) has described a number of walking band exercises that focus the warm-up on hip function which is a significant component of any ACL rehabilitation and prevention program.

To summarize the information presented, specific contraindications for exercise after ACL reconstruction include full ROM open kinetic chain leg extension exercise and closed kinetic chain exercise exceeding 90 degrees of knee flexion. For ACL reconstructions using a semitendinosus or gracilis graft, active and resistive hamstring exercise is contraindicated for the first four to six weeks; this becomes a precaution for the personal trainer during postrehabilitation resistance training and conditioning. Further, because both the patella and patellar tendon are weakened by a patellar tendon graft, caution is warranted with activities that rely on significant quadriceps use (e.g., full squats and lunges, stair stepper using deep step movements). Bicycles, elliptical trainers, stair steppers using shallow steps, and swimming are all appropriate after ACL reconstruction, regardless of the type of graft used. Table 21.7 provides movement guidelines for ACL injury.

> A comprehensive ACL prevention program will emphasize proper mechanics and include strength, balance, and plyometric exercises targeting the development of neuromuscular control during all dynamic activities.

Total Knee Arthroplasty

Years of repetitive loading on the human knee can result in degeneration and degradation of the joint surfaces of the distal femur and proximal tibia. Often the degeneration is specifically located on either the medial or the lateral side of the knee joint, based on wear patterns and more specifically the individual's lower extremity alignment. Clients who are excessively bow-legged (**genu varum**) or knock-kneed (**genu valgum**), or who have had serious injury to the knee (such as extensive fractures through the joint, meniscal pathology, or instability of the knee due to unrepaired or failed repair of ligamentous structures), are often candidates for a total knee replacement. However, the most common indication for a knee replacement, or **total knee arthroplasty (TKA)**, is advanced degenerative joint disease (osteoarthritis).

TKA requires extensive exposure of the joint with a large central incision. Prosthetic components are selected and inserted to cover the worn areas at the ends of both the femur and tibia. Rehabilitation begins immediately, with a ROM focus. Clients perform open and closed kinetic chain exercises initially in the hospital and at home prior to formal outpatient rehabilitation.

Movement and Exercise Guidelines

After discharge from formal rehabilitation, clients often have 100 to 120 degrees of knee flexion and nearly complete knee extension. Indications for exercise include cycling, swimming, and aerobic endurance–based activities that minimize joint impact loading and improve muscular and cardiovascular function and fitness levels. Specific exercises such as the leg press, multidirectional hip strengthening, calf raises, and knee flexion and extension exercises using a low resistance and high repetition format are recommended. As strength improves, and as deemed appropriate by the supervising physician, more complex movements, such as lunges onto a BOSU ball (figure 21.17), not only strengthen the knee but also improve balance and proprioception for the entire kinetic chain.

Because kneeling is generally contraindicated (because of pain and stiffness) during the first few weeks after TKA, it is necessary for clients to avoid exercises requiring that position (e.g., kneeling lat pulldown, bent-over dumbbell row using a bench) or exercises that may cause them to kneel inadvertently (e.g., lunges performed too deeply). Postures using less than 90 degrees of knee flexion are recommended in both open and closed kinetic chain exercises. Table 21.7 provides movement guidelines for clients experiencing knee pain.

> Each of the knee joint's structures requires a specific type of exercise to return the client to full function after injury or surgery; with anterior knee pain, for example, the focus is on reducing inflammation and pain, whereas after TKA the emphasis is on ROM. Quadriceps and hip strengthening is a common goal in nearly all knee injury rehabilitation and is a key to returning more normal function after injury.

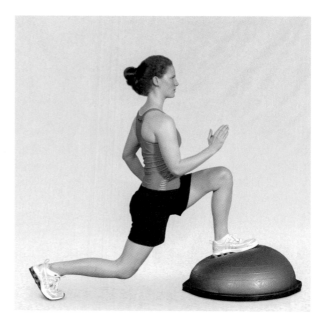

FIGURE 21.17 A lunge performed on a BOSU ball with the flat surface down will result in a greater challenge to the distal kinetic chain. An alternative method is to place the dome side of the BOSU down, resulting in a greater challenge to the proximal kinetic chain.

HIP

Although hip dysfunction does occur, personal trainers will encounter relatively few hip injuries and surgical procedures in comparison with injuries to the knee and shoulder joints. The paucity of hip pathology is primarily due to the inherent stability of the hip; although it is the same type of joint as the shoulder, the hip has a much deeper acetabulum, or socket, which provides a much more stable articulation. This stability precludes many of the abnormal wear patterns and eliminates many of the traumas the other joints experience, resulting in fewer surgical procedures. Despite its generally good fit, however, the hip joint can experience injury and may be poorly aligned, with osteoarthritis and pain as the result.

Hip Arthroscopy

The evolution of hip arthroscopy has revolutionized the management of hip injuries, particularly athletic hip injuries. Hip arthroscopy is minimally invasive and facilitates a quicker return to activity (10, 21). This surgical technique is frequently performed to remove intra-articular loose bodies or to repair a torn acetabular labrum (10). Although still considered a technique in development, current hip arthroscopic procedures have been informed by increased understanding of hip joint pathology and related pathomechanics. The development of the surgical technique has occurred far more rapidly than has the literature related to rehabilitation guidelines. However, the general approach to rehabilitation after hip arthroscopy remains consistent with that for other postsurgery rehabilitations in that it is vital and should focus on restoration of ROM, strength, and gait (21, 79). In addition, rehabilitation protocols for athletes will emphasize development of power, speed, and agility along a progressively more challenging and difficult continuum (15).

Movement and Exercise Guidelines

Although a benefit of hip arthroscopy is the relatively rapid return to activity, strict adherence to tissue healing timelines must be maintained to minimize excess and deleterious stress on the repaired tissue and joint (10, 21, 79). In general, the total time for return to activity is approximately 16 to 32 weeks, determined by the extent of the surgical procedure (i.e., loose bodies, labral tear, osteoplasty, microfracture) and the demands of the activity (10, 21, 79). However, in cases of a noncomplicated surgical procedure of a motivated individual, the timeline may be much less. For example, discharge from supervised rehabilitation around 10 to 12 weeks is not unusual and will likely coincide with the initiation of sport-specific training. As with other injuries previously discussed, a personal trainer may play a significant role in contributing to the complete return to activity of clients after hip arthroscopy. However, it is assumed that a personal trainer would likely work with a client upon discharge from rehabilitation. Thus, the client would likely present with full ROM and the ability to perform weight-bearing progressive resistance exercises.

The sport-specific training phase of postoperative recovery should involve unilateral and bilateral balance and functional activities that continue to reestab-lish dynamic rotational stability, focus on activation and strength of the gluteus medius, and emphasize progressively more difficult sport-specific skills that challenge the client in all planes of motion (15, 21, 79). Examples of activities include multidirectional lunges, lateral agility tasks, running progressions that include cuts and diagonal patterns, cariocas, and activities on unstable surfaces. Table 21.8 provides movement guidelines for hip arthroscopy.

As tissue healing advances, hip arthroscopic rehabilitation must progressively address strength, balance, and sport-specific training for the entire lower extremity.

Total Hip Arthroplasty

Commonly termed *hip replacement*, **total hip arthroplasty (THA)** is the surgical treatment of choice if nonsurgical intervention (e.g., pharmaceutical and physical therapies) for hip osteoarthritis fails. More than 100,000 prosthetic hips are implanted each year, primarily to relieve osteoarthritis pain, with pain relief typically lasting more than 15 years. There are two primary prostheses: cemented and uncemented. A variety of techniques (e.g., posterior, anterolateral, minimally invasive direct anterior, and transtrochanteric) are used during THA (44a). Each has special movement and exercise indications and contraindications.

Cemented prostheses involve affixing the femoral and acetabular components with bone cement, whereas uncemented prostheses allow direct attachment of the prosthetic components to the bone. Each type of prosthesis has its advantages and disadvantages; one of the primary differences, however, is weight-bearing restriction after surgery. Cemented prostheses allow immediate postoperative weight bearing, while uncemented prostheses require weight-bearing restrictions for anywhere from four to six weeks (44a).

TABLE 21.8 Hip Arthroscopy Movement and Exercise Guidelines

Diagnosis	Movement contraindications	Exercise contraindications	Exercise indications
Hip arthroscopy	• Forceful hip flexion • Hip abduction and rotation (early phase of rehabilitation)	Ballistic or forced stretching	• Aquatic walking • Walking • Stationary bike

Note: Contraindications and indications will vary according to the specific arthroscopic procedure performed (i.e., labral repair, microfracture, and so on).

The surgical approaches also have distinct advantages and disadvantages. Most important for the personal trainer is the movement restrictions after each method. Each technique approaches the hip joint from a different angle, thereby decreasing the strength of the hip joint's capsule at the point of entry. For example, the posterior approach—the most common approach in the United States—weakens the posterior aspect of the joint capsule, leaving the hip at increased risk of dislocation. Individuals typically adhere to restrictions for a minimum of six weeks, although this depends on the surgeon's protocols, and in some cases, they should be adhered to indefinitely.

Although varied across total hip arthroplasty surgical procedures, common movement restrictions after a posterior lateral approach during the first six weeks include the following (44a):

- No hip flexion greater than 90 degrees (may be restricted indefinitely)
- No hip adduction past neutral
- No hip internal rotation

Formal rehabilitation after THA is not prescribed as often as for the previously discussed surgical procedures. Postoperatively, individuals should progress to hip and lower extremity strengthening exercises (per surgeon's protocol) and should concentrate on improving their patterns of gait. A sample program might begin with aquatic therapy for gait training and then progress to land-based weight-bearing activities once the incision has fully healed. This sequence will decrease joint load, fear of falling, and muscle guarding.

Movement and Exercise Guidelines

When working with clients who have undergone THA, personal trainers should contact the surgeon who performed the procedure to discuss any continued movement restrictions. When prescribing exercise, the personal trainer should avoid high-impact activities (e.g., running, step aerobics, plyometrics). Lower-impact activities (e.g., swimming, walking, stair stepping, use of elliptical trainer) are indicated after surgery to improve function. Weight training is not contraindicated after THA, but some specific exercises should be modified in accordance with the physical abilities and limitations of the client. Consulting with the surgeon should be considered mandatory when in doubt about movement and exercise choices. Table 21.9 provides a list of exercise indications and contraindications after THA.

ARTHRITIS

Arthritis is a general term encompassing several different diseases. The two primary arthritis classifications are osteoarthritis and rheumatoid arthritis. Although both relate to the joint, these are two quite different diseases. **Osteoarthritis (OA)**, commonly referred to as *degenerative joint disease*, is the progressive destruction of a joint's **articular cartilage**—the cartilage covering the surface of the given joint. **Rheumatoid arthritis (RA)**, on the other hand, is a systemic inflammatory disease affecting not only the joint surface but also connective tissue (e.g., joint capsules and ligaments). In the paragraphs that follow we

TABLE 21.9 Hip Arthroplasty Movement and Exercise Guidelines

Surgical approach	Weight-bearing status*	ROM limitations	Functional movement precautions
Posterolateral	Immediate full weight bearing if cemented technique used	Flexion >90 degrees, adduction, medial rotation	Sitting in a low chair, hip flexion (putting shoes on), deep squats, bending forward to lift from floor
Anterolateral	Immediate full weight bearing if cemented technique used	Extension, adduction, lateral rotation	Turning away from surgical hip
Direct minimally invasive anterior	Immediate full weight bearing if cemented technique used	No precautions with exception of combined extension with external rotation	No functional movement precautions
Lateral/transtrochanteric	Restricted weight bearing for approximately 6 weeks	Active abduction	None

*Hip replacement techniques vary in surgical approach. Prosthetics that are inserted using a cemented fixation technique permit immediate weight bearing. Fixation techniques that do not use a cemented approach require 4-6 weeks of limited weight bearing.

provide a limited discussion of each form of arthritis and appropriate exercise choices.

Osteoarthritis

Osteoarthritis is a degenerative joint condition characterized by deterioration of the cartilaginous weight-bearing surfaces of articular joints, sclerotic changes in subchondral bone, and proliferation of new bone at the margins of joints (11, 22, 23, 53, 54). The proliferation of new bone, which often manifests itself as spurs, or osteophytes, can interfere with normal joint function and cause both pain and limited ROM. Osteoarthritis is present in 15% of adult females and 11% of adult males, and some form of OA is present in some manner in the majority of people aged 55 and older (8, 22, 53, 54).

The proposed pathophysiology of OA includes mechanical stresses that result in microfractures. This microfracturing leads to altered metabolism of chondrocytes, which then leads to a loss of cartilage, altered joint structure, and osteophyte production (11). Loss of cartilage at the joint leads to bone-on-bone contact, thereby causing inflammation and pain.

The use of dietary supplements to improve joint function is currently recommended by physicians for nearly all forms of OA. The common oral over-the-counter supplements chondroitin sulfate, glucosamine, and hyaluronic acid have been recommended for treatment of OA in weight-bearing joints (11). Further research needs to be done to bring about better understanding of both the mechanism and the stage at which these supplements are most beneficial to individuals with OA.

Movement and Exercise Guidelines

Exercise indications for individuals with OA include low-resistance, high-repetition programs of exercise that minimize loading of articular surfaces. Research indicates that training with loads as low as 30% of the 1RM can promote substantial increases in strength and hypertrophy provided the sets are performed with a high intensity of effort (75a). One modality that is particularly helpful in clients with OA is aquatic exercise. The naturally buoyant properties of water allow individuals to exercise with significantly less joint loading than with other forms of activity (81, 83). Additional indications for exercise are the inclusion of cardiovascular training activities with limited weight bearing such as biking, use of the elliptical trainer, and swimming to protect the joint surfaces and minimize impact loading. Weight management, as well as localized muscular endurance that is improved via cardiovascular exercise is of great benefit to the client with OA (table 21.10).

For the upper extremity, resistance exercise programs using predominantly open kinetic chain exercises are recommended. Closed kinetic chain exercises such as push-ups are contraindicated because of to the compressive nature of the exercise at the glenohumeral joint. In the lower extremity, open kinetic chain exercises are typically indicated, with the exception of full ROM leg extension exercises for the individual with patellofemoral OA. As discussed previously, modifications for this open kinetic chain leg extension exercise would include partial ROM arcs either from 90 to 45 degrees or from 0 to 30 degrees of knee motion, where patellofemoral compressive forces are the least damaging (51).

Clients can perform lightweight closed kinetic chain exercises for the lower extremities based on the presence of pain and the individual's general tolerance. Inclusion of balance training to enhance proprioception and motor control for the client with OA is another recommendation. This is particularly effective for training older individuals, who frequently have problems with balance.

Rheumatoid Arthritis

Rheumatoid arthritis is an inflammatory autoimmune disease affecting many joints and often several body systems. Although it may be caused by a bacterial or viral precipitant, the etiology of RA is as of

TABLE 21.10 Osteoarthritis Movement and Exercise Guidelines

Movement contraindications	Exercise contraindications	Exercise indications
High-impact activities	• Running • Snow skiing • Jogging • Plyometrics	• Bicycle • Stair stepper • Elliptical trainer • Aquatics, swimming

yet unknown. The most likely cause is the aberrant regulation of T cells, leading to the inflammation and destruction of joints (8, 22, 23, 61).

Rheumatoid arthritis involves the inflammation and **proliferation** of a joint's synovial lining. This proliferation, or thickening, increases joint pressure and, in concert with rheumatoid pannus (a tissue that dissolves collagen), leads to poor nutrient delivery to the joint, joint swelling, and muscular inhibition. The inflammatory process, swelling, and compromised nutrient delivery weaken the joint capsule and its ligamentous restraints; further, the joint surfaces (i.e., articular cartilage) deteriorate from the same causes. All of this can result in a hypermobile—or loose—and potentially unstable joint. A personal trainer who suspects a client has an unstable joint should refer the client to his or her primary medical provider for further evaluation and exercise programming. These structural changes are painful and typically cause a person with RA to limit movements to avoid pain, resulting in disuse atrophy (77, 85). This contributes to continued cartilage degeneration, increasing the pain and further weakening the joint surfaces (33, 34). So, from the primary joint deterioration, the secondary impairments of RA include decreased strength, aerobic endurance, and flexibility (54).

Presentation of RA is variable, with cycles of **exacerbation** (flare-ups with increased pain, swelling, and stiffness) and **remission** (periods of relative comfort with no outward signs of inflammation). During RA exacerbation, clients typically describe warm, swollen joints and morning stiffness. In addition to these disease cycles, RA is considered progressive. Manifestations may include osteoporosis, muscle atrophy, periarticular nodules, joint deformity, and eventual joint **ankylosis** (fixation or fusion).

Areas commonly affected by RA include the neck, shoulders, wrists, and hands. The upper and midcervical regions of the neck are common sites of inflammation, resulting in the aforementioned tissue degeneration (45, 55). Degeneration or rupture of the ligaments supporting the first two cervical vertebrae may result in a life-threatening situation. For this reason, neck-specific exercises should be considered contraindicated or should be performed only under supervision of a health care professional.

In addition to joints, RA affects muscles and bursae. Degeneration of the shoulder joints and associated structures (e.g., rotator cuff muscles and tendons) may lead to joint hyperlaxity, resulting in abnormal movement patterns and possibly an unstable shoulder joint. Rotator cuff tears occur in 30% to 40% of those with RA (26, 57). Ligamentous and capsular degeneration may result in unstable wrist joints; further, the joints of the fingers and thumbs commonly swell, causing the client to lose grip strength.

Movement and Exercise Guidelines

As in OA, the pathology of RA cannot be prevented once started. However, it may be possible to slow the debilitating effects of RA's secondary impairments (i.e., decreased strength, aerobic endurance, and flexibility). Exercise goals for clients with RA focus on improving function during daily activities, improving general health, and providing protection to the affected joints. Maintaining muscular strength, aerobic endurance, joint and musculotendinous flexibility, functional balance, and a healthy body composition addresses these goals; and these are areas that personal trainers are well equipped to deal with.

Properly designed exercise programs do not increase pain and may actually decrease it (53, 81). Resistance training is indicated for clients with RA. Both isometric and dynamic resistance training modes are appropriate (33, 34, 35, 59, 85), with isometric resistance training appropriate during periods of exacerbation (77). Further, and perhaps surprisingly, vigorous aerobic endurance exercise is not contraindicated as long as it is not high impact. In fact, not only can clients with RA tolerate high-intensity exercise, but this type of exercise may actually be anti-inflammatory and pain relieving (22, 23, 36, 53, 85). A client who is experiencing joint inflammation, however, should avoid vigorous aerobic endurance exercise. Flexibility training is another form of exercise appropriate for clients with RA (53). Although the personal trainer should emphasize not overstretching loose or unstable joints, clients with RA should perform flexibility exercises to maintain adequate joint mobility (53, 59). They should perform stretching every day and can do so in a pain-free range during flare-ups.

The commonly affected areas (i.e., cervical spine, shoulders, and wrists) require modification of exercise programming. Exercises involving the cervical spine should be avoided (e.g., stretching and manually resisted neck strengthening exercises), as should exercises that place the shoulder in an impingement-prone position (e.g., upright row) or in a position outside the safe zone shown in figure 21.11 (e.g., behind-the-neck shoulder press). A last guideline is for exercises involving the wrists and hands; clients with RA may need to have the diameter of the bar, dumbbell, or handle increased in an attempt to offset their weakened grip. For example, if a client has difficulty performing a dumbbell biceps curl, tape or padding may be applied to the dumbbell handle to build up the grip's diameter, thereby improving the client's ability to maintain his or her grasp on the dumbbell.

Because of the periods of changing pain and functional impairment, the personal trainer must select exercises and intensities for clients with RA according to individual tolerances. Clients must be aware of the occurrence of periods of exacerbation and should adjust activity and exercise accordingly; specifically, if a joint is inflamed, rest is warranted (53, 54). Table 21.11 provides a list of appropriate and inappropriate exercises for clients diagnosed with RA.

> **Clients with OA or RA both benefit from performing strengthening and aerobic exercise. The difference between the two is the body's response to activity. Exercise should not increase joint pain for either group. Particular care must be given to the client with RA during periods of exacerbation.**

CONCLUSION

Personal trainers work with a wide variety of clients, many of whom have experienced injury or have undergone surgery necessitating a modified approach to exercise prescription. When designing exercise programs for this population, it is important to understand the basic types of injury and the stages of healing that all musculoskeletal tissues follow. In concert with communication between the personal trainer and other health care practitioners, familiarity with these stages of healing and with individual injury, surgical procedures, and disease processes will assist personal trainers in implementing safe and appropriate programs of exercise for their clients.

TABLE 21.11 Rheumatoid Arthritis Movement and Exercise Guidelines

Movement contraindications	Exercise contraindications	Exercise indications
• High-impact cardiovascular exercise • Neck flexibility or strengthening in clients with history of neck instability • Movements outside the safe zone	• Running or jogging • Upper trapezius stretch • Manually resisted neck strengthening • Behind-the-neck shoulder press	• Moderate-intensity (60%-80% maximal heart rate) aerobic endurance exercise (e.g., stationary bicycle, elliptical trainer, stair stepper) • Range of motion and flexibility exercises • Isometric exercise (for the unstable joint) • Water aerobics • Stationary bicycling • Light resistance training (high reps, low weight)

Study Questions

1. Which of the following apply(ies) to the term *microtrauma*?

   I. sudden and obvious episode of tissue overload and subsequent damage

   II. results from the accumulation of tissue damage across time

   III. often referred to as an overuse injury

   IV. not always caused by repeated physical activity

   A. I only

   B. I and III only

   C. II and IV only

   D. II, III, and IV only

2. In which of the phases of healing are range of motion exercises advised?

   A. inflammation, repair, and remodeling phases

   B. remodeling phase only

   C. repair phase only

   D. repair and remodeling phases only

3. Weakness or failure of the _____ muscle to properly function does *not* contribute to subacromial impingement.

   A. upper and lower trapezius

   B. serratus anterior

   C. levator scapulae

   D. anterior deltoid

4. Which of the following exercises is contraindicated for a client following knee arthroplasty?

   A. full squat

   B. leg extension

   C. leg curl

   D. cycling

5. Which of the following activities is specifically recommended during periods of exacerbation of rheumatoid arthritis?

   A. concentric

   B. eccentric

   C. isometric

   D. plyometric

Clients With Spinal Cord Injury, Multiple Sclerosis, Epilepsy, or Cerebral Palsy

Gavin Colquitt, EdD, and Kelli M. Clark, DPT

After completing this chapter, you will be able to

- understand the basic etiology and epidemiology of spinal cord injury, multiple sclerosis, epilepsy, and cerebral palsy;

- recognize the physiological, functional, and health-related impairments caused or exacerbated by spinal cord injury, multiple sclerosis, epilepsy, and cerebral palsy;

- understand the basic physiological responses to exercise among clients with these disorders compared with others;

- recognize abnormal physiological responses to exercise in clients with these disorders;

- take necessary precautions in planning and implementing exercise and physical activity programs for clients with these disorders; and

- understand the potential functional and health benefits of regular exercise in clients with these disorders.

The many benefits of regular exercise have been well defined in apparently healthy populations. Studies have demonstrated that persons with chronic diseases and disabilities also derive significant health and fitness benefits from a regular, systematic exercise program. This chapter presents information on four chronic neuromuscular disorders: spinal cord injury, multiple sclerosis, epilepsy, and cerebral palsy. The chapter addresses the epidemiology and pathology of these diseases and disabilities as well as the exercise responses, documented benefits of exercise, and exercise testing and training guidelines in these client populations. Some individuals with these conditions may require consultation with medical providers in

The authors would like to acknowledge the significant contributions of Paul Sorace, Peter Ronai, and Tom LaFontaine to this chapter.

addition to regular intake and preassessment procedures. The primary purpose of training for clients with neuromuscular disorders should be to increase functional capacity to improve quality of life.

SPINAL CORD INJURY

Spinal cord injury (SCI) results in the impairment or loss of motor function, sensory function, or both in the trunk or limbs due to irreversible damage to neural tissues within the spinal canal (41). The various grades of SCI may be classified as either complete or incomplete. In the complete form of paralysis, if the injury occurs between the highest thoracic (T1) and highest cervical (C1) segments of the spine, impairment of the arms, trunk, legs, and pelvic organs occurs (**quadriplegia**, also called **tetraplegia**). Injury to thoracic segments T2 to T12 causes impairment in the trunk, legs, or pelvic organs or in more than one of these (**paraplegia**). Paraplegia is also the result of irreversible SCI of the lumbosacral (cauda equina) segments of the spine.

In general, the higher the injury level, the more extensive the resulting deficits. If the SCI is incomplete, the injury to the spinal cord is only partial. In comparison with the person with complete SCI, the person with incomplete SCI may have some sensation or motor function at least partially intact below the level of the injury. In these cases it is best to ask for a physician's statement regarding what muscle and sensory function remains for the individual.

Clinical Manifestations

Clinical manifestations of the acute phase of SCI are many and varied. The incidence of thromboembolic events and dysrhythmias has increased (88). Disruption of the autonomic nervous system leads to reduced vascular tone and unbalanced hyperactivity of the vagal system. Individuals with high lesions, T3-T4 and above, are prone to symptomatic **bradycardia** (low heart rate), primary cardiac arrest, and serious cardiac conduction disturbances.

More relevant to the personal trainer are clinical manifestations associated with the chronic stage of SCI. Of particular importance are potential cardiovascular problems and events. The following are common cardiovascular problems observed in persons with chronic SCI.

- Orthostatic hypotension (i.e., baroreceptor insufficiency)
- Autonomic dysreflexia

- Impaired transmission of cardiogenic pain (T4 lesion and above)
- Loss of reflex cardiac acceleration (T1 through T4 and above)
- Quadriplegic cardiac atrophy (loss of left ventricular mass)
- Atrial fibrillation and other cardiac conduction disorders
- Congestive heart failure
- Pseudomyocardial infarction (abnormal ST-wave changes)
- Sudden death due to asystole
- Atherosclerosis and its manifestations of angina pectoris and myocardial infarction

A relatively common manifestation of SCI that the personal trainer needs to be aware of is **autonomic dysreflexia (AD)**. Spinal cord injury disrupts normal neural regulation of arterial blood pressure, particularly in persons with tetraplegia and lesions above the T6 level (88). Autonomic dysreflexia results from noxious stimuli such as a distended bladder or bowel, constricted clothing, and infections that cause heightened sympathetic nervous system activity resulting in the sudden onset of hypertension. The sidebar on page 595 lists typical clinical manifestations and precipitators of AD (88).

Autonomic dysreflexia can be a life-threatening condition. To prevent AD, the personal trainer should ask clients with SCI each session if they have symptoms such as a headache, blurred vision, goose bumps, or anxiety; check blood pressure before and after the session; and be sure clients have emptied their bowels and bladders before beginning the session. The personal trainer should look for untreated high blood pressure at rest or sustained high blood pressure during recovery from exercise. Diastolic blood pressure should be back to baseline within 15 minutes.

The personal trainer needs to be alert to sudden increases in blood pressure that could reflect AD. An increase in systolic blood pressure of >20 to 40 mmHg or greater could suggest **boosting** (voluntarily inducing AD during distance racing events to improve performance). Because people with SCI generally demonstrate higher heart rates and lower blood pressures compared with others, some athletes with SCI attempt to take advantage of this phenomenon by boosting before competition. They may increase their blood pressure through maneuvers such as holding their urine to distend the bladder or pinching themselves hard enough to cause a reflex response.

AUTONOMIC DYSREFLEXIA

Autonomic dysreflexia can be life threatening. The personal trainer should look for signs of high blood pressure or boosting.

Signs and Symptoms of Autonomic Dysreflexia

- Sudden systolic blood pressure increase of >20 mmHg
- Pounding headache
- Profuse sweating and flushing of skin above level of injury, particularly of the head, neck, and shoulders
- Piloerection (goose bumps)
- Blurred vision with spots in visual fields
- Nasal congestion
- Feelings of anxiety
- Cardiac dysrhythmias—atrial fibrillation, premature ventricular depolarizations, conduction abnormalities

Common Precipitators of Autonomic Dysreflexia

- Bladder distension, urinary tract infection, bladder or kidney stones
- Epididymis or scrotal compression
- Bowel distension or impaction
- Gallstones
- Gastric ulcers, gastritis, gastric or colonic irritation, appendicitis
- Menstruation, vaginitis, pregnancy
- Intercourse or ejaculation
- Deep vein thrombosis and pulmonary emboli
- Temperature fluctuations
- Pressure sores, in-grown toenail, sunburn, burn, blisters, insect bites
- Constrictive clothing, shoes, appliances
- Pain, fracture, other trauma
- Any pain or irritating stimuli below injury level

This practice has potentially hazardous consequences and must be discouraged. Boosting is a reason for disqualification set by the International Paralympic Committee. In addition to causing pain, there are significant health risks associated with this practice, including hypertension, cerebral hemorrhage, stroke, and sudden death (110).

Preventing Injuries in Clients With Spinal Cord Injury

The most common exercise-induced injuries among persons with SCI occur at the shoulders, wrists, and elbows. They are often overuse injuries. Shoulder pain is the most common symptom among wheelchair athletes (51), and this is often due to injuries at the rotator cuff, biceps tendon, or acromioclavicular joint. Carpal tunnel syndrome (CTS) is also common among wheelchair athletes (i.e., prevalence of ~23%) (13). However, these injuries can often be prevented through training programs (30) that focus on muscular strength and mobility at the shoulder joint. Shoulder injury prevention programs that focus on strengthening and partner-assisted stretching—such as ROM in internal and external rotation; shoulder retraction strength; and internal and external rotation strength—reduce risk factors associated with injury (5, 113). Wrist injuries can also be prevented by educating clients on proper technique for wheelchair propulsion and proper positioning during functional activities such as transfers (85).

Personal trainers working with persons with SCI need to be cognizant of these and other potential injuries. Adhering to appropriate exercise technique and exercise physiology principles regarding intensity, duration, frequency, balance in exercise choice, progression, and rest and recovery in particular is essential for injury prevention and optimal physiological adaptation in this population.

> Shoulder, wrist, and elbow overuse injuries are common in persons with SCI. Conservative treatment options include physical therapy, occupational therapy, and activity modification. Therapeutic goals generally include strengthening the rotator cuff, optimizing posture via scapular stabilization, limiting compensatory movements, and stretching tight chest musculature.

Exercise Concerns in the Spinal Cord Injury Population

In addition to higher heart rate and lower blood pressure compared with others, several special concerns need to be addressed in the exercising SCI population, including temperature regulation and venous return. The personal trainer needs to be alert to potential adverse consequences of exercise in clients with SCI.

Temperature Regulation

Disorders of temperature regulation can be expected in persons with SCI, particularly those with lesions at T6 or above. In extreme hot or cold environments, SCI clients with lesions at or above T6 are unable to adequately thermoregulate through sweating or shivering (115). Adaptations that may be necessary for clients competing in these thermally challenging environments include wearing a wet suit in a cool pool or being splashed with cool water during track racing in hot, humid environments. Hot whirlpools and similar extreme temperature environments should be avoided. It is important to beware of freezer burn from cold packs or burns from heat packs.

It is crucial that persons with SCI who are exercising maintain adequate hydration and adapt gradually to environmental changes. Dehydration contributes greatly to the risk of hyper- or hypothermia. The personal trainer needs to pay special attention to ensuring good nutrition and fluid intake practices among these clients. Measures that the personal trainer can take to enhance exercise comfort include maintaining as constant an exercise environment as possible; having clients wear loose-fitting, lightweight, and breathable materials (e.g., Capilene, polypropylene), and ensuring access to cool water or sport drinks.

> Persons with SCI, particularly those with high lesions, are unable to increase skin blood flow in paralyzed areas; this impairs the ability to dissipate metabolic heat and places them at increased risk for heat-related injuries. The phenomenon also exposes them to increased risk for cold-related injuries.

Venous Return

Persons with SCI have poor venous return, particularly in the seated or upright posture, due to lower limb venous pooling secondary to lack of sympathetic tone and absence of the venous "muscle pump." This not only limits the degree of cardiovascular trainability but also can result in hypotension (low blood pressure) during exercise, with symptoms of light-headedness, faintness, and inability to maintain stroke volume and cardiac output. Studies suggest that training persons with SCI in the supine posture may minimize this problem and improve the effectiveness of upper body arm exercise (38, 73). The use of gradient-style compression hosiery may be helpful as well to prevent swelling in the lower extremities. Monitoring blood pressure during exercise is recommended.

General Health Issues of Persons With Spinal Cord Injury

Persons with SCI are at risk for several metabolic disturbances. As a consequence of relative inactivity, decreased muscle mass, and increased adiposity, a high percentage of persons with SCI have metabolic defects including abnormalities in oral carbohydrate processing, insulin resistance, and hyperinsulinemia (7). Persons with SCI also have greater incidence of dyslipidemia, hypertension, and cardiovascular disease (CVD) than do the non-SCI population (88).

Although the person with SCI may not perceive ischemic cardiac pain, other signs and symptoms such as unusual shortness of breath, excessive sweating, fatigue, light-headedness or sensation of fainting, and palpitations may occur. If any such symptom is present, an exercise session should not be started, or should be terminated, and medical follow-up should occur as soon as possible. In clients with suspected or known coronary heart disease, a physician-supervised clinical diagnostic exercise test should take place before the client starts a vigorous exercise program.

Exercise Testing and Training of Clients With Spinal Cord Injury

Persons with SCI can respond to exercise training in much the same way others do. However, problems associated with wheelchair use such as access to facilities, equipment, sidewalks, trails, and so on often make it challenging for people with SCI to engage in regular exercise. The personal trainer needs to be cognizant of these types of problems. The National Center on Health, Physical Activity, and Disability has developed a series of tools called the AIMFREE (Accessibility Instruments Measuring Fitness and Recreation Environments) for fitness professionals to assess the accessibility of facilities. In addition, a sound, basic understanding of the acute and chronic responses to exercise in this population is critical for the implementation of a safe and effective exercise program.

The functional capabilities of an individual with SCI depend on the location and completeness of the lesion. Therefore, it is recommended that clients be evaluated by a professional trained in the American Spinal Injury Association (ASIA) classification system (95). The International Standards for Neurological Classification of Spinal Cord Injury (ISNCSCI), more frequently referred to as the ASIA Impairment Scale (AIS), classifies SCI and provides vital information to the personal trainer regarding location of injury and how this relates to motor and sensory capabilities of the client.

The spine is divided into four segments: cervical, thoracic, lumbar, and sacral. The higher the lesion, the more limited the client will be in regard to functional mobility and independence. Clients with upper cervical lesions (C1-C3) typically need 24-hour care and assistance with all transfers, feeding, dressing, and hygiene tasks. They require the assistance of a ventilator for breathing and use a power chair controlled with the mouth or chin. Clients with lower cervical lesions (C4-C8) require varied amounts of assistance. Some will be able to dress and eat with the help of assistive devices and independently transfer from a power or lightweight manual chair to the bed or other surfaces. Most individuals with thoracic-level injuries can independently perform all activities of daily living, and some with lower thoracic injuries (T5-T12) are able to walk short distances with braces or a walker. Many patients with lumbar-level lesions can walk with braces, crutches, or a walker but still rely on a manual wheelchair for mobility because of the high energy expenditure needed for walking. Lastly, those with injuries at the S1-S3 level may experience muscular imbalances but can walk independently and without an assistive device.

Exercise Testing

A basic evaluation of resting measurements (e.g., heart rate and blood pressure) is required for appropriate monitoring for adverse events during exercise. However, clients with tetraplegia lack cardiac sympathetic innervation, so rating of perceived exertion is recommended for measuring exercise intensity (104) during aerobic exercise. For flexibility, static and dynamic ROM should be assessed at the shoulder and wrist, as well as lateral trunk flexion, using a goniometer. These measurements, along with information from the ASIA assessment, can indicate which tests the client will be able to perform based on the location and severity of the injury.

Because of the high risk of cardiovascular impairment in this group, maximal exercise testing should be administered only in medical settings. However, with proper screening and medical clearance, the competent personal trainer can safely administer submaximal aerobic fitness tests. Although beyond the scope of this discussion, protocols and norms for cardiovascular testing that require only upper body function have been developed for persons with SCI. The modified Åstrand test (4) and 6-minute arm test

> **Maximal exercise testing of clients with SCI should be administered only in medical settings with appropriate professional and physician supervision. However, resting and submaximal testing can provide key insight into the fitness level of individuals with SCI.**

(6MAT) can both be done using an arm ergometer, while the 6-minute push test (6MPT) can be performed using the client's own wheelchair (20).

Physical Activity and Fitness Levels in Persons With Spinal Cord Injury

Habitual physical activity is important for clients with SCI because it is related to overall health and quality of life (50). However, most individuals with SCI are not physically active, and this is often influenced by the location and severity of the injury (36, 71). For instance, physical activity rates for individuals with tetraplegia and complete lesions are much lower than those of individuals with paraplegia (102). A large-scale study found the following physical activity levels among injury severity: C1-C4, 12.68 minutes per day; C5-C8, 22.44 minutes per day; T1-S5, 30.16 minutes per day; partial impairment, 36.45 minutes per day (71). In a similar study, over half of the individuals with SCI reported no physical activity at all, whereas the rest of the participants indicated that most of their physical activity came from resistance training, aerobic exercise, and wheeling (22, 27, 54, 70).

Other researchers, however, have suggested that a significant proportion of variation in physical fitness could be attributed to neuromuscular impairment as defined by lesion level (12). One group reported that 46% of the variation in $\dot{V}O_2$peak could be explained by the level of injury, suggesting a moderate to strong relationship between neurological disruption and aerobic fitness (12). Injury severity can also affect the fitness capabilities and fitness levels of individuals with SCI because higher and more severe lesions are associated with poor maximal power output and peak oxygen uptake. Additionally, based on the type of injury, resting metabolic rates among people with SCI can be 14% to 27% lower, likely due to less overall musculature and decreased activation of the sympathetic nervous system (11).

As with other populations, there is a strong relationship between physical activity levels and both $\dot{V}O_2$peak and upper body muscle strength and endurance in persons with SCI; the greater the daily physical activity level, the greater the $\dot{V}O_2$peak and muscle strength and endurance (23, 26). Research evidence has also shown that physically active persons with SCI have 13% to 23% and 16% to 22% greater maximal cardiac outputs and stroke volumes, respectively, than their sedentary counterparts (24, 25). Thus, although there is controversy about the causes of the decreased aerobic and musculoskeletal fitness in persons with SCI, there appears to be a strong positive relationship between habitual physical activity levels and

$\dot{V}O_2$peak, muscular strength, and other measures of physical fitness.

Particularly in people with tetraplegia, it is difficult to engage enough muscle mass to adequately stress the central circulation or the heart. For example, most of the aerobic improvements with arm crank training seen in persons with tetraplegia are peripheral (increased mitochondria density, aerobic enzymes, myoglobin stores, and capillary density) (39). In deconditioned persons with tetraplegia, however, the stimulus of upper body aerobic exercise may be sufficient to modestly improve maximal cardiac output and stroke volume (37).

Tetraplegia presents unique problems for aerobic training. Particularly in the upright posture, the hemodynamic responses to arm crank ergometry are markedly reduced. Peak heart rate is usually no greater than 120 to 130 beats/min; and cardiac output, stroke volume, and blood pressure are subnormal for given levels of oxygen uptake (40). Persons with SCI, particularly those with tetraplegia, have excessive lower limb and trunk venous pooling during exercise due to autonomic impairment and lack of lower limb and trunk muscle venous pump. In addition, upper body peripheral vasodilation during exercise is not compensated adequately by concomitant lower limb vasoconstriction (39). This reduces central circulatory volume and thereby limits hemodynamic responses to exercise. This dysfunctional syndrome has been referred to as **hypokinetic circulation** (52, 53). There is some evidence that functional electrical stimulation of lower limb muscles may prevent orthostatic hypertension and circulatory hypokinesis, particularly among individuals with tetraplegia because of deficits in the autonomic nervous system (41).

Forced vital capacity (total volume of air forcefully exhaled) is reduced by 50% in persons with high tetraplegia (69). Resistive inspiratory muscle training (RIMT) may improve pulmonary function in people with tetraplegia in the short term (92) and may be beneficial as part of a more comprehensive training program.

Exercise Prescription

The most important considerations when selecting exercises for clients with SCI are the location and severity of the injury. Therefore, it is important that the personal trainer consider the motor, sensory, and autonomic functional capabilities of the client. Table 22.1 provides an overview of activities typical of a person with an ASIA spinal cord injury who is motor, sensory, and autonomically complete (104). The first column represents areas of function and the second

TABLE 22.1 Motor, Sensory, and Autonomic Functions Specific to Injury Level

	C1-3	C4	C5	C6	C7-C8	T1-T5	T6-T12	L2-L3	L4-L5	S2-4
VOLUNTARY MOTOR FUNCTION										
Functional Grasp	None	None	None	Reduced	Normal	Normal	Normal	Normal	Normal	Normal
Mobility	Power wheelchair (mouth, chin, or voice controlled)	Power wheelchair (mouth, chin, or voice controlled)	Power wheelchair (arm or hand controlled or hand-rim propelled wheelchair)	Power wheelchair (arm or hand controlled or hand-rim propelled wheelchair)	Hand-rim propelled wheelchair	Hand-rim propelled wheelchair	Hand-rim propelled wheelchair	Hand-rim propelled wheelchair	Hand-rim propelled wheelchair or walking (limited)	Walking* or hand-rim propelled wheelchair (long distance)
Transfers: chair bench or floor chair	Fully dependent for both	Fully dependent for both	Some assistance: chair bench; Dependent floor chair	Some assistance chair-bench and floor-chair	Independent for both	Independent for both	Independent for both	Independent for both	Independent for both	Independent for both
Lying to sitting	Dependent	Dependent	Moderate assistance	Independent	Independent	Independent	Independent	Independent	Independent	Independent
Sitting	Dependent for quiet sitting	Dependent for quiet sitting	Moderate assistance	Independent for quiet sitting but trunk support required for exercising	Independent for quiet sitting but trunk support required for exercising	Independent for quiet sitting but trunk support required for exercising	Independent for quiet sitting but trunk support required for exercising	Independent	Independent	Independent
Driving	No	No	Yes	Yes	Yes	Yes	Yes	Yes	Yes	Yes
Respiratory Function	Ventilator dependent	Unassisted breathing (diaphragm)	Unassisted breathing (diaphragm)	Unassisted breathing (diaphragm)	Unassisted breathing (diaphragm)	Unassisted breathing (diaphragm and some intercostal)	Normal or near	Normal	Normal	Normal
SENSORY FUNCTION										
Includes light touch, pain, proprioception, and temperature	Present in head and neck	Present in head, neck, and parts of arms	Present in head, neck, and parts of arms	Present in head, neck, and parts of arms	Present in head, neck, and parts of arms	Present in head, arms, and parts of the trunk	Present in head, arms, and parts of the trunk	Present in head, arms, trunk, and parts of the legs	Present in head, arms, trunk, and parts of the legs	Present in head, arms, trunk, and parts of the legs

(continued)

TABLE 22.1 *(continued)*

		C1-3	C4	C5	C6	C7-C8	T1-T5	T6-T12	L2-L3	L4-L5	S2-4
AUTONOMIC FUNCTION	Sudomotor and piloerector function	Normal above the level of the injury and absent below the level of the injury	Normal above the level of the injury and	Normal above the level of the injury and	Normal above the level of the injury and	Normal above the level of the injury and	Normal above the level of the injury and	Normal above the level of the injury and	Normal above the level of the injury and	Normal above the level of the injury and	Normal above the level of the injury and
	Sympathetic vasomotor function	Reduced in arms; absent in splanchnic bed and legs	Reduced in arms; absent in splanchnic bed and legs	Reduced in arms; absent in splanchnic bed and legs	Reduced in arms; absent in splanchnic bed and legs	Reduced in arms; absent in splanchnic bed and legs	Normal in arms; absent in splanchnic bed and legs	Normal in arms; reduced in splanchnic bed; absent in legs	Normal in arms; reduced in splanchnic bed; absent in legs	Normal in arms and splanchnic bed; reduced in legs	Normal in arms and splanchnic bed; reduced in legs
	Sympathetic cardiac innervation	None	None	None	None	None	Reduced	Normal	Normal	Normal	Normal
	Blood pressure responses	Impaired: susceptible to OH, EH, and AD	Impaired: susceptible to OH, EH, and AD	Impaired: susceptible to OH, EH, and AD	Impaired: susceptible to OH, EH, and AD	Impaired: susceptible to OH, EH, and AD	Possible OH, EH, or AD	Normal	Normal	Normal	Normal

Note: Spinal cord injury (SCI) segmental levels in the header row indicate the lowest intact segment or segments.

OH = orthostatic hypotension; EH = exercise-induced hypotension; AD = autonomic dysreflexia.

*Requires lower limb orthoses.

Reprinted by permission from Tweedy et al. (2017)

column represents specific functional abilities within each area. The third column begins with the highest level of injury and each additional column presents a profile of a lower level of injury.

The latest evidenced-based guidelines presented by Tweedy and colleagues (104) cover volume and type of aerobic, muscular strength, and flexibility exercise. These guidelines (see table 22.2; 104) are

TABLE 22.2 Exercise Guidelines for People With SCI

Exercise component	Volume of exercise	Type	Comments
Aerobic exercise	• ≥30 min of moderate exercise on ≥5 days/week or ≥20 min of vigorous exercise on ≥3 days/week or a combination of moderate and vigorous exercise on ≥3-5 days/week • Can be accumulated in bouts of ≥10 min	• Exercise modes involving rhythmic contraction and relaxation of the largest available muscle groups (e.g., wheelchair pushing, hand cycling, or swimming for people who cannot use their legs for exercise) • Wheelchair users who are able to use their legs for exercise should be encouraged to do so in order to maximize the cardiorespiratory demand and reduce physical strain on the upper limbs	• Moderate intensity: 3-6 METs or 12-13 on RPE scale or 40%-59% HRR • Vigorous intensity: 6-8.8 METs or 14-15 on RPE scale or 60%-89% HRR
Resistance exercise	• ≥2 days/week • Exercises covering the major muscle groups, if possible • 4-5 upper limb exercises • 3 sets of each exercise (8-12 repetitions per set) with 2-3 min recovery between each set • Moderate intensity (60%-70% of the 1RM or 12-13 on RPE scale) • Strengthen scapular stabilizers and muscles of posterior shoulder girdle to protect against overuse injuries	Free weights, pin-loaded weights, bodyweight elastic bands or tubing, hydraulic resistance	• Innervation of scapular stabilizers and posterior shoulder girdle is normal in people with PP and progressively decreases with higher lesion level in TP • Strength movements should be pain-free where possible • When pain is pre-existing, it should be monitored and exercise discontinued if pain is exacerbated • Where possible, ensure agonists and antagonists are in balance • Avoid internal shoulder rotation when in ≥90 degrees abduction to limit impingement
Flexibility	• ≥2 days/week • Address the major muscle groups, including those of the neck, upper limbs, trunk, and lower limbs • Hold each static stretch for 10-30 s and complete 60 s of total stretching time for each flexibility exercise (e.g., 2 × 30 s or 4 × 15 s) • Static stretching (active or passive) should be done to a point in the range where there is a feeling of tightness or slight discomfort, or when sensation is impaired, to a point in the range at which resistance begins to increase • Focus areas: stretching internal and external shoulder rotators, chest, and anterior shoulders	Static stretching (described in this guideline) but also dynamic stretching	• To limit impingement, avoid internal shoulder rotation when completing an overhead range of motion • Use caution when stretching paralyzed lower limbs in long-term wheelchair users because of increased incidence of sublesional osteopenia or osteoporosis • Do not stretch the finger and thumb flexors of people with TP who use a tenodesis grip

Note: These volumes of aerobic, strength, and flexibility exercise are required in order for people with SCI to achieve good cardiometabolic health, physical fitness, and functioning.

MET = metabolic equivalent; RPE = rating of perceived exertion; HRR = heart rate reserve.

Reprinted by permission from Tweedy et al. (2017).

similar to those for the general population but incorporate specific recommendations and modifications based on studies of individuals with SCI. These new guidelines also take a preventive approach to secondary conditions associated with SCI such as wheelchair ambulation performance, prevention of shoulder and wrist injury, and transfers.

When training a client with SCI, the certified personal trainer must be aware of the side effects of the most commonly used medications and their effects on exercise. For example, anticholinergic drugs (e.g., oxybutynin hydrochloride, phenoxybenzamine) block the action of acetylcholine and help prevent autonomic dysreflexia (i.e., sudden onset of hypertension) and manage neurogenic bladder. However, these medications may increase heart rate (**tachycardia**), decrease blood pressure (hypotension), and decrease sweat rates, potentially increasing the risk of overheating in warmer environments or during higher-intensity exercise. Antispastic medications (e.g., baclofen, diazepam, cyclobenzaprine, dantrolene) are commonly used to decrease spasticity and reduce tremors. Because of the muscular relaxation effect of these drugs, reductions in heart rate (bradycardia), hypotension, muscle weakness, general fatigue, and sedation may be present. In addition, antiinflammatories (e.g., ibuprofen, naproxen), antibiotics (e.g., sulfamethoxazole, trimethoprim), and antidepressants (e.g., selective serotonin reuptake inhibitors) are often prescribed to help with pain management, prevent common infections, and help individuals cope with a traumatic life-changing event, respectively. The side effects of these drugs include nausea, weight gain, fatigue, constipation, dizziness, weakness, and confusion. Thus, when training a client with SCI, the personal trainer must take additional precautions for increased fall risks, GI issues, and fatigue. It is recommended that blood pressure and rating of perceived exertion (RPE) be monitored throughout exercise because heart rate and blood pressure can be affected by these commonly prescribed medications.

In summary, persons with SCI can benefit from a systematic and progressive comprehensive exercise program. For a comprehensive overview of exercise recommendations for people with SCI, see Tweedy and colleagues (104).

MULTIPLE SCLEROSIS

Multiple sclerosis (MS) is a disease that disrupts communication between the central nervous system and other parts of the body (82). The National Institute of Neurological Disorders and Stroke (NINDS) within the National Institutes of Health (NIH) has many resources for patients, caregivers, and clinicians, based on the latest research on causes of the disease, symptoms, and treatments. As the disease progresses, the body attacks the myelin sheath surrounding the axons (white matter) while also damaging nerve cells in the gray matter in the brain (79). This results in the formation of scar tissue (also called *scleroses* or *plaques*) in the white matter. These scleroses or plaques are the result of the brain sending signals from the immune system to the myelin sheath. Similar to rheumatoid arthritis and lupus, MS is an autoimmune disease whereby the body attacks healthy cells. The symptoms associated with MS depend on the severity of the condition and the location of the sclerosis in the central nervous system.

According to the National Institutes of Health (79), people with MS experience significant variation in the intensity, timing, and severity of symptoms. Symptoms can be mild to severe, begin in a single day or develop over a period of months, and can end abruptly or continue for extended periods of time. Common terminology associated with the symptoms include *exacerbation, remission,* and *relapse*. An **exacerbation** is the onset of symptoms, sometimes referred to as an *attack*. **Remission** refers to the termination of symptoms, while **relapse** refers to the return of symptoms. Table 22.3 contains an overview of the initial and late-stage symptoms of MS (82), and table 22.4 describes the clinical classifications of MS (82).

Clients with MS typically take prescription medications (e.g., corticosteroids and beta interferons) to help reduce the severity of an exacerbation, slow the progression of the disease, decrease spasticity, and relieve pain. When training these clients, the personal trainer should be mindful of common side effects such as fatigue, weight gain, depression, increased sweat rates, seizures, muscle weakness, dizziness, and hypotension. It is recommended that blood pressure and RPE be monitored throughout exercise and overexertion be avoided to decrease risk of an MS attack.

Exercise Testing and Training of Clients With Multiple Sclerosis

People with MS experience many barriers to physical activity, including disease symptoms, psychosocial factors, fatigue, lack of knowledge of exercise, and environmental factors (e.g., cost and transportation) (91). The personal trainer should be aware of these barriers and plan a training program that proactively accounts for them and includes approaches to prevent potential symptoms.

TABLE 22.3   Initial and Late-Stage Symptoms of MS

Common early symptoms of MS	Vision problems such as blurred or double vision or optic neuritis, which causes pain in the eye and a rapid loss of vision
	Weak, stiff muscles, often with painful muscle spasms
	Tingling or numbness in the arms, legs, trunk, or face
	Clumsiness, particularly difficulty staying balanced when walking
	Bladder control problems, either inability to control the bladder or urgency
	Dizziness that does not go away
Common later symptoms of MS	Mental or physical fatigue that accompanies the initial symptoms during an attack
	Mood changes such as depression or euphoria
	Changes in the ability to concentrate or to multitask effectively
	Difficulty making decisions, planning, or prioritizing at work or in private life

Data from National Institutes of Health, National Institute of Neurological Disorders and Stroke (82).

TABLE 22.4   Major Clinical Classifications and Characteristics of Multiple Sclerosis

Classification	Characteristics
Relapsing-remitting MS (RRMS)	RRMS is characterized by periods of exacerbations or attacks followed by full or almost full recovery. This is often the initial stage of the disease.
Primary-progressive MS (PPMS)	PPMS progresses slowly and steadily from its onset. Symptoms continue from the start and steadily worsen without periods of remission and relapse. This type of MS usually coincides with a later onset, around the age of 40.
Secondary-progressive MS (SPMS)	SPMS often develops in people who have RRMS and then transition into a primary progressive course. Most individuals with RRMS will progress to SPMS without treatment.

Source: Jackson and Mulcare (56).

Exercise can greatly improve function (48, 89) and quality of life for people with MS. Aerobic endurance training in persons with MS can improve $\dot{V}O_2$peak, upper and lower body strength, body composition, and risk factors for CVD (21, 56, 75a, 99a, 101a, 101b). Additionally, exercise can improve specific symptoms associated with MS such as balance (48), muscular strength (62), and fatigue (89).

Many persons with MS experience heat sensitivity that is often associated with a transient increase in clinical signs and symptoms. This may preclude or deter persons with MS from participating in a regular exercise program in which metabolic heat is increased. Therefore, it is important that the personal trainer conduct testing in a cool, climate-controlled room. Additionally, it is important that the personal trainer be aware of all potential symptoms associated with MS and that these are monitored during exercise testing and training. Fatigue is common, so testing should be performed earlier in the day. Because of potential decreases in function as the disease progresses, testing should focus on functional assessments such as static and dynamic balance, strength, and muscular endurance as well as other functional tests such as the sit-to-stand and timed up and go (TUG) tests. A slow, progressive warm-up is also recommended before exercise testing.

> Heat may exacerbate symptoms of MS. A comfortable environment for exercise can enhance the physiological benefits and increase adherence. Proper hydration is critical for maintaining temperature balance during exercise in persons with MS.

Exercise Testing

Exercise testing of persons with MS should be administered with extreme caution. People with MS who have or are at risk for CVD must be screened and administered a clinical exercise test under the supervision of a physician to rule out ischemia and coronary heart disease before starting an exercise program. However, with proper medical clearance, the personal trainer can safely administer a submaximal aerobic exercise test to establish a baseline for future comparisons. Because of incoordination and possible balance deficits, leg or arm ergometry is the preferred modality. Some clients may benefit from seated recumbent stepping ergometers that use upper and lower extremity movements. Some of these devices are equipped with stabilization kits that would allow clients with MS to use this modality without limitations or postural or trunk control. Submaximal tests for these devices, such as the modified Åstrand, are advised (4).

Because of their relationship to function, flexibility and mobility are important test considerations. Abnormal muscle tone and spasticity can lead to long-term loss of mobility at specific joints. Therefore, mobility and ROM at joints in the upper and lower extremities should be tested with a goniometer. Before prescribing resistance training, the personal trainer should assess the health history of the individual and assess any potential limb weaknesses, spastic muscles, and **contractures** (permanent shortening of muscles and tendons). In the absence of these conditions, multiple RM tests for each major muscle group, following the guidelines in chapter 15, will help the personal trainer develop an appropriate exercise prescription for resistance training. Functional testing such as the TUG test and five times sit-to-stand test are also important considerations because they correlate with activities of daily living, gait, and balance (50).

Resistance Training

Resistance training has many benefits for clients with MS. A lower extremity progressive resistance training program can improve both muscle strength and functional capacity among the MS population (21). For example, after engaging in an eight-week progressive resistance training program consisting of 1 set of 8 to 15 repetitions at 50% to 70% of maximal voluntary contraction (MVC) strength, subjects improved knee extension, plantar flexion, and stepping performance by 7.4%, 52%, and 8.7%, respectively (111). Likewise, after participating in a six-month randomized con-

trolled exercise program consisting of one aerobic conditioning and three resistance training sessions per week, participants with MS have demonstrated significant improvements in walking speed, knee flexion strength, and upper extremity muscle endurance (96). It is recommended that clients engage in resistance training two days per week, initially performing 1 set of 10 to 15 repetitions at 60% to 80% of the estimated 1RM using various exercise modalities (67). However, performance of 1RM testing may not be safe or feasible for this population. Multiple RM testing may provide a more practical and accurate method of appropriately prescribing intensity for 10 to 15 repetitions.

Goals of resistance training should be based on the needs of the client. Exercises should be selected with movement patterns that are similar to activities of daily living. The modalities of the exercise (e.g., machine, free weights, body weight, or resistance bands) should balance the need to focus on the function, coordinative capabilities, and resistance training status of the client. Multijoint free-weight exercises have many potential benefits but should not be attempted until the client has developed a strong conditioning base using bodyweight exercises, selectorized machines, and manual resistance.

Aerobic Conditioning

Individuals with MS have poorer aerobic capacity than do people without disability, but aerobic training offers many health benefits for those with MS (65). The response of persons with MS to submaximal aerobic exercise appears to vary depending on the stage and severity of the disease progression. Moderate-intensity aerobic exercise improves physical fitness (8), mobility (60, 101), walking speed and capacity (96), and exercise tolerance (93); reduces fatigue (72); and decreases disability (60, 93) among individuals with MS. Progressive high-intensity aerobic exercise may also serve as a protective factor for brain function, potentially improving gray matter and preventing relapse (66).

This research illustrates the need to carefully prescribe aerobic exercise intensity to ensure a light to moderate workload that progresses to higher intensities. The goals of an aerobic conditioning program for persons with MS are to improve cardiorespiratory function, reduce the risks for CVD, and reduce activity-induced fatigue. It is recommended that deconditioned people with MS begin exercising two days per week at 40% of HRR, in sessions of at least 10 minutes, progressing to 30 minutes of moderate intensity two days per week and incorporating strengthening exercises for all major muscle groups two times per week (67). Exercise tolerance may be affected by poor aerobic functioning or MS symptoms (e.g., fatigue); however, many people with MS can engage in aerobic exercise. The potential for adaptations is based on current disability status, disease severity, and disease type.

> **Many people with MS can engage in aerobic exercise. The potential for adaptations is based on current disability status, disease severity, and disease type.**

Some precautions and guidelines for exercise testing and training of clients with MS are as follows (21, 56, 75a):

- Complex skill-oriented exercises should be avoided in persons with MS who experience loss of proprioception.
- The energy cost of walking may be two to three times higher than normal for people with MS, particularly those with advanced disease; thus, adjustments in workloads should be made to maintain the desired heart rate, which should be frequently monitored.
- Persons with MS are thermosensitive and therefore at an increased risk for both heat- and cold-related injuries; this emphasizes the need to ensure adequate hydration and to have persons with MS exercise in thermoneutral environments. In addition, dehydration during exercise could be exacerbated in persons with MS who have bladder dysfunction (incontinence or sense of urgent need to urinate or both) and sometimes limit their fluid intake.
- Strapping may be necessary if more severe spasticity is present.
- Recumbent bicycling may be preferred over upright cycling in clients with balance problems.
- Imbalances between agonist and antagonist muscles are common.
- Some clients may have cognitive deficits and require visual supports, multiple demonstrations, and verbal explanation.

- The variable nature of MS symptoms and progression requires that the personal trainer adjust the exercise program on a daily basis.
- It is advisable to monitor heart rate before, during, and after aerobic exercise to ensure the appropriate metabolic intensity and stimulus.
- Regular follow-ups to monitor progress are highly recommended with persons who have MS in order to facilitate compliance and to adjust the exercise prescription appropriately.
- In the case of an exacerbation, exercise should be discontinued until complete remission. The client should be referred to a clinician and may resume after medical clearance.
- If the client has incoordination in either the upper or the lower limbs, the use of a synchronized leg and arm ergometer may improve exercise performance by allowing the arms or legs to assist the weaker limbs.
- Resistance training should be performed on non–aerobic-endurance training days to prevent fatigue.
- Resistance training should be done in the seated position initially if balance is impaired.
- Flexibility exercises should be performed from either a seated or a lying position.

General exercise session programming guidelines are listed in table 22.5 (21, 49).

EPILEPSY

Epilepsy is defined medically as two or more unprovoked, recurring seizures (59). A **seizure** is an uncontrolled, paroxysmal electrical discharge within any part of the brain that causes physical or mental symptoms and may or may not be associated with convulsions. Seizures result in loss of consciousness (LOC) or involuntary alteration in movement, sensation, perception, or cognitive behavior, or some combination of these. Table 22.6 defines classifications of seizures with characteristic signs and symptoms (19). Currently, 2.3 million adults and 450,000 children and adolescents in the United States live with epilepsy, with an estimated 150,000 new diagnoses each year (81).

Status epilepticus is defined as a seizure that is abnormally long or where a person does not regain consciousness between seizures (81). This is a medical emergency, necessitating activation of emergency

TABLE 22.5 Program Design Guidelines for Clients With MS

Mode	Frequency	Intensity	Volume
RESISTANCE TRAINING			
• Machines and free weights • Body weight • Resistance bands	2 days/week	60%-80% of the 1RM or multiple RM testing	1-2 sets of 10-15 repetitions
AEROBIC TRAINING			
• Treadmill • Cycling • Arm and leg cycling • Rowing • Aquatic exercise	2-5 days/week	40%-70% HRR, RPE of 12-15	Begin with 10-min sessions while progressing to 30-60 min as tolerated
FLEXIBILITY			
Static stretching for all major muscle groups	5-7 days/week, 1 or 2 times/day	Point of mild discomfort	Hold 30-60 s; perform 2-4 repetitions

Adapted by permission from Jacobs et al. (2018, p. 271). Data from Halabchi et al. (44) and Dalgas et al. (45).

TABLE 22.6 Classification and Common Signs and Symptoms of Seizure Disorders and Approximate Percentage of Cases

TYPE OF SEIZURE		SIGNS AND SYMPTOMS
Focal seizures (occur in one part of the brain)		60% of people with epilepsy have focal seizures.
		The person may maintain consciousness but experience sensory or emotional irregularities.
		The seizure may result in a change of consciousness or a dreamlike experience.
		These seizures can be mistaken for other disorders such as narcolepsy, fainting, or mental illness.
GENERALIZED SEIZURES (OCCUR ON BOTH SIDES OF THE BRAIN)	**Absence**	These seizures are characterized by staring and subtle body movement and can cause a brief (2-15 s) loss of consciousness.
	Myoclonic	These seizures usually appear as sudden, ultrashort jerks or twitches of the arms and legs.
	Tonic–clonic (grand mal)	The most intense of all types of seizures, these are characterized by a loss of consciousness, body stiffening and shaking, and loss of bladder control.
	Atonic	Also known as *drop attacks*, these brief (<15 s) seizures may cause clients to lose normal muscle tone and to suddenly collapse or fall down.
	Tonic	These seizures result in stiffening muscles, usually the back, legs, and arms.
	Clonic	These seizures cause repetitive, jerking movements on both sides of the body.

Adapted from Commission on Classification and Terminology of the International League Against Epilepsy (19).

protocols including calling 911 or another local emergency number and transporting to a hospital emergency department. It is important that the personal trainer understand and recognize common precipitants (causes or triggers) in clients with idiopathic or secondary seizures. Table 22.7 summarizes some known precipitants and recommendations for exercise session modification.

Anecdotal reports suggest that physical activity may be a precipitant of seizure (63, 100). However, systematic studies have shown that physical activity and sport have no adverse effects on seizure occurrence in the majority of clients with epilepsy and, in fact, may contribute to better seizure control (77, 78).

The consensus of experts is that exercise and sport participation in persons with epilepsy should not be restricted; in fact, it should be encouraged (42). A review of the literature indicates that exercise could be an alternative treatment for epilepsy with the following benefits: reduced seizure susceptibility, reduced anxi-

TABLE 22.7   Precipitants of Seizures and Exercise Modifications

Common precipitants of seizures	Suggested exercise modifications
Emotional stress	Modify intensity to lower level.
Hyperventilation	Teach breathing techniques and control.
Menstruation	Modify intensity to lower level.
Sleep deprivation	Avoid exercise.
Fever	Avoid exercise.
Photic stimulation (e.g., strobe lights, TV)	Avoid situations during exercise.
Alcohol excess or withdrawal	Modify intensity to lower level.

ety and depression, and improved quality of life (3). The personal trainer should gently encourage clients with epilepsy to increase their physical activity levels.

> **Exercise could be an alternative treatment for epilepsy with the following benefits: reduced seizure susceptibility, reduced anxiety and depression, and improved quality of life.**

For approximately 70% of people with epilepsy, prescription medications can control the occurrence of seizures. Approximately 20 drugs are prescribed to treat epilepsy, with many having similar side effects such as dizziness, fatigue, and weight gain (81). Common seizure medications relevant to the personal trainer include brivaracetam, diazepam (Valium), lorazepam (Ativan), and similar tranquilizers such as clonazepam. These medications can cause severe drowsiness and fatigue as well as decreases in balance, coordination, and motor control. For most individuals, a monotherapy approach is recommended because combining medications can amplify side effects. Thus, the personal trainer should be aware of the type and number of seizure medications taken by the client. Although most individuals on antiseizure medications can exercise safely, monitoring changes (whether dosage or addition of a new prescription) is necessary because these modifications can lead to the onset of side effects. The personal trainer should continuously monitor tolerance to physical activity and exercise, provide spotting or support, and modify movements that require balance or coordination, as needed.

FIRST AID FOR SEIZURES

1. Keep client prone—lying face down if possible.
2. Remove eyeglasses and other items that may break and cause injury.
3. Loosen any tight clothing, particularly around the neck.
4. Do not restrain the client.
5. Keep objects out of client's path.
6. Do not place anything in the client's mouth.
7. After the seizure, turn the client to his or her side in recovery position (refer to CPR guidelines) to prevent aspiration.
8. Observe the client until he or she is fully awake.
9. Alert the client's physician and family.
10. The client may be able to return to exercise, but evaluate this with the client's physician on a case-by-case basis.

Exercise Testing and Training of Clients With Epilepsy

It is clear that physical activity and exercise are safe, feasible, and appropriate for individuals with epilepsy (112). In the past, people with epilepsy were discouraged from exercising or participating in physical activity because of concerns about potential inducement of a seizure. New research has overwhelmingly refuted this notion, yet some people with epilepsy are significantly less active than their counterparts

(105). It has been suggested that false notions surrounding exercise-induced seizures may propagate fear and serve as a barrier to exercise among people with epilepsy (17) and that fear of seizures may lead to poorer quality of life and mental health (103). It is important that the personal trainer be aware of these false notions and be able to refute them to support clients as they achieve their fitness goals.

The personal trainer can apply the same exercise principles for persons with epilepsy as are recommended for apparently healthy populations. A gradual and progressive approach to physical activity and weight control is recommended. With proper medical clearance and adherence to standard guidelines, it is safe to administer submaximal exercise testing to establish baseline aerobic fitness, muscle strength and endurance, flexibility, and body composition. With regard to weight control, note that even a modest weight loss of 10 pounds (4.5 kg) may affect the biological availability of antiseizure medications and thus increase the risk of side effects.

Finally, the personal trainer needs to be aware of the symptoms of a seizure and the proper first aid procedures, particularly for the tonic–clonic (grand mal) type. "First Aid for Seizures" describes basic steps to take during a seizure and the **postictal state** (the period immediately after the seizure).

> A weight loss of 10 pounds (4.5 kg) can increase the bioavailability of antiseizure medications and thus increase the risk of side effects.

CEREBRAL PALSY

Cerebral palsy (CP) refers to many neurological disorders that result in permanent motor impairment (80) that can worsen without intervention. It is the most common movement disability among children (1), and its prevalence has remained stable at an average of 2.11 in 1,000 live births (84). CP is a non-progressive yet persistent group of disorders caused by damage to the developing fetal or infant brain. Symptoms include "disturbances in sensation, perception, cognition, communication, and behavior, epilepsy and secondary musculoskeletal problems" (97, p. 9). It is common for individuals with CP to experience spasticity and dystonia (14, 43, 94). **Spasticity** is caused by disruptions within the motor neurons that manifest as a speed-dependent stretch reflex that is hyperexcited, resulting in stiffness, cramping, or spasms (10, 33, 55, 64, 99). **Dystonia** is caused by a similar disruption of motor neurons, but it results in involuntary contractions and muscle movements due to disrupted communication between the central and peripheral nervous systems, which is a result of damage to the brain (14, 45, 94).

As previously stated, CP is not a progressive disease because the brain damage does not worsen. However, secondary conditions such as spasticity can and often do worsen if not well managed, leading to further loss of joint motion and mobility and potential contractures.

CP is often classified using a topographical classification scheme based on the limbs affected. See table 22.8 for an overview of these categories (59a). The American Academy for Cerebral Palsy and Developmental Medicine has developed a comprehensive classification scheme for the diagnosis and definition of cerebral palsy (97). The classification scheme involves four key areas: motor abnormalities, accompanying impairments, anatomical and neuroimaging findings, and causation and timing.

Table 22.9 (97) provides definitions of each component of cerebral palsy classification. The set of motor abnormalities can often be complex, with several co-occurring symptoms. See the "Definitions of Cerebral Palsy–Related Terms" sidebar for a definition of these symptoms. These underlying symptoms often result in muscle weakness and poor selective motor control. However, the impact of these symptoms varies depending on the functional classification of the individual.

TABLE 22.8 Topographical Classification Categories of Cerebral Palsy

Monoplegia	Involvement of one extremity
Diplegia	Bilateral lower body involvement, with minor involvement of the upper body
Hemiplegia	Unilateral upper and lower body involvement
Triplegia	Involvement of three extremities
Double hemiplegia	Involvement of all four extremities, with increased spasticity in the upper body
Quadriplegia	Involvement of all four extremities plus the head, neck, and trunk

Adapted by permission from Kendall et al. (2015).

TABLE 22.9   Components of Cerebral Palsy Classification

Motor abnormalities	
Nature and typology	The observed tonal abnormalities assessed on examination (e.g., hypotonia, hypertonia) as well as the diagnosed movement disorders present such as spasticity, ataxia, dystonia, athetosis
Functional motor abilities	The extent to which the individual is limited in his or her motor function, including oromotor and speech function
Accompanying impairments	The presence or absence of later-developing musculoskeletal problems or accompanying nonmotor neurodevelopmental or sensory problems (such as seizures; hearing or vision impairments; or attentional, behavior, communicative, or cognitive deficits) and the extent to which impairments interact in individuals with cerebral palsy
Anatomical and neuroimaging findings	
Anatomical distribution	The parts of the body (e.g., limbs, trunk, bulbar region of the brain [cerebellum, medulla, and pons]) affected by motor impairments or limitations
Neuroimaging findings	The neuroanatomic findings on CT or MRI imaging such as ventricular enlargements, white matter loss, or brain anomaly
Causation and timing	Where there is a clearly identified cause, as is usually the case with postnatal CP (e.g., meningitis, head injury) or when brain malformations are present, and the presumed period during which the injury occurred, if known

Reprinted by permission from Rosenbaum et al. (2007).

DEFINITIONS OF CEREBRAL PALSY–RELATED TERMS

apraxia—Inability to perform coordinated voluntary gross and fine motor skills.

ataxia—Uncoordinated voluntary movements; clients with ataxia often have a wide-based gait with genu recurvatum, or hyperextended knee, and may exhibit mild intention tremors.

athetosis—Slow, writhing, contortion-like motions of the appendicular musculature.

chorea—State of excessive, spontaneous movements, irregularly timed, that are nonrepetitive and abrupt; client is unable to maintain voluntary muscle contractions.

dyskinesis—Impairment of voluntary movement resulting in incomplete movements.

dystonia—Sustained muscle contractions that result in twisting and repetitive movements or abnormal posture.

spasticity—An increase in resistance to an external force, often due to a hyperactive stretch reflex.

Individuals with CP are most often classified based on function within the lower extremities, or upper extremities, or both. Lower extremity function is classified according to the Gross Motor Function Classification System–Expanded and Revised (GMFCS-ER), which contains five levels and is based on mobility (98). Because walking is a fundamental movement pattern that develops as the individual matures, there are different versions based on age. The following levels are for an adult with CP.

Level I: Walks without limitations

Level II: Walks with limitations

Level III: Walks using a handheld mobility device

Level IV: Self-mobility with limitations; may use powered mobility

Level V: Transported in a manual wheelchair

Similar to the GMFCS-ER, the Manual Ability Classification System (MACS) (32) defines upper extremity function in the context of activities of daily living. The MACS contains the follow functional categories.

Level I: Handles objects easily and successfully

Level II: Handles most objects but with somewhat reduced quality or speed of achievement

Level III: Handles objects with difficulty; needs help to prepare or modify activities

Level IV: Handles a limited selection of easily managed objects in adapted situations

Level V: Does not handle objects and has severely limited ability to perform even simple actions

Finally, individual function can also be classified using the Cerebral Palsy International Sports and Recreation Association (CPISRA) Functional Classification categories, which take into account symptoms, functional ability, and movement capabilities. Classification for each of these categories is done by a trained medical examiner for each sport before participation. The CPISRA classification system provides the personal trainer with an overview of potential capabilities regarding exercise. For more information on the classifications of CP for sports, please see the CPISRA manual at www.cpisra.org.

> **CP is not a progressive disease because the brain damage does not worsen. However, secondary conditions such as spasticity can and often do worsen if not well managed, leading to further loss of joint motion and mobility and potential contractures.**

Exercise Testing and Training of Clients With Cerebral Palsy

All persons with CP should be screened properly for musculoskeletal abnormalities, CVD, and risk factors for chronic diseases such as atherosclerosis, diabetes, arthritis, and hypertension (2). High-risk clients with two or more risk factors for CVD (hypertension, dyslipidemia, tobacco use, sedentary lifestyle, age greater than 40, obesity, diabetes) or with symptoms of CVD (chest pain, dyspnea, increasing weakness or fatigue, palpitations) should undergo a clinical examination, including an electrocardiographically monitored graded exercise test supervised by a professional team including a physician. The client must obtain medical clearance before starting a moderate-intensity exercise program.

Guidelines for exercise testing for children and adolescents with CP have been established and are also suitable for adults (107). All guidelines are based on the functional abilities of the individual, specifically GMFCS status. Table 22.10 (98) provides an overview of expert consensus of specific maximal, submaximal, and anaerobic tests recommended for people with CP. Maximal exercise testing among most individuals with CP is safe and effective (107) as long as proper safety protocols are followed (86). In addition to the recommendations presented in table 22.10, NSCA guidelines for resistance training can be followed for many people with CP (74). For example, 1RM testing has been found to be safe and feasible for children (34) and may also be used in some individuals with CP who possess the underlying coordinative abilities to perform the exercise. However, although clients with CP may be able to do these tests, the personal trainer

TABLE 22.10 Core Set of Exercise Tests for People With Cerebral Palsy

Exercise test	Mode of testing	GMFCS levels I & II	GMFCS level III	GMFCS level IV
SUBMAXIMAL				
6MWT	Walking (field test)	+	+	−
Arm crank ergometer protocol	Arm cranking (lab test)	−	+	−
MAXIMAL				
10 m SRT (SRT-I and SRT-II)	Walking (field test)	+	−	−
McMaster all-out protocol cycle test	Cycling (lab test)	+	+	+
	Arm cranking (lab test)	−	+	+
7.5 m SRT (SRT-II protocol)	Walking (field test)	−	+	−
ANAEROBIC				
Muscle power sprint test	Walking (field test)	+	−	−
30 s Wingate cycle test	Cycling (lab test)	+	+	−
	Arm cranking (lab test)	−	+	+

GMFCS = Gross Motor Function Classification System; MWT = minute walk test; SRT = shuttle run test.

Adapted from Rosenbaum et al. (98).

should stick to more conservative methods of testing and recommendations established within chapter 15. The benefits do not outweigh the risks for this type of testing in this special population.

In ambulatory persons with CP, the leg ergometer and the arm and leg ergometer are preferred modalities for exercise testing. The treadmill may be used in persons with CP who have good balance and coordination. Because of spasticity or athetosis, the client's feet may need to be strapped to the pedals, and sufficient practice is necessary to ensure good performance. In nonambulatory persons with CP, the arm crank ergometer and wheelchair ergometer, if available, are the preferred modalities for submaximal testing. Clients should wear gloves to prevent skin abrasions, particularly if they use a wheelchair. To assess aerobic endurance, the 6- to 12-minute walk or wheelchair push may be appropriate. These tests, however, assume maximal effort—the objective is for clients to travel as much distance as they can in the timed period. Therefore, this test should be administered only to low-risk and properly screened clients.

Common tests of flexibility and muscle function such as the sit and reach and 1RM can be safely administered. Finally, skinfold thickness measurements can be taken at several sites, preferably on noninvolved body parts, and totaled for a score to establish a baseline for assessing changes in body composition. Although valid equations for predicting body fat percentage from skinfold measurements are limited in this population, the total thickness of seven to eight sites can be used for monitoring progress.

> **Many people with CP are not active because they lack the functional ability to be physically active. It is important that the personal trainer focus on improving functional capacity in order to increase the potential for physical activity participation.**

Although all individuals with CP should strive to meet the physical activity guidelines regarding moderate to vigorous physical activity, some people with CP possess functional limitations that make this difficult or impossible (6, 9, 83, 108, 109). Recommendations for exercise testing, exercise prescription, and physical activity are based on the functional ability of the individual (i.e., his or her GMFCS level). In general, the personal trainer should have two related goals for clients with CP. First, exercise testing and prescription

should focus on maximizing function. This requires a review of the current functional abilities of the client as well as current symptoms. The personal trainer can then modify or adapt exercise to overcome any deficits or imbalances in muscle strength as well as deficits in selective motor control. Second, the personal trainer should prescribe exercises that will lead to improved capabilities to engage in physical activity. The potential benefits of all types of exercises are well established among people with CP and have the potential to both improve function and increase physical activity.

Personal trainers should be aware that initial mode and intensity of exercise will vary greatly according to functional ability, specifically GMFCS status. Overall, research has found that people with CP who have greater mobility experience a greater benefit from aerobic training because they can engage in larger doses of training (108) and can therefore expend more energy. Personal trainers should choose exercise modalities with assistive rails, arm or leg cycle ergometers, or recumbent steppers that are best suited for the individual based on overall mobility and function of the upper extremities. Some individuals with CP may require short doses or practice sessions because of muscle weakness or poor selective motor control in some limbs. Specific recommendations for aerobic exercise prescription can be found in table 22.11 (108).

Resistance training exercise can improve function and other condition-specific symptoms among individuals with CP (22, 27, 54, 70). Muscular strength is a major factor of overall muscle performance, leading to the belief that muscle weakness may be the biggest cause for activity limitation in those with CP (74). Multiple factors could contribute to muscle weakness including muscle deformity (47), spasticity, cocontraction (31), and disuse of the impaired limb (35). However, resistance training is not contraindicated for people with spastic CP (108).

The relationship between strength and function is established in the research and has indicated that improvements in strength may lead to improvements in function among individuals with CP (22, 31). Therefore, exercise selection should focus on functional movements that have the potential to transfer to activities of daily living. Because of potential muscle weaknesses, single-joint or machine-based exercises may be necessary at the beginning of the training program for some individuals. Proper technique should be emphasized during the initial phase of the training program. The personal trainer needs to observe the client's ability to perform various tasks and progress

TABLE 22.11 Recommendations for Exercise and Physical Activity Prescription Among People With Cerebral Palsy

Mode	Recommendation
AEROBIC EXERCISE	
Frequency	1 or 2 sessions a week, gradually progressing to 3 sessions a week
Intensity	>60% of peak heart rate, or >40% of HRR, or between 46% and 90% $\dot{V}O_2$peak
Time	A minimum of 20 min per session for at least 8 or 16 consecutive weeks, depending on frequency (2 or 3 times a week)
Type	Regular, purposeful exercise that involves major muscle groups and is continuous and rhythmic in nature
RESISTANCE EXERCISE	
Frequency	2-4 times a week on nonconsecutive days
Intensity	1-3 sets of 6-15 repetitions at 50%-85% of the 1RM
Time	No specific duration of training has been identified for effectiveness; training period should last at least 12-16 consecutive weeks
Type	Progression in mode from primarily single-joint, machine-based resistance exercises to machine plus free-weight, multijoint (and closed kinetic chain) resistance exercises; single-joint resistance training may be more effective for very weak muscles or for children, adolescents, or adults who tend to compensate when performing multijoint exercises, or at the beginning of the training
DAILY PHYSICAL ACTIVITY	
Physical activity (moderate to vigorous)	
Frequency	≥5 days/week
Intensity	Moderate to vigorous physical activity
Time	60 min
Type	A variety of activities
Physical activity (sedentary)	
Frequency	7 days/week
Intensity	Sedentary (<1.5 METs)
Time	<2 h/day or break up sitting for 2 min every 30-60 min
Type	Nonoccupational, leisure-time sedentary activities such as watching television, using a computer, and playing video games

Reprinted by permission from Verschuren et al. (2016).

to more advanced exercises. Specific recommendations for resistance training prescription can be found in table 22.11.

Resistance training with a velocity component has been examined as a new training method for people with CP. Power training may offer unique benefits for individuals with CP compared with normal resistance training (74). Current guidelines for power training among youth provide dosing parameters. The delivery of the power training should follow NSCA guidelines for youth (34) (see chapter 18) as a starting point, ensuring that the individual has developed a sound general conditioning base that allows for exercises to be performed accurately in a full range of motion (74, 75). For power training, the NSCA recommends a volume of ≥3 sets of ≤6 repetitions at an intensity range between 30% and 80% of the 1RM, with progression toward the higher end of the range (34). Both concentric and eccentric movement phases should be performed through a full range of motion, with the concentric phase performed as fast as possible. However, novices should start at slower velocities in the initial training program. There is also some evidence that ergometry may be a feasible and effective way to deliver a power training program for individuals with severe CP, as Colquitt and colleagues (18) found that ski ergometry results in significantly improved power output as well as improvement in some secondary conditions such as pain.

Because of potential muscle tone issues among individuals with CP, flexibility training should be approached cautiously. Sustained stretching for longer durations may be more beneficial in reducing spasticity and improving range of motion (90). However, sustained stretching combined with active movement may be more effective (114). Additionally, there is some evidence that resistance training combined with stretching is more effective among individuals with spastic CP (58) for improving joint ROM and strength. Therefore, it is recommended that the personal trainer follow NSCA guidelines for incorporating stretching as part of a complete program that includes a warm-up, a cool-down, and resistance training to maximize potential benefits.

The following list shows research outcomes related to exercise among people with CP:

- Improved capacity to perform activities of daily life (61)
- Improved sense of wellness, physical fitness, and quality of life (15, 106)
- Apparent lessening of severity of spasticity and improved standing balance (43)
- Increased aerobic performance (15)
- Improved walking ability, lower body strength, and balance (87)
- Increased self-concept and social acceptance (28)
- Improved gross motor function (16)
- Improved maximal aerobic capacity and oxygen utilization (68)
- Increased muscle size, strength, and functional capacity (46)
- Increased muscle size and strength (45)

> **Persons with CP can expect a systematic program of physical exercise to yield health and fitness benefits similar to those obtained by persons without CP.**

Several medications can be used to manage the common side effects of CP. For instance, most CP medications are prescribed to decrease muscle stiffness or tightness, including antispastics, anticonvulsants, and anticholinergics. When training clients taking antispastics (e.g., baclofen, dantrolene, botuli-

num toxin, cyclobenzaprine), it is important to modify exercises where tone compromises ROM. All exercises should be performed through a comfortable ROM, as tone and spasms may vary. Anticonvulsants (e.g., Depakene, Epival, Klonopin, Topomax, Neurontin) are used to prevent seizure activity; however, these medications may cause drowsiness, headaches, weight gain, nausea, and general fatigue. Clients with CP may also use anticholinergics, which reduce muscle spasms and rigidity by blocking neurotransmitter pathways that activate skeletal and smooth muscle tissue. The personal trainer should therefore monitor reductions in resting and exercise heart rate and blood pressure throughout the training session if the client is prescribed these medications.

CONCLUSION

The scope of practice of personal trainers is expanding rapidly. Accumulating evidence supports the application of exercise training to numerous special populations, including persons with several neuromuscular disorders. Increasing and sustaining moderate to high levels of physical activity among persons with SCI, MS, CP, and epilepsy is strongly encouraged. The functional and health benefits of regular exercise for these populations are similar to those for other persons when the activities are performed safely and effectively. Many persons in these groups are at an increased risk for chronic metabolic disorders, partially because of the high frequency of physical inactivity among these populations.

Personal trainers working under the guidance of health care professionals should make an effort to promote their services to populations with the disorders covered in this chapter. The intrinsic rewards of working with persons who have these neuromuscular disorders, as well as others such as Parkinson's disease, muscular dystrophy, and post-polio syndrome, are many and certainly as meaningful as those derived from working with other clients, both non-athletic and athletic. Finally, three key references that should become part of the library of any personal trainer working with special populations are *ACSM's Exercise Management for Persons With Chronic Diseases and Disabilities* (29), *NSCA's Essentials of Training Special Populations* (57), and *ACSM's Resources for Clinical Exercise Physiology* (76).

Study Questions

1. A *complete* spinal cord injury occurring between which vertebrae can lead to quadriplegia?

   I. C1 to T1

   II. T2 to T12

   III. L4 to L5

   IV. L1 to L4

   A. I only

   B. II only

   C. II, III, and IV only

   D. I, III, and IV only

2. Which of the following is *incorrect* regarding persons with spinal cord injuries (SCI) exercising in the cold?

   A. Dehydration contributes greatly to the risk of hypothermia.

   B. Persons with SCI may be unable to adequately shiver.

   C. Beware of burns from heat packs.

   D. Persons with SCI can be unable to decrease skin blood flow in paralyzed areas.

3. Persons with spinal cord injury can suffer from a dysfunctional syndrome called hypokinetic circulation. This occurs when, during upper body exercise, upper body peripheral _____ during exercise is not compensated adequately by concomitant lower limb _____.

   A. vasodilation; vasodilation

   B. vasodilation; vasoconstriction

   C. vasoconstriction; vasodilation

   D. vasoconstriction; vasoconstriction

4. What frequency of stretching is recommended for individuals with multiple sclerosis (MS)?

   A. 1-2 days/week, 1 time/day

   B. 2-3 days/week, 1 time/day

   C. 3-4 days/week, 1 time/day

   D. 5-7 days/week, 1 or 2 times/day

5. What is the minimum amount of time in minutes recommended for aerobic exercise for people with cerebral palsy (CP)?

   A. 10

   B. 20

   C. 30

   D. 40

CHAPTER 23

Resistance Training for Clients Who Are Athletes

Joseph J. Bonyai, MEd, and Tyler D. Williams, PhD

After completing this chapter, you will be able to

- understand how to apply overload and specificity to a resistance training program for a client who is training for a sport;

- understand the value, role, and application of a periodized training program;

- describe the cycles and phases of a periodized training program;

- understand how load and repetitions are manipulated in a traditional and an undulating periodization model;

- implement strength testing protocols to determine an athlete's current strength level, future training loads, and progress made throughout training; and

- design a traditional and an undulating periodized training plan.

Personal trainers have the opportunity to work with a large variety of populations. Many clients have sedentary lifestyles with limited recreational pursuits and are sometimes deconditioned to the extent that they develop cardiometabolic medical conditions. On the opposite end of the wellness continuum, some clients are very physically active, both in their jobs and in their personal time, with each having competition-based goals and aspirations. The training needs of these athletic clients are much different from those of the general population. Building upon the basic resistance training program design principles detailed in chapter 15, this chapter describes how to develop a more advanced periodized program that will help clients with athletic aspirations meet their competitive goals.

FACTORS IN PROGRAM DESIGN

Resistance training programs have been used for many years as an integral part of a total exercise program to enhance athletic performance. Research has shown the effectiveness of carefully planned resistance training programs as a method of improving body development and sport performance (1, 28, 29, 44, 53, 65). Significant benefits can be gained from the systematic and proper application of the overload and specificity principles, the two primary tenets of resistance training. Combined with the principles of periodization to optimize the exercise stimulus, resistance training provides one of the most potent and effective methods to increase muscular performance capabilities,

The authors would like to acknowledge the significant contributions of David R. Pearson, and John F. Graham to this chapter.

improve sport performance, and reduce the potential risk of injury (12, 15, 19).

Overload Principle

The **overload principle** is based on the concept that the athlete will adapt in response to the demands of the physiological stressors placed on the neuromuscular system. Thus, the training stress placed on the muscles must be progressively increased for adaptations to continue to occur (15, 19, 58). As explained in chapter 15, the personal trainer can apply overload by increasing the amount of weight lifted in an exercise (i.e., intensity), incorporating more workouts in a week (i.e., frequency), including more (or more difficult) exercises (i.e., variation), or adding sets to one or more exercises in a workout (i.e., volume).

Specificity of Training

Specificity refers to the fact that specific methods of training produce specific changes or results. In particular, the more similar the training activity is to the actual sport movement, the greater the likelihood of a positive transfer to that sport (6, 15, 26, 59, 64, 65). Although athletes may enhance their speed and power with a non–sport-specific program (41), the most effective program will match the metabolic and biomechanical characteristics of the training program to the sport activity. This level of specificity will train the appropriate metabolic systems and will also include exercises that duplicate the joint velocities and angular movements of the sport. Therefore, the personal trainer should design the resistance training

program to include at least one exercise that mimics the movement pattern of each primary skill of the athlete's sport (see table 23.1 for examples).

Although an increase in maximum strength is a common outcome of all programs that involve lifting heavy loads, improving an athlete's ability to generate force at very rapid speeds requires training at high velocities (21). Thus, improving maximum strength by conventional slow-velocity heavy resistance training does not ensure the improvement of force development in ballistic sport movements (e.g., basketball jump shot, baseball pitch, volleyball spike). Instead, the personal trainer should select power exercises and assign moderate loads to allow the athlete to perform the movements explosively (53).

> The more similar the training activity is to the actual sport movement, the greater the likelihood of a positive transfer to that sport. Therefore, the personal trainer should design the resistance training program to include at least some exercises that mimic the movement pattern of each primary skill of the athlete's sport.

TRAINING LOAD: RESISTANCE AND REPETITIONS

The training **load**, or the amount of weight to be used, is one of the most important factors to consider in the design of a training program. There are many ways

TABLE 23.1 Examples of Sport-Specific Exercises

Sport skill	Related sport-specific exercises*
Ball passing	Medicine ball chest pass, push-up, bench press
Ball kicking	Split squat, split squat jump, hip flexion, knee extension, cable hip abduction, cable hip adduction
Freestyle swimming	Lat pulldown, straight-arm pulldown, vertical jump, squat
Jumping	Depth jump, hurdle jump, box jump, back squat, power clean, power snatch
Racket stroke	Dumbbell bench press, push-up, dumbbell fly, row variations, reverse fly, wrist curl, reverse wrist curl, wrist supination, wrist pronation
Rowing	Clean pull, squat, deadlift, leg press, dumbbell row, machine row, suspension trainer row
Running or sprinting	Uphill sprint, resisted and assisted sprints, single-arm alternate-leg bounding, jumping, hopping, power clean, power snatch, back squat, step-up, lunge
Throwing or pitching	Medicine ball rotational throws, medicine ball slams, lateral bounding, lunge

*This is not an exhaustive list: Many other sport-specific exercises can be included.

to determine the training load. The assigned load will exert a large impact on the number of repetitions that can be performed and ultimately the types of physiological and performance adaptations stimulated. Ultimately the interplay between load and **volume** (repetitions × sets × resistance) is dictated by the type of training program established and the intended goals of the program.

Before assigning the training load and the repetitions to be performed in each set, the personal trainer must perform baseline testing of the client. The purpose of this testing is to determine the client's abilities to handle specific loads in a series of selected exercises. Once the personal trainer establishes these abilities, he or she can assign training loads.

Influential Factors

The load, the number of repetitions, and the targeted outcomes of a resistance training program are strongly related. For example, higher loads performed for fewer repetitions tends to lead to a greater development of muscular strength (50), while lifting lighter loads for higher repetitions often results in greater improvements in muscular endurance (51). In its most basic form, a client's training program would address specific goals and target them with selected repetition and load relationships. This, however, is a gross simplification of the training process. Regardless of the client's goals, the training plan should include periods in which muscular endurance, strength, and, often, power are developed. Sequencing different repetition and loading schemes will magnify training adaptations and provide a greater chance of accomplishing the client's goals (23, 42, 59).

Percentage of 1-Repetition Maximum Relationship

The **repetition maximum (RM)** is the maximum load the client can handle in a specific exercise for specific number of repetitions. As the load becomes heavier, the number of repetitions the client can perform will decrease. Eventually the load will become so heavy that the client can perform only 1 repetition; this is the **1-repetition maximum (1RM)**. Conversely, the lighter the load, the more repetitions the client can perform. This association between 1RM and repetitions has been termed the percentage of 1RM (%1RM)–repetition relationship.

Load assignments are best accomplished by using percentages of the 1RM (18, 53, 55) or of a specified

targeted maximum repetition range. For example, table 23.2 (6, 8, 13, 36, 53) indicates that if a client's 1RM is 200 pounds (90.9 kg), he or she should be able to perform 8 repetitions with 160 pounds (72.7 kg). (According to table 23.2, 8 repetitions completed corresponds with 80% 1RM. Therefore, 200 pounds × 0.80 = 160 pounds [72.7 kg]).

As another example, if a client's 5RM is 120 pounds (54.5 kg), his or her 1RM is estimated to be around 138 pounds (62.7 kg). (Based on table 23.2, a 5RM corresponds with 87% 1RM. Thus, 120 pounds divided by 0.87 = 137.9 pounds [62.7 kg]).

By using these relationships, the personal trainer can estimate the training loads to prescribe for the client. It is important to note that the numbers in table 23.2 are only estimates and that these values can vary depending on the exercises used in the program and the training status of the client (10, 47, 54).

An alternative method is to use an intensity that allows for performance of a specific number of repetitions, or what is known as an **RM target**. With use

TABLE 23.2 Percentage of 1-Repetition Maximum–Repetition Relationship

% 1-repetition maximum (1RM)	Estimated number of repetitions performed
100	1
95	2
93	3
90	4
87	5
85	6
83	7
80	8
77	9
75	10
70	11
67	12
65	15
60	20

Note: The number of repetitions that can be performed at a given percent of the 1RM and the percent of the 1RM that can be lifted for a given number of repetitions will vary depending on the type of exercise and the training status of the client.

Adapted from Sheppard and Triplett (53), Bompa and Buzzichelli (6), Brzycki (8), Epley (13), and Mayhew et al. (36).

of this method, the client lifts the heaviest load he or she can for the selected repetition scheme (15, 18, 30). For example, if the client were to perform 3 sets at a 12RM load, he or she would use the heaviest weight that would allow him or her to perform 3 sets with no less or more than 12 repetitions.

A similar method, using what is called the **RM target zone**, is to assign a range such as 3RM to 5RM (15). When an RM target zone is prescribed, the client uses the heaviest weight he or she can lift to perform the exercise for the number of repetitions within the range. The RM target and RM target zone methods for assigning load may be problematic because in both instances the client is required to train to muscular failure. The scientific literature suggests that training to failure does not lead to greater strength improvements versus not training to failure and may lead to greater fatigue accumulation, resulting in impaired neuromuscular performance for the subsequent training sessions (11, 39).

Limitations in the Percent 1-Repetition Maximum Relationship

Although the %1RM–repetition relationship is an excellent tool for prescribing intensities in resistance training for athletic clients, it is important to realize several limitations that may affect its accuracy.

1. There appears to be a relationship between the %1RM and the number of repetitions that can be performed, but several studies suggest the relationship is not as robust as once thought (24, 32, 34, 35, 36, 37).

2. Training status appears to influence the relationship between repetitions and %1RM, with trained individuals being able to perform more repetitions at a given %1RM (24, 25, 35, 54, 60).

3. When working with the %1RM–repetition relationship, it is important to remember that the number of repetitions performed at a specific %1RM is related only to a single set and not to multiple sets. With multiple sets, fatigue will cause a reduction in the number of repetitions that can be performed in later sets, thus altering the %1RM–repetition relationship (49).

4. The %1RM–repetition association is, for the most part, based on research on the bench press, back squat, and power clean (15, 60). The relationship between %1RM and repetitions likely does not apply to all exercises (24, 25, 54) and should be applied with care when working with clients.

5. The mode of resistance training appears to affect the number of repetitions that can be performed at a given %1RM. Generally, more repetitions can be performed at any given %1RM with machine-based exercises (e.g., vertical chest press) than with free-weight exercises (e.g., bench press) (24, 25).

6. More repetitions can be performed at any given %1RM for core exercises compared with assistance exercises (25, 54).

7. The order of exercises may also affect the number of repetitions that can be performed at any given %1RM. Whether it is a core or assistance exercise, placing an exercise toward the end of the workout results in a decrease in the number of repetitions (56).

When using the %1RM–repetition relationships presented in table 23.2, the personal trainer will probably have greater success estimating with loads of ≥75% of 1RM performed with ≤10 repetitions (8, 9, 33, 61), because the %1RM–repetition relationship becomes increasingly inaccurate as the load decreases and the number of repetitions increases (53, 61). Therefore, the information presented in table 23.2 should be used only as a guide and not to derive hard and fast rules.

Guidelines for Assessing Load Capabilities

Before assigning training loads, the personal trainer must perform some form of assessment to estimate the client's capabilities. The following are methods for accomplishing this:

- Directly assessing the 1RM
- Estimating the 1RM
- Using a percentage of the client's body weight for testing
- Repetition maximum testing

One or more of these methods can be used depending on the client's training status, the client's technical proficiency, and the type of exercise being tested (53).

Assessing the 1-Repetition Maximum

The personal trainer must determine the 1RM to use the %1RM–repetition relationships presented in table 23.2. As a general rule, the 1RM test poses minimal risks to both clinical and athletic clients (48, 52); and it is considered the gold standard of muscular strength assessments (3). The biggest issue with the 1RM test is whether the client has the technique needed to perform the exercise correctly with increasing loads. If technique is lacking, it may be best to use other methods. Although a test-established 1RM is the most accurate way to determine loading, it is also possible to use a submaximal load to estimate the 1RM (9, 53, 25). It is important to note that using estimations from submaximal loads may result in overestimation of the 1RM (31, 36, 37, 45, 62), which could lead to problems for prescribing training intensities.

As a rule, clients who are classified as untrained, have been recently injured, or are under medical supervision should not perform a 1RM test. It may be prudent to reserve this type of testing for more advanced clients who have developed the appropriate technical base and can perform the test exercise using appropriate technique with various loads (see chapter 15 for more information).

In selecting the exercises to be tested with a 1RM, the personal trainer should choose only those exercises that can be performed safely, accurately, and consistently (53). In general, large muscle multijoint core exercises are best suited for 1RM testing because heavy loads are better tolerated with these exercises. As a rule, 1RM testing should not be used with assistance exercises because of the large physiological stress placed on the smaller muscle groups and soft tissue structures across a single joint (2). Therefore, it is important to use sound judgment when selecting exercises for a 1RM test.

As one example, even though the lunge and step-up are large muscle multijoint exercises, they are not typically used with 1RM testing because of the uneven loads they place on the lower body. The uneven loads and large balance demands can increase the potential for injury and accidents. The bent-over row is another exercise that is not well-suited for 1RM testing. Although this exercise does incorporate the large muscle joints of the upper back and functions across several joints, it is likely that during a 1RM test the smaller, supporting musculature of the lower back may not be able to maintain appropriate body positions, which would result in an inaccurate assessment of strength, as well as increase the risk of injury. Once an exercise has been deemed acceptable for testing and the client can be classified as having intermediate or advanced training status, the personal trainer should use the appropriate 1RM testing protocol as explained in chapter 11.

Estimating the 1-Repetition Maximum

If the client is unable to perform an actual 1RM test, there are two ways the 1RM can be estimated. Such estimation procedures can be used to develop the loading structure and resistance training plan.

1. Use of RM testing

2. Use of prediction equations

One way to estimate a client's 1RM is to use an RM test, which then can be used to estimate the 1RM. The best means of ensuring accuracy is to use lower numbers of repetitions, such as a 6RM or 10RM (i.e., the heaviest load the client can lift 6 or 10 times with proper technique). As a basic rule, the RM should be determined within three testing sets.

Repetition maximum testing is very similar to the test for determining the 1RM; the main difference is that each testing set includes more repetitions. Since the number of repetitions is greater, the load changes across testing sets should be smaller (~50% of the amounts suggested for 1RM testing in chapter 11).

Once the client's 6RM, for example, has been determined, table 23.3 can be used to estimate the 1RM. The personal trainer will look at the row titled "Max repetitions" and move across that row to find the notation for 6 repetitions, which is 85% of the 1RM. Once this column is located, the personal trainer can move down the column looking for the number closest to (but not greater than) the client's 6RM. For example, if the client's 6RM for the leg press is 140 pounds (63.5 kg), the estimated 1RM will be 165 pounds (74.8 kg). This estimated 1RM load will then be used to determine the client's actual training loads.

The results of the RM test can also be used with prediction equations to determine the 1RM. A number of these equations, which use repetitions to failure to estimate 1RM, have been published (table 23.4; 35) (1, 8, 13, 31, 35, 36, 40). In general, the accuracy of these equations is greater when heavier relative loads are used (1). Therefore, the recommendation is to use heavier loads performed for fewer repetitions than the 10RM when using prediction equations (1, 7, 9, 33, 61). The phase of the training plan also affects the accuracy of these equations (6, 53). If the client has been training with high volumes, such as sets of 10 to 15 repetitions, the equations will become less accurate. Conversely, a prediction equation becomes more robust if the client is using lower volumes and heavier weights.

TABLE 23.3 Estimating a 1-Repetition Maximum (1RM) From a Training Load

	Max repetitions												
	1	2	3	4	5	6	7	8	9	10	12	15	20
	% of 1RM												
	100	95	93	90	87	85	83	80	77	75	67	65	60
10	10	9	9	9	9	8	8	8	8	7	7	6
15	14	14	14	13	13	12	12	12	11	10	10	9
20	19	19	18	17	17	17	16	15	15	13	13	12
25	24	23	23	22	21	21	20	19	19	17	16	15
30	29	28	27	26	26	25	24	23	23	20	20	18
35	33	33	32	30	30	29	28	27	26	23	23	21
40	38	37	36	35	34	33	32	31	30	27	26	24
45	43	42	41	39	38	37	36	35	34	30	29	27
50	48	47	45	44	43	42	40	39	38	34	33	30
55	52	51	50	48	47	46	44	42	41	37	36	33
60	57	56	54	52	51	50	48	46	45	40	39	36
65	62	60	59	57	55	54	52	50	49	44	42	39
70	67	65	63	61	60	58	56	54	53	47	46	42
75	71	70	68	65	64	62	60	58	56	50	49	45
80	76	74	72	70	68	66	64	62	60	54	52	48
85	81	79	77	74	72	71	68	65	64	57	55	51
90	86	84	81	78	77	75	72	69	68	60	59	54
95	90	88	86	83	81	79	76	73	71	64	62	57
100	95	93	90	87	85	83	80	77	75	67	65	60
105	100	98	95	91	89	87	84	81	79	70	68	63
110	105	102	99	96	94	91	88	85	83	74	72	66
115	109	107	104	100	98	95	92	89	86	77	75	69
120	114	112	108	104	102	100	96	92	90	80	78	72
125	119	116	113	109	106	104	100	96	94	84	81	75
130	124	121	117	113	111	108	104	100	98	87	85	78
135	128	126	122	117	115	112	108	104	101	90	88	81
140	133	130	126	122	119	116	112	108	105	94	91	84
145	138	135	131	126	123	120	116	112	109	97	94	87
150	143	140	135	131	128	125	120	116	113	101	98	90
155	147	144	140	135	132	129	124	119	116	104	101	93
160	152	149	144	139	136	133	128	123	120	107	104	96
165	157	153	149	144	140	137	132	127	124	111	107	99
170	162	158	153	148	145	141	136	131	128	114	111	102
175	166	163	158	152	149	145	140	135	131	117	114	105
180	171	167	162	157	153	149	144	139	135	121	117	108

LOAD IN POUNDS OR KILOGRAMS

					Max repetitions							
1	2	3	4	5	6	7	8	9	10	12	15	20
					% of 1RM							
100	95	93	90	87	85	83	80	77	75	67	65	60
185	176	172	167	161	157	154	148	142	139	124	120	111
190	181	177	171	165	162	158	152	146	143	127	124	114
195	185	181	176	170	166	162	156	150	146	131	127	117
200	190	186	180	174	170	166	160	154	150	134	130	120
205	195	191	185	178	174	170	164	158	154	137	133	123
210	200	195	189	183	179	174	168	162	158	141	137	126
215	204	200	194	187	183	178	172	166	161	144	140	129
220	209	205	198	191	187	183	176	169	165	147	143	132
225	214	209	203	196	191	187	180	173	169	151	146	135
230	219	214	207	200	196	191	184	177	173	154	150	138
235	223	219	212	204	200	195	188	181	176	157	153	141
240	228	223	216	209	204	199	192	185	180	161	156	144
245	233	228	221	213	208	203	196	189	184	164	159	147
250	238	233	225	218	213	208	200	193	188	168	163	150
255	242	237	230	222	217	212	204	196	191	171	166	153
260	247	242	234	226	221	216	208	200	195	174	169	156
265	252	246	239	231	225	220	212	204	199	178	172	159
270	257	251	243	235	230	224	216	208	203	181	176	162
275	261	256	248	239	234	228	220	212	206	184	179	165
280	266	260	252	244	238	232	224	216	210	188	182	168
285	271	265	257	248	242	237	228	219	214	191	185	171
290	276	270	261	252	247	241	232	223	218	194	189	174
295	280	274	266	257	251	245	236	227	221	198	192	177
300	285	279	270	261	255	249	240	231	225	201	195	180
305	290	284	275	265	259	253	244	235	229	204	198	183
310	295	288	279	270	264	257	248	239	233	208	202	186
315	299	293	284	274	268	261	252	243	236	211	205	189
320	304	298	288	278	272	266	256	246	240	214	208	192
325	309	302	293	283	276	270	260	250	244	218	211	195
330	314	307	297	287	281	274	264	254	248	221	215	198
335	318	312	302	291	285	278	268	258	251	224	218	201
340	323	316	306	296	289	282	272	262	255	228	221	204
345	328	321	311	300	293	286	276	266	259	231	224	207
350	333	326	315	305	298	291	280	270	263	235	228	210
355	337	330	320	309	302	295	284	273	266	238	231	213
360	342	335	324	313	306	299	288	277	270	241	234	216

LOAD IN POUNDS OR KILOGRAMS*

(continued)

TABLE 23.3 *(continued)*

	Max repetitions												
1	2	3	4	5	6	7	8	9	10	12	15	20
					% of 1RM							
100	95	93	90	87	85	83	80	77	75	67	65	60
365	347	339	329	318	310	303	292	281	274	245	237	219
370	352	344	333	322	315	307	296	285	278	248	241	222
375	356	349	338	326	319	311	300	289	281	251	244	225
380	361	353	342	331	323	315	304	293	285	255	247	228
385	366	358	347	335	327	320	308	296	289	258	250	231
390	371	363	351	339	332	324	312	300	293	261	254	234
395	375	367	356	344	336	328	316	304	296	265	257	237
400	380	372	360	348	340	332	320	308	300	268	260	240
405	385	377	365	352	344	336	324	312	304	271	263	243
410	390	381	369	357	349	340	328	316	308	275	267	246
415	394	386	374	361	353	344	332	320	311	278	270	249
420	399	391	378	365	357	349	336	323	315	281	273	252
425	404	395	383	370	361	353	340	327	319	285	276	255
430	409	400	387	374	366	357	344	331	323	288	280	258
435	413	405	392	378	370	361	348	335	326	291	283	261
440	418	409	396	383	374	365	352	339	330	295	286	264
445	423	414	401	387	378	369	356	343	334	298	289	267
450	428	419	405	392	383	374	360	347	338	302	293	270
455	432	423	410	396	387	378	364	350	341	305	296	273
460	437	428	414	400	391	382	368	354	345	308	299	276
465	442	432	419	405	395	386	372	358	349	312	302	279
470	447	437	423	409	400	390	376	362	353	315	306	282
475	451	442	428	413	404	394	380	366	356	318	309	285
480	456	446	432	418	408	398	384	370	360	322	312	288
485	461	451	437	422	412	403	388	373	364	325	315	291
490	466	456	441	426	417	407	392	377	368	328	319	294
495	470	460	446	431	421	411	396	381	371	332	322	297
500	475	465	450	435	425	415	400	385	375	335	325	300
505	480	470	455	439	429	419	404	389	379	338	328	303
510	485	474	459	444	434	423	408	393	383	342	332	306
515	489	479	464	448	438	427	412	397	386	345	335	309
520	494	484	468	452	442	432	416	400	390	348	338	312
525	499	488	473	457	446	436	420	404	394	352	341	315
530	504	493	477	461	451	440	424	408	398	355	345	318
535	508	498	482	465	455	444	428	412	401	358	348	321

LOAD IN POUNDS OR KILOGRAMS

	Max repetitions												
	1	2	3	4	5	6	7	8	9	10	12	15	20
	% of 1RM												
	100	95	93	90	87	85	83	80	77	75	67	65	60
LOAD IN POUNDS OR KILOGRAMS*	540	513	502	486	470	459	448	432	416	405	362	351	324
	545	518	507	491	474	463	452	436	420	409	365	354	327
	550	523	512	495	479	468	457	440	424	413	369	358	330
	555	527	516	500	483	472	461	444	427	416	372	361	333
	560	532	521	504	487	476	465	448	431	420	375	364	336
	565	537	525	509	492	480	469	452	435	424	379	367	339
	570	542	530	513	496	485	473	456	439	428	382	371	342
	575	546	535	518	500	489	477	460	443	431	385	374	345
	580	551	539	522	505	493	481	464	447	435	389	377	348
	585	556	544	527	509	497	486	468	450	439	392	380	351
	590	561	549	531	513	502	490	472	454	443	395	384	354
	595	565	553	536	518	506	494	476	458	446	399	387	357
	600	570	558	540	522	510	498	480	462	450	402	390	360

*Whenever possible, round down to the nearest 5 lb or 2.5 kg increment.

TABLE 23.4 Sample 1-Repetition Maximum Prediction Equations

Reference	Equation
Bean and Adams (5)	$1RM = RepWt \div (1 - 0.02 \times RTF)$
Brown (7)	$1RM = (Reps \times 0.0338 + 0.9849) \times RepWt$
Mayhew et al. (34)	$1RM = RepWt \div (0.522 + 0.419\ e^{-0.055 \times RTF})$
O'Connor et al. (40)	$1RM = 0.025\ (RepWt \times RTF) + RepWt$

1RM = 1-repetition maximum; RepWt = repetition weight (i.e., a load lighter than the 1RM to perform repetitions); RTF = repetitions to failure.

Adapted from Mayhew et al. (35).

PERIODIZATION OF RESISTANCE TRAINING

One of the most important developments in the theory of sport training has been the advancement of concepts related to periodization. **Periodization** is the systematic process of planned variations in a resistance training program over a training cycle (15, 19, 57, 58). The primary goals of periodization are met by appropriately manipulating volume and intensity and by effectively selecting exercises. Research indicates that this concept promotes training adaptations (14, 28). One of the primary advantages of this training approach is the reduced risk of overtraining because of the purposeful time devoted to physical and mental recovery (15, 58). Typically, only core exercises are periodized, but all exercises can be varied for intensity and volume (15, 19, 58).

> **Periodization is the systematic process of planned variations in a resistance training program over a training cycle.**

Cycles and Phases

Periodized programs are typically divided into three distinct cycles. The **macrocycle** is the largest division; it typically constitutes an entire training year but may also be a period of up to four years (e.g., for an Olympic athlete). Macrocycles typically comprise two or more **mesocycles** divided into several weeks to a few months. The number of mesocycles is dependent on the goals of the athlete and, if applicable, the number of sport competitions contained within the period. Each mesocycle is divided into **microcycles**, ranging from one week to four weeks, that include daily and weekly training variations (15, 58).

In 1981, Stone and colleagues (57) developed an American model for strength and power sports by modifying the periodization program that had been created by the Soviet Union and Eastern European countries (19, 65). This approach divides a resistance training program into five mesocycles, each with a primary goal or focus:

- **Hypertrophy phase**: to develop a muscular and metabolic base for more intense future training using a resistance training program that includes sport-specific or non–sport-specific exercises performed at a high volume and a low intensity.

- **Strength phase**: to increase maximal muscle force by following a resistance training program that focuses on sport-specific exercises of moderate volume and intensity.

- **Strength/power phase**: to increase the speed of force development and power by integrating sport-specific power/explosive exercises of low volume and high intensity.

- **Competition or peaking phase**: to attain peak strength and power by performing a very-high-intensity and very-low-volume sport-specific resistance training program.

- **Active rest phase**: to allow physiological and mental recovery through limited low-volume and low-intensity resistance training or the performance of physical activities unrelated to one's sport.

It has been hypothesized that greater strength and power gains can be achieved by repeating this set of five mesocycles more than once per year (15, 57). The concept of variation is a vital factor that explains a potential advantage of performing the entire set of training phases multiple times in a single year instead of only once (15, 57).

Variation in Exercise Selection

Some evidence suggests that variations in exercise selection for the same muscle group result in greater increases in strength and power than a program with no variation in exercises (16). This does not mean the personal trainer needs to vary the exercises performed in every training session or that all exercises must be changed when one change is made. However, changes

in exercises may be made every two or three weeks, or some exercises can be varied every other training session (i.e., with two somewhat different training sessions performed alternately). Still, maintaining certain core exercises throughout the training program may allow for continuous progress because of the complex motor demands of the major exercises (4).

> **Variations in exercise selection for the same muscle group result in greater increases in strength and power than a program with no variation in exercises.**

TRADITIONAL AND UNDULATING MODELS OF PERIODIZED RESISTANCE TRAINING

The classic **traditional periodization** model, often mistermed *linear periodization*, consists of gradual increases in training intensity and reductions in training volume from one mesocycle to the next. If there is variation in the loading within the week or microcycle, the number of sets and repetitions for a given exercise does not change across the workouts. A variation on the traditional model involves within-week or microcycle fluctuations in both the assigned training load and the training volume for most (or all) core exercises. This type of periodization model is referred to as **undulating** (2, 15, 43).

Traditional Periodization Model

For the traditional model, weekly fluctuations in the core exercises occur such that the full RM load (i.e., 100% of the assigned training load) is performed on one day (referred to as the heavy day). Subsequent training in the same week for the same exercise is performed at a light level (10%-30% lighter loads than on the RM day), or a moderate or medium level (5%-10% lighter loads than on the RM day), or both (depending on whether there are two or three workouts in a week)—all with the same set and repetition assignments. Advancing a traditional periodized program involves a gradual increase in intensity over multiple weeks (or microcycles) of training. Usually, the length of time devoted to a particular intensity load ranges from two to four weeks. The program ends with an active rest phase before the start of another complete training cycle or an in-season (competitive) period.

> A traditional periodization program involves gradual increases in training intensity and gradual decreases in training volume from one mesocycle to the next. Within a microcycle, training intensity fluctuates based on alterations in training loads, but no variation occurs in the assigned number of sets and repetitions.

Sample Traditional Periodization Program

Before starting the periodized program, the personal trainer should recommend that the athlete complete a lower-intensity four- to six-week base training program. This introductory program will allow the athlete to learn exercise technique, gain an initial adaptation to resistance exercise stress, and prepare for the first training cycle. Loads are typically very light (e.g., 15RM-20RM). This base program is especially important for beginners and may or may not be used with experienced, trained athletes.

- *Hypertrophy/Endurance phase:* This two- to four-week phase formally starts a periodized program. The personal trainer should direct the athlete to perform 3 to 5 sets of each exercise at an intensity that allows ≥6 repetitions (about 6RM-30RM) per set, with at least 2 minutes of rest between sets and exercises for core exercises and 60 to 90 seconds of rest for single-joint exercises. This will create a higher-volume, lower-intensity stimulus.

- *Strength phase:* Using the same length cycle of two to four weeks, the athlete performs 3 to 5 sets of 1 to 6 repetitions per exercise with an intensity of about 85% of the 1RM. A 3- to 5-minute rest period is allowed between sets and exercises.

- *Strength/Power phase:* For the next two to four weeks, the athlete performs exercises that allow only 1 to 6 repetitions for 3 to 5 sets at 85% to 95% of the 1RM. The personal trainer also includes power exercises (e.g., push press, power clean) with somewhat lighter loads (53) to permit rapid and explosive movements. A longer rest period between sets is recommended for adequate recovery.

- *Competition phase:* During a two- or three-week period, the personal trainer further increases the load so that it allows only 1 to 3 repetitions at ≥93% of the 1RM (slightly lighter loads for power exercises [53]). The athlete performs 3 or 4 sets of each exercise with a 3- to 5-minute rest period between sets and exercises. This phase allows for the peaking of strength and power abilities, which is especially important for sports that require maximal strength and rapid force development.

- *Active rest phase:* At this point, the athlete moves into the competitive season after a week of active rest or formally completes a one- to three-week active rest period before returning to the hypertrophy phase to repeat the periodized program.

A summary of the parameters of the traditional periodization phases is included in table 23.5, and a sample program is shown in table 23.6 (15, 19, 38, 53, 59).

TABLE 23.5   Summary of the Program Design of a Traditional Periodization Program (Core Exercises)

Phase	Length (weeks)	Sets	Goal (repetitions)	Rest period (time)	Assigned load
Hypertrophy	2-3	3-5	6-30+	≥2 min; 60-90 s for single-joint exercises	≤85% 1RM; 80%-100% 6RM-30RM
Strength	2-3	3-5	1-6	2-5 min	≥85% 1RM; 80%-100% 1RM-6RM
Strength/Power	2-3	3-5	1-6	2-5 min	85%-95% 1RM; 80%-100% 1RM-6RM*
Competition	2-3	1-4	1-3	3-5 min	≥93% 1RM; 80%-100% 1RM-3RM*
Active rest	1	No resistance training	No resistance training	No resistance training	No resistance training

1RM = maximum weight for 1 repetition; RM = maximum weight for the assigned repetition number. These guidelines apply to core exercises only.

*The loads for power exercises (e.g., push press, power clean) may need to be reduced to permit explosive and rapid movements.

Based on Medicine ACoS (38), Sheppard and Triplett (53), Haff (19), Fleck and Kraemer (15), and Stone et al. (59).

TABLE 23.6 Sample Three-Day Traditional Periodized Program

Phase	Week	Sets	Goal reps	Rest period length (minutes)	Monday — Heavy day — 100% of the assigned training load	Wednesday — Light day — 80% of the assigned training load[c]	Friday — Medium day — 90% of the assigned training load[c]
Hypertrophy	1	3	12	2	67% 1RM; 100% 12RM	54% 1RM; 80% 12RM	60% 1RM; 90% 12RM
	2	3	10	2	75% 1RM; 100% 10RM	60% 1RM; 80% 10RM	68% 1RM; 90% 10RM
	3	4	8	2	80% 1RM; 100% 8RM	64% 1RM; 80% 8RM	72% 1RM; 90% 8RM
Strength	4	3	6	3[a]	85% 1RM; 100% 6RM	68% 1RM; 80% 6RM	77% 1RM; 90% 6RM
	5	4	5	3[a]	87% 1RM; 100% 5RM	70% 1RM; 80% 5RM	78% 1RM; 90% 5RM
	6	5	5	3[a]	87% 1RM; 100% 5RM	70% 1RM; 80% 5RM	78% 1RM; 90% 5RM
Strength/Power	7	3	4	3[a]	90% 1RM; 100% 4RM[b]	72% 1RM; 80% 4RM	81% 1RM; 90% 4RM
	8	4	3	3[a]	93% 1RM; 100% 3RM[b]	74% 1RM; 80% 3RM	84% 1RM; 90% 3RM
	9	5	3	3[a]	93% 1RM; 100% 3RM[b]	74% 1RM; 80% 3RM	84% 1RM; 90% 3RM
Competition	10	3	2	5	95% 1RM; 100% 2RM[b]	76% 1RM; 80% 2RM	86% 1RM; 90% 2RM
	11	4	2	5	95% 1RM; 100% 2RM[b]	76% 1RM; 80% 2RM	86% 1RM; 90% 2RM
	12	4	1	5	100% 1RM; 100% 1RM[b]	80% 1RM; 80% 1RM	90% 1RM; 90% 1RM
Active rest	13	No resistance training					

1RM = maximum weight for 1 repetition; RM = maximum weight for the assigned repetition number. These guidelines apply to core exercises only.

[a]Some exercises or situations may require up to 5 min rest.

[b]The loads for power exercises (e.g., push press, power clean) need to be somewhat lighter to permit rapid and explosive movements.

[c]The athlete should complete the same number of goal repetitions—not more simply because the loads are lighter. This applies also to the power exercises whose loads were lightened from the heavy day assignments. The %1RMs shown for the light and medium days were calculated by multiplying the %1RMs of the heavy day by 0.80 and 0.90 (respectively).

Based on ACSM (38), Sheppard and Triplett (53), Haff (19), Fleck and Kraemer (15), and Stone et al. (59).

Caveat for Coinciding Periodization Phases With Sport Seasons

When applying the traditional periodization phases to an athlete's sport seasons, the personal trainer needs to realize it would be inappropriate to have an athlete cycle through each phase over a 12-week period, especially if the athlete is in the middle of the in-season. For instance, an athlete would not want to complete a high-volume hypertrophy phase of training during the in-season because this may lead to fatigue and reduced performance. Instead, the personal trainer should design the resistance training program so the periodization phases coincide with the athlete's sport seasons. Thus, the athlete should continue strength and power training with low volumes during the in-season to maintain performance and manage fatigue. (For a more detailed discussion see Haff; 19.)

Undulating Periodization Model

An undulating periodization model varies the training phases throughout the week by manipulating the intensity (load) and volume of the core exercises. This contrasts with the traditional periodization model that modulates the load but keeps the sets and repetitions intact. For example, the phasic variations of a four-day undulating program could be 3 sets of 5 repetitions at 85% of the 1RM (strength) on Monday, 2 sets of 15 at 60% of the 1RM (light) on Tuesday, 4 sets of 3 high-velocity repetitions at 60% of 1RM (power) on Thursday, and 3 sets of 8 repetitions at 75% of the 1RM (moderate) on Friday. This continues for a given period before the athlete begins a competition period or a one- or two-week active rest phase.

> An undulating periodization program involves within-week or microcycle fluctuations in training phases by manipulating the assigned training load and volume.

Sample Undulating Periodization Program

As recommended before the start of the traditional periodization program, the athlete may need to complete a four- to six-week base training program that incorporates many repetitions with light loads (e.g., 15RM-20RM) to reinforce proper exercise technique and provide a foundation for later phases. An undulating program can use the same time frame as a traditional periodization model (i.e., 12-16 weeks). The different training sessions are sequenced or rotated within a seven-day (or longer) microcycle. The characteristics of undulating periodization workouts are listed in table 23.7, and a sample program is shown in table 23.8 (15, 19, 38, 53, 59).

- *Monday (heavy day):* This workout emphasizes muscular strength by assigning 3 or 4 sets of each exercise with a 3RM to 6RM load. To promote recovery, the personal trainer should allow a 3- to 5-minute rest period.
- *Tuesday (light day):* The lighter loads of this workout permit more repetitions, but they are still repetition maximums (e.g., 10RM-30RM). The athlete performs 2 to 4 sets of each exercise with a 1- to 2-minute rest period between sets and exercises.
- *Thursday (power day):* There are two load and repetition schemes for this workout, depending on the exercise. For power exercises, the athlete performs 3 or 4 sets of 2 to 4 repetitions at high movement velocities with 30% to 70% of the 1RM; all

TABLE 23.7   Summary of the Program Design of an Undulating Periodization Program (Core Exercises)

Phase	Sets	Goal repetitions	Rest period length	Assigned load
Heavy	3-4	3-6	3-5 min	85%-93% 1RM; 90%-100% 3RM-6RM
Light	2-4	10-30	1-2 min	≤75% 1RM; 80%-100% 10RM-30RM
Power	3-4	1-6	2-5 min	Power exercises 30%-70% 1RM* 50%-80% 1RM-6RM Other core exercises 85%-95% 1RM* 80%-100% 1RM-6RM
Moderate	2-4	6-10	≥2 min	75%-85% 1RM; 80%-100% 6RM-10RM

1RM = maximum weight for 1 repetition; RM = maximum weight for the assigned repetition number. These guidelines apply to core exercises only.

*For power exercises, the personal trainer should assign loads at 30% to 70% of the 1RM to allow the athlete to perform them explosively; consult Kawamori and Haff (27) for details about assigning loads for power exercises. Other core exercises should be assigned 1RM to 6RM loads.

Based on Medicine ACoS (38), Sheppard and Triplett (53), Haff (19), Fleck and Kraemer (15), and Stone et al. (59).

TABLE 23.8 Sample Four-Day Undulating Periodization Program

Week	Day 1 Heavy day				Day 2 Light day				Day 3 Power day					Day 4 Moderate day			
	Sets	Goal reps	Rest (min)	Load	Sets	Goal reps	Rest (min)	Load	Sets	Goal reps	Rest[a] (min)	Load[b] (power)	Load[b] (other)	Sets	Goal reps	Rest (min)	Load[c]
1	3	6	4	85% 1RM or 90% 6RM	2	15	1	65% 1RM or 80% 15RM	3	4	3	30% 1RM or 50% 4RM	90% 1RM or 90% 4RM	2	10	2	75% 1RM or 80% 10RM
2	3	6	4	85% 1RM or 95% 6RM	3	15	1	65% 1RM or 82.5% 15RM	3	4	3	32.5% 1RM or 52.5% 4RM	90% 1RM or 92.5% 4RM	3	10	2	75% 1RM or 82.5% 10RM
3	4	6	4	85% 1RM or 100% 6RM	3	15	1	65% 1RM or 85% 15RM	4	4	3	35% 1RM or 55% 4RM	90% 1RM or 95% 4RM	3	10	2	75% 1RM or 85% 10RM
4	3	5	5	87% 1RM or 92.5% 5RM	4	15	1	65% 1RM or 87.5% 15RM	4	4	3	37.5% 1RM or 57.5% 4RM	90% 1RM or 97.5% 4RM	4	10	2	75% 1RM or 87.5% 10RM
5	3	5	5	87% 1RM or 95% 5RM	4	15	1	65% 1RM or 90% 15RM	4	4	3	40% 1RM or 60% 4RM	90% 1RM or 100% 4RM	4	10	2	75% 1RM or 90% 10RM
6	4	5	5	87% 1RM or 97.5% 5RM	2	12	1.5	67% 1RM or 80% 12RM	3	3	3	45% 1RM or 65% 3RM	93% 1RM or 90% 3RM	2	9	2.5	77% 1RM or 80% 9RM
7	4	5	5	87% 1RM or 100% 5RM	3	12	1.5	67% 1RM or 82.5% 12RM	3	3	3	47.5% 1RM or 67.5% 3RM	93% 1RM or 92.5% 3RM	2	9	2.5	77% 1RM or 82.5% 9RM
8	3	4	5	90% 1RM or 92.5% 4RM	3	12	1.5	67% 1RM or 85% 12RM	4	3	3	50% 1RM or 70% 3RM	93% 1RM or 95% 3RM	3	9	2.5	77% 1RM or 85% 9RM
9	3	4	5	90% 1RM or 95% 4RM	4	12	1.5	67% 1RM or 87.5% 12RM	4	3	3	52.5% 1RM or 72.5% 3RM	93% 1RM or 97.5% 3RM	4	9	2.5	77% 1RM or 87.5% RM
10	4	4	5	90% 1RM or 97.5% 4RM	4	12	1.5	67% 1RM or 90% 12RM	4	3	3	55% 1RM or 75% 3RM	93% 1RM or 100% 3RM	4	9	2.5	77% 1RM or 90% 9RM
11	4	4	5	90% 1RM or 100% 4RM	2	10	1.5	75% 1RM or 80% 10RM	3	2	3	50% 1RM or 70% 2RM	95% 1RM or 90% 2RM	2	8	3	80% 1RM or 80% 8RM
12	3	3	5	93% 1RM or 92.5% 3RM	3	10	1.5	75% 1RM or 82.5% 10RM	3	2	3	52.5% 1RM or 72.5% 2RM	95% 1RM or 92.5% 2RM	3	8	3	80% 1RM or 82.5% 8RM
13	3	3	5	93% 1RM or 95% 3RM	3	10	1.5	75% 1RM or 85% 10RM	4	2	3	55% 1RM or 75% 2RM	95% 1RM or 95% 2RM	3	8	3	80% 1RM or 85% 8RM
14	4	3	5	93% 1RM or 97.5% 3RM	4	10	1.5	75% 1RM or 87.5% 10RM	4	2	3	57.5% 1RM or 77.5% 2RM	95% 1RM or 97.5% 2RM	4	8	3	80% 1RM or 87.5% 8RM
15	4	3	5	93% 1RM or 100% 3RM	4	10	1.5	75% 1RM or 90% 10RM	4	2	3	60% 1RM or 80% 2RM	90% 1RM or 100% 2RM	4	8	3	80% 1RM or 90% 8RM
16	Active rest																

1RM = maximum weight for 1 repetition; RM = maximum weight for the assigned repetition number. These guidelines apply to core exercises only.

[a] Some exercises or situations may require up to a 5-min rest.

[b] For power exercises, the personal trainer should assign loads at 30% to 70% of the 1RM to allow the athlete to perform them explosively. (For further information about determining training loads for power exercises, refer to Kawamori and Haff [27]). Other core exercises should be assigned 1RM to 6RM loads.

[c] Or loads 5% to 10% less than the heavy day loads.

Based on Medicine ACoS (38), Sheppard and Triplett (53), Haff (19), Fleck and Kraemer (15), and Stone et al. (59).

other core exercises are assigned the same number of sets but use 1RM to 6RM loads. In addition, the personal trainer can include plyometric power exercises (e.g., with a medicine ball) to develop the power component in the training program of trained and experienced athletes. A 2- to 5-minute rest period between sets is recommended to allow adequate rest for the power exercises.

- *Friday (moderate day):* This session uses loads 5% to 10% lighter than on the heavy day, or at least a sufficiently reduced intensity that allows 6 to 10 repetitions for 2 to 4 sets of each exercise. At least a 2-minute rest period is recommended between sets and exercises.

An example of a three-day undulating periodization program is to perform 3 sets of 10 repetitions at 70% of the 1RM on the first training day of the week (hypertrophy focus), 5 sets of 3 high-velocity repetitions at 60% of the 1RM on the next training day (power focus), and 4 sets of 5 repetitions at 85% of the 1RM on the last training day (strength focus) (66). Again, both the load and volume are modified throughout the week.

Effectiveness of Traditional and Undulating Periodized Programs

The effectiveness of a periodized program is attributed to the systematic variation that allows the athlete to adequately recover from the assigned loads and repetitions. Often the undulating method of periodization is used so that training can continue through the season. This is especially important for sports with long seasons (e.g., tennis, wrestling, basketball, hockey). Typically, during the in-season program, the frequency of training is reduced and the volume of exercise is modulated in relation to the amount of competition and volume of sport practice. The key element of this type of training is the variation and ability to allow rest after a training or competition period (18).

Further, there is much debate whether the traditional model or an undulating model is more effective for promoting muscular adaptations. Collectively, the current evidence suggests that there is little difference between traditional and undulating periodization models when training for strength and hypertrophy (17, 22). Since each periodized model contains training variation at differing levels, using a traditional or undulating periodized plan is a superior approach to training athletes rather than a nonperiodized training plan (46, 63).

> **During the in-season, training frequency is reduced and the volume of exercise is modulated in relation to the number of competitive events and the volume of sport practice.**

CONCLUSION

Since one type of workout will not benefit every athlete in the same way, a training program should blend existing exercise science knowledge (e.g., adhering to the specificity and overload principles) with the practical requirements of administering an individualized exercise program. To this end, a personal trainer can design a periodized resistance training program that meets the needs of the athlete and attends to the specific demands of that individual's sport.

Study Questions

1. Which of the following is *incorrect* regarding the *overload* principle?

   A. The training stress placed on the muscles must be progressively increased for adaptations to continue to occur.

   B. When athletes experience overload, they are burned out and their performance is reduced.

   C. Overload can be induced by increasing the weight lifted.

   D. Overload can be induced by increasing the training frequency.

2. The %1RM–repetition relationship is, for the most part, based on research on three exercises. Which of the following exercises is the relationship *not* based on?

   A. bench press

   B. lat pulldown

   C. back squat

   D. power clean

3. The _____ is typically divided into several weeks to a few months.

   A. megacycle

   B. macrocycle

   C. mesocycle

   D. microcycle

4. What is the recommended rest period during a strength/power phase in a *traditional* periodization model?

   A. 1 min

   B. 60-90 s

   C. 1-2 min

   D. 3-5 min

5. Which of the following periodization models is typically used in sports with long seasons (e.g. tennis, wrestling, basketball, hockey) because it allows training to continue through the season?

   A. linear periodization

   B. traditional periodization

   C. undulating periodization

   D. fluctuating periodization

CHAPTER 24

Facility and Equipment Layout and Maintenance

Jamie L. Aslin, MS, and Chat Williams, MS

After completing this chapter, you will be able to

- understand the facility design and planning process, facility specification guidelines, the exercise equipment selection process, and spacing requirements of a health and fitness facility;

- understand the special considerations given to equipment layout needs for a home exercise facility; and

- identify the appropriate maintenance and cleaning guidelines for all aspects of an exercise facility and the exercise equipment.

Essential components of personal training involve health risk appraisal, proper selection of fitness assessments, accurate administration of assessments and interpretation of the results, designing appropriate exercise programs, and safe and effective instruction and coaching. In addition, personal trainers are frequently responsible for design of a health and fitness facility, as well as the maintenance of exercise equipment used within the facility. This chapter discusses the topics of facility design and equipment layout and maintenance.

FACILITY DESIGN AND PLANNING

An effective facility design requires painstaking effort and a well-organized plan. Designing and planning a facility includes four main phases: predesign, design, construction, and preoperation (8). These phases are commonly identified whether the committee is considering building a new facility or adding to or updating an existing facility. Before any of the phases begin, a facility design committee should be formed. The committee should consist of various levels of professionals including, but not limited to, administrators, facility management personnel, an architect, a contractor, a lawyer, a representative number of prospective users of the facility, and a personal trainer (8).

> A personal trainer should be involved in the four major phases of designing and planning a health and fitness facility: predesign, design, construction, and preoperation.

The authors would like to acknowledge the significant contributions of Shinya Takahashi and Mike Greenwood to this chapter.

Predesign Phase

In the **predesign phase**, the committee conducts a needs analysis and a feasibility study. The committee also creates a master plan, selects an architect, and outlines possible future expansion and alternative uses of the areas within the facility.

When conducting a **needs analysis**, the committee should ask the following questions (8, 11):

- Who are or will be the clientele of the facility?
- What is the maximum number of prospective users? What is an expected number of users for the first year and beyond?
- Where should the facility be located? What are the geographic characteristics of the location (e.g., downtown, residential, close to a busy street, near competitors)?
- What programs and services are needed?
- What is the available budget?
- What are the specific needs of the potential clientele?
- What is the main focus of the facility?
- Who supervises and keeps up the facility?
- When is the facility to be constructed and functionally operational?
- What is the expected longevity of the facility?

When the committee finds that a need exists, the next step is to conduct a **feasibility study**, which will determine whether the project should be undertaken. As part of the feasibility study, the committee determines the cost, facility location, program needs, and projected usage of the facility. A **SWOT analysis**—an analysis of strengths, weaknesses, opportunities, and threats—is often conducted as part of a feasibility study (8).

If the results of the needs analysis and feasibility study are positive, the committee develops a **master plan**, which will explain in detail the project goals and the procedures needed to achieve those goals. The committee should state the major objective of the new facility (11) and write minor objectives such as equipment requirements—how much and what types of cardiovascular, free-weight, selectorized, testing, and rehabilitation equipment will be needed. As part of this process, the group will need to gather and analyze information on currently available equipment and facilities (11). If facility expansion is a main goal, this information should be especially useful when updates are necessary.

An architect with excellent credentials and a strong work record should be selected. The selection should be based on a bid process in which the committee evaluates costs and experience (8).

As part of the process, the committee should consider future expansion or alternative uses of the areas within the facility. This could be a part of the master plan and might include future expansion sites within or next to the facility as well as alternative future usage of the projected rooms. A common mistake is to plan the facility based on current needs and not consider and plan for future ones (8, 21).

Design Phase

The **design phase** may take several months, and the final result should be a detailed blueprint of the new facility. The committee will accomplish the detailed blueprint of the facility design by working closely with an architect from the committee as well as other facility management, facility design, and health and fitness professionals, including a personal trainer. The design should take into account equipment and facility spacing and local health, safety, and legal codes.

Construction Phase

The **construction phase** takes the most time. Throughout this phase, the facility design committee should oversee the construction and monitor the proceedings to ensure the master plan and project deadlines are being fulfilled in a timely manner (8).

Preoperation Phase

Staffing and staff development for a facility are the focus of the **preoperation phase**. The following questions may need to be considered (8):

- How many staff members will the facility need (professional staff, part-time staff, maintenance staff, interns, and so on)?
- What level of qualifications will the job positions require?
- How will positions be advertised and staff recruited?
- What interview process will be used?
- How will staff be scheduled?
- How will staff be trained?

FACILITY SPECIFICATION GUIDELINES

Personal trainers should be familiar with the structural specifications of a health and fitness facility. The following are guidelines for the design of a health and fitness facility, first for the facility as a whole and then for the resistance training room in particular.

General Health and Fitness Facility Guidelines

Many guidelines apply to the facility as a whole, including the cardiovascular machine area, resistance training room, stretching area, and other fitness areas or rooms.

- *Passageways.* According to the Americans with Disabilities Act (ADA), passageway width must be at least 36 inches (91.4 cm) to accommodate wheelchairs (8, 22). Hallways and circulation passages need to be at least 60 inches (152.4 cm) in width (22). The floor should remain level through door entrances (i.e., the door threshold on the floor should not be raised above floor level). If the threshold exceeds 0.5 inches (1.3 cm), the facility must have a ramp or lift with a slope of 1 foot (30.5 cm) for every inch (2.5 cm) of elevation change to accommodate access to the facility (8). Emergency exit signage must be free of obstructions and have clear visibility (e.g., sufficient lighting) (8).

- *Natural lighting and windows.* Natural lighting tends to increase motivation when a person is exercising (20), so it is desirable to locate cardiovascular machines next to or facing windows. An open feeling and natural lighting are positives for people doing aerobic exercise. However, if higher windows or skylights are installed, it is essential to carefully evaluate their location (15). If glare is a problem, it can be significantly reduced by window tinting, shades, or blinds.

- *Repair and maintenance shop.* It is desirable to locate a repair and maintenance shop adjacent to or near a fitness room (15) for convenience when large, heavy equipment needs to be transferred to the shop.

- *Water fountain.* The recommendation is to have a water fountain installed close to the entrance of the main fitness rooms or other convenient locations for easy access. However, it should not be located where it could be a distraction to clients or block the flow of traffic. The ADA requires that all water fountains be installed at a height that can be reached by a person in a wheelchair (22).

- *Emergency first aid kit and automated external defibrillator (AED).* It is desirable to install an emergency first aid kit, as well as an AED, within or near fitness rooms for immediate access. The AEDs in a facility should be located within a 1.5-minute walk of a potential incident site (22). The ADA requires all AED devices to be at a height that can be reached by a person in a wheelchair (22).

- *Background music and noise.* It is recommended that health and fitness facilities be designed to maintain background noise levels below 70 decibels and never exceed 90 decibels (22). In addition, the recommended time-weighted average (TWA) exposure for occupational noise is 85 decibels per 8-hour time period (17). An exposure at or above this level is considered hazardous. To provide balanced sound distribution for music, speakers should be installed high in all corners of the rooms (19). When a room has a high ceiling and noise disturbance is prominent, sound panel installation to reduce this problem may be considered. In the resistance training room, another source of noise is the weights themselves. Urethane-coated free weights are more expensive than metal weights but may significantly reduce the noise.

- *Electrical requirements.* It is generally recommended that a fitness facility have both 110- and 220-volt outlets because some types of cardiovascular equipment run on 220 volts (15). To ensure meeting the electrical requirements, planners must consult with manufacturing companies before making a final decision on the equipment to purchase. Additional outlets around fitness rooms would be convenient for vacuuming, scrubbing, and other purposes. In addition, ground-fault circuit interrupters are essential safety devices for automatically shutting down power in the event of an electrical short due to water or insulation problems (15, 22).

- *Temperature and humidity control.* A recommended temperature range for the strength and conditioning facility is 72 to 78 °F (22-26 °C) (1). Other temperature recommendations range between 68 and 72 °F (20-22 °C) (22). Temperature can vary dramatically depending on the structure of the facility as well as usage level (e.g., windows, doors, insulation, and number of exercisers). In addition, the amount of motorized equipment being used at the same time may affect the temperature. Therefore, a zone heating and cooling system may be the most cost-effective and user friendly (15). The capacity of the ventilation systems should be at least 8 to 10 air exchanges per hour, and an optimal range is 12 to 15 air exchanges per hour (15). Further, it is desirable to have a sufficient mix of external fresh air and recirculated internal air moving through the facility (8). Optimal air circulation may be achieved by ceiling fans. For example, two or more fans can facilitate air circulation in a 1,200-square-foot (111.5 m²) facility. The optimal humidity level of a fitness area is 50% or less and no higher than 60% (22). In addition, air fresheners can be used where excessive odor is present.

- *Signage.* Signage should be installed to clearly display operational policies, facility rules, safety guidelines, entrances, exits, rest rooms, and so on (21, 22).

- *Communication boards.* Communication boards or display monitors can be used to display information on upcoming events, announcements, and educational materials. These should be located near the front entrance of the facility where people can view them without blocking the flow of traffic.

- *Telephones.* Telephones should be located in the supervisor's office for emergency purposes. Additional phones may be installed at the front entrance and should be mounted at a maximum height of 4 feet (1.2 m) to accommodate persons in a wheelchair (22).

- *Suggestion box.* A comment and suggestion box may be placed near the main entrance of a health and fitness facility.

Resistance Training Room Guidelines

Resistance training rooms have unique characteristics that require specific guidelines.

- *Location of resistance training room.* An ideal location for a resistance training room is on the ground floor near locker rooms and a service entrance so that delivery of equipment to and from the room is convenient (15). It is desirable to locate a resistance training room away from areas that require privacy and minimal noise,

such as classrooms, laboratories, computer rooms, libraries, or hotel guest rooms.

- *Space for supervisors.* A supervisor's office is ideally located inside the resistance training room so that the supervisor can view the entire room, or at least in the proximity of the room so that he or she is easily accessible. If the supervisor's office is located inside the resistance training room, large windows with an unobstructed view (e.g., no large exercise equipment in front of the windows) are recommended.

- *Staff-to-member ratios.* At least one qualified health and fitness professional should be available to assist members with any questions, to provide guidance, and to respond in case of emergency. Currently there is no standard ratio, but it is recommended that a facility not exceed 100 participants per qualified health and fitness professional (23).

- *Ceiling height.* The desirable ceiling height ranges from 12 to 14 feet (3.7 to 4.3 m) (15). A common mistake when selecting a ceiling height for a resistance training room is not allowing sufficient space for heating and cooling air ducts, light fixtures, utility cables, wires, and plumbing structures (15).

- *Windows.* Windows in the resistance training room should be a minimum of 20 inches (50.8 cm) above the floor (15). This will help decrease the chance of breakage from a rolling barbell plate or dumbbell. If possible, it is best to avoid placing windows where spotters or exercisers would be likely to lean against them (15).

- *Doors.* It is desirable to have double doors with removable center posts for more convenient transfer of large, heavy exercise equipment (15). In addition, when a major deep cleaning is scheduled, the large opening to the resistance training room facilitates moving cleaning and exercise equipment in and out.

- *Lighting.* It is desirable for lighting to be brighter than would be required for a classroom or office (i.e., 50 foot-candles or 538 lux). The recommendation for lighting in the resistance training room is 75 to 100 foot-candles or 807 to 1,076 lux (16, 22). The ADA requires all light switches to be at a height accessible by a person in a wheelchair (22).

- *Storage area.* A resistance training room requires more storage space than one might expect (8). Storage may be needed for cleaning supplies and equipment, staff apparel, towels, small equipment, and exercise equipment accessories.

■ *Mirrors.* Mirrors in the resistance training room should be installed at least 20 inches (50.8 cm) above the floor so they are not damaged by barbell plates or dumbbells rolling against them or barbell plates leaning against them (the diameter of a typical 45-pound [20 kg] Olympic barbell plate is approximately 18 inches or 46 cm) (15). Dumbbell racks and all other weight equipment should be placed at least 6 inches (15.2 cm) away from the mirrors to decrease the chance of breakage (15). If dumbbell racks are located close to mirrors and tend to get moved, it may be necessary to secure them (i.e., bolt them down). Protective rails or special protective padding can be anchored to the base of the wall or floor to help protect the mirrors (1). There are benefits to having mirrors in the resistance training room. A mirror provides a client with immediate feedback during an exercise. In addition, it provides feedback to a personal trainer on exercise technique via blindside viewing of a client's body during an exercise. Mirrors are also motivational because clients can see improvements and changes in their physical characteristics. Furthermore, mirrors enhance the look of the resistance training room and make it appear more spacious. However, mirrors have potential negative effects as well. Clients can become distracted watching the mirror and fail to concentrate on proper exercise technique. Also, some clients do not want to see themselves in a mirror.

■ *Floor.* For flooring material in the resistance training room, carpet is the least expensive choice; carpets also come in a wide range of colors and may have an attractive appearance (4). Interlocking rubber mats usually provide more cushion and durability than carpet; however, dirt, sand, and other debris are more likely to become trapped in the interlocking spaces between mats (13). Darker colors are typically recommended for a floor because they are less likely to show dirt and stains (4). Although a poured rubber surface is the most expensive choice, it is the best flooring option because it is seamless and provides more cushion and durability (13). Another option to consider is indoor turf for performing plyometrics, speed and agility drills, and ground-based resisted movements (such as sled pushes and pulls) (10). A wood floor is the best flooring choice for Olympic platforms because the smooth, flat surface provides better foot contact (1). The surface of a floor should have the proper level of shock absorption and traction to minimize the risk of high-impact- or fall-related injuries. A suspended floor or rubber mats are appropriate for plyometric exercises. Hard surfaces, including concrete, asphalt, tile, and hardwood floors, are not proper surfaces for high-impact activities (9). If a resistance training room is not located on the ground floor, a load-bearing capacity of at least 100 pounds per square foot (488.2 kg/m²) is desirable to accommodate heavier exercise equipment and to prevent any structural damage from dropped heavy weights (19, 21).

■ *Walls.* The walls of a resistance training room with high traffic flow or high activity must be free of obstructions such as extended bars, cables, light bulbs, broken or unsecured mirrors, shelves, and other fixtures (7).

> **In order to provide a safe and effective exercise environment, personal trainers should be familiar with all aspects of health and fitness facility specifications.**

SELECTING EXERCISE EQUIPMENT

Evaluating exercise equipment for a health and fitness facility involves three phases: developing functional criteria for the equipment, evaluating the specifications and the effectiveness of the equipment, and evaluating the manufacturers' business practices (12). In addition to this process, two other planning tools are used—a tentative floor plan and a priority list (13). The **tentative floor plan** reflects all major and minor objectives of the facility design. It should also specify the types and amounts of equipment needed (13). The **priority list** should be developed based on the facility's needs analysis. The highest priority in any health and fitness facility is safety and prevention of injuries.

> **Personal trainers should be involved in all three phases of the exercise equipment selection process: developing functional criteria, evaluating specifications and effectiveness, and evaluating the manufacturers' business practices.**

Phase 1: Develop Functional Criteria for the Equipment

The first step in selecting exercise equipment is to develop criteria that meet users' functional needs for the equipment. When selecting resistance exercise equipment, it is critical to understand the mechanics of the equipment (e.g., cam system; leverage system; resistance systems including water pressure, air pressure, weight stacks, barbell plates, springs, hydraulic and electromagnetic equipment). In addition, planners should analyze the types of movements that will be used (e.g., dynamic constant external resistance [DCER], isokinetic single plane vs. multiplane, and isolateral and bilateral) before making a final decision.

On the other hand, when selecting cardiovascular equipment, it is essential to consider choosing the most versatile and popular types of equipment to meet the needs of a variety of targeted populations (e.g., a treadmill can be used for various speeds of walking and running; some elliptical machines can change the stride lengths).

Phase 2: Evaluate Specifications and Effectiveness of the Equipment

Based on the facility's needs analysis, the following questions can be used in the exercise equipment selection process.

- What age groups and fitness levels characterize the individuals who will be using the equipment?
- Are there any priorities to be considered for purchasing the exercise equipment (e.g., cardiovascular vs. resistance training equipment)?
- Are there any unique selling points of the facility to be considered?
- How can color coordination be achieved?
- How much should the equipment cost?
- What is the warranty on the equipment?
- Does the company provide maintenance training sessions?
- Does the company provide periodic maintenance services?
- How fast can replacement parts for the equipment arrive?

For resistance training equipment, the following specification categories should be considered:

- Structural materials (i.e., size and gauge of the steel)
- Connecting materials (e.g., welds, bolts, nuts, sleeves, collars, gaskets, washers, clamps)
- Materials that affect functionality (e.g., bearings, bushings, rails, pulleys, cables, belts, handles, springs, insulators, lubricators, paint, upholstery, plating, grinding, and filing)

It is critical to estimate how many pieces of equipment a health and fitness facility needs before making purchasing decisions. In most cases, cardiovascular equipment is an essential component of a health and fitness facility, and the decision on how many pieces of cardiovascular equipment are needed should be a first priority. In the fitness industry, there are no specific standards or guidelines for estimating the correct amount of cardiovascular equipment, but it is common practice to follow several steps. The first step is to determine how many members will be using the facility during any given 2-hour period, by taking 25% of the total membership (22). The second step is to determine the total number of members who will be daily users, by taking 33% of the 25% figure arrived at in step 1. The third step uses a previously established standard for how many pieces of equipment the facility will have for a given number of daily users. For example, if the facility has established a standard of one piece of cardiovascular equipment for every five daily users, a facility that has 2,000 members should have a total of 33 cardiovascular machines.

To maximize the use of floor space, cordless cardiovascular equipment may be advantageous. Whereas equipment with a power cord is limited as to location, cordless equipment can be installed anywhere in the facility. Several manufacturers make an attachable TV monitor for cardiovascular equipment. Some offer computer consoles that display TV channels, connect to the internet, and so on; these of course are more expensive. Installing multiple large TV monitors on walls or hanging them from the ceiling in front of a cardiovascular area is a less expensive option. If the machine requires a cable to connect to cable or satellite TV, the location choices may be limited. If a computerized exercise tracking system is being considered for each weight training machine as well as the cardiovascular machines, additional wiring and outlets may be required.

Although there are no standards or guidelines for how much or what types of resistance training equipment a facility should have, this can be determined based on the total facility space, the members' demographic characteristics (e.g., age, sex, physical abilities), the members' needs and preferences, and their patterns of usage. A common recommendation is to provide at least one circuit weight training area for every 1,000 users (22).

It is ideal to see and use equipment if possible before making a final decision. If the equipment under consideration as a top choice is used at a local facility, it is common practice to visit the facility to further evaluate the equipment. In some cases manufacturing companies, as well as local health and fitness dealers, are willing to provide a demo unit to try out. Attending exercise equipment trade shows or health fitness conferences is another way to see equipment and meet a company's sales representatives to obtain more information. There may be a special conference discount rate available.

It is also advisable to ask if an exercise equipment company or its dealer has a trade-in option to help lower the cost on a new purchase. A leasing option could also be considered.

Phase 3: Evaluate Manufacturers' Business Practices

The first step in evaluating exercise equipment manufacturers' business practices is to review the companies' business records, the quality of their products, their customer service, and overall reputation. To accomplish this task, it is critical to contact as many sales representatives as possible from a variety of companies to find out about specific products and services. The manufacturers or dealers should be able to provide a list of facilities that have the specific equipment being considered. In addition, making calls to references for further evaluation of the equipment and services may be beneficial. Any equipment manufacturers or dealers with poor-quality products, poor customer service, or other unacceptable business practices should be eliminated from consideration (13).

If keeping expenses low is a priority, it is ideal to purchase most, if not all, pieces of equipment from the same company, as a volume discount may be available. In addition, shipping costs can be lowered if a large quantity of equipment is ordered from one company since shipping costs are determined on a volume basis according to weight. However, since each manufacturer has its own specialties, it is almost impossible to purchase the best quality of all equipment that a facility needs from one manufacturer.

After specifications for all the equipment are determined, the committee should ask selected manufacturers, dealers, or both to provide bids. After all bids are obtained, the committee evaluates the bids and determines the best proposal (i.e., the best price for best quality of the equipment). A purchase order may be required. It is not uncommon to make a down payment of 50% at the time the order is placed (2). It is critical to have a clear understanding of a contract with the manufacturer or dealer including delivery date, installation obligations, and payment methods.

DELIVERY AND ARRIVAL OF NEW EXERCISE EQUIPMENT

After new exercise equipment is ordered, a definite delivery date and time should be established (21). It is common for the manufacturer to hire a shipping company to deliver the equipment, especially with large quantities. It is essential to contact both the manufacturer and the shipping company to confirm the delivery date and time. A shipping company's primary responsibility is delivering the equipment, not installing it. It is important to establish which party will be responsible for installation of new equipment upon delivery. This should be clarified when the equipment is ordered.

Consideration needs to be given to the number of staff needed at the time of delivery, how the equipment will be transported to specific areas of the facility, whether the facility or part of the facility needs to be closed during the delivery process, and whether additional tools or equipment such as carts and pallet jacks will be required. As soon as the new equipment is installed, it should be inspected carefully; any defects should be documented and also photographed if possible. The manufacturer or dealer should be contacted as soon as possible regarding the appropriate actions for exchanging defective equipment. Recording and filing the serial and model numbers of the equipment for inventory is a good practice.

FLOOR PLAN AND EQUIPMENT ORGANIZATION

Three general types of equipment are used in a health and fitness facility: equipment for resistance training, for aerobic training, and for stretching and bodyweight exercise. The following are methods of organizing equipment and relevant considerations:

- Arrange the facility so that the areas for cardiovascular machines, selectorized machines, free weights, Olympic lift platforms, stretching, bodyweight exercise, and rehabilitation are separate.

- Group the resistance training equipment in separate locations in the resistance training room based on the body part they target (e.g., chest, shoulders, back, arms, legs, abdomen). A color coding system (e.g., different upholstery colors) can help users easily identify which selectorized machines are for which muscles or muscle groups. In addition, a map can be displayed to show where particular resistance training machines are located.

- A circuit weight training area can be arranged so that all major muscles or muscle groups can be trained in a time-efficient way.

- Resistance training equipment and cardiovascular machines can be arranged based on brands or manufacturers. When a large quantity of equipment is purchased from more than two companies, this type of equipment arrangement may be preferable.

- Cardiovascular machines can be arranged based on their types, such as treadmills, elliptical machines, bikes, rowing machines, and stair steppers. Arrangement options can be affected by whether a machine requires a power outlet or not.

- Special considerations, such as accessibility and an inclusive environment for persons with disabilities, should enter into organizing the equipment.

- Depending on the facility's size and targeted audience, organizing the exercise areas based on equipment type creates an efficient use of space (15). Larger facilities that serve more clients have more and a greater variety of equipment, so clustering equipment based on the body part targeted improves functionality and accessibility.

> Personal trainers should be familiar with all aspects of equipment placement and spacing guidelines in order to provide effective supervision as well as a safe exercise environment.

Equipment Placement

The following general guidelines should be followed for equipment placement in an exercise facility. More specific examples are listed in table 24.1, "Guidelines for Equipment User Space and Safety Cushion."

- Exercise equipment that requires a spotter should be located away from windows, mirrors, and doors to prevent distraction or collision with other clients; instead, this type of equipment should be placed in areas that are easily supervised and accessible.

- Taller machines (e.g., lat pulldown, cable column) or pieces of equipment (e.g., squat racks, power racks) should be placed along the walls or pillars to allow better visibility. Also, they may need to be bolted to the walls or floors for increased stability and safety.

- Dumbbell racks and weight trees are typically placed against the walls. Shorter or smaller pieces of equipment should be placed in the middle of the room to improve visibility and maximize use of space. Single-tier and multi-tier dumbbell racks are available on the market. A decision should be made on how much space can be used for this purpose and how many dumbbells need to be available for the clients.

- For circuit weight training, resistance training machines are typically placed in an order such that large muscle groups are trained earlier and small muscle groups later (20). In addition, arranging the circuit in such a way that a user can train the muscles or muscle groups in an alternate fashion may minimize the length of breaks needed between the exercises (e.g., chest press, then leg press).

- A separate designated space for stretching should be set up in an area that has less traffic or is quieter. In addition to the stretching area, in a larger facility it may be desirable to have individual stretching mats for convenience (e.g., a user may be able to take a mat and find another spot when the stretching area is too crowded).

- Cardiovascular machines that require clients to be in an upright position or that are taller (e.g., treadmills, stair climbers, elliptical trainers) should be placed behind the cardiovascular machines that require clients to be lower to the ground (e.g., rowing machines, stationary bikes, semirecumbent cycles). With this placement, the taller machines will not impair the visual field (e.g., for television watching) of clients using machines that are lower to the ground.

- Treadmills and any other cardiovascular machines with outside moving parts exposed should have sufficient surrounding room for safety reasons. In addition, treadmills should not be placed near or next to medicine balls or stability balls. A ball left on the floor can potentially be sucked under a treadmill belt and cause serious injury.

- All exercise equipment should be placed at least 6 inches (15.2 cm) from mirrors.

TABLE 24.1 Guidelines for Equipment User Space and Safety Cushion

Type of exercise or equipment	Needed user space and safety cushion for stand-alone pieces of equipment
Supine and prone exercises (e.g., bench press, lying triceps extension)	**Formula** (Actual weight bench length [a user space length of 6-8 ft] + a safety space cushion of 3 ft on each side[a]) *multiplied by* (Actual bar length [a user space width of 4-7 ft] + a safety space cushion of 3 ft on each side[a]) **Example** If a client is using a 6 ft weight bench for the bench press exercise with an Olympic bar: (6 ft + 3 ft + 3 ft) $\times$ (7 ft + 3 ft + 3 ft) = 156 ft^2
Standing exercises (e.g., biceps curl, upright row)	**Formula** (User space length for a standing exercise of 4 ft + a safety space cushion of 3 ft on each side[a]) *multiplied by* (Actual bar length [a user space width of 4-7 ft] + a safety space cushion of 3 ft on each side[a]) **Example** If a client is performing the (standing) biceps curl using a 4 ft bar: (4 ft + 3 ft + 3 ft) $\times$ (4 ft + 3 ft + 3 ft) = 100 ft^2
Standing exercises from or in a rack (e.g., back squat, shoulder press)	**Formula** (User space length for a standing exercise [in a rack] of 4-6 ft + a safety space cushion of 3 ft on each side[a]) *multiplied by* (Olympic bar length [a user space width of 7 ft] + a safety space cushion of 3 ft on each side[a]) **Example** If a client is performing the back squat exercise in a 4 ft^2 power rack using an Olympic bar: (4 ft + 3 ft + 3 ft) $\times$ (7 ft + 3 ft + 3 ft) = 130 ft^2
Olympic lifting area (e.g., power clean, lunge[b]; step-up[b])	**Formula** (Lifting platform length [a user space length of typically 8 ft] + a safety space cushion of 3-4 ft on each side[a]) *multiplied by* (Lifting platform width [a user space width of typically 8 ft] + a safety space cushion of 3-4 ft on each side[a]) **Example** If a client is performing the power clean exercise on an Olympic lifting platform with a 4 ft safety space cushion: (8 ft + 4 ft + 4 ft) $\times$ (8 ft + 4 ft + 4 ft) = 256 ft^2
Stretching and warm-up activities	**Formula** (A user space length of 7 ft) *multiplied by* (A user space width of 7 ft) **Example** If a client is performing a modified Hurdler's stretch: (7 ft) $\times$ (7 ft) = 49 ft^2
Aerobic and resistance training exercise machines	**Formula** (The length of the actual machine [a user space length of 3-8 ft] + a safety space cushion of 3 ft on each side[a]) *multiplied by* (The width of the actual machine [a user space length of 1.5-6 ft] + a safety space cushion of 3 ft on each side[a]) **Examples** If a client is running on a treadmill: (7 ft + 3 ft + 3 ft) $\times$ (3 ft + 3 ft + 3 ft) = 117 ft^2 If a client is performing the machine seated chest press exercise: (5 ft + 3 ft + 3 ft) $\times$ (4 ft + 3 ft + 3 ft) = 110 ft^2
In a home exercise facility: Aerobic dance, kickboxing, calisthenics, bodyweight exercises	**Formula** (A user space length of 5-7 ft) *multiplied by* (A user space width of 5-7 ft) **Example** If a client is exercising to an aerobic dance videotape in a home facility: (6 ft) $\times$ (6 ft) = 36 ft^2

[a]If this exercise or piece of equipment was placed in a group of similar equipment, then the safety space cushion would be only 3 ft on one side because the adjacent piece of equipment would provide the safety space cushion on the other side. Therefore, the space calculations would be (User space length + 3 ft) multiplied by (User space width + 3 ft).

[b]Although the lunge and step-up are not explosive or power exercises and therefore do not have to be performed on a platform, the "moving" or "traveling" nature of these exercises and others like them would benefit from the segregation provided by an Olympic platform. Thus, from a safety standpoint they are included in this category.

Adapted by permission from Greenwood and Greenwood (2008, p. 551).

Equipment Spacing

Proper equipment spacing will allow easy access to the machines, better traffic flow, and safer execution of an exercise. Proper equipment spacing also allows for a personal trainer to supervise the facility and interact with the clients safely and effectively.

There are two major functions of proper equipment spacing. First, appropriate spacing of equipment improves the personal trainer's supervisory ability and provides sufficient room for clients to perform each exercise safely (called the **user space**). Second, proper spacing should also facilitate access between each piece of equipment (called the **safety space cushion**) and enhance the flow of traffic. The fitness area should provide between 25 and 50 square feet (2.3-4.6 m²) per piece of equipment on the floor (22). To effectively serve clients who use wheelchairs, more than 3 feet (0.9 m) around the equipment may be needed. The ADA requires that each piece of equipment have an adjacent clear floor space of at least 30 by 48 inches (76.2 cm by 121.9 cm) (22).

Table 24.1 shows the total space requirements (i.e., the user space plus a safety space cushion) for various types of exercise equipment (15, 22). The following guidelines for equipment spacing are suggested by the National Strength and Conditioning Association (4, 8).

Facility Traffic Flow

- Sufficient traffic flow around the perimeter of resistance and cardiovascular machine areas is required to allow clients and personal trainers easy access to the equipment. Different colors or patterns of flooring or carpet can be used to identify walkways through the facility. To effectively serve clients who use wheelchairs, more than 3 feet (0.9 m) of space may be needed.

- At least one walkway should bisect the room to provide quick and easy access in and out of the facility in an emergency.

> A personal trainer should be familiar with home exercise equipment purchases, special considerations for the home gym environment, and home gym space and equipment arrangements.

- An unobstructed pathway of 3 feet (0.9 m) wide should be maintained in the facility at all times as stipulated by federal, state, and local laws. No exercise machines or equipment should block or hinder the flow of traffic in the facility.

- Although ceiling height does not affect traffic flow on the floor, the ceiling should be free of all low-hanging items (e.g., beams, pipes, lighting, signs) and high enough to allow clients to perform overhead and jumping exercises. A minimum of 12 feet (3.7 m) is recommended.

Stretching and Bodyweight Exercise Area

- An area for stretching that allows 40 to 60 square feet (3.7-5.6 m²) of space per user is reasonable (22), with 49 square feet (4.6 m²) considered optimal (7).

- A larger area may be needed if a personal trainer assists a client with stretching (e.g., proprioceptive neuromuscular facilitation exercises).

Resistance Training Machine Area

- All resistance training machines and equipment must be spaced at least 2 feet (0.6 m), preferably 3 feet (0.9 m), apart.

- If a free-weight exercise will be performed in a resistance training machine area (e.g., a circuit training workout area), a 3-foot (0.9 m) safety space cushion is needed between the ends of the barbell and all adjacent stations (15).

- Multistation machines may be a better choice for some facilities because of the shape of the resistance training room, arrangement of the equipment, and amount of space available. The different sizes and configurations of available space in a facility provide a variety of options. If possible, more than the 3-foot (0.9 m) spacing is recommended between multistation machines and single-station machines.

Resistance Training Free-Weight Area

- The ends of all Olympic bars and fixed-weight barbells on racks should be spaced 3 feet (0.9 m) apart.

- The area designated for free weights should be able to accommodate three or four people.

- If resistance training equipment does not have weight racks (e.g., squat racks and power racks typically have weight racks), weight trees should be placed close to plate-loaded equipment and benches but not closer than 3 feet (0.9 m).

- Dumbbell racks should be placed at least 6 inches (15.2 cm) away from a mirror to decrease the chance of breakage (15). The racks may need to be bolted down if they constantly shift toward the mirror. This shifting can occur when dumbbells are reracked by users.

Olympic Lifting Area

- Perimeter walkways around the platform area should be 3 to 4 feet (0.9-1.2 m) wide (8).
- Space needed for the Olympic lifting area is 36 square feet (3.3 m^2) (14).

Aerobic Exercise Area

- An ideal safety space cushion of 3 feet (0.9 m) should be provided on all sides of the aerobic exercise machines (placement too close to walls should be avoided) to allow clients and supervising personal trainers easy access as well as for safety reasons.
- Table 24.1 (17b) gives precise space guidelines, but common recommendations are 24 square feet (2.2 m^2) for stationary bikes and stair machines, 6 square feet (0.6 m^2) for skiing machines, 40 square feet (3.7 m^2) for rowing machines, and 45 square feet (4.2 m^2) for treadmills (6). These spacing recommendations include the safety space cushion between the machines.

SPECIAL CONSIDERATIONS FOR A HOME FACILITY

In a home exercise facility, there are special considerations because of the smaller space available. Considerations that apply to the commercial setting, with respect to available space and equipment, also apply to a home exercise facility but typically on a smaller scale. It is still essential to provide sufficient space for effective instruction and a safe environment. In many cases, the client may look to a personal trainer for advice on purchasing home equipment. Clients and personal trainers need to address potential hazards that may exist in a home exercise facility, such as environmental issues (e.g., lighting, temperature, humidity) and the safety of children and pets.

Home Exercise Equipment Purchases

The purchase of appropriate home exercise equipment is one of the greatest challenges the personal trainer and client face. A thorough analysis and evaluation of the equipment is necessary to make a final decision, and the following aspects of the home exercise equipment purchasing process should be taken into consideration.

Some critical decisions must be made before exercise equipment for a home environment is purchased. The first consideration is the needs of the client along with a predetermined budget. The next is the amount of available exercise space, including ceiling height, door width, and any other structural aspects of the home. Third is the abundance of home exercise equipment available from reputable companies that provide attractive warranties. The Internet is an excellent way to find equipment, but it is a good practice to try out the equipment if it is available at a local store. Also, since most exercise equipment is heavy, the shipping and handling fees should enter into the final decision. Fourth, cost is always an important factor, but variety, diversity, portability, and space efficiency are also necessary considerations. Some personal trainers warn against the purchase of exercise equipment that can be dismantled and stored out of sight because this practice can create a barrier to accessing the equipment and reaching exercise goals.

Home Environment Issues

A home exercise facility presents additional safety concerns that revolve around the access to the exercise area by children and pets. Electrical concerns are another safety issue.

- To prevent serious injury, children and pets should be kept a safe distance from electrical outlets and any exercise equipment.
- A see-through gate placed in the entryway can help promote a safer home exercise environment.
- If doors or windows provide access to the exercise area, they should be locked when the equipment is not in use. To ensure that the living environment is safe, it may be necessary to disable some types of equipment (i.e., unplug cords to treadmills,

remove accessory attachments for resistance machines, remove weight pins from machines, remove weight plates from bars, place bars out of the flow of traffic).

■ The client and personal trainer should also make sure the home exercise facility has a sufficient electrical supply to accommodate the additional equipment (20).

■ When possible, outlets should have 110- and 220-voltage capabilities and be protected with ground-fault circuit interrupters (GFCIs) so that power is automatically shut down in the event of an electrical overload (15). Additional electrical outlets should be available for vacuum cleaners and other electric equipment and tools.

■ The client should use a padded mat for floor exercises to help reduce perspiration accumulation on any permanent carpeted surface.

Home Equipment Layout

Because a home exercise facility is smaller, has less equipment, and serves fewer people than a commercial facility, all fixed equipment (e.g., aerobic exercise machines and dumbbell racks) is typically arranged along the perimeter of the room fairly close to the walls. Use common sense to prevent injuries and structural damage to the home facility (see figure 24.1).

■ The space cushion around equipment is often reduced (e.g., 18 inches [45.7 cm] instead of 3 feet [0.9 m]).

■ The recommendation for space for activities such as aerobic dance, kickboxing, calisthenics, and bodyweight exercises is 25 to 49 square feet (2.3-4.6 m²) (22).

■ Entertainment equipment such as televisions, DVD players, radios, CD players, or newer technologies in the exercise area can be installed on a wall or the ceiling so the client can view instructional exercise videos and listen to music or news (22).

FACILITY AND EQUIPMENT MAINTENANCE

Facility and equipment maintenance can easily become reactive rather than proactive. In order to provide a safe exercise environment, preventive maintenance procedures need to be a focus. Regular maintenance and cleaning procedures not only provide a safe environment but also increase the longevity of exercise equipment. Personal trainers should follow the CDC guidelines for disinfecting exercise equipment and spaces for virus control. A systematic daily, weekly, and monthly inspection, maintenance, and cleaning schedule should be established. This will

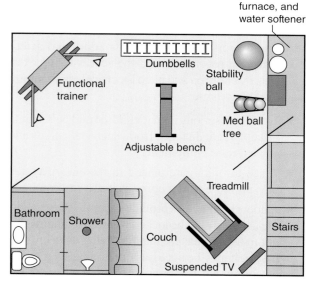
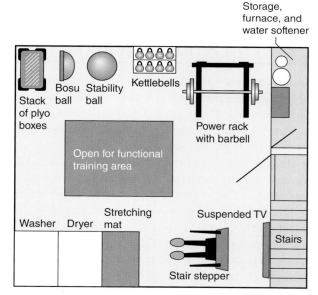

FIGURE 24.1 Two examples of home exercise facility floor plans.

ensure safety for clients and proper functioning of the equipment. Personal trainers must be familiar with all aspects of inspection, maintenance, and cleaning procedures for the equipment to safeguard their clients against potential injuries and avoid litigation.

> **Proper facility and equipment maintenance not only promotes a safe exercise environment but also increases longevity of the facility and equipment.**

Facility Maintenance

In many cases, a majority of members use a resistance training room for their main workouts; therefore the resistance training room becomes a representation of the entire facility. Areas such as those under and between equipment may be difficult to clean thoroughly. Therefore maintaining and cleaning health and fitness facilities should begin with an assessment of the types of surfaces that are present and the maintenance and cleaning difficulties that could arise in each area.

Refer to "NSCA's Safety Checklist for Exercise Facility and Equipment Maintenance" at the end of this chapter for a cleaning schedule and list of facility and equipment maintenance tasks.

- Personal trainers should frequently assess the condition of walls, floors, and ceilings, as well as the accessibility and safe placement of equipment.
- Cleaning of the commercial exercise facility is often handled by both custodial staff and the personal training staff. Another option is to hire a professional cleaning company.
- Cleaning of the home facility can be handled by the owner of the house or by the personal trainer. If a personal trainer uses a client's home gym (on-site personal training), the cleaning obligations should be discussed and determined with the client.

Floor

- The personal trainer needs to inspect, maintain, and clean the floor regularly.
- Wooden flooring must be kept free of splinters, holes, protruding nails, uneven boards, and loose screws. Inspection of these potential problem areas should occur daily during regular cleaning.

- Tile flooring should be treated with antifungal and antibacterial agents, especially in the aerobic exercise area. Tile floors should also be resistant to slipping and moisture and should be free of chalk and dirt buildup.
- Resilient rubber flooring in the free-weight and machine areas should be treated with antifungal and antibacterial agents in the same manner as the flooring in the aerobic exercise area. Rubber flooring must be kept free of large gaps, cuts, and worn spots.
- Interlocking mats must be secure, free from protruding tabs, and arranged so as not to pull apart or become wrinkled.
- The stretching area must be kept free of accumulated dust. Mats or carpets should be nonabsorbent and should contain antifungal and antibacterial agents.
- Carpeting must be kept free of tears, and walkways and high-traffic areas should be protected with additional mats. All areas must be swept and vacuumed or mopped according to designated cleaning schedules.
- Flooring must be kept glued and fastened down properly, and all fixed equipment must be attached (bolted) securely to the floor.

Walls

- The personal trainer needs to inspect, maintain, and clean walls regularly. Wall surfaces include mirrors, windows, exits, storage areas, and shelves. Wall surfaces should be cleaned two or three times a week or as needed.

Ceiling

- The personal trainer needs to inspect, maintain, and clean the ceiling. Maintenance and cleaning of ceilings in the exercise facility are often overlooked. This duty includes ceiling fixtures and attachments such as lights, air-conditioning units, heating units, air ducts, sprinkler heads and pipes, speakers, TV monitors, and ceiling fans.
- Tiled ceilings must be kept clean, and any damaged or missing tiles should be replaced as needed. Open ceilings with exposed pipes and ducts do not require regular dust removal but should be cleaned as needed.

Equipment Maintenance

Keeping the equipment functional, clean, and safe to use is a critical part of a personal trainer's daily duties. Equipment that is constantly used and not consistently cleaned or maintained is potentially dangerous to the client and the personal trainer.

- In a commercial exercise facility, the maintenance staff, personal trainers, and local equipment representatives should clean and maintain the exercise equipment regularly.

- Providing disposable cleaning towelettes and a cleaning solution bottle with rags near the exercise equipment may encourage users to clean the equipment before and after use. In addition, when bodily fluids such as sweat are cleaned off a machine, wearing disposable latex or latex-free gloves is recommended. These should be readily available at the facility. If this is not an option, hand washing with soap and water should be required after equipment has been cleaned of sweat or any other bodily fluids.

- Minor cleaning of exercise equipment in a health and fitness facility can be handled by a client; however, it is the personal trainer's responsibility to maintain and clean this equipment regularly and properly.

Stretching Area

Equipment commonly used for stretching includes padded mats, stretching sticks, elastic cords, and wall ladders.

- Mats in stretching areas should be cleaned and disinfected daily and in a timely manner.

- The mats should be free of cracks and tears.

- Areas between mats should be swept or vacuumed regularly to prevent dust and dirt buildup.

- The stretching area should be free of benches, dumbbells, and other equipment that may create clutter and may tear mat surfaces. All equipment should be stored after use, and elastic cords should be secured to a base, checked for wear, and replaced when necessary.

- Cleaning solution bottles and rags for cleaning mats after use may be considered. Such items should be close to the stretching mat but located so as not to represent a hazard.

Bodyweight Exercise Area

Stability balls, medicine balls, plyometric boxes, ladders, cones, balance training equipment, utility benches, hyperextension benches, and jump ropes are typically used in the bodyweight exercise area.

- All mats and bench upholstery should be disinfected daily and should be free of cracks and tears.

- The tops and bottoms of plyometric boxes should have nonslip surfaces for safe use and should be inspected monthly for excessive wear.

- Other equipment and accessories should be inspected regularly for functional safety and should be cleaned on a regular basis to extend their life span.

Resistance Training Machine Area

A large variety of resistance training machines on the market (e.g., cam, pulley, cable, belt, chain, plate loaded, selectorized, pneumatic, isokinetic) are available in both single-station or multistation designs.

- Bench upholstery and machine surfaces that come into contact with skin should be cleaned and disinfected daily and should be free of cracks and tears.

- Guide rods on selectorized machines should be cleaned and lubricated two or three times per week.

- No machine should have loose bolts, screws, cables, chains, or protruding or worn parts that need replacement or removal. In addition, if machines are bolted down to the floor or wall, the bolts should be inspected for safety monthly.

- Weight plates on resistance training machines should be inspected weekly for cracks.

- Extra L- or T-shaped pins designed for the selectorized machines and belts should be kept in stock so that clients do not try to improvise with unsafe substitutes.

- Chains, cables, belts, and pulleys should be adjusted for proper alignment, tension, and smooth function on a weekly basis because even minor misalignments can cause premature wearing and damage to belts and cables.

Free-Weight Resistance Area

Free-weight resistance exercises involve the use of various types of bars, benches (with and without uprights or racks), squat or power racks, barbells, dumbbells, kettlebells, and weight trees for barbell plates.

- All equipment, including safety equipment (e.g., belts, straps, wraps, pads, chains, gloves, locks, safety bars), should be returned to proper storage areas after use to prevent pathway obstruction.

- All bench and rack welds should be inspected monthly or as needed.

- In and around squat and power racks, the floor should be nonslip and should be cleaned regularly.

- Dumbbells should be checked frequently for loose hex nuts or broken welds.

- An "out of order" sign should be clearly posted on nonfunctional or broken equipment (even in a home facility), or a sheet can be placed over the nonfunctional equipment to prevent user access; or, more desirably, such equipment should be removed from the area or locked out of service.

- All protective padding and upholstery should be free of cracks and tears and cleaned and disinfected daily.

Olympic Lifting Area

Not all facilities have an Olympic lifting area, but those that do commonly have a segregated wooden lifting platform, Olympic bars, bumper plates, racks, locks, and chalk bins. Maintenance and cleaning of this area should occur regularly.

- Olympic bars and curl bars should be properly lubricated and tightened to maintain the rotating bar ends.

- Any defective Olympic bars or curl bars should be replaced immediately.

- The knurling (rough area for hand placement) on Olympic bars should be kept free of debris and chalk buildup by means of occasional cleaning and brushing. A wire brush can be used to brush off the accumulated chalk residue on the knurling.

- The platform should be inspected for gaps, cuts, slits, and splinters (depending on the type of surface) and properly swept or mopped to remove chalk. A protective coating material (e.g., urethane) on a wooden platform may be reapplied if it is worn.

- The platform area should be free of benches, boxes, and other clutter to give the client sufficient room to safely perform power and explosive exercises.

Aerobic Exercise Area

Aerobic equipment is among the most popular within a health and fitness facility and should be a priority for facility expansion (23). A great variety of cardiovascular machines are available on the market, including stationary bikes, treadmills, rowing machines, semirecumbent bikes, sprint machines, stair steppers, elliptical trainers, and skiing machines.

- Equipment surfaces that come into contact with skin should be cleaned and disinfected frequently. This is particularly true during and after periods of heavy use. Cleaning and disinfecting not only protects clients from unsanitary conditions but also extends the life of equipment surfaces and maintains their appearance. Personal trainers should follow the CDC guidelines for disinfecting exercise equipment and spaces for virus control. There are commercially available holders for cleaning solution bottles. If heavy usage of exercise equipment is expected, it may be appropriate to install holders and supply rags so that people can clean the equipment after exercising. Placing floor mats or rugs to trap water, sand, dirt, and other unwanted debris in front of each entrance may help maximize the cleanliness and appearance of the facility.

- All moving parts (e.g., belts, chains, joints, flywheels) should be properly lubricated and cleaned two or three times weekly or when needed.

- During the cleaning process, straps, belts, connective bolts, and screws need to be checked for tightness or wear and replaced if necessary.

- Measurement devices such as RPM (revolutions per minute) meters should be properly maintained; the manufacturer usually does this, but wiping off sweat and dirt regularly will extend the life of the equipment.

A well-written emergency response plan identifies the roles and responsibilities of the employees and the specific actions each employee should take to minimize injuries and facility damage. In the event of an emergency, personal trainers notify all parties affected by the situation, maintain communication with the proper emergency professionals until they arrive on the scene, identify actions to take to alleviate the situation, and assist when needed.

There are three scenarios when encountering an active shooter, in this order: Run, hide, or fight. As a last option and only if lives are in danger, the personal trainer should act with physical aggression, attempting to disarm the shooter and fight. Throwing items and yelling loudly may provide a distraction.

- Equipment parts such as seats and benches should be easy to adjust.
- If budget allows, keeping extra equipment parts for prompt replacement can be a good practice. This will eliminate the time for contacting a dealer or manufacturing company to order a part and waiting for the part to arrive.

EMERGENCY RESPONSE PLAN

Personal trainers and fitness professionals should implement an emergency response plan to protect employees and clients. The emergency response plan may include steps to protect individuals from injury, property loss, or loss of life in the event of major disasters including but not limited to fire, environmental disasters, medical situations, and security threats. A well-written emergency response plan lays out the roles and responsibilities of the employees and the specific actions each employee should take to minimize injuries and facility damage (18).

In the event of an emergency, personal trainers should notify all parties affected by the situation, maintain communication with the proper emergency professionals until they arrive on the scene, identify actions to take to alleviate the situation, and assist when needed. During a fire emergency, employees should take a few simple steps to ensure safety: The fire alarm should be sounded, the fire department should be contacted, and employees should exit the building via the nearest exit and return only after being cleared by the fire department. Because there are multiple types of environmental disasters, personal trainers should first determine the type and notify the proper authorities of the situation. Alert all employees who might be affected so that medical attention can be provided if needed. Cleanup may begin once the area has been contained and emergency professionals have completed a full assessment.

When creating an emergency response plan for medical situations, personal trainers should consider all the parties involved and develop a plan specific to their facility. Roles should be assigned to staff members, members should be educated on the facility action plan, and equipment used during emergencies should be assessed. The personal trainer and staff should have access to a phone, be familiar with 911 availability in the area, and maintain up-to-date training. Staff roles include providing immediate care to the individual, retrieving medical equipment, calling 911, directing medical personnel once they arrive on the scene, and maintaining crowd control. Staff

training and education includes recognizing an emergency, maintaining scene safety, CPR/AED training, blood-borne pathogen training, ongoing training on implementing the emergency action plan, and testing medical equipment to ensure it is in good condition and operating efficiently. Training protocols should be practiced and modified yearly so that all new and current staff are familiar with the plan (3).

In case of an active shooter or security threat, personal trainers must first decide on the most rational way to protect themselves, the staff, and the members. If opportunity presents itself, contact law enforcement and provide the location and number of victims in the facility, number of assailants and physical descriptions, and the type of weapons involved.

There are three scenarios when encountering an active shooter, in this order: Run, hide, or fight. If there is time to run and safely exit, everyone should do so, leaving personal items behind and keeping hands visible so that any law enforcement officers on sight can identify that no weapon is present. If running is not an option, the next step is to hide in a secure area, blocking and locking any doors and remaining out of sight of the shooter. As a last option and only if the lives of any staff or members are in danger, the personal trainer should act with physical aggression and attempt to disarm the shooter. Throwing items and yelling loudly may provide a distraction. Once law enforcement arrives on the scene, all staff and members should immediately raise their hands and spread their fingers. Keeping hands visible at all times, individuals move toward law enforcement officers, following their directions and avoiding any quick movements (5).

After developing an emergency response plan for fire, environmental disasters, medical situations, and security threats, the personal trainer and staff should have annual meetings to review and update the information to ensure the safety of the employees, members, and facility.

CONCLUSION

Painstaking effort and systematic planning are the key elements of a successful facility design. The four main phases in designing the health and fitness facility are predesign, design, construction, and preoperation. Personal trainers should be familiar with all facility specification guidelines in order to design a safe and functional facility. Selecting exercise equipment for a facility is a multifaceted process. The three main phases of selecting exercise equipment are developing functional criteria, evaluating the specifications and the effectiveness of the equipment, and evaluating the manufacturers' business practices. A tentative floor plan and a priority list should be used to finalize the selection of the right equipment for a facility. Creating appropriate spaces between exercise equipment promotes better traffic flow, safer execution of exercises, more effective supervision of a facility, and better interaction with clients. Although a smaller scale of facility design and equipment arrangement applies to a home exercise facility, clients and personal trainers need to address various aspects of potential hazards that may exist, such as environmental issues and the safety of children and pets.

Facility and equipment maintenance can easily become reactive rather than proactive. Proper facility and equipment maintenance can promote not only a sanitized and safe environment but also increased longevity of the facility and equipment. An emergency response plan is critical to minimize injuries, fatalities, and facility damage. In addition, developing and regularly practicing an active shooter plan will prepare the employees and emergency professionals on how to respond.

Study Questions

1. Which of the four phases of designing and planning a health and fitness facility includes a needs analysis?

   A. predesign

   B. design

   C. construction

   D. preoperation

2. It is recommended that health and fitness facilities be designed to maintain background noise levels below _____ decibels.

   A. 70

   B. 80

   C. 90

   D. 100

3. Which of the following combinations of equipment are *not* recommended to be grouped together?

   A. treadmills and ellipticals

   B. machine leg extension and machine chest press

   C. Olympic lifting platforms and stretching equipment

   D. dumbbells and barbells

4. What is the typical space cushion around fitness equipment in a home equipment layout, as opposed to the 3 feet (0.9 m) in a commercial facility?

   A. 6 inches (15.2 cm)

   B. 12 inches (30.5 cm)

   C. 18 inches (45.7 cm)

   D. 24 inches (61.0 cm)

5. Which of the following is the correct order of responses that should be followed when dealing with an active shooter?

   A. fight, run, hide

   B. run, hide, fight

   C. run, fight, hide

   D. hide, run, fight

NSCA'S SAFETY CHECKLIST FOR EXERCISE FACILITY AND EQUIPMENT MAINTENANCE

EXERCISE FACILITY

Floor

- ❏ Inspected and cleaned daily
- ❏ Wooden flooring free of splinters, holes, protruding nails, and loose screws
- ❏ Tile flooring resistant to slipping; no moisture or chalk accumulation
- ❏ Rubber flooring free of cuts, slits, and large gaps between pieces
- ❏ Interlocking mats secure and arranged with no protruding tabs
- ❏ Nonabsorbent carpet free of tears; wear areas protected by throw mats
- ❏ Area swept and vacuumed or mopped on a regular basis
- ❏ Flooring glued or fastened down properly

Walls

- ❏ Wall surfaces cleaned two or three times a week (or more often if needed)
- ❏ Walls in high-activity areas free of protruding appliances, equipment, or wall hangings
- ❏ Mirrors and shelves securely fixed to walls
- ❏ Mirrors and windows cleaned regularly (especially in high-activity areas, such as around drinking fountains and in doorways)
- ❏ Mirrors placed a minimum of 20 inches (50.8 cm) off the floor in all areas
- ❏ Mirrors not cracked or distorted (replace immediately if damaged)

Ceiling

- ❏ All ceiling fixtures and attachments dusted regularly
- ❏ Ceiling tile kept clean
- ❏ Damaged or missing ceiling tile replaced as needed
- ❏ Open ceilings with exposed pipes and ducts cleaned as needed

EXERCISE EQUIPMENT

Stretching and Bodyweight Exercise Area

- ❏ Mat area free of weight benches and equipment
- ❏ Mats and bench upholstery free of cracks and tears
- ❏ No large gaps between stretching mats
- ❏ Area swept and disinfected daily
- ❏ Equipment properly stored after use
- ❏ Elastic cords secured to base with safety knot and checked for wear
- ❏ Surfaces that contact skin treated with antifungal and antibacterial agents daily
- ❏ Nonslip material on the top surface and bottom or base of plyometric boxes
- ❏ Ceiling height sufficient for overhead exercises (12 feet [3.7 m] minimum) and free of low-hanging apparatus (beams, pipes, lighting, signs, etc.)

Resistance Training Machine Area

- ❏ Easy access to each station (a minimum of 2 feet [0.6 m] between machines; 3 feet [0.9 m] is optimal)
- ❏ Area free of loose bolts, screws, cables, and chains
- ❏ Proper selectorized pins used
- ❏ Securing straps functional
- ❏ Parts and surfaces properly lubricated and cleaned
- ❏ Protective padding free of cracks and tears
- ❏ Surfaces that contact skin treated with antifungal and antibacterial agents daily
- ❏ No protruding screws or parts that need tightening or removal
- ❏ Belts, chains, and cables aligned with machine parts
- ❏ No worn parts (frayed cable, loose chains, worn bolts, cracked joints, etc.)

Resistance Training Free Weight Area

- ❏ Easy access to each bench or area (a minimum of 2 feet [0.6 m] between machines; 3 feet [0.9 m] is optimal)
- ❏ Olympic bars properly spaced (3 feet [0.9 m]) between ends
- ❏ All equipment returned after use to prevent obstruction of pathway
- ❏ Safety equipment (belts, collars, safety bars) used and returned
- ❏ Protective padding free of cracks and tears
- ❏ Surfaces that contact skin treated with antifungal and antibacterial agents daily
- ❏ Securing bolts and apparatus parts (collars, curl bars) tightly fastened
- ❏ Nonslip mats on squat rack floor area
- ❏ Olympic bars turn properly and are properly lubricated and tightened
- ❏ Benches, weight racks, standards, and the like secured to the floor or wall
- ❏ Nonfunctional or broken equipment removed from area or locked out of service
- ❏ Ceiling height sufficient for overhead exercises (12 feet [3.7 m] minimum) and free of low-hanging apparatus (beams, pipes, lighting, signs, etc.)

Olympic Lifting Platform Area

- ❏ Olympic bars properly spaced (3 feet [0.9 m]) between ends
- ❏ All equipment returned after use to prevent obstruction of lifting area
- ❏ Olympic bars rotate properly and are properly lubricated and tightened
- ❏ Bent Olympic bars replaced; knurling clear of debris
- ❏ Collars functioning
- ❏ Sufficient chalk available
- ❏ Wrist straps, belts, and knee wraps available, functioning, and stored properly
- ❏ Benches, chairs, boxes kept at a distance from lifting area
- ❏ No gaps, cuts, slits, splinters in mat
- ❏ Area properly swept and mopped to remove splinters and chalk
- ❏ Ceiling height sufficient for overhead exercises (12 feet [3.7 m] minimum) and free of low-hanging apparatus (beams, pipes, lighting, signs, etc.)

Aerobic Exercise Area

- ❏ Easy access to each station (minimum of 2 feet [0.6 m] between machines; 3 feet [0.9 m] is optimal)
- ❏ Bolts and screws tight
- ❏ Functioning parts easily adjustable
- ❏ Parts and surfaces properly lubricated and cleaned
- ❏ Foot and body straps secure and not ripped
- ❏ Measurement devices for tension, time, and revolutions per minute properly functioning
- ❏ Surfaces that contact skin treated with antifungal and antibacterial agents daily

FREQUENCY OF MAINTENANCE AND CLEANING TASKS

Daily

- ❏ Inspect all flooring for damage or wear.
- ❏ Clean (sweep, vacuum, or mop and disinfect) all flooring.
- ❏ Clean and disinfect upholstery.
- ❏ Clean and disinfect drinking fountain.
- ❏ Inspect fixed equipment's connection with floor.
- ❏ Clean and disinfect equipment surfaces that contact skin.
- ❏ Clean mirrors.
- ❏ Clean windows.
- ❏ Inspect mirrors for damage.
- ❏ Inspect all equipment for damage; wear; loose or protruding belts, screws, cables, or chains; insecure or nonfunctioning foot and body straps; improper functioning or improper use of attachments, pins, or other devices.
- ❏ Clean and lubricate moving parts of equipment.
- ❏ Inspect all protective padding for cracks and tears.
- ❏ Inspect nonslip material and mats for proper placement, damage, and wear.
- ❏ Remove trash and garbage.
- ❏ Clean light covers, fans, air vents, clocks, and speakers.
- ❏ Ensure that equipment is returned and stored properly after use.

Two or Three Times per Week

- ❏ Clean and lubricate aerobic machines and the guide rods on selectorized resistance machines.

Once per Week

- ❏ Clean (dust) ceiling fixtures and attachments.
- ❏ Clean ceiling tile.

As Needed

- ❏ Replace light bulbs.
- ❏ Clean walls.
- ❏ Replace damaged or missing ceiling tiles.
- ❏ Clean open ceilings with exposed pipes or ducts.
- ❏ Remove (or place sign on) broken equipment.
- ❏ Fill chalk boxes.
- ❏ Clean bar knurling.
- ❏ Clean rust from floor, plates, bars, and equipment with a rust-removing solution.

From *NSCA's Essentials of Personal Training,* 3rd ed., edited for the National Strength and Conditioning Association by B. Schoenfeld and R. Snarr (Champaign, IL: Human Kinetics, 2022).

CHAPTER 25

Professional, Legal, and Ethical Responsibilities of Personal Trainers

Anthony A. Abbott, EdD, and Georgia H. Goslee, Esq.

After completing this chapter, you will be able to

- appreciate, understand, and explain basic aspects of the law, particularly tort law, and the legal system as they are applicable to the delivery of personal training services;

- define negligence and identify the four elements that an injured client must prove in a lawsuit against a personal trainer based on negligence;

- identify the professional, legal, and ethical responsibilities of a personal trainer and understand the consequences of those responsibilities; and

- adopt and implement risk management strategies to minimize the risks of claims and litigation in personal training.

This chapter explores the legal aspects of personal training, which are not novel or unique legal principles of law. These legal aspects draw upon traditional and substantive areas of the law applied to a set of facts involving inappropriate conduct by personal trainers and fitness facilities. It concentrates on the accepted **standard of care** owed to fitness clients by personal trainers, as well as service delivery issues for these professionals (18). The chapter focuses on those essential services and protective actions that not only help to insulate the personal trainer against litigation but also promote professionalism. Even more importantly, those services provide safe and effective programming for the personal trainer's clientele.

While this chapter primarily focuses on concepts of tort and contract law, we also review certain aspects of criminal law. Federal laws are enacted by the U.S. Congress whereas state laws are enacted by state legislative bodies. For our purpose in this chapter, we principally rely upon concepts of state law.

Laws in place in other countries are different from those applicable in the United States. As a consequence, personal trainers providing services in other countries should seek legal advice as necessary. The chapter also addresses risk management strategies to avoid becoming embroiled in litigation. *The materials presented in this chapter or in other sources are no substitute for the professional legal advice that*

The authors would like to acknowledge the significant contributions of David L. Herbert and JoAnn Eickhoff-Shemek to this chapter.

personal trainers should seek in individual situations and cases.

Risk management in this context is the identification of various risks applicable to personal training activities as obtained through audit. These risks are then analyzed in an effort to eliminate and reduce those risks to improve the safe delivery of services, the chances of untoward events, and related claims and lawsuits. Risk avoidance and minimization strategies focus on the safe and effective screening of fitness clients, the proper recommendation or prescription of activity, the appropriate provision and supervision of training exercises, and the effective delivery of emergency response when necessary—all in accordance with accepted standards and guidelines as promulgated by industry leaders. Once personal trainers understand the legal requirements associated with their delivery of service to clients and once they appreciate the fact that their negligent acts or omissions may well lead to client harm and potential claims and suits against them, they will be better equipped to minimize risks to their clients while reducing their own legal exposure arising out of professional activities (14).

The concept of negligence is examined so that personal trainers are more aware of their conduct as it relates to the elements of negligence. **Lines of defense** are also presented so that personal trainers may be able to protect themselves from unforeseen events or problems that lead to lawsuits. These lines of defense include adherence to professional standards and guidelines and the use of protective legal documents with clients, such as assumption of risk forms, prospectively executed waivers of liability or releases, or both. The protections provided by liability insurance are also of importance and represent yet another line of defense for personal trainers to protect or insulate them from client claims and lawsuits.

> **Personal trainers should use the principles of risk management to ensure the safety of clients and to prevent costly lawsuits.**

We begin with an actual court case in which the first author was retained as an expert witness, a case wherein factual names have been replaced with comical names to protect the privacy of all individuals.

Bailiff: "Here ye, here ye, the Circuit Court for Anywhere, USA, is now in session, the honorable Justus Wright presiding."

Judge Wright: "Mr. Bailiff, please call the first case."

Bailiff: "The first case on the docket, Your Honor, is Grumble v. Traynor in a lawsuit in which the plaintiff alleges that the defendant was negligent in providing personal trainer services."

Judge Wright: "Counsel, please identify yourselves for the record."

Plaintiff's lawyer: "For the record, my name is Lye Belle Proffet, of the law firm Goodman, Goldman, and Gotchya, and I represent Ima Dees Grumble in her claim of negligence against Sue Mee Traynor and the Ms. Fit Factory, a personal training studio for women."

Defendant's lawyer: "For the record, my name is Stan Bye Yurman, of the law firm Schyster, Schuckster, and Schwindler, and I represent Sue Mee Traynor, owner and operator of the Ms. Fit factory, in her defense of this claim."

Judge Wright: "Very well, counselors, are there any preliminary matters?"

Ms. Proffet: "No, Your Honor."

Mr. Yurman: "No, Your Honor."

Judge Wright: "All right, Ms. Proffet, you may begin with a brief opening statement followed by Mr. Yurman's opening statement, and then Ms. Proffet, please call your first witness."

Ms. Profett: "Your Honor, ladies and gentlemen of the jury, the plaintiff will prove that on Friday, February 28, 2020, Ima Dees Grumble suffered an unnecessary and severe injury that has left her permanently disabled, an injury that resulted from inappropriate and unsafe exercise instruction provided by the defendant, Sue Mee Traynor. At approximately 10:00 a.m. on this day, Ms. Grumble, not having been properly screened and tested regarding her capacity for exercise, was instructed, for the first time, to perform an exercise called a lunge with weights or dumbbells in her hands. The defendant demonstrated a perfunctory example of this exercise without weights and without sufficient cautionary instruction or guidance relating to exercise progression. When Ms. Grumble lost her balance, the defendant was not in a position to assist or "spot" her, and therefore, Ms. Grumble, dropping her weights, fell to the tile surface, at which time she tried to break her fall with her right hand, thereby leading to a compound fracture of the wrist. After numerous surgeries, lost time on the job, and great inconvenience to her family, not to mention the pain and suffering,

Ms. Grumble continues to be burdened by a limited range of motion of her wrist as well as fingers and, therefore, has received a medical disability regarding her capacity to effectively perform many activities of daily living to include an inability to carry out some very basic hygienic tasks."

After reviewing the evidence, the court rendered a verdict in favor of the plaintiff and awarded damages in the amount $100,000 plus attorney fees and court costs.

THE PERILS OF LITIGATION

Hopefully, the reader will never find himself or herself named as a defendant in such a lawsuit. The costs are more than monetary and the psychological stress also exacts a lasting toll. However, the current escalation of litigation would appear to be a reflection of a serious industry problem regarding client expectations versus service delivery. Movies and television may lead one to believe that litigation is an exciting event, but this is a media myth. The reality is that for plaintiffs and defendants alike, lawsuits are time consuming, expensive, and emotionally traumatic.

Increased Litigation

In a society that is becoming more litigious with every passing year, the personal trainer must recognize the reality of a potential lawsuit. Unfortunately, many personal trainers, like the proverbial ostrich hiding its head in the sand, do choose to ignore this possibility, a fact evidenced by the large percentage who fail to carry liability insurance. This "ignorance is bliss" attitude is also reflected in the low attendance at legal issues and risk management presentations often conducted for personal trainers at national conferences by professional fitness associations.

Over the past 30 to 40 years, the fitness boom has come of age; and with it, facilities such as clubs, gyms, and spas have advertised the availability of "professional" fitness instruction, which implies safe and effective exercise programming for the public. In reality, few fitness facilities, to include personal training studios, have stringent education, certification, and experience requirements for their instructors and personal trainers. In those instances where training for instructor personnel is provided, it is often on-the-job training by in-house instructor-trainers who frequently lack appropriate credentials themselves. This is both unfortunate and

unnecessary, for professional standards and rigorous certification programs are available through fitness industry leaders such as the NSCA and American College of Sports Medicine (ACSM). This absence of professional standards for fitness instructors and personal trainers often results in a lack of basic knowledge of screening, testing, planning, organizing, leading, and supervising groups as well as teaching individuals, safely and effectively. However, it would seem reasonable, from the standpoint of public safety, to expect some level of competence before fitness instructors and personal trainers are permitted to work with the public.

The significance of the problem centers around the public's right to be protected from unsafe practices, particularly in an area associated with the health promotion industry. Unfortunately, there are no licensure or certification requirements mandating stringent training programs for health facility fitness instructors and personal trainers. Who can deny the grave responsibility that one has in assisting people in vigorous exercise programs. This problem has endured for many years during which time no state has enacted licensure or mandated professional training requirements for fitness instructors and personal trainers.

Many health care professionals and fitness authorities are deeply concerned about the qualifications, or rather lack of qualifications, on the part of exercise instructors and personal trainers. Understandably, college and university educators contend that the physical education and exercise science profession has been bypassed in the growth of the fitness industry; and as a result, quality instruction and training have been generally ignored. In an effort to keep their overhead down, many facility owners and managers frequently hire minimum wage staff while dismissing college-educated physical education and exercise science majors as "overqualified."

Apparently, many fitness facility entrepreneurs have jumped on the fitness bandwagon for financial gain at the expense of their clientele's health and safety. In other words, many such entrepreneurs are more sales oriented than service oriented. Unfortunately, this same entrepreneurial fever and greed that has led to the hiring of untrained staff within the fitness industry has also led to disappointment within the arena of fitness instructor and personal trainer certification. It has been estimated that there are over 300 certification programs, most conducted by self-appointed fitness authorities who have no formal or very limited training in exercise science themselves. One must remember that a certificate is no more valuable than the training behind it and the standards used for awarding such a credential.

Training and Certification

Becoming a truly qualified personal trainer requires an in-depth knowledge of human anatomy, basic physiology, kinesiology, exercise science, and practical training and testing under the direction of knowledgeable and experienced instructors. This cannot be achieved through weekend cram courses and certification programs during which students are typically primed for specific questions to which they regurgitate the answers on an examination. Although many certifying associations will forward candidates' study materials in advance for which they are responsible, there is rarely sufficient time for practical training and comprehensive testing to ensure candidates are capable of safe and effective exercise programming for the public.

Distance learning vocational programs cannot provide the practical experience that is essential to developing the skills and ability to be a competent personal trainer. Although most academic concepts can be conveyed through online or home-study programs, extremely important technical skills and safety proficiency cannot be delivered through this type of learning experience. Whether the ability to administer a submaximal stress test while monitoring heart rate and blood pressure or the ability to demonstrate the safe operation of exercise equipment as well as identifying and remedying client errors in a timely manner, these skills can only be learned and perfected with hands-on experience.

To develop the knowledge, skills, and abilities of a competent personal trainer, one must undergo formal instruction in exercise science through an accredited university or a credible vocational program that provides comprehensive academic instruction and extensive practical training taught by qualified exercise physiologists. Upon completion of academic instruction coupled with substantial practical training in the areas of health assessment, fitness testing, performance evaluation, program design, and client supervision, serious and knowledgeable students will seek certification through truly nonprofit, professional associations such as the NSCA and the ACSM. Most graduates of an athletic training program from an accredited university will usually seek certification through the National Athletic Trainers' Association (NATA).

Over the years various research and informal studies have indicated that there exists a wide disparity in the standards among certifying organizations. Additionally, it has been suggested that years of experience in the fitness field alone have not enabled personal trainers to achieve the knowledge base and skill levels required of a competent personal trainer. Research has supported these observations by concluding that formal education in exercise science coupled with certification from either ACSM or NSCA, versus other certifications, were strong predictors of a personal trainer's exercise knowledge base, whereas years of experience was not related to such knowledge (20).

In years past, individuals injured at fitness facilities would accept the blame themselves and rarely hold others responsible. The injured would attribute their strained muscles and tendons, sprained ligaments, or shoulder and low back pain to just being out of shape and, therefore, would feel embarrassed to bring their injuries to anyone's attention other than their doctors. Today, however, the public has become more aware of this lack of professionalism within the fitness industry and is beginning to hold health facilities, fitness instructors, and personal trainers accountable for unsafe instruction and inadequate supervision. Consequently, we have witnessed an upsurge in personal injury and death case lawsuits against facilities, instructors, and personal trainers with an understandable, concurrent rise in liability insurance. Even with an effort to deter with waivers and releases, the public appears more willing to take their grievances to court.

Significance of Understanding Legal Aspects

With the acceptance of personal trainers as a viable form of fitness instruction, and the accompanying growth of personal trainers within the fitness industry, it is predictable that more lawsuits will be filed against these individuals. Because many personal trainers operate out of their own studios, provide service within their clients' homes, and offer online training, injured parties may have no recourse other than to bring legal action against the individual personal trainer. The personal trainer operating out of a fitness facility often finds that an injured party will pursue a claim against the facility rather than the personal trainer since the facility is viewed as having deeper pockets or more financial resources. In many instances, judgments have been granted against the health facility as well as the personal trainer in the same lawsuit. Noteworthy is the fact that since personal trainers are presumed to have unique instructional skills and special technical abilities along with obvious fiduciary relationships with their clients, it would be anticipated that they be held to a higher standard of care than the average fitness instructor.

Therefore, it should be obvious to personal trainers that it is incumbent upon them to be aware of the basic structure and function of our legal system. Knowledge of this system may be an asset or a liability to the personal trainer's operation, enabling the personal trainer to take advantage of potentially protective mechanisms while avoiding those pitfalls that can undermine their business. The significance of understanding the legal aspects of personal training is addressed and examined in light of professional competency and risk management. Personal trainers will be held to the standard of care as promulgated by the industry leaders.

> **Knowledge of and respect for the legal system enables one to become a more competent personal trainer and enables one to assist in defending himself or herself in a lawsuit.**

THE LEGAL SYSTEM

The origin of our law stems from statutory law, or governmental enactments, and from common law. The two broad categories of our laws are civil law and criminal law.

Divisions of Law

Common law is that collection of unwritten laws based upon customs, general usages, and court decisions. It is more frequently referred to as **case law** since it is typically arrived at through judicial decisions of past cases to which lawyers will refer or which they will cite when attempting to persuade the court of their position.

Statutory law, on the other hand, is enacted and authorized by a legislative body such as Congress and state and local legislatures. Consequently, it is often referred to as **codified law**, for it is written into law by acts of local, state, and federal governmental bodies. Codified or statutory laws typically impose duties or

restrictions upon individuals; but sometimes, such laws may even grant immunity such as the "Good Samaritan" law (13).

Civil law applies to one's private rights and, therefore, personal responsibilities or obligations that individuals must recognize and observe when dealing with others. Hence, this division of law addresses grievances between individuals as well as groups, corporations, and other entities and attempts to resolve such differences, often via monetary judgments. Civil law also comprises a system of remedies for violations of one's rights or the rights of a collective body. With respect to the personal trainer, the realm of civil law dealing with contracts and tort law are the areas in which most liability for personal trainers arise and which will be covered more extensively in this chapter.

Criminal Law, in contrast, governs an individual's or group's conduct to society as a whole, rather than to individuals per se or to collective bodies. When individuals violate societal prohibitions or deviate from these laws, they are subject to governmental punishment including fines, imprisonment, or both. Although the personal trainer is less likely to become embroiled in a criminal violation, there always exists the possibility of the unlawful practice of medicine or some allied health profession, as in attempting to diagnose and prescribe medicine or rehabilitative exercise. This unauthorized practice of an allied health profession may even include going beyond one's scope of practice by providing dietary counseling to clients.

Contract Law

The **law of contracts** governs the legal rights and obligations between individuals, legal entities, and collective bodies that consent to a valid agreement. Agreements generate legal obligations to perform or not to perform some undertaking. While there are other legal requirements, basically, there is an offer proposed by one party, and an acceptance of that offer by the other party. This agreement, or contract, reflects a promise for an exchange, which in personal training usually amounts to a service (exercise instruction) for money (financial remuneration).

Ideally, the terms and conditions of a **personal service contract** will be agreed upon, set forth in writing, and signed by the client and the personal trainer. Contractual requirements are established when it is documented that a written agreement exists that memorializes the mutual terms of the parties. There are many other types of contracts to be found within the fitness industry; contracts used not only by exercise facilities but also by personal trainers. Other client contracts include releases, waivers, express assumptions of risk, informed consents, and generally any type of exculpatory agreement that tends to lessen the potential for legal liability. The many contracts about which a personal trainer should be knowledgeable are covered more extensively in the section "Protective Legal Documents."

Additionally, contracts are often generated between business partners or associate personal trainers as well as between personal trainers and independent contractors who work with them. Frequently, personal trainers work as independent contractors for fitness facilities with whom they have such contracts. The legal litmus test for an independent contractor is "control." If the personal trainer works "for" someone and that person or employer has control over the personal trainer's conduct, time, and activities during the scope of his or her service, then he or she is considered an employee, not an independent contractor. The IRS sets the legal standards for the independent contractor, not the fitness facility.

Tort Law

The **law of torts** governs the legal rights and obligations between individuals as well as between collective bodies in relationship to civil wrongs or injuries. By definition, a **tort** is any wrongful act that does not involve a breach of contract and, therefore, may be cause for a civil suit for which a court of law can award compensation in the form of damages. Following are the basic elements of a successful tort: If a (1) legal duty has been created and (2) a breach occurs, (3) which is the actual or proximate cause (4) of an injury, then compensation or monetary damages (5) may be awarded.

Tortious acts are primarily subdivided into two major categories, intentional and negligent conduct. As the name implies, an **intentional tort** reflects conduct that purposely brought about a given consequence such as a physical injury or a damaged reputation. However, unless there is sufficient evidence of an intentional tort, courts generally give the benefit of the doubt to the defendant and presume that torts are of the negligent type.

A negligence suit may be brought against one for failure to conform one's conduct to a generally accepted standard. **Negligence** is defined as a failure to exercise a reasonable degree of care under the existing circumstances that prevailed at the time of assault or injury. As relates to the personal trainer, this would signify a failure to act with due care (**omission**) or to act with substandard performance of a duty owed (**commission**). When a duty has been created, a court of law will evaluate a personal trainer's performance in relationship to established standards and guidelines published by peer professional associations such as the NSCA and ACSM. Then, if this omission or commission is determined to be the proximate cause of a proven assault or injury, damages may be awarded.

> **Personal trainers are likely to be sued for a claim of negligence due to substandard performance, which is an area of tort law.**

Additionally, there is a third tortious act referred to as **strict liability**, which is the concept of "liability regardless of fault." Imposition of liability without fault is based upon an ideology of social justice that demands compensation to the injured. The rationale for strict liability is that even if there is no negligence, "public policy demands that responsibility be fixed wherever it will most effectively reduce the hazards to life and health inherent in defective products that reach the market" (13, p. 192). As relates to the personal trainer, documented defective equipment responsible for an injury or death may lead to a judgment against the manufacturer rather than the personal trainer who provides instruction on such equipment.

ANATOMY OF A LAWSUIT

One can understand the anatomy of a lawsuit by considering the sequence of events that occur during a typical personal injury claim (14). If a fitness client feels that he or she has been injured because of the negligence of a personal trainer, that person may retain counsel, who may attempt to negotiate a settlement or initiate a lawsuit against the personal trainer. In legal terminology, the injured party is then designated as the **plaintiff**, or the moving party bringing the lawsuit. The personal trainer now becomes the **defendant**, or the party against whom the lawsuit is brought. The personal trainer will notify his or her insurance carrier, who in turn may instruct the personal trainer to also retain counsel. Frequently the insurance company will assist the personal trainer in locating and securing counsel. At this point, the insurance provider for the defendant personal trainer may begin an investigation in hopes of preventing the suit from going forward or possibly facilitating an early settlement, thereby limiting or minimizing the insurance company's payout.

If an early termination to the suit cannot be achieved, then the lengthy process of discovery ensues. During discovery, most documents pertaining to the client–personal trainer relationship will be produced, inspected, and analyzed. Documents such as personal service contracts, medical history, lifestyle questionnaire, physical exam reports, blood lab results, physician clearance forms, informed consents, waivers (release forms), assumption of risk, fitness profiles, program design, workout logs, personal notes and any other documents must be made available for scrutiny by both lawyers. During this pretrial phase, interrogatories and depositions of plaintiff and defendant may be taken along with those of other witnesses who have knowledge of or involvement with the incident in question. During deposition of the personal trainer, opposing counsel will not only query the personal trainer about the specific events leading to the injury but also ask about his or her formal education in exercise science, certifications, licenses, practical experience, continuing education, and anything relating to the defendant's qualifications as a competent personal trainer as well as previous acts of incompetence or other lawsuits.

A key witness in negligence cases involving personal trainers is frequently an **expert witness**. An expert witness may be used by either party. That witness is a specialist in the field of exercise science and will review all documents in the case and render an expert's opinion as to whether the defendant did or did not violate the standard of care. These experts are well trained, are highly educated, and serve to assist the judge or jury in reaching a correct decision about liablity.

> **During their depositions, personal trainers must document their qualifications and competencies.**

It is also important to understand the three types of burdens of proof in our judicial system. The most difficult burden of proof is "beyond a reasonable doubt," applied only in criminal trials. Civil trials have either a burden of proof called by a "preponderance of the evidence," which means a slight advantage to one of the parties, or by "clear and convincing evidence," which means more than a slight advantage but not as much as beyond a reasonable doubt.

In many instances parties to a lawsuit submit to arbitration or the court may order **mediation** in hopes of settling the matter out of court. This avoids any further legal expenses to the parties involved as well as to the legal forum having jurisdiction. When arbitration or mediation is unsuccessful, a jury trial or a court trial is elected and scheduled in order that the parties may present their cases for adjudication. In a court trial, the judge alone determines liability and damages.

NEGLIGENCE

Negligence should be a primary concern for all personal trainers and employers (e.g., managers or owners of fitness facilities) of personal trainers. Employers can be found vicariously liable for the negligent acts of their personal trainers through a legal doctrine called **respondeat superior**, meaning "let the master answer" (14). Under this doctrine, if a client is injured because of the conduct of a personal trainer, the client can sue both the personal trainer and the personal trainer's employer for negligence if the client can prove all the essential elements of the doctrine of respondeat superior. Therefore, it is essential for personal trainers and their employers to understand the concept of negligence and know what steps they can take to minimize liability. If the personal trainer is not an actual employee but is considered an independent contractor, the employer may still be vicariously liable.

Not all injuries are caused by the negligence (or "ordinary" negligence) of a personal trainer or his or her employer. Other causes include "inherent" injuries, which are due to accidents that are not preventable and are no one's fault, and "extreme forms of negligence," which are due to gross negligence, willful and wanton behavior, reckless conduct, or the failure of the defendant to exercise even scant care (14). Injured individuals can also contribute to their own injury through their own negligence. Negligence as discussed in this chapter is often referred to by the law as "ordinary" negligence, distinguishing it from extreme forms of negligence.

Definitions

Negligence is the failure to conform one's conduct to a generally accepted standard or the failure to act as a reasonably prudent person would act under similar circumstances (14). Negligence can occur by omission, or a failure to perform a task with application, knowledge, skills, and ability (e.g., the personal trainer does not have the client complete a preparticipation screening form), or by commission, that is, performance in a negligent manner (e.g., the personal trainer teaches an exercise incorrectly or in an unsafe manner).

> ▶ **Negligence is the failure to conform one's conduct to a generally accepted standard.**

In a negligence lawsuit, the plaintiff has the burden of proof. The plaintiff must prove all of the following four elements:

1. **Duty**: an obligation recognized by law requiring the defendant (e.g., the personal trainer) to conform to a certain conduct that reflects the standard of care
2. **Breach of duty**: the conduct of the personal trainer that was not consistent with the standard of care
3. **Causation**: the connection between the breach of duty and the injury; the breach of duty must be the factual or proximal cause of the injury
4. **Damages**: the monetary loss due to the injury, which can include both economic damages (e.g., medical costs, lost wages) and noneconomic damages (e.g., pain and suffering)

Economic and noneconomic damages are considered **compensatory damages**—those that compensate the plaintiff for his or her actual loss or injury. For example, compensatory damages can be awarded to the plaintiff for ordinary negligence. Courts can also award the plaintiff **punitive damages**—those over and above the compensatory damages—to punish the defendant for acting willfully, maliciously, or fraudulently or to set an example for similar wrongdoers. For example, punitive damages could be awarded for extreme forms of negligence on the part of the defendant.

Regarding damages, most states now have comparative negligence statutes that have replaced contributory negligence. Under **contributory negligence**, a plaintiff would be barred from recovering any damages if he or she contributed in any way to his or her injury. Under **comparative negligence**, negligence is measured in terms of percentages, and damages allowed are diminished in proportion to the amount of negligence attributable to the person for whose injury recovery is sought. For example, if the damages totaled $100,000 and the plaintiff contributed 25% to the

injury whereas the defendant contributed 75%, then the plaintiff would only receive $75,000 in damages.

Duty and the Personal Trainer

The court or jury makes a factual determination as to whether the defendant personal trainer breached the duty owed to the client in two ways: By comparing the personal trainer's conduct to the accepted standard of care (practice) and comparing his or her conduct to the standards of practice developed and published by professional organizations and the state's tort law of negligence. If the personal trainer's conduct falls beneath either, he or she may be liable to the client for damages.

Standards of Practice

Standards of practice published by professional organizations are commonly referred to as standards, guidelines, position statements, and recommendations. Many organizations in the fitness field have published standards of practice to provide benchmarks of desirable practices for professionals. Two sets of standards of practice that have been peer reviewed and have achieved industry-wide consensus include

1. the NSCA Strength and Conditioning Professional Standards and Guidelines (28) and
2. ACSM's Health/Fitness Facility Standards and Guidelines (27).

These publications define standards and guidelines in a similar fashion. **Standards** are levels of quality or attainment, a set pattern or model for guidance conforming to a measurement of value or a model of authority. Standards require particular procedures, the adherence to which complies with that level of accomplishment, whereas **guidelines** are recommended procedures that are not intended to reflect the standard of care but are designed to further enhance the quality and safety of services provided. The NSCA published the following nine areas of potential exposure to legal liability and promulgates nine standards and 14 guidelines within those nine areas that can create a risk of injury to a personal trainer's clients.

1. Preparticipation screening and clearance
2. Personnel qualifications
3. Program supervision and instruction
4. Facility and equipment setup, inspection, maintenance, repair, and signage

5. Emergency planning and response
6. Records and record keeping
7. Equal opportunity and access
8. Participation in strength and conditioning activities by children
9. Supplements, ergogenic aids, and drugs

The ACSM published eight standards and 37 guidelines. The eight standards address the following areas:

1. Preactivity screening
2. Orientation, education, and supervision
3. Risk management and emergency policies
4. Professional staff and independent contractors
5. Operating practices
6. Facility design and construction
7. Facility equipment
8. Signage

It is essential that all fitness professionals, including personal trainers, familiarize themselves with these published standards of practice and implement them within the daily operations of fitness facilities and programs or services. Published standards of practice can serve as a shield (minimize liability associated with negligence) for the personal trainer who adheres to them. However, they can also serve as a sword (increase liability associated with negligence) for the personal trainer who does not adhere to them.

Published standards of practice can be introduced as evidence (via expert witness testimony) in determining whether the personal trainer breached his or her duty. Published standards often help the court determine whether or not the defendant's conduct reflected the current standard of care owed to the plaintiff. If there is no breach of duty, there can be no negligence. However, if one's conduct is inconsistent with published standards of practice, it can be viewed as a breach of duty that can then lead to negligence. The prudent personal trainer adheres to the most stringent standards and practices embodied in those promulgated by the NSCA and ACSM. As these associations are routinely viewed as the "gold standard" in the fitness industry and as previous legal opinions have adopted these standards, they should be viewed as a safe harbor for personal trainers.

Ethics

In addition to standards of practice, many organizations have published ethical standards. These ethical standards may also be introduced into a court of law as evidence of duty. For example, the NSCA established the following four principles within their Code of Ethics, each of which has multiple subprinciples (21):

1. Professionals shall respect the rights, welfare, and dignity of all individuals in the context of their professional practice.
2. Professionals shall comply with all applicable laws, policies, and regulations in the context of their professional practice.
3. Professionals shall maintain and promote high standards.
4. Professionals shall not engage in any behavior or form of conduct that adversely reflects on the NSCA.

Ethics are external standards based on right and wrong, fairness, a framework for acceptable behavior based on a reasonable and prudent individual. While a court does not view ethical considerations as an element of a claim, courts may take them into consideration and allow them to carry different weight than substantive evidence in arriving at a decision. While there may be a slight or even greater distinction between ethics and morality, the essence of both connote right from wrong, a sense of fair and reasonable judgment, and a code of appropriate conduct, tolerance and behavior accepted by society.

Morality Versus Legality: A Fitness Challenge

As stated earlier, the current escalation of litigation is a reflection of a serious industry problem regarding client expectations and service delivery. Far too often, individuals pursuing a healthier lifestyle are injured or may die as a result of personal trainers not being truly qualified professionals. These injuries and deaths are typically a result of insufficient screening, ineffective instruction, and improper supervision, which are often compounded by an inadequate emergency response. Just because one is a certified personal trainer does not mean that he or she is a qualified personal trainer. Although one may have been awarded a credible certification reflecting that he or she ought to be qualified, this credential does not necessarily mean that he or she was justified in their conduct (2).

As an attorney with a special interest in health club law and as the founder of the *Exercise Standards and Malpractice Reporter*, David Herbert wrote a fictional legal thriller entitled *The Personal Trainer: A Tale of Pain, Gain, Greed & Lust* (17). This book, based upon his years of experience in dealing with the fitness industry and awareness of practices founded on unscrupulous financial gain, portrays how an unqualified personal trainer, responsible for a client's death, is confronted with the legal system. Flaws in the fitness industry and the legal system are exposed along with the ramifications of a personal trainer's practicing the trade without sound ethics, education, and training, thereby making the personal trainer ill prepared to work safely and effectively with his or her client.

In the fitness industry, lack of supervision throughout a facility reflects a failure on the part of management to have in mind the best interests of the membership. The first priority of any facility should be the health and safety of its members; however, frequently such a priority remains subordinate to generating revenue and to achieving the highest profitability. For example, providing supervision of a swimming pool would require additional personnel and consequent funding. However, this could be avoided legally because county ordinances may only require the visibility of cautionary signage such as "Swim at your own risk, no lifeguard on duty." Similarly, management may take the attitude that supervision of steam rooms, saunas, and whirlpools would be too costly when cautionary signage would meet legal requirements. Too often, management fails to feel responsible and to recognize that morality should supersede legality (1) (figure 25.1).

Special Relationship

Another way courts can determine whether the personal trainer breached his or her duty is by examining the special relationship that exists between the personal trainer and the client. Courts may determine that this is a fiduciary relationship. **Fiduciary relationships** exist when one person trusts in and relies upon another (e.g., an attorney and client, a broker and principal, a trustee and beneficiary, a doctor and patient, a health care provider and patient, and perhaps a personal trainer and client). In a personal trainer–client relationship, the client trusts and relies upon the personal trainer's fitness expertise.

In this type of special relationship, the personal trainer has additional responsibilities involving honest intent, confidentiality, truthfulness, and frankness toward clients (14). A breach of these duties could make the personal trainer liable. Because of these responsibilities, the personal trainer could be held to a higher

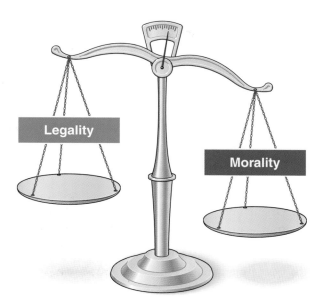

FIGURE 25.1 Morality should supersede legality.

standard of care than other fitness professionals such as group exercise leaders. Also, given the additional training, education, and credible certifications that many rehabilitative trainers and personal trainers have coupled with their higher client fees, these types of trainers are likely to be held to a higher standard of care (18).

> **The trust and bond between client and personal trainer help define legal responsibilities.**

Duties and Responsibilities of Personal Trainers

In a negligence lawsuit the court will determine whether the personal trainer breached his or her duty to the client. In making that determination the court will evaluate whether the personal trainer adhered to the standard of care set forth by the industry's leading associations such as the NSCA and ACSM. The personal trainer is required to understand and meet substantive criteria related to standards of practice in properly discharging his or her duty to the client. It is the imposition of this criteria and complementary aspects of honesty and integrity that form the basis of the personal trainer's duty, which is a legal obligation established by law.

Qualifications

The competence of a personal trainer will be evaluated and determined in a negligence lawsuit. The qualifications (or lack of qualifications) of the personal trainer will be used in determining negligence. Therefore, it is wise for personal trainers to obtain the appropriate qualifications. However, there are no state or federal laws requiring any specific qualifications such as a degree, certification, or licensure in personal training. Education, whether it is a degreed exercise science program or a credible vocational program coupled with commensurate work experience, is an important factor in determining the competence of the personal trainer.

Even if a personal trainer has a high level of qualifications, this does not mean that he or she could never be liable for negligence. A personal trainer's conduct could fall below the standard of care despite the number of degrees, experience, and certifications in the fitness field. As previously stated, personal trainers could be certified and qualified but not justified in their conduct with a client. However, when personal trainers obtain and apply proper knowledge, skills, and abilities, it is less likely that their conduct will fall below the standard of care.

Preparticipation Screening and Medical Clearance

The primary purpose of screening members before permitting them to engage in physical activity is to determine whether they ought to have a physical exam, perhaps including a clinical stress test, and whether they need medical clearance. **Preactivity screening** is the procedure by which a facility can identify those members who are at an increased risk for experiencing exercise-related cardiovascular incidents as well as musculoskeletal problems. The present standard of care dictates that screening procedures be practiced without exception. Both the NSCA (28) and ACSM (27) require participants to undergo preparticipation screening before engaging in an exercise program.

Any exercise programming should be initiated with a screening process that provides knowledge of a member's past and present health history as well as lifestyle considerations. Before an exercise program is undertaken, it is prudent to complete a **health risk appraisal** or **medical history questionnaire** to determine whether there are any medical contraindications to exercise that could necessitate a physician's clearance prior to any exercise and fitness programming. Contraindications of primary concern are the following:

- Cardiovascular disease (heart attack, stroke, hypertension, aneurysm, claudication, and severe mitral valve prolapse)
- Pulmonary disease (bronchitis, emphysema, and asthma)
- Metabolic disease (diabetes mellitus, thyroid disorders, and renal complications)
- Musculoskeletal problems (fractures, sprains, strains, hernias, arthritis, and structural limitations)
- Any condition placing the client at higher than normal risk

The personal trainer involved with the screening process should become familiar with the exercise-related ramifications of these conditions. The preactivity screening process is a vital step in the health and fitness continuum. It enables personal trainers to begin on a safer footing as they prepare to test and create a program for clients. Additionally, it establishes a baseline of health parameters that serve as markers for monitoring future progress. As such, it becomes invaluable as a motivational tool. It should never be overlooked or bypassed.

A health appraisal allows the personal trainer to better assess the suitability of exercise for clients. It minimizes the risk of injury, disability, or even death while lessening the potential for litigation. It also establishes the appropriateness of the next step in this process: the fitness assessment. During the health appraisal, it is typical to acquire demographic information, complete a medical history, and administer a lifestyle questionnaire. All this information contributes to the goal of client screening, which is to classify the client in one of the following categories:

- People who should be excluded from exercise because of medical contraindications
- People with known disease conditions who require referral to a medically supervised exercise program
- People with known disease, symptoms, or risk factors that require further medical evaluation and clearance before starting an exercise program
- People with special needs for safe and effective exercise programming
- People who may begin traditional exercise programs

High blood pressure is a major risk factor for heart disease, stroke, and kidney failure; approximately one-third of Americans have hypertension, and almost one-third of these individuals are not aware they have this silent killer. It therefore stands to reason that personal trainers should administer blood pressure testing as part of the screening process. However, personal trainers must not go beyond their scope of practice when screening clients and taking blood pressure. A blood pressure assessment only enables personal trainers to suspect the need of a medical diagnosis or to determine whether medical clearance is necessary (12).

All states have statutes that authorize certain licensed health care professionals to diagnose and treat patients. A violation of these statutes by unauthorized individuals such as personal trainers could result in criminal prosecution. Although personal trainers may feel that a particular diagnosis such as hypertension is likely, they are not legally authorized to make medical diagnoses or prescribe treatment. Personal trainers must understand that they are "suspecticians," not diagnosticians.

> **Personal trainers are "suspectitians," not diagnosticians; that is, although they may feel that a particular diagnosis is likely, they may not make medical diagnoses or prescribe treatment.**

Another potential legal problem regarding health history forms may arise when a personal trainer obtains information and then either does not use it properly or does not have the knowledge or background needed to decipher it or realize what it may require. This type of conduct could be used against the personal trainer to demonstrate his or her deviation from the standards of practices and standard of care, thereby breaching his or her duty owed to the client. Therefore, it is important for personal trainers to have adequate knowledge and experience to understand, interpret, and use health history data appropriately.

Fitness Testing

Many personal trainers routinely perform physical fitness assessments to determine a client's level of physical fitness as it pertains to disease prevention and health promotion. Proper procedures to identify and test only appropriate individuals are as important as preactivity screening. People undergo voluntary fitness-related physical assessments for several reasons. ACSM has identified the following four purposes for fitness testing:

1. Collecting baseline data and educating participants about their health and fitness status relative to health-related standards and age- and sex-norms

2. Providing data that are helpful in development of individualized exercise programs to address all health and fitness components

3. Collecting follow-up data that allow evaluation of progress following an exercise prescription and long-term monitoring as participants age

4. Motivating participants by establishing reasonable and attainable health and fitness goals (6)

Before members arrive for testing, they should be given written instructions regarding how to prepare for the tests. Explicit instructions are necessary to ensure testing validity and accuracy. The testing environment is critical for test validity and reliability, especially concerning constancy of environment (temperature and humidity) for accurate follow-up testing.

Testing procedures should be thoroughly explained beforehand, and any tendency to rush through the battery of tests should be avoided. During pretest instructions, all clients should be required to read and sign an **informed consent** for exercise testing. The informed consent may provide an assumption of risk defense against potential liability. Prior to undertaking fitness testing, personal trainers are advised to obtain legally sufficient informed consent documents (for their state) to provide their clients with court-tested documents that can withstand judicial scrutiny. Typically, an informed consent addresses these topics:

- Purpose and explanation of the test
- Attendant risks and discomforts
- Responsibilities of the client
- Benefits to be expected
- Client inquiries about testing procedures
- Use of testing data and confidentiality
- Freedom of consent to engage in testing

The specific tests to be administered will vary from one person to another depending on the screening process and determination of the client's health status. Typically, tests assess the five components of health-related physical fitness: aerobic endurance, muscular strength, muscular endurance, flexibility, and body composition. Some personal trainers may go beyond health-related fitness testing and even provide physical performance–related fitness tests to those clients who are more athletically inclined, testing such components as agility, balance, coordination, power, quickness, and speed.

Evaluation

Upon completing the fitness assessments, the personal trainer must evaluate the data from the fitness tests along with the health appraisal and be prepared to share such information with the client. Typically, the initial evaluation of data for each test is based on classification scales for sex and age. However, the personal trainer must be careful not to get locked into a mere comparison with the normative data. To evaluate members strictly upon this basis is to overlook the important principle of individual differences. Failing to recognize these differences violates this basic principle that client needs must be understood in order to design tailor-made programs that improve the chances of success without risk of injury.

When going over testing data with a member, it is essential to conduct the process in a professional setting and in a motivational manner. In the privacy of an office or similar sanctum, the personal trainer establishes a relationship with the client that reflects the air of confidentiality that must exist between the two. The personal trainer accepts the responsibility of being proficient in the science of exercise programming and therefore being knowledgeable about the appropriate stresses to be applied to the client. Suitable stress that will bring about positive physiological changes (training effects) without negative physiological consequences (injury) can most effectively be determined if the personal trainer has access to the information found within both the health appraisal and the fitness assessment.

Program Design and Scope of Practice

Although the term *exercise prescription* is frequently found within textbooks and scientific literature, it is not the most appropriate wording when dealing with the average client. The term *prescription* has clinical connotations, and people associate this word with sick individuals in need of medical assistance. The term *exercise prescription* may discourage some clients. Additionally, the word *prescription* may make a disgruntled member more likely to pursue litigation based on the results of the personal trainer's recommendations. The personal trainer should instead discuss the personal trainer's recommendations in terms of program design.

Program design typically has five components: exercise mode, intensity, duration, frequency, and progression. These five components can be applied not only to aerobic training but also to resistance training and flexibility activities. The challenge for the personal trainer is to ensure that these components of program design are based on the information gleaned from the health appraisal and fitness assessment.

If the personal trainer attempts to "diagnose" medical conditions from the data obtained from the health history, or "treat" a medical condition through an exercise program for a client, he or she will likely be violating the unauthorized practice of medicine statute. A personal trainer can tell clients that their individualized exercise program will help them achieve their health and fitness goals; but if the personal trainer attempts to diagnose and prescribe, then he or she is practicing a vocation beyond their limitations and endangering the clients. Therefore, when developing the exercise program for the client, it is incumbent upon the personal trainer to design the program within his or her scope of practice. To do otherwise not only threatens the client's health but also places the personal trainer at risk for a liability lawsuit as well as the potential for the criminal offense of practicing medicine without a license.

In addition to clients relying on their personal trainers for their expertise in designing exercise programs, clients often want nutrition advice or want their personal trainers to put them on a special diet. Again, to avoid problems with the unauthorized practice of medicine or the unauthorized practice of an allied health profession (e.g., a licensed or registered dietitian), personal trainers should refrain from recommending any special diet or specific supplements. They should limit their nutrition education or advice to general information on healthy and lifelong eating habits as outlined in textbooks (23) as well as those recommendations outlined by the Academy of Nutrition and Dietetics and the U.S. Department of Agriculture and Health and Human Services in their Dietary Guidelines for Americans (29). The personal trainer should never write out a specific meal plan for a client unless he or she is a licensed or registered dietitian; and if this is not the case, then the personal trainer should refer clients to such allied health professionals (25).

Because of the special relationship created between the personal trainer and the client, clients may share personal problems, such as financial or relationship difficulties, with their personal trainer. In this situation the personal trainer should not attempt to "counsel" the client, for this act could be considered outside the scope of practice. Rather the personal trainer could refer clients to a qualified counselor or therapist. The general rule is that any time the interests or needs of the client exceed the recognized expertise or qualifications of the personal trainer, the personal trainer should refer the client to the appropriate health care provider. Regarding the personal information of a client that is available to the personal trainer, it must be remembered that such information is confidential. The Health Insurance Portability and Accountability Act (HIPAA) requires that all information gathered about a client's health status must be kept confidential, such as in a personal trainer's client file. The HIPAA Privacy Rule provides federal protections for personal health information held by health care providers to include personal trainers (7).

> The proper scope of practice for personal trainers includes assessing, motivating, educating, and training clients to help achieve their fitness and health goals; it does not entail diagnosing, treating, or counseling, which are responsibilities of licensed health care providers. Health information garnered from a client must be kept confidential in accordance with the HIPAA Privacy Rule.

Supervision and Instruction

Supervision refers to observing and directing activities in order to ensure their success. The failure to properly supervise and instruct clients creates significant exposure to liability and is the most common allegation of negligence. Specific supervision requires that the personal trainer be with the client continuously throughout the training session and attentively observe the client's exercise performance. During the exercise session, this would mean constant attentiveness to a client's exercise regimen and the ability to promptly recognize ineffective or unsafe movements requiring timely correction. Attentive monitoring includes watching for the following:

1. Signs and symptoms of overexertion
2. Maintaining appropriate intensity levels
3. Proper form and execution of each exercise (including spotting)

The ability to relate well to clients, communicate effectively, motivate sufficiently, and move to action appropriately is the hallmark of the professional personal trainer. This means being able to deal with all types of personalities and encouraging clients to achieve success. Consequently, personal trainers must understand not only the science of exercise but also the art of influencing human behavior. Social skills combined with a sincere concern for clients, an appropriate knowledge base, exercise expertise, and a conscientious commitment to the job provide the essentials for successful programming.

Frequently personal trainers working at a fitness facility either as a staff member or an independent contractor may be required to provide some floor supervision. General floor supervision requires at least one qualified personal trainer capable of answering any member questions, instructing beginners on equipment operation, providing guidance as needed, and responding to any potential emergency situations. Personal trainers must be alert to potentially unsafe activities. Safe floor monitoring requires that all areas be readily visible to staff personnel or personal trainers on duty; there must be no blind spots in which a member who is in danger could be unobserved. Floor supervision requirements at facilities can become an asset because competent personal trainers may influence members to engage a supervisor as a personal trainer.

As an aside, but of extreme importance, is the fact that at facilities supervision is frequently lacking in locker rooms and wet areas. All too often, members develop cardiovascular complications in the locker room, and the only people present, if any, are other members. Therefore, a locker room attendant should be available at all times. An attendant can be providing housekeeping services while simultaneously monitoring members and remaining available to provide an emergency response. It is not uncommon to witness sauna, steam, and whirlpool or jacuzzi rooms completely unattended. There are numerous reports and documentation of people being discovered dead in saunas and steam rooms or drowned in whirlpools or jacuzzis (1). Not only should these areas be under constant surveillance but facility staff, reinforced with appropriate signage, should also ensure that members limit their exposure time to about 10 minutes. In addition to being a source of unnecessary expense and maintenance difficulties, wet areas are a potential area for litigation.

Supervision begins with the first client contact and ends with a client's termination of the relationship. Therefore, a personal trainer may be liable of faulty supervision if he or she fails to screen clients for risk factors before undertaking exercise programs, fails to provide fitness profiles determining clients' capacity for exercise, fails to design exercise programs befitting clients' levels of health and fitness, fails to educate clients about safety concerns relating to exercise, or fails to attentively supervise clients' exercise programs. In addition, faulty supervision is epitomized by the lack of recognizing a potential medical emergency and responding in a timely and effective manner.

Equipment and Facility Safety

The law classifies members and clients of fitness facilities as business invitees because of the mutual benefit that exists between them and the landowner or occupier (13). Landowners or occupiers have a duty to act reasonably toward invitees regarding the activities and conditions on their property. This involves reasonable inspection of the property for danger and reasonable repairing or warning of dangers. Eickhoff-Shemek and colleagues list the following responsibilities to meet this duty (14):

1. Inspect the premises and equipment regularly to determine if any condition(s) might be considered dangerous.

2. Document that the inspections have taken place and file the documents in a secure place.

3. If a condition could be considered "dangerous" by an invitee, it is necessary to correct the condition (e.g., repair or remove the condition) or warn the invitee of the possible danger (e.g., post proper warning signage that an invitee will see and understand).

Although this is a primary duty of the owner or occupier of the facility, a personal trainer who is an independent contractor could be viewed as taking on such responsibilities. The same responsibilities will apply if a personal trainer works with clients in their homes, even though the client in this case would not be classified as an invitee. However, the personal trainer must ensure that the home in which the client is being trained provides a safe environment.

Numerous lawsuits have resulted from injury to individuals using exercise equipment. Clients injured on exercise equipment can sue the personal trainer, the equipment manufacturer, the facility or all three. When it is established that there is no faulty equipment but rather the fault lies with the personal trainer, the client can sue both the personal trainer and the facility under the concept of vicarious liability (13).

The personal trainer can minimize equipment-related negligence by implementing the many standards of practice as outlined by the NSCA and ACSM in their standards and guidelines publications. These standards and guidelines reflect issues that often arise in equipment-related lawsuits, such as not properly instructing or supervising clients who use the equipment; not properly inspecting equipment before client use; and not properly warning clients of risks when using equipment (e.g., using a lat pulldown machine with an S hook).

The personal trainer has numerous responsibilities, and each one represents an area of vulnerability and possible exposure to liability. If personal trainers can remember the acronym "STEPS" (figure 25.2), they will go a long way toward preventing the distressing experience of litigation. When a personal trainer is

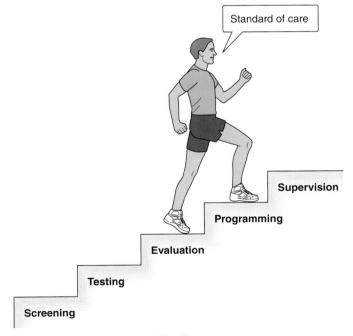

FIGURE 25.2 STEPS to success in avoiding legal liability.

continually attentive to applying the standard of care to each of these five steps, then successful navigation through these potentially litigious waters is more likely—it is almost assured.

Emergency Plan

Regarding health and safety standards for fitness facilities, there is the common recognition among professional associations that a comprehensive **emergency response plan (ERP)** is of paramount importance and, therefore, a standard to which all facilities must adhere. As stated in the NSCA executive summary concerning professional standards and guidelines, "strength and conditioning professionals must develop a written, venue-specific emergency response plan to deal with injuries and reasonably foreseeable untoward events within each facility" (28, p. 12). Similar to this NSCA standard, both ACSM and IHRSA share an identical standard that states: "A club/facility must be able to respond in a timely manner to any reasonably foreseeable emergency event that threatens the health and safety of club/facility users. Toward this end, a club/facility must have an appropriate emergency plan that can be executed by qualified personnel in a timely manner" (19, p. 1; 27, p. 18).

When a "Code Blue" is called over the PA system, personal trainers, whether staff or independent contractors, are expected to respond to emergencies along with other staff members. Frequently, because of the higher expectations of personal trainers, these personnel are relied upon to deliver the bulk of the emergency response necessary to effect a successful rescue. Without question, a successful rescue depends heavily upon a well-conceived and implemented emergency response plan.

Obviously a number of considerations and procedures are necessary to constitute a comprehensive emergency response plan. For by its very nature, the ERP must consist of numerous and succinct strategies to handle untoward events that may occur without warning. The plan should be written and cover not only environmental situations but also life-threatening and non–life-threatening situations in order to provide a guideline for proper procedures to be followed (26). All facility personnel involved with executing the plan should sign off on the fact that they have read, understood, and agree to comply with all actions outlined. This plan should include an emergency procedures sheet not only highlighting the sequence of events to be followed but also listing important emergency agencies and their phone numbers. This sheet can be posted at convenient and strategic locations throughout a facility, thereby permitting periodic review by the entire staff. Knowledge of agencies and numbers are worthless if phones are not readily available and rapidly operable. Whether a large health and fitness facility or a small personal training studio, these requirements of an emergency action plan remain the same.

Typical facility emergencies to be anticipated are such events as heat-related illnesses, physical injuries, heart attacks, and even a sudden cardiac arrest (SCA). The emergency plan is designed to ensure that minor problems do not escalate to major incidents and that major incidents do not intensify to fatal events. Heat exhaustion dealt with promptly and effectively can forestall heatstroke, a severe laceration with appropriate administration of first aid can prevent a bleed out, and a myocardial infarction (MI) responded to with emergency cardiac care can stave off an SCA (12). Even in the case of an SCA, effective CPR coupled with the swift application of an automated external defibrillator (AED) can convert the victim to a life-saving rhythm.

Emergency plans must guarantee the fastest available access to emergency medical personnel and facilities. To this end, a good plan outlines specific roles for staff members such as who should recognize an untoward event, activate the emergency medical services (EMS) system, alert staff of the incident, attend to the victim, secure first aid equipment, assist the principle caregiver(s), verify responders are en route, take charge of crowd control, guide emergency responders to the scene, and most importantly, take responsibility for the coordination of the overall effort. Additionally, other assigned duties are for staff to notify the victim's family, record the incident, write up the after-action report, collect the names of witnesses, and follow through with corrective actions for those tasks that were not handled expeditiously and correctly (12).

From the initial recognition of the emergency to the final corrective actions report, there are numerous steps that must be followed to maximize the health and safety of clientele. Each step needs to be analyzed with regard to the uniqueness of the facility, the qualifications of the personnel, and the physical and financial resources available. For example, in alerting staff to a potential heart attack or cardiac arrest by calling a "Code Blue," would it be most advantageous to announce to the entire membership that an emergency of this type was in progress? Probably not. It might be more appropriate to have a code word that would alert staff but not members in order to avoid curious onlookers who would only create more confusion. Again, each facility or personal training studio is unique; and therefore, owners, managers, and personal trainers must analyze what procedures would serve their clientele best.

The proper handling of untoward events will often require the use of special emergency equipment; and therefore, a first aid kit or multiple kits, depending upon the size of the facility, must be available. It is crucial that kits be properly marked, identifiable, accessible, and easily transportable as well as stocked according to foreseeable events and the skills of responders. Consequently, kits must be periodically checked, at least once a month, to verify that contents match an enclosed recommended list of supplies and that contents are not outdated. Equipment and supplies must be used according to manufacturer's and recognized professional guidelines; and when using these materials, it is imperative that precautions for preventing disease transmission be followed as outlined by the CDC and OSHA.

Emergencies entail not only the previously cited accidents and injuries one might anticipate but also crises such as fires, floods, tornadoes, earthquakes, hurricanes, severe storms, bomb threats, and even terrorist activities. Crises could also include sexual harassment, intoxicated clients, hazardous spills, thievery, unruly behavior, parking lot accidents, and other health concerns or life-threatening events that may be peculiar to a given site. Fire evacuation plans, severe weather contingencies, and even procedures for handling and ejecting disruptive patrons are important considerations the personal trainer might have to encounter.

Emergency plans must be practiced and rehearsed with regularity. Ideally, mock emergencies should be conducted at least on a quarterly basis if not more often or as often as necessary to ensure a rapid and effective response. Some of these rehearsals and drills should be undertaken on an unannounced basis. Responsible critiques and corrective actions of such rehearsals will only improve the plan. The emergency response plan, to include rehearsals, should be evaluated by facility risk managers, legal advisors, and medical providers to ensure that timely and effective procedures are being followed as well as modified when needed. It is recommended that facilities enlist a medical liaison to keep the emergency plan updated and to periodically evaluate the skills and ability of personnel, including personal trainers (12).

> **Emergency response plans should be rehearsed (announced and unannounced) on a regular basis and followed up with timely critiques and corrective actions.**

"The frequency of rehearsals should not be a locked-in number, but must vary depending upon the type of facility, number of staff, and turnover of personnel. Emergency plans must be rehearsed with a frequency that ensures that not only will all personnel have the opportunity to participate in drills on both an announced and unannounced basis but more importantly that they will be able to respond rapidly and effectively" (1a, p. 38).

The question is: "Are staff, instructors, and personal trainers throughout the fitness industry maintaining their first aid and CPR/AED certifications as well as retaining their skills?" The answer is a resounding "No." Again, it has been recognized that just because a fitness instructor or personal trainer is certified does not mean that he or she is qualified (2). This inconsistency applies not only to a lack of knowledge and skills related to exercise instruction but also to an inability to respond to emergencies.

It is true that most fitness instructor and personal trainer certification programs require that candidates possess CPR/AED certification. Notwithstanding this fact that most fitness instructors and personal trainers are CPR/AED certified, this does not correspond with their being qualified to administer CPR and deploy an AED. It is common for instructors and personal trainers to undergo cursory, perfunctory, and hurried CPR and AED instruction such as a four-hour AHA Heartsaver course (10). "This shortcoming, coupled with the fact that instructors and personal trainers rarely receive ongoing training and evaluation through rehearsals and drills, results in certified but unqualified CPR responders. Couple this with the sad fact that CPR and AED awareness and skills deteriorate very rapidly after initial training, and it is no wonder that potential rescuers fail to recognize and respond to SCA" (1a, p. 39).

The retention of CPR/AED information and skills is short lived and fleeting. A study reported in PubMed and published in the *European Resuscitation Journal* reflected that adults who participated in Heartsaver courses experienced significant performance decline in their CPR skills after a post-training interval of only two months. Of extreme concern was the fact that CPR skill retention for students declined on some measures to the level of untrained controls (15). Insight Instructional Media reviewed 19 published studies on CPR/AED skill retention, all of which reflected that these skills were lost very rapidly. The investigators determined that, on average, 66% of subjects were unable to pass a skills test three months after their instructor-led training program. After one year, 90% of subjects failed skill testing based on national CPR and AED standards (3).

One of the biggest concerns has been the inability of fitness instructors and personal trainers to recognize an individual experiencing an SCA and immediately respond with CPR and AED deployment. This inability to recognize an SCA has been a common issue in many of the death cases in fitness facilities resulting in lawsuits. Although the AHA and the American Red Cross (ARC) manuals outline the signs indicative of a cardiac arrest, why are instructors and personal trainers typically unable to meet this challenge and save lives? The answer is that obviously their CPR training was inadequate, coupled with a lack of rehearsals and drills.

A most important component of ongoing training to be addressed in rehearsals and drills is to emphasize this common issue of failing to recognize the signs of cardiac arrest. So often, SCA victims are mistaken to be having a seizure because of their abnormal breathing pattern. Abnormal breathing is frequently **agonal breathing** and is a sign of cardiac arrest. As described in AHA and ARC student workbooks, agonal breathing may be present in the first few minutes after an SCA.

These workbooks highlight the concept of agonal breathing with a "cautionary" note stating, "A person who gasps usually looks like he is drawing air in very quickly. The mouth may be open and the jaw, head, or neck may move with gasps. Gasps may appear forceful or weak. Some time may pass between gasps because they usually happen at a slow rate. The gasp may sound like a snort, snore, or groan. Gasping is not normal breathing. It is a sign of cardiac arrest" (10, p. 4). Consequently, it requires immediate CPR followed with a rapid deployment of an AED.

As stated, professional personal trainers should be certified in both first aid and CPR to include an AED. Although precautionary measures, these are important considerations; and a lack of these credentials truly reflects professional irresponsibility. Informal surveys reflect that although personal trainers are typically certified in CPR, most do not have certification in first aid. Of those with CPR, many are certified in only adult CPR and this without training in AEDs.

For those personal trainers operating out of small studios or servicing clients within the home, the responsibility of an emergency response falls solely upon their shoulders. Therefore, it is even more incumbent upon the personal trainer that he or she be highly trained and extremely competent in delivering first aid, CPR, and the deployment of an AED. Fortunately, the AHA is not restricted to just CPR/AED courses but for years has also offered first aid, CPR, and AED courses (11). Personal trainers might also consider becoming certified as a "first responder" who is capable of using certain adjunctive equipment as well as administering oxygen.

There are obvious reasons why personal trainers should be capable of providing first aid. From minor cuts to major lacerations, simple contusions to severe concussions, heat cramps to heatstroke, mild hypoglycemia to insulin shock, the "professional personal trainer" ought to be able to respond to these emergencies. Notwithstanding the importance of such emergencies, it would seem appropriate to address the most serious concern likely to confront the personal trainer, a cardiovascular complication, perhaps a severe MI or an SCA. The question is whether the fitness facility, personal trainer, or both are prepared to make the difference between life and death.

The fact is that medical complications due to exercise are a reality; and of greatest concern are cardiovascular complications. It has been well documented that coronary incidents are transiently increased with vigorous exercise in comparison with everyday, spontaneous occurrences (6). For those free of coronary artery disease, the relative risk of vigorous exercise is extremely low. Unfortunately, coronary artery disease is very prevalent among older, sedentary individuals, many of whom are now joining fitness facilities and availing themselves of personal training services. It should be noted that many of the people joining fitness facilities today are over 55 years old.

When a mild to moderate MI is suspected (e.g., tightness of the chest, radiating pain), activation of the emergency medical services system is essential. In addition to making the member or client as comfortable as possible and keeping him or her calm, the personal trainer should immediately administer emergency oxygen if it is available. In addition to activation of EMS, supplemental oxygen is probably the most important step that can be taken in treating the suspected MI. The fact is that any victim of a potentially life-threatening illness or injury, and this is without exception, should receive emergency medical oxygen.

When individuals experience the discomfort of an MI, it is a very common reaction to deny the possibility of their having a heart attack, thereby preventing or delaying the arrival of EMS. This denial is not limited to the victim as it may also persuade the potential rescuer, such as a personal trainer, that this discomfort is due to other conditions. "The tendency of people involved in an emergency to deny or downplay the serious nature of the presenting problem is a natural one that must be overcome to provide rapid intervention and maximize the victim's chance of survival" (8, p. 29). Denial of the serious nature of the symptoms not only may lead to serious heart damage before the victim is medically treated but also increases the risk of death.

When an SCA occurs within the fitness facility, the personal trainer's studio, or the client's home, the prognosis is poor unless an AED is available. In the United States, SCA strikes an estimated 350,000 people each year outside of the hospital environment, and approximately 90% die (9). Rapid defibrillation is the only definitive treatment. Because of the unavoidable response time of paramedics, defibrillation by EMS personnel is usually too late to provide successful resuscitation. Once blood stops circulating, every minute without defibrillation decreases the chances of survival by approximately 7% to 10% (8). The only solution to this dilemma is the availability of an AED on the premises, an AED that can be immediately applied to the victim.

> **Having first aid equipment, oxygen, and an AED available reflects a professional commitment to an emergency response.**

Some lawyers will argue that the use of AEDs and oxygen may increase fitness facilities' exposure to litigation by having them held to a higher standard of care. There is likely little merit to this argument, especially when considering position stands by professional associations like the American Heart Association (AHA) and the ACSM. In early 2002, these associations came out with the AHA/ACSM Scientific Statement on automated external defibrillators in health and fitness facilities, a supplement to their previous recommendations for emergency policies at facilities. In this statement, a public access defibrillation (PAD) plan with AED is "encouraged" in fitness centers servicing a general membership and even "strongly encouraged" in centers with memberships

over 2,500 as well as those with programs for clinical populations (4). It should be noted that the ACSM has gone beyond encouraging the use of AEDs in fitness facilities and currently in their *Health/Fitness Facility Standards and Guidelines* text recognizes a PAD program as a "standard" (27). Prudence should also dictate that facilities be equipped with emergency oxygen that can be administered by properly trained staff. The really important question to ask is: "Will the availability of oxygen and AEDs save lives?" The answer to this question is a resounding "Yes!"

The AHA's guidelines contain clear CPR guidelines as well as an even stronger commitment to the concept of "public access defibrillation" through AEDs, which have been hailed as the most significant breakthrough in CPR since the advent of mouth-to-mouth rescue breathing. It is the goal of the AHA that victims of an SCA be defibrillated within 5 minutes of onset. For this reason, the AHA recommends that AEDs be placed in locations where there is a reasonable probability of one SCA occurring every five years. Certainly fitness facilities fall within this category (4).

In order to provide the gift of life as well as health to members and individual clients, facilities and personal trainers should have AEDs and oxygen readily available. This emergency equipment is essential in order to give the victims of MI and SCA a fighting chance. It stands to reason that personal trainers should encourage the training for and the use of such equipment within their respective fitness facilities; and if personal trainers are operating out of their own individual studios or within clients' homes, then they should invest in this equipment and its associated training.

As discussed earlier, many people over 55 are joining fitness facilities and availing themselves of personal trainers. With age comes many more risk factors and the potential for untoward events to which facility staff and personal trainers must respond. The fact is that frequently those over 55 fall within the category of being a special population or clients with specific disabilities or chronic diseases, or both. The personal trainer has to be prepared to work with populations that have received medical clearance to exercise in nonclinical settings but are living with hypertension, heart disease, stroke, diabetes, end-stage renal disease, chronic obstructive pulmonary disease, peripheral arterial disease, neurological disorders, orthopedic concerns, and their associated risks. Fortunately a number of professional associations are providing training and certification to work with these special populations. For example, the NSCA has published a textbook entitled *NSCA's Essentials of Training Special Populations* (22), the ACSM published *ACSM's Exercise Management for Persons with Chronic Diseases and Disabilities* (5); and the American Council on Exercise published *ACE's Medical Exercise Specialist Manual* (24). As most personal trainers are currently working with some higher than normal risk clients, it makes sense that personal trainers undertake additional education and certification in this field of special populations not only to work more safely with their clients but also to lessen their possibilities of litigation.

Record Keeping and Confidentiality

Record keeping is an integral part of any successful business. Obviously, records will vary in number and type depending upon the size of an operation, clientele serviced, and programs conducted. Record keeping is essential in order to know where one has been, where one is currently, and where one is going in the future. Written documentation of the operations of a fitness facility, a personal training studio, or an individual personal trainer's business is not only important to the financial success of that enterprise but also may be critical to the defense of a potential lawsuit. Notwithstanding the significance of typical business records, this section will deal only with those documents likely to be discoverable in a lawsuit, whether by subpoena or service.

When a discovery "Request for Production of Documents" is served on the defendant, he or she must be forthcoming with any and all records relating to the case. The following documents and memoranda are likely to be considered relevant in determining whether or not the four essential elements of a tort can be met and, therefore, a negligence claim can prevail. For that reason, it is recommended that the personal trainer maintain a filing system with the following records.

Initial interview notes can substantiate the type of arrangement that is anticipated or agreed upon by the personal trainer and his or her client. During the initial interview or a later meeting, a personal service contract may be drafted and finalized that further legitimizes the responsibilities of both parties. If there are any addendums to this contract, then they should be attached to the initial agreement.

After the contractual arrangement has been finalized, the personal trainer will normally provide the client with a self-administered medical history form to be filled out by the client at home and then

later reviewed with the personal trainer. After going through the medical history form with the client, the personal trainer may have the client sign off on this form, swearing—under the penalties of perjury—that the information is true and accurate to the best of his or her knowledge. It is crucial that a client's signature be witnessed, preferably by someone other than the personal trainer. Ideally, the client will be required to complete a comprehensive medical history form; however, as a bare minimum and only if the client is limited to moderate exercise, the personal trainer may just require the Par-Q+, Physical Activity Readiness Questionnaire for Everyone. To assist with this health appraisal, it is also recommended that the personal trainer walk the client through a lifestyle questionnaire that will provide a more comprehensive picture of the client's health status.

Depending upon the client's health status as well as age and goals, the personal trainer may or may not require that the client be medically examined and a physician clearance form be completed and returned to the personal trainer. Additionally, it is helpful for the personal trainer to have copies of any physical exam reports inclusive of stress test results along with lab results and blood profiles. For this information to be released to the personal trainer, he or she must provide the client with a release of medical information form. If the personal trainer is relying upon information received from a phone contact with a doctor or his or her medical staff within the office, then the personal trainer should document this communication by means of medical notes reflecting the date, to whom he or she spoke, and the exact nature of the conversation.

If the client is to be scheduled for fitness testing, then this will be noted in the personal trainer's appointment book or log, and the client will be provided with an appointment letter that includes preparation directions for testing. Prior to testing, an informed consent will be read by the client and explained to the client by the personal trainer. After ascertaining that any questions have been answered to the complete satisfaction of the client, the personal trainer will ensure that the consent form is dated, signed, and witnessed. After testing, a fitness profile should be provided to the client, and a fitness testing record sheet should be kept by the personal trainer.

With the information garnered from the health appraisal and fitness testing, the personal trainer is then ready to generate a program design or exercise prescription. Again, prior to training, an informed consent should be executed. With the assistance of a lawyer, the personal trainer may draft other **exculpatory documents** in the form of anticipatory waivers, releases of liability, disclaimers, and express assumptions of risk. Exculpatory agreements are designed to move the personal trainer out of or away from liability and to remove or reduce legal responsibility.

In addition to the written program design or exercise prescription, it is in the best legal interest of the personal trainer to record any educational materials provided to the client and educational sessions attended by the client that have been acknowledged in writing by the client. The personal trainer should keep a training log on each client to document workouts and reflect client progress. Progress notes from the observation of training logs as well as follow-up fitness testing ought to be shared with the client as well as recorded in his or her file. Any other congratulatory letters or motivational messages need to be photocopied and placed within the client's file. Any written correspondence to the personal trainer from the client should also be retained and filed appropriately.

Fitness facilities as well as personal training studios are required to maintain suitable signage for locker rooms, wet areas (steam room, whirlpool, and sauna), racquetball courts, pools, cardiovascular areas, and weight rooms. It is mandatory that the signage (often in the form of instructions or directives) exhibited on equipment is not removed.

When equipment is defective or broken, it should be removed from the floor or appropriate signs placed on the equipment to alert clients that it is not to be used. Records of manufacturer operational manuals, equipment instructions, and "out of order" signs may be helpful in the event of an incident related to an equipment injury. It can also be advantageous to have staff sign off on an **agreement to comply form**, indicating they have read, understood, and agree to comply with manufacturer's instructions for the operation of specific equipment.

Regarding liability concerns with exercise equipment, it is important to document that equipment has been installed (installation record) according to the manufacturer's directives and, of particular importance, that unstable equipment has been secured to the floor in order to avoid its falling on clients. Every facility or studio needs to create and make use of a preventive maintenance schedule for equipment; and this schedule can be verified through inspection logs along with corrective maintenance forms.

In line with the earlier discussion of untoward events or emergencies and crises that could occur, it is mandatory that facilities and studios have a written emergency response plan, which would include a risk management plan that allows for inspections and corrective action. Emergency plans provide for rehearsals and both announced and unannounced drills, which are followed up with critique sheets and, again, corrective action forms. Also, as mentioned before, emergency procedures sheets are to be placed at convenient and strategic locations throughout the facility or studio to assist in emergency response as well as permit periodic review by staff.

It is obvious that numerous records must be kept by the professional personal trainer. Consequently, he or she must create a filing system to organize the various records for immediate availability. Additionally, the personal trainer must generate a separate file for each client; and within this file, there should be subfiles for the various documents and memoranda to be kept. After terminating a client and personal trainer relationship, it is recommended that files be retained for at least four years if not an indefinite period of time.

It is appropriate that the subject of confidentiality be again addressed, particularly in light of the numerous records just discussed. Obviously, personal trainers are going to have at their disposal very personal information about their clients. Not only for ethical reasons but legal concerns as well, the personal trainer must be very sensitive to how this information and data are handled and secured, especially as it concerns a client's health and the HIPAA Privacy Rule (7).

If the personal trainer wishes to use a client's name, such as for referrals or marketing purposes (e.g., "before and after" pictures), then it is important that he or she obtain a signed and witnessed release form from the client. If the personal trainer wishes to use data for statistical or marketing purposes from a client's fitness profiles (e.g., baseline and follow-up measurements), then this should be stated in the informed consent the client signs before fitness testing.

Finally, it must be remembered that the client and personal trainer relationship has to be kept on a professional basis at all times. Because the personal trainer is privy to information about the client's personal habits as well as medical and physical condition, the personal trainer must treat this information with the utmost privacy and respect. Additionally, when talking with the client, the personal trainer should not encourage disclosure but rather make every effort to avoid learning personal details other than those relating to medical, fitness, motivational, and business concerns. In the same token, the personal trainer does not need to share his or her own personal problems with the client. Because of the very nature of the personal trainer and client relationship, the sharing of personal and intimate details with a client may lead to romantic interests that will only undermine the personal trainer's effectiveness in training the client and, perhaps, sabotage his or her business as well. Discretion is the byword for the professional personal trainer.

Finally, it is not uncommon for personal trainers to work with underage clients, not only teens but also preteens. The personal trainer needs to recognize that the maturity level of these clients is such that they often see events in a very different light than the personal trainer does, and therefore tremendous potential for misunderstanding exists. The personal trainer must be overly cautious when working with these young clients; and because of issues surrounding the age of consent the personal trainer would do well to schedule sessions in open areas and public environments where training can be observed by other adults. Additionally, training young clients in small groups may lessen the chance of false accusations, especially when one is working with the opposite sex.

STRATEGIES FOR MINIMIZING LEGAL LIABILITY ASSOCIATED WITH NEGLIGENCE

Personal trainers may use three major risk management strategies to minimize legal liability associated with negligence:

1. Implement procedures that reflect the duties and responsibilities discussed in the preceding section.
2. Implement the use of waivers.
3. Purchase appropriate liability insurance.

Risk management is a proactive administrative process, meaning the personal trainer should address all three of these strategies before starting a personal training practice.

By implementing procedures that reflect legal duties and responsibilities, personal trainers provide themselves with a first line of defense if they are ever sued for negligence. Remember, the plaintiff will have to first prove that the personal trainer had a particular duty and that the personal trainer breached that duty. It may be easy for a plaintiff to prove that a duty existed by virtue of his or her relationship with the personal trainer. However, if the personal trainer can show that

he or she did indeed implement the proper procedures within his or her practice, it will be more difficult for the plaintiff to prove that there was any breach of duty even though the plaintiff was injured. If there is no breach of duty, negligence cannot be established, and the case will typically be dismissed.

A second line of defense for personal trainers is to have all clients sign a prospective release (waiver) prior to participation in the training program. Though a waiver should never be used as a substitute for implementing procedures that reflect a personal trainer's responsibilities, it can be used to protect personal trainers from their own negligence. There are numerous factors to consider before implementing a waiver, as discussed in the next section, "Protective Legal Documents."

A third and final line of defense is to have liability insurance. If a court rules that a defendant was negligent, the insurance company, as opposed to the defendant, may pay the damages up to the limits established in the policy. Personal trainers who are employees of a fitness facility may be included under the **general liability insurance** covering the facility and its employees for general acts of negligence. Personal trainers who are employees of a business, as well as those who are self-employed, can purchase **professional liability insurance**, often available at relatively inexpensive group rates. When purchasing liability insurance, it is important to consult with legal and insurance experts to help ensure that the insurance purchased will cover all activities conducted during personal training sessions. For example, if training sessions are held outdoors, typical general and professional liability insurance may not cover these activities.

PROTECTIVE LEGAL DOCUMENTS

Several different types of protective legal documents exist, but the following three are commonly used in the fitness field:

1. Informed consent
2. Agreement to participate
3. Prospective release (waiver)

Before discussion of the type of legal protection afforded by such documents, it will be helpful to review three of the causes of injury or death most frequently associated with physical activity:

1. **Inherent**: injuries due to accidents that are not preventable and are no one's fault

2. **Negligence**: injuries due to the fault of the defendant (sometimes the plaintiff)

3. **Extreme forms of negligence**: injuries due to the gross negligence, willful and wanton, or reckless conduct of the defendant (13)

For lawsuits arising from injuries caused by inherent risks, an **informed consent** or an **agreement to participate** may provide the best legal protection through what is called an assumption of risk defense (13). Within each of these documents is a section informing the participant of the potential risks associated with the activity (e.g., type of injuries [death] that can occur). This consent form helps serve as evidence of the assumption of risk defense, meaning that the client knew and fully understood the risks, appreciated those risks, and voluntarily assumed them. Generally, the law does not allow individuals to recover for injuries they have assumed (e.g., participation in an obstacle challenge or race).

For lawsuits arising from negligence of the personal trainer, a **prospective release**, or **waiver**, may provide the best protection. Within the waiver is a key section that includes an exculpatory clause—that clause explicitly stating that the client releases the personal trainer from any liability associated with negligence on part of the personal trainer. This clause may provide evidence that the client forfeited (waived) his or her right to pursue a successful negligent lawsuit against the personal trainer, but it must be written and administered carefully to be enforceable. The exculpatory clause does not provide protection for lawsuits arising from inherent injuries. Therefore, an **assumption of risk** section is often added to provide this protection, outlining the specific dangers of an activity undertaken (e.g., plyometric box jumps).

Validity of waivers vary from state to state, and therefore a personal trainer may find himself or herself with a waiver that provides greater protection in one state than another. Because validity is determined by each state, the personal trainer should retain a lawyer that is familiar with that state's laws to ensure that the most protective waiver possible is used. In line with this concept, the content in this chapter is for educational purposes only; and therefore, you are advised to seek competent counsel in your state or jurisdiction for legal advice.

There are generally no legal documents to protect personal trainers in lawsuits arising from extreme forms of negligence. A few states may allow the use of a waiver to protect from such conduct, but most do not. Extreme forms of negligence can occur when a

> **Although waivers are generally protective in most states regarding general negligence, law firms may obtain judgments against personal trainers by documenting "gross" negligence, or an extreme departure from the standard of care or the failure to provide even scant care.**

defendant had prior knowledge that a danger or risk existed but took no corrective action to prevent the danger or risk; for example, a personal trainer has prior knowledge that a certain exercise can put a client at risk for an injury but has the client perform that exercise anyway. It is important to realize that this type of conduct could subject the personal trainer to punitive damages, which are rarely covered by liability insurance (16).

Enforceability of Protective Documents

Protective legal documents signed by the client, prior to participation in the training program, may provide important "evidence" in a court of law that either strengthens the defense of the personal trainer or defeats the plaintiff's claim entirely. For example, if the personal trainer had a client sign a legally sufficient and properly administered waiver, this document may serve as evidence that the injured client waived his or her right to sue for negligence.

Depending on a court's rules of civil procedure the personal trainer would, in response to the plaintiff's complaint for negligence, file a motion to dismiss and assert the affirmative defense of waiver (13). The rules may require him or her to assert this defense in addition to filing the normal answer to the plaintiff's complaint. Either way, whether the court hears the motion before the trial or defers it until later, the purpose of the waiver is to defeat the plaintiff's claim.

An affirmative defense is a statutory defense raised by the defendant in a civil lawsuit designed to defeat the plaintiff's claim (13). There are many such defenses such as contributory or comparative negligence, fraud, assumption of the risk, and many more. The most commonly recognized affirmative defense is the statute of limitations (13). For example, if in a particular state the statute of limitations for negligence is three years and the plaintiff files a lawsuit one day after or one year after the expiration of the statutory period, the plaintiff is barred from filing the claim. The plaintiff has relinquished the right to pursue the claim because the time period has lapsed. Be mindful that there are exceptions to nearly every rule in court. Sometimes, for good cause shown or other extenuating circumstances, the court may allow the plaintiff to go forward even though the statute of limitations has lapsed. One of the most critical questions in determining whether the statute of limitations has lapsed is to know when it began to run, which of course may vary from state to state.

The general belief that a fitness facility is not liable for the negligent acts of personal trainers working in their facilities needs to be explained in context of the legal doctrine of respondeat superior ("let the master answer"). As explained on page 656, the legal doctrine that a party who has a specific superior legal relationship (e.g., an employer) to another, and who has the right, ability, or duty to control the activities of that person, is responsible for, and is vicariously liable for, the acts of their agents. This applies to the employee but not the independent contractor. An employee is the agent of the employer.

Often the distinction is not clear as to who is or is not an employee and who is an independent contractor. If the personal trainer is legally classified as an employee, then the employer may be liable for the personal trainer's negligent acts. If, however, the personal trainer is legally classified as an independent contractor, the employer is not likely to be held responsible for that personal trainer's negligent acts.

An employer typically has control over personal trainers' activities when he or she sets hours of a work period; requires the personal trainers to punch a time clock when they arrive and leave work; assigns a specific job title and description; pays a weekly or biweekly wage; and sees that federal and state taxes and other deductions are withheld from the personal trainers' paychecks.

When a fitness facility enters into an agreement with a personal trainer to allow the personal trainer to use its facilities to train his or her client in, but does not dictate the terms of his or her work; does not control his or her schedule or other activities, and does not pay the personal trainer a wage, then that personal trainer is typically described as an independent contractor. In many instances the personal trainer pays the facility owner. If the facility owner pays the personal trainer for some service rendered while in the facility, the facility owner provides the personal trainer with a Form 1099 at the end of each year.

The legal litmus test, however, for the status of the personal trainer is "control" as defined by the Internal Revenue Service and not the contract between the facility owner and the personal trainer. In other words, the contract with the personal trainer as an independent contractor could formally identify the personal trainer as an independent contractor and, at the same time, enumerate his or her job title and description, work hours, lunch break, and so on. That becomes a problem because the description attempts to create one relationship while the terms of the agreement provide for control of the activities of the personal trainer, which creates another relationship. In that situation the court is most likely to rule that the personal trainer is an employee and hold the employer liable for the negligent acts of the personal trainer.

The employee or agent must be within the course and scope of his or her employment and in furtherance of the employer's business at the time of the negligent incident. Under this theory, courts impute liability to the employer for misconduct of the employee. The employer owes a duty of care and loyalty to the employee to take reasonable steps to ensure a safe working environment and to maintain equipment in proper condition. The employee's duty is to operate within the standard of care, in furtherance of the employer's business.

Regarding risk management for the personal trainer, Eickhoff-Shemek summarized the principle concerns for which a personal trainer must be aware to avoid a lawsuit and protect himself or herself. These concerns are addressed through seven lines of defense, which are as follows (14):

1. Provide a professional environment.
2. Know and adhere to the law and published standards of practice.
3. Develop the knowledge, skills, and abilities to become a qualified and competent personal trainer.
4. Develop and comply with written policies and procedures related to preactivity screening, fitness testing, program design, client instruction, client supervision, exercise equipment, and facility risks.
5. Adopt, follow, and regularly rehearse emergency response plans.
6. Adopt waiver/release and assumption of risk documents.
7. Secure professional liability insurance.

CONCLUSION

Understanding the legal aspects of personal training and implementing them into a personal trainer's daily routine ensures that exposure to legal liability is reduced. It also places the personal trainer in a much better position to assist legal counsel in defending a lawsuit for negligence in the event one occurs. To be successful an individual must pursue the profession of personal training with a spirit of conscientiousness and a dedication to integrity. When personal trainers become thoroughly prepared and truly committed to providing the most effective exercise programs and the safest training environments, then this vocational pursuit will deserve the recognition of an allied health care profession. However, to become acknowledged as professionals, personal trainers must be willing to undergo formal instruction in exercise science through accredited university programs or credible vocational programs in order to receive not only comprehensive theoretical education but also extensive practical training taught by qualified exercise physiologists. As a result of developing the appropriate knowledge, skills, and abilities of an exercise professional, coupled with a sincere concern for clients, one can ascend the "STEPS to success" and enjoy not only a personally rewarding and financially profitable career as a personal trainer but also a bright and sunny future free from the ominous clouds of litigation.

Study Questions

1. Which of these is defined as the standard that is owed to fitness clients by personal trainers?
   - A. standard of litigation
   - B. standard of defense
   - C. standard of professionalism
   - D. standard of care

2. Which of the following is defined as a legal situation in which the personal trainer acts with substandard care that results in an injury?
   - A. intentional tort
   - B. negligence
   - C. unintentional tort
   - D. strict liability

3. Which of the following is defined as the monetary loss due to the injury, which can include both economic damages (e.g., medical costs, lost wages) and noneconomic damages (e.g., pain and suffering)?
   - A. duty
   - B. breach of duty
   - C. causation
   - D. damages

4. Which of the following is *true* regarding equipment and facility safety?
   - A. A personal trainer working as an independent contractor cannot be considered responsible for facility equipment.
   - B. Clients in their own homes cannot be considered invitees.
   - C. A personal trainer is responsible for a safe environment if that environment is the client's own home.
   - D. Clients of fitness facilities are *not* considered business invitees.

5. A plaintiff *cannot* move forward with a case once the statute of limitations has passed, under any circumstances.
   - A. true
   - B. false

Name: _____ *(please print)*

1. PURPOSE AND EXPLANATION OF TESTING

I hereby consent to voluntarily engage in an exercise test to determine my circulatory and respiratory fitness. I also consent to the taking of samples of my exhaled air during exercise to properly measure my oxygen consumption. I also consent, if necessary, to have a small blood sample drawn by needle from my arm for blood chemistry analysis and to the performance of lung function and body fat (skinfold pinch) tests. It is my understanding that the information obtained will help me evaluate future physical activities and sports activities in which I may engage.

Before I undergo the test, I certify to the program that I am in good health and have had a physical examination conducted by a licensed medical physician within the last _____ months. Further, I hereby represent and inform the program that I have completed the pretest history interview presented to me by the program staff and have provided accurate responses to the questions as indicated on the history form or as supplied to the interviewer. It is my understanding that I will be interviewed by a physician or other person prior to my undergoing the test who will, in the course of interviewing me, determine if there are any reasons that would make it undesirable or unsafe for me to take the test. Consequently, I understand that it is important that I provide complete and accurate responses to the interviewer and recognize that my failure to do so could lead to possible unnecessary injury to myself during the test.

The test I will undergo will be performed on a motor-driven treadmill or bicycle ergometer with the amount of effort gradually increasing. As I understand it, this increase in effort will continue until I feel and verbally report to the operator any symptoms such as fatigue, shortness of breath, or chest discomfort that may appear. It is my understanding and I have been clearly advised that it is my right to request that a test be stopped at any point if I feel unusual discomfort or fatigue. I have been advised that I should, immediately upon experiencing any such symptoms or if I so choose, inform the operator that I wish to stop the test at that or any other point. My wishes in this regard shall be absolutely carried out.

It is further my understanding that prior to beginning the test, I will be connected by electrodes and cables to an electrocardiographic recorder, which will enable the program personnel to monitor my cardiac (heart) activity. It is my understanding that during the test itself, a trained observer will monitor my responses continuously and take frequent readings of blood pressure, the electrocardiogram, and my expressed feelings of effort. I realize that a true determination of my exercise capacity depends on progressing the test to the point of my fatigue.

Once the test has been completed, but before I am released from the test area, I will be given special instructions about showering and recognition of certain symptoms that may appear within the first 24 hours after the test. I agree to follow these instructions and promptly contact the program personnel or medical providers if such symptoms develop.

2. RISKS

I understand and have been informed that there exists the possibility of adverse changes during the actual test. I have been informed that these changes could include abnormal blood pressure, fainting, disorders of heart rhythm, stroke, and very rare instances of heart attack or even death. I have been told that every effort will be made to minimize these occurrences by preliminary examination and by precautions and observations taken during the test. I have also been informed that emergency equipment and personnel are readily available to deal with these unusual situations should they occur. I understand that there is a risk of injury, heart attack, or even death as a result of my performance of this test, but knowing those risks, it is my desire to proceed to take the test as herein indicated.

3. BENEFITS TO BE EXPECTED AND AVAILABLE ALTERNATIVES TO THE EXERCISE TESTING PROCEDURE

The results of this test may or may not benefit me. Potential benefits relate mainly to my personal motives for taking the test, that is, knowing my exercise capacity in relation to the general population, understanding my fitness for certain sports and recreational activities, planning my physical conditioning program, or evaluating the effects of my recent physical activity habits. Although my fitness might also be evaluated by alternative means, for example, a bench step test or an outdoor running test, such tests do not provide as accurate a fitness assessment as the treadmill or bike test, nor do those options allow equally effective monitoring of my responses.

4. CONFIDENTIALITY AND USE OF INFORMATION

I have been informed that the information obtained in this exercise test will be treated as privileged and confidential and will consequently not be released or revealed to any person without my express written consent. I do, however, agree to the use of any information for research or statistical purposes so long as same does not provide facts that could lead to my identification. Any other information obtained, however, will be used only by the program staff to evaluate my exercise status or needs.

5. INQUIRIES AND FREEDOM OF CONSENT

I have been given an opportunity to ask certain questions as to the procedures. Generally, these requests have been noted by the testing staff, and the responses are as follows:

_____

_____

_____

_____

_____

I further understand that there are also other remote risks that may be associated with this procedure. Despite the fact that a complete accounting of all these remote risks has not been provided to me, I still desire to proceed with the test.

I acknowledge that I have read this document in its entirety or that it has been read to me if I have been unable to read same.

I consent to the rendition of all services and procedures as explained herein by all program personnel.

Date: _____

Participant's signature: _____

Witness' signature: _____

Test supervisor's signature: _____

The law varies from state to state. No form should be adopted or used by any program without individualized legal advice.

From *NSCA's Essentials of Personal Training,* 3rd ed., edited for the National Strength and Conditioning Association by B. Schoenfeld and R. Snarr (Champaign, IL: Human Kinetics, 2022).

Name: _____ *(please print)*

1. PURPOSE AND EXPLANATION OF THE PROCEDURE

I hereby consent to voluntarily engage in an acceptable plan of personal fitness training. I also give consent to be placed in personal fitness training program activities that are recommended to me for improvement of my general health and well-being. These may include dietary education, stress management, and health/fitness education activities. The levels of exercise I perform will be based on my cardiorespiratory (heart and lungs) and muscular fitness. I understand that I may be required to undergo a graded exercise test as well as other fitness tests prior to the start of my personal fitness training program in order to evaluate and assess my present level of fitness. I will be given exact personal instructions regarding the amount and kind of exercise I should do. I agree to participate three times per week in the formal program sessions. Professionally trained personal fitness trainers will provide leadership to direct my activities, monitor my performance, and otherwise evaluate my effort. Depending on my health status, I may or may not be required to have my blood pressure and heart rate evaluated during these sessions to regulate my exercise within desired limits. I understand that I am expected to attend every session and to follow staff instructions with regard to exercise, diet, stress management, and other health/fitness-related programs. If I am taking prescribed medications, I have already so informed the program staff and further agree to so inform them promptly of any changes my doctor or I make with regard to use of these. I will be given the opportunity for periodic assessment and evaluation at regular intervals after the start of my program.

I have been informed that during my participation in this personal fitness training program, I will be asked to complete the physical activities unless symptoms such as fatigue, shortness of breath, chest discomfort, or similar occurrences appear. At that point, I have been advised that it is my complete right to decrease or stop exercise and that it is my obligation to inform the personal fitness training program personnel of my symptoms. I hereby state that I have been so advised and agree to inform the personal fitness training program personnel of my symptoms, should any develop.

I understand that while I exercise, a personal fitness trainer will periodically monitor my performance and perhaps measure my pulse and blood pressure or assess my feelings of effort for the purposes of monitoring my progress. I also understand that the personal fitness trainer may reduce or stop my exercise program when any of these findings so indicate that this should be done for my safety and benefit.

I also understand that during the performance of my personal fitness training program, physical touching and positioning of my body may be necessary to assess my muscular and bodily reactions to specific exercises, as well as to ensure that I am using proper technique and body alignment. I expressly consent to the physical contact for these reasons.

2. RISKS

I understand and have been informed that there exists the remote possibility of adverse changes occurring during exercise including, but not limited to, abnormal blood pressure, fainting, dizziness, disorders of heart rhythm, and very rare instances of heart attack, stroke, or even death. I further understand and I have been informed that there exists the risk of bodily injury including, but not limited to, injuries to the muscles, ligaments, tendons, and joints of the body. I have been told that every effort will be made to minimize these occurrences by proper staff assessments of my condition before each exercise session, by staff supervision during exercise, and by my own careful control of exercise efforts. I fully understand the risks associated with exercise, including the risk of bodily injury, heart attack, stroke, or even death, but knowing these risks, it is my desire to participate as herein indicated.

3. BENEFITS TO BE EXPECTED AND AVAILABLE ALTERNATIVES TO EXERCISE

I understand that this program may or may not benefit my physical fitness or general health. I recognize that involvement in the exercise sessions and personal fitness training sessions will allow me to learn proper ways to perform conditioning exercises, use fitness equipment, and regulate physical effort. These experiences should benefit me by indicating how my physical limitations may affect my ability to perform various physical activities. I further understand that if I closely follow the program's instructions, I will likely improve my exercise capacity and fitness level after a period of three to six months.

4. CONFIDENTIALITY AND USE OF INFORMATION

I have been informed that the information obtained in this personal fitness training program will be treated as privileged and confidential and will consequently not be released or revealed to any person without my express written consent. I do, however, agree to the use of any information that is not personally identifiable with me for research and statistical purposes so long as same does not identify me or provide facts that could lead to my identification. I also agree to the use of any information for the purpose of consultation with other health/fitness professionals, including my doctor. Any other information obtained, however, will be used by the program staff in the course of prescribing exercise for me and evaluating my progress in the program.

5. INQUIRIES AND FREEDOM OF CONSENT

I have been given an opportunity to ask certain questions as to the procedures of this program. Generally, these requests have been noted by the interviewing staff, with the responses as follows:

_____

_____

_____

_____

_____

I further understand that there are also other remote risks that may be associated with this personal fitness training program. Despite the fact that a complete accounting of all these remote risks has not been provided to me, it is still my desire to participate.

I acknowledge that I have read this document in its entirety or that it has been read to me if I have been unable to read same.

I expressly consent to the rendition of all services and procedures as explained herein by all program personnel.

Date: _____

Client's signature: _____

Authorized representative's signature: _____

[Club name]

[Address]

[Address]
The law varies from state to state. No form should be adopted or used by any program without individualized legal advice.

From *NSCA's Essentials of Personal Training,* 3rd ed., edited for the National Strength and Conditioning Association by B. Schoenfeld and R. Snarr (Champaign, IL: Human Kinetics, 2022).

PURPOSE OF THIS BINDING AGREEMENT

By reading and signing this document, "You," the undersigned, sometimes also referred to as "User" or "I," will agree to release and hold _____ [Club name] ("Club" or "We") harmless from, and assume all responsibility for, all claims, demands, injuries, damages, actions, or causes of action to persons or property, arising out of or connected with your use of the Club's facilities, premises, or services. The agreement and release is for the benefit of the Club, its employees, agents, independent contractors, other users of the Club, and all persons on the Club's premises. This agreement includes your release of these persons from responsibility for injury, damage, or death to yourself because of those acts or omissions claimed to be related to the ordinary negligence of these persons. This agreement also includes your representations as to important matters that the Club will rely upon.

A. REPRESENTATIONS

The undersigned, You, represent (a) that you understand that use of the Club premises, facilities, equipment, services, and programs includes an inherent risk of injury to persons and property; (b) that you are in good physical condition and have no disabilities, illnesses, or other conditions that could prevent you from exercising and using the Club's equipment/facilities without injuring yourself or impairing your health; and (c) that you have consulted a physician concerning an exercise program that will not risk injury to yourself or impairment of your health. Such risk of injury includes, but is not limited to, injuries arising from or relating to use by you or others of exercise equipment and machines, locker rooms, spa and other wet areas, and other Club facilities; injuries arising from or relating to participation by you or others in supervised or unsupervised activities or programs through the Club; injuries and medical disorders arising from or relating to use of the Club's facilities including heart attacks, sudden cardiac arrests, strokes, heat stress, sprains, strains, broken bones, and torn muscles, tendons, and ligaments, among others; and accidental injuries occurring anywhere in the Club including lobbies, hallways, exercise areas, locker rooms, steam rooms, pool areas, Jacuzzis, saunas, and dressing rooms. Accidental injuries include those caused by you, those caused by other persons, and those of a "slip-and-fall" nature. If you have any special exercise requirements or limitations, you agree to disclose them to the Club before using the Club's facilities; and when seeking help in establishing an exercise program, you hereby agree that all exercise and use of the Club's facilities, services, programs, and premises are undertaken by you at your sole risk. As used herein, the terms "include," "including," and words of similar import are descriptive only, and are not limiting in any manner.

You also acknowledge and represent that you realize and appreciate that access to and use of the Club's facilities during nonsupervised times increases and enhances certain risks to you. You realize that if you use the Club during nonsupervised hours, any emergency response to you in the event of need for same may be impossible or delayed. While we encourage you to use the Club's facility with a partner during nonsupervised times, you may choose to do so without a partner, therefore enhancing and increasing the risks to you as to the provision of first aid and emergency response. You realize that a delay in the provision of first aid and/or emergency response may result in greater injury and disability to you and may cause or contribute to your death. Use of the Club with no one else present to supervise or watch your activities is not recommended and would not be allowed unless you agree to assume all risks of injury, whether known or unknown to you.

You do hereby further declare yourself to be physically sound and suffering from no condition, impairment, disease, infirmity, or other illness that would prevent your participation or use of equipment or machinery except as hereinafter stated. You do hereby acknowledge that you have been informed of the need for a physician's approval for your participation in an exercise/fitness activity or in the use of exercise equipment and machinery. You also acknowledge that it has been recommended that you have a yearly or more frequent physical examination and consultation with your physician as to physical activity, exercise, and use of exercise and training equipment so that you might have his or her recommendations concerning these fitness activities and equipment use. You acknowledge either that you have had a physical examination and have been given your physician's permission to participate, or that you have decided to participate in activity and use of equipment and machinery without the approval of your physician and do hereby assume all responsibility for your participation and activities, and use of equipment and machinery in your activities.

YOU HAVE READ THE FOREGOING, ACKNOWLEDGE THAT YOU UNDERSTAND THE TERMS AND CONDITIONS SET FORTH IN THE PRECEDING PARAGRAPHS, AND AGREE TO SAME.

Initials: _____

B. EXPRESS ASSUMPTION OF ALL RISKS

You have represented to us and acknowledged that you understand and appreciate all of the risks associated with your participation in various activities at the Club and in the use of equipment or facilities at the Club, including the risks of injury, disability, and death. You have also acknowledged that there are greater, enhanced, and even other risks to you if you decide to use the Club's facility during nonsupervised times. Knowing and appreciating all of these risks and enhanced risks, you have knowingly and intelligently determined to expressly assume all risks associated with all of your activities and use of equipment/facilities at the Club.

You understand and are aware that strength, flexibility, and aerobic exercise, including the use of equipment, is a potentially hazardous activity. You also understand that fitness activities involve the risk of injury and even death, and that you are voluntarily participating in these activities and using equipment and machinery with knowledge of the dangers involved. We have also reviewed the risks with you on the date when you signed this Agreement and answered any questions that you may have had. You hereby agree to expressly assume and accept any and all risks of injury or death including those related to your use of or presence at this facility, your use of equipment, and your participation in activity, including those risks related to the ordinary negligence of those released by this Agreement and including all claims related to ordinary negligence in the selection, purchase, setup, maintenance, instruction as to use, and use and/or supervision of use, if any, associated with all equipment and facilities.

YOU HAVE READ THE FOREGOING, ACKNOWLEDGE THAT YOU UNDERSTAND THE TERMS AND CONDITIONS SET FORTH IN THE PRECEDING PARAGRAPHS, AND AGREE TO SAME.

Initials: _____

C. AGREEMENT AND RELEASE OF LIABILITY

In consideration of being allowed to participate in the activities and programs of the Club and to use its equipment/facilities and machinery in addition to the payment of any fee or charge, you do hereby waive, release, and forever discharge the Club and its directors, officers, agents, employees, representatives, successors and assigns, administrators, executors, and all others from any and all responsibilities or liability from injuries or damages resulting from your participation in any activities or your use of equipment/facilities or machinery in the previously mentioned activities. You do also hereby release all of those mentioned and any others acting upon their behalf from any responsibility or liability for any injury or damage to yourself, including those caused by the negligent act or omission of any of those mentioned or others acting on their behalf or in any way arising out of or connected with your participation in any activities of the Club. This provision shall apply to ordinary acts of negligence but shall not apply to gross acts/omissions of negligence, willful or wanton acts/omissions, or those of an intentional/criminal nature.

YOU HAVE READ THE FOREGOING, ACKNOWLEDGE THAT YOU UNDERSTAND THE TERMS AND CONDITIONS SET FORTH IN THE PRECEDING PARAGRAPHS, AND AGREE TO SAME.

Initials: _____

D. LOSS OR THEFT OF PROPERTY

The Club is not responsible for lost or stolen articles. You should keep any valuables with you at all times while using the facilities. Storage space or lockers do not always protect valuables. Consequently, by executing this Agreement and any accompanying documents, you do hereby agree to assume all responsibility for your own property and that of any dependent(s) and to insure that property against risk of loss as you see fit. By the execution hereof, you expressly, on behalf of yourself and any dependents, do hereby knowingly agree to forego, waive, release, and prospectively give up any right to institute any claim or action against the Club relating to lost or stolen property, including property lost or stolen due to the negligent act or omission of the Club. You agree to indemnify and save the Club and all of its personnel harmless from any action, claim, suit, or subrogated claim or suit instituted at any time hereafter against the Club related to the theft or loss of your or your dependents' property at the Club. The Club shall be indemnified by you for all costs, expenses, and fees, including attorney fees, incurred by the Club or its personnel by reason of any such action.

YOU HAVE READ THE FOREGOING, ACKNOWLEDGE THAT YOU UNDERSTAND THE TERMS AND CONDITIONS SET FORTH IN THE PRECEDING PARAGRAPHS, AND AGREE TO SAME.

Initials: _____

User shall receive a copy of the foregoing Agreement at the time of its initialing and signing and hereby acknowledges User's receipt of same.

YOU HAVE READ THE FOREGOING, ACKNOWLEDGE THAT YOU UNDERSTAND THE TERMS AND CONDITIONS SET FORTH IN THE PRECEDING PARAGRAPHS, AND AGREE TO SAME.

Initials: _____

This Agreement shall be interpreted according to the laws of the State of _____ . If any part of this Agreement should ever be determined by a court of final jurisdiction to be invalid, the remaining portions hereof shall be deemed to be valid and enforceable.

YOU HAVE READ THE FOREGOING, ACKNOWLEDGE THAT YOU UNDERSTAND THE TERMS AND CONDITIONS SET FORTH IN THE PRECEDING PARAGRAPHS, AND AGREE TO SAME.

Initials: _____

ACKNOWLEDGMENT

I have read and received a completed copy of this Agreement and all of its Exhibits, as well as any Rules and Regulations of the Club, which are incorporated herein by reference. I agree to be bound by the terms and conditions of the Agreement and the Rules and Regulations of the Club, as same exist or as same may be amended from time to time hereafter. This Agreement shall be binding upon me and my spouse, my heirs, my estate, my executors, my administrators, and my successors and/or assigns. I realize that this Agreement is designed to prevent me and/or them from filing any personal injury or other lawsuit based upon ordinary negligence, including negligent battery, or even negligent wrongful death, loss of consortium, or any other similar lawsuit arising out of any injury to me which I or they may possess hereafter.

The undersigned, on behalf of myself and my heirs, executors, administrators, successors, and assigns, hereby agrees to indemnify the Club and all those hereby released and to hold them absolutely harmless if anyone, including the undersigned, should hereafter file suit against the Club or those released hereby for any matter intended to be released by this Agreement, including claims based upon ordinary negligence such as but not limited to personal injury, wrongful death, loss of consortium, or other similar actions.

Signature: _____ Date: _____

Print name: _____

Address: _____

Phone number: (_____) _____ - _____

From *NSCA's Essentials of Personal Training*, 3rd ed., edited for the National Strength and Conditioning Association by B. Schoenfeld and R. Snarr (Champaign, IL: Human Kinetics, 2022).

The Business of Personal Training

Mark A. Nutting, BS and Robert Linkul, MS

Building a successful career as a personal trainer requires more than knowing exercise science and programming. It requires understanding the business side of the fitness industry. Personal trainers need to know what options exist for employment. They could choose to work for a fitness studio, club, or other organization, or become independent contractors and work for themselves. Personal trainers should also choose a specific population they would like to work with, which will help them decide what kinds of programs to offer and how to price, market, and sell those offerings. The following sections cover these items with the intent of giving personal trainers the knowledge needed to build successful businesses and careers.

One of the first and most important decisions personal trainers should make about building their business is what specific population or target market they wish to work with. Defining the type of clients the personal trainer wishes to serve will help determine many of the business decisions to follow, and the more specific that market, the easier those decisions will be. For example, if a personal trainer decides to pursue golf conditioning as a focus or niche, the type of program to offer, where to offer it, how to market it, and even how much to charge will be influenced by having chosen golf conditioning. It would benefit a personal trainer to be even more specific about the target market, such as choosing to work with women golfers, or even women golfers over 50 years of age. At the same time, clients with a specific goal prefer to work with a specialist versus someone who does a little of everything. This makes a personal trainer whose niche is golf conditioning for women over 50 more desirable to that demographic. Each of these specifics helps the personal trainer home in on the answers to many of the business particulars. It is important to note that in choosing a niche, the personal trainer needs to make sure there is enough of that target market available to build and sustain the business. Using the golf training example, if there are no golf courses or enthusiasts nearby, that specialty would likely be too limiting to build a viable business.

Personal trainers new to the industry may not be sure what type of client they wish to work with. If so, it might be best for the personal trainer to seek employment in a facility that allows the opportunity to work with many different types of clients. From the experience gained, the personal trainer can then determine which population he or she finds most rewarding to work with.

EMPLOYMENT OPTIONS FOR THE PERSONAL TRAINER

Once certified, personal trainers have two main options of employment. They can choose to become an employee of an established organization that typically has set business practices, umbrella insurance coverage, established standards of professional growth, and guidelines for training practices by which the employee will be managed. The second option is to operate on their own as an independent contractor without regulation or direction of a management department, under their own insurance coverage, and with their own guidelines for training and business development. Each of these options has its advantages and disadvantages that personal trainers should weigh when selecting which situation best suits their needs and allows them the opportunity to become successful.

Employee-Based Personal Trainers

There are many reasons why working as an **employee** might be beneficial for a personal trainer. Working for others can allow a personal trainer to train various client types, discover a preferred target market, learn from peers and management, and even move into management. All these opportunities could be enormously valuable in building a career while working for others or as an entrepreneur should the personal trainer choose to pursue his or her own business.

Common Business Models

There are multiple business models within the fitness industry that personal trainers may want to consider as they pursue their choice of employment. The four most common business models where personal trainers can find employment are fitness studios, not-for-profit and community centers, commercial gyms or health clubs, and corporate fitness facilities. Each of these business models is likely to have different operating procedures and requirements for employment. No matter which business model the personal trainer ultimately decides to pursue, there are some general expectations that go along with being an employee.

Fitness Studios Fitness studios are typically independently owned and operated (i.e., not a franchise) and will have their own designated business practices and requirements for hiring employees or offering independent contractors a place to rent. Studios typically offer one or more of the following: personal training, small group training, large group training, and group fitness. Many are open by appointment or class only. Some private studios serve a specific demographic, such as older adults, youth sport performance, or postrehabilitation. Others may cater to a more general health and fitness population. Fitness studios can be great career options for intermediate- or entry-level personal trainers who know their target demographic and are ready to build a solid following and committed clientele.

Not-for-Profit and Community Fitness Centers Not-for-profit and community centers (e.g., YMCAs, Jewish Community Centers, city-run recreation departments) typically hire employees to work under the designated business practices of that establishment. Independent contractors are not commonly hired because these organizations like to maintain control over the actions of those working at their facilities. These centers are geared toward family involvement, often offering personal training sessions, classes, health promotion events, and community outreach programs for people of all ages. This is a great avenue for entry-level personal trainers because their area of interest (target demographic) may not be known at the point of hiring. These organizations provide many learning opportunities, allowing new employees to find an area of expertise they want to pursue.

Commercial Gym or Health Club Commercial gym models range from smaller equipment-only gyms that offer no classes or additional member activities to supersized clubs with pools, tennis courts, basketball courts, and more. The equipment-only gyms are more likely to hire an independent contractor because they

often lack the staff needed to manage an employee-based personal training department. Larger commercial facilities tend to bring on personal trainers as employees and recognize them as an important revenue source. Small or large, these are membership-driven facilities that typically encourage members to purchase extensive personal training packages. Personal trainers can grow a successful business inside commercial clubs but may have restrictions placed on their professional growth depending on the imposed business model. Restrictions can include the number of clients trained, hours worked, and commissions earned.

Corporate Fitness Facilities Corporate fitness facilities are health and wellness programs typically located inside large businesses that offer fitness and personal training programs for their employees. The corporate fitness model is designed to proactively pursue health improvements of employees as a strategy to reduce health care costs, workers' compensation, and absenteeism, and to increase productivity. Many businesses are realizing significant returns on investment from their corporate fitness programs, which has paved the way for personal training employment opportunities.

An Overview of Being an Employee

Every business has its own business practices, guidelines, requirements, and professional standards for its personal trainers to adhere to. This section discusses the typical advantages and disadvantages of working as an employee with the understanding that some or all of these may differ depending on the company and its offerings. These offerings include professional requirements, the hiring process, general and professional liability insurance, compensation and benefits, work duties and responsibilities, and sales and marketing guidelines.

Expectations of Being an Employee Every business has its own business practices, guidelines, requirements, and standards for its employed personal trainers. These include professional requirements, the hiring process, general or professional liability insurance, compensation and benefits, work duties, responsibilities, and sales and marketing guidelines.

Professional Requirements Most facilities have set professional requirements for their employees to maintain under the terms of their employment. These requirements may include obtaining and maintaining their accredited personal training certification, obtaining and maintaining cardiopulmonary resuscitation (CPR) certification, and abiding by the professional code of conduct in their employee guidelines.

Hiring Process   Potential employees will typically find job openings on online employment websites or the individual website of the facility in which they want to work, or they may simply walk into a particular facility and inquire about employment. In regard to posted openings, the description will outline the basic requirements of the position and how to go about applying. This often includes a resume and a cover letter detailing the following:

- *Work objective:* The work objective is typically a sentence or two detailing the intentions of the individual seeking employment, what position he or she is applying for, and, in short, why he or she may be a qualified candidate for the position.
- *Education and certification:* This includes formal education (e.g., high school, college, masters) and an accredited personal training certification as well as any additional certificates earned.
- *Work experience and expertise:* Work experience should outline the candidate's work history. This may include working at multiple locations and progressions in job title (e.g., personal trainer in training, employed personal trainer, head personal trainer, fitness director). Expertise refers to a demographic or specific style of training the candidate has chosen as a primary focus. This can include general fitness, older adults, youth, sport development, physical limitations, prenatal, and many more.
- *References and resources:* References can include two or three individuals who can speak to the candidate's competency, work ethic, and overall nature because they have worked with or previously employed the candidate. Resources can refer to any educational pieces or work experiences the candidate can share to showcase his or her services (e.g., articles published, programs designed and successfully implemented).

A **cover letter** is a brief introduction page that comes with the resume. This page is a longer version of the aforementioned work objective of the resume in which candidates detail their intentions to apply for a specific position. This includes why they are qualified for the position, how they meet the requirements for the position, what experience and added value they can offer to the business, and any other pertinent information that may highlight their abilities. For highly sought-after positions that attract hundreds of applicants (e.g., corporate fitness, management positions), a high-quality cover letter is vitally important because it is often scrutinized to get a more detailed overall impression of the candidate.

Once the resume and cover letter have been created and the application has been completed, the candidate should return the forms in the manner the potential employer prefers. Follow-ups may be needed to confirm receipt of the paperwork, to answer any other questions the potential employer may have, or to schedule an interview (e.g., in person, online via video chat, phone conversation).

Professional Liability Insurance   Typically, employed personal trainers are provided professional and general liability insurance coverage under the umbrella of the employer's insurance plan. Personal trainers should ask if this is indeed the case or if they need to purchase their own coverage. Most insurance plans have some form of coverage for bodily injury (for the employee, the client, or both), property damage, sexual harassment, claims of negligence, loss of personal information, or other legal issues (4). There can be gray areas of coverage depending on the type of insurance purchased by the employer, and the personal trainer may need to purchase additional umbrella coverage if the employer's is found to be incomplete. Personal trainers should review all insurance coverage policies to ensure their protection as an employee is up to date and understood.

Compensation and Benefits   As of July 2020, the annual salary for personal trainers working in the United States ranges from $44,400 and $75,600, with average earnings of $61,600 (6). Most clubs either pay personal trainers a percentage of the client fee or a flat fee for service. Either way, the personal trainer's compensation typically falls within the 40% to 60% range. The Association of Fitness Studios reported that 76% of personal trainers are being compensated hourly versus receiving a salary; of those receiving an hourly wage, 53% are compensated between $20 and $39 per hour (1).

Some facilities offer benefits to qualified employees. Eligibility is typically awarded when the employee obtains full-time status, working 30 to 40 hours per week on a consistent basis. The specific number of hours required to achieve full-time employment status can vary by the state in which the business is located; typically, a consistent number of work hours must be logged in three consecutive months without change. Benefits can include medical insurance, dental insurance, vision insurance, childcare, sick leave, vacation time, continued education, a retirement plan (e.g., a 401(k) account), facility membership (single or family), and other amenities.

Work Duties and Responsibilities   Work duties and responsibilities are dictated by the owner or general manager of the facility and must fall within professional guidelines of the job. Duties and responsibilities vary from facility to facility and can include but are not limited to assessment techniques, coaching cues, exercise progressions, program design blueprints or templates, required uniform and attire, grooming and appearance requirements, scheduled office hours, scheduled floor hours, and scheduled facility management hours (e.g., organizing equipment, folding towels). All duties and responsibilities, however, must follow a code of conduct in which the employee is not asked to do anything that does not fall within standard industry practice (e.g., cleaning restrooms, cleaning windows).

Marketing and Sales Guidelines Employed personal trainers are typically marketed by the facility but have the ability to market their services outside the facility as well (e.g., business cards, flyers, social media) per the facility's approval. Employees typically have sales requirements or financial goals set by their manager. As a general rule, employees may be asked to sell memberships and personal training sessions or packages as part of their job duties. The prices for training services are set by ownership and are typically not negotiable by the personal trainer; thus, personal trainers cannot attempt to undersell other employees or make deals with a client to earn business. In addition, personal trainers may be asked to sell supplements, merchandise (e.g., shirts, foam rollers), and other facility services (e.g., massage, group classes, education courses) as dictated by management.

Techniques for Building a Client Base Organizations use many different business practices and techniques to create business for their personal trainers. Some of these include the following:

- *Working floor hours:* Employee-based personal trainers can perform floor hours at the beginning of their employment, allowing them to earn a minimum hourly rate while interacting with members. Some facilities require that floor hours be worked throughout personal trainers' employment. Personal trainers can use these member interactions to build rapport, find out more about a member's needs and goals, and determine if the member is a potential client. These interactions can include answering questions, offering quick tutorials, spotting a lift, or simply offering casual conversation. Floor hours might also require maintaining the facility and can include folding and stacking towels, wiping down equipment, creating general fitness programs, teaching introductory fitness class, coaching introductory sessions on equipment use, and maintaining the general and overall cleanliness and professionalism of the fitness area.

- *Referral programs:* Referral programs are typically designed and implemented by management in hopes of further developing new business leads and opportunities for their employees. They often include reward incentives (e.g., free T-shirt, training sessions, workout towel and water bottle) for current clients who recruit new customers from their friends, family, or coworkers. Referral programs can include lead-generating events like "bring a friend to work out" day, community or charity events (e.g., food drive), fitness challenges, holiday-themed group workouts, and more. These events, often complimentary, are designed to introduce potential new customers to a health and fitness experience with a personal trainer, showcasing the personal trainer's personality and knowledge.

- *Educational offerings:* Offering educational courses gives members an opportunity to learn about specific health and fitness topics. They also showcase the personal trainer's personality, knowledge, and skill set. Courses can focus on topics such as preventing lower back injuries, improving posture, developing more power in your golf game, reaping the benefits of resistance training, preventing osteoporosis, and more. Educational offerings are a great way to create opportunity for personal trainers to speak directly to their target demographic in hopes of earning new business.

Professional Growth and Development In most cases entry-level personal trainers will work floor hours to earn new business. Often the floor hours are tapered back once the personal trainer obtains and maintains a designated number of client sessions. The personal trainer's regular working schedule is then opened up, facilitating the ability to fill his or her schedule as needed with paid client sessions. Personal trainers can grow their businesses by obtaining more one-on-one clients; offering partner and small group training sessions and group fitness classes; hosting workshops and bootcamps; and so on.

Positive employee performance reviews may lead to higher commission (income) splits, an increase in flat session rates, or health benefits (if the company offers them). Positive reviews may also offer professional advancement opportunities, which could include monies for further education or position promotions such as to head personal trainer, assistant fitness director, fitness director, or assistant general manager.

Independent Contractor Personal Trainers

Independent contractor personal trainers typically run their businesses by one of the following means:

- Opening their own studio or small gym
- Subleasing designated space inside another facility to house and use their own equipment

- Paying rent to use the space and equipment provided in an established facility
- Training clients in their homes or offices

As an independent contractor, personal trainers would have the freedom to set their own rates, select their own work hours, and create their own program designs as best they see fit; however, they also have responsibilities that employees do not have. Liability insurance, business licensing, ongoing expenses of operation (overhead), health benefits, payroll, marketing, referral programs, and facility maintenance are all professional responsibilities that fall on the independent contractor (business owner) in order to operate legally and successfully.

Professional Requirements

Independent contractor personal trainers are required to manage the reporting and filing of taxes, uphold state business codes of conduct, and work within the business laws established by each state. Although not required, personal trainers can take additional steps to elevate their standing within the profession. These include the following:

- Obtaining and maintaining an accredited certified personal training certification
- Obtaining and maintaining accredited first aid, CPR, and automated external defibrillator (AED) certifications
- Earning annual continuing education credits (CECs) or units (CEUs) to maintain a good standing within their certifying agency
- Establishing a professional business entity such as a limited liability corporation (LLC) or sole proprietorship that the business will be insured and operated under
- Obtaining and maintaining in good standing professional liability insurance that will cover themselves, their clients, and all practices inside the facility in which they operate (*Note:* insurance policies are often designated to one specific location and do not travel with the personal trainer.)
- Keeping proper client records including initial interview and consultation packets, assessments, reassessment and review packets, payment information, emergency contact forms, lability waivers, physical activity readiness questionnaires (e.g., PAR-Q+), incident report forms (e.g., injury, complaint), and client termination forms (e.g., end of service)

The Process of Starting a Business

Whether working as an independent contractor in their own building, subleasing space, or renting equipment inside another facility, independent contractor personal trainers are starting their own business. As mentioned previously, independent contractors should consider obtaining a business license to separate their business and personal liabilities before opening. Outside of business licensing, personal trainers must address many other business development considerations before opening their doors to new business.

Creating a business plan detailing how the operation will be financed is vitally important to the business's success. The addition of a timeline can be useful to frame out the progression of the business, including when all financials are received, when equipment will be purchased, when the tenant is granted access to the location, and when the equipment is to be delivered and installed. Standard operating procedures detail daily operating requirements such as the steps for opening, closing, and dealing with emergencies.

Once the basic paperwork, licensing, and finances are completed, the task of designing the facility and purchasing, delivering, and installing the equipment becomes the focus. Purchasing the office supplies, toiletries, cleaning supplies, sweat towels, hydration stations, internet, phone, and security system are also topics to be addressed. The design of initial interview and consultation forms, personal trainer–client agreements, personal trainer–client–facility agreements, liability forms, assessment forms, membership data collection, financial reporting forms (or software), daily workout program designs, and warm-up and cooldown program designs are some other considerations that independent contractor personal trainers (business owners) must consider as part of operating a business at a successful level.

Note: These requirements and suggestions are relevant to independent contractor personal trainers who choose to train within their clients' homes, who sublease or rent from multiple facilities, or who coach clients online. There are multiple business models or combinations of business models in the personal training industry that can be followed; however, they all share similar responsibilities and recommendations for opening, owning, and operating.

Professional Liability Insurance

Independent contractors are responsible for carrying their own **professional liability insurance** when subleasing space or when renting equipment inside another facility. Full facility coverage only safeguards employee-based personal trainers working under the business licensed in the space being used. Independent contractors are operating as their own entity and thus do not (typically) qualify under any other professional liability insurance plans in effect inside the same space.

An independent contractor's insurance should have coverage for the use and function of equipment as well as those who may be injured using it. Professional liability insurance is designed to cover and protect independent contractors, their clients, and their business. Liability and legal issues can occur with overlapping insurance plans because the facility's insurance company and the independent contractor's insurance company can and should differ. Liability for legal action and fault depends on many different factors. Because of the complexities and ranges of legal actions that can occur, it is suggested that independent contractors purchase personalized professional liability insurance plans that cover the demands of their business model; establish themselves as their own entity by registering as an LLC or as a sole proprietor; and obtain and maintain an accredited personal trainer designation and first aid, CPR, and AED certifications.

Compensation and Benefits

Independent contractors are typically compensated by collecting fees from their clients. They are responsible for filing their own taxes (e.g., quarterly, semiannually, annually) and must budget accordingly to be able to pay those taxes. Independent contractors are not employees and therefore have to pay rent for the use of the facility. There are two typical payment options in this regard: Pay the owner for the use of a facility and its available equipment, or pay for the use of a designated space in a gym and bring their own equipment. Independent contractors and the facility owner will typically negotiate and come to an agreement on a flat rate to be paid each month (e.g., $800) or a commission share based on the success of the business (e.g., 30% of their total gross income each month).

Independent contractors are responsible for purchasing their own benefits. Benefits can include medical insurance, dental insurance, vision insurance, and retirement options (e.g., IRA). Independent contractors can also set up their own relief packages, which could include saving funds for sick leave, vacation time, paid time off, continued education, and other professional development opportunities.

Work Duties and Responsibilities

The work duties and responsibilities of an independent contractor typically consist of three primary components. First is the financial agreement made between the personal trainer and facility owner outlining the fee for the use of the facility. Second is the agreement to operate the business within a professional code of conduct outlining the use of legitimate paperwork, payment processing, and record keeping. Third is the agreement to operate the business within a professional code of ethics outlining an assurance to treat clients and coworkers with respect and in a professional manner at all times.

Outside of these requirements, independent contractors have minimal responsibilities to the facility or facility owner because the agreement to be an independent contractor allows the freedom to run the business as they see fit. This includes setting their own prices, providing and managing paperwork, collecting payments, carrying professional liability insurance, selecting and wearing uniforms, and writing workouts.

Marketing and Sales Guidelines

Independent contractors are responsible for their own marketing campaigns and materials. This includes everything from creating and managing their website, local networking, e-marketing campaigns, social media posts, and other publicity-related efforts. Marketing and sales strategies should be geared toward the personal trainer's target demographic. These strategies will be discussed in greater detail later in this appendix.

DETERMINING PERSONAL TRAINING OFFERINGS

When personal training was a new profession, sessions lasted 60 minutes and were typically sold in 10-session packages. Although the goals of clients would vary, the way sessions were packaged and sold was not. Today, leaders in the fitness industry recognize that people prefer a variety of training options and have responded accordingly.

Personal trainer offerings may vary in the following:

- Number of clients in each session
- Length of the sessions
- Focused goals of a package or program
- Combinations of session types included in a program
- Duration of a package or program (number of weeks)
- Number of sessions in a package or program

Number of Clients in Each Session

One-on-one personal training and group fitness classes used to be the only options available to individuals seeking professional supervision. Now several additional options are available. The numbers of participants and the names of these options vary greatly from facility to facility, so personal trainers can define and set their own group size. In general, there is semiprivate training (2-5 participants), small group training (2-15 participants), and large group training or group fitness classes (12+ participants).

Length of the Sessions

As mentioned previously, sessions used to be a standard 60 minutes. Now sessions are offered in a variety of time increments, with 30, 45, and 60 minutes being the most common.

Focused Goals of a Package or Program

Personal trainers can create packages of sessions (of any length) to be sold without a particular predefined goal. This has been a standard for many years, whereby clients buy X number of sessions to work on their individual needs and goals. Personal trainers can also create predefined programs. These typically have a specific goal with set start and end dates, days of the week to be held, time of day, number of participants, and so on. An example might be an eight-week Bridal Conditioning program. It could have a 15-participant maximum enrollment and might include three boot camp–style classes, two resistance training sessions, and one nutrition education class each week. Having a very specific program offering like this makes marketing the program simpler because the personal trainer knows exactly who their target market is. Knowing that specific target market helps define where and how to inform people about the program.

Combinations of Session Types

When putting together a specific program, a personal trainer needs to consider if a single session type is sufficient or if a mix of session types would give the client the best results. For example, a personal trainer who wants to offer a Zero to 5K program might decide the client would be best served by three 30-minute walk/run sessions per week. Alternatively, the personal trainer may decide the client would be better served by doing two 30-minute walk/run sessions, two 30-minute resistance training sessions, and one 60-minute walk/run small group session. Ultimately, the personal trainer should choose the most effective combination of offerings for each program. Then, the personal trainer can set the price of the program based on that structure.

Duration of a Package or Program

This is simply the number of weeks the program will run. It should be long enough to attain the desired results, but not so long that it seems too big a time commitment to the client. Many programs run in the 4-week to 12-week range.

Number of Sessions in a Package or Program

Ultimately, when pricing a package or program, the personal trainer needs to consider the type and number of sessions for the whole program, however long it runs.

SETTING APPROPRIATE PRICING

Setting prices for the services a personal trainer offers is not a simple process and there is no one best approach. Personal trainers must consider a number of variables in order to come up with the appropriate prices for their offerings.

It is important to note that what clients are charged is not the same as what the personal trainer is compensated. As mentioned previously, most clubs either pay personal trainers a percentage of the client fee or a flat fee falling between 40% and 60% of the service cost. Even when working as independent contractors or sole proprietors, it would be prudent for personal trainers to use a payroll service and pay themselves only a certain percentage, withhold estimated taxes, and save the remainder to go toward business expenses and maintaining a positive cash flow. Table 1 (1, 2, 3, 7) lists examples of personal trainer compensation; of those, only IDEA (7) listed average client session rates.

A personal trainer may decide that semiprivate or small group training may be the best offering for his or her target market. The structure of these offerings can vary greatly as well as the pricing and personal trainer compensation. A general guideline for determining an appropriate price would be to base the group price on a percentage of what is being charged for one-on-one sessions. Since the client gets less personal attention, they necessarily should pay less. Often this works out to be between 60% and 75% of the price of a one-on-one session. The more clients are added to the session, the smaller the percentage can be, but personal trainers need to understand they are not simply splitting that cost among the participants. Training more clients at the same time is more challenging for the personal trainer; thus the personal trainer, as well as the club or studio, should earn more for that session.

Setting one-on-one personal training prices is not as simple as extrapolating fees from the national averages seen in table 1. Rather, the personal trainer needs to consider other factors that affect pricing. These include the following (5):

- Operating expenses
- Target market
- Competition
- Unique selling proposition
- Perceived value
- Self-value
- Time

TABLE 1 Examples of Personal Training Session Rates and Compensation

	Bureau of Labor Statistics (BLS)	Association of Fitness Studios (AFS)	International Health, Racquet & Sportsclub Association (IHRSA)	IDEA Health & Fitness Association
Reporting year	2019	2018	2015	2015
Average client session rates				
30 min				$37.50
45 min				$51.50
60 min				$60.75
90 min				$90.25
Personal trainer compensation (per hour)	$19.42*	$20-$39	$29.55	$30.50
Reference	(2)	(1)	(3)	(7)

*This is a combination of both personal trainers' and group fitness instructors' average hourly rate.

Operating Expenses

One of the major considerations in pricing is that once a personal trainer has built his or her business to a desired workload (that could be 30 training hours per week), the associated income should cover all expenses and provide enough additional income for the personal trainer to live the kind of life he or she wishes. This means the prices of the chosen offerings need to be high enough to cover the costs of equipment, rent, utilities, transportation, licensing fees, marketing expenses, payroll, and whatever else may be needed. If the prices of the offerings do not cover these expenses, then they have been set too low.

Target Market

Whatever target market the personal trainer has chosen, those individuals need to be able to afford the services offered. This means that if the personal trainer has chosen to work with the underprivileged or low-income individuals, the offering has to be low enough for that population to be able to afford it. This can be challenging because choosing a low-priced model may not allow the personal trainer to cover operating costs and payroll. This may necessitate transition from offering one-on-one sessions to small group alternatives in order to keep prices down while allowing the personal trainer to earn a fair wage.

Competition

Although fees charged by the competition should not necessarily dictate what a personal trainer decides to charge, it does help to know what the current market supports as a "normal" price. If a personal trainer perceives his or her services to be equal to or better than the competition, the competition's fees can serve as a minimal pricing option. A personal trainer who decides to charge more than the competition should be able to justify why his or her services are worth the higher price.

Unique Selling Proposition

A personal trainer's **unique selling proposition,** often referred to as a USP, is what differentiates him or her from the competition, and it may also be what makes him or her stand out to the target market. A personal trainer's credentials and experience might set him or her above the competition, but so will a high level of service and a caring attitude. The personal trainer's niche and expertise may create a greater drawing card for potential clients. Looking back to the example of a personal trainer who specializes in golf conditioning for women over 50 years old, that particular market is very specific. A USP like that can help catch the attention of that target market.

Perceived Value

This factor ties in closely to what the personal trainer's competition charges and his or her USP. As mentioned previously, a personal trainer does not need to charge what the competition does; however, what the competition charges may set a perceived value on personal training services. This is why many clubs, studios, and personal trainers do not give specific prices over the phone. If a potential client only hears price and cannot experience the value, the choice of who they use may come down to who offers the lowest price. Here is when it is critical to show the personal trainer's USP so that the potential client understands why these services may be worth more. Most people also understand that specialists, in all fields, may cost more than a generalist, and personal trainers with expertise in a particular area tend to have a higher perceived value than those who do not.

Self-Value

A personal trainer's perceived value by potential clients is important, but so is the personal trainer's own sense of value. This is important for setting pricing for a couple of reasons. Personal trainers who set prices that are lower than their perception of worth will never be happy with the day-to-day delivery of services. The same will be true if the set prices are more than the personal trainer perceives he or she is worth. This personal trainer will feel guilty, believing the price is higher than the value. Unfortunately, this feeling of the price being higher than the value is often based in the mindset of pricing strictly for the time with the client as opposed to pricing for the expertise the personal trainer offers the client.

Time

There are a limited number of hours in a day that a personal trainer can work. Within a given working week, a personal trainer needs to generate enough income to meet expenses and personal income needs. Personal trainers can typically choose how many hours per week they work, but the fewer the hours worked, the more money they need to make per hour. There are also nontraining hours that need to be planned for within the pricing model, including transportation time and expenses (e.g., gas, public transportation fees) as well as session planning time.

With all of these variables taken into consideration, personal trainers should be able to create initial programs and pricing structures that will work with their business models. Once these are set, the personal trainer can move on to how to market and sell the programs.

MARKETING PERSONAL TRAINING SERVICES

Marketing is the process that brings a target market from awareness of products or services to becoming a customer or client. For the personal trainer, marketing begins by understanding the target clients. What do they like to do? Where do they like to go? What do they read? Where do they get their information? The answers to questions like these will help the personal trainer locate potential clients. For example, if a personal trainer seeks to train women golfers over 50, connecting with country clubs,

golf courses, golf instructors, golf publications, and so on can be an inroad to creating relationships with that demographic. Businesses, organizations, and publications are unlikely to simply give personal trainers access to their members, clients, or readership. Businesses and individuals want to do business with those they know, like, and trust. So personal trainers must find ways to build appropriate relationships.

No matter what method of marketing is used, the key to getting potential clients to know, like, and trust a personal trainer is to create a relationship with them. With this in mind, personal trainers should seek to help where they can, answer questions whenever possible, and provide value to potential clients before they try to sell their services.

Meeting Face to Face

There are many ways for a personal trainer to connect with the target market. One of the most effective ways is to meet potential clients in person. It is said that a picture is worth a thousand words, but video tells a bigger story. With the ability to see and hear an individual's expressions, mannerisms, and voice, viewers can get an even greater sense of who someone is. Meeting up in person goes one step farther than video because now there can be a conversation between people. This makes meeting face to face the best way for a personal trainer to maximize the opportunity to connect and build a relationship.

There are a number of ways a personal trainer can accomplish face-to-face meetings. The personal trainer can do the following:

- Join organizations that serve the target market.
- Volunteer for those organizations. This can be in the form of volunteering for fundraisers or charity events or offering to do a presentation or workshop on a topic of interest for them.
- Attend and network at public events that the personal trainer's target market will also attend.
- Create an event that the target market would be interested in attending. This could include a charity event, an open house, a presentation, a workshop, or even just a social gathering.

Connecting Online

Although it may not be as effective as meeting in person, personal trainers can connect to their target markets through social media and email. Some online tools are popular with one demographic and not with another. Personal trainers should be selective and focus on the most popular ones for their specific demographic. Once again, the personal trainer should seek out pages and groups that are popular with the target demographic as well as key individuals who can help act as connectors. In the case of the women golfers over 50, this might be golf course owners and managers, golf instructors, and even caddies.

UNDERSTANDING AND IMPLEMENTING SALES

For the sake of this section, marketing is considered as all actions that inform and create interest in potential clients up to the point that they meet with the personal trainer or salesperson. **Selling** is the sum of the interactions that lead up to a financial commitment for services by the clients.

Misunderstanding Sales

One hurdle facing many personal trainers comes from the belief that selling is somehow disreputable. With that notion in mind, personal trainers also often feel they should not have to sell. Both of these viewpoints can make it challenging to acquire new clients. The sales process is critical for getting a commitment from a potential client, and it is actually very simple and natural once the personal trainer understands the process.

The Sales Process

The ideal opportunity for personal trainers to sell their services is during the initial meeting or consultation with the potential client. The review of a medical health history, lifestyle questionnaire, and individual goals is a time of discovery. If the personal trainer is not in a location where holding that interview is possible or does not have the time at that moment, an effort should be made to set up a meeting in the future. For example, people may approach a personal trainer at a social gathering or at the grocery store, where it would be inappropriate to hold an in-depth interview. In such cases, the personal trainer should seek to set up an interview appointment with the potential client.

The Components of a Client Consultation

A **client consultation** is usually the first opportunity for a personal trainer to get to know the prospective client. This meeting, if performed properly, has the potential to help the individual get started on a journey toward better health and fitness. However, if the meeting is performed improperly, it could turn potential clients off on the idea of getting professional assistance, which could lead them to struggle and fail in reaching their goals. Personal trainers should practice the skills needed for the various components of the consultation.

The Greeting

First impressions do matter, and the personal trainer should do his or her best to make the potential client feel comfortable. The personal trainer should greet the potential client warmly, with a gentle smile and direct eye contact that matches the pressure the individual exerts. The personal trainer should then guide the prospective client to a private area where the consultation will take place. The individual should be invited to relax in a seat and get comfortable.

The Interview

Once the individual gets comfortable, the personal trainer should ask him or her to fill out the appropriate medical health history and lifestyle questionnaire. The interview is an opportunity for the personal trainer to find out as much as possible about the potential client's medical health and fitness status, lifestyle behaviors, and habits, and to help clarify his or her goals. It is also a time to create rapport with the individual. This is accomplished by listening intently while using active listening techniques, such as offering acknowledgement like "I see" or "Yes" and verbally paraphrasing or repeating key points, such as, "So, you want to lower your cholesterol level." The personal trainer should also ask open-ended questions that invite the potential client to talk more about a topic (e.g., "How would your life be different if you reached your goal?"). The personal trainer's act of listening and the individual's sense of "being heard" set up a trusting relationship.

The Recommendation

After concluding the interview portion of the consultation, the personal trainer will be able to make a well-informed recommendation as to the potential client's best course of action going forward. This recommendation is based on the information gathered and is the personal trainer's honest opinion as to how to proceed. The personal trainer should explain what program he or she is recommending, with explanations as to how it will solve problems the client may have had in the past and handle obstacles that may come up in the future.

Asking for Client Commitment

After making the recommendation, the personal trainer asks for a commitment from the potential client. This can be as simple as asking, "Does that sound like something you would be interested in?" or "Is this something you'd like to do?"

If the response is "yes," then the personal trainer can follow up with an acknowledgement and suggest moving forward by saying something such as, "That's great! When would you like to get started?" If the personal trainer has explained how the recommendation fit the potential client's needs and goals in a way that demonstrated the value of the program, price may not even come up until it is time to pay for the program.

If the potential client's response is "no," the personal trainer should inquire what it is about the recommendation that is not suitable. Maybe there is a simple clarification that can be made by the personal trainer, but sometimes potential clients believe they can do it on their own. The fact that a prospective client wants to work on his or her own should not upset the personal trainer. Rather, the best thing the personal trainer can do is provide more information, giving the individual the best chance of succeeding; for example, "Okay. If you're going to try this on your own, here are the things you need to keep in mind." Then the personal trainer should list the steps it will take for the potential client to achieve his or her goals. The personal trainer should end the conversation by wishing the person luck and asking if it would be okay to check back in a week to see how things are going. The check-up call serves two purposes. It gives potential clients a week to find out whether they can or cannot do this on their own, and it shows that the personal trainer cares about how they are doing. It is important to note that even when people decide not to work with a personal trainer at the initial consultation, they may change their minds later on, and if the interactions were positive, they may also refer others to that personal trainer.

That is the sales process. It involves creating a relationship with a potential client by delivering a warm greeting, listening actively, asking open-ended questions, making the most appropriate recommendation, and asking for a confirmation that the individual wants to take part. This process is the best way a personal trainer can help someone in need of guidance, and personal trainers should look forward to those opportunities.

CONCLUSION

It is essential that personal trainers be knowledgeable in exercise science and programming to effectively help their clients reach their health and wellness goals. It is also essential that personal trainers understand the business side of personal training. Without that, no matter how good at fitness programming they are, they will have difficulty getting clients and building a career as a personal trainer.

Determining a target demographic is a great start that will help guide the personal trainer on many of the decisions that follow. Based on who the personal trainer wants to work with, he or she can then choose the work status (employee or independent contractor) and work environment (type of facility) that best suits the chosen career direction. Regardless of whether the personal trainer decides to work as an employee or become an independent contractor, he or she will need to adapt to each scenario and its own unique duties and responsibilities.

Working as an employee most often means the choice of types of services and prices are up to the facility owner or manager. As an independent contractor, the personal trainer will need to decide what type of session or program to offer clients and what the pricing structure will look like. No matter what work environment the personal trainer chooses, building a business relies on the ability to build relationships with the target demographic. The personal trainer then needs to be able to create an opportunity to sit down with potential clients; learn about their needs, wants, and past obstacles; and devise a recommendation as to the best course of action to reach the desired goals. Once the recommendation is presented, the personal trainer then asks for a commitment from the individual to complete the sale.

Knowing business basics is just the beginning. Just like knowing the basics of exercise science, personal trainers need to commit to ongoing learning in all areas that will make them better, more effective personal trainers.

Study Questions

1. In which business model are facilities typically independently owned and operated (i.e., not a franchise)?

   A. commercial gyms

   B. corporate fitness facilities

   C. fitness studios

   D. not-for-profit and community centers

2. Which of the following is *incorrect* regarding marketing and sales guidelines at an employee-based facility?

   A. Personal trainers may be asked to sell supplements.

   B. Personal trainers can earn extra business by reducing personal training prices below those of their colleagues.

   C. Employees typically have sales requirements or financial goals.

   D. Personal trainers are typically marketed by the facility but have the ability to market their services outside the facility as well.

3. What is generally the most popular length (in minutes) of a personal training session?

   A. 20

   B. 30

   C. 45

   D. 60

4. _____ is the sum of the interactions that lead up to a financial commitment for services by the clients.

   A. Advertising

   B. Marketing

   C. Selling

   D. Branding

5. Which of the following statements about being a personal trainer is *incorrect*?

   A. A personal trainer must determine a target demographic.

   B. Working as an employee most often means that the choice of types of services and their prices are up to the facility owner or manager.

   C. If working as an independent contractor, the personal trainer will need to decide what type of session or program to offer clients and what the pricing structure will look like.

   D. Being knowledgeable regarding exercise science is all a personal trainer needs to be successful.

ANSWERS TO STUDY QUESTIONS

Chapter 1
1. A; 2. A; 3. D; 4. A; 5. B

Chapter 2
1. C; 2. D; 3. C; 4. B; 5. D

Chapter 3
1. C; 2. B; 3. C; 4. B; 5. C

Chapter 4
1. D; 2. A; 3. B; 4. C; 5. C

Chapter 5
1. B; 2. B; 3. B; 4. A; 5. B

Chapter 6
1. A; 2. A; 3. A; 4. D; 5. C

Chapter 7
1. B; 2. A; 3. B; 4. C; 5. B

Chapter 8
1. D; 2. D; 3. B; 4. D; 5. B

Chapter 9
1. C; 2. C; 3. C; 4. B; 5. C

Chapter 10
1. B; 2. C; 3. C; 4. C; 5. C

Chapter 11
1. C; 2. B; 3. B; 4. A; 5. A

Chapter 12
1. B; 2. B; 3. D; 4. B; 5. B

Chapter 13
1. A; 2. C; 3. A; 4. D; 5. A

Chapter 14
1. D; 2. D; 3. B; 4. D; 5. A

Chapter 15
1. A; 2. D; 3. C; 4. D; 5. A

Chapter 16
1. C; 2. B; 3. B; 4. B; 5. C

Chapter 17
1. D; 2. B; 3. B; 4. C; 5. B

Chapter 18
1. D; 2. A; 3. C; 4. C; 5. B

Chapter 19
1. C; 2. C; 3. C; 4. B; 5. B

Chapter 20
1. D; 2. D; 3. D; 4. C; 5. B

Chapter 21
1. D; 2. D; 3. D; 4. A; 5. C

Chapter 22
1. A; 2. D; 3. B; 4. D; 5. B

Chapter 23
1. B; 2. B; 3. C; 4. D; 5. C

Chapter 24
1. A; 2. A; 3. C; 4. C; 5. B

Chapter 25
1. D; 2. B; 3. D; 4. C; 5. B

Appendix
1. C; 2. B; 3. D; 4. C; 5. D

REFERENCES

Chapter 1

1. Beck, TW, Housh, TJ, Johnson, GO, Schmidt, RJ, Housh, DJ, Coburn, JW, Malek, MH, and Mielke, M. Effects of a protease supplement on eccentric exercise-induced markers of delayed-onset muscle soreness and muscle damage. *J Strength Cond Res* 21: 661-667, 2007.

1a. Behnke, RS. *Kinetic Anatomy.* 3rd ed. Champaign, IL: Human Kinetics, 2012.

2. Cheung, K, Hume, P, and Maxwell, L. Delayed onset muscle soreness: Treatment strategies and performance factors. *Sports Med* 33: 145-164, 2003.

3. Colliander, EB, and Tesch, PA. Effects of eccentric and concentric muscle actions in resistance training. *Acta Physiol Scand* 140: 31-39, 1990.

4. Conroy, BP, Kraemer, WJ, Maresh, CM, Fleck, SJ, Stone, MH, Fry, AC, Miller, PD, and Dalsky, GP. Bone mineral density in elite junior Olympic weightlifters. *Med Sci Sports Exerc* 25: 1103-1109, 1993.

5. Duncan, CS, Blimkie, CJ, Cowell, CT, Burke, ST, Briody, JN, and Howman-Giles, R. Bone mineral density in adolescent female athletes: relationship to exercise type and muscle strength. *Med Sci Sports Exerc* 34: 286-294, 2002.

6. Hawkins, SA, Schroeder, ET, Wiswell, RA, Jaque, SV, Marcell, TJ, and Costa, K. Eccentric muscle action increases site-specific osteogenic response. *Med Sci Sports Exerc* 31: 1287-1292, 1999.

7. Henneman, E, Somjen, G, and Carpenter, DO. Functional significance of cell size in spinal motoneurons. *J Neurophysiol* 28: 560-580, 1965.

8. Higbie, EJ, Cureton, KJ, Warren III, GL, and Prior, BM. Effects of concentric and eccentric training on muscle strength, cross-sectional area, and neural activation. *J Appl Physiol* 81: 2173-2181, 1996.

9. Huxley, HE. The mechanism of muscular contraction. *Science* 164: 1356-1365, 1969.

9a. Kenney, WL, Wilmore, JH, and Costill, DL. *Physiology of Sport and Exercise.* 7th ed. Champaign, IL: Human Kinetics, 2020.

10. Knight, CA, and Kamen, G. Adaptations in muscular activation of the knee extensor muscles with strength training in young and older adults. *J Electromyogr Kinesiol* 11: 405-412, 2001.

11. Leong, B, Kamen, G, Patten, C, and Burke, JR. Maximal motor unit discharge rates in the quadriceps muscles of older weight lifters. *Med Sci Sports Exerc* 31: 1638-1644, 1999.

12. Milner-Brown, HS, Stein, RB, and Yemm, R. Changes in firing rate of human motor units during linearly changing voluntary contractions. *J Physiol* 230: 371-390, 1973.

13. Nguyen, D, Brown, LE, Coburn, JW, Judelson, DA, Eurich, AD, Khamoui, AV, and Uribe, BP. Effect of delayed-onset muscle soreness on elbow flexion strength and rate of velocity development. *J Strength Cond Res* 23: 1282-1286, 2009.

14. Schroeder, ET, Hawkins, SA, and Jaque, SV. Musculoskeletal adaptations to 16 weeks of eccentric progressive resistance training in young women. *J Strength Cond Res* 18: 227-235, 2004.

15. Triplett, NT. Structure and function of body systems, In *Essentials of Strength Training and Conditioning.* 4th ed. Haff, GG, and Triplett, NT, eds. Champaign, IL: Human Kinetics, 1-18, 2016.

Chapter 2

1. Guyton, AC, and Hall, JE. *Textbook of Medical Physiology.* Philadelphia: Elsevier Saunders, 2006.

2. Kenney, WL, Wilmore, JH, and Costill, DL. *Physiology of Sport and Exercise.* 7th ed. Champaign, IL: Human Kinetics, 2020.

3. Nelson, DL, and Cox, MM. *Lehninger Principles of Biochemistry.* New York: W.H. Freeman, 2008.

3a. Triplett, NT. Structure and function of body systems. In *Essentials of Strength and Conditioning.* 4th ed. Haff, GG, and Triplett, NT, eds. Champaign, IL: Human Kinetics, 1-18, 2016.

4. Wagner, PD. Determinants of maximal oxygen transport and utilization. *Annu Rev Physiol* 58:21-50, 1996.

5. West, JB. *Respiratory Physiology: The Essentials.* Philadelphia: Wolters Kluwer Health/Lippincott Williams & Wilkins, ix., 2008.

Chapter 3

1. Achten, J, and Jeukendrup, AE. Maximal fat oxidation during exercise in trained men. *Int J Sports Med* 24:603-608, 2003.

2. Alghannam, AF, Gonzalez, JT, and Betts, JA. Restoration of muscle glycogen and functional capacity: Role of post-exercise carbohydrate and protein co-ingestion. *Nutrients* 10:253, 2018.

3. Baker, JS, McCormick, MC, and Robergs, RA. Interaction among skeletal muscle metabolic energy systems during intense exercise. *J Nutr Metab*, 2010. [e-pub]

4. Brooks, GA, Fahey, TD, and Baldwin, KM. *Exercise Physiology: Human Bioenergetics and Its Applications.* 4th ed. New York: Wiley, 31-42, 59-180, 213-240, 2005.

5. Brooks, GA, and Mercier, J. Balance of carbohydrate and lipid utilization during exercise: The "crossover" concept. *J Appl Physiol* 76:2253-2261, 1994.

6. Burke, DG, Chilibeck, PD, Parise, G, Candow, DG, Mahoney, D, and Tarnopolsky, M. Effect of creatine and weight training on muscle creatine and performance in vegetarians. *Med Sci Sports Exerc* 35:1946-1955, 2003.

7. Butts, J, Jacobs, B, and Silvis, M. Creatine use in sports. *Sports Health* 10:31-34, 2018.

7a. Cramer, JT. Bioenergetics of Exercise and Training, In *Essentials of Strength Training and Conditioning.* 3rd ed. Baechle, TR, and Earle, RW, eds. Champaign, IL: Human Kinetics, 41-64, 2008.

8. DeBold, EP. Recent insights into muscle fatigue at the cross-bridge level. *Frontiers Physiol* 3, 2012. [e-pub]

9. Emhoff, CW, Messonnier, LA, Horning, MA, Fattor, JA, Carlson, TJ, and Brooks, GA. Gluconeogenesis and hepatic glycogenolysis during exercise at the lactate threshold. *J Appl Physiol* 114:297-306, 2013.

10. Gastin, PB. Energy system interaction and relative contribution during maximal exercise. *Sports Med* 31:725-741, 2001.

11. Goforth, HW Jr, Laurent, D, Prusaczyk, WK, Schneider, KE, Petersen, KF, and Shulman, GI. Effects of depletion exercise and light training on muscle glycogen supercompensation in men. *Am J Physiol Endocrinol Metab* 285:E1304-1311, 2003.

12. Ghosh, AK. Anaerobic threshold: Its concept and role in endurance sport. *Malaysian J Med Sci* 11:24-36, 2004.

12a. Herda, TJ, and Cramer, JT. Bioenergetics of Exercise and Training, In *Essentials of Strength Training and Conditioning.* 4th ed. Haff, GG, and Triplett, NT, eds. Champaign, IL: Human Kinetics, 43-63, 2016.

12b. Kenney, WL, Wilmore, JH, and Costill, DL. *Physiology of Sport and Exercise.* 7th ed. Champaign, IL: Human Kinetics, 2020.

13. Knuiman, P, Hopman MTE, and Mensink, M. Glycogen availability and skeletal muscle adaptations with endurance and resistance exercise. *Nutr Metab* 12, 2015. [e-pub]

14. Kreider, RB, Kalman, DS, Antonio, J, Ziegenfuss, TN, Wildman, R, Collins, R, Candow, DG, Kleiner, SM, Almada, AL, and Lopez, HL. International Society of Sports Nutrition position stand: Safety and efficacy of creatine supplementation in exercise, sport, and medicine. *J Int Soc Sports Nutr* 14:18, 2017. [e-pub]

15. Levenhagen, DK, Gresham, JD, Carlson, MG, Maron, DJ, Borel, MJ, and Flakoll, PJ. Postexercise nutrient intake timing in humans is critical to recovery of leg glucose and protein homeostasis. *Am J Physiol Endocrinol Metab* 280:E982-993, 2001.

16. Purdom, T, Kravitz, L, Dokladny, K, and Mermier, C. Understanding the factors that affect maximal fat oxidation. *J Int Soc Sports Nutr* 15:3, 2018. [e-pub]

17. Rennie, MJ, and Tipton, KD. Protein and amino acid metabolism during and after exercise and the effects of nutrition. *Ann Rev Nutr* 20:457-483, 2000.

18. Robergs, RA, Ghiasvand, F, and Parker, D. Biochemistry of exercise-induced metabolic acidosis. *Am J Physiol: Regul Integr Comp Physiol* 287:R502-516, 2004.

19. Sahlin, K, and Harris, RC. The creatine kinase reaction: A simple reaction with functional complexity. *Amino Acids* 40:1363-1367, 2011.

20. Sahlin, K, Tonkonogi, M, and Soderlund, K. Energy supply and muscle fatigue in humans. *Acta Physiol Scand* 162:261-266, 1998.

21. Spriet, LL. New insights into the interaction of carbohydrate and fat metabolism during exercise. *Sports Med* 44 (Suppl 1):S87-S96, 2014.

22. Stallknecht, B, Vissing, J, and Galbo, H. Lactate production and clearance in exercise. Effects of training: A mini review. *Scand J Med Sci Sports* 8:127-131, 1998.

23. Tipton, KD, and Wolfe, RR. Exercise-induced changes in protein metabolism. *Acta Physiol Scand* 162:377-387, 1998.

Chapter 4

1. An, KN, Hui, FC, Morrey, BF, Linscheid, RL, and Chao, EY. Muscles across the elbow joint: A biomechanical analysis. *J Biomech* 14(10):659-661, 1981.

2. Andersen, LL, Andersen, JL, Magnusson, SP, Suetta, C, Madsen, JL, Christensen, LR, and Aagaard, P. Changes in the human muscle force-velocity relationship in response to resistance training and subsequent detraining. *J Appl Physiol* 99(1):87-94, 1985.

3. Bassett, RW, Browne, AO, Morrey, BF, and An, KN. Glenohumeral muscle force and moment mechanics in a position of shoulder instability. *J Biomech* 23(5):405-415, 1990.

4. Blackard, DO, Jensen, RL, and Ebben, WP. Use of EMG analysis in challenging kinetic chain terminology. *Med Sci Sports Exerc* 31(3):443-448, 1999.

5. Bodine, SC, Roy, RR, Eldred, E, and Edgerton, VR. Maximal force as a function of anatomical features of motor units in the cat tibialis anterior. *J Neurophysiol* 57(6):1730-1745, 1987.

6. Bosco, C, Viitasalo, JT, Komi, PV, and Luhtanen, P. Combined effect of elastic energy and myoelectrical potentiation during stretch-shortening cycle exercise. *Acta Physiol Scand* 114(4):557-565, 1982.

7. Caulfield, BS, and Berninger, D. Exercise technique for free weight and machine training, In *Essentials of Strength Training and Conditioning.* 4th ed. Haff, GG, and Triplett, NT, eds. Champaign, IL: Human Kinetics, 351-408, 2016.

8. Chiu, LZ, and Salem, GJ. Comparison of joint kinetics during free weight and flywheel resistance exercise. *J Strength Cond Res* 20(3):555-562, 2006.

9. Elliott, BC, Wilson, GJ, and Kerr, GK. A biomechanical analysis of the sticking region in the bench press. *Med Sci Sports Exerc* 21(4):450-462, 1989.

10. Enoka, RM. *Neuromechanical Basis of Human Movement.* Champaign, IL: Human Kinetics, 1994.

11. Escamilla, RF, Fleisig, GS, Zheng, N, Barrentine, SW, Wilk, KE, and Andrews, JR. Biomechanics of the knee during closed kinetic chain and open kinetic chain exercises. *Med Sci Sports Exerc* 30(4):556-569, 1998.

12. Finni, T, Ikegawa, S, Lepola, V, and Komi, PV. Comparison of force-velocity relationships of vastus lateralis muscle in isokinetic and in stretch-shortening cycle exercises. *Acta Physiol Scand* 177(4):483-491, 2003.

13. Folland, J, and Morris, B. Variable-cam resistance training machines: Do they match the angle-torque relationship in humans? *J Sports Sci* 26(2):163-169, 2008.

14. Garhammer, J, and McLaughlin, T. Power output as a function of load variation in Olympic and power lifting. *Journal of Biomechanics* 13(2):198, 1980.

15. Harman, E. Resistive torque analysis of 5 nautilus exercise machines. *Journal of Biomechanics* 15(2):113, 1983.

16. Harman, EA, Johnson, M, and Frykman, PN. A movement-oriented approach to exercise prescription. *NSCA Journal* 14(1):47-54, 1992.

17. Hather, BM, Tesch, PA, Buchanan, P, and Dudley, GA. Influence of eccentric actions on skeletal muscle adaptations to resistance training. *Acta Physiol Scand* 143(2):177-185, 1991.

18. Knuttgen, H, and Kraemer, WJ. Terminology and measurement in exercise performance. *J Appl Sport Sci Res* 1(1):1-10, 1987.

19. *Le Système International d'Unités.* Sevres, France: Bureau International des Poids et Mesures, 2006.

20. Lieber, RL. *Skeletal Muscle Structure and Function: Implications for Rehabilitation and Sports Medicine.* Baltimore: Williams & Wilkins, 1992.

21. Maganaris, CN, Baltzopoulos, V, Ball, D, and Sargeant, AJ. In vivo specific tension of human skeletal muscle. *J Appl Physiol* 90(3):865-872, 1985.

22. McBride, J. Biomechanics of Resistance Training, In *Essentials of Strength Training and Conditioning.* 4th ed. Haff, GG, and Triplett, NT, eds. Champaign, IL: Human Kinetics, 19-42, 2016.

23. McGill, SM. *Low Back Disorders: Evidence-Based Prevention and Rehabilitation.* Champaign, IL: Human Kinetics, 2007.

24. Moritani, T, and deVries, HA. Neural factors versus hypertrophy in the time course of muscle strength gain. *Am J Phys Med* 58(3):115-130, 1979.

25. Neumann, DA. *Kinesiology of the Musculoskeletal System: Foundations of Rehabilitation.* St. Louis: Mosby, 2010.

26. Perrin, DH. *Isokinetic Exercise and Assessment.* Champaign, IL: Human Kinetics, 1993.

27. Perrine, JJ, and Edgerton, VR. Muscle force-velocity and power-velocity relationships under isokinetic loading. *Med Sci Sports Exerc* 10(3):159-166, 1978.

28. Simoneau, GG, Bereda, SM, Sobush, DC, and Starsky, AJ. Biomechanics of elastic resistance in therapeutic exercise programs. *J Orthop Sports Phys Ther* 31(1):16-24, 2001.

29. Steindler, LA. *Kinesiology of the Human Body Under Normal and Pathologic Conditions.* Springfield, IL: Charles C Thomas, 63, 1973.

30. Steinkamp, LA, Dillingham, MF, Markel, MD, Hill, JA, and Kaufman, KR. Biomechanical considerations in patellofemoral joint rehabilitation. *Am J Sports Med* 21(3):438-444, 1993.

31. Thein, JM, and Brody, LT. Aquatic-based rehabilitation and training for the elite athlete. *J Orthop Sports Phys Ther* 27(1):32-41, 1998.

32. Thorstensson, A, Karlsson, J, Viitasalo, JH, Luhtanen, P, and Komi, PV. Effect of strength training on EMG of human skeletal muscle. *Acta Physiol Scand* 98(2):232-236, 1976.

33. Whiting, WC, and Rugg, S. *Dynatomy: Dynamic Human Anatomy.* Champaign, IL: Human Kinetics, 2006.

34. Whiting, WC, and Zernicke, RF. *Biomechanics of Musculoskeletal Injury.* Champaign, IL: Human Kinetics, 2008.

35. Zajac, FE, and Gordon, ME. Determining muscle's force and action in multi-articular movement. *Exerc Sport Sci Rev* 17:187-230, 1989

36. Zajac, FE. Muscle coordination of movement: A perspective. *J Biomech* 26(Suppl 1):109-124, 1993.

37. Zatsiorsky, VM. *Kinematics of Human Motion.* Champaign, IL: Human Kinetics, 1998.

Chapter 5

1. American College of Sports Medicine position stand. Osteoporosis and exercise. *Med Sci Sports Exerc* 27:i-vii, 1995.

2. Abe, T, Brechue, WF, Fujita, S, and Brown, JB. Gender differences in FFM accumulation and architectural characteristics of muscle. *Med Sci Sports Exerc* 30:1066-1070, 1998.

3. Ahtiainen, JP, Hulmi, JJ, Kraemer, WJ, Lehti, M, Nyman, K, Selanne, H, Alen, M, Pakarinen, A, Komulainen, J, Kovanen, V, Mero, AA, and Häkkinen, K. Heavy resistance exercise training and skeletal muscle androgen receptor expression in younger and older men. *Steroids* 76:183-192, 2011.

4. Alen, M, Pakarinen, A, Häkkinen, K, and Komi, PV. Responses of serum androgenic-anabolic and catabolic hormones to prolonged strength training. *Int J Sports Med* 9:229-233, 1988.

5. Antonio, J, and Gonyea, WJ. Skeletal muscle fiber hyperplasia. *Med Sci Sports Exerc* 25:1333-1345, 1993.

6. Balshaw, TG, Massey, GJ, Maden-Wilkinson, TM, Lanza, MB, and Folland, JP. Neural adaptations after 4 years vs 12 weeks of resistance training vs untrained. *Scand J Med Sci Sports* 29:348-359, 2019.

7. Bamman, MM, Petrella, JK, Kim, JS, Mayhew, DL, and Cross, JM. Cluster analysis tests the importance of myogenic gene expression during myofiber hypertrophy in humans. *J Appl Physiol (1985)* 102:2232-2239, 2007.

8. Bathgate, KE, Bagley, JR, Jo, E, Talmadge, RJ, Tobias, IS, Brown, LE, Coburn, JW, Arevalo, JA, Segal, NL, and Galpin, AJ. Muscle health and performance in monozygotic twins with 30 years of discordant exercise habits. *Eur J Appl Physiol* 118:2097-2110, 2018.

9. Beck, BR, Daly, RM, Singh, MA, and Taaffe, DR. Exercise and Sports Science Australia (ESSA) position statement on exercise prescription for the prevention and management of osteoporosis. *J Sci Med Sport* 20:438-445, 2017.

10. Bellemare, F, Woods, JJ, Johansson, R, and Bigland-Ritchie, B. Motor-unit discharge rates in maximal voluntary contractions of three human muscles. *J Neurophysiol* 50:1380-1392, 1983.

11. Benli Kucuk, E, Ozyemisci Taskiran, O, Tokgoz, N, and Meray, J. Effects of isokinetic, isometric, and aerobic exercises on clinical variables and knee cartilage volume using magnetic resonance imaging in patients with osteoarthritis. *Turk J Phys Med Rehabil* 64:8-16, 2018.

12. Bickel, CS, Cross, JM, and Bamman, MM. Exercise dosing to retain resistance training adaptations in young and older adults. *Med Sci Sports Exerc* 43:1177-1187, 2011.

12a. Bird, SP, Tarpenning, KM, and Marino, FE. Designing resistance training programmes to enhance muscular fitness. *Sports Med* 35:841-851, 2005.

13. Bishop, P, Cureton, K, and Collins, M. Sex difference in muscular strength in equally-trained men and women. *Ergonomics* 30:675-687, 1987.

14. Booth, FW, Laye, MJ, and Roberts, MD. Lifetime sedentary living accelerates some aspects of secondary aging. *J Appl Physiol (1985)* 111:1497-1504, 2011.

14a. Borde, R, Hortobágyi, T, and Granacher, U. Dose–response relationships of resistance training in healthy old adults: A systematic review and meta-analysis. *Sports Med* 45:1693-1720, 2015.

15. Bouchard, C, Rankinen, T, and Timmons, JA. Genomics and genetics in the biology of adaptation to exercise. *Compr Physiol* 1:1603-1648, 2011.

16. Braith, RW, Graves, JE, Leggett, SH, and Pollock, ML. Effect of training on the relationship between maximal and submaximal strength. *Med Sci Sports Exerc* 25:132-138, 1993.

17. Broeder, CE, Burrhus, KA, Svanevik, LS, and Wilmore, JH. The effects of either high-intensity resistance or endurance training on resting metabolic rate. *Am J Clin Nutr* 55:802-810, 1992.

18. Cadegiani, FA, and Kater, CE. Hormonal aspects of overtraining syndrome: A systematic review. *BMC Sports Sci Med Rehabil* 9:14, 2017.

19. Cardinale, M, and Stone, MH. Is testosterone influencing explosive performance? *J Strength Cond Res* 20:103-107, 2006.

20. Carroll, KM, Bazyler, CD, Bernards, JR, Taber, CB, Stuart, CA, DeWeese, BH, Sato, K, and Stone, MH. Skeletal muscle fiber adaptations following resistance training using repetition maximums or relative intensity. *Sports (Basel)* 7, 2019.

21. Churchward-Venne, TA, Tieland, M, Verdijk, LB, Leenders, M, Dirks, ML, de Groot, LC, and van Loon, LJ. There are no nonresponders to resistance-type exercise training in older men and women. *J Am Med Dir Assoc* 16:400-411, 2015.

22. Clarkson, PM, Devaney, JM, Gordish-Dressman, H, Thompson, PD, Hubal, MJ, Urso, M, Price, TB, Angelopoulos, TJ, Gordon, PM, Moyna, NM, Pescatello, LS, Visich, PS, Zoeller, RF, Seip, RL, and Hoffman, EP. ACTN3 genotype is associated with increases in muscle strength in response to resistance training in women. *J Appl Physiol (1985)* 99:154-163, 2005.

23. Contessa, P, De Luca, CJ, and Kline, JC. The compensatory interaction between motor unit firing behavior and muscle force during fatigue. *J Neurophysiol* 116:1579-1585, 2016.

24. Costill, DL, Daniels, J, Evans, W, Fink, W, Krahenbuhl, G, and Saltin, B. Skeletal muscle enzymes and fiber composition in male and female track athletes. *J Appl Physiol* 40:149-154, 1976.

25. Costill, DL, Fink, WJ, and Pollock, ML. Muscle fiber composition and enzyme activities of elite distance runners. *Med Sci Sports* 8:96-100, 1976.

26. Cotofana, S, Ring-Dimitriou, S, Hudelmaier, M, Himmer, M, Wirth, W, Sanger, AM, and Eckstein, F. Effects of exercise intervention on knee morphology in middle-aged women: A longitudinal analysis using magnetic resonance imaging. *Cells Tissues Organs* 192:64-72, 2010.

27. Couppe, C, Kongsgaard, M, Aagaard, P, Hansen, P, Bojsen-Moller, J, Kjaer, M, and Magnusson, SP. Habitual loading results in tendon hypertrophy and increased stiffness of the human patellar tendon. *J Appl Physiol (1985)* 105:805-810, 2008.

28. Crewther, B, Cronin, J, and Keogh, J. Possible stimuli for strength and power adaptation: Acute metabolic responses. *Sports Med* 36:65-78, 2006.

29. Cullinen, K, and Caldwell, M. Weight training increases fat-free mass and strength in untrained young women. *J Am Diet Assoc* 98:414-418, 1998.

30. Daly, RM, Dalla Via, J, Duckham, RL, Fraser, SF, and Helge, EW. Exercise for the prevention of osteoporosis in postmenopausal women: An evidence-based guide to the optimal prescription. *Braz J Phys Ther* 23:170-180, 2019.

31. Damas, F, Phillips, SM, Libardi, CA, Vechin, FC, Lixandrao, ME, Jannig, PR, Costa, LA, Bacurau, AV, Snijders, T, Parise, G, Tricoli, V, Roschel, H, and Ugrinowitsch, C. Resistance training-induced changes in integrated myofibrillar protein synthesis are related to hypertrophy only after attenuation of muscle damage. *J Physiol* 594:5209-5222, 2016.

32. DeFreitas, JM, Beck, TW, Stock, MS, Dillon, MA, and Kasishke, PR, 2nd. An examination of the time course of training-induced skeletal muscle hypertrophy. *Eur J Appl Physiol* 111:2785-2790, 2011.

33. Del Vecchio, A, Casolo, A, Negro, F, Scorcelletti, M, Bazzucchi, I, Enoka, R, Felici, F, and Farina, D. The increase in muscle force after 4 weeks of strength training is mediated by adaptations in motor unit recruitment and rate coding. *J Physiol* 597:1873-1887, 2019.

34. DeLuca, CJ. The use of surface electromyography in biomechanics. *J Appl Biomech* 13:135-163, 1997.

35. Dons, B, Bollerup, K, Bonde-Petersen, F, and Hancke, S. The effect of weight-lifting exercise related to muscle fiber composition and muscle cross-sectional area in humans. *Eur J Appl Physiol Occup Physiol* 40:95-106, 1979.

36. Enoka, RM. *Neuromechanical Basis of Kinesiology.* 2nd ed. Champaign, IL: Human Kinetics, 1994.

37. Enoka, RM, and Duchateau, J. Rate coding and the control of muscle force. *Cold Spring Harb Perspect Med* 7, 2017.

38. Farthing, JP, and Chilibeck, PD. The effects of eccentric and concentric training at different velocities on muscle hypertrophy. *Eur J Appl Physiol* 89:578-586, 2003.

39. Fatouros, IG, Kambas, A, Katrabasas, I, Nikolaidis, K, Chatzinikolaou, A, Leontsini, D, and Taxildaris, K. Strength training and detraining effects on muscular strength, anaerobic power, and mobility of inactive older men are intensity dependent. *Br J Sports Med* 39:776-780, 2005.

40. Fiatarone, MA, O'Neill, EF, Ryan, ND, Clements, KM, Solares, GR, Nelson, ME, Roberts, SB, Kehayias, JJ, Lipsitz, LA, and Evans, WJ. Exercise training and nutritional supplementation for physical frailty in very elderly people. *N Engl J Med* 330:1769-1775, 1994.

41. Folland, JP, and Williams, AG. The adaptations to strength training: Morphological and neurological contributions to increased strength. *Sports Med* 37:145-168, 2007.

41a. French, D. Adaptations to anaerobic training programs. In *Essentials of Strength Training and Conditioning.* 4th ed. Haff, GG, and Triplett, NT, eds. Champaign, IL: Human Kinetics, 91, 2016.

42. Frontera, WR, Meredith, CN, O'Reilly, KP, and Evans, WJ. Strength training and determinants of VO$_2$max in older men. *J Appl Physiol (1985)* 68:329-333, 1990.

43. Frontera, WR, Meredith, CN, O'Reilly, KP, Knuttgen, HG, and Evans, WJ. Strength conditioning in older men: Skeletal muscle hypertrophy and improved function. *J Appl Physiol (1985)* 64:1038-1044, 1988.

44. Frontera, WR, Suh, D, Krivickas, LS, Hughes, VA, Goldstein, R, and Roubenoff, R. Skeletal muscle fiber quality in older men and women. *Am J Physiol Cell Physiol* 279:C611-618, 2000.

45. Fry, AC, and Kraemer, WJ. Resistance exercise overtraining and overreaching. Neuroendocrine responses. *Sports Med* 23:106-129, 1997.

46. Fry, AC, Kraemer, WJ, van Borselen, F, Lynch, JM, Marsit, JL, Roy, EP, Triplett, NT, and Knuttgen, HG. Performance decrements with high-intensity resistance exercise overtraining. *Med Sci Sports Exerc* 26:1165-1173, 1994.

47. Fry, AC, Schilling, BK, Staron, RS, Hagerman, FC, Hikida, RS, and Thrush, JT. Muscle fiber characteristics and performance correlates of male Olympic-style weightlifters. *J Strength Cond Res* 17:746-754, 2003.

48. Fry, AC, Webber, JM, Weiss, LW, Harber, MP, Vaczi, M, and Pattison, NA. Muscle fiber characteristics of competitive power lifters. *J Strength Cond Res* 17:402-410, 2003.

49. Garfinkel, S, and Cafarelli, E. Relative changes in maximal force, EMG, and muscle cross-sectional area after isometric training. *Med Sci Sports Exerc* 24:1220-1227, 1992.

50. Gomiero, AB, Kayo, A, Abraao, M, Peccin, MS, Grande, AJ, and Trevisani, VF. Sensory-motor training versus resistance training among patients with knee osteoarthritis: Randomized single-blind controlled trial. *Sao Paulo Med J* 136:44-50, 2018.

51. Grandou, C, Wallace, L, Impellizzeri, FM, Allen, NG, and Coutts, AJ. Overtraining in resistance exercise: An exploratory systematic review and methodological appraisal of the literature. *Sports Med*, 2019.

52. Gratzke, C, Hudelmaier, M, Hitzl, W, Glaser, C, and Eckstein, F. Knee cartilage morphologic characteristics and muscle status of professional weight lifters and sprinters: A magnetic resonance imaging study. *Am J Sports Med* 35:1346-1353, 2007.

53. Graves, JE, Pollock, ML, Leggett, SH, Braith, RW, Carpenter, DM, and Bishop, LE. Effect of reduced training frequency on muscular strength. *Int J Sports Med* 9:316-319, 1988.

54. Green, H, Goreham, C, Ouyang, J, Ball-Burnett, M, and Ranney, D. Regulation of fiber size, oxidative potential, and capillarization in human muscle by resistance exercise. *Am J Physiol* 276:R591-596, 1999.

55. Groennebaek, T, and Vissing, K. Impact of resistance training on skeletal muscle mitochondrial biogenesis, content, and function. *Front Physiol* 8:713, 2017.

56. Häkkinen, K, and Komi, PV. Electromyographic changes during strength training and detraining. *Med Sci Sports Exerc* 15:455-460, 1983.

57. Häkkinen, K, Pakarinen, A, Alen, M, Kauhanen, H, and Komi, PV. Neuromuscular and hormonal adaptations in athletes to strength training in two years. *J Appl Physiol (1985)* 65:2406-2412, 1988.

58. Häkkinen, K, Pakarinen, A, Kraemer, WJ, Newton, RU, and Alen, M. Basal concentrations and acute responses of serum hormones and strength development during heavy resistance training in middle-aged and elderly men and women. *J Gerontol A Biol Sci Med Sci* 55:B95-B105, 2000.

59. Hansen, M, Miller, BF, Holm, L, Doessing, S, Petersen, SG, Skovgaard, D, Frystyk, J, Flyvbjerg, A, Koskinen, S, Pingel, J, Kjaer, M, and Langberg, H. Effect of administration of oral contraceptives in vivo on collagen synthesis in tendon and muscle connective tissue in young women. *J Appl Physiol (1985)* 106:1435-1443, 2009.

60. Haun, CT, Vann, CG, Mobley, CB, Osburn, SC, Mumford, PW, Roberson, PA, Romero, MA, Fox, CD, Parry, HA, Kavazis, AN, Moon, JR, Young, KC, and Roberts, MD. Pre-training skeletal muscle fiber size and predominant fiber type best predict hypertrophic responses to 6 weeks of resistance training in previously trained young men. *Front Physiol* 10:297, 2019.

61. Haun, CT, Vann, CG, Osburn, SC, Mumford, PW, Roberson, PA, Romero, MA, Fox, CD, Johnson, CA, Parry, HA, Kavazis, AN, Moon, JR, Badisa, VLD, Mwashote, BM, Ibeanusi, V, Young, KC, and Roberts, MD. Muscle fiber hypertrophy in response to 6 weeks of high-volume resistance training in trained young men is largely attributed to sarcoplasmic hypertrophy. *PLOS One* 14:e0215267, 2019.

62. Haun, CT, Vann, CG, Roberts, BM, Vigotsky, AD, Schoenfeld, BJ, and Roberts, MD. A critical evaluation of the biological construct skeletal muscle hypertrophy: Size matters but so does the measurement. *Front Physiol* 10:247, 2019.

63. Heden, T, Lox, C, Rose, P, Reid, S, and Kirk, EP. One-set resistance training elevates energy expenditure for 72 h similar to three sets. *Eur J Appl Physiol* 111:477-484, 2011.

64. Henriksen, M, Klokker, L, Graven-Nielsen, T, Bartholdy, C, Schjodt Jorgensen, T, Bandak, E, Danneskiold-Samsoe, B, Christensen, R, and Bliddal, H. Association of exercise therapy and reduction of pain sensitivity in patients with knee osteoarthritis: A randomized controlled trial. *Arthritis Care Res (Hoboken)* 66:1836-1843, 2014.

65. Hermann, A, Holsgaard-Larsen, A, Zerahn, B, Mejdahl, S, and Overgaard, S. Preoperative progressive explosive-type resistance training is feasible and effective in patients with hip osteoarthritis scheduled for total hip arthroplasty—a randomized controlled trial. *Osteoarthritis Cartilage* 24:91-98, 2016.

66. Hickson, RC, Dvorak, BA, Gorostiaga, EM, Kurowski, TT, and Foster, C. Potential for strength and endurance training to amplify endurance performance. *J Appl Physiol (1985)* 65:2285-2290, 1988.

67. Hoff, J, Helgerud, J, and Wisloff, U. Maximal strength training improves work economy in trained female cross-country skiers. *Med Sci Sports Exerc* 31:870-877, 1999.

68. Hong, AR, and Kim, SW. Effects of resistance exercise on bone health. *Endocrinol Metab (Seoul)* 33:435-444, 2018.

69. Hornberger, TA. Mechanotransduction and the regulation of mTORC1 signaling in skeletal muscle. *Int J Biochem Cell Biol* 43:1267-1276, 2011.

70. Hortobagyi, T, Houmard, JA, Stevenson, JR, Fraser, DD, Johns, RA, and Israel, RG. The effects of detraining on power athletes. *Med Sci Sports Exerc* 25:929-935, 1993.

71. Hunter, GR, Wetzstein, CJ, Fields, DA, Brown, A, and Bamman, MM. Resistance training increases total energy expenditure and free-living physical activity in older adults. *J Appl Physiol (1985)* 89:977-984, 2000.

72. Ikai, M, and Steinhaus, AH. Some factors modifying the expression of human strength. *J Appl Physiol* 16:157-163, 1961.

73. Jan, MH, Lin, JJ, Liau, JJ, Lin, YF, and Lin, DH. Investigation of clinical effects of high- and low-resistance training for patients with knee osteoarthritis: A randomized controlled trial. *Phys Ther* 88:427-436, 2008.

74. Jenkins, NDM, Miramonti, AA, Hill, EC, Smith, CM, Cochrane-Snyman, KC, Housh, TJ, and Cramer, JT. Greater neural adaptations following high- vs. low-load resistance training. *Front Physiol* 8:331, 2017.

75. Johnson, MB, and Thiese, SM. A review of overtraining syndrome—recognizing the signs and symptoms. *J Athl Train* 27:352-354, 1992.

76. Kongsgaard, M, Aagaard, P, Kjaer, M, and Magnusson, SP. Structural Achilles tendon properties in athletes subjected to different exercise modes and in Achilles tendon rupture patients. *J Appl Physiol (1985)* 99:1965-1971, 2005.

77. Kraemer, WJ, Noble, B, Culver, B, and Lewis, RV. Changes in plasma proenkephalin peptide F and catecholamine levels during graded exercise in men. *Proc Natl Acad Sci U S A* 82:6349-6351, 1985.

78. Kraemer, WJ, and Ratamess, NA. Hormonal responses and adaptations to resistance exercise and training. *Sports Med* 35:339-361, 2005.

79. Kraemer, WJ, Staron, RS, Hagerman, FC, Hikida, RS, Fry, AC, Gordon, SE, Nindl, BC, Gothshalk, LA, Volek, JS, Marx, JO, Newton, RU, and Häkkinen, K. The effects of short-term resistance training on endocrine function in men and women. *Eur J Appl Physiol Occup Physiol* 78:69-76, 1998.

80. Lambert, CP, and Flynn, MG. Fatigue during high-intensity intermittent exercise: Application to bodybuilding. *Sports Med* 32:511-522, 2002.

81. Langberg, H, Rosendal, L, and Kjaer, M. Training-induced changes in peritendinous type I collagen turnover determined by microdialysis in humans. *J Physiol* 534:297-302, 2001.

82. MacDougall, JD, Gibala, MJ, Tarnopolsky, MA, MacDonald, JR, Interisano, SA, and Yarasheski, KE. The time course for elevated muscle protein synthesis following heavy resistance exercise. *Can J Appl Physiol* 20:480-486, 1995.

83. MacDougall, JD, Ray, S, Sale, DG, McCartney, N, Lee, P, and Garner, S. Muscle substrate utilization and lactate production. *Can J Appl Physiol* 24:209-215, 1999.

84. Maclaren, DP, Gibson, H, Parry-Billings, M, and Edwards, RH. A review of metabolic and physiological factors in fatigue. *Exerc Sport Sci Rev* 17:29-66, 1989.

85. Martyn-St James, M, and Carroll, S. Progressive high-intensity resistance training and bone mineral density changes among premenopausal women: Evidence of discordant site-specific skeletal effects. *Sports Med* 36:683-704, 2006.

86. Masuda, K, Masuda, T, Sadoyama, T, Inaki, M, and Katsuta, S. Changes in surface EMG parameters during static and dynamic fatiguing contractions. *J Electromyogr Kinesiol* 9:39-46, 1999.

87. McBride, JM, Triplett-McBride, T, Davie, AJ, Abernethy, PJ, and Newton, RU. Characteristics of titin in strength and power athletes. *Eur J Appl Physiol* 88:553-557, 2003.

88. Merton, PA. Voluntary strength and fatigue. *J Physiol* 123:553-564, 1954.

89. Miller, BF, Olesen, JL, Hansen, M, Dossing, S, Crameri, RM, Welling, RJ, Langberg, H, Flyvbjerg, A, Kjaer, M, Babraj, JA, Smith, K, and Rennie, MJ. Coordinated collagen and muscle protein synthesis in human patella tendon and quadriceps muscle after exercise. *J Physiol* 567:1021-1033, 2005.

90. Milner-Brown, HS, Stein, RB, and Lee, RG. Synchronization of human motor units: Possible roles of exercise and supraspinal reflexes. *Electroencephalogr Clin Neurophysiol* 38:245-254, 1975.

91. Mitchell, CJ, Churchward-Venne, TA, Bellamy, L, Parise, G, Baker, SK, and Phillips, SM. Muscular and systemic correlates of resistance training-induced muscle hypertrophy. *PLoS One* 8:e78636, 2013.

92. Mobley, CB, Haun, CT, Roberson, PA, Mumford, PW, Kephart, WC, Romero, MA, Osburn, SC, Vann, CG, Young, KC, Beck, DT, Martin, JS, Lockwood, CM, and Roberts, MD. Biomarkers associated with low, moderate, and high vastus lateralis muscle hypertrophy following 12 weeks of resistance training. *PLOS One* 13:e0195203, 2018.

93. Moritani, T, and deVries, HA. Neural factors versus hypertrophy in the time course of muscle strength gain. *Am J Phys Med* 58:115-130, 1979.

94. Muddle, TWD, Colquhoun, RJ, Magrini, MA, Luera, MJ, DeFreitas, JM, and Jenkins, NDM. Effects of fatiguing, submaximal high- versus low-torque isometric exercise on motor unit recruitment and firing behavior. *Physiol Rep* 6:e13675, 2018.

95. Mujika, I, and Padilla, S. Muscular characteristics of detraining in humans. *Med Sci Sports Exerc* 33:1297-1303, 2001.

96. Neumann, AJ, Gardner, OF, Williams, R, Alini, M, Archer, CW, and Stoddart, MJ. Human articular cartilage progenitor cells are responsive to mechanical stimulation and adenoviral-mediated overexpression of bone morphogenetic protein 2. *PLOS One* 10:e0136229, 2015.

97. Ni, GX, Zhou, YZ, Chen, W, Xu, L, Li, Z, Liu, SY, Lei, L, and Zhan, LQ. Different responses of articular cartilage to strenuous running and joint immobilization. *Connect Tissue Res* 57:143-151, 2016.

98. Ochiai, S, Watanabe, A, Oda, H, and Ikeda, H. Effectiveness of thermotherapy using a heat and steam generating sheet for cartilage in knee osteoarthritis. *J Phys Ther Sci* 26:281-284, 2014.

99. Ohno, Y, Ando, K, Ito, T, Suda, Y, Matsui, Y, Oyama, A, Kaneko, H, Yokoyama, S, Egawa, T, and Goto, K. Lactate stimulates a potential for hypertrophy and regeneration of mouse skeletal muscle. *Nutrients* 11, 2019.

100. Ohno, Y, Oyama, A, Kaneko, H, Egawa, T, Yokoyama, S, Sugiura, T, Ohira, Y, Yoshioka, T, and Goto, K. Lactate increases myotube diameter via activation of MEK/ERK pathway in C2C12 cells. *Acta Physiol (Oxf)* 223:e13042, 2018.

101. Osternig, LR, Hamill, J, Lander, JE, and Robertson, R. Co-activation of sprinter and distance runner muscles in isokinetic exercise. *Med Sci Sports Exerc* 18:431-435, 1986.

102. Ozaki, H, Loenneke, JP, Thiebaud, RS, and Abe, T. Resistance training induced increase in VO$_2$max in young and older subjects. *Eur Rev Aging Phys A* 10:107-116, 2013.

103. Paavolainen, L, Häkkinen, K, Hamalainen, I, Nummela, A, and Rusko, H. Explosive-strength training improves 5-km running time by improving running economy and muscle power. *J Appl Physiol (1985)* 86:1527-1533, 1999.

104. Parcell, AC, Woolstenhulme, MT, and Sawyer, RD. Structural protein alterations to resistance and endurance cycling exercise training. *J Strength Cond Res* 23:359-365, 2009.

105. Pastor, T, Frohlich, S, Sporri, J, Schreiber, T, and Schweizer, A. Cartilage abnormalities and osteophytes in the fingers of elite sport climbers: An ultrasonography-based cross-sectional study. *Eur J Sport Sci* 20:1-8, 2019.

106. Petersen, SR, Haennel, RG, Kappagoda, CT, Belcastro, AN, Reid, DC, Wenger, HA, and Quinney, HA. The influence of high-velocity circuit resistance training on VO$_2$max and cardiac output. *Can J Sport Sci* 14:158-163, 1989.

107. Philippe, AG, Lionne, C, Sanchez, AMJ, Pagano, AF, and Candau, R. Increase in muscle power is associated with myofibrillar ATPase adaptations during resistance training. *Exp Physiol* 104:1274-1285, 2019.

108. Prince, FP, Hikida, RS, and Hagerman, FC. Human muscle fiber types in power lifters, distance runners and untrained subjects. *Pflugers Arch* 363:19-26, 1976.

109. Psek, JA, and Cafarelli, E. Behavior of coactive muscles during fatigue. *J Appl Physiol (1985)* 74:170-175, 1993.

110. Robergs, RA, Pearson, DR, Costill, DL, Fink, WJ, Pascoe, DD, Benedict, MA, Lambert, CP, and Zachweija, JJ. Muscle glycogenolysis during differing intensities of weight-resistance exercise. *J Appl Physiol (1985)* 70:1700-1706, 1991.

111. Roberts, MD, Haun, CT, Mobley, CB, Mumford, PW, Romero, MA, Roberson, PA, Vann, CG, and McCarthy, JJ. Physiological differences between low versus high skeletal muscle hypertrophic responders to resistance exercise training: Current perspectives and future research directions. *Front Physiol* 9:834, 2018.

112. Roberts, MD, Mobley, CB, Vann, CG, Haun, CT, Schoenfeld, BJ, Young, KC, and Kavazis, AN. Synergist ablation-induced hypertrophy occurs more rapidly in the plantaris than soleus muscle in rats due to different molecular mechanisms. *Am J Physiol Regul Integr Comp Physiol* 318:R360-R368, 2019.

113. Roberts, MD, Romero, MA, Mobley, CB, Mumford, PW, Roberson, PA, Haun, CT, Vann, CG, Osburn, SC, Holmes, HH, Greer, RA, Lockwood, CM, Parry, HA, and Kavazis, AN. Skeletal muscle mitochondrial volume and myozenin-1 protein differences exist between high versus low anabolic responders to resistance training. *PeerJ* 6:e5338, 2018.

114. Roos, EM, and Dahlberg, L. Positive effects of moderate exercise on glycosaminoglycan content in knee cartilage: A four-month, randomized, controlled trial in patients at risk of osteoarthritis. *Arthritis Rheum* 52:3507-3514, 2005.

115. Sale, DG, MacDougall, JD, Upton, AR, and McComas, AJ. Effect of strength training upon motoneuron excitability in man. *Med Sci Sports Exerc* 15:57-62, 1983.

116. Sampson, SL, Sylvia, M, and Fields, AJ. Effects of dynamic loading on solute transport through the human cartilage endplate. *J Biomech* 83:273-279, 2019.

117. Schoenfeld, BJ, Grgic, J, Ogborn, D, and Krieger, JW. Strength and hypertrophy adaptations between low- vs. high-load resistance training: A systematic review and meta-analysis. *J Strength Cond Res* 31:3508-3523, 2017.

118. Schuenke, MD, Mikat, RP, and McBride, JM. Effect of an acute period of resistance exercise on excess post-exercise oxygen consumption: Implications for body mass management. *Eur J Appl Physiol* 86:411-417, 2002.

119. Schwab, R, Johnson, GO, Housh, TJ, Kinder, JE, and Weir, JP. Acute effects of different intensities of weight lifting on serum testosterone. *Med Sci Sports Exerc* 25:1381-1385, 1993.

120. Staron, RS, Karapondo, DL, Kraemer, WJ, Fry, AC, Gordon, SE, Falkel, JE, Hagerman, FC, and Hikida, RS. Skeletal muscle adaptations during early phase of heavy-resistance training in men and women. *J Appl Physiol (1985)* 76:1247-1255, 1994.

121. Staron, RS, Leonardi, MJ, Karapondo, DL, Malicky, ES, Falkel, JE, Hagerman, FC, and Hikida, RS. Strength and skeletal muscle adaptations in heavy-resistance-trained women after detraining and retraining. *J Appl Physiol (1985)* 70:631-640, 1991.

122. Stec, MJ, Kelly, NA, Many, GM, Windham, ST, Tuggle, SC, and Bamman, MM. Ribosome biogenesis may augment resistance training-induced myofiber hypertrophy and is required for myotube growth in vitro. *Am J Physiol Endocrinol Metab* 310:E652-E661, 2016.

123. Sterczala, AJ, Herda, TJ, Miller, JD, Ciccone, AB, and Trevino, MA. Age-related differences in the motor unit action potential size in relation to recruitment threshold. *Clin Physiol Funct Imaging* 38:610-616, 2018.

124. Stock, MS, Mota, JA, DeFranco, RN, Grue, KA, Jacobo, AU, Chung, E, Moon, JR, DeFreitas, JM, and Beck, TW. The time course of short-term hypertrophy in the absence of eccentric muscle damage. *Eur J Appl Physiol* 117:989-1004, 2017.

125. Teichtahl, AJ, Wluka, AE, Forbes, A, Wang, Y, English, DR, Giles, GG, and Cicuttini, FM. Longitudinal effect of vigorous physical activity on patella cartilage morphology in people without clinical knee disease. *Arthritis Rheum* 61:1095-1102, 2009.

126. Tesch, PA, Komi, PV, and Häkkinen, K. Enzymatic adaptations consequent to long-term strength training. *Int J Sports Med* 8 Suppl 1:66-69, 1987.

127. Tesch, PA, Thorsson, A, and Colliander, EB. Effects of eccentric and concentric resistance training on skeletal muscle substrates, enzyme activities and capillary supply. *Acta Physiol Scand* 140:575-580, 1990.

127a. Tesch, PA, Thorsson, A, and Essen-Gustavsson, B. Enzyme activities of FT and ST muscle fibers in heavy-resistance trained athletes. *J Appl Physiol* 67:83-87, 1989.

128. Thalacker-Mercer, A, Stec, M, Cui, X, Cross, J, Windham, S, and Bamman, M. Cluster analysis reveals differential transcript profiles associated with resistance training-induced human skeletal muscle hypertrophy. *Physiol Genomics* 45:499-507, 2013.

129. Thepaut-Mathieu, C, Van Hoecke, J, and Maton, B. Myoelectrical and mechanical changes linked to length specificity during isometric training. *J Appl Physiol (1985)* 64:1500-1505, 1988.

130. Thulkar, J, Singh, S, Sharma, S, and Thulkar, T. Preventable risk factors for osteoporosis in postmenopausal women: Systematic review and meta-analysis. *J Midlife Health* 7:108-113, 2016.

131. Turner, CH, Owan, I, and Takano, Y. Mechanotransduction in bone: Role of strain rate. *Am J Physiol* 269:E438-E442, 1995.

132. Vissing, K, Brink, M, Lonbro, S, Sorensen, H, Overgaard, K, Danborg, K, Mortensen, J, Elstrom, O, Rosenhoj, N, Ringgaard, S, Andersen, JL, and Aagaard, P. Muscle adaptations to plyometric vs. resistance training in untrained young men. *J Strength Cond Res* 22:1799-1810, 2008.

132a. Weir, JP, and Brown, LE. Resistance training adaptations, In *NSCA's Essentials of Personal Training.* 2nd ed. Coburn, JW, and Malek, MH, eds. Champaign, IL: Human Kinetics, 76, 2012.

133. Weir, JP, Housh, DJ, Housh, TJ, and Weir, LL. The effect of unilateral concentric weight training and detraining on joint angle specificity, cross-training, and the bilateral deficit. *J Orthop Sports Phys Ther* 25:264-270, 1997.

134. Weir, JP, Housh, TJ, Evans, SA, and Johnson, GO. The effect of dynamic constant external resistance training on the isokinetic torque-velocity curve. *Int J Sports Med* 14:124-128, 1993.

135. Weir, JP, Housh, TJ, and Weir, LL. Electromyographic evaluation of joint angle specificity and cross-training after isometric training. *J Appl Physiol (1985)* 77:197-201, 1994.

136. Weir, JP, Housh, TJ, Weir, LL, and Johnson, GO. Effects of unilateral isometric strength training on joint angle specificity and cross-training. *Eur J Appl Physiol Occup Physiol* 70:337-343, 1995.

137. Werkhausen, A, Albracht, K, Cronin, NJ, Paulsen, G, Bojsen-Moller, J, and Seynnes, OR. Effect of training-induced changes in Achilles tendon stiffness on muscle-tendon behavior during landing. *Front Physiol* 9:794, 2018.

138. Westh, E, Kongsgaard, M, Bojsen-Moller, J, Aagaard, P, Hansen, M, Kjaer, M, and Magnusson, SP. Effect of habitual exercise on the structural and mechanical properties of human tendon, in vivo, in men and women. *Scand J Med Sci Sports* 18:23-30, 2008.

139. Wiesinger, HP, Kosters, A, Muller, E, and Seynnes, OR. Effects of increased loading on in vivo tendon properties: A systematic review. *Med Sci Sports Exerc* 47:1885-1895, 2015.

140. Wilson, JM, Loenneke, JP, Jo, E, Wilson, GJ, Zourdos, MC, and Kim, JS. The effects of endurance, strength, and power training on muscle fiber type shifting. *J Strength Cond Res* 26:1724-1729, 2012.

141. Woolstenhulme, MT, Conlee, RK, Drummond, MJ, Stites, AW, and Parcell, AC. Temporal response of desmin and dystrophin proteins to progressive resistance exercise in human skeletal muscle. *J Appl Physiol (1985)* 100:1876-1882, 2006.

142. Zhang, YY, Yang, M, Bao, JF, Gu, LJ, Yu, HL, and Yuan, WJ. Phosphate stimulates myotube atrophy through autophagy activation: Evidence of hyperphosphatemia contributing to skeletal muscle wasting in chronic kidney disease. *BMC Nephrol* 19:45, 2018.

Chapter 6

1. Armstrong, LE, and VanHeest, JL. The unknown mechanism of the over-training syndrome: Clues from depression and psychoneuroimmunology. *Sports Med* 32(3):185-209, 2002.

2. Barbier, J, Ville, N, Kervio, G, Walther, G, and Carre, F. Sports-specific features of athlete's heart and their relation to echocardiographic parameters. *Herz* 31(6):531-543, 2006.

3. Bouchard, C, Dionne, FT, Simoneau, JA, and Boulay, MR. Genetics of aerobic and anaerobic performances. *Exerc Sport Sci Rev* 20:27-58, 1992.

4. Broeder, CE, Burrhus, KA, Svanevik, LS, Volpe, J, and Wilmore, JH. Assessing body composition before and after resistance or endurance training. *Med Sci Sports Exerc* 29(5):705-712, 1997.

5. Buckwalter, JA, and Woo, SL-Y. Effects of repetitive motion on the musculoskeletal tissues. In *Orthopaedic Sports Medicine: Principles and Practice.* Vol. 1. DeLee, JC, and Drez, D, eds. Philadelphia: Saunders, 60-72, 1994.

6. Cavanaugh, DJ, and Cann, CE. Brisk walking does not stop bone loss in postmenopausal women. *Bone* 9(4):201-204, 1988.

7. Coggan, AR. Plasma glucose metabolism during exercise in humans. *Sports Med* 11(2):102-124, 1991.

8. Colberg, SR, Albright, A, Blissmer, B, Braun, B, Chasen-Taber, L, Fernhall, B, Regensteiner, J, Rubin, R, and Signal, R. American College of Sports Medicine position stand. Exercise and type 2 diabetes. *Med Sci Sports Exerc* 42(12):2282-2303, 2010.

9. Costill, DL, Fink, WJ, Hargreaves, M, King, DS, Thomas, R, and Fielding, R. Metabolic characteristics of skeletal muscle during detraining from competitive swimming. *Med Sci Sports Exerc* 17(3):339-343, 1985.

10. Coyle, EF, Martin III, WH, Sinacore, DR, Joyner, MJ, Hagberg, JM, and Holloszy, JO. Time course of loss of adaptations after stopping prolonged intense endurance training. *J Appl Physiol* 57(6):1857-1864, 1984.

11. Dart, AM, Meredith, IT, and Jennings, GL. Effects of 4 weeks endurance training on cardiac left ventricular structure and function. *Clin and Exper Pharm and Physiol* 19(11):777-783, 1992.

12. Davies, CT, and Few, JD. Effects of exercise on adrenocortical function. *J Appl Physiol* 35(6):887-891, 1973.

13. Dempsey, JA. J.B. Wolffe memorial lecture. Is the lung built for exercise? *Med Sci Sports Exerc* 18(2):143-155, 1986.

14. Dempsey, JA, Harms, CA, and Ainsworth, DM. Respiratory muscle perfusion and energetics during exercise. *Med Sci Sports Exerc* 28(9):1123-1128, 1996.

15. Donnelly, JE, Blair, SN, Jakicic, JM, Manore, MM, Rankin, JW, and Smith, BK. American College of Sports Medicine position stand. Appropriate physical activity intervention strategies for weight loss and prevention of weight regain for adults. *Med Sci Sports Exerc* 41(2):459-471, 2009.

16. Duncker, DJ, and Bache, RJ. Regulation of coronary blood flow during exercise. *Physiol Rev* 88(3):1009-1086, 2008.

17. Ebeling, P, Bourey, R, Koranyi, L, Tuominen, JA, Groop, LC, Henriksson, J, Mueckler, M, Sovijarvi, A, and Koivisto, VA. Mechanism of enhanced insulin sensitivity in athletes. Increased blood flow, muscle glucose transport protein (GLUT-4) concentration, and glycogen synthase activity. *J Clin Invest* 92(4):1623-1631, 1993.

18. Emter, CA, and Laughlin, MH. Adaptations to cardiorespiratory exercise training. In *ACSM's Resource Manual for Guidelines for Exercise Testing and Prescription.* 7th ed. Swain, DP, ed. Philadelphia: Lippincott Williams & Wilkins, 496-510, 2014.

19. Faude, O, Kindermann, W, and Meyer, T. Lactate threshold concepts: How valid are they? *Sports Med* 39(6):469-490, 2009.

20. Garber, CE, Blissmer, B, Deschenes, M, Franklin, B, Lamonte, M, Lee, I, Nieman, D, and Swain, D. American College of Sports Medicine position stand. Quantity and quality of exercise for developing and maintaining cardiorespiratory, musculoskeletal, and neuromotor fitness in apparently healthy adults: Guidance for prescribing exercise. *Med Sci Sports Exerc* 43(7):1334-1359, 2011.

21. Halson, SL, and Jeukendrup, AE. Does overtraining exist? An analysis of overreaching and overtraining research. *Sports Med* 34(14):967-981, 2004.

22. Harms, CA, Babcock, MA, McClaran, SR, Pegelow, DF, Nickele, GA, Nelson, WB, and Dempsey, JA. Respiratory muscle work compromises leg blood flow during maximal exercise. *J Appl Physiol* 82(5):1573-1583, 1997.

23. Hartley, LH, Mason, JW, Hogan, RP, Jones, LG, Kotchen, TA, Mougey, EH, Wherry, FE, Pennington, LL, and Ricketts, PT. Multiple hormonal responses to graded exercise in relation to physical training. *J Appl Physiol* 33(5):602-606, 1972.

24. Haskell, WL, Lee, IM, Pate, RR, Powell, KE, Blair, SN, Franklin, BA, Macera, CA, Heath, GW, Thompson, PD, and Bauman, A. Physical activity and public health: Updated recommendation for adults from the American College of Sports Medicine and the American Heart Association. *Med Sci Sports Exerc* 39(8):1423-1434, 2007.

25. Hawley, JA, and Lessard, SJ. Exercise training-induced improvements in insulin action. *Acta Physiol* 192(1):127-135, 2008.

26. Hennessy, LC, and Watson, AWS. The interference effects of training for strength and endurance simultaneously. *J Strength Condit Res* 8(1):12-19, 1994.

27. Henriksen, EJ. Invited review: Effects of acute exercise and exercise training on insulin resistance. *J Appl Physiol* 93(2):788-796, 2002.

28. Hickson, RC. Skeletal muscle cytochrome c and myoglobin, endurance, and frequency of training. *J Appl Physiol* 51(3):746-749, 1981.

29. Higginbotham, MB, Morris, KG, Williams, RS, McHale, PA, Coleman, RE, and Cobb, FR. Regulation of stroke volume during submaximal and maximal upright exercise in normal man. *Circ Res* 58(2):281-291, 1986.

30. Holloszy, JO, and Coyle, EF. Adaptations of skeletal muscle to endurance exercise and their metabolic consequences. *J Appl Physiol* 56(4):831-838, 1984.

31. Hoppeler, H. Exercise-induced ultrastructural changes in skeletal muscle. *Int J Sports Med* 7(4):187-204, 1986.

32. Horowitz, JF. Regulation of lipid mobilization and oxidation during exercise in obesity. *Exerc and Sport Sci Rev* 29(1):42-46, 2001.

33. Hughes, JM, Petit, M, and Scibora, L. Exercise prescription for patients with osteoporosis. In *ACSM's Resource Manual for Guidelines for Exercise Testing and Prescription.* 7th ed. Swain, DP, ed. Philadelphia: Lippincott Williams & Wilkins. 699-712, 2014.

34. Hunter, GR, Demment, R, and Miller, D. Development of strength and maximum oxygen uptake during simultaneous training for strength and endurance. *J Sports Med Phys Fit* 27(3):269-275, 1987.

35. Hurley, BF, Nemeth, PM, Martin III, WH, Hagberg, JM, Dalsky, GP, and Holloszy, JO. Muscle triglyceride utilization during exercise: Effect of training. *J Appl Physiol* 60(2):562-567, 1986.

36. Jacks, DE, Sowash, J, Anning, J, McGloughlin, T, and Andres, F. Effect of exercise at three exercise intensities on salivary cortisol. *J Strength Condit Res* 16(2):286-289, 2002.

37. Janicki, JS, Sheriff, DD, Robotham, JL, and Wise, RA. Cardiac output during exercise: Contributions of the cardiac, circulatory, and respiratory systems. In *Section 12: Exercise: Regulation and Integration of Multiple Systems.* Rowell, LB, and Shepherd, JT, eds. New York: Oxford University Press, 651-704, 1996.

38. Jozsa, L, and Kannus, P. *Human Tendons: Anatomy, Physiology, and Pathology.* Champaign, IL: Human Kinetics, 1-574, 1997.

39. Kenney, WL, Wilmore J, and Costill, D. *Physiology of Sport and Exercise.* 7th ed. Champaign, IL: Human Kinetics, 2020.

39a. Kenney, WL, Wilmore J, and Costill, D. *Physiology of Sport and Exercise.* 6th ed. Champaign, IL: Human Kinetics, 2015.

40. Kenney, MJ, and Seals, DR. Postexercise hypotension. Key features, mechanisms, and clinical significance. *Hypertension* 22(5):653-664, 1993.

41. Kiens, B, Essen-Gustavsson, B, Christensen, NJ, and Saltin B. Skeletal muscle substrate utilization during submaximal exercise in man: Effect of endurance training. *J Physiol* 469:459-478, 1993.

42. King, DS, Baldus, PJ, Sharp, RL, Kesl, LD, Feltmeyer, TL, and Riddle, MS. Time course for exercise-induced alterations in insulin action and glucose tolerance in middle-aged people. *J Appl Physiol* 78(1):7-22, 1995.

43. Kohrt, WM, Bloomfield, SA, Little, KD, Nelson, ME, and Yingling VR. American College of Sports Medicine position stand: Physical activity and bone health. *Med Sci Sports Exerc* 36(11):1985-1996, 2004.

44. Kraemer, WJ, Patton, JF, Gordon, SE, Harman, EA, Deschenes, MR, Reynolds, K, Newton, RU, Triplett, NT, and Dziados, JE. Compatibility of high-intensity strength and endurance training on hormonal and skeletal muscle adaptations. *J Appl Physiol* 78(3):976-989, 1995.

45. Laughlin, MH, Korthuis, RJ, Duncker, DJ, and Bache, RJ. Control of blood flow to cardiac and skeletal muscle during exercise. In *Section 12: Exercise: Regulation and Integration of Multiple Systems.* Rowell, LB, and Shepherd, JT, eds. New York: Oxford University Press, 705-769, 1996.

46. Lehmann, M, Foster, C, and Keul, J. Overtraining in endurance athletes: A brief review. *Med Sci Sports Exerc* 25(7):854-862, 1993.

47. Mangine, B, Nuzzo, G, and Harrelson, GL. Physiologic factors of rehabilitation. In *Physical Rehabilitation of the Injured Athlete.* 3rd ed. Andrews, JR, Harrelson, GL, and Wilk, KE, eds. Philadelphia: Saunders, 13-33, 2004.

48. McArdle, WD, Katch, FI, and Katch, VL. *Exercise Physiology: Nutrition, Energy, and Human Performance.* 7th ed. Philadelphia: Lippincott Williams & Wilkins, 94, 136, 138, 163, 162-163, 186, 206, 215, 237, 240, 261, 272, 322, 344, 345, 417, 441, 441-442, 445, 468, 471, 491, 493, 820, 2010.

49. McCarthy, JP, Agre, JC, Graf, BK, Pozniak, MA, and Vailas, AC. Compatibility of adaptive responses with combining strength and endurance training. *Med Sci Sports Exerc* 27(3):429-436, 1995.

50. McCarthy, JP, Pozniak, MA, and Agre, JC. Neuromuscular adaptations to concurrent strength and endurance training. *Med Sci Sports Exerc* 34(3):511-519, 2002.

51. McGuire, DK, Levine, BD, Williamson, JW, Snell, PG, Blomqvist, CG, Saltin, B, and Mitchell, JH. A 30-year follow-up of the Dallas Bedrest and Training Study: II. Effect of age on cardiovascular adaptation to exercise training. *Circulation* 104(12):1358-1366, 2001.

52. Michel, BA, Lane, NE, Bjorkengren, A, Bloch, DA, and Fries, JF. Impact of running on lumbar bone density: A 5-year longitudinal study. *J Rheumatol* 19(11):1759-1763, 1992.

53. Mier, CM, Turner, MJ, Ehsani, AA, and Spina RJ. Cardiovascular adaptations to 10 days of cycle exercise. *J Appl Physiol* 83(6):1900-1906, 1997.

54. Mikines, KJ, Sonne, B, Farrell, PA, Tronier, B, and Galbo, H. Effect of physical exercise on sensitivity and responsiveness to insulin in humans. *Am J Physiol-Endoc M* 254(3):248-259, 1988.

55. Nichols, DL, Sanborn, CF, and Essery, EV. Bone density and young athletic women. An update. *Sports Medicine* 37(11):1001-1014, 2007.

56. Nordin, M, Lorenz, T, and Campello, M. Biomechanics of tendons and ligaments. In *Basic Biomechanics of the Musculoskeletal System.* 3rd ed. Nordin, M, and Frankel, VH, eds. Baltimore: Lippincott, Williams & Wilkins, 102-125. 2001.

57. Ogden, CL, Carroll, MD, Curtin, LR, McDowell, MA, Tabak, CJ, and Flegal, KM. Prevalence of overweight and obesity in the United States, 1999-2004. *J Am Med Assoc* 295(13):1549-1555, 2006.

58. Pescatello, LS, Franklin, BA, Fagard, R, Farquhar, WB, Kelley, GA, and Ray, CA. American College of Sports Medicine position stand. Exercise and hypertension. *Med Sci Sports Exerc* 36(3):533-553, 2004.

59. Plowman, SA, and Smith, DL. *Exercise Physiology for Health, Fitness, and Performance.* 5th ed. Philadelphia: Wolters Kluwer, 499, 501, 503, 2017.

60. Powers, SK, and Howley, ET. *Exercise Physiology: Theory and Application to Fitness and Performance.* 10th ed. New York: McGraw Hill Education, 81, 114-120, 208, 240, 300, 301, 303, 2018.

61. Rasmussen, B, Klausen, K, Clausen, JP, and Trap-Jensen, J. Pulmonary ventilation, blood gases, and blood pH after training of the arms or the legs. *J Appl Physiol* 38(2):250-256, 1975.

62. Rico-Sanz, J, Rankinen, T, Joanisse, DR, Leon, AS, Skinner, JS, Wilmore, JH, Rao, DC, and Bouchard, C. Familial resemblance for muscle phenotypes in the HERITAGE Family Study. *Med Sci Sports Exerc* 35(8):1360-1366, 2003.

63. Rubal, BJ, Al-Muhailani, AR, and Rosentswieg, J. Effects of physical conditioning on the heart size and wall thickness of college women. *Med Sci Sports Exerc* 19(5):423-429, 1987.

64. Saks, V, Dzeja, P, Schlattner, U, Vendelin, M, Terzic, A, and Wallimann, T. Cardiac system bioenergetics: Metabolic basis of the Frank-Starling law. *J Physiol* 571(2):253-273, 2006.

65. Sawka, MN, Convertino, VA, Eichner, ER, Schnieder, SM, and Young, AJ. Blood volume: Importance and adaptations to exercise training, environmental stresses, and trauma/sickness. *Med Sci Sports Exerc* 32(2):332-348, 2000.

66. Scruggs, KD, Martin, NB, Broeder, CE, Hofman, Z, Thomas, EL, Wambsgans, KC, and Wilmore, JH. Stroke volume during submaximal exercise in endurance-trained normotensive subjects and in untrained hypertensive subjects with beta blockade (propranolol and pindolol). *Am J Cardiol* 67(5):416-421, 1991.

67. Shimamura, C, Iwamoto, J, Takeda, T, Ichimura, S, Abe, H, and Toyama, Y. Effect of decreased physical activity on bone mass in exercise-trained young rats. *J Orthop Sci* 7(3):358-363, 2002.

68. Stiegler, P, and Cunliffe, A. The role of diet and exercise for the maintenance of fat-free mass and resting metabolic rate during weight loss. *Sports Med* 36(3):239-262, 2006.

69. Urhausen, A, and Kindermann, W. Diagnosis of overtraining: What tools do we have? *Sports Med* 32(2):95-102, 2002.

70. Vogiatzis, I, Athanasopoulos, D, Boushel, R, Guenette, JA, Koskolou, M, Vasilopoulou, M, Wagner, H, Roussos, C, Wagner, PD, and Zakynthinos, S. Contribution of respiratory muscle blood flow to exercise-induced diaphragmatic fatigue in trained cyclists. *J Physiol* 586(22):5575-5587, 2008.

71. Widdowson, WM, Healy, ML, Sönksen, PH, and Gibney, J. The physiology of growth hormone and sport. *Growth Horm IGF Res* 19(4):308-319, 2009.

72. Wilmore, JH, Stanforth, PR, Hudspeth, LA, Gagnon, J, Daw, EW, Leon, AS, Rao, DC, Skinner, JS, and Bouchard, C. Alterations in resting metabolic rate as a consequence of 20 wk of endurance training: The HERITAGE Family Study. *Am J Clin Nutr* 68(1):66-71, 1998.

73. Zouhal, H, Jacob, C, Delamarche, P, and Gratas-Delamarche, A. Catecholamines and the effects of exercise, training and gender. *Sports Med* 38(5):401-423, 2008.

Chapter 7

1. Ahlborg, B, Bergstrom, J, Brohult, J, Ekelund, L, Hultman, E, and Maschio, G. Human muscle glycogen content and capacity for prolonged exercise after different diets. *Foersvarsmedicine* 3:85-99, 1967.

2. Alabama State Board of Examiners in Dietetics & Nutritionists. Rules and regulations. Title 34: Dietetics / Nutrition Practice Act, chapter 34. www.boed.alabama.gov/rules.aspx. Accessed October 15, 2019.

3. American College of Sports Medicine. Position stand. Exercise and fluid replacement. *Med Sci Sports Exerc* 28:i-vii, 1996.

4. American Dietetic Association. Dietetics practitioner state licensure provisions. 2009. www.eatright.org/ada/files/State_Licensure_Summary_without_dfns_011409.pdf. Accessed April 30, 2010.

5. Antonio, J, Ellerbroek, A, Silver, T, Orris, S, Scheiner, M, Gonzalez, A, and Peacock, CA. A high protein diet (3.4 g/kg/d) combined with a heavy resistance training program improves body composition in healthy trained men and women—a follow-up investigation. *J Int Soc Sport Nutr* 12:39, 2015.

6. Bailey, RL, Gahche, JJ, Miller, PE, Thomas, PR, and Dwyer, JT. Why US adults use dietary supplements. *JAMA Intern Med* 173(5):355-61, 2013.

7. Balsom, PD, Wood, K, Olsson, P, and Ekblom, B. Carbohydrate intake and multiple sprint sports: With special reference to football (soccer). *Int J Sports Med* 20:48-52, 1999.

8. Barry, MJ, and Edgman-Levitan, S. Shared decision making—pinnacle of patient-centered care. *New Engl J Med* 366(9):780-781, 2012.

9. Below, PR, Mora-Rodriguez, R, Gonzalez-Alonso, J, and Coyle, EF. Fluid and carbohydrate ingestion independently improve performance during 1 h of intense exercise. *Med Sci Sports Exerc* 27:200-210, 1995.

10. Borghi, L, Meschi, T, Amato, F, Briganti, A, Novarini, A, and Giannini, A. Urinary volume, water, and recurrences in idiopathic calcium nephrolithiasis: A 5-year randomized prospective study. *J Urol* 155:839-843, 1996.

11. Brown, RC, and Cox, CM. Effects of high fat versus high carbohydrate diets on plasma lipids and lipoproteins in endurance athletes. *Med Sci Sports Exerc* 30:1677-1683, 1998.

12. Burke, LM. Nutritional needs for exercise in the heat. *Comp Biochem Physiol* 128:735-748, 2001.

13. Burke, LM, Collier, GR, Beasley, SK, Davis, PG, Fricker, PA, Heeley, P, Walder, K, and Hargreaves, M. Effect of coingestion of fat and protein with carbohydrate feedings on muscle glycogen storage. *J Appl Physiol* 78:2187-2192, 1995.

14. Burke, LM, Lundy, B, Fahrenholtz, IL, and Melin, AK. Pitfalls of conducting and interpreting estimates of energy availability in free-living athletes. *Int J Sport Nutr Exerc Metab* 28(4):350-363, 2018.

15. Campbell, B, Kreider, RB, Ziegenfuss, T, La Bounty, P, Roberts, M, Burke, D, Landis, J, Lopez, H, and Antonio, J. International Society of Sports Nutrition position stand: Protein and exercise. *J Int Soc Sport Nutr* 4:8, 2007.

16. Costill, DL, Sherman, WM, Fink, WJ, Maresh, C, Witten, M, and Miller, JM. The role of dietary carbohydrates in muscle glycogen resynthesis after strenuous running. *Am J Clin Nutr* 34:1831-1836, 1981.

17. Davis, B. Essential fatty acids in vegetarian nutrition. *Vegetarian Diet* 7:5-7, 1998.

18. Ernst, ND, Sempos, CT, Briefel, RR, and Clark, MB. Consistency between US dietary fat intake and serum total cholesterol concentrations: The National Health and Nutrition Examination Surveys. *Am J Clin Nutr* 66(Suppl):S965-S972, 1997.

19. Fogelholm, GM, Koskinen, R, Laakso, J, Rankinen, T, and Ruokonen, I. Gradual and rapid weight loss: Effects on nutrition and performance in male athletes. *Med Sci Sports Exerc* 25:371-373, 1993.

20. Food and Agriculture Organization (FAO). *Human Energy Requirements.* Report of a Joint FAO/WHO/UNU Expert Consultation. Food and Nutrition Technical Report Series 1. Rome: Author, 2004.

21. Goday, A, Bellido, D, Sajoux, I, Crujeiras, AB, Burguera, B, García-Luna, PP, Oleaga, A, Moreno, B, and Casanueva, FF. Short-term safety, tolerability and efficacy of a very low-calorie-ketogenic diet interventional weight loss program versus hypocaloric diet in patients with type 2 diabetes mellitus. *Nutr Diabetes* 6(9):e230, 2016.

22. Grandjean, AC, Reimers, KJ, Bannick, KE, and Haven, MC. The effect of caffeinated, non-caffeinated, caloric and non-caloric beverages on hydration. *J Am Coll Nutr* 19:591-600, 2000.

23. Grandjean, AC, Reimers, KJ, and Ruud, JS. Dietary habits of Olympic athletes. In *Nutrition in Exercise and Sport.* Wolinsky, I, ed. Boca Raton, FL: CRC Press, 421-430, 1998.

24. Greene, DA, Varley, BJ, Hartwig, TB, Chapman, P, and Rigney, M. A low-carbohydrate ketogenic diet reduces body mass without compromising performance in powerlifting and Olympic weightlifting athletes. *J Strength Cond Res* 32(12):3373-3382, 2018.

25. Helms, ER, Aragon, AA, and Fitschen, PJ. Evidence-based recommendations for natural bodybuilding contest preparation: nutrition and supplementation. *J Int Soc Sport Nutr* 11:20, 2014.

26. Helms, ER, Zinn, C, Rowlands, DS, and Brown, SR. A systematic review of dietary protein during caloric restriction in resistance trained lean athletes: A case for higher intakes. *Int J Sport Nutr Exerc Met* 24(2):127-138, 2014.

27. Horswill, CA. Effective fluid replacement. *Int J Sport Nutr* 8:175-195, 1998.

28. Hudson, JL, Wang, Y, Bergia III, RE, and Campbell, WW. Protein intake greater than the RDA differentially influences whole-body lean mass responses to purposeful catabolic and anabolic stressors: A systematic review and meta-analysis. *Adv Nutr* 11:548-558, 2020.

29. Iraki, J, Fitschen, P, Espinar, S, and Helms, E. Nutrition recommendations for bodybuilders in the off-season: A narrative review. *Sports (Basel)* 7(7):E154, 2019.

30. Jacobs, KA, and Sherman, WM. The efficacy of carbohydrate supplementation and chronic high-carbohydrate diets for improving endurance performance. *Int J Sport Nutr* 9:92-115, 1999.

31. Johnstone, AM, Horgan, GW, Murison, SD, Bremner, DM, and Lobley, GE. Effects of a high-protein ketogenic diet on hunger, appetite, and weight loss in obese men feeding ad libitum. *Am J Clin Nutr* 87(1):44-55, 2008.

32. Jospe, MR, Brown, RC, Williams, SM, Roy, M, Meredith-Jones, KA, and Taylor, RW. Self-monitoring has no adverse effect on disordered eating in adults seeking treatment for obesity. *Obes Sci Pract* 2018 4(3):283-288, 2018.

33. Kephart, WC, Pledge, CD, Roberson, PA, Mumford, PW, Romero, MA, Mobley, CB, Martin, JS, Young, KC, Lowery, RP, Wilson, JM, Huggins, KW, and Roberts, MD. The three-month effects of a ketogenic diet on body composition, blood parameters, and performance metrics in CrossFit trainees: A pilot study. *Sports (Basel)* 6(1):E1, 2018.

34. Kim, JS. Examining the effectiveness of solution-focused brief therapy: A meta-analysis. *Res Soc Work Prac* 18(2):107-116, 2008.

35. Kochan, RG, Lamb, DR, Lutz, SA, Perrill, CV, Reimann, EM, and Schlende, KK. Glycogen synthase activation in human skeletal muscle: Effects of diet and exercise. *Am J Physiol* 236:E660-E666, 1979.

36. Leitzmann, MF, Willett, WC, Rimm, EB, Stampfer, MJ, Spiegelman, D, Colditz, GA, and Giovannucci, E. A prospective study of coffee consumption and the risk of symptomatic gallstone disease in men. *J Am Med Assoc* 281:2106-2112, 1999.

37. Lemon, PWR. Effects of exercise on dietary protein requirements. *Int J Sport Nutr* 8:426-447, 1998.

38. Levinson, CA, Fewell, L, and Brosof, LC. My Fitness Pal calorie tracker usage in the eating disorders. *Eat Behav* 27:14-16, 2017.

39. Licensure for Arizona RDs. Arizona Dietetic Association. www.eatrightarizona.org/Licensurehandout.pdf. Accessed January 1, 2010.

40. Linardon, J, and Messer, M. My Fitness Pal usage in men: Associations with eating disorder symptoms and psychosocial impairment. *Eat Behav* 33:13-17, 2019.

41. Linseisen, J, Welch, AA, Ock, M, Amiano, P, Agnoli, C, Ferrari, P, Sonestedt, E, Chaj, V, Bueno-de-Mesquita, HB, Kaaks, R, Weikert, C, Dorronsoro, M, Rodr, L, Ermini, I, Mattieloo, A, van der Schouw, YT, Manjer, J, Nilsson, S, Jenab, M, Lund, E, Brustad, M, Halkj, J, Jakobsen, MU, Khaw, KT, Crowe, F, Georgila, C, Misirli, G, Niravong, M, Touvier, M, Bingham, S, Riboli, E, and Slimani, N. Dietary fat intake in the European Prospective Investigation into Cancer and Nutrition: Results from the 24-h dietary recalls. *Eur J Clin Nutr 63*:S61-S80, 2009.

42. Loria-Kohen, V, Gómez-Candela, C, Fernández-Fernández, C, Pérez-Torres, A, García-Puig, J, and Bermejo, LM. Evaluation of the usefulness of a low-calorie diet with or without bread in the treatment of overweight/obesity. *Clin Nutr* 31(4):455-461, 2012.

43. MacDougall, JD, Ward, GR, Sale, DG, and Sutton, JR. Muscle glycogen repletion after high intensity intermittent exercise. *J Appl Physiol* 42:129-132, 1977.

44. Maughan, RJ, Leiper, JB, and Shirreffs, SM. Restoration of fluid balance after exercise-induced dehydration: Effects of food and fluid intake. *Eur J Appl Physiol* 73:317-325, 1996.

45. Maughan, RJ, Owen, JH, Shirreffs, SM, and Leiper, JB. Post-exercise rehydration in man: Effects of electrolyte addition to ingested fluids. *Eur J Appl Physiol* 69:209-215, 1994.

46. Michaud, DS, Spiegelman, D, Clinton, SK, Rimm, EB, Curhan, GC, Willett, WC, and Giovannucci, EL. Fluid intake and the risk of bladder cancer in men. *New Engl J Med* 340:1390-1397, 1999.

47. Mitchell, JB, DiLauro, PC, Pizza, FX, and Cavender, DL. The effect of pre-exercise carbohydrate status on resistance exercise performance. *Int J Sport Nutr* 7:185-196, 1997.

48. Morton, RW, Murphy, KT, McKellar, SR, Schoenfeld, BJ, Henselmans, M, Helms, E, Aragon, AA, Devries, MC, Banfield, L, Krieger, JW, and Phillips, SM. A systematic review, meta-analysis and meta-regression of the effect of protein supplementation on resistance training-induced gains in muscle mass and strength in healthy adults. *Brit J Sport Med* 52(6):376-384, 2018.

49. Mountjoy, M, Sundgot-Borgen, JK, Burke, LM, Ackerman, KE, Blauwet, C, Constantini, N, Lebrun, C, Lundy, B, Melin, AK, Meyer, NL, Sherman, RT, Tenforde, AS, Klungland Torstveit, M, and Budgett, R. IOC consensus statement on relative energy deficiency in sport (RED-S): 2018 update. *Brit J Sport Med* 52(11):687-697, 2018.

50. Muller, MJ, Enderle, J, and Bosy-Westphal, A. Changes in energy expenditure with weight gain and weight loss in humans. *Curr Obes Rep* 5(4):413-423, 2016.

51. Muoio, DM, Leddy, JJ, Horvath, PJ, Awad, AB, and Pendergast, DR. Effect of dietary fat on metabolic adjustments to maximal VO$_2$ and endurance in runners. *Med Sci Sports Exerc* 26:81-88, 1994.

52. National Academy of Sciences Institute of Medicine, Food and Nutrition Board. *Dietary Reference Intakes for Energy, Carbohydrate, Fiber, Fat, Fatty Acids, Cholesterol, Protein, and Amino Acids (Macronutrients).* Washington, DC: National Academies Press, 2005.

53. Ogden, J, and Whyman, C. The effect of repeated weighing on psychological state. *Eur Eat Disord Rev* 5(2):121-130, 1997.

54. Pendergast, DR, Horvath, PJ, Leddy, JJ, and Venkatraman, JT. The role of dietary fat on performance, metabolism, and health. *Am J Sports Med* 24:S53-S58, 1996.

55. Phillips, SM, Chevalier, S, and Leidy, HJ. Protein "requirements" beyond the RDA: Implications for optimizing health. *Appl Physiol Nutr Metab* 41(5):565-572, 2016.

56. Phinney, SD, Bistrian, BR, Evans, WJ, Gervino, E, and Blackburn, GL. The human metabolic response to chronic ketosis without caloric restriction: Preservation of submaximal exercise capability with reduced carbohydrate oxidation. *Metabolis* 32:769-776, 1983.

57. Piehl, KS, Adolfsson, S, and Nazar, K. Glycogen storage and glycogen synthase activity in trained and untrained muscle of man. *Acta Physiol Scand* 90:779-788, 1974.

58. Reimers, KJ. Evaluating a healthy, high performance diet. *Strength Cond* 16:28-30, 1994.

59. Roberts, J, Zinchenko, A, Mahbubani, K, Johnstone, J, Smith, L, Merzbach, V, Blacutt, M, Banderas, O, Villasenor, L, Vårvik, FT, and Henselmans, M. Satiating effect of high protein diets on resistance-trained individuals in energy deficit. *Nutrients* 11(1):56, 2019.

60. Rolls, BJ, Castellanos, VH, Halford, JC, Kilara, A, Panyam, D, Pelkman, CL, Smith, GP, and Thorwart, M. Volume of food consumed affects satiety in men. *American Journal of Clin Nutr* 67:1170-1177, 1998.

61. Santana, JC, Dawes, J, Antonio, J, and Kalman, DS. The role of the fitness professional in providing sports/exercise nutrition advice. *Strength Cond J* 29(30):69-71, 2007.

62. Sawka, MN, Burke, LM, Eichner, ER, Maughan, RJ, Montain, SJ, and Stachenfeld, NS. Exercise and fluid replacement position stand. *Med Sci Sports Exerc* 39(2):377-389, 2007.

63. Sherman, WM. Metabolism of sugars and physical performance. *Am J Clin Nutr* 62(Suppl):S228-S241, 1995.

64. Sherman, WM, Doyle, JA, Lamb, DR, and Strauss, RH. Dietary carbohydrate, muscle glycogen, and exercise performance during 7 d of training. *Am J Clin Nutr* 57:27-31, 1993.

65. Sherman, WM, and Wimer, GS. Insufficient carbohydrate during training: Does it impair performance? *Int J Sport Nutr* 1(1): 28-44, 1991.

66. Shirreffs, SM, Taylor, AJ, Leiper, JB, and Maughan RJ. Post-exercise rehydration in man: Effects of volume consumed and drink sodium content. *Med Sci Sports Exerc* 28:1260-1271, 1996.

67. Simpson, CC, and Mazzeo, SE. Calorie counting and fitness tracking technology: Associations with eating disorder symptomatology. *Eat Behav* 26:89-92, 2017.

68. Slater, GJ, Dieter, BP, Marsh, DJ, Helms, ER, Shaw, G, and Iraki, J. Is an energy surplus required to maximize skeletal muscle hypertrophy associated with resistance training? *Front Nutr* 6:131, 2019.

69. Sugiura, K, and Kobayashi, K. Effect of carbohydrate ingestion on sprint performance following continuous and intermittent exercise. *Med Sci Sports Exerc* 30:1624-1630, 1998.

70. Symons, JD, and Jacobs, I. High-intensity exercise performance is not impaired by low intramuscular glycogen. *Med Sci Sports Exerc* 21:550-557, 1989.

71. Taren, DL, Tobar, M, Hill, A, Howell, W, Shisslak, C, Bell, I, and Ritenbaugh, C. The association of energy intake bias with psychological scores of women. *Eur J Clin Nutr* 53(7):570-578, 1999.

72. Ting, R, Dugré, N, Allan, GM, and Lindblad, AJ. Ketogenic diet for weight loss. *Can Fam Physician* 64(12):906, 2018.

73. USDA MyPlate. www.ChooseMyPlate.gov. Accessed June 26, 2011.

74. Vandenberghe, K, Hespel, P, Eynde, BV, Lysens, R, and Richter, EA. No effect of glycogen level on glycogen metabolism during high intensity exercise. *Med Sci Sports Exerc* 27:1278-1283, 1995.

75. Vargas, S, Romance, R, Petro, JL, Bonilla, DA, Galancho, I, Espinar, S, Kreider, RB, and Benítez-Porres, J. Efficacy of ketogenic diet on body composition during resistance training in trained men: A randomized controlled trial. *J Int Soc Sport Nutr* 15(1):31, 2018.

76. Volek, JS, Kraemer, WJ, Bush, JA, Incledon, T, and Boetes, M. Testosterone and cortisol in relationship to dietary nutrients and resistance exercise. *J Appl Physiol* 82:49-54, 1997.

77. von Loeffelholz, C, and Birkenfeld, A. The role of non-exercise activity thermogenesis in human obesity. In Feingold, KR, Anawalt, B, Boyce, A, Chrousos, G, de Herder, W, Dungan, K, Grossman, A, Hershman, JM, Hofland, J, Kaltsas, G, Koch, C, Kopp, P, Korbonits, M, McLachlan, R, Morley, JE, New, M, Purnell, J, Singer, F, Stratakis, CA, Trence, DL, and Wilson, DP., editors. *Endotext* [Internet]. South Dartmouth, MA: MDText.com, 2018.

78. Walberg, JL, Leidy, MK, Sturgill, DJ, Hinkle, DE, Ritchey, SJ, and Sebolt, DR. Macronutrient needs in weight lifters during caloric restriction. *Med Sci Sports Exerc* 19:S70, 1987.

79. Wardlaw, GM, and Insel, PM. *Perspectives in Nutrition.* St. Louis: Mosby Year Book, 76, 1996.

80. Westenhoefer, J, Engel, D, Holst, C, Lorenz, J, Peacock, M, Stubbs, J, Whybrow, S, and Raats, M. Cognitive and weight-related correlates of flexible and rigid restrained eating behaviour. *Eat Behav* 14(1):69-72, 2013.

81. Wilmore, JH, Morton, AR, Gilbey, HJ, and Wood, RJ. Role of taste preference on fluid intake during and after 90 min of running at 60% of VO$_2$max in the heat. *Med Sci Sports Exerc* 30:587-595, 1998.

82. World Health Organization. *Protein and Amino Acid Requirements in Human Nutrition.* WHO Technical Report Series. Geneva: WHO Press, 2007. http://whqlibdoc.who.int/trs/WHO_TRS_935_eng.pdf. Accessed April 20, 2010.

Chapter 8

1. Armstrong, CA, Sallis, JF, Howell, MF, and Hofstetter, CR. Stages of change, self-efficacy, and the adoption of vigorous exercise: A prospective analysis. *J Sport Exerc Psy* 15:390-402, 1993.

2. Bahrke, MS, and Morgan, WP. Anxiety reduction following exercise and meditation. *Cognit Ther Res* 2:323-333, 1978.

3. Bandura, A. *Self-Efficacy: The Exercise of Control.* San Francisco: Freeman, 1997.

4. Bartholomew, JB, and Linder, DE. State anxiety following resistance exercise: The role of gender and exercise intensity. *J Behav Med* 21:205-219, 1988.

5. Bixby, WR, Spalding, TW, and Hatfield, BD. Temporal dynamics and dimensional specificity of the affective response to exercise of varying intensity: Differing pathways to a common outcome. *J Sport Exerc Psy* 23:171-190, 2001.

6. Blair, SN, Dunn AN, Marcus, BG, Carpenter, RA, and Jaret, P. *Active Living Every Day.* Champaign, IL: Human Kinetics, 2001.

7. Blumenthal, JA, Babyak, MA, Moore, KA, Craighead, WE, Herman, S, Khatri, P, Waugh, R, Napolitano, MA, Forman, LM, Applebaum, M, Doraiswamy, M, and Krishman R. Effects of exercise training on older patients with major depression. *Arch Intern Med* 159:2349-2356, 1999.

8. Bonvallet, M, and Bloch, V. Bulbar control of cortical arousal. *Science* 133:1133-1134, 1961.

9. Brajendra, B, and Rajesh, T. Stress management techniques for athletes during sports: A critical review. *J Drug Deliv Ther* 8:67-72, 2018.

10. Brown, TC, Fry, MD, and Moore, EWG. A motivational climate intervention and exercise-related outcomes: A longitudinal perspective. *Motiv Sci* 3:337-353, 2017.

11. Buckworth, J, and Dishman, RK. *Exercise Psychology.* Champaign, IL: Human Kinetics, 2002.

12. Calfas, KJ, and Taylor, WC. Effects of physical activity on psychological variables in adolescents. *Pediatric Exerc Science* 6:406-423, 1994.

13. Cannon, WB. *Bodily Changes in Pain, Hunger, Fear, and Rage: An Account of Recent Researches Into the Function of Emotional Excitement.* 2nd ed. New York: Appleton, 1929.

14. Cardinal, BJ. The stages of exercise scale and stages of exercise behavior in female adults. *J Sports Med Phys Fitness* 35:87-92, 1995.

15. Cardinal, BJ. Predicting exercise behavior using components of the transtheoretical model of behavior change. *J Sport Behav* 20:272-283, 1997.

16. Chaouloff, F. The serotonin hypothesis. In *Physical Activity and Mental Health.* Morgan, WP, ed. Washington, DC: Taylor & Francis, 179-198, 1997.

17. Courneya, KS. Perceived severity of the consequences of physical inactivity across the stages of change in older adults. *J Sport Exerc Psy* 17:447-457, 1995.

18. Conn, VS. Depressive symptom outcomes of physical activity interventions: Meta-analysis finds. *Ann Behav Med* 39:128-138, 2010.

19. Cox, RH. *Sport Psychology: Concepts and Applications.* 5th ed. Boston: McGraw-Hill, 2002.

20. Craft, LL, and Landers, DM. The effect of exercise on clinical depression and depression resulting from mental illness: A meta-analysis. *J Sport Exerc Psy* 20:339-357, 1988.

21. Davidson, RJ. Cerebral asymmetry and emotion: Conceptual and methodological conundrums. *Cogn Emot* 7:115-138, 1993.

21a. Deci, EL, Koestner, R, and Ryan, RM. A meta-analytic review of experiments examining the effects of extrinsic rewards on intrinsic motivation. *Psychological Bulletin* 125:627-668, 1999.

22. Deci, EL, and Ryan, RM. *Intrinsic Motivation and Self-Determination in Human Behavior.* New York: Plenum Press, 1985.

23. Deci, EL, and Ryan, RM. A motivational approach to self: Integration in personality. In *Nebraska Symposium on Motivation 1991: Vol. 38. Perspectives on Motivation: Current Theory and Research in Motivation.* Dienstbier, RA, ed. Lincoln: University of Nebraska Press, 237-288, 1991.

24. Dishman, RK. The norepinephrine hypothesis. In *Physical Activity and Mental Health.* Morgan, WP, ed. Washington, DC: Taylor & Francis, 199-212, 1997.

25. Druckman, D, and Swets, JA. *Enhancing Human Performance: Issues, Theories and Techniques.* Washington, DC: National Academy Press, 1988.

26. Duda, JL. Relationships between task and ego orientation and the perceived purpose of sport among high school athletes. *J Sport Exerc Psy* 11:318-335, 1989.

27. Duda, JL, and Nicholls, JG. Dimensions of achievement motivation in schoolwork and sport. *J Educ Psychol* 84:290-299, 1992.

28. Dunn, AL, Trivedi, MH, Kampert, JB, Clark, CG, and Chambliss, HO. Exercise treatment for depression: Efficacy and dose response. *Am J Prev Med* 28:1-8, 2005.

29. Dustman, RE, Emmerson, RY, Ruhling, RO, Shearer, DE, Steinhaus, LA, Johnson, SC, Bonekat, HW, and Shigeoka, JW. Age and fitness effects on EEG, ERPs, visual sensitivity, and cognition. *Neurobiol of Aging* 11:193-200, 1990.

30. Ekkekakis, P, Hall, EE, and Petruzzello, SJ. The relationship between exercise intensity and affect responses demystified: To crack the 40-year-old nut replace the 40-year-old nutcracker! *Ann Behav Med* 35:136-149, 2008.

31. Ekkekakis, P, Parfitt, G, and Patruzzello, SJ. The pleasure and displeasure people feel when they exercise at different intensities: Decennial update and progress towards a tripartite rationale for exercise intensity prescription. *Sports Med* 41:641-671, 2011.

31a. Ettman, CK, Abdalla, SM, Cohen, GH, Sampson, L, Vivier, PM, and Galea, S. Prevalence of depression symptoms in US adults before and during the COVID-19 pandemic. *JAMA Network Open* 3:e2019686, 2020.

32. Fitzsimmons, PA, Landers, DM, Thomas, JR, and Van Der Mars, H. Does self-efficacy predict performance in experienced weightlifters? *Res Q Exerc Sport* 62:424–431, 1991.

33. Fry, MD, and Moore, EWG. Motivation in sport: Theory and application. In *APA Handbook of Sport and Exercise Psychology I.* Anshel, MH, ed. Washington, DC: American Psychological Association, 273-299, 2019.

34. Golding, J, and Ungerleider, S. *Beyond Strength: Psychological Profiles of Olympic Athletes.* Madison, WI: Brown and Benchmark, 1992.

35. Hall, HK, and Kerr, AW. Goal setting in sport and physical activity: Tracing empirical developments and establishing conceptual direction. In *Advances in Motivation in Sport and Exercise.* Roberts, GC, ed. Champaign, IL: Human Kinetics, 83-234, 2001.

36. Hart, EA, Leary, MR, and Rejeski, WJ. The measurement of social physique anxiety. *J Sport Exerc Psy* 11:94-104, 1989.

37. Hatfield, BD. Exercise and mental health: The mechanisms of exercise-induced psychological states. In *Psychology of Sports, Exercise and Fitness.* Diamant, L, ed. Washington, DC: Hemisphere, 17-50, 1991.

38. Hogue, CM, Fry, MD, and Fry, AC. The differential impact of motivational climate on adolescents' psychological and physiological stress responses. *Psychol Sport and Exerc* 30:118-127, 2017.

39. Hogue, CM, Fry, MD, Fry, AC, and Pressman, SD. The influence of a motivational climate intervention on participants' salivary cortisol and psychological responses. *J Sport Exerc Psy* 35:85-97, 2013.

40. Hogue, CM, Fry, MD, and Iwasaki, S. The impact of the perceived motivational climate in physical education classes on adolescent greater life stress, coping appraisals, and experience of shame. *Sport Exerc Perform* 8:273-289, 2019.

41. Iso-Ahola, SE, and Hatfield, BD. *Psychology of Sports: A Social Psychological Approach.* Dubuque, IA: Brown, 1986.

42. Jacobson, E. *Progressive Relaxation.* Chicago: University of Chicago Press, 1974.

43. Javnbakht, M, Hejazi, KR, and Ghasemi. M. Effects of yoga on depression and anxiety of women. *Complement Ther Clin Pract* 15:102-104, 2009.

44. Jerath, R, Edry, JW, Barnes, VA, and Jerath, V. Physiology of long pranayamic breathing: Neural respiratory elements may provide a mechanism that explains how slow deep breathing shifts the autonomic nervous system. *Med Hypotheses* 67:566-571, 2006.

45. Kugler, J, Seelback, H, and Kruskemper, GM. Effects of rehabilitation exercise programmes on anxiety and depression in coronary patients: A meta-analysis. *Brit J Clin Psychol* 33:401-410, 1994.

46. Kyllo, LB, and Landers, DM. Goal setting in sport and exercise: A research synthesis to resolve the controversy. *J Sport Exerc Psy* 17:117-137, 1995.

47. Landers, DM. The arousal-performance relationship revisited. *Res Q Exerc Sport* 51:77-90, 1980.

48. Landers, DM, and Arent, SA. Physical activity and mental health. In *Handbook of Sport Psychology.* 2nd ed. Singer, RN, Hausenblas, HA, and Janelle, CM, eds. New York: Wiley, 740-765, 2001.

49. Landers, DM, and Arent, SA. Physical activity and mental health. In *Handbook of Sport Psychology.* 3rd ed. Tenenbaum, G, and Eklund, RC, eds. New York: Wiley, 469-491, 2007.

50. Landers, DM, and Petruzzello, SJ. Physical activity, fitness, and anxiety. In *Physical Activity, Fitness, and Health.* Bouchard, C, Shepard, RJ, and Stevens, T, eds. Champaign, IL: Human Kinetics, 868-882, 2007.

51. Lim, S, and Lipman, L. Mental practice and memorization of piano music. *J Gen Psychol* 118:21-30, 1991.

52. Long, BC, and Van Stavel, R. Effects of exercise training on anxiety: A meta-analysis. *J Appl Sport Psychol* 7:167-189, 1995.

53. Marcus, BH, Eaton, CA, Rossi, JS, and Harlow, LL. Self-efficacy, decision making, and stages of change: An integrative model of physical exercise. *J Applied Soc Psychol* 24:489-508, 1994.

54. Martens, R. *Social Psychology and Physical Activity.* New York: Harper & Row, 1975.

55. McDonald, DG, and Hodgdon, JA. *The Psychological Effects of Aerobic Fitness Training: Research and Theory.* New York: Springer-Verlag, 1991.

56. Meijer, EH, Smulders, FTY, and Hatfield, BD. The effects of rhythmic physical activity and the EEG. Paper submitted for presentation at the annual meeting of the Society for Psychophysiological Research, Washington, DC, 2002.

57. Moore, EWG. Strength training and sport psychology. In *Oxford Research Encyclopedia of Psychology.* Braddick, O, ed. New York: Oxford University Press, 1-32, 2017.

58. Morgan, WP. Affective beneficence of vigorous physical activity. *Med Sci Sports Exerc* 17:94-100, 1985.

59. Morgan, WP. Prescription of physical activity: A paradigm shift. *Quest* 53:366-382, 2001.

60. Neto, JMD, Silva, FB, De Oliveira, ALB, Lopes Couto, N, Dantas, EHM, and de Luca Nascimento, MA. Effects of verbal encouragement on performance of the multistage 20 m shuttle run. *Acta Sci Health Sci* 37:25-30, 2015.

61. North, TC, McCullagh, P, and Tran, ZV. Effects of exercise on depression. *Exercise Sport Sci R* 18:379-415, 1990.

62. O'Block, FR, and Evans, FH. Goal setting as a motivational technique: In *Psychological Foundations of Sport.* Silva, JM, and Weinberg, RS, eds. Champaign, IL: Human Kinetics, 188-196, 1984.

63. Petruzzello, SJ, Ekkekakis, P, and Hall, EE. Physical activity, affect and electroencephalogram studies. In *Psychobiology of Physical Activity.* Acevedo, EO, and Ekkekakis, P, eds. Champaign, IL: Human Kinetics, 91-109, 2006.

64. Petruzzello, SJ, Landers, DM, Hatfield, BD, Kubitz, KA, and Salazar, W. A meta-analysis on the anxiety-reducing effects of acute and chronic exercise. *Sports Med* 11:143-182, 1991.

65. Prochaska, JO, and Marcus, MH. The transtheoretical model: The applications to exercise. In *Advances in Exercise Adherence.* Dishman, RK, ed. Champaign, IL: Human Kinetics, 161-180, 1994.

66. Roberts, GC. Motivation in sport: Understanding and enhancing the motivation and achievement of children. In *Handbook of Research on Sport Psychology.* Singer, RN, Murphy, M, and Tennant, LK, eds. New York: Macmillan, 405-420, 1993.

67. Roberts, GC. Understanding the dynamics of motivation in physical activity: The influence of achievement goals on motivational processes. In *Advances in Motivation in Sport and Exercise.* Roberts, GC, ed. Champaign, IL: Human Kinetics, 1-50, 2001.

68. Roberts, GC, and Treasure, DC. Achievement goals, motivation climate and achievement strategies and behaviors in sport. *Int J Sport Psychol* 26:64-80, 1995.

69. Ryan, RM, Frederick, CM, Lepes, D, Rubio, N, and Sheldon, KM. Intrinsic motivation and exercise adherence. *Int J Sport Psychol* 28:335-354, 1997.

70. Sheinbein, S. Psychological effect of injury on the athlete: A recommendation for psychological intervention. *AMAA Journal* 29(3):3-10, 2016.

71. Sherwood, DE, and Selder, DJ. Cardiorespiratory health, reaction time and aging. *Med Sci Sports Exerc* 11:186-189, 1979.

72. Siedentop, D, and Ramey, G. Extrinsic rewards and intrinsic motivation. Motor skills: Theory into practice. 2:49-62, 1977.

73. Skinner, BF. *The Behavior of Organisms: An Experimental Analysis.* New York: Appleton Century Crofts, 1938.

74. Skinner, BF. *Science and Human Behavior.* New York: Macmillan, 1953.

75. Smith, SL, Fry, MD, Ethington, CA, and Yuhua, L. The effect of female athletes' perceptions of their coaches' behaviors on their perceptions of the motivational climate. *J Appl Sport Psychol* 17:170-177, 2005.

76. Solomon, RL, and Corbit, JD. An opponent-process theory of motivation: II. Cigarette addiction. *J Abnorm Psychol* 81:158-171, 1973.

77. Spielberger, CD. *Manual for the State-Trait Anxiety Inventory (Form Y).* Palo Alto, CA: Consulting Psychologists Press, 1983.

78. Spirduso, WW. Exercise and the aging brain. *Res Q Exerc Sport* 54:208-218, 1983.

79. Staub, JN, Kraemer, WJ, Pandit, AL, Haug, WB, Comstock, BA, Dunn-Lewis, C, Hooper, DR, Maresh, CM, Volek, JS, and Häkkinen, K. Positive effects of augmented verbal feedback on power production in NCAA Division I collegiate athletes. *J Strength Cond Res* 27:2067-2072, 2013.

80. Tomich, GM, Frana, DC, Diorio, ACM, Britto, RR, Sampaio, RF, Parreira, VF. Breathing pattern, thoracoabdominal motion and muscular activity during three breathing exercises. *Brazilian J Med Bio Res* 40: 1409-1417. 2007.

81. U.S. Department of Health and Human Services. *Physical Activity and Health: A Report of the Surgeon General.* Atlanta: National Center for Chronic Disease Prevention and Health Promotion, 1996.

82. Vallerand, RJ, Losier, GF. An integration analysis of intrinsic and extrinsic motivation in sport. *J Appl Sport Psychol* 11:142-169, 1999.

83. Von Euler, C, and Soderberg, V. The influence of hypothalamic thermoceptive structures on the electroencephalogram and gamma motor activity. *Electroen Clin Neuro* 9:391-408, 1957.

84. Wells, CM, Collins, D, and Hale, BD. The self-efficacy-performance link in maximum strength performance. *J Sport Sci* 11:167-175, 1993.

85. Wise, JB, Posner, AE, and Walker, GL. Verbal messages strengthen bench press efficacy. *J Strength Cond Res* 18:26-29, 2004.

86. Woo, M, Kim, S, Kim, J, and Hatfield, BD. The influence of exercise intensity on frontal electroencephalographic (EEG) asymmetry and self-reported affect. *Res Q Exerc Sport* 81:349-359, 2010.

87. Woo, M, Kim, S, Kim, J, Petruzzello, SJ, and Hatfield, BD. Examining the exercise-affect dose-response relationship: Does duration influence frontal EEG asymmetry? *Int J Psychophysiol* 72:166-172, 2009.

Chapter 9

1. Albert, CM, Mittleman, MA, Chae, CU, Lee, IM, Hennekens, CH, and Manson, JE. Triggering of sudden death from cardiac causes by vigorous exertion. *New Engl J Med* 343(19):1355-1361, 2000.

2. Almada, SL, Zonderman, AB, Shekelle, RB, Dyer, AR, Daviglus, ML, Costa Jr., PT, and Stamler, J. Neuroticism and cynicism and risk of death in middle-aged men: The Western Electric Study. *Psychosom Med* 53(2):165-175, 1991.

3. American College of Sports Medicine. *ACSM's Resource Manual for Guidelines for Exercise Testing and Prescription,* 5th ed. Baltimore: Williams & Wilkins, 2006.

4. American College of Sports Medicine. *ACSM's Guidelines for Exercise Testing and Prescription*, 11th ed. Philadelphia: Wolters Kluwer, 2022.

5. American Diabetes Association. 2. Classification and diagnosis of diabetes: *Standards of Medical Care in Diabetes—2019. Diabetes Care* 42(Suppl 1):S13-S28, 2019.

5a. Arnett, DK, Blumenthal, RS, Albert, MA, Buroker, AB, Goldberger, ZD, Hahn, EJ, Himmelfarb, CD, Khera, A, Lloyd-Jones, D, McEvoy, JW, and Michos, ED. 2019 ACC/AHA guideline on the primary prevention of cardiovascular disease: A report of the American College of Cardiology/American Heart Association Task Force on Clinical Practice Guidelines. *J Am Coll Cardiol* 74(10):e177-e232, 2019.

6. Bredin, S, Gledhill, N, and Warburton, D. The PAR-Q+ Collaboration. Revision of the physical activity readiness questionnaire (PAR-Q). *Can J Sport Sci* 17:338-345, 2011.

7. Brownson, R, Remington, P, and Davis, J, eds. *Chronic Disease Epidemiology and Control.* Washington, DC: American Public Health Association, 379-382, 1998.

8. Celli, BR, MacNee, WATS, Agusti, AATS, Anzueto, A, Berg, B, Buist, AS, Calverley, PM, Chavannes, N, Dillard, T, Fahy, B, and Fein, A. Standards for the diagnosis and treatment of patients with COPD: A summary of the ATS/ERS position paper. *Eur Respir J* 23(6):932-946, 2004.

9. Centers for Disease Control and Prevention, National Center for Chronic Disease Prevention and Health Promotion, and Office on Smoking and Health. *How Tobacco Smoke Causes Disease: The Biology and Behavioral Basis for Smoking-Attributable Disease: A Report of the Surgeon General.* Atlanta: Centers for Disease Control and Prevention, 2010.

10. Chida, Y, and Steptoe, A. Greater cardiovascular responses to laboratory mental stress are associated with poor subsequent cardiovascular risk status: A meta-analysis of prospective evidence. *Hypertension* 55(4):1026-1032, 2010.

11. Chobanian, AV, Bakris, GL, Black, HR, Cushman, WC, Green, LA, Izzo Jr, JL, Jones, DW, Materson, BJ, Oparil, S, Wright Jr, JT, and Roccella, EJ. The seventh report of the joint national committee on prevention, detection, evaluation, and treatment of high blood pressure: The JNC 7 report. *J Am Med Assoc* 289(19):2560-2571, 2003.

12. Drought, HJ. Personal training: The initial consultation. *Conditioning Instructor* 1(2):2-3, 1990.

13. Expert Panel on Detection, Evaluation, and Treatment of High Blood Cholesterol in Adults. Executive summary of the third report of the National Cholesterol Education Program (NCEP) expert panel on detection, evaluation, and treatment of high blood cholesterol in adults (Adult Treatment Panel III). *J Am Med Assoc* 285(19):2486-2497, 2001.

14. Faigenbaum, AD, and Westcott, WL. *Youth Strength Training*, 1st ed. Monterey, CA: Healthy Learning Books and Videos, 2005.

15. Fletcher, GF, Balady, G, Blair, SN, Blumenthal, J, Caspersen, C, Chaitman, B, Epstein, S, Sivarajan Froelicher, ES, Froelicher, VF, Pina, IL, and Pollock, ML. Statement on exercise: Benefits and recommendations for physical activity programs for all Americans. A statement for health professionals by the Committee on Exercise and Cardiac Rehabilitation of the Council on Clinical Cardiology, American Heart Association. *Circulation* 94(4):857-862, 1996.

16. Franklin, BA, Thompson, PD, Al-Zaiti, SS, Albert, CM, Hivert, MF, Levine, BD, Lobelo, F, Madan, K, Sharrief, AZ, and Eijsvogels, TM. American Heart Association Physical Activity Committee of the Council on Lifestyle and Cardiometabolic Health, Council on Cardiovascular and Stroke Nursing, Council on Clinical Cardiology, and Stroke Council. Exercise-related acute cardiovascular events and potential deleterious adaptations following long-term exercise training: Placing the risks into perspective–an update: A scientific statement from the American Heart Association. *Circulation* 141(13):e705-e736, 2020.

17. Gibbons, RJ, Balady, GJ, Bricker, JT, Chaitman, BR, Fletcher, GF, and Froelicher, VF. Guideline update for exercise testing: Summary article: A report of the American College of Cardiology/American Heart Association Task Force on Practice Guidelines (Committee to Update the 1997 Exercise Testing Guidelines). *Circulation* 106(14):1883-1892, 2002.

18. Glantz, SA, and Parmley, WW. Passive and active smoking. A problem for adults. *Circulation* 94(4):596-598, 1996.

19. Glovaci, D, Fan, W, and Wong, ND. Epidemiology of diabetes mellitus and cardiovascular disease. *Curr Cardiol Rep* 21(4):21, 2019.

20. Herbert, DL. Medical, legal considerations for strength training for children. *Strength Cond J* 15(6):77, 1993.

21. Herbert, DL, and Herbert, WG. *Legal Aspects of Preventative and Rehabilitative Exercise Programs,* 3rd ed. Canton, OH: Professional Reports Corporation, 1993.

22. Hubert, HB, Feinleib, M, McNamara, PM, and Castelli, WP. Obesity as an independent risk factor for cardiovascular disease: A 26-year follow-up of participants in the Framingham Heart Study. *Circulation* 67(5):968-977, 1983.

22a. Jellinger, PS, Handelsman, Y, Rosenblit, PD, Bloomgarden, ZT, Fonseca, VA, Garber, AJ, Grunberger, G, Guerin, CK, Bell, DS, Mechanick, JI, and Pessah-Pollack, R. American Association of Clinical Endocrinologists and American College of Endocrinology guidelines for management of dyslipidemia and prevention of cardiovascular disease. *Endocr Pract* 23:1-87, 2017.

23. Jensen, MD, Ryan, DH, Apovian, CM, Ard, JD, Comuzzie, AG, Donato, KA, and Yanovski, M. AHA/ACC/TOS Guidelines for the management of overweight and obesity in adults: A report of the American College of Cardiology/American Heart Association Task Force on Practice Guidelines and the Obesity Society. *Circulation* 129(25 Suppl 2):S139-S140, 2014.

24. Klieman, C, and Osborne, K. *If It Runs in Your Family: Heart Disease: Reducing Your Risk.* New York: Bantam Books, 1991.

25. Kodama, S, Saito, K, Tanaka, S, Horikawa, C, Saito, A, Heianza, Y, Anasako, Y, Nishigaki, Y, Yachi, Y, Iida, KT, and Ohashi, Y. Alcohol consumption and risk of atrial fibrillation: A meta-analysis. *J Am Coll Cardiol* 57(4):427-436, 2011.

26. Kordich, JA. Evaluating your client: Fitness assessment protocols and norms. In *Essentials of Personal Training Symposium Study Guide.* Lincoln, NE: NSCA Certification Commission, 2000.

27. Last, JM. *A Dictionary of Epidemiology,* 5th ed. New York: Oxford University Press, 2008.

28. Lubin, JH, Couper, D, Lutsey, PL, Woodward, M, Yatsuya, H, and Huxley, RR. Risk of cardiovascular disease from cumulative cigarette use and the impact of smoking intensity. *Epidemiology* 27(3):395-404, 2016.

29. Malhotra, A, Redberg, RF, and Meier, P. Saturated fat does not clog the arteries: Coronary heart disease is a chronic inflammatory condition, the risk of which can be effectively reduced from healthy lifestyle interventions. *Brit J Sport Med* 51(15):1111-1112, 2017.

30. Maron, BJ, Doerer, JJ, Haas, TS, Tierney, DM, and Mueller, FO. Sudden deaths in young competitive athletes. *Circulation: Analysis of 1866 deaths in the United States, 1980-2006* 119(8):1085-1092, 2009.

31. Maron, BJ, Estes, NM, and Maron, MS. Is it fair to screen only competitive athletes for sudden death risk, or is it time to level the playing field? *Am J Cardiol* 121(8):1008-1010, 2018.

32. Maron, BJ, Levine, BD, Washington, RL, Baggish, AL, Kovacs, RJ, and Maron, MS. Eligibility and disqualification recommendations for competitive athletes with cardiovascular abnormalities: Task force 2: Preparticipation screening for cardiovascular disease in competitive athletes: a scientific statement from the American Heart Association and American College of Cardiology. *Circulation* 132(22):e267-e272, 2015.

33. Maron, BJ, Thompson, PD, and Maron, MS. There is no reason to adopt ECGs and abandon American Heart Association/American College of Cardiology History and Physical Screening for detection of cardiovascular disease in the young. *J Am Heart Assoc* 8(14):e013007-e013007, 2019.

34. Martynov, AI, Akatova, EV, Pervichko, EI, Nikolin, OP, and Urlaeva, IV. Influence of type A behavioral activity on the development of cardiovascular disease. *CardioSomatics* 10(4):39-43, 2019.

35. McInnis, KJ, and Balady, GJ. Higher cardiovascular risk clients in health clubs. *ACSM's Health Fit J* 3(1):9-24, 1999.

35a. Mozaffarian, D, Benjamin, EJ, Go, AS, Arnett, DK, Blaha, MJ, Cushman, M, De Ferranti, S, Després, JP, Fullerton, HJ, Howard, VJ, and Huffman, MD. Heart disease and stroke statistics—2015 update: A report from the American Heart Association. *Circulation* 131(4):e29-e322, 2105.

36. Natarajan, P, Ray, KK, and Cannon, CP. High-density lipoprotein and coronary heart disease: Current and future therapies. *J Am Coll Cardiol* 55(13):1283-1299, 2010.

37. National Strength and Conditioning Association NSCA-CPT Job Analysis Committee. NSCA-CPT detailed content outline. 2018.

38. NIH Consensus Development Panel on Triglyceride, High Density Lipoprotein, and Coronary Heart Disease. Triglyceride, high-density lipoprotein, and coronary heart disease. *J Am Med Assoc* 269:505-510, 1993.

39. Pate, RR, Pratt, M, Blair, SN, Haskell, WL, Macera, CA, Bouchard, C, Buchner, D, Ettinger, W, Heath, GW, King, AC, and Kriska, A. Physical activity and public health: A recommendation from the Centers for Disease Control and Prevention and the American College of Sports Medicine. *J Am Med Assoc* 273(5):402-407, 1995.

40. Petek, BJ, and Baggish, AL. Current controversies in pre-participation cardiovascular screening for young competitive athletes. *Expert Rev Cardiovasc Ther* 18(7):435-442, 2020.

41. Physician and Sportsmedicine. *Preparticipation Physical Evaluation,* 3rd ed. Minneapolis: McGraw-Hill, 2005.

42. Pollock, ML, Lowenthal, DT, Foster, C, Pels III, AE, Rod, J, Stoiber, J, and Schmidt, D.H. Acute and chronic responses to exercise in patients treated with beta blockers. *J Cardiopulm Rehabil* 11(2):132-144, 1991.

43. Russek, LG, King, SH, Russek, SJ, and Russek, HI. The Harvard Mastery of Stress Study 35-year follow-up: Prognostic significance of patterns of psychophysiological arousal and adaptation. *Psychol Med* 52:271-285, 1990.

44. Sacks, FM, Lichtenstein, AH, Wu, JH, Appel, LJ, Creager, MA, Kris-Etherton, PM, Miller, M, Rimm, EB, Rudel, LL, Robinson, JG, and Stone, NJ. Dietary fats and cardiovascular disease: A presidential advisory from the American Heart Association. *Circulation* 136(3):e1-e23, 2017.

45. Sharkey, B, and Gaskill, S. *Fitness and Health,* 7th ed. Champaign, IL: Human Kinetics, 397-401, 2013.

46. Sims, J, and Carrol, D. Cardiovascular and metabolic activity at rest and during physical challenge in normotensives and subjects with mildly elevated blood pressure. *Psychophysiology* 27:149-160, 1990.

47. Slavich, GM, and Shields, GS. Assessing lifetime stress exposure using the Stress and Adversity Inventory for Adults (Adult STRAIN): An overview and initial validation. *Psychosom Med* 80(1):17, 2018.

48. Steptoe, A, and Kivimäki, M. Stress and cardiovascular disease. *Nat Rev Cardiol* 9(6):360-370, 2012.

49. U.S. Department of Health and Human Services. *Physical Activity Guidelines for Americans,* 2nd ed. Washington, DC: Author, 2018.

50. Verrill, D, Graham, H, Vitcenda, M, Peno-Green, L, Kramer, V, and Corbisiero, T. Measuring behavioral outcomes in cardiopulmonary rehabilitation: An AACVPR statement. *J Cardiopulm Rehabil Prev* 29(3):193-203, 2009.

51. Virani, SS, Alonso, A, Benjamin, EJ, Bittencourt, MS, Callaway, CW, Carson, AP, Chamberlain, AM, Chang, AR, Cheng, S, Delling, FN, and Djousse, L. Heart disease and stroke statistics—2020 update: A report from the American Heart Association. *Circulation* 141:e139-e596, 2020.

52. Warburton, DER, Jamnik, VK, Bredin, SSD, and Gledhill, N, on behalf of the PAR-Q+ Collaboration. The Physical Activity Readiness Questionnaire for Everyone (PAR-Q+) and Electronic Physical Activity Readiness Medical Examination (ePARmed-X+). *Health Fit J Can* 4(2):3-23, 2011.

53. Whang, W, Manson, JE, Hu, FB, Chae, CU, Rexrode, KM, Willett, WC, Stampfer, MJ, and Albert, CM. Physical exertion, exercise, and sudden cardiac death in women. *J Am Med Assoc* 295(12):1399-1403, 2006.

54. Whelton, PK, He, J, Appel, LJ, Cutler, JA, Havas, S, Kotchen, TA, Roccella, EJ, Stout, R, Vallbona, C, Winston, MC, and Karimbakas, J. Primary prevention of hypertension: Clinical and public health advisory from the National High Blood Pressure Education Program. *J Am Med Assoc* 288(15):1882-1888, 2002.

55. Zhang, X, Devlin, HM, Smith, B, Imperatore, G, Thomas, W, Lobelo, F, Ali, MK, Norris, K, Gruss, S, Bardenheier, B, and Cho, P. Effect of lifestyle interventions on cardiovascular risk factors among adults without impaired glucose tolerance or diabetes: A systematic review and meta-analysis. *PLOS One* 12(5):e0176436, 2017.

Chapter 10

1. AirNow. Air quality index (AQI) basics. www.airnow.gov/aqi/aqi-basics. Accessed December 16, 2020.

2. American College of Sports Medicine. *ACSM's Guidelines for Exercise Testing and Prescription,* 11th ed. Philadelphia: Wolters Kluwer, 2022.

3. Armstrong, LE, Casa, DJ, Millard-Stafford, M, Moran, DS, Pyne, SW, and Roberts, WO. Exertional heat illness during training and competition. *Med Sci Sports Exerc* 39(3):556-572, 2007.

4. Åstrand, I. Aerobic work capacity in men and women with special reference to age. *Acta Physiol Scand* 49(169):45-60, 1960.

5. Baechle, TR, and Earle, RW. *Weight Training: Steps to Success.* 5th ed. Champaign, IL: Human Kinetics, 2019.

6. Baechle, TR, Earle, RW, and Wathen, D. Resistance training. In *Essentials of Strength Training and Conditioning.* 3rd ed. Baechle, TR, and Earle, RW, eds. Champaign, IL: Human Kinetics, 382-412, 2008.

7. Baumgartner, TA, and Jackson, AS. *Measurement for Evaluation.* 8th ed. Boston: McGraw-Hill, 2008.

8. Bilodeau, B, Roy, B, and Boulay, M. Upper-body testing of cross-country skiers. *Med Sci Sports Exerc* 27(11):1557-1562, 1995.

9. Buono, MJ, Roby, JJ, Micale, FG, Sallis, JF, and Shepard, WE. Validity and reliability of predicting maximum oxygen uptake via field tests in children and adolescents. *Pediatr Exerc Sci* 3(3):250-255, 1991.

10. Carver, S. Injury prevention and treatment. In *Health Fitness Instructor's Handbook.* 4th ed. Howley, ET, and Franks, BD, eds. Champaign, IL: Human Kinetics. 393-420, 2003.

11. Caton, M. Equipment selection, purchase, and maintenance. *ACSM's Resource Manual for Guidelines for Exercise Testing and Prescription.* 3rd ed. Roitman, JL, ed. Baltimore: Lippincott Williams & Wilkins, 625-631, 1998.

12. Coris, E, Ramirez, A, and Van Durme, D. Heat illness in athletes: The dangerous combination of heat, humidity and exercise. *Sports Med* 34(1):9-16, 2004.

13. Daniels, J, Oldridge, N, Nagel, F, and White, B. Differences and changes in VO_2 among young runners 10-18 years of age. *Med Sci Sports* 17:200-203, 1978.

14. Deurenberg, P, and Deurenberg-Yap, M. Validity of body composition methods across ethic population groups. *Acta Diabetol* 40:S246-S249, 2003.

15. Fleck, SJ, and Kraemer, WJ. *Designing Resistance Training Programs.* 4th ed. Champaign, IL: Human Kinetics, 2014.

16. Frampton, M. Does inhalation of ultrafine particles cause pulmonary vascular effects in humans? *Inhal Toxicol* 19:75-79, 2007.

17. Fulco, CS, Rock, PB, and Cymerman, A. Maximal and submaximal exercise performance at altitude. *Aviat Space Envir Md* 69(8):793-801, 1998.

18. Gabbett, T, and Georgieff, B. Physiological and anthropometric characteristics of Australian junior national, state, and novice volleyball players. *J Strength Cond Res* 21(3):902-908, 2007.

19. Gergley, T, McArdle, W, DeJesus, P, Toner, M, Jacobowitz, S, and Spina, R. Specificity of arm training on aerobic power during swimming and running. *Med Sci Sports Exerc* 16(4):349-354, 1984.

20. Golding, LA, ed. *YMCA Fitness Testing and Assessment Manual.* Champaign, IL: Human Kinetics, 2000.

21. Hambrecht, RP, Schuler, GC, Muth, T, Grunze, MF, Marburger, CT, Niebauer, J, Methfessel, SM, and Kübler, W. Greater diagnostic sensitivity of treadmill versus cycle exercise testing of asymptomatic men with coronary artery disease. *Am J Cardiol* 70(2):141-146, 1992.

22. Herbert, DL. Legal and professional responsibilities of personal training. In *The Business of Personal Training.* Roberts, SO, ed. Champaign, IL: Human Kinetics, 53-63, 1996.

23. Heyward, VH, and Wagner, DR. *Applied Body Composition Assessment.* 2nd ed. Champaign, IL: Human Kinetics, 2004.

24. Housh, TJ, Cramer, JT, Weir, JP, Beck, TW, and Johnson, GO. *Physical Fitness Laboratories on a Budget.* Scottsdale, AZ: Holcomb Hathaway, 2009.

25. Howley, ET, and Franks, BD. *Health Fitness Instructor's Handbook.* 4th ed. Champaign, IL: Human Kinetics, 2003.

26. Katch, F, and Katch, V. The body composition profile. Techniques of measurement and applications. *Clin Sport Med* 3(1):31-63, 1984.

27. Kraemer, WJ, and Fleck, SJ. *Optimizing Strength Training.* Champaign, IL: Human Kinetics, 2007.

28. Lacy, AC, and Hastad, DN. *Measurement and Evaluation in Physical Education and Exercise Science.* 5th ed. San Francisco: Pearson Education, 2007.

29. Laughlin, N, and Busk, P. Relationships between selected muscle endurance tasks and gender. *J Strength Cond Res* 21(2):400-404, 2007.

30. Lloyd, RS, and Faigenbaum, AD. Age- and sex-related differences and their implications for resistance exercise, In *Essentials of Strength Training and Conditioning*. 4th ed. Haff, GG, and Triplett, NT, eds. Champaign, IL: Human Kinetics, 135-154, 2016.

31. Lockie, RG, Risso, FG, Giuliano, DV, Orjalo, AJ, and Jalilvand, F. Practical fitness profiling using field test data for female elite-level collegiate soccer players: A case analysis of a Division I team. *Strength Cond J* 40(3):58-71, 2018.

32. Mayhew, JL, Johnson, BD, LaMonte, MJ, Lauber, D, and Kemmler, W. Accuracy of prediction equations for determining one repetition maximum bench press in women before and after resistance training. *J Strength Cond Res* 22(5):1570-1577, 2008.

33. McArdle, WD, Katch, FI, and Katch, VL. *Exercise Physiology: Energy, Nutrition, and Human Performance*. 5th ed. Philadelphia: Lippincott Williams & Wilkins, 2001.

34. McClain, JJ, Welk, GJ, Ihmels, M, and Schaben, J. Comparison of two versions of the PACER aerobic fitness test. *J Phys Act Health* 3(Suppl 2):S47-S57, 2006.

35. McGuigan, MR. Principles of test selection and administration. In *Essentials of Strength Training and Conditioning*. 4th ed. Haff, GG, and Triplett, NT, eds. Champaign, IL: Human Kinetics, 249-258, 2016.

36. Moritani, T, and deVries, H. Neutral factors versus hypertrophy in the time course of muscle strength gain. *Am J Phys Med* 58(3):115-130, 1979.

37. Morrow Jr., JR, Kang, M, Disch, JG, and Mood, DP. *Measurement and Evaluation in Human Performance*. 5th ed. Champaign, IL: Human Kinetics, 2016.

38. Myers, J, Buchanan, N, Walsh, D, Kraemer, M, McAuley, P, Hamilton-Wessler, M, and Froelicher, VF. Comparison of the ramp versus standard exercise protocols. *J Am Coll Cardiol* 17(6):1334-1342, 1991.

39. Noonan, V, and Dean, E. Submaximal exercise testing: Clinical application and interpretation. *Phys Ther* 80(8):782-807, 2000.

40. O'Brien, CP. Are current exercise test protocols appropriate for older patients? *Coronary Artery Dis* 10:43-46, 1999.

41. Powers, SK, and Howley, ET. *Exercise Physiology: Theory and Application to Fitness and Performance*. 7th ed. Boston: McGraw-Hill, 2009.

42. Prentice, AM, and Jebb, SA. Beyond body mass index. *Obes Rev* 2:141-147, 2001.

43. Reuter, BH, and Dawes, JJ. Program design and technique for aerobic endurance training, In *Essentials of Strength Training and Conditioning*. 4th ed. Haff, GG, and Triplett, NT, eds. Champaign, IL: Human Kinetics, 559-581, 2016.

44. Rodgers, GP, Ayanian, JZ, Balady, G, Beasley, JW, Brown, KA, Gervino, EV, Paridon, S, Quinones, M, Schlant, RC, Winters Jr., WL, and Achord, JL. American College of Cardiology/American Heart Association Clinical Competence statement on stress testing: A report of the American College of Cardiology/American Heart Association/American College of Physicians—American Society of Internal Medicine Task Force on Clinical Competence. *J Am Coll Cardiol* 36(4):1441-1453, 2000.

45. Rozenek, R, and Storer, TW. Client assessment tools for the personal fitness trainer. *Strength Cond* 19:52-63, 1997.

46. Rusk, DB. Creating your own personal training business. In *The Business of Personal Training*. Roberts, SO, ed. Champaign, IL: Human Kinetics, 23-30, 1996.

47. Springer, BA, Marin, R, Chan, T, Roberts, H, and Gill, NW. Normative values for the unimpeded stance test with eyes open and closed. *J Geriatr Phys Ther* 30(1):8-15, 2007.

48. Soutine, H. Physical activity and health: Musculoskeletal issues. *Adv Physiother* 9(2):65-75, 2007.

49. Statler, T, and Brown, V. Facility policies, procedures, and legal issues. In *Essentials of Strength Training and Conditioning*. 4th ed. Haff, GG, and Triplett, NT, eds. Champaign, IL: Human Kinetics, 641-656, 2016.

50. Tan, R, and Spector, S. Exercise-induced asthma. *Sports Med* 25(1):1-6, 1998.

51. Terrados, N, and Maughan. RJ. Exercise in the heat: Strategies to minimize the adverse effects on performance. *J Sport Sci* 13:S55-S62, 1995.

52. Thomas, JR, Nelson, JK, and Silverman, SJ. *Research Methods in Physical Activity*. 7th ed. Champaign, IL: Human Kinetics, 2015.

53. Tramel, W, Lockie, RG, Lindsay, KG, and Dawes, JJ. Associations between absolute and relative lower body strength to measures of power and change of direction speed in Division II female volleyball players. *Sports* 7(7):160, 2019.

54. Turley, KR, Wilmore, JH, Simons-Morton, B, Williston, JM, Epping, JR, and Dahlstrom, G. The reliability and validity of the 9-minute run in third-grade children. *Pediatr Exerc Sci* 6:178-187, 1994.

55. van den Tillaar, R, and Ettema, G. Effect of body size and gender in overarm throwing performance. *Eur J Appl Physiol* 91(4):413-418, 2004.

56. Victor, R, Leimbach, W, Seals, D, Wallin, B, and Mark, A. Effects of the cold pressor test on muscle sympathetic nerve activity in humans. *Hypertension* 9(5):429-436, 1987.

57. Wang, Z, Heshka, S, Pierson, R, and Heymsfield, S. Systematic organization of body-composition methodology: An overview with emphasis on component-based methods. *Am J Clin Nutr* 61(3):457-465, 1995.

58. Wilmore, JH, Costill, DL, and Kenney, WL. *Physiology of Sport and Exercise*. 7th ed. Champaign, IL: Human Kinetics, 2019.

Chapter 11

1. American College of Sports Medicine. *ACSM's Guidelines for Exercise Testing and Prescription*, 11th ed. Philadelphia: Wolters Kluwer, 2022.

2. American College of Sports Medicine. *ACSM's Guidelines for Exercise Testing and Prescription*, 8th ed. Philadelphia: Lippincott Williams & Wilkins, 2010.

3. Åstrand, I. Aerobic work capacity in men and women with special reference to age. *Acta Physiol Scand* 49(Suppl):S1-S92, 1960.

4. Åstrand, P-O, and Ryhming, I. A nomogram for calculation of aerobic capacity (physical fitness) from pulse rate during submaximal work. *J Appl Physiol* 7:218-221, 1954.

5. Baumgartner, TA, Jackson, AS, Mahar, MT, and Rowe, DA. *Measurement for Evaluation in Physical Education and Exercise Science*. 8th ed. Boston: McGraw-Hill, 2007.

6. Beam, WC, and Adams, GM. *Exercise Physiology: Laboratory Manual*. 7th ed. New York: McGraw-Hill, 2014.

7. Bray, GA, and Gray, DS. Obesity. Part I—Pathogenesis. *West J Med* 149:429-441, 1988.

8. Cable, A, Nieman, DC, Austin, M, Hogen, E, and Utter, AC. Validity of leg-to-leg bioelectrical impedance measurement in males. *J Sports Med Phys Fitness* 41:411-414, 2001.

9. Canadian Society for Exercise Physiology (CSEP). *The Canadian Physical Activity, Fitness & Lifestyle Approach: CSEP-Health-Related Appraisal & Counseling Strategy*. 3rd ed. Ottawa, ON: Author, 2003.

10. Castro-Piñero, J, Girela-Rejón, MJ, González-Montesinos, JL, Mora, J, Conde-Caveda, J, Sjöström, M, and Ruiz, JR. Percentile values for flexibility tests in youths aged 6 to 17 years: Influence of weight status. *Eur J Sport Sci* 13:139-148, 2013.

10a. Chobanian, AV, Bakris, GL, Black, HR, Cushman, WC, Green, LA, Izzo, JL, Jr, Jones, DW, Materson, BJ, Oparil, S, Wright, JT, Jr, and Roccella, EJ. Joint National Committee on Prevention, Detection, Evaluation, and Treatment of High Blood Pressure. National Heart, Lung, and Blood Institute, & National High Blood Pressure Education Program Coordinating Committee. Seventh report of the Joint National Committee on Prevention, Detection, Evaluation, and Treatment of High Blood Pressure. *Hypertension* 42(6):1206–1252, 2003.

11. Chu, DA. Assessment. In *Explosive Power and Strength: Complex Training for Maximum Results*. Champaign, IL: Human Kinetics, 167-180, 1996.

12. Clemons, JM, Campbell, B, and Jeansonne, C. Validity and reliability of a new test of upper body power. *J Strength Cond Res* 24:1559-1565, 2010.

13. Deurenberg, P, Deurenberg-Yap, M, and Schouten, FJ. Validity of total and segmental impedance measurements for prediction of body composition across ethnic population groups. *Eur J Clin Nutr* 56:214-220, 2002.

14. Devries, HA, and Housh, TJ. *Physiology of Exercise for Physical Education, Athletics, and Exercise Science*. 5th ed. Madison, WI: Brown and Benchmark, 1994.

14a. Eckerson, JM, Stout, JR, Evetovich, TK, Housh, TJ, Johnson, GO, and Worrell, N. Validity of self-assessment techniques for estimating percent fat in men and women. *J Strength Cond Res* 12(4): 243-247, 1998.

15. Ehrman, JK, and American College of Sports Medicine. *ACSM's Resource Manual for Guidelines for Exercise Testing and Prescription.* 6th ed. Philadelphia: Wolters Kluwer Health/Lippincott Williams & Wilkins, 2010.

16. Ellegard, L, Bertz, F, Winkvist, A, Bosaeus, I, and Brekke, HK. Body composition in overweight and obese women postpartum: Bioimpedance methods validated by dual energy X-ray absorptiometry and doubly labeled water. *Eur J Clin Nutr* 70:1181-1188, 2016.

16a. Fukuda, DH. *Assessments for Sport and Athletic Performance.* Champaign, IL: Human Kinetics, 2019.

17. Fukuda, DH. Agility and sprinting. In *Assessments for Sport and Athletic Performance.* Champaign, IL: Human Kinetics, 107-132, 2019.

18. Fukuda, DH. Flexibility and balance. In *Assessments for Sport and Athletic Performance.* Champaign, IL: Human Kinetics, 77-106, 2019.

19. Fukuda, DH. Muscular strength and endurance. In *Assessments for Sport and Athletic Performance.* Champaign, IL: Human Kinetics, 165-207, 2019.

20. Fukuda, DH. Power. In *Assessments for Sport and Athletic Performance.* Champaign, IL: Human Kinetics, 133-164, 2019.

21. Gabbett, TJ, Nassis, GP, Oetter, E, Pretorius, J, Johnston, N, Medina, D, Rodas, G, Myslinski, T, Howells, D, Beard, A, and Ryan, A. The athlete monitoring cycle: A practical guide to interpreting and applying training monitoring data. *Br J Sports Med* 51:1451-1452, 2017.

22. Gibson, AL, Heyward, VH, and Mermier, CM. Predictive accuracy of Omron body logic analyzer in estimating relative body fat of adults. *Int J Sport Nutr Exerc Metab* 10:216-227, 2000.

23. Gibson, AL, Wagner, DR, and Heyward, VH. *Advanced Fitness Assessment and Exercise Prescription.* 8th ed. Champaign, IL: Human Kinetics, 2019.

24. Gibson, AL, Wagner, DR, and Heyward, VH. Assessing cardiorespiratory fitness. In *Advanced Fitness Assessment and Exercise Prescription.* 8th ed. Champaign, IL: Human Kinetics, 79-123, 2019.

25. Gibson, AL, Wagner, DR, and Heyward, VH. Assessing flexibility. In *Advanced Fitness Assessment and Exercise Prescription.* 8th ed. Champaign, IL: Human Kinetics, 309-329, 2019.

26. Gibson, AL, Wagner, DR, and Heyward, VH. Preliminary health screening and risk classification. In *Advanced Fitness Assessment and Exercise Prescription.* 8th ed. Champaign, IL: Human Kinetics, 29-54, 2019.

27. Gillam, GM, and Marks, M. 300 yard shuttle run. *Strength Cond J* 5:46-46, 1983.

28. Golding, LA. *YMCA Fitness Testing and Assessment Manual.* 4th ed. Champaign, IL: Human Kinetics, 2000.

29. Grenier, SG, Russell, C, and McGill, SM. Relationships between lumbar flexibility, sit-and-reach test, and a previous history of low back discomfort in industrial workers. *Can J Appl Physiol* 28:165-177, 2003.

30. Haff, GG, and Dumke, C. Anaerobic fitness measurements. In *Laboratory Manual for Exercise Physiology.* Champaign, IL: Human Kinetics, 305-360, 2012.

31. Haff, GG, and Dumke, C. Flexibility testing. In *Laboratory Manual for Exercise Physiology.* Champaign, IL: Human Kinetics, 79-114, 2012.

32. Harrison, GG, Buskirk, ER, Carter Lindsay, JE, Johnston, FE, Lohman, TG, Pollock, ML, Roche, AF, and Wilmore, JH. Skinfold thicknesses and measurement technique. In *Anthropometric Standardization Reference Manual.* Lohman, TG, Roche, AF, and Martorell, R, eds, 55-70, 1988.

33. Herrington, L, Munro, A, and Jones, P. Assessment of factors associated with injury risk. In *Performance Assessment in Strength and Conditioning.* Comfort, P, Jones, PA, and McMahon, JJ, eds. London: Routledge, 53-96, 2018.

34. Herrington, LC, and Munro, AG. A preliminary investigation to establish the criterion validity of a qualitative scoring system of limb alignment during single-leg squat and landing. *J Exerc Sports Orthop* 1:1-6, 2014.

35. Heyward, VH, and Gibson, AL. *Advanced Fitness Assessment and Exercise Prescription.* 7th ed. Champaign, IL: Human Kinetics, 2014.

36. Heyward, VH, and Wagner, DR. *Applied Body Composition Assessment.* 2nd ed. Champaign, IL: Human Kinetics, 2004.

37. Hoffman, J. Anaerobic power. In *Norms for Fitness, Performance, and Health.* Champaign, IL: Human Kinetics, 53-66, 2006.

38. Hoffman, J. Athletic performance testing and normative data. In *Physiological Aspects of Sport Training and Performance.* 2nd ed. Champaign, IL: Human Kinetics, 237-267, 2014.

38a. Hodgdon, JA. A history of the US Navy physical readiness program from 1976 to 1999. San Diego CA: Naval Health Research Center, 1999.

39. Hooper, SL, Mackinnon, LT, Howard, A, Gordon, RD, and Bachmann, AW. Markers for monitoring overtraining and recovery. *Med Sci Sports Exerc* 27:106-112, 1995.

40. Housh, TJ, Cramer, JT, Weir, JP, Beck, TW, and Johnson, GO. Muscular power. In *Physical Fitness Laboratories on a Budget.* Scottsdale, AZ: Holcomb Hathaway, 127-162, 2009.

41. Houtkooper, LB, Lohman, TG, Going, SB, and Howell, WH. Why bio-electrical impedance analysis should be used for estimating adiposity. *Am J Clin Nutr* 64:S436-S448, 1996.

42. Jackson, AS. Research design and analysis of data procedures for predicting body density. *Med Sci Sports Exerc* 16:616-622, 1984.

43. Jackson, AS, and Pollock, ML. Practical assessment of body composition. *Phys Sportsmed* 13:76-90, 1985.

44. Johnson, JC. *Postural Assessment.* Champaign, IL: Human Kinetics, 2012.

44a. Kaminsky, LA, Arena, R, and Myers, J. Reference standards for cardiorespiratory fitness measured with cardiopulmonary exercise testing: Data from the fitness registry and the importance of exercise national database. *Mayo Clinic Proceedings* 90(11):1515-1523, 2015.

44b. Kaminsky, LA, Imboden, MT, Arena, R, and Myers, J. Reference Standards for Cardiorespiratory Fitness Measured With Cardiopulmonary Exercise Testing Using Cycle Ergometry: Data From the Fitness Registry and the Importance of Exercise National Database (FRIEND) Registry. *Mayo Clinic Proceedings* 92(2): 228–233, 2017.

45. Kendall, FP, McCreary, EK, and Provance, PG. *Muscles: Testing and Function With Posture and Pain.* 5th ed. Baltimore: Lippincott Williams & Wilkins, 2005.

46. Kjaer, IG, Torstveit, MK, Kolle, E, Hansen, BH, and Anderssen, SA. Normative values for musculoskeletal- and neuromotor fitness in apparently healthy Norwegian adults and the association with obesity: A cross-sectional study. *BMC Sports Sci Med Rehabil* 8:37, 2016.

47. Kline, GM, Porcari, JP, Hintermeister, R, Freedson, PS, Ward, A, Mccarron, RF, Ross, J, and Rippe, JM. Estimation of VO$_2$max From a One-Mile Track Walk, Gender, Age, and Body-Weight. *Med Sci Sports Exerc* 19:253-259, 1987.

48. Kordich, JA. *Evaluating Your Client: Fitness Assessment and Protocol Norms.* Lincoln, NE: NSCA Certification Commission, 2002.

49. Kraemer, WJ, Ratamess, NA, Fry, AC, and French, DN. Strength training: Development and evaluation of methodology. In *Physiological Assessment of Human Fitness.* 2nd ed. Maud, PJ, and Foster, C, eds. Champaign, IL: Human Kinetics, 119-150, 2006.

50. Lee, DR, and Kim, LJ. Reliability and validity of the closed kinetic chain upper extremity stability test. *J Phys Ther Sci* 27:1071-1073, 2015.

51. Leger, L, and Thivierge, M. Heart-rate monitors—validity, stability, and functionality. *Phys Sportsmed* 16:143-151, 1988.

52. Lohman, TG. *Advances in Body Composition Assessment.* Champaign, IL: Human Kinetics, 1992.

53. Lohman, TG, Houtkooper, L, and Going, SB. Body fat measurement goes high-tech: Not all are created equal. *ACSM's Health Fit J* 1:30-35, 1997.

54. Malek, MH, Housh, TJ, Berger, DE, Coburn, JW, and Beck, TW. A new non-exercise based VO$_2$max equation for aerobically trained men. *J Strength Cond Res* 19:559-565, 2004.

55. Malek, MH, Housh, TJ, Berger, DE, Coburn, JW, and Beck, TW. A new nonexercise-based VO$_2$max equation for aerobically trained females. *Med Sci Sport Exer* 36:1804-1810, 2004.

56. McArdle, WD, Katch, FI, and Katch, VL. *Exercise Physiology: Nutrition, Energy, and Human Performance.* 7th ed. Philadelphia: Lippincott Williams & Wilkins, 2009.

57. McDowell, MA, Fryar, CD, Ogden, CL, and Flegal, KM. Anthropometric reference data for children and adults: United States, 2003–2006. *Natl Health Stat Rep* 10:5, 2008.

58. McGuigan, M. Administration, scoring, and interpretation of selected tests. In *Essentials of Strength Training and Conditioning*. 4th ed. Haff, G, and Triplett, NT, eds. Champaign, IL: Human Kinetics, 259-316, 2016.

59. McGuigan, M. Quantifying training stress. In *Monitoring Training and Performance in Athletes*. Champaign, IL: Human Kinetics, 69-102, 2017.

60. McIntosh, G, Wilson, L, and Hall, H. Trunk and lower extremity muscle endurance: Normative data for adults. *J Rehabil Outcome Meas* 2:20-39, 1998.

60a. Moon, JR, Hull, HR, Tobkin, SE, Teramoto, M, Karabulut, M, Roberts, MD, Ryan, ED. Kim, SJ, Dalbo, VJ, Walter, AA, Smith, AE, Cramer, JT, and Stout, JR. Percent body fat estimations in college women using field and laboratory methods: A three-compartment model approach. *J Int Society Sports Nutr* 4(1):1-9, 2007.

61. Morrow, JR, Jackson, AW, Disch, JG, and Mood, DP. *Measurement and Evaluation in Human Performance*. 4th ed. Champaign, IL: Human Kinetics, 2011.

62. Nieman, DC. Musculoskeletal fitness. In *Exercise Testing and Prescription: A Health-Related Approach*. 7th ed. Boston: McGraw-Hill, 136-158, 2011.

63. Patterson, DD, and Peterson, DF. Vertical jump and leg power norms for young adults. *Meas Phys Educ Exerc Sci* 8:33-41, 2004.

64. Pauole, K, Madole, K, Garhammer, J, Lacourse, M, and Rozenek, R. Reliability and validity of the T-test as a measure of agility, leg power, and leg speed in college-aged men and women. *J Strength Cond Res* 14:443-450, 2000.

65. Peterson, MD. Power. In *NSCA's Guide to Tests and Assessments*. Miller, T, ed. Champaign, IL: Human Kinetics, 217-252, 2012.

66. Pi-Sunyer, FX, Becker, DM, Bouchard, C, Carleton, RA, Colditz, GA, Dietz, WH, Foreyt, JP, Garrison, RJ, Grundy, SM, Hansen, BC, and Higgins, M. Clinical guidelines on the identification, evaluation, and treatment of overweight and obesity in adults: Executive summary. Expert Panel on the Identification, Evaluation, and Treatment of Overweight in Adults. *Am J Clin Nutr* 68:899-917, 1998.

67. Pickering, TG, Hall, JE, Appel, LJ, Falkner, BE, Graves, J, Hill, MN, Jones, DW, Kurtz, T, Sheps, SG, and Roccella, EJ, Subcommittee of Professional Public Education of the American Heart Association Council on High Blood Pressure Research. Recommendations for blood pressure measurement in humans and experimental animals: Part 1: Blood pressure measurement in humans: A statement for professionals from the Subcommittee of Professional and Public Education of the American Heart Association Council on High Blood Pressure Research. *Hypertension* 45:142-161, 2005.

68. Pollock, ML, Wilmore, JH, and Fox III, SM. *Health and Fitness Through Physical Activity*. New York: Wiley, 1978.

69. The President's Council on Fitness, Sports and Nutrition. Normative data. The President's Challenge 2010, 2010.

70. Prisant, LM, Alpert, BS, Robbins, CB, Berson, AS, Hayes, M, Cohen, ML, and Sheps, SG. American National Standard for nonautomated sphygmomanometers. Summary report. *Am J Hypertens* 8:210-213, 1995.

71. Reiman, MP, and Manske, RC. Lower extremity anaerobic power testing. In *Functional Testing in Human Performance*. Champaign, IL: Human Kinetics, 263-274, 2009.

72. Reiman, MP, and Manske, RC. Speed, agility, and quickness testing. In *Functional Testing in Human Performance*. Champaign, IL: Human Kinetics, 191-208, 2009.

73. Reiman, MP, and Manske, RC. Strength and power testing. In *Functional Testing in Human Performance*. Champaign, IL: Human Kinetics, 131-190, 2009.

74. Reynolds, JM, Gordon, TJ, and Roberts, RA. Prediction of one repetition maximum strength from multiple repetition maximum testing and anthropometry. *J Strength Cond Res* 20:584-592, 2006.

75. Ritz, P, Salle, A, Audran, M, and Rohmer, V. Comparison of different methods to assess body composition of weight loss in obese and diabetic patients. *Diabetes Res Clin Pract* 77:405-411, 2007.

76. Roush, JR, Kitamura, J, and Waits, MC. Reference values for the Closed Kinetic Chain Upper Extremity Stability Test (CKCUES) for collegiate baseball players. *N Am J Sports Phys Ther* 2:159-163, 2007.

77. Sheppard, JM, and Triplett, NT. Program design for resistance training. In *Essentials of Strength Training and Conditioning*. 4th ed. Haff, G, and Triplett, NT, eds. Champaign, IL: Human Kinetics, 439-470, 2016.

78. Tomkinson, GR, Carver, KD, Atkinson, F, Daniell, ND, Lewis, LK, Fitzgerald, JS, Lang, JJ, and Ortega, FB. European normative values for physical fitness in children and adolescents aged 9-17 years: Results from 2,779,165 Eurofit performances representing 30 countries. *Br J Sports Med* 52(22):1445-1456, 2017.

79. Triplett, NT. Speed and agility. In *NSCA's Guide to Tests and Assessments*. Miller, T, ed. Champaign, IL: Human Kinetics, 253-274, 2012.

79a. Tucci HT, Martins J, Sposito Gde C, Camarini PM, and de Oliveira, AS. Closed kinetic chain upper extremity stability test (CKCUES test): A reliability study in persons with and without shoulder impingement syndrome. *BMC Musculoskelet Disord* 15:1, 2014.

80. Utter, AC, Nieman, DC, Ward, AN, and Butterworth, DE. Use of the leg-to-leg bioelectrical impedance method in assessing body-composition change in obese women. *Am J Clin Nutr* 69:603-607, 1999.

81. van Marken Lichtenbelt, WD, Hartgens, F, Vollaard, NB, Ebbing, S, and Kuipers, H. Body composition changes in bodybuilders: A method comparison. *Med Sci Sports Exerc* 36:490-497, 2004.

82. Ward, LC, Heitmann, BL, Craig, P, Stroud, D, Azinge, EC, Jebb, S, Cornish, BH, Swinburn, B, O'Dea, K, Rowley, K, McDermott, R, Thomas, BJ, and Leonard, D. Association between ethnicity, body mass index, and bioelectrical impedance. Implications for the population specificity of prediction equations. *Ann NY Acad Sci* 904:199-202, 2000.

83. Wathen, D. Load selection. In *Essentials of Strength and Conditioning*. 1st ed. Baechle, TR, ed. Champaign, IL: Human Kinetics, 435-436, 1994.

84. Whelton, PK, Carey, RM, Aronow, WS, Casey Jr., DE, Collins, KJ, Dennison Himmelfarb, C, DePalma, SM, Gidding, S, Jamerson, KA, Jones, DW, MacLaughlin, EJ, Muntner, P, Ovbiagele, B, Smith Jr., SC, Spencer, CC, Stafford, RS, Taler, SJ, Thomas, RJ, Williams Sr., KA, Williamson, JD, and Wright Jr., JT. 2017 ACC/AHA/AAPA/ABC/ACPM/AGS/APhA/ASH/ASPC/NMA/PCNA guideline for the prevention, detection, evaluation, and management of high blood pressure in adults: A report of the American College of Cardiology/American Heart Association Task Force on Clinical Practice Guidelines. *Hypertension* 71:e13-e115, 2018.

Chapter 12

1. Alemdaroglu, U, Koklu, Y, and Koz, M. The acute effect of different stretching methods on sprint performance in taekwondo practitioners. *J Sport Med Phys Fit* 57:1104-1110, 2016.

2. Amako, M, Oda, T, Masuoka, K, Yokoi, H, and Campisi, P. Effect of static stretching on prevention of injuries for military recruits. *Mil Med* 168(6):442-446, 2003.

3. Avloniti, A, Chatzinikolaou, A, Fatouros, IG, Avloniti, C, Protopapa, M, Draganidis, D, Stampoulis, T, Leontsini, D, Mavropalias, G, Gounelas, G, and Kambas, A. The acute effects of static stretching on speed and agility performance depend on stretch duration and conditioning level. *J Strength Cond Res* 30:2767-2773, 2016.

4. Ayala, F, Calderón-López, A, Delgado-Gosálbez, JC, Parra-Sánchez, S, Pomares-Noguera, C, Hernández-Sánchez, S, López-Valenciano, A, and De Ste Croix, M. Acute effects of three neuromuscular warm-up strategies on several physical performance measures in football players. *PLOS One* 12(1):1-17, 2017.

5. Barroso, R, Tricoli, V, Santos Gil, SD, Ugrinowitsch, C, and Roschel, H. Maximal strength, number of repetitions, and total volume are differently affected by static-, ballistic-, and proprioceptive neuromuscular facilitation stretching. *J Strength Cond Res* 26:2432-2437, 2012.

6. Behm, D, Blazevich, A, Kay, A, and McHugh, M. Acute effects of muscle stretching on physical performance, range of motion, and injury incidence in healthy active individuals: A systematic review. *App Physiol Nutr Me* 41(1):1-11, 2016.

7. Behm, DG, and Chaouachi, A. A review of the acute effects of static and dynamic stretching on performance. *Eur J Appl Physiol* 111:2633-2651, 2011.

8. Behm, DG, Leonard, AM, Young, WB, Bonney, AC, and MacKinnon, SN. Trunk muscle electromyographic activity with unstable and unilateral exercises. *J Strength Cond Res* 19(1):193-201, 2005.

9. Bergouignan, A, Rudwill, F, Simon, C, and Blanc, S. Physical inactivity as the culprit of metabolic inflexibility: Evidence from bed-rest studies. *J Appl Physiol* 111(4):1201-1210, 2011.

10. Blackburn, JT, Bell, DR, Norcross, MF, Hudson, JD, and Kimsey, MH. Sex comparison of hamstring structural and material properties. *Clin Biomech* 24:65-70, 2009.

11. Bradley, PS, Olsen, PD, and Portas, MD. The effect of static, ballistic, and proprioceptive neuromuscular facilitation stretching on vertical jump performance. *J Strength Cond Res* 21:223-226, 2007.

12. Calatayud, J, Borreani, S, Colado, JC, Martin, FF, Rogers, ME, Behm, DG, and Andersen, LL. Muscle activation during push-ups with different suspension training systems. *J Sport Sci Med* 13(3):502-510, 2014.

13. Carter, JM, Beam, WC, McMahan, SG, Barr, MK, and Brown, LE. The effects of stability ball training on spinal stability in sedentary individuals. *J Strength Cond Res* 20(2):429-435, 2006.

14. Chidi-Ogbolu, N, and Baar, K. Effect of estrogen on musculoskeletal performance and injury risk. *Front Physiol* 9:1834, 2019.

15. Cho, M, and Kim, JY. Changes in physical fitness and body composition according to the physical activities of Korean adolescents. *J Exerc Rehabil* 13(5):568-572, 2017.

16. Chulvi-Medrano, I, Rial, T, Cortell-Tormo, JM, Alakhdar, Y, La Scala Teixeira, CV, Masiá-Tortosa, L, and Dorgo, S. Manual resistance versus conventional resistance training: Impact on strength and muscular endurance in recreationally trained men. *J Sport Sci Med* 16(3):343-349, 2017.

17. Clark, DR, Lambert, MI, and Hunter, AM. Contemporary perspectives of core stability training for dynamic athletic performance: A survey of athletes, coaches, sports science and sports medicine practitioners. *Sports Med* 4(1):32, 2018.

18. Cosio-Lima, LM, Reynolds, KL, Winter, C, Paolone, V, and Jones, MT. Effects of physical ball and conventional floor exercises. *J Strength Cond Res* 17:475-483, 2003.

19. Dallas, G, Smirniotou, A, Tsiganos, G, Tsopani, D, Di Cagno, A, and Tsolakis, C. Acute effect of different stretching methods on flexibility and jumping performance in competitive artistic gymnasts. *J Sport Med Phys Fit* 54:683-690, 2014.

20. Dawes, J. *Complete Guide to TRX® Suspension Training®*. Champaign, IL: Human Kinetics, 2017.

21. de Oliveira, UF, de Araújo, LC, de Andrade, PR, Dos Santos, HH, Moreira, DG, Sillero-Quintana, M, and de Almeida Ferreira, JJ. Skin temperature changes during muscular static stretching exercise. *J Exerc Rehabil* 14(3):451-459, 2018.

22. Eiling, E, Bryant, AL, Petersen, W, Murphy, A, and Hohmann, E. Effects of menstrual-cycle hormone fluctuations on musculotendinous stiffness and knee joint laxity. *Knee Surg Sports Tr A* 15:126-132, 2007.

23. Ferreira, MG, Bertor, WRR, de Carvalho, AR, and Bertolini, GRF. Effects of static, ballistic, and proprioceptive neuromuscular facilitation stretching on vertical jump variables. *Sci Med* 25(4):2, 2015.

24. Funk, D, Swank, AM, Adams, KJ, and Treolo, D. Efficacy of moist heat pack application over static stretching on hamstring flexibility. *J Strength Cond Res* 15(1):123-126, 2001.

25. Grieco, C. PNF stretching-training tips—proprioceptive neuromuscular facilitation. *American Fitness* July-August, 2002.

26. Hamlyn, N, Behm, DG, and Young, WB. Trunk muscle activation during dynamic weight-training exercises and isometric instability activities. *J Strength Cond Res* 21(4):1108-1112, 2007.

27. Harris, S, Ruffin, E, Brewer, W, and Ortiz, A. Muscle activation patterns during suspension training Exercises. *Int J Sports Phys Ther* 12(1):42-52, 2017.

28. Huxel Bliven, KC, and Anderson, BE. Core stability training for injury prevention. *Sports Health* 5(6):514-522, 2013.

29. Jaggers, JR, Swank, AM, Frost, KL, and Lee, CD. The acute effects of dynamic and ballistic stretching on vertical jump height, force, and power. *J Strength Cond Res* 22:1844-1849, 2008.

30. Jakubek, MD. Stability balls: Reviewing the literature regarding their use and effectiveness. *Strength Cond J* 29(5):58-63, 2007.

31. Jeffreys, I. *The Warm-Up*. Human Kinetics: Champaign, IL, 2019.

32. Jeffreys, I. Warm-up revisited: The ramp method of optimizing warm-ups. *Strength Cond J* (6):12-18, 2007.

33. Kemmler, W, von Stengel, S, Kohl, M, and Bauer, J. Impact of exercise changes on body composition during the college years—a five year randomized controlled study. *BMC Public Health* 16:50, 2016.

34. Kjaer, M, and Hansen, M. The mystery of female connective tissue. *J Appl Physiol* 105:1026-1027, 2008.

35. Koshida, S, Urabe, Y, Miyashita, K, Iwai, K, and Kagimori, A. Muscular outputs during dynamic bench press under stable versus unstable conditions. *J Strength Cond Res* 22(5):1584-1588, 2008.

36. Ladwig, MA. The psychological effects of a pre-workout warm-up: An exploratory study. *J Multidiscipl Res* 5(3):79-87, 2013.

37. Marshall, PWM, and Murphy, BA. Core stability on and off a Swiss ball. *Arch Phys Med Rehab* 86:242-249, 2005.

38. Marshall, PWM, and Murphy, BA. Increased deltoid and abdominal muscle activity during Swiss ball bench press. *J Strength Cond Res* 20(4):745-750, 2006.

39. McHugh, MP, Magnusson, SP, Gleim, GW, and Nicholas, JA. Viscoelastic stress relaxation in human skeletal muscle. *Med Sci Sports Exerc* 24(12):1375-1382, 1992.

40. Melrose, D, and Dawes, J. Resistance characteristics of the TRX® suspension training system at different angles and distances from the hanging point. *J Athl Enhancement* 4(1):2-5, 2015.

41. Milanović, Z, Pantelić, S, Trajković, N, Sporiš, G, Kostić, R, and James, N. Age-related decrease in physical activity and functional fitness among elderly men and women. *Clin Interv Aging* 8:549, 2013.

42. Mistry, GS, Vyas, NJ, and Sheth, MS. Comparison of hamstrings flexibility in subjects with chronic low back pain versus normal individuals. *J Clin Exp Res* 2:85, 2014.

43. Monteiro, WD, Simão, R, Polito, MD, Santana, CA, Chaves, RB, Bezerra, E, and Fleck, SJ. Influence of strength training on adult women's flexibility. *J Strength Cond Res* 22:672-677, 2008.

44. Nakamura, K, Kodama, T, and Mukaino, Y. Effects of active individual muscle stretching on muscle function. *J Phys Ther Sci* 26(3):341-344, 2014.

45. Nepocatych, S, Ketcham, CJ, Vallabhajosula, S, and Balilionis, G. The effects of unstable surface balance training on postural sway, stability, functional ability and flexibility in women. *J Sport Med Phys Fit* 58:27-34, 2018.

46. Nimphius, S, McGuigan, MR, and Newton, RU. Changes in muscle architecture and performance during a competitive season in female softball players. *J Strength Cond Res* 26:2655-2666, 2012.

47. Nuzzo, JL, McCaulley, GO, Cormie, P, Cavill, MJ, and McBride, JM. Trunk muscle activity during stability ball and free weight exercises. *J Strength Cond Res* 22(1):95-102, 2008.

48. Page, P. Current concepts in muscle stretching for exercise and rehabilitation. *Int J Sports Phys Ther* 7:109-119, 2012.

49. Palmer, TB, Jenkins, ND, Thompson, BJ, and Cramer, JT. Influence of stretching velocity on musculotendinous stiffness of the hamstrings during passive straight-leg raise assessments. *Musculoskelet Sci Pract* 30:80-85, 2017.

50. Pardeiro, M, and Yanci, J. Warm-up effects on physical performance and psychological perception in semiprofessional soccer players. *Rev Int Cienc Deporte* 13(48):104-116, 2017.

51. Petrofsky, JS, Laymon, M, and Lee, H. Effect of heat and cold on tendon flexibility and force to flex the human knee. *Med Sci Monitor* 19:661-667, 2013.

52. Purton, J, Humphries, B, and Warman, G. Comparison of peak muscular activation between Ab-roller and exercise ball. Honors thesis, Central Queensland University, Rockhampton, Queensland. 2001.

53. Raceinais, S, Cocking, S, and Periard, JD. Sports and environmental temperature: From warming-up to heating-up. *Temperature* 4(3):227-257, 2017.

54. Rees, S, Murphy, AJ, Watsford, ML, McLachlan, KA, and Coutts, AJ. Effects of proprioceptive neuromuscular facilitation stretching on stiffness and force-producing characteristics of the ankle in active women. *J Strength Cond Res* 21(2):572-577, 2007.

55. Ryan, ED, Beck, TW, Herda, TJ, Hull, HR, Hartman, MJ, Costa, PB, Defreitas, JM, Stout, JR, and Cramer, JT. The time course of musculotendinous stiffness responses following different durations of passive stretching. *J Orthop Sport Phys* 38(10):632-639, 2008.

56. Ryan, ED, Herda, TJ, Costa, PB, Walter, AA, Hoge, KM, Stout, JR, and Cramer, JT. Viscoelastic creep in the human skeletal muscle-tendon unit. *Eur J Appl Physiol* 108(1):207-211, 2010.

57. Santana, JC, and Fukuda, DH. Unconventional methods, techniques, and equipment for strength and conditioning in combat sports. *Strength Cond J* 33(6):64-70, 2011.

58. Sato, K, and Mokha, M. Does core strength training influence running kinetics, lower extremity stability, and 5000-m performance in runners? *J Strength Cond Res* 23(1):133-140, 2008.

59. Schibek, JS, Guskiewicz, KM, Prentice, WE, Mays, S, and Davis, JM. The effect of core stabilization training on functional performance in swimming. Master's thesis, University of North Carolina, Chapel Hill. 1999.

60. Schleip, R, and Müller, DG. Training principles for fascial connective tissues: Scientific foundation and suggested practical applications. *J Bodyw Mov Ther* 17:103-115, 2013.

61. Schwarz, N, Harper, S, Waldhelm, A, McKinley-Barnard, SK, Holden, SL, and Kovaleski, JE. A Comparison of machine versus free-weight squats for the enhancement of lower-body power, speed, and change-of-direction ability during an initial training phase of recreationally active women. *Sports* 7(10):215, 2019.

62. Sharman, MJ, Cresswell, AG, and Riek, S. Proprioceptive neuromuscular facilitation stretching: Mechanisms and clinical implications. *Sports Med* 36:929-939, 2006.

63. Shellock, FG, and Prentice, WE. Warming-up and stretching for improved physical performance and prevention of sports-related injuries. *Sports Med* 2(4):267-278, 1985.

64. Simão, R, Lemos, A, Salles, B, Leite, T, Oliveira, E, Rhea, M, and Reis, VM. The influence of strength, flexibility, and simultaneous training on flexibility and strength gains. *J Strength Cond Res* 25:1333-1338, 2011.

65. Snarr, RL, and Esco, MR. Electromyographic comparison of traditional and suspension push-ups. *J Hum Kinet* 39:75-83, 2013.

66. Snarr, RL, and Esco, MR. Electromyographical comparison of plank variations performed with and without instability devices. *J Strength Cond Res* 28(11):3298-3305, 2014.

67. Snarr, RL, Casey, JC, Hallmark, AV, and Eckert, RM. Instability device training: Helpful or Hype? *PTQ* 2(1):4-8, 2015.

68. Snarr, RL, Hallmark, AV, Nickerson, BS, and Esco, MR. Electromyographical analysis of pike variations with and without instability devices. *J Strength Cond Res* 30(12):3436-3442, 2016.

69. Stanton, R, Reaburn, PR, and Humphries, B. The effect of short-term Swiss ball training on core stability and running economy. *J Strength Cond Res* 18(3):522-528, 2004.

70. Stathokostas, L, Little, RM, Vandervoort, AA, and Paterson, DH. Flexibility training and functional ability in older adults: A systematic review. *J Aging Res* 2012:306818-306818, 2012.

71. Sternlight, E, Rugg, S, Fujii, L, Tomomitsu, K, and Seki, M. Electromyographic comparison of a stability ball crunch with a traditional crunch. *J Strength Cond Res* 21(2):506-509, 2007.

72. Stricker, T, Malone, T, and Garrett, WE. The effects of passive warming on muscle injury. *Am J Sport Med* 18(2):141-145, 1990.

73. Stutchfield, B, and Coleman, S. The relationships between hamstring flexibility, lumbar flexion, and low back pain in rowers. *Eur J Sport Sci* 6(4):255-260, 2006.

74. Tancred, T, and Tancred, B. An examination of the benefits of warm-up: A review. *New Stud Athletics* 10(4):35-41, 1995.

75. Thomas, M. The functional warm-up. *Strength Cond J* 22(2):51-53, 2000.

76. Trindade, TB, Prestes, J, Neto, LO, Medeiros, RMV, Tibana, RA, de Sousa, NMF, and Dantas, PMS. Effects of pre-exhaustion versus traditional resistance training on training volume, maximal strength, and quadriceps hypertrophy. *Front Physiol* 10:1424, 2019.

77. Vera-Garcia, FJ, Grenuer, SG, and McGill, S. Abdominal muscle response during curl-ups on both stable and unstable surfaces. *Phys Ther* 80:564-569, 2000.

78. Wahl, JM, and Behm, DG. Not all instability training devices enhance muscle activation in highly resistance-trained individuals. *J Strength Cond Res* 22(4):1360-1370, 2008.

79. Weerapong, P, Hume, PA, and Kolt, GS. Stretching: Mechanisms and benefits for sport performance and injury prevention. *Phys Ther Rev* 9:189-206, 2004.

80. Willardson, J. Core stability training: Applications to sports conditioning programs. *J Strength Cond Res* 21(3):979-985, 2007.

Chapter 13

1. Barnes, M, and Cinea, KE. Explosive movements. In *Strength Training*, Brown, LE, ed. Champaign, IL: Human Kinetics.

2. Barnes, M, and Cinea, KE. Lower body exercises. In *Strength Training*, Brown, LE, ed. Champaign, IL: Human Kinetics.

3. Barnes, M, and Cinea, KE. Torso exercises. In *Strength Training*, Brown, LE, ed. Champaign, IL: Human Kinetics.

4. Barnes, M, and Cinea, KE. Upper body exercises. In *Strength Training*, Brown, LE, ed. Champaign, IL: Human Kinetics.

5. Caulfield, S, and Berninger, D. Exercise technique for free weight and machine training. In *Essentials of Strength Training and Conditioning*, 4th ed. Haff, GG, and Triplett, NT, eds. Champaign, IL: Human Kinetics.

6. Chen, W, Wu, H, Lo, S, Chen, H, Yang, W, Huang, C, and Liu, C. Eight-week battle rope training improves multiple physical fitness dimensions and shooting accuracy in collegiate basketball players. *J Strength Cond Res* 32(10):2715-2724, 2018.

7. Cholewicki, J, Juluru, K, and McGill, S. Intra-abdominal pressure mechanism for stabilizing the lumbar spine. *J Biomech* 32(1):13-17, 1999.

8. Delavier, F. *Strength Training Anatomy*. Champaign, IL: Human Kinetics, 2006.

9. Eckert, R, and Snarr, RL. Exercise technique: Kettlebell thruster. *Strength Cond J* 36(4):73-76, 2014.

10. Eckert, RM, and Snarr, RL. Barbell hip thrust. *J Sport Hum Perf* 2(2):1-9, 2014.

11. Faigenbaum, A, and Westcott, W. *Youth Strength Training*. Champaign, IL: Human Kinetics, 2009.

12. Fountaine, CJ, and Schmidt, BJ. Metabolic cost of rope training. *J Strength Cond Res* 29(4):889-893, 2015.

13. Graham, JF. Exercise technique: Power clean. *Strength Cond J* 22(6):63-65, 2000.

14. Graham, JF. Exercise technique: Barbell lunge. *Strength Cond J* 24(5):30-32, 2002.

15. Graham, JF. Exercise technique: Front squat. *Strength Cond J* 24(3):75-76, 2002.

16. Graham, JF. Exercise technique: Barbell bench press. *Strength Cond J* 25(3):50-51, 2003.

17. Graham, JF. Exercise technique: Barbell upright row. *Strength Cond J* 26(5):60-61, 2004.

18. Graham, JF. Exercise technique: Leg curl. *Strength Cond J* 27(1):59-60, 2005.

19. Graham, JF. Exercise technique: Barbell overhead press. *Strength Cond J* 30(3):70-71, 2008.

20. Graham, JF. Resistance exercise techniques and spotting. In *Conditioning for Strength and Human Performance*. Chandler, TJ, and Brown, LE, eds. Philadelphia: Lippincott Williams & Wilkins, 2008.

21. Harman, EA, Rosenstein, RM, Frykman, PN, and Nigro, GA. Effects of a belt on intra-abdominal pressure during weightlifting. *Med Sci Sports Exerc* 21(2):186-190, 1989.

22. Haff, GG, Berninger, D, and Caulfield, S. Exercise technique for alternative modes and nontraditional implement training. In *Essentials of Strength Training and Conditioning*, 4th ed. Haff, GG, and Triplett, NT, eds. Champaign, IL: Human Kinetics, 2016.

23. Hoffman, JR, and Ratamess, NA. *A Practical Guide to Developing Resistance Training Programs*. Monterey, CA: Coaches Choice, 2006.

24. Lander, JE, Hundley, JR, and Simonton, RL. The effectiveness of weight-belts during multiple repetitions of the squat exercise. *Med Sci Sports Exerc* 24(5):603-609, 1990.

25. Lander, JE, Simonton, RL, and Giacobbe, JKF. The effectiveness of weight-belts during the squat exercise. *Med Sci Sports Exerc* 22(1):117-126, 1990.

26. Langford, EL, Wilhoite, SW, Collum, C, Weekley, H, Cook, JS, Adams, KA, and Snarr, RL. Exercise technique: Battle rope conditioning. *Strength Cond J* 41(6):115-121, 2019.

27. Lanham, S, Cooper, J, Chrysosferidis, P, Szekely, B, Langford, E, and Snarr, RL. Exercise technique: Deficit deadlift. *Strength Cond J* 41(1):115-119, 2019.

28. Martino, M, and Dawes, J. Battling ropes: A dynamic training tool for the tactical athlete. *J Aust Strength Cond* 20(3):52-56, 2012.

29. McMaster, DT, Cronin, J, and McGuigan, MR. Forms of variables resistance training. *Strength Cond J* 31(1):50-64, 2009.

30. McMaster, DT, Cronin, J, and McGuigan, MR. Quantification of rubber and chain-based resistance modes. *J Strength Cond Res* 24(8):2056-2064, 2010.

30a. National Strength and Conditioning Association. *Essentials of Strength Training and Conditioning*, 4th ed. Haff, GG, and Triplett, NT, eds. Champaign, IL: Human Kinetics, 2016.

31. Newton, H. *Explosive Lifting for Sports*. Champaign, IL: Human Kinetics, 2002.

32. NSCA Certification Commission. *Exercise Technique Manual for Resistance Training*, 3rd ed. Champaign, IL: Human Kinetics, 2016.

33. Raaj, MKP, and Rosario, CK. Impact of battle rope training on selected physical fitness components and performance variables among volleyball players. *Indian J Res* 6(4):579-580, 2018.

34. Snarr, L, Eckert, RM, and Abbott, P. A comparative analysis and technique of the lat pull-down. *Strength Cond J* 37(5):21-25, 2015.

35. Snarr, RL, and McGinn, W. Addressing weaknesses in squat patterns. *J Sport Hum Perf* 3(1):1-12, 2015.

36. Snarr, RL, Esco, MR, and Eckert, RM. Exercise highlight: Single-leg squat. *J Aust Strength Cond* 22(4):37-44, 2014.

37. Snarr, RL, and Eckert, RM. Exercise highlight: Reverse lunge to plyometric sprinter start. *J Aust Strength Cond* 22(1):5-13, 2013.

Chapter 14

1. American College of Sports Medicine. *ACSM's Guidelines for Exercise Testing and Prescription*. 10th ed. Philadelphia: Wolters Kluwer, 85-86, 2017.

2. American Council on Exercise. *Group Fitness Instructor Manual*. 4th ed. San Diego: Author, 4, 2016.

3. American Red Cross. *Swimming and Water Safety*. Yardley, PA: StayWell, 94, 2009.

4. Aquatic Exercise Association. *Aquatic Fitness Programming: Standards and Guidelines*. Nokomis, FL: Author, 4, 11, 2018. https://aeawave.org/Portals/0/AEA_Cert_Docs/AEA_Standards_Guidlines_2020.pdf?ver=2019-12-18-131623-417&timestamp=1576696862726. Accessed January 12, 2020.

5. Barker, AL, Talevski, J, Morello, RT, Brand, CA, Rahmann, AE, and Urquhart, DM. Effectiveness of aquatic exercise for musculoskeletal conditions: A meta-analysis. *Arch Phys Med Rehab* 95(9):1776-1786, 2014.

6. Bonzheim, SC, Franklin, BA, DeWitt, C, Marks, C, Goslin, B, Jarski, R, and Dann, S. Physiologic responses to recumbent versus upright cycle ergometry, and implications for exercise prescription in patients with coronary artery disease. *Am J Cardiol* 69(1):40-44, 1992.

7. Bricker, K, and Bonelli, S. *Traditional Aerobics and Step Training*. 2nd ed. Monterey, CA: Coaches Choice, 6, 2007.

8. Costigan, PA, Deluzio, KJ, and Wyss, UP. Knee and hip kinetics during normal stair climbing. *Gait & Posture* 16(1):31-37, 2002.

9. Deschodt, VJ, Arsac, LM, and Rouard, AH. Relative contribution of arms and legs in humans to propulsion in 25-m sprint front-crawl swimming. / Contribution relative des bras et des jambes de l'homme a la propulsion lors du crawl en sprint. *Eur J Appl Physio Occup Physiol* 80(3):192-199, 1999.

10. Evans, M. *Endurance Athlete's Edge*. Champaign, IL: Human Kinetics, 75-77, 93, 1997.

11. Gibala, MJ, Little, JP, van Essen, M, Wilkin, GP, Burgomaster, KA, Safdar, A, Raha, S, and Tarnopolsky, MA. Short-term sprint interval versus traditional endurance training: Similar initial adaptations in human skeletal muscle and exercise performance. *J Physiol* 575(3): 901-911, 2006.

12. Glover, B, and Florence, SL. *The Competitive Runner's Handbook*. Rev. ed. New York: Penguin, 336-337, 1999.

13. Hagberg, JM, Mullin, JP, Giese, MD, and Spitznagel, E. Effect of pedaling rate on submaximal exercise responses of competitive cyclists. *J Appl Physiol Respir Environ Exerc Physiol* 51(2):447-451, 1981.

14. Hall, C, Figueroa, A, Fernhall, B, and Kanalay, JA. Energy expenditure of walking and running: Comparison with prediction equations. *Med Sci Sports Exerc* 36(12):2128-2134, 2004.

15. Hobson, W, Campbell, C, and Vickers, M. *Swim, Bike, Run*. Champaign, IL: Human Kinetics, 45-54, 2001.

16. Jones, AM, and Doust, JH. A 1% treadmill grade most accurately reflects the energetic cost of outdoor running. *J Sports Sci* 14(4):321-327, 1996.

17. Lepers, R, Millet, GY, Maffiuletti, NA, Hausswirth, C, and Brisswalter, J. Effect of pedalling rates on physiological response during endurance cycling. *Eur J Appl Physiol* 85(3-4):392-395, 2001.

18. Lucia, A, Hoyos, J, and Chicharro, JL. Preferred pedalling cadence in professional cycling. *Med Sci Sports Exerc* 33(8):1361-1366, 2001.

18a. Maglischo, EW. *Swimming Fastest*. Champaign, IL: Human Kinetics, 181, 2003.

19. Michaud, TJ, Rodriguez-Zayas, J, Armstrong, C, and Hartnig, M. Ground reaction forces in high impact and low impact aerobic dance. *J Sport Med Phys Fit* 33(4):359-366, 1993.

20. Neff, A, Leary, M, and Sherlock, L. Developing strength in an aquatic environment—research summary and sample workout. Aquatic Exercise Association. https://aeawave.org/Portals/0/Research/Developing%20Strength%20in%20an%20Aquatic%20Environment..pdf?ver=2019-06-17-161859-973&timestamp=1560802880264, 2019. Accessed January 12, 2020.

21. Quesada, JIP, Perez-Soriano, P, Lucas-Cuevas, AG, Palmer, RS, and Cibrian Ortiz de Anda, RM. Effect of bike-fit in the perception of comfort, fatigue and pain. *J Sports Sci* 35(14):1459-1465, 2017.

22. Reilly, DT, and Martens, M. Experimental analysis of the quadriceps muscle force and patello-femoral joint reaction force for various activities. *Acta Orthop Scand* 43(2):126-137, 1972.

23. Scharff-Olson, M, and Williford, HN. Step aerobics fulfills its promise: High on fitness, low on impact. *ACSMS Health Fit J* 2:32-37, 1998.

23a. Shih, J, Wang, YT, and Moeinzadeh, MH. Effect of speed and experience on kinetic and kinematic factors during exercise on a stair-climbing machine. *J Sport Rehabil* 5(3): 224-233, 1996.

24. Takaishi, T, Yasuda, Y, Ono, T, and Moritani, T. Optimal pedaling rate estimated from neuromuscular fatigue for cyclists. *Med Sci Sports Exerc* 28(12):1492-1497, 1996.

25. Wang, SY, Chenfu, H, and Yang, CH. Biomechanical analysis of high-low impact aerobic dance and step aerobics. *20th International Symposium on Biomechanics in Sports* 179-182, 2002.

Chapter 15

1. Abadie, BR, and Wentworth, M. Prediction of 1-RM strength from a 5-10 repetition submaximal test in college aged females. *J Exerc Physiol (Online)* 3:1-5, 2000.

2. Adams, GM. *Exercise Physiology Laboratory Manual*, 3rd ed. Boston: McGraw-Hill, 1998.

3. American College of Sports Medicine. Position stand. Progression models in resistance training for healthy adults. *Med Sci Sports Exerc* 41:687-708, 2009.

4. Baker, D, and Nance, S. The relation between running speed and measures of strength and power in professional rugby league players. *J Strength Cond Res* 13:230-235, 1999.

5. Baz-Valle, E, Fontes-Villalba, M, and Santos-Concejero, J. Total number of sets as a training volume quantification method for muscle hypertrophy: A systematic review. *J Strength Cond Res* 35(3):870-878, 2021.

6. Baz-Valle, E, Schoenfeld, BJ, Torres-Unda, J, Santos-Concejero, J, and Balsalobre-Fernández C. The effects of exercise variation in muscle thickness, maximal strength and motivation in resistance trained men. *PLOS One* 14(12):e0226989, 2019.

7. Berger, RA. Effect of varied weight training programs on strength. *Res Quar* 33:168-181, 1962.

8. Bompa, TO, and Haff, GG. *Periodization: Theory and Methodology of Training*, 5th ed. Champaign, IL: Human Kinetics, 2009.

9. Burd, NA, Andrews, RJ, West, DW, Little, JP, Cochran, AJ, Hector, AJ, Cashaback, JG, Gibala, MJ, Potvin, JR, Baker, SK, and Phillips, SM. Muscle time under tension during resistance exercise stimulates differential muscle protein sub-fractional synthetic responses in men. *J Physiol* 590(2):351-362, 2012.

10. Campos, GE, Luecke, TJ, Wendeln, HK, Toma, K, Hagerman, FC, Murray, TF, Ragg, KE, Ratamess, NA, Kraemer, WJ, and Staron, RS. Muscular adaptations in response to three different resistance-training regimens: Specificity of repetition maximum training zones. *Eur J Appl Physiol* 88(1-2):50-60, 2002.

11. Caserotti, P, Aagaard, P, Buttrup Larsen, J, and Puggaard, L. Explosive heavy-resistance training in old and very old adults: Changes in rapid muscle force, strength, and power. *Scand J Med Sci Spor* 18:773-782, 2008.

12. Coyle, EF, Feiring, DC, Rotkis, TC, Cote, RWD, Roby, FB, Lee, W, and Wilmore, JH. Specificity of power improvements through slow and fast isokinetic training. *J Appl Physiol* 51:1437-1442, 1981.

13. Craig, BW. Variation: An important component of training. *Strength Cond J* 22:22-23, 2000.

14. Dudley, GA, Tesch, PA, Miller, BJ, and Buchanan, P. Importance of eccentric actions in performance adaptations to resistance training. *Aviat Space Envir Md* 62:543-550, 1991.

15. Earle, RW, and Baechle, TR. Resistance training program design. In *NSCA's Essentials of Personal Training.* Baechle, TR, and Earle, RW, eds. Champaign, IL: Human Kinetics, 361-398, 2004.

16. Fleck, SJ. Periodized strength training: A critical review. *J Strength Cond Res* 13:82-89, 1999.

17. Fleck, S, and Kraemer, WJ. *Designing Resistance Training Programs,* 3rd ed. Champaign, IL: Human Kinetics, 375, 2004.

18. Fry, AC, and Kraemer, WJ. Resistance exercise overtraining and over-reaching. *Sports Med* 23(2):106-129, 1997.

18a. Grandou, C, Wallace, L, Impellizzeri, FM, Allen, NG, and Coutts, AJ. Overtraining in resistance exercise: An exploratory systematic review and methodological appraisal of the literature. *Sports Med* 50(4):815-828, 2020.

19. Grgic, J, Lazinica, B, Mikulic, P, Krieger, JW, and Schoenfeld, BJ. The effects of short versus long inter-set rest intervals in resistance training on measures of muscle hypertrophy: A systematic review. *Eur J Sport Sci* 17(8):983-993, 2017.

20. Grgic, J, Schoenfeld, BJ, Davies, TB, Lazinica, B, Krieger, JW, and Pedisic, Z. Effect of resistance training frequency on gains in muscular strength: A systematic review and meta-analysis. *Sports Med* 48(5):1207-1220, 2018.

21. Haff, GG, Burgess, S, and Stone, MH. Cluster training: Theoretical and practical applications for the strength and conditioning professional. *Prof Strength Cond* 12:12-17, 2008.

22. Haff, GG, Hobbs, RT, Haff, EE, Sands, WA, Pierce, KC, and Stone, MH. Cluster training: A novel method for introducing training program variation. *Strength Cond J* 30:67-76, 2008.

23. Haff, GG, Kraemer, WJ, O'Bryant, HS, Pendlay, G, Plisk, S, and Stone, MH. Roundtable discussion: Periodization of training-part 1. *Strength Cond J* 26:50-69, 2004.

24. Haff, GG, Whitley, A, McCoy, LB, O'Bryant, HS, Kilgore, JL, Haff, EE, Pierce, K, and Stone, MH. Effects of different set configurations on barbell velocity and displacement during a clean pull. *J Strength Cond Res* 17:95-103, 2003.

25. Häkkinen, K. Neuromuscular adaptations during strength training, aging, detraining, and immobilization. *Crit Rev Phys Rehabil Med* 6:161-198, 1994.

26. Häkkinen, K, Alen, M, and Komi, PV. Changes in isometric force- and relaxation-time, electromyographic and muscle fibre characteristics of human skeletal muscle during strength training and detraining. *Acta Physiol Scand* 125:573-585, 1985.

27. Häkkinen, K, Pakarinen, A, Alen, M, Kauhanen, H, and Komi, PV. Neuromuscular and hormonal responses in elite athletes to two successive strength training sessions in one day. *Eur J Appl Physiol* 57:133-139, 1988.

28. Harris, GR, Stone, MH, O'Bryant, HS, Proulx, CM, and Johnson, RL. Short-term performance effects of high power, high force, or combined weight-training methods. *J Strength Cond Res* 14:14-20, 2000.

29. Hazell, T, Kenno, K, and Jakobi, J. Functional benefit of power training for older adults. *J Aging Phys Activ* 15:349-359, 2007.

30. Helms, ER, Cronin, J, Storey, A, and Zourdos, MC. Application of the repetitions in reserve-based rating of perceived exertion scale for resistance training. *Strength Cond J* 38(4):42-49, 2016.

31. Henwood, TR, Riek, S, and Taaffe, DR. Strength versus muscle power-specific resistance training in community-dwelling older adults. *J Gerontol A-Biol* 63:83-91, 2008.

32. Henwood, TR, and Taaffe, DR. Short-term resistance training and the older adult: The effect of varied programmes for the enhancement of muscle strength and functional performance. *Clin Physiol Funct I* 26:305-313, 2006.

33. Hickson, RC, Dvorak, BA, Gorostiaga, EM, Kurowski, TT, and Foster, C. Potential for strength and endurance training to amplify endurance performance. *J Appl Physiol* 65:2285-2290, 1988.

34. Hickson, RC, Hidaka, K, and Foster, C. Skeletal muscle fiber type, resistance training, and strength-related performance. *Med Sci Sports Exerc* 26:593-598, 1994.

35. Hunter, GR, McCarthy, JP, and Bamman, MM. Effects of resistance training on older adults. *Sports Med* 34:329-348, 2004.

36. Issurin, V. *Block Periodization: Breakthrough in Sports Training.* Yessis, M, ed. Muskegan, MI: Ultimate Athlete Concepts, 213, 2008.

37. Issurin, V. Block periodization versus traditional training theory: A review. *J Sport Med Phys Fit* 48:65-75, 2008.

38. Izquierdo, M, Ibanez, J, Gonzalez-Badillo, JJ, Häkkinen, K, Ratamess, NA, Kraemer, WJ, French, DN, Eslava, J, Altadill, A, Asiain, X, and Gorostiaga, EM. Differential effects of strength training leading to failure versus not to failure on hormonal responses, strength, and muscle power gains. *J Appl Physiol* 100:1647-1656, 2006.

39. Kraemer, WJ, and Ratamess, NA. Fundamentals of resistance training: Progression and exercise prescription. *Med Sci Sports Exerc* 36:674-688, 2004.

40. Kraemer, WJ, Vingren, JL, Hatfield, DL, Spiering, BA, and Fragala, MS. Resistance training programs. In *ACSM's Resources for the Personal Trainer,* 2nd ed. Thompson, WR, ed. Baltimore: Lippincott Williams & Wilkins, 372-403, 2007.

41. Kramer, JB, Stone, MH, O'Bryant, HS, Conley, MS, Johnson, RL, Nieman, DC, Honeycutt, DR, and Hoke, TP. Effects of single vs. multiple sets of weight training: Impact of volume, intensity, and variation. *J Strength Cond Res* 11:143-147, 1997.

42. Lasevicius, T, Ugrinowitsch, C, Schoenfeld, BJ, Roschel, H, Tavares, LD, De Souza, EO, Laurentino, G, and Tricoli, V. Effects of different intensities of resistance training with equated volume load on muscle strength and hypertrophy. *Eur J Sport Sci* 18(6):772-780, 2018.

43. Pearson, D, Faigenbaum, A, Conley, M, and Kraemer, WJ. The National Strength and Conditioning Association's basic guidelines for the resistance training of athletes. *Strength Cond J* 22:14-27, 2000.

44. Peterson, MD, Rhea, MR, and Alvar, BA. Maximizing strength development in athletes: A meta-analysis to determine the dose-response relationship. *J Strength Cond Res* 18:377-382, 2004.

45. Plisk, SS, and Stone, MH. Periodization strategies. *Strength Cond J* 25:19-37, 2003.

46. Poliquin, C. Five steps to increasing the effectiveness of your strength training program. *Strength Cond J* 10:34-39, 1988.

47. Ralston, GW, Kilgore, L, Wyatt, FB, and Baker, JS. The effect of weekly set volume on strength gain: A meta-analysis. *Sports Med* 47(12):2585-2601, 2017.

48. Ratamess, NA, Falvo, MJ, Mangine, GT, Hoffman, JR, Faigenbaum, AD, and Kang, J. The effect of rest interval length on metabolic responses to the bench press exercise. *Eur J Appl Physiol* 100:1-17, 2007.

49. Rhea, MR, and Alvar, BA. Aerobic endurance exercise techniques and programming. In *NSCA's Essentials of Tactical Strength and Conditioning.* Alvar, BA, Sell, K, and Deuster, PA, eds. Champaign, IL: Human Kinetics, 393-412, 2017.

50. Rhea, MR, Alvar, BA, Burkett, LN, and Ball, SD. A meta-analysis to determine the dose response for strength development. *Med Sci Sports Exerc* 35:456-464, 2003.

51. Robertson, RJ. *Perceived Exertion for Practitioners: Rating Effort With The OMNI Picture System.* Champaign, IL: Human Kinetics, 49, 2004.

52. Robinson, JM, Stone, MH, Johnson, RL, Penland, CM, Warren, BJ, and Lewis, RD. Effects of different weight training exercise/rest intervals on strength, power, and high intensity exercise endurance. *J Strength Cond Res* 9:216-221, 1995.

53. Schoenfeld, BJ, Contreras, B, Vigotsky, AD, and Peterson, M. Differential effects of heavy versus moderate loads on measures of strength and hypertrophy in resistance-trained men. *J Sports Sci Med* 15(4):715, 2016.

54. Schoenfeld, BJ, Contreras, B, Willardson, JM, Fontana, F, and Tiryaki-Sonmez, G. Muscle activation during low-versus high-load resistance training in well-trained men. *Eur J Appl Physiol* 114(12):2491-2497, 2014.

55. Schoenfeld, BJ, Grgic, J, Ogborn, D, and Krieger, JW. Strength and hypertrophy adaptations between low-vs. high-load resistance training: A systematic review and meta-analysis. *J Strength Cond Res* 31(12):3508-3523, 2017.

56. Schoenfeld, BJ, Ogborn, D, and Krieger, JW. Dose-response relationship between weekly resistance training volume and increases in muscle mass: A systematic review and meta-analysis. *J Sports Sci* 35(11):1073-1082, 2017.

57. Schoenfeld, BJ, Peterson, MD, Ogborn, D, Contreras, B, and Sonmez, GT. Effects of low-vs. high-load resistance training on muscle strength and hypertrophy in well-trained men. *J Strength Cond Res* 29(10):2954-2963, 2015.

58. Schoenfeld, BJ, Ratamess, NA, Peterson, MD, Contreras, B, Sonmez, GT, and Alvar, BA. Effects of different volume-equated resistance training loading strategies on muscular adaptations in well-trained men. *J Strength Cond Res* 28(10):2909-2918, 2014.

59. Senna, G, Salles, BF, Prestes, J, Mello, RA, and Roberto, S. Influence of two different rest interval lengths in resistance training sessions for upper and lower body. *J Sport Sci Med* 8(2):197, 2009.

60. Sheppard, JM, and Triplett, NT. Program design for resistance training. In *Essentials of Strength and Conditioning,* 4th ed. Haff, GG, and Triplett, NT. Champaign, IL: Human Kinetics, 439-470, 2016.

61. Sperandei, S, Vieira, MC, and Reis, AC. Adherence to physical activity in an unsupervised setting: Explanatory variables for high attrition rates among fitness center members. *J Sci Med Sport* 19:916–920, 2016.

62. Stone, MH, and Borden, RA. Modes and methods of resistance training. *J Strength Cond Res* 19:18-23, 1997.

63. Stone, MH, Keith, R, Kearney, JT, Wilson, GD, and Fleck, SJ. Overtraining: A review of the signs and symptoms of overtraining. *J Appl Sport Sci Res* 5:35-50, 1991.

64. Stone, MH, and O'Bryant, HO. *Weight Training: A Scientific Approach.* Edina, MN: Burgess, 1987.

65. Stone, MH, Pierce, K, Sands, WA, and Stone, M. Weightlifting: Program design. *Strength Cond J* 28:10-17, 2006.

66. Stone, MH, Sands, WA, Pierce, KC, Newton, RU, Haff, GG, and Carlock, J. Maximum strength and strength training: A relationship to endurance? *Strength Cond J* 28:44-53, 2006.

67. Stone, MH, Stone, ME, and Sands, WA. *Principles and Practice of Resistance Training.* Champaign, IL: Human Kinetics, 376, 2007.

68. Testa, M, Noakes, TD, and Desgorces, FD. Training state improves the relationship between rating of perceived exertion and relative exercise volume during resistance exercises. *J Strength Cond Res* 26(11):2990-2996, 2012.

69. Willardson, JM. A brief review: Factors affecting the length of the rest interval between resistance exercise sets. *J Strength Cond Res* 20:978-984, 2006.

70. Willardson, JM, and Burkett, LN. A comparison of 3 different rest intervals on the exercise volume completed during a workout. *J Strength Cond Res* 19:23-26, 2005.

71. Willardson, JM, and Burkett, LN. The effect of rest interval length on the sustainability of squat and bench press repetitions. *J Strength Cond Res* 20:400-403, 2006.

72. Young, WB, James, R, and Montgomery, I. Is muscle power related to running speed with changes of direction? *J Sports Med Phys Fit* 42:282-288, 2002.

73. Zatsiorsky, VM, and Kraemer, WJ. *Science and Practice of Strength Training,* 2nd ed. Champaign, IL: Human Kinetics, 251, 2006.

74. Zourdos, MC, Klemp, A, Dolan, C, Quiles, JM, Schau, KA, Jo, E, Helms, E, Esgro, B, Duncan, S, Merino, SG, and Blanco, R. Novel resistance training–specific rating of perceived exertion scale measuring repetitions in reserve. *J Strength Cond Res* 30(1):267-275, 2016.

Chapter 16

1. Ainsworth, B, Haskell, W, Herrmann, S, Meckes, N, Bassett, D, Tudor-Locke, C, Greer, J, Vezina, J, Whitt-Glover, M, and Leon, A. 2011 Compendium of physical activities: A second update of codes and MET values. *Med Sci Sports Exerc* 43:1575-1581, 2011.

2. American College of Sports Medicine. *ACSM's Guidelines for Exercise Testing and Prescription,* 11th ed. Philadelphia: Wolters Kluwer, 2022.

3. Arnett, DK, Blumenthal, RS, Albert, MA, Buroker, AB, Goldberger, ZD, Hahn, EJ, Himmelfarb, CD, Khera, A, Llooyd-Jones, D, McEvoy, JW, Michos, ED, Miedema, MD, Munoz, D, Smith, SC, Virani, SS, Williams, KA, Yeboah, J, and Ziaeian, B. 2019 ACC/AHA Guideline on the Primary Prevention of Cardiovascular Disease: Executive summary: A report of the American College of Cardiology/American Heart Association Task Force on Clinical Practice Guidelines. *Circulation* 140:e563-e595, 2019.

4. Åstrand, I, Åstrand, P-O, Christensen, EH, and Hedman, R. Intermittent muscular work. *Acta Physiol Scand* 48:448-453, 1960.

5. Åstrand, PO. *Experimental Studies of Physical Working Capacity in Relation to Sex and Age.* Copenhagen: Munksgaard, 1952.

6. Åstrand, P-O, and Rodahl, K. *Textbook of Work Physiology: Physiological Bases of Exercise.* 2nd ed. New York: McGraw-Hill, 1977.

7. Bell, GJ, Petersen, SR, Wessel, J, Bagnall, K, and Quinney, HA. Physiological adaptations to concurrent endurance training and low velocity resistance training. *Int J Sports Med* 12:384-390, 1991.

8. Bell, GJ, Petersen, SR, Wessel, J, Bagnall, K, and Quinney, HA. Adaptations to endurance and low velocity resistance training performed in a sequence. *Can J Sport Sci* 16:186-192, 1991.

9. Ben-Ezra, V, Lacy, C, and Marshall, D. Perceived exertion during graded exercise: Treadmill vs step ergometry. *Med Sci Sports Exerc* 24, 1992.

10. Ben-Ezra, V, and Verstraete, R. Step ergometry: Is it task-specific training? *Eur J Appl Physiol* 63:261-264, 1991.

11. Bressel, E, Heise, GD, and Bachman, G. A neuromuscular and metabolic comparison between forward and reverse pedaling. *J Appl Biomech* 14:401-411, 1998.

12. Christensen, EH, Hedman, R, and Saltin, B. Intermittent and continuous running (a further contribution to the physiology of intermittent work). *Acta Physiol Scand* 50:269-286, 1960.

13. Chtara, M, Chamari, K, Chaouachi, M, Chaouachi, A, Koubaa, D, Feki, Y, Millet, G, and Amri, M. Effects of intra-session concurrent endurance and strength training sequence on aerobic performance and capacity. *Br J Sports Med* 39:555-560, 2005.

14. Chtara, M, Chaouachi, A, Levin, GT, Chaouachi, M, Chamari, K, Amri, M, and Laursen, PB. Effect of concurrent endurance and circuit resistance training sequence on muscular strength and power development. *J Strength Cond Res* 22:1037-1045, 2008.

15. Costill, DL. *Inside Running: Basics of Sports Physiology.* Indianapolis: Benchmark Press, 1986.

16. Craig, BW, Lucas, J, Pohlman, R, and Stelling, H. The effects of running, weightlifting and a combination of both on growth hormone release. *J Strength Cond Res* 5:198, 1991.

17. Daniels, J. Training distance runners—a primer. *Gatorade Sports Sci Exch* 1:1-5, 1989.

18. Ebisu, T. Splitting the distance of endurance running: On cardiovascular endurance and blood lipids. *Jpn J Phys Educ* 30:37-43, 1985.

19. Esfarjani, F, and Laursen, PB. Manipulating high-intensity interval training: Effects on VO_2max, the lactate threshold and 3000 m running performance in moderately trained males. *J Sci Med Sport* 10:27-35, 2007.

20. Eston, RG, and Brodie, DA. Responses to arm and leg ergometry. *Br J Sports Med* 20:4-6, 1986.

21. Faigenbaum, A, and McFarland, JE. Guidelines for implementing a dynamic warm-up for physical education. *J Phys Educ Recreat Dance JOPERD* 78:25-28, 2007.

22. Fleck, SJ, and Kramer, WJ. *Designing Resistance Training Programs.* 3rd ed. Champaign, IL: Human Kinetics, 2004.

23. Fox, SM, Naughton, JP, and Haskell, WL. Physical activity and the prevention of coronary heart disease. *Ann Clin Res* 3:404-432, 1971.

24. Franklin, BA. Aerobic exercise training programs for the upper body. *Med Sci Sports Exerc* 21:S141-S148, 1989.

25. Franklin, BA, Vander, L, Wrisley, D, and Rubenfire, M. Aerobic requirements of arm ergometry: Implications for exercise testing and training. *Phys Sportsmed* 11:81-90, 1983.

26. Garber, C, Blissmer, B, Deschenes, M, Franklin, B, Lamonte, M, Lee, I-M, Nieman, D, and Swain, D. Quantity and quality of exercise for developing and maintaining cardiorespiratory, musculoskeletal, and neuromotor fitness in apparently healthy adults: Guidance for prescribing exercise. *Med Sci Sports Exerc* 43:1334-1359, 2011.

27. Glass, SC, Knowlton, RG, and Becque, MD. Perception of effort during high-intensity exercise at low, moderate and high wet bulb globe temperatures. *Eur J Appl Physiol* 68:519-524, 1994.

28. Goldberg, L, Elliot, DL, and Kuehl, KS. Assessment of exercise intensity formulas by use of ventilatory threshold. *Chest* 94:95-98, 1988.

29. Green, JH, Cable, NT, and Elms, N. Heart rate and oxygen consumption during walking on land and in deep water. *J Sports Med Phys Fitness* 30:49-52, 1990.

30. Gulati, M, Shaw, LJ, Thisted, RA, Black, HR, Bairey Merz, CN, and Arnsdorf, MF. Heart rate response to exercise stress testing in asymptomatic women: The St. James Women Take Heart Project. *Circulation* 122:130-137, 2010.

31. Gutin, B, Stewart, K, Lewis, S, and Kruper, J. Oxygen consumption in the first stages of strenuous work as a function of prior exercise. *J Sports Med Phys Fitness* 16:60-65, 1976.

32. Haennel, R, Teo, KK, Quinney, A, and Kappagoda, T. Effects of hydraulic circuit training on cardiovascular function. *Med Sci Sports Exerc* 21:605-612, 1989.

33. Hanson, JM. *The Relationship Between Personal Incentives for Exercise and the Selection of Activity Among Patrons of Fitness Centers and Recreation Centers.* Eugene: University of Oregon, International Institute for Sport and Human Performance: Microform Publications, 1994.

34. Hardman, AE. Issues of fractionization of exercise (short vs long bouts). *Med Sci Sports Exerc* 33:S421-S427; discussion S452-453, 2001.

35. Hennessy, LC, and Watson, AWS. The interference effects of training for strength and endurance simultaneously. *J Strength Cond Res* 8:12, 1994.

36. Hickson, RC. Interference of strength development by simultaneously training for strength and endurance. *Eur J Appl Physiol* 45:255-263, 1980.

37. Hickson, RC, Dvorak, BA, Gorostiaga, EM, Kurowski, TT, and Foster, C. Strength training and performance in endurance-trained subjects. *Med Sci Sports Exerc* 20, 1988.

38. Hickson, RC, Dvorak, BA, Gorostiaga, EM, Kurowski, TT, and Foster, C. Potential for strength and endurance training to amplify endurance performance. *J Appl Physiol Bethesda Md 1985* 65:2285-2290, 1988.

39. Hickson, RC, Foster, C, Pollock, ML, Galassi, TM, and Rich, S. Reduced training intensities and loss of aerobic power, endurance, and cardiac growth. *J Appl Physiol Bethesda Md 1985* 58:492-499, 1985.

40. Hickson, RC, Kanakis, C, Davis, JR, Moore, AM, and Rich, S. Reduced training duration effects on aerobic power, endurance, and cardiac growth. *J Appl Physiol* 53:225-229, 1982.

41. Hickson, RC, and Rosenkoetter, MA. Reduced training frequencies and maintenance of increased aerobic power. *Med Sci Sports Exerc* 13:13-16, 1981.

42. Hickson, RC, Rosenkoetter, MA, and Brown, MM. Strength training effects on aerobic power and short-term endurance. *Med Sci Sports Exerc* 12:336-339, 1980.

43. Howley, ET. You asked for it: Question authority. *ACSM's Health Fit J* 4:6, 2000.

44. Hunter, G, Demment, R, and Miller, D. Development of strength and maximum oxygen uptake during simultaneous training for strength and endurance. *J Sports Med Phys Fitness* 27:269-275, 1987.

45. Hurley, BF, Seals, DR, Ehsani, AA, Cartier, LJ, Dalsky, GP, Hagberg, JM, and Holloszy, JO. Effects of high-intensity strength training on cardiovascular function. *Med Sci Sports Exerc* 16:483-488, 1984.

46. Jakicic, J, Clark, K, Coleman, E, Donnelly, J, Foreyt, J, Melanson, E, Volek, J, and Volpe, S. Appropriate intervention strategies for weight loss and prevention of weight regain for adults. *Med Sci Sports Exerc* 33:2145-2156, 2001.

47. Kang, J, Chaloupka, EC, Mastrangelo, MA, and Angelucci, J. Physiological responses to upper body exercise on an arm and a modified leg ergometer. *Med Sci Sports Exerc* 31:1453-1459, 1999.

48. Karvonen, J, and Vuorimaa, T. Heart rate and exercise intensity during sports activities. Practical application. *Sports Med Auckl NZ* 5:303-311, 1988.

49. Karvonen, MJ, Kentala, E, and Mustala, O. The effects of training on heart rate: A longitudinal study. *Ann Med Exp Biol Fenn* 35:307-315, 1957.

50. Kearney, JT, Stull, GA, Ewing, JL, and Strein, JW. Cardiorespiratory responses of sedentary college women as a function of training intensity. *J Appl Physiol* 41:822-825, 1976.

51. Kramer, J. Performance benefits of the warm-up. *Olymp Coach* 12:8-9, 2002.

52. Lamb, DR. Basic principles for improving sport performance. *Sports Science Exchange* 8:1-5, 1995.

53. Levin, GT, Mcguigan, MR, and Laursen, PB. Effect of concurrent resistance and endurance training on physiologic and performance parameters of well-trained endurance cyclists. *J Strength Cond Res* 23:2280-2286, 2009.

54. Liang, MTC, Alexander, JF, Taylor, HL, Serfass, RC, and Leon, AS. Aerobic training threshold: Intensity, duration and frequency of exercise. *Scand J Sports Sci* 4:5-8, 1982.

55. Londeree, BR, and Ames, SA. Trend analysis of the % VO$_2$ max-HR regression. *Med Sci Sports* 8:122-125, 1976.

56. Londeree, BR, and Moeschberger, ML. Effect of age and other factors on maximal heart rate. *Res Q Exerc Sport* 53:297-304, 1982.

57. Mahon, AD, Stolen, KQ, and Gay, JA. Differentiated perceived exertion during submaximal exercise in children and adults. *Pediatr Exerc Sci* 13:145-153, 2001.

58. Marcinik, EJ, Potts, J, Schlabach, G, Will, S, Dawson, P, and Hurley, BF. Effects of strength training on lactate threshold and endurance performance. *Med Sci Sports Exerc* 23:739-743, 1991.

59. Marigold, EA. The effects of training at predetermined heart rate levels for sedentary college women. *Med Sci Sports* 6:14-19, 1974.

60. McArdle, WD, Katch, FI, and Katch, VL. *Exercise Physiology: Energy, Nutrition, and Human Performance.* 7th ed. Philadelphia: Lippincott Williams & Wilkins, 2009.

61. McConell, GK, Costill, DL, Widrick, JJ, Hickey, MS, Tanaka, H, and Gastin, PB. Reduced training volume and intensity maintain aerobic capacity but not performance in distance runners. *Int J Sports Med* 14:33-37, 1993.

62. McKenzie, DC, Fox, EL, and Cohen, K. Specificity of metabolic and circulatory responses to arm or leg interval training. *Eur J Appl Physiol* 39:241-248, 1978.

63. Monteiro, AG, Alveno, DA, Prado, M, Monteiro, GA, Ugrinowitsch, C, Aoki, MS, and Picarro, IC. Acute physiological responses to different circuit training protocols. *J Sports Med Phys Fitness* 48:438-442, 2008.

64. Moyna, NM, Robertson, RJ, Meckes, CL, Peoples, JA, Millich, NB, and Thompson, PD. Intermodal comparison of energy expenditure at exercise intensities corresponding to the perceptual preference range. *Med Sci Sports Exerc* 33:1404-1410, 2001.

65. Murphy, MH, and Hardman, AE. Training effects of short and long bouts of brisk walking in sedentary women. *Med Sci Sports Exerc* 30:152-157, 1998.

66. Nieman, DC. *Exercise Testing and Prescription.* 5th ed. Boston: McGraw-Hill, 2003.

67. O'Toole, ML, Douglas, PS, and Hiller, WD. Applied physiology of a triathlon. *Sports Med Auckl NZ* 8:201-225, 1989.

68. Potteiger, JA. Aerobic endurance exercise training. In *Essentials of Strength Training and Conditioning.* Baechle, TR, and Earle, RW, eds. Champaign, IL: Human Kinetics, 495-509, 2000.

69. Powers, SK, and Howley, ET. *Exercise Physiology: Theory and Application to Fitness and Performance.* 7th ed. New York: McGraw-Hill, 2008.

70. Raasch, CC, and Zajac, FE. Locomotor strategy for pedaling: Muscle groups and biomechanical functions. *J Neurophysiol* 82:515-525, 1999.

71. Reybrouck, T, Heigenhauser, GF, and Faulkner, JA. Limitations to maximum oxygen uptake in arms, leg, and combined arm-leg ergometry. *J Appl Physiol* 38:774-779, 1975.

72. Rhodes, RE, Martin, AD, Taunton, JE, Rhodes, EC, Donnelly, M, and Elliot, J. Factors associated with exercise adherence among older adults. An individual perspective. *Sports Med Auckl NZ* 28:397-411, 1999.

73. Riddle, S, and Orringer, C. Measurement of oxygen consumption and cardiovascular response during exercise on the Stairmaster 4000PT versus the treadmill. *Med Sci Sports Exerc* 22 (2 Suppl): S65, 1990.

74. Riebe, D, Ehrman, JK, Liguori, G, and Magal, M. *ACSM's Guidelines for Exercise Testing and Prescription.* 10th ed. Philadelphia: Lippincott Williams & Wilkins, 2018.

75. Robertson, RJ, and Noble, BJ. Perception of physical exertion: Methods, mediators, and applications. *Exerc Sport Sci Rev* 25:407-452, 1997.

76. Ryan, RM, Frederick, CM, Lepes, D, Rubio, N, and Sheldon, KM. Intrinsic motivation and exercise adherence. *Int J Sport Psychol* 28:335-354, 1997.

77. Saltin, B, Hartley, LH, Kilbom, A, and Åstrand, I. Physical training in sedentary middle-aged and older men. II. Oxygen uptake, heart rate, and blood lactate concentration at submaximal and maximal exercise. *Scand J Clin Lab Invest* 24:323-334, 1969.

78. Sharkey, B. Intensity and duration of training and the development of cardiorespiratory endurance. *Med Sci Sports* 2:197-202, 1970.

79. Shellock, FG, and Prentice, WE. Warming-up and stretching for improved physical performance and prevention of sports-related injuries. *Sports Med Auckl NZ* 2:267-278, 1985.

80. Shephard, RJ. Intensity, duration and frequency of exercise as determinants of the response to a training regime. *Int Z Für Angew Physiol Einschließlich Arbeitsphysiologie* 26:272-278, 1968.

81. Skinner, JS, Gaskill, SE, Rankinen, T, Leon, AS, Rao, DC, Wilmore, JH, and Bouchard, C. Heart rate versus %VO_2max: Age, sex, race, initial fitness, and training response—HERITAGE. *Med Sci Sports Exerc* 35:1908-1913, 2003.

82. Springer, C, Barstow, TJ, Wasserman, K, and Cooper, DM. Oxygen uptake and heart rate responses during hypoxic exercise in children and adults. *Med Sci Sports Exerc* 23:71-79, 1991.

83. Stone, MH, Fleck, SJ, Triplett, NT, and Kraemer, WJ. Health- and performance-related potential of resistance training. *Sports Med Auckl NZ* 11:210-231, 1991.

84. Swain, DP, Abernathy, KS, Smith, CS, Lee, SJ, and Bunn, SA. Target heart rates for the development of cardiorespiratory fitness. *Med Sci Sports Exerc* 26:112-116, 1994.

85. Swain, DP, and Leutholtz, BC. Heart rate reserve is equivalent to %VO_2 reserve, not to %VO_2max. *Med Sci Sports Exerc* 29:410-414, 1997.

86. Tanaka, H, Monahan, KD, and Seals, DR. Age-predicted maximal heart rate revisited. *J Am Coll Cardiol* 37:153-156, 2001.

87. Thomas, TR, Ziogas, G, Smith, T, Zhang, Q, and Londeree, BR. Physiological and perceived exertion responses to six modes of submaximal exercise. *Res Q Exerc Sport* 66:239-246, 1995.

88. Tulppo, MP, Mäkikallio, TH, Laukkanen, RT, and Huikuri, HV. Differences in autonomic modulation of heart rate during arm and leg exercise. *Clin Physiol Oxf Engl* 19:294-299, 1999.

89. Turcotte, L, Byrnes, W, Frykman, P, Freedson, P, and Katch, F. The effects of hydraulic resistive training on maximal oxygen uptake and anaerobic threshold. *Med Sci Sports Exerc* 16: S183, 1984.

90. U.S. Department of Health and Human Services. *Physical Activity Guidelines Advisory Committee Scientific Report.* Washington, DC: U.S. Department of Health and Human Services, 2018.

91. Van De Graaff, KM, and Fox, SI. *Concepts of Human Anatomy and Physiology.* 5th ed. Boston: WCB/McGraw-Hill, 1999.

92. Velasquez, KS, and Wilmore, JH. Changes in cardiorespiratory fitness and body composition after a 12-week bench step training program. *Med Sci Sports Exerc* 24, 1993.

93. Wells, CL, Pate, RR, Lamb, DR, and Murray, R. Training for performance of prolonged exercise. In *Perspectives in Exercise Science and Sports Medicine.* Lamb, DR, and Murray, R, eds. Indianapolis: Benchmark Press, 357-388.

94. Whaley, MH, Kaminsky, LA, Dwyer, GB, Getchell, LH, and Norton, JA. Predictors of over- and underachievement of age-predicted maximal heart rate. *Med Sci Sports Exerc* 24:1173-1179, 1992.

95. White, LJ, Dressendorfer, RH, Muller, SM, and Ferguson, MA. Effectiveness of cycle cross-training between competitive seasons in female distance runners. *J Strength Cond Res* 17:319-323, 2003.

96. Wilber, RL, Moffatt, RJ, Scott, BE, Lee, DT, and Cucuzzo, NA. Influence of water run training on the maintenance of aerobic performance. *Med Sci Sports Exerc* 28:1056-1062, 1996.

97. Wilmore, JH, and Costill, DL. *Physiology of Sport and Exercise.* 4th ed. Champaign, IL: Human Kinetics, 2007.

98. Yamaji, K, Greenley, M, Northey, DR, and Hughson, RL. Oxygen uptake and heart rate responses to treadmill and water running. *Can J Sport Sci* 15:96-98, 1990.

99. Zeni, AI, Hoffman, MD, and Clifford, PS. Energy expenditure with indoor exercise machines. *J Am Med Assoc* 275:1424-1427, 1996.

100. Zimmermann, CL, Cook, TM, Bravard, MS, Hansen, MM, Honomichl, RT, Karns, ST, Lammers, MA, Steele, SA, Yunker, LK, and Zebrowski, RM. Effects of stair-stepping exercise direction and cadence on EMG activity of selected lower extremity muscle groups. *J Orthop Sports Phys Ther* 19:173-180, 1994.

101. Zupan, MF, and Scott Petosa, P. Aerobic and resistance cross-training for peak triathlon performance. *Strength Cond J* 17:7, 1995.

Chapter 17

1. Asmussen E and Bonde-Petersen F. Storage of elastic energy in skeletal muscles in man. *Acta Physiologica Scandinavica* 91: 385-392, 1974.

2. Aura O and Vitasalo JT. Biomechanical characteristics of jumping. *International Journal of Sport Biomechanics* 5: 89-97, 1989.

3. Berg K, Latin RW, and Baechle T. Physical fitness of NCAA Division I football players. *Strength & Conditioning Journal* 14: 68-73, 1992.

4. Bobbert MF, Gerritsen KG, Litjens MC, and Van Soest AJ. Why is countermovement jump height greater than squat jump height? *Medicine and science in sports and exercise* 28: 1402-1412, 1996.

5. Borkowski J. Prevention of pre-season muscle soreness: Plyometric exercise. *J Athletic Train* 25: 122, 1990.

6. Bosco C, Ito A, Komi P, Luhtanen P, Rahkila P, Rusko H, and Viitasalo J. Neuromuscular function and mechanical efficiency of human leg extensor muscles during jumping exercises. *Acta Physiologica Scandinavica* 114: 543-550, 1982.

7. Bosco C, Komi PV, and Ito A. Prestretch potentiation of human skeletal muscle during ballistic movement. *Acta Physiologica Scandinavica* 111: 135-140, 1981.

8. Bosco C, Viitasalo J, Komi P, and Luhtanen P. Combined effect of elastic energy and myoelectrical potentiation during stretch-shortening cycle exercise. *Acta Physiologica Scandinavica* 114: 557-565, 1982.

9. Brown L, Ferrigno V, and Santana J. *Training for Speed, Agility and Quickness.* Champaign, IL: Human Kinetics, 2000.

10. Cavagna GA, Dusman B, and Margaria R. Positive work done by a previously stretched muscle. *Journal of applied physiology* 24: 21-32, 1968.

11. Cavagna GA, Saibene FP, and Margaria R. Effect of negative work on the amount of positive work performed by an isolated muscle. *Journal of applied physiology* 20: 157-158, 1965.

12. Chambers C, Noakes T, Lambert E, and Lambert M. Time course of recovery of vertical jump height and heart rate versus running speed after a 90-km foot race. *Journal of sports sciences* 16: 645-651, 1998.

13. Chimera NJ, Swanik KA, Swanik CB, and Straub SJ. Effects of plyometric training on muscle-activation strategies and performance in female athletes. *Journal of athletic training* 39: 24, 2004.

14. Chmielewski TL, Myer GD, Kauffman D, and Tillman SM. Plyometric exercise in the rehabilitation of athletes: physiological responses and clinical application. *Journal of Orthopaedic & Sports Physical Therapy* 36: 308-319, 2006.

15. Chu D and Korchemny R. Sprinting stride actions: Analysis and evaluation. *National Strength and Conditioning Association Journal* 11: 6-8, 82-85, 1989.

16. Chu D and Plummer L. Jumping into plyometrics: The language of plyometrics. *National Strength and Conditioning Association Journal* 6: 30-31, 1984.

17. Chu DA. *Jumping into plyometrics.* Champaign, IL: Human Kinetics, 1998.

18. Cissik JM. Technique and speed development for running. *NSCA's Performance Training Journal* 1: 18-21, 2002.

19. Cissik JM. Means and methods of speed training, part I. *Strength & Conditioning Journal* 26: 24-29, 2004.

20. Cissik JM. Means and methods of speed training: Part II. *Strength and conditioning journal* 27: 18, 2005.

21. Clark M and Wallace T. Plyometric training with elastic resistance, in: *The Scientific and Clinical Application of Elastic Resistance*. P Page, TS Ellenbecker, eds. Champaign, IL: Human Kinetics, 2003.

22. Committee CE. Coaching Education Program: Level II Course (Sprints, Hurdles, Relays). USA Track and Field, 2001, pp 8-17, 33-42.

23. Costello F. Speed: Training for speed using resisted and assisted methods. *National Strength and Conditioning Association Journal* 7: 74-75, 1985.

24. Cronin J and Hansen KT. Resisted sprint training for the acceleration phase of sprinting. *Strength and conditioning journal* 28: 42, 2006.

25. de Villarreal ESS, González-Badillo JJ, and Izquierdo M. Low and moderate plyometric training frequency produces greater jumping and sprinting gains compared with high frequency. *The Journal of Strength & Conditioning Research* 22: 715-725, 2008.

26. De Vos NJ, Singh NA, Ross DA, Stavrinos TM, Orr R, and Fiatarone Singh MA. Optimal load for increasing muscle power during explosive resistance training in older adults. *The Journals of Gerontology Series A: Biological Sciences and Medical Sciences* 60: 638-647, 2005.

27. Dick FW. *Sprints and Relays*. London: British Amateur Athletic Board, 1987.

28. Dillman CJ, Fleisig GS, and Andrews JR. Biomechanics of pitching with emphasis upon shoulder kinematics. *Journal of Orthopaedic & Sports Physical Therapy* 18: 402-408, 1993.

29. Dintiman GB, Ward RD, and Tellez T. *Sports Speed*. Champaign, IL: Human Kinetics, 1998.

30. Ebben WP. Practical guidelines for plyometric intensity. *NSCA's Performance training Journal* 6: 12-16, 2007.

31. Enoka RM. *Neuromechanical basis of kinesiology*. Champaign, IL: Human Kinetics, 1994.

32. Faigenbaum AD. Plyometrics for kids: Facts and fallacies. *NSCA's Performance Training Journal* 5: 13-16, 2006.

33. Faigenbaum AD, Kraemer WJ, Blimkie CJ, Jeffreys I, Micheli LJ, Nitka M, and Rowland TW. Youth resistance training: updated position statement paper from the national strength and conditioning association. *The Journal of Strength & Conditioning Research* 23: S60-S79, 2009.

34. Feltner M and Dapena J. Dynamics of the shoulder and elbow joints of the throwing arm during a baseball pitch. *Journal of Applied Biomechanics* 2: 235-259, 1986.

35. Fleck S. Interval training: Physiological basis. *National Strength and Conditioning Association Journal* 5: 40, 57-63, 1983.

36. Fleck S and Kraemer W. *Designing Resistance Training Programs*. Champaign, IL: Human Kinetics, 2014.

37. Fleisig GS, Barrentine SW, Zheng N, Escamilla RF, and Andrews JR. Kinematic and kinetic comparison of baseball pitching among various levels of development. *Journal of biomechanics* 32: 1371-1375, 1999.

38. Fowler NE, Lees A, and Reilly T. Spinal shrinkage in unloaded and loaded drop-jumping. *Ergonomics* 37: 133-139, 1994.

39. Fowler NE, Lees A, and Reilly T. Changes in stature following plyometric drop-jump and pendulum exercises. *Ergonomics* 40: 1279-1286, 1997.

40. Franchi MV, Monti E, Carter A, Quinlan JI, Herrod PJJ, Reeves ND, and Narici MV. Bouncing Back! Counteracting Muscle Aging With Plyometric Muscle Loading. *Frontiers in Physiology* 10, 2019.

41. Gambetta V, Wincklet G, Rogers J, Orognen J, Seagrave L, and Jolly S. Sprints and relays., in: *TAC Track and Field Coaching Manual*. TD Committees, V Gambetta, eds. Champaign, IL: Leisure Press, 1989.

42. Gamble P. Approaching Physical Preparation for Youth Team-Sports Players. *Strength & Conditioning Journal* 30: 29-42, 2008.

43. Gottschall JS and Kram R. Ground reaction forces during downhill and uphill running. *Journal of Biomechanics* 38: 445-452, 2005.

44. Guyton AC and Hall JE. *Textbook of Medical Physiology*. Philadelphia: Saunders, 2000.

45. Hewett TE, Stroupe AL, Nance TA, and Noyes FR. Plyometric training in female athletes: decreased impact forces and increased hamstring torques. *The American journal of sports medicine* 24: 765-773, 1996.

46. Hill AV. *First and last experiments in muscle mechanics*. Cambridge, England: Cambridge Univ. Press, 1970.

47. Holcomb WR, Kleiner DM, and Chu DA. Plyometrics: Considerations for safe and effective training. *Strength & Conditioning Journal* 20: 36-41, 1998.

48. Jakalski K. The pros and cons of using resisted and assisted training methods with high school sprinters: parachutes, tubing and towing. *Track Coach* 144: 4585-4589, 1998.

49. Jarver J. *Sprints and Relays: Contemporary Theory, Technique and Training*. Los Altos, CA: Tafnews Press, 1990.

50. Judge LW. Developing speed strength: In-season training program for the collegiate thrower. *Strength and Conditioning Journal* 29: 42, 2007.

51. Kaeding CC and Whitehead R. Musculoskeletal injuries in adolescents. *Primary Care: Clinics in Office Practice* 25: 211-223, 1998.

52. Kilani H, Palmer S, Adrian M, and Gapsis J. Block of the stretch reflex of vastus lateralis during vertical jumps. *Human Movement Science* 8: 247-269, 1989.

53. Kotzamanidis C. Effect of plyometric training on running performance and vertical jumping in prepubertal boys. *Journal of strength and conditioning research* 20: 441, 2006.

54. Kraemer WJ, Mazzetti SA, Nindl BC, Gotshalk LA, Volek JS, Bush JA, Marx JO, Dohi K, Gomez AL, and Miles M. Effect of resistance training on women's strength/power and occupational performances. *Medicine & Science in Sports & Exercise* 33: 1011-1025, 2001.

55. LaChance P. Plyometric exercise. *Strength & Conditioning Journal* 17: 16-23, 1995.

56. Lipp EJ. Athletic physeal injury in children and adolescents. *Orthopaedic Nursing* 17: 17, 1998.

57. Markovic G and Mikulic P. Neuro-Musculoskeletal and Performance Adaptations to Lower-Extremity Plyometric Training. *Sports medicine* 40: 859-895, 2010.

58. Matthews P. The knee jerk: Still an enigma? *Can J Physiol Pharmacol* 68: 347-354, 1990.

59. Maulder PS, Bradshaw EJ, and Keogh JW. Kinematic alterations due to different loading schemes in early acceleration sprint performance from starting blocks. *The Journal of Strength & Conditioning Research* 22: 1992-2002, 2008.

60. McBride JM, McCaulley GO, and Cormie P. Influence of preactivity and eccentric muscle activity on concentric performance during vertical jumping. *The Journal of Strength & Conditioning Research* 22: 750-757, 2008.

61. McNeely E. Introduction to plyometrics: Converting strength to power. *NSCA's Performance Training Journal* 6: 19-22, 2005.

62. Mero A, Komi P, and Gregor R. Biomechanics of sprint running. *Sports medicine* 13: 376-392, 1992.

63. Miller JM, Hilbert SC, and Brown LE. Speed, quickness, and agility training for senior tennis players. *Strength & Conditioning Journal* 23: 62, 2001.

64. Moravec P, Ruzicka J, Susanka P, Dostal E, Kodejs M, and Nosek M. The 1987 International Athletic Foundation/IAAF scientific project report: time analysis of the 100 metres events at the II world championships in athletics. *New studies in Athletics* 3: 61-96, 1988.

65. Myer GD, Ford KR, McLean SG, and Hewett TE. The effects of plyometric versus dynamic stabilization and balance training on lower extremity biomechanics. *The American journal of sports medicine* 34: 445-455, 2006.

66. Myer GD, Paterno MV, Ford KR, and Hewett TE. Neuromuscular training techniques to target deficits before return to sport after anterior cruciate ligament reconstruction. *The Journal of Strength & Conditioning Research* 22: 987-1014, 2008.

67. Newman B. Speed development through resisted sprinting. *NSCA Journal* (3) pp: 9-13, 2007.

68. Newton RU, Murphy AJ, Humphries BJ, Wilson GJ, Kraemer WJ, and Häkkinen K. Influence of load and stretch shortening cycle on the kinematics, kinetics and muscle activation that occurs during explosive upper-body movements. *European journal of applied physiology and occupational physiology* 75: 333-342, 1997.

69. NSCA. Position statement: Explosive/plyometric exercises. *National Strength and Conditioning Association Journal* 15: 16, 1993.

70. Pappas AM, Zawacki RM, and Sullivan TJ. Biomechanics of baseball pitching: a preliminary report. *The American journal of sports medicine* 13: 216-222, 1985.

71. Phelps SM. Speed Training. *Strength & Conditioning Journal* 23: 57, 2001.

72. Piper T. Organizational and Motivational Strategies for Prepubescent Athletes. *Strength & Conditioning Journal* 25: 54-57, 2003.

73. Potteiger JA, Lockwood RH, Haub MD, Dolezal BA, Almuzaini KS, Schroeder JM, and Zebas CJ. Muscle power and fiber characteristics following 8 weeks of plyometric training. *The Journal of Strength & Conditioning Research* 13: 275-279, 1999.

74. Radcliffe JC and Farentinos RC. *Plyometrics: explosive power training.* Champaign, IL: Human Kinetics, 1985.

75. Radcliffe JC and Farentinos RC. *High-powered plyometrics.* Champaign, IL: Human Kinetics, 1999.

76. Sandler R and Robinovitch S. An analysis of the effect of lower extremity strength on impact severity during a backward fall. *Journal of biomechanical engineering* 123: 590-598, 2001.

77. Santos EJ and Janeira MA. Effects of complex training on explosive strength in adolescent male basketball players. *The Journal of Strength & Conditioning Research* 22: 903-909, 2008.

78. Schmolinsky G. *Track and Field: The East German Textbook of Athletics.* Toronto: Sports Books, 2000.

79. Shiner J, Bishop T, and Cosgarea A. Integrating low-intensity plyometrics into strength and conditioning programs. *Strength and Conditioning Journal* 27: 10-20, 2005.

80. Siff M. *Supertraining.* Denver, CO: Supertraining Institute, 2000.

81. Sinnett AM, Berg K, Latin RW, and Noble JM. The relationship between field tests of anaerobic power and 10-km run performance. *Journal of strength and conditioning research* 15: 405-412, 2001.

82. Svantesson U, Grimby G, and Thomee R. Potentiation of concentric plantar flexion torque following eccentric and isometric muscle actions. *Acta physiologica scandinavica* 152: 287-293, 1994.

83. Turner AM, Owings M, and Schwane JA. Improvement in running economy after 6 weeks of plyometric training. *The Journal of Strength & Conditioning Research* 17: 60-67, 2003.

84. Verkhoshansky Y and Tatyan V. Speed-strength preparation of future champions. *Soviet Sports Rev* 18: 166-170, 1983.

85. Vetrovsky T, Steffl M, Stastny P, and Tufano JJ. The Efficacy and Safety of Lower-Limb Plyometric Training in Older Adults: A Systematic Review. *Sports Medicine* 49: 113-131, 2019.

86. Voight M, Draovitch P, and Tippett S. Plyometrics, in: *Eccentric Muscle Training in Sports and Orthopaedics.* M Albert, ed. New York, NY: Churchill Livingstone, 1995.

87. Warpeha J. Principles of speed training. *NSCA's Performance Training Journal* 6: 6-7, 2007.

88. Wathen D. Literature review: Plyometric exercises. *National Strength and Conditioning Association Journal* 15: 17-19, 1993.

89. Wilk KE and Voight M. Plyometrics for the overhead athlete, in: *The Athletic Shoulder.* JR Andrews, KE Wilk, eds. New York, NY: Churchill Livingstone, 1993.

90. Wilk KE, Voight ML, Keirns MA, Gambetta V, Andrews JR, and Dillman CJ. Stretch-shortening drills for the upper extremities: theory and clinical application. *Journal of Orthopaedic & Sports Physical Therapy* 17: 225-239, 1993.

91. Wilson GJ, Murphy AJ, and Giorgi A. Weight and plyometric training: effects on eccentric and concentric force production. *Canadian Journal of Applied Physiology* 21: 301-315, 1996.

92. Wilt F. Training for competitive running, in: *Exercise Physiology.* HB Falls, ed. New York, NY: Academic Press, 1968, pp 395-414.

93. Witzke KA and Snow CM. Effects of polymetric jump training on bone mass in adolescent girls. *Medicine and science in sports and exercise* 32: 1051-1057, 2000.

94. Zazulak B, Cholewicki J, and Reeves PN. Neuromuscular control of trunk stability: clinical implications for sports injury prevention. *JAAOS-Journal of the American Academy of Orthopaedic Surgeons* 16: 497-505, 2008.

Chapter 18

Preadolescent Youth Section

1. Abrignani, M, Lucà, F, Favilli, S, Benvenuto, M, Rao, C, Di Fusco, S, Gabrielli, D, Gulizia, M, Cardiovascular Prevention Area Young Cardiologists Area, Paediatric Cardiology Task Force of the Associazione Nazionale Medici Cardiologi Ospedalieri (ANMCO), and Heart Care Foundation. Lifestyles and cardiovascular prevention in childhood and adolescence. *Pediatr Cardiol* 40:1113-1125, 2019.

2. Anderson, P, Butcher, K, and Schanzenbach, D. Understanding recent trends in childhood obesity in the United States. *Econ Human Biol* 34:16-25, 2019.

3. Aubert, S, Barnes, J, Abdeta, C, Abi Nader, P, Adeniyi, A, Aguilar-Farias, N, Andrade Tenesaca, D, Bhawra, J, Brazo-Sayavera, J, Cardon, G, Chang, C, Delisle Nyström, C, Demetriou, Y, Draper, C, Edwards, L, Emeljanovas, A, Gába, A, Galaviz, K, González, S, Herrera-Cuenca, M, Huang, W, Ibrahim, I, Jürimäe, J, Kämppi, K, Katapally, T, Katewongsa, P, Katzmarzyk, P, Khan, A, Korcz, A, Kim, Y, Lambert, E, Lee, E, Löf, M, Loney, T, López-Taylor, J, Liu, Y, Makaza, D, Manyanga, T, Mileva, B, Morrison, S, Mota, J, Nyawornota, V, Ocansey, R, Reilly, J, Roman-Viñas, B, Silva, D, Saonuam, P, Scriven, J, Seghers, J, Schranz, N, Skovgaard, T, Smith, M, Standage, M, Starc, G, Stratton, G, Subedi, N, Takken, T, Tammelin, T, Tanaka, C, Thivel, D, Tladi, D, Tyler, R, Uddin, R, Williams, A, Wong, S, Wu, C, Zembura, P, and Tremblay, M. Global Matrix 3.0 physical activity report card grades for children and youth: Results and analysis from 49 countries. *J Phys Act Health* 15:S251-S273, 2018.

4. Baquet, G, Van Praagh, E, and Berthoin, S. Endurance training and aerobic fitness in young people. *Sports Med* 33:1127-1143, 2003.

5. Bar-Or, O. *Sports Medicine for the Practitioner.* New York: Springer-Verlag, 1983.

6. Behm, D, Young, J, Whitten, J, Reid, J, Quigley, P, Low, J, Li, Y, Lima, C, Hodgson, D, Chaouachi, A, Prieske, O, and Granacher, U. Effectiveness of traditional strength versus power training on muscle strength, power and speed with youth: A systematic review and meta-analysis. *Front Physiol* 8:423, 2017.

7. Bergeron, M, Mountjoy, M, Armstrong, N, Chia, M, Côté, J, Emery, C, Faigenbaum, A, Hall, G, Kriemler, S, Léglise, M, Malina, R, Pensgaard, A, Sanchez, A, Soligard, T, Sundgot-Borgen, J, van Mechelen, W, Weissensteiner, J, and Engebretsen, L. International Olympic Committee consensus statement on youth athletic development. *Brit J Sport Med* 49:843-851, 2015.

8. Cicone, Z, Holmes, C, Fedewa, M, MacDonald, H, and Esco, M. Age-based prediction of maximal heart rate in children and adolescents: A systematic review and meta-analysis. *Res Q Exercise Sport* 90:417-428, 2019.

9. Collins, H, Booth, J, Duncan, A, and Fawkner, S. The effect of resistance training interventions on fundamental movement skills in youth: A meta-analysis. *Sports Med Open* 5:17, 2019.

10. Collins, H, Booth, J, Duncan, A, Fawkner, S, and Niven, A. The effect of resistance training interventions on 'the self' in youth: A systematic review and meta-analysis. *Sports Med Open* 5:29, 2019.

11. Collins, H, Fawkner, S, Booth, J, and Duncan, A. The effect of resistance training interventions on weight status in youth: A meta-analysis. *Sports Med Open* 4:41, 2018.

12. Ding, D, Lawson, K, Kolbe-Alexander, T, Finkelstein, E, Katzmarzyk, P, van Mechelen, W, and Pratt, M. The economic burden of physical inactivity: A global analysis of major non-communicable diseases. *Lancet* 388:1311-1324, 2016.

13. Dishman, R, Motl, R, Saunders, R, Felton, G, Ward, D, Dowda, M, and Pate, R. Enjoyment mediates effects of a school-based physical activity intervention. *Med Sci Sports Exerc* 37:478-487, 2005.

14. Donnelly, J, Hillman, C, Castelli, D, Etnier, J, Lee, S, Tomporowski, P, Lambourne, K, and Szabo-Reed, A. Physical activity, fitness, cognitive function, and academic achievement in children: A systematic review. *Med Sci Sports Exerc* 48:1197-1222, 2016.

15. Eddolls, W, McNarry, M, Stratton, G, Winn, C, and Mackintosh, K. High-intensity interval training interventions in children and adolescents: A systematic review. *Sports Med* 47:2326-2374, 2017.

16. Faigenbaum, A, and Bruno, L. A fundamental approach for treating pediatric dynapenia in kids. *ACSMS Health Fit J* 21:18-24, 2017.

17. Faigenbaum, A, Kraemer, W, Blimkie, C, Jeffreys, I, Micheli, L, Nitka, M, and Rowland, T. Youth resistance training: Updated position statement paper from the National Strength and Conditioning Association. *J Strength Cond Res* 23:S60-S79, 2009.

18. Faigenbaum, A, Lloyd, R, MacDonald, J, and Myer, G. Citius, altius, fortius: Beneficial effects of resistance training for young athletes: Narrative review. *Brit J Sport Med* 50:3-7, 2016.

19. Faigenbaum, A, Lloyd, R, Oliver, J, and American College of Sports Medicine. *Essentials of Youth Fitness.* Champaign, IL: Human Kinetics, 2020.

20. Faigenbaum, A, and Myer, G. Resistance training among young athletes: Safety, efficacy and injury prevention effects. *Brit J Sport Med* 44:56-63, 2010.

21. Faigenbaum, A, and Rial Rebullido, T. Understanding physical literacy in youth. *Strength Cond J* 40:90-94, 2018.

22. Faigenbaum, A, Rial Rebullido, T, Pena, J, and Chulvi-Medrano, I. Resistance exercise for the prevention and treatment of pediatric dynapenia. *J Sci Sport Exerc* 1(3):208-216, 2019.

23. Faigenbaum, A, and Westcott, WL. *Youth Strength Training.* Champaign, IL: Human Kinetics, 2009.

24. García-Hermoso, A, Ramírez-Campillo, R, and Izquierdo, M. Is muscular fitness associated with future health benefits in children and adolescents? A systematic review and meta-analysis of longitudinal studies. *Sports Med* 49(7):1079-1094, 2019.

25. Goldfield, G, Kenny, G, Alberga, A, Tulloch, H, Doucette, S, Cameron, J, and Sigal, R. Effects of aerobic or resistance training or both on health related quality of life in youth with obesity: The HEARTY trial. *Appl Physiol Nutr Me* 42:361-370, 2017.

26. Jung, H, Jeon, S, Lee, N, Kim, K, Kang, M, and Lee, S. Effects of exercise intervention on visceral fat in obese children and adolescents. *J Sport Med Phys Fit* 59:1045-1057, 2019.

27. Laursen, J, Andersen, T, and Andersen, L. Strength training as superior, dose-dependent and safe prevention of acute and overuse sports injuries: A systematic review, qualitative analysis and meta-analysis. *Brit J Sport Med* 52:1557-1563, 2018.

28. Laursen, J, Bertelsen, D, and Andersen, L. The effectiveness of exercise interventions to prevent sports injuries: A systematic review and meta-analysis of randomised controlled trials. *Brit J Sport Med* 48:871-877, 2014.

29. Legerlotz, K, Marzilger, R, Bohm, S, and Arampatzis, A. Physiological adaptations following resistance training in youth athletes: A narrative review. *Pediatr Exerc Sci* 28:501-520, 2016.

30. Lesinski, M, Prieske, O, and Granacher, U. Effects and dose–response relationships of resistance training on physical performance in youth athletes: A systematic review and meta-analysis. *Brit J Sport Med* 50:781-795, 2016.

31. Lloyd, R, Cronin, J, Faigenbaum, A, Haff, G, Howard, R, Kraemer, W, Micheli, L, Myer, G, and Oliver, J. The National Strength and Conditioning Association position statement on long-term athletic development. *J Strength Cond Res* 30:1491-1509, 2016.

32. Lloyd, R, Faigenbaum, A, Stone, M, Oliver, J, Jeffreys, I, Moody, J, Brewer, C, Pierce, K, McCambridge, T, Howard, R, Herrington, L, Hainline, B, Micheli, L, Jaques, R, Kraemer, W, McBride, M, Best, T, Chu, D, Alvar, B, and Myer, G. Position statement on youth resistance training: The 2014 International Consensus. *Brit J Sport Med* 4:498-505, 2014.

33. Lloyd, R, and Oliver, J, eds. *Strength and Conditioning for Young Athletes.* Oxon: Routledge, 2020.

34. Logan, K, Cuff, S, and Council on Sports Medicine and Fitness. Organized sports for children, preadolescents, and adolescents. *Pediatrics* 143(6):e20190997, 2019.

35. Mayer-Davis, E, Lawrence, J, Dabelea, D, Divers, J, Isom, S, Dolan, L, Imperatore, G, Linder, B, Marcovina, S, Pettitt, D, Pihoker, C, Saydah, S, Wagenknecht, L, and SEARCH for Diabetes in Youth Study. Incidence trends of type 1 and type 2 diabetes among youths, 2002-2012. *New Engl J Med* 37:1419-1429, 2017.

36. Myer, G, Faigenbaum, A, Edwards, E, Clark, J, Best, T, and Sallis, R. 60 minutes of what? A developing brain perspective for activation children with an integrative approach. *Brit J Sport Med* 49:1510-1516, 2015.

37. Myer, G, Jayanthi, N, DiFiori, J, Faigenbaum, A, Kiefer, A, Logerstedt, D, and Micheli, L. Sports specialization, part II: Alternative solutions to early sport specialization in youth athletes. *Sports Health* 8:65-73, 2016.

38. Myer, G, Quatman, C, Khoury, J, Wall, E, and Hewett, T. Youth vs. adult "weightlifting" injuries presented to United States Emergency Rooms: Accidental vs. non-accidental injury mechanisms. *J Strength Cond Res* 23:2054-2060, 2009.

39. Nadeau, K, Anderson, B, Berg, E, Chiang, J, Chou, H, Copeland, K, Hannon, T, Huang, T, Lynch, J, Powell, J, Sellers, E, Tamborlane, W, and Zeitler, P. Youth-onset type 2 diabetes consensus report: Current status, challenges, and priorities. *Diab Care* 39:1635-1642, 2016.

40. Pate, R, Hillman, C, Janz, K, Katzmarzyk, P, Powell, K, Torres, A, and Whitt-Glover, M. Physical activity and health in children younger than 6 years: A systematic review. *Med Sci Sports Exerc* 51:1282-1291, 2019.

41. Petushek, E, Sugimoto, D, Stoolmiller, M, Smith, G, and Myer, G. Evidence-based best-practice guidelines for preventing anterior cruciate ligament injuries in young female athletes: A systematic review and meta-analysis. *Am J Sport Med* 47:1744-1753, 2019.

42. Poitras, V, Gray, C, Borghese, M, Carson, V, Chaput, J, Janssen, I, Katzmarzyk, P, Pate, R, Gorber, S, Kho, M, Sampson, M, and Tremblay, M. Systematic review of the relationships between objectively measured physical activity and health indicators in school-aged children and youth. *Appl Physiol Nutr Me* 41:S197-S239, 2016.

43. Rodriguez-Ayllon, M, Cadenas-Sánchez, C, Estévez-López, F, Muñoz, N, Mora-Gonzalez, J, Migueles, J, Molina-García, P, Henriksson, H, Mena-Molina, A, Martínez-Vizcaíno, V, Catena, A, Löf, M, Erickso, K, Lubans, D, Ortega, F, and Esteban-Cornejo, I. Role of physical activity and sedentary behavior in the mental health of preschoolers, children and adolescents: A systematic review and meta-analysis. *Sports Med* 49:1383-1410, 2019.

44. Rothman, L, Macpherson, A, Ross, T, and Buliung, R. The decline in active school transportation (AST): A systematic review of the factors related to AST and changes in school transport over time in North America. *Prev Med* 111:314-322, 2018.

45. Rowland, T. *Children's Exercise Physiology.* Champaign, IL: Human Kinetics, 2005.

46. Ruiz, R, Sommer, E, Tracy, D, Banda, J, Economos, C, JaKa, M, Evenson, K, Buchowski, M, and Barkin, S. Novel patterns of physical activity in a large sample of preschool-aged children. *BMC Public Health* 18:242, 2018.

47. Sigal, R, Alberga, A, Goldfield, G, Prud'homme, D, Hadjiyannakis, S, Gougeon, R, Phillips, P, Tulloch, H, Malcolm, J, Doucette, S, Wells, G, Ma, J, and Kenny, G. Effects of aerobic training, resistance training, or both on percentage body fat and cardiometabolic risk markers in obese adolescents: The healthy eating aerobic and resistance training in youth randomized clinical trial. *JAMA Pediatr* 168:1006-1014, 2014.

48. Skinner, A, Ravanbakht, S, Skelton, J, Perrin, E, and Armstrong, S. Prevalence of obesity and severe obesity in US children, 1999-2016. *Pediatrics* 141(3):e20173459, 2018.

49. Smith, J, Eather, N, Morgan, P, Plotnikoff, R, Faigenbaum, A, and Lubans, D. The health benefits of muscular fitness for children and adolescents: A systematic review and meta-analysis. *Sports Med* 44:1209-1223, 2014.

50. Smith, J, Eather, N, Weaver, R, Riley, N, Beets, M, and Lubans, D. Behavioral correlates of muscular fitness in children and adolescents: A systematic review. *Sports Med* 49(6):887-904, 2019.

51. Society of Health and Physical Educators. *National Standards & Grade Level Outcomes for K-12 Physical Education.* Champaign, IL: Human Kinetics Publishers, 2014.

52. Stricker, P, Faigenbaum, A, McCambridge, T, and Council on Sports Medicine and Fitness. Resistance training for children and adolescents. *Pediatrics* 145(6):e20201011, 2020.

53. Tarp, J, Child, A, White, T, Westgate, K, Bugge, A, Grøntved, A, Wedderkopp, N, Andersen, L, Cardon, G, Davey, R, Janz, K, Kriemler, S, Northstone, K, Page, A, Puder, J, Reilly, J, Sardinha, L, van Sluijs, E, Ekelund, U, Wijndaele, K, Brage, S, and International Children's Accelerometry Database (ICAD) Collaborators. Physical activity intensity, bout-duration, and cardiometabolic risk markers in children and adolescents. *Int J Obesity* 42:1639-1650, 2018.

54. Telama, R, Yang, X, Leskinen, E, Kankaanpää, A, Hirvensalo, M, Tammelin, T, Viikari, J, and Raitakari, O. Tracking of physical activity from early childhood through youth into adulthood. *Med Sci Sports Exerc* 46:955-962, 2014.

55. Thorborg, K, Krommes, K, Esteve, E, Clausen, M, Bartels, E, and Rathleff, M. Effect of specific exercise-based football injury prevention programmes on the overall injury rate in football: A systematic review and meta-analysis of the FIFA 11 and 11+ programmes. *Brit J Sport Med* 51:562-571, 2017.

56. United States Department of Health and Human Services. *Physical Activity Guidelines for Americans.* Washington, DC: Department of Health and Human Services, 2018.

57. Valkenborghs, S, Noetel, M, Hillman, C, Nilsson, M, Smith, J, Ortega, F, and Lubans, D. The impact of physical activity on brain structure and function in youth: A systematic review. *Pediatrics* 144:e20184032, 2019.

58. Webster, K, and Hewett, T. Meta-analysis of meta-analyses of anterior cruciate ligament injury reduction training programs. *J Orthop Res* 36:2696-2708, 2018.

59. Wibaek, R, Vistisen, D, Girma, T, Admassu, B, Abera, M, Abdissa, A, Mudie, K, Kæstel, P, Jørgensen, M, Wells, J, Michaelsen, K, Friis, H, and Andersen, G. Body mass index trajectories in early childhood in relation to cardiometabolic risk profile and body composition at 5 years of age. *Am J Clin Nutr* 110(5):1175-1185, 2019.

60. World Health Organization. *Global Action Plan on Physical Activity 2018-2030: More Active People for a Healthier World.* Geneva: Author, 2018.

61. Yang, L, Cao, C, Kantor, E, Nguyen, L, Zheng, X, Park, Y, Giovannucci, E, Matthews, C, Colditz, G, and Cao, Y. Trends in sedentary behavior among the US population, 2001-2016. *J Am Med Assoc* 321:1587-1597, 2019.

62. Yogman, M, Garner, A, Hutchinson, J, Hirsh-Pasek, K, Golinkoff, R, Committee on Psychological Aspects of Child and Family Health, and Council on Communications and Media. The power of play: A pediatric role in enhancing development in young children. *Pediatrics* 142:e20182058, 2018.

Older Adults Section

1. American College of Sports Medicine Position Stand. Exercise and physical activity for older adults. *Med Sci Sports Exerc* 41:1510-1530, 2009.

2. American College of Sports Medicine. *ACSM's Guidelines for Exercise Testing and Prescription.* 10th ed. Philadelphia: Wolters Kluwer, 2018.

3. Annesi, J, and Westcott, WL. Relationship of feeling states after exercise and total mood disturbance over 10 weeks in formerly sedentary women. *Percep Motor Skills* 99:107-115, 2004.

4. Anton, M, Cortez-Cooper, M, Devan, A, Neidre, DB, Cook, JN, and Tanaka, H. Resistance training increases basal limb blood flow and vascular conductance in aging humans. *J Appl Physiol* 101(5):1351-1355, 2006.

5. Baechle, TR, and Westcott, WL. *Fitness Professional's Guide to Strength Training Older Adults.* Champaign, IL: Human Kinetics, 23, 2010.

6. Barry, B, and Carson, R. The consequences of resistance training for movement control in older adults. *J Gerontol A-Biol* 59:730-754, 2004.

7. Bemben, D, Fetters, N, Bemben, M, Nabavi, N, and Koh, E. Musculoskeletal response to high and low intensity resistance training in early postmenopausal women. *Med Sci Sports Exerc* 32:1949-1957, 2000.

8. Best, JR, Chiu, BK, Hsu, CL, Nagamatsu, LS, and Liu-Ambrose, T. Long term effects of resistance exercise training on cognition and brain volume in older women: Results from a randomized controlled trial. *J Int Neuropsychol Soc* 21(10):745-756, 2015.

9. Bircan, C, Karasel, SA, Akgun, B, El, O, and Alper, S. Effects of muscle strengthening versus aerobic exercise program in fibromyalgia. *Rheumatol Int* 28:527-532, 2008.

10. Blair, SN, Kohl 3rd, HW, Paffenbarger Jr., RS, Clark, DG, Cooper, KH, and Gibbons, LW. Physical fitness and all-cause mortality: A prospective study of healthy men and women. *J Am Med Assoc* 262:2395-2401, 1989.

11. Boyle, J. Projection of the year 2050 burden of diabetes in the US adult population: Dynamic modeling of incidence, mortality, and prediabetes prevalence. *Pop Health Met* 8(1):29, 2010.

12. Brierley, EJ, Johnson, MA, James, OF, and Turnbull, DM. Effects of physical activity and age on mitochondrial function. *QJM* 89:251-258, 1996.

13. Brosseau, L, Wells, GA, Tugwell, P, Egan, M, Wilson, KG, Dubouloz, CJ, Casimiro, L, Robinson, VA, McGowan, J, Busch, A, Poitras, S, Moldofsky, H, Harth, M, Finestone, HM, Nielson, W, Haines-Wangda, A, Russell-Doreleyers, M, Lambert, K, Marshall, AD, and Veilleux, L. Ottawa panel evidence-based clinical practical guidelines for strengthening exercises in the management of fibromyalgia: Part 2. *Phys Ther* 88:873-886, 2008.

14. Bweir, S, Al-Jarrah, M, Almalty, AM, Maayah, M, Smirnova, IV, Novikova, L, Stehno-Bittel, L. Resistance exercise training lowers HbA1c more than aerobic training in adults with type 2 diabetes. *Diab Metab Syndr* 1:27, 2009.

15. Campbell, W, Crim, M, Young, V, and Evans, W. Increased energy requirements and changes in body composition with resistance training in older adults. *Am J Clin Nutri* 60(2):167-175, 1994.

16. Carpinelli, R, and Otto, R. Strength training: Single versus multiple sets. *Sports Med* 26:73-84, 1998.

17. Cassilhas, R, Viana, V, Grasmann, V, Santos, RT, Santos, RF, Tufik, S, and Mello, M. The impact of resistance exercise on the cognitive function of the elderly. *Med Sci Sports Exerc* 39:1401-1407, 2007.

18. Castaneda, C, Layne, JE, Munez-Orians, L, Gordon, PL, Walsmith, J, Foldvari, M, Roubenoff, R, Tucker, KL, and Nelson, ME. A randomized controlled trial of resistance exercise training to improve glycemic control in older adults with type 2 diabetes. *Diab Care* 25(12):2335-2341, 2002.

19. Castillo, EM, Goodman-Gruen, D, Kritz-Silverstein, D, Morton, DJ, Wingard, DL, Barrett-Connor, E. Sarcopenia in elderly men and women: The Rancho Bernardo study. *Am J Prev Med* 25:226-231, 2003.

20. Chilibeck, P, Calder, A, Sale, D, and Webber, C. A comparison of strength and muscle mass increases during resistance training in young women. *Eur J Appl Physiol O* 77:170-175, 1997.

21. Chodzko-Zajko, W, and Schwinggel, A. Older adults: Ages 65 and older. In *American College of Sports Medicine Complete Guide to Health & Fitness.* Bushman, B, ed. Champaign, IL: Human Kinetics, 223-246, 2011.

22. Colcombe, SJ, Erickson, KI, Scalf, PE, Kim, JS, Prakash, R, McAuley, E, Elavsky, S, Marquez, DX, Hu, L, and Kramer, AF. Aerobic exercise increases brain volume in aging humans. *J Gerontol A-Biol* 297(16):1819-1822, 2006.

23. Colcombe, S, and Kramer, A. Fitness effects on the cognitive function of older adults: A meta-analytic study. *Psychol Sci* 14:125-130, 2003.

24. Cornelissen, V, and Fagard, R. Effect of resistance training on resting blood pressure: A meta-analysis of randomized controlled trials. *J Hyperten* 23(2):251-259, 2005.

25. DeMichele, P, Pollock, M, Graves, J, Foster, D, Carpenter, D, Garzarella, L, Brechue, W, and Fulton, M. Isometric torso rotation strength: Effect of training frequency on its development. *Arch Phys Med Rehab* 78:64-69, 1997.

26. Doherty, TJ, Vandervoort, AA, Taylor, AW, and Brown, WF. Effects of motor unit losses on strength in older men and women. *J Appl Physiol* 74:868-874, 1993.

27. Fahlman, M, Boardly, D, Lambert, C, and Flynn, M. Effects of endurance training and resistance training on plasma lipoprotein profiles in elderly women. *J Gerontol A-Biol* 57(2):B54-B60, 2002.

28. Faigenbaum, A, Skrinar, G, Cesare, W, Kraemer, W, and Thomas, H. Physiologic and symptomatic responses of cardiac patients to resistance exercise. *Arch Phys Med Rehab* 70:395-398, 1990.

29. Flack, KD, Davy, KP, Hulver, MW, Winett, RA, Frisard, MI, and Davy, BM. Aging, resistance training, and diabetes prevention. *J Aging Res* 127315, 2011. doi.org/10.4061/2011/127315, 2011

30. Fox, SM, Naughton, JP, and Gorman, PA. Physical activity and cardiovascular health. *Mod Con Cardio Health* 41:20, 1972.

31. Fragala, MS, Cadore, EL, Dorgo, S, Izquierdo, M, Kraemer, WJ, Peterson, MD, and Ryan, ED. Resistance training for older adults: Position Statement from the National Strength and Conditioning Association. *J Strength Cond Res* 33(8):2019-2052, 2019.

32. Frontera, WR, Hughes, VA, Fiatarone, MA, Fielding, RA, Evans, WJ, and Roubenoff, R. Aging of skeletal muscle: A 12-yr longitudinal study. *J Appl Physiol* 88:1321-1326, 2000.

33. Galvao, DA, Nosaka, K, Taaffe, DR, Spry, N, Kristjanson, LJ, McGuigan, MR, Suzuki, K, Yamaya, K, and Newton, RU. Resistance training and reduction of treatment side effects in prostate cancer patients. *Med Sci Sports Exerc* 38(12):2045-2052, 2006.

34. Gordon, NF, Gulanick, M, Costa, F, Fletcher, G, Franklin, BA, Roth, EJ, and Shephard, T. Physical activity and exercise recommendations for stroke survivors: An American Heart Association scientific statement from the Council on Clinical Cardiology, Subcommittee on Exercise, Cardiac Rehabilitation, and Prevention; the Council on Cardiovascular Nursing; the Council on Nutrition, Physical Activity, and Metabolism; and the Stroke Council. *Stroke* 35:1230-1240, 2004.

35. Graham, J. Resistance training exercise technique. In *NSCA's Essentials of Personal Training,* 2nd ed. Coburn, J, and Malek, M, eds. Champaign, IL: Human Kinetics, 289, 2012.

36. Graves, J, Pollock, M, Jones, A, Colvin, A, and Leggett, S. Specificity of limited range of motion variable resistance training. *Med Sci Sports Exerc* 21(1):84-89, 1989.

37. Green, JS, Stanforth, PR, Rankinen, T, Leon, AS, Rao, D, Skinner, JS, Bouchard, C, and Wilmore, JH. The effects of exercise training on abdominal visceral fat, body composition, and indicators of the metabolic syndrome in postmenopausal women with and without estrogen replacement therapy: The HERITAGE family study. *Metabolis* 53:1192-1196, 2004.

38. Hackney, KJ, Engels, HJ, and Gretebeck, RJ. Resting energy expenditure and delayed-onset muscle soreness after full-body resistance training with an eccentric concentration. *J Strength Cond Res* 22(5):1602-1609, 2008.

39. Heden, T, Lox, C, Rose, P, Reid, S, and Kirk, E. One-set resistance training elevates energy expenditure for 72 hours similar to three sets. *Euro J Appl Physiol* 111:477-484, 2011.

40. Holviala, JH, Sullivan, JM, Kraemer, WJ, Alen, M, and Häkkinen, K. Effects of strength training on muscle strength characteristics, functional capabilities, and balance in middle-aged and older women. *J Strength Cond Res* 20:336-344, 2006.

41. Hunter, G, Bickel, C, Fisher, G, Neumeier, W, and McCarthy, J. Combined aerobic and strength training and energy expenditure in older women. *Med Sci Sports Exerc* 45:1386-1393, 2013.

42. Hunter, G, Wetzstein, C, Fields, D, Brown, A, and Bamman, M. Resistance training increases total energy expenditure and free-living physical activity in older adults. *J Appl Physiol* 89(3):977-984, 2000.

43. Hurley, BF, Hanson, ED, and Sheaff, AK. Strength training as a countermeasure to aging muscle and chronic disease. *Sports Med* 41:289-306, 2011.

44. Jellinger, RS, Davidson, JA, and Blonde, I. Road maps to achieve glycemic control in type 2 diabetes mellitus: ACE/AACE Diabetes Road Map Task Force. *Endoc Pract* 13:260-268, 2007.

45. Kelley, G, and Kelley, K. Impact of progressive resistance training on lipids and lipoproteins in adults: A meta-analysis of randomized controlled trials. *Prevent Med* 48:9-19, 2009.

46. Kemmler, WS, Von Stengel, S, Weineck, J, Lauber, D, Kalender, W, Engelke, K. Exercise effects on menopausal risk factors of early postmenopausal women: 3-yr Erlangen fitness osteoporosis prevention study results. *Med Sci Sports Exerc* 37:194-203, 2005.

47. Kerr, D, Ackland, T, Maslen, B, Morton, A, and Prince, R. Resistance training over 2 years increases bone mass in calcium-replete postmenopausal women. *J Bone Miner Res* 16:175-181, 2001.

48. King, L, Birmingham, T, Kean, C, Jones, J, Bryant, D, and Griffin, J. Resistance training for medial compartment knee osteoarthritis and malalignment. *Med Sci Sports Exerc* 40:1376-1384, 2008.

49. Koffler, K, Menkes, A, Redmond, A, Whitehead, W, Pratley, R, and Hurley, B. Strength training accelerates gastrointestinal transit in middle-aged and older men. *Med Sci Sports Exerc* 24:415-419, 1992.

50. Kohrt, WM, Kirwan, JP, Staten, MA, Bourey, RE, King, DS, and Holloszy, JO. Insulin resistance in aging is related to abdominal obesity. *Diabetes* 42(2):273-281, 1993.

51. Krieger, J. Single versus multiple sets of resistance exercise: A meta-regression. *J Strength Cond Res* 23:1890-1901, 2009.

52. Lange, A, Vanwanseele, B, and Fiatarone Singh, M. Strength training for treatment of osteoarthritis of the knee: A systematic review. *Arth Rheum* 59:1488-1494, 2008.

53. Larsson, L, Sjodin, B, and Karlsson, J. Histochemical and biochemical changes in human skeletal muscle with age in sedentary males, age 22-65 years. *Acta Physiol Scand* 103:31-39, 1978.

54. Lee, IM, Hsieh, CC, and Paffenbarger Jr., RS. Exercise intensity and longevity in men. The Harvard Alumni Health Study. *J Am Med Assoc* 273:1179-1184, 1995.

55. Leitzmann, MF, Park, Y, Blair, A, Ballard-Barbash, R, Mouw, T, Hollenbeck, AR, and Schatzkin, A. Physical activity recommendations and decreased risk of mortality. *Arch Intern Med* 167:2453-2460, 2007.

56. Li, R, Xia, J, Zhang, X, Gathirua-Mwangi, WG, Guo, J, Li, Y, McKenzie, S, and Song, Y. Associations of muscle mass and strength with all-cause mortality among US older adults. *Med Sci Sports Exerc* 50(3):458-467, 2018.

57. Liu, Y, Lee, DC, Li, Y, Zhu, W, Zhang, R, Sui, X, Lavie, CJ, and Blair, SN. Associations of resistance exercise with cardiovascular disease morbidity and mortality. *Med Sci Sports Exerc* 51(3):499-508, 2019.

58. Marcell, TJ. Sarcopenia: Causes, consequences, and preventions. *J Gerontol A-Biol* 58(10):M911-M916, 2003.

59. Melov, S, Tarnopolsky, M, Beckman, K, Felkey, K, and Hubbard, A. Resistance exercise reverses aging in human skeletal muscle. *PLOS One* 2:e465, 2007.

60. Miranda, H, Fleck, S, Simão, R, Barreto, A, Dantas, E, and Novaes, J. Effect of two different rest period lengths on the number of repetitions performed during resistance training. *J Strength Cond Res* 21:1032-1036, 2007.

61. Munn, J, Herbert, R, Hancock, M, and Gandevia, S. Resistance training for strength: Effect of number of sets and contraction speed. *Med Sci Sports Exerc* 37:1622-1626, 2005.

62. Nelson, ME, Fiatarone, M, Morganti, C, Trice, I, Greenberg, RA, and Evans, WJ. Effects of high-intensity strength training on multiple risk factors for osteoporotic fractures. *J Am Med Assoc* 272:1909-1914, 1994.

63. Pescatello, LS, Franklin, BA, Fagard, R, Farquhar, WB, Kelley, GA, and Ray, CA. American College of Sports Medicine position stand. Exercise and hypertension. *Med Sci Sports Exerc* 36:533-553, 2004.

64. Peters, RK, Cady Jr., LD, Bischoff, DP, Bernstein, L, and Pike, MC. Physical fitness and subsequent myocardial infarction in healthy workers. *J Am Med Assoc* 249:3052-3056, 1983.

65. Phillips, SM. Resistance exercise: Good for more than just grandma and grandpa's muscles. *Appl Physiol Nutr Me* 32:1198-1205, 2007.

66. Pollock, ML, Franklin, BA, Balady, GJ, Chaitman, BL, Fleg, JL, Fletcher, B, Limacher, M, Piña, IL, Stein, RA, Williams, M, Bazzarre, T, and AHA Science Advisory. Resistance exercise in individuals with and without cardiovascular disease: Benefits, rationale, safety, and prescription: An advisory from the Committee on Exercise, Rehabilitation, and Prevention, Council on Clinical Cardiology, American Heart Association; Position paper endorsed by the American College of Sports Medicine. *Circulation* 101:828-833, 2000.

67. Pratley, R, Nicklas, B, Rubin, M, Miller, J, Smith, A, Smith, M, Hurley, B, and Goldberg, A. Strength training increases resting metabolic rate and norepinephrine levels in healthy 50- to 65-year-old men. *J Appl Physiol* 76(1):133-137, 1994.

68. Rhea, M, Alvar, B, and Burkett, L. A meta-analysis to determine the dose response for strength development. *Med Sci Sports Exerc* 35:456-464, 2003.

69. Risch, S, Norvell, N, Polock, M, Risch, R, Langer, H, Fulton, M, Graves, M, and Leggett, S. Lumbar strengthening in chronic low back pain patients. *Spine* 18:232-238, 1993.

70. Schlicht, J, Camaione, D, and Owen, S. Effect of intense strength training on standing balance, walking speed, and sit-to-stand performance in older adults. *J Gerontol A-Biol* 56:M281-M286, 2001.

71. Schoenfeld, BJ, Peterson, MD, Ogborn, D, Contreras, B, and Sommez, GT. Effects of low-versus high-load resistance training on muscle strength and hypertrophy in well-trained men. *J Strength Cond Res* 29(10):2954-2963, 2015.

72. Shephard, R. Maximal oxygen intake and independence in old age. *Brit J Sport Med* 43:342-346, 2009.

73. Sigal, RJ, Kenny, GP, Wasserman, DH, Castaneda-Sceppa, C, and White, RD. Physical activity/exercise and type 2 diabetes: A consensus statement from the American Diabetes Association. *Diab Care* 29:1433-1438, 2006.

74. Singh, N, Clements, K, and Fiatarone, M. A randomized controlled trial of progressive resistance exercise in depressed elders. *J Gerontol A-Biol* 52:M27-M35, 1997.

75. Skelton, DA, Greig, CA, Davies, JM, and Young, A. Strength, power, and related functional ability of healthy people aged 65-89 years. *Age Ageing* 23:371-377, 1994.

76. Strasser, B, and Schobersberger, W. Evidence of resistance training as a treatment therapy in obesity. *J Obes* 2011:482564, 2011.

77. Strasser, B, Siebert, U, and Schobersberger, W. Resistance training in the treatment of metabolic syndrome. *Sports Med* 40(5):397-415, 2010.

78. Sui, X, Lamonte, MJ, Laditka, JN, Hardin, JW, Chase, N, Hooker, SP, and Blair, SN. Cardiorespiratory fitness and adiposity as mortality predictors in older adults. *J Am Med Assoc* 298:2507-2516, 2007.

79. Taaffe, D, Pruitt, L, Pyka, G, Guido, D, and Marcus, R. Comparative effects of high and low intensity resistance training on thigh muscle strength, fiber area, and tissue composition in elderly women. *Clin Physiol* 16:381-392, 1996.

80. Thompson, PD, Buchner, D, Pina, IL, Balady, GJ, Williams, MA, Marcus, BH, Berra, K, Blair, SN, Costa, F, Franklin, B, Fletcher, GF, Gordon, NF, Pate, RR, Rodriguez, BL, Yance, AK, Wenger, NK; American Heart Association Council on Clinical Cardiology Subcommittee on Exercise, Rehabilitation, and Prevention; American Heart Association Council on Nutrition, Physical Activity, and Metabolism Subcommittee on Physical Activity. Exercise and physical activity in the prevention and treatment of atherosclerotic cardiovascular disease: A statement from the Council on Clinical Cardiology (Subcommittee on Exercise, Rehabilitation, and Prevention) and the Council on Nutrition, Physical Activity, and Metabolism (Subcommittee on Physical Activity). *Circulation* 107:3109-3116, 2003.

81. Trappe, S, Gallagher, P, Harber, M, Carrithers, J, Fluckey, J, and Trappe, T. Single muscle fibre contractile properties in young and old men and women. *J Physiol* 552:47-58, 2003.

82. Treuth, MS, Hunter, GR, Kekes-Szabo, T, Weinsier, RL, Goran, MI, and Berland, L. Reduction in intra-abdominal adipose tissue after strength training in older women. *J Appl Physiol* 78:1425-1431, 1995.

83. Troiano, RP, Berrigan, D, Dodd, KW, Masse, LC, Tilert, T, and McDowell, M. Physical activity in the United States measured by accelerometer. *Med Sci Sports Exerc* 40(1):181-188, 2008.

83a. Watson, SL, Weeks, BK, Weis, LJ, Harding, AT, Horan, SA, and Beck, BR. High-intensity resistance and impact training improves bone mineral density and physical function in postmenopausal women with osteopenia and osteoporosis: The LIFTMOR randomized controlled trial. *J Bone Miner Res* 33(2):211-220, 2018.

83b. Westcott, WL. *Building Strength and Stamina,* 2nd ed. Champaign, IL: Human Kinetics, 9, 2003.

84. Westcott, WL. Combining strength and endurance exercise. *Fit Manage* 21(1):24-27, 2005.

85. Westcott, WL. Strength training for frail older adults. *J Act Aging* 8:52-59, 2009.

86. Westcott, WL. Resistance training is medicine: Effects of strength training on health. *Curr Sports Med Rep* 11(4):209-216, 2012.

87. Westcott, WL. Older adults. In *NSCA's Essentials of Training Special Populations.* Jacobs, PJ, ed. Champaign, IL: Human Kinetics, 383-401, 2018.

87b. Westcott, WL, and Baechle, TR. *Fitness Professional's Guide to Strength Training Older Adults,* 2nd ed. Champaign, IL: Human Kinetics, 22, 2010.

88. Westcott, WL, Winett, RA, Annesi, JJ, Wojcik, JR, Anderson, ES, and Madden, PJ. Prescribing physical activity: Applying the ACSM protocols for exercise type, intensity, and duration across 3 training frequencies. *Phys Sportsmed* 2(37):51-58, 2009.

89. Wilson, G, Newton, R, Murphy, A, and Humphries, B. The optimal training load for the development of dynamic athletic performance. *Med Sci Sports Exerc* 25:1279-1286, 1993.

90. Wolfe, I, Van Cronenbourg, J, Kemper, H, Kostense, PJ, and Twisk, JW. The effect of exercise training programs on bone mass: A meta-analysis of published controlled trials in pre and post-menopausal women. *Osteoporosis Int* 9:1-12, 1999.

Pregnant Women Section

1. American College of Obstetricians and Gynecologists, Committee on Obstetric Practice. Committee opinion: Physical activity and exercise during pregnancy and the postpartum period. *Obstet Gynecol* 135: e178-e188, 2020.

2. American College of Obstetricians and Gynecologists, Committee on Obstetric Practice. Committee opinion: Optimizing postpartum care. *Obstet Gynecol* 131:e140-e150, 2018.

2a. American College of Obstetricians and Gynecologists, Committee on Obstetric Practice. Committee opinion: Physical activity and exercise during pregnancy and the postpartum period. *Obstet Gynecol* 126:e135-e142, 2015.

3. American College of Sports Medicine. *ACSM's Guidelines for Exercise Testing and Prescription,* 11th ed. Philadelphia: Wolters Kluwer, 2022.

4. Beetham, K, Giles, C, Noetel, M, Clifton, V, Jones, J, and Naughton, G. The effects of vigorous intensity exercise in the third trimester of pregnancy: A systematic review and meta-analysis. *BMC Pregnancy Childb* 19:281, 2019.

5. Bø, K, Artal, R, Barakat, R, Brown, W, Davies, G, Dooley, M, Evenson, K, Haakstad, L, Kayser, B, Kinnunen, T, Larsen, K, Mottola, M, Nygaard, I, van Poppel, M, Stuge, B, and Khan, K. Exercise and pregnancy in recreational and elite athletes: 2016/2017 evidence summary from the IOC expert group meeting, Lausanne. Part 5. Recommendations for health professionals and active women. *Brit J Sport Med* 52:1080-1085, 2018.

6. Clapp, J, Kim, H, Burciu, B, Schmidt, S, Petry, K, and Lopez, B. 2002. Continuing regular exercise during pregnancy: Effect of exercise volume on fetoplacental growth *Am J Obstet Gynecol* 186:142-147, 2002.

7. Connolly, C, Conger, S, Montoye, A, Marshall, M, Schlaff, R, Badon, S, and Pivarnik, J. Walking for health during pregnancy: A literature review and considerations for future research. *J Sport Health Sci* 8:410-411, 2019.

8. Dipietro, L, Evenson, K, Bloodgood, B, Sprow, K, Troiano, R, Piercy, K, Vaux-Bjerke, A, and Powell, K. 2018 Physical Activity Guidelines Advisory Committee. Benefits of physical activity during pregnancy and postpartum: An umbrella review, *Med Sci Sports Exerc* 51:1292-1302, 2019.

9. Hesketh, K, and Evenson, K. Prevalence of U.S. pregnant women meeting 2015 ACOG physical activity guidelines. *Am J Prevent Med* 51:e87-e89, 2015.

10. Kelly, A. 2005. Practical exercise advice during pregnancy. *Phys Sportsmed* 33:24-31, 2005.

11. Koletzko, B, Godfrey, K, Poston, L, Szajewska, H, van Goudoever, J, de Waard, M, Brands, B, Grivell, R, Deussen, R, Dodd, M, Patro-Golab, B, and Zalewski, B. Early Nutrition Project Systematic Review Group. Nutrition during pregnancy, lactation and early childhood and its implications for maternal and long-term child health: The early nutrition project recommendations. *Annals Nutr Metab* 74:93-106, 2019.

12. Mottola, M, Davenport, M, Ruchat, S, Davies, G, Poitras, V, Gray, C, Jaramillo Garcia, A, Barrowman, N, Adamo, K, Duggan, M, Barakat, R, Chilibeck, P, Fleming, K, Forte, M, Korolnek, J, Nagpal, T, Slater, L, Stirling, D, and Zehr, L. Canadian guideline for physical activity throughout pregnancy. *Brit J Sport Med* 52(21):1339-1346, 2019.

13. Mudd, L, Owe, K, Mottola, M, and Pivarnik, J. Health benefits of physical activity during pregnancy: An international perspective. *Med Sci Sports Exerc* 45:268-277, 2013.

14. Pivarnik, J, Chambliss, H, Clapp, J, Dugan, S, Hatch, M, Lovelady, C, Mottola, M, and Williams, M. Impact of physical activity during pregnancy and postpartum on chronic disease risk. *Med Sci Sports Exerc* 38:989-1006, 2006.

15. Russo, L, Nobles, C, Ertel, K, Chasan-Tabeer, L, and Whitcomb, B. Physical activity interventions in pregnancy and risk of gestational diabetes mellitus. *Obstet Gynecol* 125:576-582, 2015.

16. Sytsma, T, Zimmerman, K, Manning, J, Jenkins, S, Nelson, N, Clark, M, Boldt, K, and Borowski, K. Perceived barriers to exercise in the first trimester of pregnancy. *J Perinat Educ* 27(4):198-206, 2018.

17. Wang, J, Wen, D, Liu, X, and Liu, Y. Impact of exercise on maternal gestational weight gain: An updated meta-analysis of randomized controlled trials. *Medicine (Baltimore)* 98:e16199, 2019.

18. Woodley, S, Boyle, R, Cody, J, Mørkved, S, and Hay-Smith, E. Pelvic floor muscle training for prevention and treatment of urinary and faecal incontinence in antenatal and postnatal women. *Cochrane Db Syst Rev* 12(4):CD007471, 2017.

Chapter 19

1. Alberti, KG, Zimmet, P, and Shaw, J. Metabolic syndrome—a new worldwide definition. A consensus statement from the international diabetes federation. *Diabetic Med* 23:469-480, 2006.

2. American College of Sports Medicine. *ACSM's Guidelines for Exercise Testing and Prescription*, 11th ed. Philadelphia: Wolters Kluwer, 2022.

3. American College of Sports Medicine. Position stand: The female athlete triad. *Med Sci Sports Exerc* 39(10):1867-1882, 2007.

4. American College of Sports Medicine. Position stand: Appropriate physical activity intervention strategies for weight loss and prevention of weight regain for adults. *Med Sci Sports Exerc* 41(2):459-471, 2009.

5. American College of Sports Medicine and American Diabetes Association. Position stand: Exercise and type 2 diabetes. *Med Sci Sports Exerc* 42(12):2282-2303, 2010.

6. American Diabetes Association. Standards of medical care in diabetes—2012. *Diabetes Care* 35(Suppl 1):S11-S63, 2012.

7. American Heart Association. Cholesterol management guide for health care practitioners. 2018. https://professional.heart.org/-/media/files/health-topics/cholesterol/cholesterol-guide-for-hc-practitioners-english.pdf?la=en. Accessed November 10, 2019.

8. American Psychiatric Association. *Diagnostic and Statistical Manual of Mental Disorders (DSM-IV)*, 4th ed. Washington, DC: Author, 1994.

9. Ang, LW, Ma, S, Cutter, J, Chew, SK, Tan, CE, and Tai, ES. The metabolic syndrome in Chinese, Malays and Asian Indians. Factor analysis of data from the 1998 Singapore National Health Survey. *Diabetes Res Clin Pract* 67(1):53-62, 2005.

10. Arnett, DK, Blumenthal, RS, Albert, MA, Buroker, AB, Goldberger, ZD, Hahn, EJ, Himmelfarb, CD, Khera, A, Lloyd-Jones, D, McEvoy, JW, Michos, ED, Miedema, MD, Muñoz, D, Smith Jr., SC, Virani, SS, Williams Sr., KA, Yeboah, J, and Ziaeian, B. 2019 ACC/AHA guideline on the primary prevention of cardiovascular disease: A report of the American College of Cardiology/American Heart Association Task Force on Clinical Practice Guidelines. *Circulation* 140(11):e596-e646, 2019.

11. Balducci, S, Zanuso, S, Fernando, F, Fallucca, F, Fallucca, S, and Pugliese, G. Physical activity/exercise training in type 2 diabetes: The role of the Italian diabetes and exercise study. *Diabetes Metab Res* 25:S29-S33, 2009.

12. Bandyopadhyay, D, Qureshi, A, Ghosh, S, Ashish, K, Heise, LR, Hajra, A, and Ghosh, RK. Safety and efficacy of extremely low LDL-cholesterol levels and its prospects in hyperlipidemia management. *J Lipids* 2018:8598054, 2018.

13. Baker, C, and Brownell, KD. Physical activity and maintenance of weight loss: Physiological and psychological mechanisms. In *Physical Activity and Obesity*, Bouchard, C. ed. Champaign, IL: Human Kinetics, 311-328, 2000.

14. Benjamin, EJ, Blaha, MJ, Chiuve, SE, Cushman, M, Das, SR, Deo, R, de Ferranti, SD, Floyd, J, Fornage, M, Gillespie, C, Isasi, CR, Jiménez, MC, Jordan, LC, Judd, SE, Lackland, D, Lichtman, JH, Lisabeth, L, Liu, S, Longenecker, CT, Mackey, RH, Matsushita, K, Mozaffarian, D, Mussolino, ME, Nasir, K, Neumar, RW, Palaniappan, L, Pandey, DK, Thiagarajan, RR, Reeves, MJ, Ritchey, M, Rodriguez, CJ, Roth, GA, Rosamond, WD, Sasson, C, Towfighi, A, Tsao, CW, Turner, MB, Virani, SS, Voeks, JH, Willey, JZ, Wilkins, JT, Wu, JH, Alger, HM, Wong, SS, and Muntner, P; American Heart Association Statistics Committee and Stroke Statistics Subcommittee. Heart disease and stroke statistics—2017 Update: A report from the American Heart Association. *Circulation* 135:e1-e458, 2017.

15. Berkman, ND, Brownley, KA, Peat, CM, Lohr, KN, Cullen, KE, Morgan, LC, Bann, CM, Wallace, IF, and Bulik, CM, eds. Management and outcomes of binge-eating disorder. Rockville (MD): Agency for Healthcare Research and Quality. 15(16)-EHC030-EF, 2015.

16. Blair, SN, Kampert, JB, Kohl, HW, Barlow, CE, Macera, CA, Paffenbarger, RS, and Gibbons, LW. Influences of cardiorespiratory fitness and other precursors on cardiovascular disease and all-cause mortality in men and women. *J Am Med Assoc* 276(3):205-210, 1996.

17. Blair, S, and Nichaman, MZ. The public health problem of increasing prevalence rates of obesity and what should be done about it. *Mayo Clin Proc* 77:109-113, 2002.

18. Bouchard, C. Introduction. In *Physical Activity and Obesity*, Bouchard, C, ed. Champaign, IL: Human Kinetics, 3-19, 2000.

19. Bowen, KJ, Sullivan, VK, Kris-Etherton, PM, and Petersen, KS. Nutrition and cardiovascular disease: An update. *Curr Atheroscler Rep* 20(2):8, 2018.

20. Broekhuizen, LN, Boekholdt, SM, Arsenault, BJ, Despres, JP, Stroes, ES, Kastelein, JJ, Khaw, KT, and Wareham, NJ. Physical activity, metabolic syndrome, and coronary risk: The EPIC-Norfolk prospective population study. *Eur J Cardiov Prev R* 18(2):209-217, 2011.

21. Call, C, Walsh, BT, and Attia, E. From *DSM-IV* to *DSM-5*: Changes to eating disorder diagnoses. *Curr Opin Psychiatr* 26(6):532-536, 2013.

22. Colberg, SR, and Swain, DP. Exercise and diabetic control. *Physician Sportsmed* 28(4):63-81, 2000.

23. Colberg, SR, Sigal, RJ, Yardley, JE, Riddell, MC, Dunstan, DW, Dempsey, PC, Horton, ES, Castorino, K, and Tate, DF. Physical activity/exercise and diabetes: A position statement of the American Diabetes Association. *Diabetes Care* 39(11):2065-2079, 2016.

24. Conley, MS, and Rozenek, R. National Strength and Conditioning Association position statement: Health aspects of resistance exercise and training. *Strength Cond J* 23(6):9-23, 2001.

25. Daily, JP, and Stumbo, JR. Female athlete triad. *Primary Care* 45(4):615-624, 2018.

26. Delva, J, Johnston, LD, and O'Malley, PM. The epidemiology of overweight and related lifestyle behaviors: Racial/ethnic and socioeconomic status differences among American youth. *Am J Prev Med* 33(4S):S178-S186, 2007.

27. DeSalvo, KB, Olson, R, and Casavale, KO. Dietary guidelines for Americans. *J Am Med Assoc* 315(5):457-458, 2016.

28. De Pietro, L, Dziura, J, Yeckel, CW, and Neufer, PD. Exercise and improved insulin sensitivity in older women: Evidence of the enduring benefits of higher intensity training. *J Appl Physiol* 100:142-149, 2006.

29. De Souza, MJ, Koltun, KJ, and Williams, NI. The role of energy availability in reproductive function in the female athlete triad and extension of its effects to men: An initial working model of a similar syndrome in male athletes. *Sports Med* 49:125-137, 2019.

30. Despres, JP, and Lamarche, B. Physical activity and the metabolic complications of obesity. In *Physical Activity and Obesity*, Bouchard, C, ed. Champaign, IL: Human Kinetics, 329-354, 2000.

31. Despres, JP, Lemieux, I, and Prud'homme, D. Treatment of obesity: Need to focus on high risk abdominally obese patients. *Brit Med J* 322:716-720, 2001.

32. Devrim, A, Bilgic, P, and Hongu, N. Is there any relationship between body image perception, eating disorders, and muscle dysmorphic disorders in male bodybuilders? *Am J Mens Health* 12(5):1746-1758, 2018.

33. Drazin, MB. Type 1 diabetes and sports participation. *Physician Sportsmed* 28(12):49-66, 2002.

34. Eickhoff-Shemek, J. Scope of practice. *ACSM's Health Fit J* 6(5):28-31, 2002.

35. Estruch, R, Ros, E, Salas-Salvadó, J, Covas, MI, Corella, D, Arós, F, Gómez-Gracia, E, Ruiz-Gutiérrez, V, Fiol, M, Lapetra, J, Lamuela-Raventos, RM, Serra-Majem, L, Pintó, X, Basora, J, Muñoz, MA, Sorlí, JV, Martínez, JA, and Martínez-González, MA; PREDIMED Study Investigators. Primary prevention of cardiovascular disease with a Mediterranean diet supplemented with extra-virgin olive oil or nuts. *N Engl J Med*. 368(14):1279-1290, 2013.

36. Fabiani, R, Naldini, G, and Chiavarini, M. Dietary patterns and metabolic syndrome in adult subjects: A systematic review and meta-analysis. *Nutrients* 11(9):E2056, 2019.

37. Ford, ES, Giles, WH, and WH. Dietz. Prevalence of the metabolic syndrome among US adults: Findings from the Third National Health and Nutrition Examination Survey. *J Am Med Assoc* 287:356-359, 2002.

38. Fryar, CD, Carroll, MD, and Ogden, CL. Prevalence of overweight, obesity, and extreme obesity among adults aged 20 and over: United States, 1960-1962 through 2011-2014. Atlanta: National Center for Health Statistics. Centers for Disease Control and Prevention, 2016.

39. Galmiche, M, Déchelotte, P, Lambert, G, and Tavolacci, MP. Prevalence of eating disorders over the 2000-2018 period: A systematic literature review. *Am J Clin Nutr* 109(5):1402-1413, 2019.

40. Gennuso, KP, Gangnon, RE, Thraen-Borowski, KM, and Colbert, LH. Dose response relationships between sedentary behavior and the metabolic syndrome and its components. *Diabetologia* 58:485-492, 2015.

41. Go, AS, Mozaffarian, D, Roger, VL, Benjamin, EJ, Berry, JD, Blaha, MJ, Dai, S, Ford, ES, Fox, CS, Franco, S, Fullerton, HJ, Gillespie, C, Hailpern, SM, Heit, JA, Howard, VJ, Huffman, MD, Judd, SE, Kissela, BM, Kittner, SJ, Lackland, DT, Lichtman, JH, Lisabeth, LD, Mackey, RH, Magid, DJ, Marcus, GM, Marelli, A, Matchar, DB, McGuire, DK, Mohler 3rd, ER, Moy, CS, Mussolino, ME, Neumar, RW, Nichol, G, Pandey, DK, Paynter, NP, Reeves, MJ, Sorlie, PD, Stein, J, Towfighi, A, Turan, TN, Virani, SS, Wong, ND, Woo, D, and Turner, MB; American Heart Association Statistics Committee and Stroke Statistics Subcommittee. Heart disease and stroke statistics—2014 update: A report from the American Heart Association. *Circulation* 129(3):e28-e292, 2014.

42. Goldberg, L, Elliott, DL, Schutz, RW, and Kloster, FE. Changes in lipid and lipoprotein levels after weight training. *J Am Med Assoc* 252:504-506, 1984.

43. Grundy, SM, Brewer Jr., HB, Cleeman, JI, Smith Jr., SC, and Lenfant, C. Definition of metabolic syndrome: Report of the National Heart, Lung, and Blood Institute/American Heart Association conference on scientific issues related to definition. *Circulation* 109:433-438, 2004.

44. Grundy, SM, Hansen, B, Smith Jr. SC, Cleeman, JI, and Kahn, RA. Clinical management of metabolic syndrome: Report of the American Heart Association/National Heart, Lung, and Blood Institute/American Diabetes Association conference on scientific issues related to management. *Circulation* 109:551-556, 2004.

45. Grundy, SM, Stone, NJ, Bailey, AL, Beam, C, Birtcher, KK, Blumenthal, RS, Braun, LT, de Ferranti, S, Faiella-Tommasino, J, Forman, DE, Goldberg, R, Heidenreich, PA, Hlatky, MA, Jones, DW, Lloyd-Jones, D, Lopez-Pajares, N, Ndumele, CE, Orringer, CE, Peralta, CA, Saseen, JJ, Smith Jr., SC, Sperling, L, Virani, SS, and Yeboah, J. 2018 AHA/ACC/AACVPR/AAPA/ABC/ACPM/ADA/AGS/APhA/ASPC/NLA/PCNA guideline on the management of blood cholesterol: Executive summary: A report of the American College of Cardiology/American Heart Association task force on clinical practice guidelines. *J Am Coll Cardiol* 73(24):3168-3209, 2019.

45a. Hales, CM, Carroll, MD, Fryar, CD, and Ogden, CL. Prevalence of obesity and severe obesity among adults: United States, 2017-2018. *NCHS Data Brief*, (360), 1-8, 2020.

46. Hamer, M, Stamatakis, E, and Steptoe, A. Effects of substituting sedentary time with physical activity on metabolic risk. *Med Sci Sports Exerc* 46:1946-1950, 2014.

47. Hurley, BF, Hagberg, JM, Goldberg, AP, Seals, DR, Ehsani, AA, Brennan, RE, and Holloszy, JO. Resistive training can reduce coronary risk factors without altering VO$_2$max or percent body fat. *Med Sci Sports Exerc* 20(2):150-154, 2005.

48. Ibañez, J, Izquierdo, M, Argüelles, I, Forga, L, Larrión, JL, García-Unciti, M, Idoate, F, and Gorostiaga, EM. Twice-weekly progressive resistance training decreases abdominal fat and improves insulin sensitivity in older men with type 2 diabetes. *Diabetes Care* 28:662-667, 2005.

49. Jensen, MD, Ryan, DH, Apovian, CM, Ard, JD, Comuzzie, AG, Donato, KA, Hu, FB, Hubbard, VS, Jakicic, JM, Kushner, RF, Loria, CM, Millen, BE, Nonas, CA, Pi-Sunyer, FX, Stevens, J, Stevens, VJ, Wadden, TA, Wolfe, BM, Yanovski, SZ, Jordan, HS, Kendall, KA, Lux, LJ, Mentor-Marcel, R, Malik, VS, and Hu, FB. Sugar-sweetened beverages and cardiometabolic health: An update of the evidence. *Nutrients* 11(8):E1840, 2019.

50. Kelley, G. Dynamic resistance exercise and resting blood pressure in adults: A meta-analysis. *J Appl Physiol* 82(5):1559-1565, 1997.

51. Klem, ML, Wing, RR, McGuire, MT, Seagle, HM, and Hill, JO. A descriptive study of individuals successful at long-term maintenance of substantial weight loss. *Am J Clin Nutr* 66:239-246, 1997.

52. Kokkinos, PF, and Fernhall, B. Physical activity and high density lipoprotein cholesterol levels. *Sports Med* 28:307-314, 1999.

53. Lavie, CJ, Milani, RV, Artham, SM, Patel, DA, and Ventura, HO. The obesity paradox, weight loss, and coronary disease. *Am J Med* 122(12):1106-1114, 2009.

53a. Leavitt, N. A call for the CDC to track eating disorders. Harvard T.H. Chan School of Public Health, 2017. www.hsph.harvard.edu/news/features/cdc-eating-disorders-tracking. Accessed October 23, 2020.

54. Mack, LR, and Tomich, PG. Gestational diabetes: Diagnosis, classification, and clinical care *Obstet Gyn Clin N Am* 44(2):207-217, 2017.

55. Magrann, S, and Radford Keagy, S. *Weight Control and Eating Disorders.* Eureka, CA: Nutrition Dimension, 2001.

56. Maughan, RJ, Watson, P, Cordery, PA, Walsh, NP, Oliver, SJ, Dolci, A, Rodriguez-Sanchez, N, and Galloway, SD. A randomized trial to assess the potential of different beverages to affect hydration status: Development of a beverage hydration index. *Am J Clin Nutr* 103(3):717-723, 2016.

57. McElroy, SL, and Guerdjikova, AI. Understanding and coping with binge eating disorder: The patient's perspective. *J Clin Psychiat* 76(8):e1044, 2015.

57a. Moholdt, T, Lavie, CJ, and Nauman, J. Sustained physical activity, not weight loss, associated with improved survival in coronary heart disease. *J Am Coll Cardiol* 71(10):1094-1101, 2018.

58. Morgan, LC, Trisolini, MG, Wnek, J, Anderson, JL, Halperin, JL, Albert, NM, Bozkurt, B, Brindis, RG, Curtis, LH, DeMets, D, Hochman, JS, Kovacs, RJ, Ohman, EM, Pressler, SJ, Sellke, FW, Shen, WK, Smith Jr., SC, Tomaselli, GF; American College of Cardiology/American Heart Association Task Force on Practice Guidelines; and Obesity Society. 2013 AHA/ACC/TOS guideline for the management of overweight and obesity in adults: A report of the American College of Cardiology/American Heart Association Task Force on Practice Guidelines and the Obesity Society. *Circulation* 129(25 Suppl 2):S102-S138, 2014.

59. Mountjoy, M, Sundgot-Borgen, JK, Burke, LM, Ackerman, KE, Blauwet, C, Constantini, N, Lebrun, C, Lundy, B, Melin, AK, Meyer, NL, Sherman, RT, Tenforde, AS, Klungland Torstveit, M, and Budgett, R. IOC consensus statement on relative energy deficiency in sport (RED-S): 2018 update. *Brit J Sport Med* 52(11):687-697, 2018.

60. Mozaffarian, D, Appel, LJ, and Van Horn, L. Components of a cardioprotective diet: New insights. *Circulation* 123(24):2870-2891, 2011.

61. Murray, SB, Rieger, E, Hildebrandt, T, Karlov, L, Russell, J, Boon, E, Dawson, RT, and Touyz, SW. A comparison of eating, exercise, shape, and weight related symptomatology in males with muscle dysmorphia and anorexia nervosa. *Body Image* 9(2):193-200, 2012.

61a. National Eating Disorders Association, www.nationaleatingdisorders.org/warning-signs-and-symptoms, www.nationaleatingdisorders.org/learn/by-eating-disorder/anorexia, www.nationaleatingdisorders.org/learn/by-eating-disorder/bulimia, www.nationaleatingdisorders.org/learn/by-eating-disorder/bed. Accessed October 23, 2020.

61b. National Heart, Lung, and Blood Institute. *Managing Overweight and Obesity in Adults: Systematic Evidence Review From the Obesity Expert Panel, 2013.* Washington, DC: U.S. Department of Health and Human Services, National Institutes of Health, 55, 2013. www.nhlbi.nih.gov/sites/default/files/media/docs/obesity-evidence-review.pdf. Accessed October 23, 2020.

62. National Institutes of Health and National Heart, Lung, and Blood Institute. *Clinical Guidelines on the Identification, Evaluation, and Treatment of Overweight and Obesity in Adults.* NIH Pub. No. 98-4083, 1998. www.nhlbi.nih.gov/guidelines/obesity/ob_gdlns.pdf. Accessed January 13, 2003.

63. National Institutes of Health and National Heart, Lung, and Blood Institute. *The Practical Guide: Identification, Evaluation, and Treatment of Overweight and Obesity in Adults.* NIH Pub. No. 00-4084, 2000. www.nhlbi.nih.gov/guidelines/obesity/prctgd_c.pdf. Accessed November 21, 2002.

64. National Institutes of Health and National Heart, Lung, and Blood Institute. *Third Report of the National Cholesterol Education Program (NCEP) Expert Panel on Detection, Evaluation, and Treatment of High Blood Cholesterol in Adults (Adult Treatment Panel III) Executive Summary.* NIH Pub. No. 01-3670, 2001. www.nhlbi.nih.gov/guidelines/cholesterol/atp3xsum.pdf. Accessed November 21, 2002.

65. National Task Force on the Prevention and Treatment of Obesity, National Institutes of Health. Very low-calorie diets. *J Am Med Assoc* 270:967-974, 1993.

66. Norris, R, Carroll, D, and Cochrane, R. The effect of aerobic and anaerobic training on fitness, blood pressure, and psychological stress and well-being. *J Psychosom Res* 34:367-375, 1990.

67. Ogden, CL, Carroll, MD, McDowell, MA, and Flegal, KM. Obesity among adults in the United States—no statistically significant change since 2003-2004. *NCHS Data Brief* (1):1-8,2007.

68. Pate, RR, Pratt, M, Blair, SN, Haskell, WL, Macera, CA, Bouchard, C, Buchner, D, Ettinger, W, Heath, GW, and King, AC. Physical activity and public health: A recommendation from the Centers for Disease Control and Prevention and the American College of Sports Medicine. *J Am Med Assoc* 273:402-407, 1995.

69. Piercy, KL, Troiano, RP, Ballard, RM, Carlson, SA, Fulton, JE, Galuska, DA, George, SM, and Olson, RD. The Physical Activity Guidelines for Americans. *J Am Med Assoc* 320(19):2020-2028, 2018.

70. Pollock, ML, Franklin, BA, Balady, GJ, Chaitman, BL, Fleg, JL, Fletcher, B, Limacher, M, Pi-a, I, Stein, RA, Williams, M, and Bazzarre, T. AHA Science Advisory. Resistance exercise in individuals with and without cardiovascular disease: Benefits, rationale, safety, and prescription. *Circulation* 101(7):828-833, 2000.

71. Proctor, MH, Moore, LL, Gao, D, Cupples, LA, Bradlee, ML, Hood, MY, and Ellison, RC. Television viewing and change in body fat from preschool to early adolescents: The Framingham Children's Study. *Int J Obes Relat Metab Disord* 27:827-833, 2003.

72. Pronk, NP, and Wing, RR. Physical activity and long-term maintenance of weight loss. *Obes Res* 2:587-599, 1994.

73. Ross, R, and Despres, FP. Abdominal obesity, insulin resistance, and the metabolic syndrome: Contribution of physical activity/exercise. *Obesity* 17:S1-S2, 2009.

74. Sacks, FM, Lichtenstein, AH, Wu, JHY, Appel, LJ, Creager, MA, Kris-Etherton, PM, Miller, M, Rimm, EB, Rudel, LL, Robinson, JG, Stone, NJ, Van Horn, LV; American Heart Association. Dietary fats and cardiovascular disease: A presidential advisory from the American Heart Association. *Circulation* 136(3):e1-e23, 2017.

75. Same, RV, Feldman, DI, Shah, N, Martin, SS, Al Rifai, M, Blaha, MJ, Graham, G, and Ahmed, HM. Relationship between sedentary behavior and cardiovascular risk. *Curr Cardiol Rep* 18:6, 2016.

76. Sangha, S, Oliffe, JL, Kelly, MT, and McCuaig, F. Eating disorders in males: How primary care providers can improve recognition, diagnosis, and treatment. *Am J Mens Health* 13(3):1-12, 2019.

77. Sperling, LS, Mechanick, JI, Neeland, IJ, Herrick, CJ, Després, JP, Ndumele, CE, Vijayaraghavan, K, Handelsman, Y, Puckrein, GA, Araneta, MR, Blum, QK, Collins, KK, Cook, S, Dhurandhar, NV, Dixon, DL, Egan, BM, Ferdinand, DP, Herman, LM, Hessen, SE, Jacobson, TA, Pate, RR, Ratner, RE, Brinton, EA, Forker, AD, Ritzenthaler, LL, and Grundy, SM. The cardiometabolic health alliance: Working toward a new care model for the metabolic syndrome. *J Am Coll Cardiol* 66(9):1050-1067, 2015.

78. Steffen, LM, Dai, S, Fulton, JE, and Labarthe, DR. Overweight in children and adolescents associated with TV viewing and parental weight. *Am J Prev Med* 37:S50-S55, 2009.

79. Storlie, J, and Jordan, HA, eds. *Behavioral Management of Obesity.* Champaign, IL: Human Kinetics, 1984.

80. Tenforde, AS, Barrack, MT, Nattiv, A, and Fredericson, M. Parallels with the female athlete triad in male athletes. *Sports Med* 46(2):171-182, 2016.

81. U.S. Department of Health and Human Services. Historical background, terminology, evolution of recommendations, and measurement, Appendix B, NIH consensus conference statement. In *Physical Activity and Health: A Report of the Surgeon General.* Atlanta: U.S. Department of Health and Human Services, Centers for Disease Control and Prevention, National Center for Chronic Disease Prevention and Health Promotion, 47, 1996.

82. U.S. Department of Health and Human Services. *Overweight and Obesity: At a Glance: The Surgeon General's Call to Action to Prevent and Decrease Overweight and Obesity.* Washington, DC: U.S. Department of Health and Human Services, Office of the Surgeon General, 2007.

83. U.S. Department of Health and Human Services. *Overweight and Obesity: Health Consequences: The Surgeon General's Call to Action to Prevent and Decrease Overweight and Obesity.* Washington, DC: U.S. Department of Health and Human Services, Office of the Surgeon General, 2007.

84. Vanderwater, EA, and Haung, X. Parental weight status as a moderator of the relationship between television viewing and childhood overweight. *Arch Pediat Adol Med* 160:622-627, 2006.

85. Vega, CL. Taking small steps . . . to big changes. *IDEA Today* 2:20-22, 1991.

86. Westerberg, DP, and Waitz, M. Binge-eating disorder. *Osteopathic Family Physician* 5(6):230-233, 2013.

87. World Health Organization. *Overweight and Obesity.* Report of a WHO Consultation on Obesity. Geneva: Author, 2018.

88. Yen, CF, Hsiao, RC, Ko, CH, Yen, JY, Huang, CF, Liu, SC, and Wang, SY. The relationships between body mass index and television viewing, internet use and cellular phone use: The moderating effects of sociodemographic characteristics and exercise. *Int J Eat Disorder* 43(6):565-571, 2010.

Chapter 20

1. Aggarwal, B, Mulgirigama, A, and Berend, N. Exercise-induced bronchoconstriction: Prevalence, pathophysiology, patient impact, diagnosis and management. *NPJ Prim Care Respir Med* 28(1):1-8, 2018.

2. Akinbami, LJ, Moorman, JE, Bailey, C, Zahran, HS, King, M, Johnson, CA, and Liu, X. Trends in asthma prevalence, health care use, and mortality in the United States, 2001-2010. *NCHS Data Brief* 94:1-8, 2012.

3. Ali, Z, Norsk, P, and Ulrik, CS. Mechanisms and management of exercise-induced asthma in elite athletes. *J Asthma* 49:480-486, 2012.

4. American College of Sports Medicine. *Exercise Management for Persons With Chronic Diseases and Disabilities,* 4th ed. Champaign, IL: Human Kinetics, 2016.

5. American College of Sports Medicine. *ACSM's Guidelines for Exercise Testing and Prescription,* 11th ed. Philadelphia: Wolters Kluwer, 2022.

6. American Heart Association. Exercise standards for testing and training: A statement for healthcare professionals from the American Heart Association. *Circulation* 104(14):1694-1740, 2001.

7. American Lung Association. Create an asthma action plan. www.lung.org/lung-health-and-diseases/lung-disease-lookup/asthma/living-with-asthma/managing-asthma/create-an-asthma-action-plan.html. Accessed March 6, 2020.

8. American Lung Association. *How serious is COPD?* www.lung.org/lung-health-and-diseases/lung-disease-lookup/copd/learn-about-copd/how-serious-is-copd.html. Accessed October 16, 2019.

9. American Thoracic Society, European Respiratory Society. Skeletal muscle dysfunction in chronic obstructive pulmonary disease. *Am J Respir Crit Care* 159(4 Pt 2):S1-S40, 1999.

10. Anderson, GP. Endotyping asthma: New insights into key pathogenic mechanisms in a complex, heterogeneous disease. *Lancet* 372:1107-1119, 2008.

11. Andras, A, and Ferket, B. Screening for peripheral arterial disease. *Cochrane Db Syst Rev* Apr 7(4):CD010835, 2014.

12. Arakawa, K. Effect of exercise on hypertension and associated complications. *Hypertens Res* 19(Suppl 1):S87-S91, 1996.

13. Asthma and Allergy Foundation of America. Asthma action plan. www.aafa.org/asthma-treatment-action-plan. Accessed June 1, 2019.

14. Benjamin, EJ, Muntner, P, and Bittencourt, MS. Heart disease and stroke statistics-2019 update: A report from the American Heart Association. *Circulation* 139(10):e56-e528, 2019.

15. Billinger, SA, Arena, R, Bernhardt, J, Eng, JJ, Franklin, BA, Johnson, CM, MacKay-Lyons, M, Macko, RF, Mead, GE, Roth, EJ, and Shaughnessy, M. Physical activity and exercise recommendations for stroke survivors: A statement for healthcare professionals from the American Heart Association/American Stroke Association. *Stroke* 45(8):2532-2553, 2014.

16. Blumenthal, JA, Thyrum, ET, Gullette, ED, Sherwood, A, and Waugh, R. Do exercise and weight loss reduce blood pressure in patients with mild hypertension? *N C Med J* 56(2):92-95, 1995.

17. Borhani, NO. Significance of physical activity for prevention and control of hypertension. *J Hum Hypertens* 10(Suppl 2):S7-S11, 1996.

18. Burdon, JG, Juniper, EF, Killian, KJ, Hargreave, FE, and Campbell, EJ. The perception of breathlessness in asthma. *Am Rev Respir Dis* 126:825-828, 1982.

19. Centers for Disease Control and Prevention. Asthma action plan. www.cdc.gov/asthma/actionplan.html. Accessed October 1, 2019.

20. Centers for Disease Control and Prevention. Peripheral arterial disease (PAD). www.cdc.gov/heartdisease/PAD.htm. Accessed June 1, 2019.

21. Chetta, A, Castagnaro, A, Foresi, A, Del Donno, M, Pisi, G, Malorgio, R, and Olivieri, D. Assessment of breathlessness perception by Borg scale in asthmatic patients: Reproducibility and applicability to different stimuli. *J Asthma* 40:323-329, 2003.

22. Chobanian, AV, Bakris, GL, Black, HR, Cushman, WC, Green, LA, Izzo Jr., JL, Jones, DW, Materson, BJ, Oparil, S, Wright Jr., JT, Roccella, EJ; National Heart, Lung, and Blood Institute Joint National Committee on Prevention, Detection, Evaluation, and Treatment of High Blood Pressure; National High Blood Pressure Education Program Coordinating Committee. The seventh report of the joint national committee on prevention, detection, evaluation, and treatment of high blood pressure: The JNC 7 report. *J Am Med Assoc* 289(19):2560-2572, 2003.

23. Conley, M, and Rozeneck, R. Health aspects of resistance exercise and training: NSCA position statement. *Strength Cond J* 23(6):9-23, 2001.

24. Dias, FD, Sampaio, LMM, da Silva, GA, Gomes, ÉLD, do Nascimento, ESP, Alves, VLS, Stirbulov, R, and Costa, D. Home-based pulmonary rehabilitation in patients with chronic obstructive pulmonary disease: A randomized clinical trial. *Int J Chronic Obstruc* 8:537-544, 2013.

25. Engstrom, G, Hedblad, B, and Janzon, L. Hypertensive men who exercise regularly have lower rate of cardiovascular mortality. *J Hypertens* 17(6):737-742, 1999.

26. Fauci, AS, Braunwald, E, Isselbacher, KJ. Disorders of the cardiovascular system. In *Harrison's Principles of Internal Medicine,* 14th ed. New York: McGraw-Hill, 1345-1352, 1998.

27. Fokkenrood, HJ, Bendermacher, BL, Lauret, GJ, Willigendael, EM, Prins, MH, and Teijink, JA. Supervised exercise therapy versus non-supervised exercise therapy for intermittent claudication. *Cochrane Db Syst Rev* Aug 23(8):2013.

28. Gotshall, RW. Airway response during exercise and hyperpnoea in non-asthmatic and asthmatic individuals. *Sports Med* 36:513-527, 2006.

29. Haas, TL, Lloyd, PG, Yang, H-T, and Terjung, RL. Exercise training and peripheral arterial disease. *Comp Physiol* 2(4):2933-3017, 2012.

30. Hagberg, JM, Ehsoni, AA, and Goldring, D. Effect of weight training on blood pressure and haemodynamics in hypertensive adolescents. *J Pediatr* 104:147-151, 1984.

31. Hagberg, JM, Park, JJ, and Brown, MD. The role of exercise training in the treatment of hypertension: An update. *Sports Med* 30(3):193-206, 2000.

32. Halbert, JA, Silagy, CA, Withers, RT, Hamdorf, PA, and Andrews, GR. The effectiveness of exercise in lowering blood pressure: A meta-analysis of randomized controlled trials of 4 weeks or longer. *J Hum Hypertens* 11(10):641-649, 1997.

33. Harris, KA, and Holly, RG. Physiological responses to circuit weight training in borderline hypertensive subjects. *Med Sci Sports Exerc* 19:246-252, 1987.

34. Holland, AE, Mahal, A, Hill, CJ, Lee, AL, Burge, AT, Cox, NS, Moore, R, Nicolson, C, O'Halloran, P, Lahham, A, and Gillies, R. Home-based rehabilitation for COPD using minimal resources: A randomised, controlled equivalence trial. *Thorax* 72:57-65, 2017.

35. Iepsen, UW, Jorgensen, KJ, Ringbaek, T, Lange, P. A systematic review of endurance, resistance and combined exercise training in COPD. *Eur Resp J* 44(Suppl 58):3033, 2014.

36. Kelley, G. Dynamic resistance exercise and resting blood pressure in adults: A meta-analysis. *J Appl Physiol* 82(5):1559-1565, 1997.

37. Kelley, GA, and Kelley, KA. Progressive resistance exercise and resting blood pressure: A meta-analysis of randomized controlled trials. *Hypertension* 35(3):838-843, 2000.

38. Khakban, A, Sin, DD, FitzGerald, JM, McManus, BM, Ng, R, Hollander, Z, and Sadatsafavi, M. The projected epidemic of chronic obstructive pulmonary disease hospitalizations over the next 15 years. A population-based perspective. *Am J Respir Crit Care* 195:287-291, 2017.

39. Khan, DA. Exercise-induced bronchoconstriction: Burden and prevalence. *Allergy Asthma Proc* 33:1-6, 2012.

40. Kokkinos, PF, and Papademetriou, V. Exercise and hypertension. *Coronary Artery Dis* 11(2):99-102, 2000.

41. Krafczyk, MA, and Asplund, CA. Exercise-induced bronchoconstriction: Diagnosis and management. *Am Fam Physician* 84(4):427-434, 2011.

42. Laslovich, SM, and Laslovich, JM. Exercise and asthma: A review. *Strength Cond J* 35(4):38-48, 2013.

43. Liao, WH, Chen, JW, Chen, X, Lin, L, Yan, HY, Zhou, YQ, and Chen, R. Impact of resistance training in subjects with COPD: A systematic review and meta-analysis. *Resp Care* 60:1130-1145, 2015.

44. Majahalme, S, Turjanmaa, V, Tuomisto, M, Kautiainen, H, and Uusitalo, A. Intra-arterial blood pressure during exercise and left ventricular indices in normotension and borderline and mild hypertension. *Blood Pressure* 6(1):5-12, 1997.

45. Manolas, J. Patterns of diastolic abnormalities during isometric stress in patients with systemic hypertension. *Cardiology* 88(1):36-47, 1997.

46. McDermott, MM. The magnitude of the problem of peripheral arterial disease: Epidemiology and clinical significance. *Clev Clin J Med* 73(4 Suppl):S2:7, 2006.

47. National Vital Statistics Reports. Deaths: Final data for 2019. www.cdc.gov/nchs/data/nvsr/nvsr70/nvsr70-08-508.pdf. Accessed September 29, 2021.

48. Norgren, L, Hiatt, WR, Dormandy, JA, Nehler, MR, Harris, KA, and Fowkes, FGR. Inter-society consensus for the management of peripheral arterial disease (TASC II). *J Vasc Surg* 45(1):S5-S67, 2007.

49. Papademetriou, V, and Kokkinos, PF. The role of exercise in the control of hypertension and cardiovascular risk. *Curr Opin Nephrol Hy* 5(5):459-462, 1996.

50. Parsons, JP, Craig, TJ, Stoloff, SW, Hayden, ML, Ostrom, NK, Eid, NS, and Colice, GL. Impact of exercise-related respiratory symptoms in adults with asthma: Exercise-Induced Bronchospasm Landmark National Survey. *Allergy Asthma Proc* 32:431-437, 2011.

51. Parsons, JP, Hallstrand, TS, Mastronarde, JG, Kaminsky, DA, Rundell, KW, Hull, JH, Storms, WW, Weiler, JM, Cheek, FM, Wilson, KC, and Anderson, SD. An official American Thoracic Society clinical practice guideline: Exercise induced bronchoconstriction. *Am J Resp Crit Care* 187(9):1016-1027, 2013.

52. Pascoe, CD, Wang, L, Syyong, HT, and Paré, PD. A brief history of airway smooth muscle's role in airway hyperresponsiveness. *J Allergy* (Cairo) 2012:768982. www.ncbi.nlm.nih.gov/pmc/articles/PMC3483821. Accessed June 6, 2019.

53. Ries, AL, Bauldoff, GS, Carlin, BW, Casaburi, R, Emery, CF, Mahler, DA, Make, B, Rochester, CL, Zuwallack, R, and Herrerias, C. Pulmonary rehabilitation: Joint ACCP/AACVPR evidence-based clinical practice guidelines. *Chest* 131(5 Suppl):4S-42S, 2007.

54. Roberts, S. Resistance training: Guidelines for individuals with heart disease. *Conditioning Instructor* 2(3):4-6, 1992.

55. Ronai, P, and Sorace, P. Exercise and stroke. *Strength Cond J* 37(1):50-55, 2015.

56. Roos, RJ. The Surgeon General's report: A prime source for exercise advocates. *Physician Sportsmed* 25(4):122-131, 1997.

57. Sallis, RE. *Essentials of Sports Medicine.* St. Louis: Mosby Yearbook, 1997.

58. Sallis, RE, Allen, M, and Massimino, F. *Sports Medicine Review.* St. Louis: Mosby Yearbook, 1997.

59. Tulio, S, Egle, S, and Greily, G. Blood pressure response to exercise of obese and lean hypertensive and normotensive male adolescents. *J Hum Hypertens* 9(12):953-958, 1995.

60. U.S. National Center for Health Statistics. National Vital Statistics Reports. www.cdc.gov/nchs/products/nvsr.htm. Accessed September 29, 2021.

61. Weiler, JM, Brannan, JD, Randolph, CC, Hallstrand, TS, Parsons, J, Silvers, W, Storms, W, Zeiger, J, Bernstein, DI, Blessing-Moore, J, and Greenhawt, M. Exercise-induced bronchoconstriction update. *J Allergy Clin Immun* 138:1292-1295, 2016.

62. Whelton, PK. ACC/AHA/AAPA/ABC/ACPM/AGS/APhA/ASH/ASPC/NMA/PCNA guideline for the prevention, detection, evaluation, and management of high blood pressure in adults: Executive summary: A report of the American College of Cardiology/American Heart Association Task Force on Clinical Practice Guidelines. *Hypertension* 71(6):e136-e139, 2017.

63. Winstein, CJ, Stein, J, Arena, R, Bates, B, Cherney, LR, Cramer, SC, Deruyter, F, Eng, JJ, Fisher, B, Harvey, RL, and Lang, CE. Guidelines for adult stroke rehabilitation and recovery: A guideline for healthcare professionals from the American Heart Association/American Stroke Association. *Stroke,* 47(6):e98-e169, 2016.

64. Wust, RC, and Degresn, H. Factors contributing to muscle wasting and dysfunction in COPD patients. *Int J Chronic Obstruc* 2:289-300, 2007.

65. Wyrwich, KW, Nelson, HS, Tierney, WM, Babu, AN, Kroenke, K, and Wolinsky, FD. Clinically important differences in health-related quality of life for patients with asthma: An expert consensus panel report. *Ann Allergy Asthma Im* 91:148-153, 2003.

Chapter 21

1. Amadio, PC. Tendon and ligament. In *Wound Healing: Biochemical and Clinical Aspects.* Cohen, IK, Diegelmann, RF, and Lindblad, WJ, eds. Philadelphia: Saunders, 384, 1992.

2. Anderson, AF, Snyder, RB, and Lipscomb Jr, AB. Anterior cruciate ligament reconstruction. A prospective randomized study of three surgical methods. *Am J Sport Med* 29(3):272-279, 2001.

3. Barrett, D. Proprioception and function after anterior cruciate reconstruction. *J Bone Joint Surg Br* 73:833-837, 1991.

4. Barrett, GR, Noojin, FK, Hartzog, CW, and Nash, CR. Reconstruction of the anterior cruciate ligament in females: A comparison of hamstring versus patellar tendon autograft. *Arthroscopy* 18(1):46-54, 2002.

5. Berkowitz, M, and Greene, C. Disability expenditures. *Am Rehabil* 15(1):7, 1989.

6. Blackburn, TA, McLeod, WE, White, B, and Wofford, L. EMG analysis of posterior rotator cuff exercises. *J Athl Train* 25:40-45, 1990.

7. Boden, BP, Dean, GS, Feagin, JA, and Garrett, WE. Mechanisms of anterior cruciate ligament injury. *Orthopedics* 23(6):573-578, 2000.

8. Breedveld, FC. New insights in the pathogenesis of rheumatoid arthritis. *J Rheumatol* (Suppl)53:3-7, 1998.

9. Burkhart, SS, Diaz Pagan, DL, Wirth, MA, and Athanasiou, KA. Cyclic loading of anchor-based rotator cuff repairs. *Arthroscopy* 13(2):720-724, 1997.

10. Byrd, JWT. The role of hip arthroscopy in the athletic hip. *Clin Sport Med* 25:255-278, 2006.

11. Carfagno, D, and Ellenbecker, TS. Osteoarthritis of the glenohumeral joint: Nonsurgical treatment options. *Physician Sportsmed* 30:19-32, 2002.

11a. Chaconas, E, Kolber, MJ, Hanney, WJ, Daugherty, ML, Wilson, SH, and Sheets, C. Shoulder external rotator eccentric training versus general shoulder exercise for subacromial pain syndrome: A randomized controlled trial. *Int J Sports Phys Ther* 12:1121-1133, 2017.

12. Clisby, EF, Bitter, NL, Sandow, MJ, Jones, MA, Magarey, ME, and Jaberzadeh, S. Relative contributions of infraspinatus and deltoid during external rotation with symptomatic subacromial impingement. *J Shoulder Elb Surg* 17(1 Suppl):S87-S92, 2008.

13. Cook, G. *Athletic Body in Balance.* Champaign, IL: Human Kinetics, 2003.

14. Curwin, S, and Stanish, W. *Tendinitis: Its Etiology and Treatment.* Lexington, MA: Collamore Press, 1984.

15. DePalma, B. Rehabilitation of the groin, hip, and thigh. In *Techniques in Musculoskeletal Rehabilitation,* 1st ed. Prentice, WE, and Voight, ML, eds. New York: McGraw-Hill, 2001.

16. Dodds, JA, and Arnoczky, SP. Anatomy of the anterior cruciate ligament: A blueprint for repair and reconstruction. *Arthroscopy* 10(2):132-139, 1994.

17. Earl, JE, and Vetter, CS. Patellofemoral pain. *Phys Med Rehabil Cli* 18:439-458, 2007.

18. Ellenbecker, TS. Rehabilitation of shoulder and elbow injuries in tennis players. *Clin Sport Med* 14(1):87-110, 1995.

19. Ellenbecker, TS. Postrehabilitation: Shoulder conditioning for tennis. *IDEA Personal Trainer* (March):18-27, 2000.

20. Ellenbecker, TS, and Davies, GJ. *Closed Kinetic Chain Rehabilitation.* Champaign, IL: Human Kinetics, 2001.

21. Enseki, KR, Martin, RL, Draovitch, P, Kelly, BT, Philippon, MJ, and Schenker, ML. The hip joint: Arthroscopic procedures and postoperative rehabilitation. *J Orthop Sport Phys* 36(7):516-525, 2006.

22. Feldmann, M, Brennan, FM, and Maini, RN. Rheumatoid arthritis. *Cell* 85(3):307-310, 1996.

23. Feldmann, SV. *Exercise for the Person With Rheumatoid Arthritis. Rehabilitation of Persons With Rheumatoid Arthritis.* Gaithersburg, MD: Aspen, 1996.

24. Feller, JA, Webster, KE, and Gavin, B. Early post-operative morbidity following anterior cruciate ligament reconstruction: Patellar tendon versus hamstring graft. *Knee Surg Sport Tr A* 9:260-266, 2001.

25. Freeman, M, Dean, M, and Hanham, I. The etiology and prevention of functional instability of the foot. *J Bone Joint Surg* 47B:669-677, 1965.

26. Friedman, RJ. Total shoulder arthroplasty in rheumatoid arthritis. In *Shoulder Reconstruction.* Neer, CS, and Demarest, RJ, eds. Philadelphia: Saunders, 158, 1990.

27. Galin, JI, Goldstein, IM, and Snyderman, R. *Inflammation: Basic Principles and Clinical Correlates.* New York: Raven Press, 1988.

28. Gambetta, V. *Athletic Development: The Art and Science of Functional Sports Conditioning.* Champaign, IL: Human Kinetics, 2007.

29. Giladi, M, Milgrom, C, Simkin, A, and Danon, Y. Stress fractures: Identifiable risk factors. *Am J Sport Med* 19(6):647-652, 1991.

30. Gregory, PL. "Overuse"—an overused term. *Brit J Sport Med* 36:83-84, 2002.

31. Gross, ML, Brenner, SL, Esformes, I, and Sonzogni, JJ. Anterior shoulder instability in weight lifters. *Am J Sport Med* 21(4):599-603, 1993.

32. Guskiewicz, KM, and Perrin, DH. Effect of orthotics on postural sway following inversion ankle sprain. *J Orthop Sport Phys* 23(5):326-331, 1996.

33. Häkkinen, A, Häkkinen, K, and Hannonen, P. Effects of strength training on neuromuscular function and disease activity in patients with recent-onset inflammatory arthritis. *Scand J Rheumatol* 23(5):237-242, 1994.

34. Häkkinen, A, Sokka, T, Kotaniemi, A, Kautiainen, H, Jappinen, I, Laitinen, L, and Hannonen, P. Dynamic strength training in patients with early rheumatoid arthritis increases muscle strength but not bone density. *J Rheumatol* 26:1257-1263, 1999.

35. Harkcom, TM, Lampman, RM, Banwell, BF, and Castor, CW. Therapeutic value of graded aerobic exercise training in rheumatoid arthritis. *Arthritis Rheum* 28(1):32-39, 1985.

36. Hazes, JM, and van den Ende, CHM. How vigorously should we exercise our rheumatoid arthritis patients? *Ann Rheum Dis* 55:861-862, 1996.

37. Hensinger, RN. Spondylolysis and spondylolisthesis in children and adolescents. *J Bone Joint Surg* 71A:1098-1107, 1989.

38. Hewett, TE. *Understanding and Preventing Noncontact ACL Injuries.* Hewett, T, Shultz, S, and Griffin, L, eds. Champaign, IL: Human Kinetics, 2007.

39. Hides, JA, Richardson, CA, and Jeull, GA. Multifidus muscle recovery is not automatic after resolution of acute, first-episode low back pain. *Spine* 21(23):2763-2769, 1996.

40. Hoshina, H. Spondylolysis in athletes. *Physician Sportsmed* 8(9):75-79, 1980.

41. Hunter, S, and Prentice, WE. Rehabilitation of the ankle and foot. In *Techniques in Musculoskeletal Rehabilitation.* Prentice, WE, and Voight, ML, eds. New York: McGraw-Hill, 2001.

42. Ireland, ML, Willson, JD, Ballantyne, BT, and Davis, IM. Hip strength in females with and without patellofemoral pain. *J Orthop Sport Phys* 33(11):671-676, 2003.

43. Johansson, H, Sjolander, P, and Soljka, P. A sensory role for the cruciate ligaments. *Clin Orthop Relat R* 268:161-178, 1991.

44. Kibler, WB. Biomechanical analysis of the shoulder during tennis activities. *Clin Sport Med* 14:79-85, 1995.

44a. Kolber, MJ. Hip osteoarthrosis. In *Orthopedic Management of the Hip and Pelvis.* Cheatham, SW, and Kolber, MJ, eds. St. Louis: Elsevier, 2016.

44b. Kolber, MJ, Corrao, M, and Hanney, WJ. Characteristics of anterior shoulder instability in the weight-training population. *J Strength Cond Res* 27:1333-1339, 2013.

44c. Kolber, MJ, Hanney, WJ, Cheatham, SW, Salamh, PA, Masaracchio, M, and Xinliang, L. Shoulder joint and muscle characteristics among weight-training participants with and without impingement syndrome. *J Strength Cond Res* 31:1024-1032, 2017.

45. Kramer, J, Jolesz, F, and Kleefield, J. Rheumatoid arthritis of the cervical spine. *Rheum Dis Clin N Am* 17:757, 1991.

46. Kraus, DR, and Shapiro, D. The symptomatic lumbar spine in the athlete. *Clin Sport Med* 8:59-69, 1989.

47. Kuland, DN. The injured athletes' pain. *Curr Concept Pain* 1:3-10, 1983.

48. Leadbetter, WB. Cell-matrix response in tendon injury. *Clin Sport Med* 11(3):533-578, 1992.

49. MacDougall, JD, Elder, GCB, Sale, DG, Moroz, JR, and Sutton, JR. Effect of strength training and immobilization on human muscle fibers. *Eur J Appl Physiol* 43:25-34, 1980.

50. Mandelbaum, BR, Silvers, HJ, Watanabe, DS, Knarr, JF, Thomas, SD, Griffin, LY, Kirkendall, DT, and Garrett Jr, W. Effectiveness of a neuromuscular and proprioceptive training program in preventing anterior cruciate ligament injuries in female athletes: 2-year follow-up. *Am J Sport Med* 33 (7): 1003-1010, 2005.

51. McConnell, J. Patellofemoral joint complications and considerations. In *Knee Ligament Rehabilitation*, 2nd ed. Ellenbecker, TS, ed. Philadelphia: Churchill Livingstone, 2000.

52. McGuine, TA, and Keene, JS. The effect of a balance training program on the risk of ankle sprains in high school athletes. *Am J Sport Med* 34(7):1103-1111, 2006.

53. Minor, MA, Hewett, JE, Webel, RR, Anderson, SK, and Kay, DR. Efficacy of physical conditioning exercises in patients with rheumatoid arthritis and osteoarthritis. *Arthritis Rheum* 32:1396-1405, 1989.

54. Minor, MA, and Kay, DR. Arthritis. In *ACSM's Exercise Management for Persons With Chronic Diseases and Disabilities*, 2nd ed. Durstine, JL, and Moore, GE, eds. Champaign, IL: Human Kinetics, 2003.

55. Moncur, D, and Williams, HJ. Cervical spine management in patients with rheumatoid arthritis. *Phys Ther* 68:509, 1988.

56. Muller, EA. Influence of training and of inactivity on muscle strength. *Arch Phys Med Rehab* 51:449-462, 1970.

57. Neer, CS, Weston, KC, and Stanton, FJ. Recent experience in total shoulder replacement. *J Bone Joint Surg* 64A:319, 1982.

58. Neitzel, JA, Kernozek, T, and Davies, GJ. Loading response following ACL reconstruction during parallel squat exercise. *Clin Biomech* 17:551-554, 2002.

59. Nieman, DC. Exercise soothes arthritis joint effects. *ACSMS Health Fit J* 4:20-27, 2000.

60. Nies-Byl, N, and Sinnott, PL. Variations in balance and body sway in middle-aged adults: Subjects with healthy backs compared with subjects with low-back dysfunction. *Spine* 16:325-330, 1991.

61. Panayi, GS. T-cell-dependent pathways in rheumatoid arthritis. *Curr Opin Rheumatol* 9(3):236-240, 1997.

62. Panjabi, MM. The stabilizing system of the spine. Part I Function, dysfunction, adaptation, and enhancement. *J Spinal Disord* 5:383-389, 1992.

63. Parsons, IM, Apreleva, M, Fu, FH, and Woo, SL. The effect of rotator cuff tears on reaction forces at the glenohumeral joint. *J Orthop Res* 20:439-446, 2002.

64. Petersen, T, Kryger, P, Ekdahl, C, Olsen, S, and Jacobsen, S. The effect of McKenzie therapy as compared with that of intensive strengthening training for the treatment of patients with subacute or chronic low back pain: A randomized controlled trial. *Spine* 27(16):1702-1709, 2002.

65. Porterfield, JA, and DeRosa, C. *Mechanical Low Back Pain: Perspectives in Functional Anatomy*, 2nd ed. Philadelphia: Saunders, 1998.

66. Potach, DH, and Borden, R. Rehabilitation and reconditioning. In *Essentials of Strength Training and Conditioning*, 2nd ed. Baechle, TR, and Earle, RW, eds. Champaign, IL: Human Kinetics, 2000.

67. Prentice, WE. *Arnheim's Principles of Athletic Training*, 12th ed. New York: McGraw-Hill, 2006.

68. Rack, PMH, and Westbury, DR. The short range stiffness of active mammalian muscle and its effect on mechanical properties. *J Physiol* 240:331-350, 1974.

69. Radcliffe, JC. *High-Powered Plyometrics*. Champaign, IL: Human Kinetics, 1999.

70. Radcliffe, JC. *Functional Training for Athletes at All Levels*. Berkeley, CA: Ulysses Press, 2007.

71. Richardson, CA, Snijders, CJ, Hides, JA, Damen, L, Pas, MS, and Storm, J. The relationship between the transversus abdominis muscles, sacroiliac joint mechanics, and low back pain. *Spine* 27(4):399-405, 2002.

72. Rotella, RJ. Psychological care of the injured athlete. In *The Injured Athlete*, 2nd ed. Kuland, D, ed. Philadelphia: Lippincott, 1985.

73. Saal, J. The role of inflammation in lumbar pain. *Spine* 20:1821-1827, 1995.

74. Safran, MR, Benedetti, RS, Bartolozzi 3rd, AR, and Mandelbaum, BR. Lateral ankle sprains: A comprehensive review part 1: Etiology, pathoanatomy, histopathogenesis, and diagnosis. *Med Sci Sports Exerc* 31:S429-S437, 1999.

75. Safran, MR, Benedetti, RS, Bartolozzi 3rd, AR, and Mandelbaum, BR. Lateral ankle sprains: A comprehensive review part 2: Treatment and rehabilitation with emphasis on the athlete. *Med Sci Sports Exerc* 31: S438-S447, 1999.

75a. Schoenfeld, BJ, Grgic, J, Ogborn, D, and Krieger, JW. Strength and hypertrophy adaptations between low-vs. high-load resistance training: A systematic review and meta-analysis. *J Strength Cond Res* 31(12):3508-3523, 2017.

76. Scovazzo, ML, Browne, A, Pink, M, Jobe, FW, and Kerrigan, J. The painful shoulder during freestyle swimming. An electromyographic cinematographic analysis of twelve muscles. *Am J Sport Med* 19(6):577-582, 1991.

77. Semble, EL, Loeser, RF, and Wise, CM. Therapeutic exercise for rheumatoid arthritis and osteoarthritis. *Semin Arthritis Rheu* 20:32-40, 1990.

78. Shelbourne, KD, and Trumper, RV. Anterior cruciate ligament reconstruction: Evolution of rehabilitation. In *Knee Ligament Rehabilitation*, 2nd ed. Ellenbecker, TS, ed. Philadelphia: Churchill Livingstone, 2000.

79. Stalzer, S, Wahoff, M, and Scanlan, M. Rehabilitation following hip arthroscopy. *Clin Sport Med* 25:337-357, 2003.

80. Standaert, CJ. Spondylolysis in the adolescent athlete. *Clin J Sport Med* 12(2):119-122, 2002.

81. Stenstrom, C. Therapeutic exercise in rheumatoid arthritis. *Arthrit Care Res* 7:190-197, 1994.

82. Thacker, SB, Stroup, DF, Branche, CM, Gilchrist, J, Goodman, RA, and Weitman, EA. The prevention of ankle sprains in sports. *Am J Sport Med* 27(6):753-760, 1999.

83. Thein, JM, and Thein-Brody, L. Aquatic therapy. In *Knee Ligament Rehabilitation*, 2nd ed. Ellenbecker, TS, ed. Philadelphia: Churchill Livingstone, 2000.

84. Valovich-McLeod, TC. The effectiveness of balance training programs on reducing the incidence of ankle sprains in adolescent athletes. *J Sport Rehabil* 17:1-8, 2008.

85. van den Ende, CHM, Hazes, JMW, le Cessie, S, Mulder, WJ, Belfor, DG, Breedveld, FC, and Dijkmans, BA. Comparison of high and low intensity training in well controlled rheumatoid arthritis. Results of a randomized clinical trial. *Ann Rheum Dis* 55:798-805, 1996.

86. Warner, MJ, and Amato, HK. The mind: An essential healing tool for rehabilitation. *Athlet Ther Today* (May):37-41, 1997.

87. Wilk, KE, and Andrews, JR. The effects of pad placement and angular velocity on tibial displacement during isokinetic exercise. *J Orthop Sport Phys* 17(1):24-30, 1990.

88. Wilk, KE, Davies, GJ, and Mangine, RE. Patellofemoral disorders: A classification system and clinical guidelines for non-operative rehabilitation. *J Orthop Sport Phys* 28:307-322, 1998.

89. Williams, MM, Hawley, JA, McKenzie, RA, and van Wijmen, PM. A comparison of the effects of two sitting postures on back and referred pain. *Spine* 16(10):1185-1191, 1991.

90. Young, A, Stokes M, and Iles, JF. Effects of joint pathology on muscle. *Clin Orthop Relat R* 47:678-685, 1987.

Chapter 22

1. Accardo, P, ed. *Capute and Accardo's Neurodevelopmental Disabilities in Infancy and Childhood*. Baltimore, MD: Brookes, 2008.

2. Anderson, MA, and Laskin, JJ. Cerebral palsy. In *ACSM's Resources for Clinical Exercise Physiology: Musculoskeletal, Neuromuscular, Neoplastic, Immunologic, and Hematologic Conditions*. Myers, J, and Nieman, DC, eds. Philadelphia: Wolters Kluwer Health/Lippincott Williams & Wilkins Health, 19-33, 2010.

3. Arida, RM, de Almeida, A-CG, Cavalheiro, EA, and Scorza, FA. Experimental and clinical findings from physical exercise as complementary therapy for epilepsy. *Epilepsy Behav* 26:273-278, 2013.

4. Åstrand, PO, and Ryhming, I. A nomogram for calculation of aerobic capacity (physical fitness) from pulse rate during sub-maximal work. *J Appl Physiol* 7:218-221, 1954.

5. Aytar, A, Zeybek, A, Pekyavas, NO, Tigli, AA, and Ergun, N. Scapular resting position, shoulder pain and function in disabled athletes. *Prosthet Orthot Int* 39:390-396, 2015.

6. Balemans, AC, Van Wely, L, De Heer, SJ, Van den Brink, J, De Koning, JJ, Becher, JG, and Dallmeijer, AJ. Maximal aerobic and anaerobic exercise responses in children with cerebral palsy. *Med Sci Sports Exerc* 45:561-568, 2013.

7. Bauman, WA, and Spungen, AM. Metabolic changes in persons after spinal cord injury. *Phys Med Rehabil Clin* 11:109-140, 2000.

8. Bjarnadottir, O, Konradsdottir, A, Reynisdottir, K, and Olafsson, E. Multiple sclerosis and brief moderate exercise. A randomised study. *Mult Scler J* 13:776-782, 2007.

9. Bjornson, KF, Belza, B, Kartin, D, Logsdon, R, and McLaughlin, JF. Ambulatory physical activity performance in youth with cerebral palsy and youth who are developing typically. *Phys Ther* 87:248-257, 2007.

10. Brashear, A, and Elovic, E. *Spasticity: Diagnosis and Management*. New York: Demos, 2016.

11. Buchholz, AC, and Pencharz, PB. Energy expenditure in chronic spinal cord injury. *Curr Opin Clin Nutr* 7:635-639, 2004.

12. Burkett, L, Chisum, J, Stone, W, and Fernhall, B. Exercise capacity of untrained spinal cord injured individuals and the relationship of peak oxygen uptake to level of injury. *Spinal Cord* 28:512-521, 1990.

13. Burnham, RS, and Steadward, RD. Upper extremity peripheral nerve entrapments among wheelchair athletes: Prevalence, location, and risk factors. *Arch Phys Med Rehabil* 75:519-524, 1994.

14. Christensen, D, Van Naarden Braun, K, Doernberg, NS, Maenner, MJ, Arneson, CL, Durkin, MS, Benedict, RE, Kirby, RS, Wingate, MS, Fitzgerald, R, and Yeargin-Allsopp, M. Prevalence of cerebral palsy, co-occurring autism spectrum disorders, and motor functioning—Autism and Developmental Disabilities Monitoring Network, USA, 2008. *Dev Med Child Neurol* 56:59-65, 2014.

15. Cleary, SL, Taylor, NF, Dodd, KJ, and Shields, N. An aerobic exercise program for young people with cerebral palsy in specialist schools: A phase I randomized controlled trial. *Dev Neurorehabil* 20:331-338, 2017.

16. Clutterbuck, G, Auld, M, and Johnston, L. Active exercise interventions improve gross motor function of ambulant/semi-ambulant children with cerebral palsy: A systematic review. *Disabil Rehabil* 41:1131-1151, 2019.

17. Collard, SS, and Ellis-Hill, C. How do you exercise with epilepsy? Insights into the barriers and adaptations to successfully exercise with epilepsy. *Epilepsy Behav* 70:66-71, 2017.

18. Colquitt, G, Kiely, K, Caciula, M, Li, L, Vogel, RL, and Moreau, NG. Community-based upper extremity power training for youth with cerebral palsy: A pilot study. *Phys Occup Ther Pediatr* 40:31-46, 2020.

19. Commission on Classification and Terminology of the International League Against Epilepsy. Proposal for revised classification of epilepsies and epileptic syndromes. *Epilepsia* 30:389-399, 1989.

20. Cowan, RE, Callahan, MK, and Nash, MS. The 6-min push test is reliable and predicts low fitness in spinal cord injury. *Med Sci Sports Exerc* 44:1993-2000, 2012.

21. Dalgas, U, Stenager, E, Jakobsen, J, Petersen, T, Hansen, HJ, Knudsen, C, Overgaard, K, and Ingemann-Hansen, T. Resistance training improves muscle strength and functional capacity in multiple sclerosis. *Neurology* 73:1478-1484, 2009.

22. Damiano, DL, and Abel, MF. Functional outcomes of strength training in spastic cerebral palsy. *Arch Phys Med Rehabil* 79:119-125, 1998.

23. Davis, G, Shephard, R, and Jackson, R. Cardio-respiratory fitness and muscular strength in the lower-limb disabled. *Can J Appl Sport Sci* 6:159-165, 1981.

24. Davis, GM, and Shephard, RJ. Cardiorespiratory fitness in highly active versus inactive paraplegics. *Med Sci Sports Exerc* 20:463-468, 1988.

25. Davis, GM, Shephard, RJ, and Leenen, FH. Cardiac effects of short term arm crank training in paraplegics: Echocardiographic evidence. *Eur J Appl Physiol O* 56:90-96, 1987.

26. Davis, GM, Tupling, SJ, and Shephard, RJ. Dynamic strength and physical activity in wheelchair users. Presented at 1984 Olympic Scientific Congress—Sports and Disabled Athletes, Champaign, IL, 1984.

27. Dodd, KJ, Taylor, NF, and Graham, HK. A randomized clinical trial of strength training in young people with cerebral palsy. *Dev Med Child Neurol* 45:652-657, 2003.

28. Dodd, KJ, Taylor, NF, and Graham, HK. Strength training can have unexpected effects on the self-concept of children with cerebral palsy. *Pediatr Phys Ther* 16:99-105, 2004.

29. Durstine, JL, Moore, GE, Painter, PL, and American College of Sports Medicine. *ACSM's Exercise Management for Persons With Chronic Diseases and Disabilities*. Champaign, IL: Human Kinetics, 2016.

30. Dutton, RA. Medical and musculoskeletal concerns for the wheelchair athlete: A review of preventative strategies. *Curr Sports Med Rep* 18:9-16, 2019.

31. Elder, GC, Kirk, J, Stewart, G, Cook, K, Weir, D, Marshall, A, and Leahey, L. Contributing factors to muscle weakness in children with cerebral palsy. *Dev Med Child Neurol* 45:542-550, 2003.

32. Eliasson, AC, Krumlinde-Sundholm, L, Rosblad, B, Beckung, E, Arner, M, Ohrvall, AM, and Rosenbaum, P. The Manual Ability Classification System (MACS) for children with cerebral palsy: Scale development and evidence of validity and reliability. *Dev Med Child Neurol* 48:549-554, 2006.

33. Elovic, EP, Munin, MC, Kanovsky, P, Hanschmann, A, Hiersemenzel, R, and Marciniak, C. Randomized, placebo-controlled trial of inco-botulinumtoxina for upper-limb post-stroke spasticity. *Muscle Nerve* 53:415-421, 2016.

34. Faigenbaum, AD, Kraemer, WJ, Blimkie, CJ, Jeffreys, I, Micheli, LJ, Nitka, M, and Rowland, TW. Youth resistance training: Updated position statement paper from the national strength and conditioning association. *J Strength Cond Res* 23:S60-79, 2009.

35. Feltham, MG, Ledebt, A, Deconinck, FJ, and Savelsbergh, GJ. Assessment of neuromuscular activation of the upper limbs in children with spastic hemiparetic cerebral palsy during a dynamical task. *J Electromyogr Kinesiol* 20:448-456, 2010.

36. Fernhall, B, Heffernan, K, Jae, SY, and Hedrick, B. Health implications of physical activity in individuals with spinal cord injury: A literature review. *J Health Hum Serv Adm* 30:468-502, 2008.

37. Figoni, S. Circulorespiratory effects of arm training and detraining in one C5-6 quadriplegic man. Presented at the annual conference of the American Physical Therapy Association, Chicago, 1986.

38. Figoni, S, Gupta, C, and Glaser, RM. Effects of posture on arm exercise performance of adults with tetraplegia. *J Clin Exerc Physiol* 1:74-85, 1999.

39. Figoni, SF. Exercise responses and quadriplegia. *Med Sci Sports Exerc* 25:433-441, 1993.

40. Figoni, SF, Boileau, RA, Massey, BH, and Larsen, JR. Physiological responses of quadriplegic and able-bodied men during exercise at the same Vo2. *Adapt Phys Act Q* 5:130-139, 1988.

41. Gater Jr., DR, Dolbow, D, Tsui, B, and Gorgey, AS. Functional electrical stimulation therapies after spinal cord injury. *NeuroRehabilitation* 28:231-248, 2011.

42. Gates, JR, and Spiegel, RH. Epilepsy, sports and exercise. *Sports Medicine* 15:1-5, 1993.

43. Gatica-Rojas, V, Cartes-Velásquez, R, Méndez-Rebolledo, G, Guzman-Muñoz, E, and Lizama, LEC. Effects of a Nintendo Wii exercise program on spasticity and static standing balance in spastic cerebral palsy. *Dev Neurorehabil* 20:388-391, 2017.

44. Geister, TL, Quintanar-Solares, M, Martin, M, Aufhammer, S, and Asmus, F. Qualitative development of the 'Questionnaire on Pain caused by Spasticity (QPS),' a pediatric patient-reported outcome for spasticity-related pain in cerebral palsy. *Qual Life Res* 23:887-896, 2014.

45. Gillett, JG, Boyd, RN, Carty, CP, and Barber, LA. The impact of strength training on skeletal muscle morphology and architecture in children and adolescents with spastic cerebral palsy: A systematic review. *Res Dev Disabil* 56:183-196, 2016.

46. Gillett, JG, Lichtwark, GA, Boyd, RN, and Barber, LA. Functional anaerobic and strength training in young adults with cerebral palsy. *Med Sci Sports Exerc* 50:1549-1557, 2018.

47. Gough, M, and Shortland, AP. Could muscle deformity in children with spastic cerebral palsy be related to an impairment of muscle growth and altered adaptation? *Dev Med Child Neurol* 54:495-499, 2012.

48. Gunn, H, Markevics, S, Haas, B, Marsden, J, and Freeman, J. Systematic review: The effectiveness of interventions to reduce falls and improve balance in adults with multiple sclerosis. *Arch Phys Med Rehabil* 96:1898-1912, 2015.

49. Halabchi, F, Alizadeh, Z, Sahraian, MA, and Abolhasani, M. Exercise prescription for patients with multiple sclerosis; potential benefits and practical recommendations. *BMC Neurol* 17:185, 2017.

50. Hetz, SP, Latimer, AE, and Ginis, KA. Activities of daily living performed by individuals with SCI: Relationships with physical fitness and leisure time physical activity. *Spinal Cord* 47:550-554, 2009.

51. Heyward, OW, Vegter, RJK, de Groot, S, and van der Woude, LHV. Shoulder complaints in wheelchair athletes: A systematic review. *PLOS One* 12:e0188410, 2017.

52. Hjeltnes, N. Oxygen uptake and cardiac output in graded arm exercise in paraplegics with low level spinal lesions. *Scand J Rehabil Med* 9:107-113, 1977.

53. Hjeltnes, N. Control of medical rehabilitation of para-and tetraplegics by repeated evaluation of endurance capacity. *Int J Sport Med* 5:S171-S174, 1984.

54. Horvat, M. Effects of a progressive resistance training program on an individual with spastic cerebral palsy. *Am Correct Ther J* 41:7-11, 1987.

55. Hughes, C, and Howard, IM. Spasticity management in multiple sclerosis. *Phys Med Rehabil Cli* 24:593-604, 2013.

56. Jackson, K, and Mulcare, J. Multiple sclerosis. In *ACSM's Resources for Clinical Exercise Physiology,* 2nd ed. Myers, J, and Nieman, D, eds. Baltimore: Lippincott Williams & Wilkins, 34-43, 2009.

57. Jacobs, PL, and National Strength & Conditioning Association (U.S.). *NSCA's Essentials of Training Special Populations.* Champaign, IL: Human Kinetics, 2018.

58. Kalkman, BM, Holmes, G, Bar-On, L, Maganaris, CN, Barton, GJ, Bass, A, Wright, DM, Walton, R, and O'Brien, TD. Resistance training combined with stretching increases tendon stiffness and is more effective than stretching alone in children with cerebral palsy: A randomized controlled trial. *Front Pediatr* 7:1-10, 2019.

59. Kammerman, S, and Wasserman, L. Seizure disorders: Part 1. Classification and diagnosis. *Western J Med* 175:99, 2001.

59a. Kendall, K, Colquitt, G, and Hyde, P. Therapeutic physical activities for individuals with cerebral palsy. In *Therapeutic Physical Activity.* Li, L, and Zhang, S, eds. Hauppauge, NY: Nova Science Publishers, 2015.

60. Kileff, J, and Ashburn, A. A pilot study of the effect of aerobic exercise on people with moderate disability multiple sclerosis. *Clin Rehabil* 19:165-169, 2005.

61. Kim, B-J, Kim, S-M, and Kwon, H-Y. The effect of group exercise program on the self-efficacy and activities of daily living in adults with cerebral palsy. *J Phys Ther Sci* 29:2184-2189, 2017.

62. Kjolhede, T, Vissing, K, and Dalgas, U. Multiple sclerosis and progressive resistance training: A systematic review. *Mult Scler* 18:1215-1228, 2012.

63. Korczyn, A. Participation of epileptic patients in sports. *J Sport Med Phys Fit* 19(2):195-198, 1979.

64. Lance, J, Feldman, R, Young, R, and Koela, W, eds. *Spasticity: Disorder Motor Control.* Chicago: Year Book Medical Publishers, 1980.

65. Langeskov-Christensen, M, Heine, M, Kwakkel, G, and Dalgas, UJSM. Aerobic capacity in persons with multiple sclerosis: A systematic review and meta-analysis. *Sports Med* 45:905-923, 2015.

66. Langeskov-Christensen, M, Hvid, LG, Nygaard, MKE, Ringgaard, S, Jensen, HB, Nielsen, HH, Petersen, T, Stenager, E, Eskildsen, SF, and Dalgas, UJC. Efficacy of high-intensity progressive aerobic exercise on brain atrophy measures in multiple sclerosis: A randomized, controlled, cross-over, phase-2 trial. *Lancet* 1-37, 2019.

67. Latimer-Cheung, AE, Martin Ginis, KA, Hicks, AL, Motl, RW, Pilutti, LA, Duggan, M, Wheeler, G, Persad, R, and Smith, KM. Development of evidence-informed physical activity guidelines for adults with multiple sclerosis. *Arch Phys Med Rehabil* 94:1829-1836.e1827, 2013.

68. Lauglo, R, Vik, T, Lamvik, T, Stensvold, D, Finbråten, A-K, and Moholdt, T. High-intensity interval training to improve fitness in children with cerebral palsy. *BMJ Open Sport Exerc Med* 2:e000111, 2016.

69. Linn, W, Spungen, A, Gong Jr., H, Adkins, R, Bauman, A, and Waters, R. Forced vital capacity in two large outpatient populations with chronic spinal cord injury. *Spinal Cord* 39:263-268, 2001.

70. MacPhail, HE, and Kramer, JF. Effect of isokinetic strength-training on functional ability and walking efficiency in adolescents with cerebral palsy. *Dev Med Child Neurol* 37:763-775, 1995.

71. Martin Ginis, KA, Latimer, AE, Arbour-Nicitopoulos, KP, Buchholz, AC, Bray, SR, Craven, BC, Hayes, KC, Hicks, AL, McColl, MA, Potter, PJ, Smith, K, and Wolfe, DL. Leisure time physical activity in a population-based sample of people with spinal cord injury part I: Demographic and injury-related correlates. *Arch Phys Med Rehabil* 91:722-728, 2010.

72. McCullagh, R, Fitzgerald, AP, Murphy, RP, and Cooke, G. Long-term benefits of exercising on quality of life and fatigue in multiple sclerosis patients with mild disability: A pilot study. *Clin Rehabil* 22:206-214, 2008.

73. McLean, KP, Jones, PP, and Skinner, JS. Exercise prescription for sitting and supine exercise in subjects with quadriplegia. *Med Sci Sports Exer* 27:15-21, 1995.

74. Moreau, NG, and Gannotti, ME. Addressing muscle performance impairments in cerebral palsy: Implications for upper extremity resistance training. *J Hand Ther* 28:91-99; quiz 100, 2015.

75. Moreau, NG, Holthaus, K, and Marlow, N. Differential adaptations of muscle architecture to high-velocity versus traditional strength training in cerebral palsy. *Neurorehab Neural Re* 27:325-334, 2013.

75a. Mulcare, JA. Multiple sclerosis. In *ACSM's Exercise Management for Persons With Chronic Diseases and Disabilities.* Durstine, JL, ed. Champaign, IL: Human Kinetics, 267-272, 2002.

76. Myers, J, Nieman, DC, and American College of Sports Medicine. *ACSM's Resources for Clinical Exercise Physiology: Musculoskeletal, Neuromuscular, Neoplastic, Immunologic, and Hematologic Conditions.* Philadelphia: Wolters Kluwer Health/Lippincott Williams & Wilkins Health, 2010.

77. Nakken, K, Bjørholt, P, Johannessen, S, LoSyning, T, and Lind, E. Effect of physical training on aerobic capacity, seizure occurrence, and serum level of antiepileptic drugs in adults with epilepsy. *Epilepsia* 31:88-94, 1990.

78. Nakken, KO. Clinical research physical exercise in outpatients with epilepsy. *Epilepsia* 40:643-651, 1999.

79. National Institutes of Health, National Institute of Neurological Disorders and Stroke. *Multiple Sclerosis: Hope Through Research.* Bethesda, MD: National Institutes of Health, 2012.

80. National Institutes of Health, National Institute of Neurological Disorders and Stroke. *Hope Through Research: Cerebral Palsy.* Bethesda, MD: National Institutes of Health, 2013.

81. National Institutes of Health, National Institute of Neurological Disorders and Stroke. *Epilepsy: Hope Through Research.* Bethesda, MD: National Institutes of Health, 2015.

82. National Institutes of Health, National Institute of Neurological Disorders and Stroke. Multiple sclerosis information page. 2019. www.ninds.nih.gov/Disorders/All-Disorders/Multiple-Sclerosis-Information-Page. Accessed January 14, 2020.

83. Nooijen, C, Slaman, J, van der Slot, W, Stam, H, Roebroeck, M, van den Berg-Emons, R, and Learn2Move Research, G. Health-related physical fitness of ambulatory adolescents and young adults with spastic cerebral palsy. *J Rehabil Med* 46:642-647, 2014.

84. Oskoui, M, Coutinho, F, Dykeman, J, Jette, N, and Pringsheim, T. An update on the prevalence of cerebral palsy: A systematic review and meta-analysis. *Dev Med Child Neurol* 55:509-519, 2013.

85. Paralyzed Veterans of America Consortium for Spinal Cord, Medicine. Preservation of upper limb function following spinal cord injury: A clinical practice guideline for health-care professionals. *J Spinal Cord Med* 28:434-470, 2005.

86. Paridon, SM, Alpert, BS, Boas, SR, Cabrera, ME, Caldarera, LL, Daniels, SR, Kimball, TR, Knilans, TK, Nixon, PA, Rhodes, J, Yetman, AT, American Heart Association Council on Cardiovascular Disease in the Young, CoAH, and Obesity in Youth. Clinical stress testing in the pediatric

age group: A statement from the American Heart Association Council on Cardiovascular Disease in the Young, Committee on Atherosclerosis, Hypertension, and Obesity in Youth. *Circulation* 113:1905-1920, 2006.

87. Peungsuwan, P, Parasin, P, Siritaratiwat, W, Prasertnu, J, and Yamauchi, J. Effects of combined exercise training on functional performance in children with cerebral palsy: A randomized-controlled study. *Pediatr Phys Ther* 29:39-46, 2017.

88. Phillips, WT, Kiratli, BJ, Sarkarati, M, Weraarchakul, G, Myers, J, Franklin, BA, Parkash, I, and Froelicher, V. Effect of spinal cord injury on the heart and cardiovascular fitness. *Curr Probl Cardiol* 23:641-716, 1998.

89. Pilutti, LA, Greenlee, TA, Motl, RW, Nickrent, MS, and Petruzzello, SJ. Effects of exercise training on fatigue in multiple sclerosis: A meta-analysis. *Psychosom Med* 75:575-580, 2013.

90. Pin, T, Dyke, P, and Chan, M. The effectiveness of passive stretching in children with cerebral palsy. *Dev Med Child Neurol* 48:855-862, 2006.

91. Ploughman, M. Breaking down the barriers to physical activity among people with multiple sclerosis—a narrative review. *Phys Ther Rev* 22:124-132, 2017.

92. Postma, K, Haisma, JA, Hopman, MTE, Bergen, MP, Stam, HJ, and Bussmann, JB. Resistive inspiratory muscle training in people with spinal cord injury during inpatient rehabilitation: A randomized controlled trial. *Phys Ther* 94:1709-1719, 2014.

93. Rampello, A, Franceschini, M, Piepoli, M, Antenucci, R, Lenti, G, Olivieri, D, and Chetta, A. Effect of aerobic training on walking capacity and maximal exercise tolerance in patients with multiple sclerosis: A randomized crossover controlled study. *Phys Ther* 87:545-555, 2007.

94. Rice, J, Skuza, P, Baker, F, Russo, R, and Fehlings, D. Identification and measurement of dystonia in cerebral palsy. *Dev Med Child Neurol* 59:1249-1255, 2017.

95. Roberts, TT, Leonard, GR, and Cepela, DJ. Classifications in brief: American Spinal Injury Association (ASIA) impairment scale. *Clin Orthop Relat R* 475:1499-1504, 2017.

96. Romberg, A, Virtanen, A, Ruutiainen, J, Aunola, S, Karppi, SL, Vaara, M, Surakka, J, Pohjolainen, T, and Seppanen, A. Effects of a 6-month exercise program on patients with multiple sclerosis: A randomized study. *Neurology* 63:2034-2038, 2004.

97. Rosenbaum, P, Paneth, N, Leviton, A, Goldstein, M, Bax, M, Damiano, D, Dan, B, and Jacobsson, B. A report: The definition and classification of cerebral palsy. *Dev Med Child Neurol Suppl* 109:8-14, 2007.

98. Rosenbaum, PL, Palisano, RJ, Bartlett, DJ, Galuppi, BE, and Russell, DJ. Development of the Gross Motor Function Classification System for cerebral palsy. *Dev Med Child Neurol* 50:249-253, 2008.

99. Rush, R, and Kumbhare, D. Spasticity. *Can Med Assoc J* 187:436, 2015.

99a. Sadovnick, AD, Baird, PA, and Ward, RH. Multiple sclerosis: Updated risks for relatives. *Am J Med Genet* 29:533-541, 1988.

100. Schmitt, B, Thun-Hohenstein, L, Vontobel, H, and Boltshauser, E. Seizures induced by physical exercise: Report of two cases. *Neuropediatrics* 25:51-53, 1994.

101. Snook, EM, and Motl, RW. Effect of exercise training on walking mobility in multiple sclerosis: A meta-analysis. *Neurorehabil Neural Re* 23:108-116, 2009.

101a. Sutherland, GJ, and Anderson, MB. Exercise and multiple sclerosis: Physiological, psychological, and quality of life issues. *J Sport Med Phys Fit* 41:421-432, 2001.

101b. Svenson, B, Gerdle, B, and Elert, L. Endurance training in patients with multiple sclerosis: Five case studies. *Phys Ther* 74:1017-1026, 1994.

102. Tasiemski, T, Bergstrom, E, Savic, G, and Gardner, BP. Sports, recreation and employment following spinal cord injury—a pilot study. *Spinal Cord* 38:173-184, 2000.

103. Tedrus, G, Sterca, GS, and Pereira, RB. Physical activity, stigma, and quality of life in patients with epilepsy. *Epilepsy Behav* 77:96-98, 2017.

104. Tweedy, SM, Beckman, EM, Geraghty, TJ, Theisen, D, Perret, C, Harvey, LA, and Vanlandewijck, YC. Exercise and Sports Science Australia (ESSA) position statement on exercise and spinal cord injury. *J Sci Med Sport* 20:108-115, 2017.

105. Vancampfort, D, Ward, PB, and Stubbs, B. Physical activity and sedentary levels among people living with epilepsy: A systematic review and meta-analysis. *Epilepsy Behav* 99:106390, 2019.

106. Verschuren, O, Ketelaar, M, Gorter, JW, Helders, PJM, Uiterwaal, CSPM, and Takken, T. Exercise training program in children and adolescents with cerebral palsy: A randomized controlled trial. *Arch Pediatr Adoles Med* 161:1075-1081, 2007.

107. Verschuren, O, Ketelaar, M, Keefer, D, Wright, V, Butler, J, Ada, L, Maher, C, Reid, S, Wright, M, Dalziel, B, Wiart, L, Fowler, E, Unnithan, V, Maltais, DB, van den Berg-Emons, R, and Takken, T. Identification of a core set of exercise tests for children and adolescents with cerebral palsy: A Delphi survey of researchers and clinicians. *Dev Med Child Neurol* 53:449-456, 2011.

108. Verschuren, O, Peterson, MD, Balemans, AC, and Hurvitz, EA. Exercise and physical activity recommendations for people with cerebral palsy. *Dev Med Child Neurol* 58:798-808, 2016.

109. Verschuren, O, and Takken, T. Aerobic capacity in children and adolescents with cerebral palsy. *Res Dev Disabil* 31:1352-1357, 2010.

110. Wan, D, and Krassioukov, AV. Life-threatening outcomes associated with autonomic dysreflexia: A clinical review. *J Spinal Cord Med* 37:2-10, 2014.

111. White, LJ, McCoy, SC, Castellano, V, Gutierrez, G, Stevens, JE, Walter, GA, and Vandenborne, K. Resistance training improves strength and functional capacity in persons with multiple sclerosis. *Mult Scler* 10:668-674, 2004.

112. Willis, J, Hoping, L, Mahlberg, N, and Ronen, GM. Youth with epilepsy: Their insight into participating in enhanced physical activity study. *Epilepsy Behav* 89:63-69, 2018.

113. Wilroy, J, and Hibberd, E. Evaluation of a shoulder injury prevention program in wheelchair basketball. *J Sport Rehabil* 27:554-559, 2018.

114. Wu, YN, Hwang, M, Ren, Y, Gaebler-Spira, D, and Zhang, LQ. Combined passive stretching and active movement rehabilitation of lower-limb impairments in children with cerebral palsy using a portable robot. *Neurorehabil Neural Re* 25:378-385, 2011.

115. Yamasaki, M, Kim, KT, Choi, SW, Muraki, S, Shiokawa, M, and Kurokawa, T. Characteristics of body heat balance of paraplegics during exercise in a hot environment. *J Physiol Anthropol Appl Human Sci* 20:227-232, 2001.

Chapter 23

1. Abadie, BR, and Wentworth, MC. Prediction of one repetition maximal strength from a 5-10 repetition submaximal strength test in college-aged females. *J Exerc Physiol* 3:1-5, 2000.

2. Baechle, TR, and Earle, RW. *Weight Training: Steps to Success,* 5th ed. Champaign, IL: Human Kinetics, 2019.

3. Bayles, MP. Muscular fitness and assessment. In *ACSM's Resource Manual for Guidelines for Exercise Testing and Prescription,* 7th ed. Baltimore: Lippincott Williams & Wilkins, 2014.

4. Baz-Valle, E, Schoenfeld, BJ, Torres-Unda, J, Santos-Concejero, J, and Balsalobre-Fernández, C. The effects of exercise variation in muscle thickness, maximal strength and motivation in resistance trained men. *PLOS One* 14:e0226989, 2019.

5. Beam, W, and Adams, G. *Exercise Physiology Laboratory Manual,* 8th ed. New York: McGraw-Hill Higher Education, 2019.

6. Bompa, TO, and Buzzichelli, C. *Periodization: Theory and Methodology of Training,* 6th ed. Champaign, IL: Human Kinetics, 2018.

7. Brown, H. *Lifetime Fitness.* Scottsdale, AZ: Gorsuch Scarisbrick, 1992.

8. Brzycki, M. Strength testing—predicting a one-rep max from reps-to-fatigue. *J Phys Educ Recreat Dance* 64:88-90, 1993.

9. Chapman, PP, Whitehead, JR, and Binkert, RH. The 225-lb reps-to-fatigue test as a submaximal estimate of 1-RM bench press performance in college football players. *J Strength Cond Res* 12:258-261, 1998.

10. Cooke, DM, Haischer, MH, Carzoli, JP, Bazyler, CD, Johnson, TK, Varieur, R, Zoeller, RF, Whitehurst, M, and Zourdos, MC. Body mass and femur length are inversely related to repetitions performed in the back squat in well-trained lifters. *J Strength Cond Res* 33:890-895, 2019.

11. Davies, T, Orr, R, Halaki, M, and Hackett, D. Effect of training leading to repetition failure on muscular strength: A systematic review and meta-analysis. *Sports Med* 46:487-502, 2016.

12. DeLorme, TL. Restoration of muscle power by heavy-resistance exercises. *J Bone Joint Surg* 27:645-667, 1945.

13. Epley, B. *The Path to Athletic Power: The Model Conditioning Program for Championship Performance.* Champaign, IL: Human Kinetics, 2004.

14. Fleck, SJ. Periodized strength training: A critical review. *J Strength Cond Res* 13:82-89, 1999.

15. Fleck, SJ, and Kraemer, W. *Designing Resistance Training Programs,* 4th ed. Champaign, IL: Human Kinetics, 2014.

16. Fonseca, RM, Roschel, H, Tricoli, V, de Souza, EO, Wilson, JM, Laurentino, GC, Aihara, AY, de Souza Leão, AR, and Ugrinowitsch, C. Changes in exercises are more effective than in loading schemes to improve muscle strength. *J Strength Cond Res* 28:3085-3092, 2014.

17. Grgic, J, Mikulic, P, Podnar, H, and Pedisic, Z. Effects of linear and daily undulating periodized resistance training programs on measures of muscle hypertrophy: A systematic review and meta-analysis. *PeerJ* 5:e3695, 2017.

18. Haff, GG. Roundtable discussion: Periodization of training—part 1. *Strength Cond J* 26:50-69, 2004.

19. Haff, GG. Periodization. In *Essentials of Strength Training and Conditioning,* 4th ed. Haff, GG, and Triplett, TT, eds. Champaign, IL: Human Kinetics, 2016, 583-604.

20. Haff, GG and Triplett, TT. *Essentials of Strength Training and Conditioning,* 4th ed. Champaign, IL: Human Kinetics, 2016.

21. Häkkinen, K, Komi, PV, Alén, M, and Kauhanen, H. EMG, muscle fibre and force production characteristics during a 1 year training period in elite weight-lifters. *Eur J Appl Physiol Occup Physiol* 56:419-427, 1987.

22. Harries, SK, Lubans, DR, and Callister, R. Systematic review and meta-analysis of linear and undulating periodized resistance training programs on muscular strength. *J Strength Cond Res* 29:1113-1125, 2015.

23. Harris, GR, Stone, MH, O'Bryant, HS, Proulx, CM, and Johnson, RL. Short-term performance effects of high power, high force, or combined weight-training methods. *J Strength Cond Res* 14:14-20, 2000.

24. Hoeger, WW, Barette, SL, Hale, DF, and Hopkins, DR. Relationship between repetitions and selected percentages of one repetition maximum. *J Strength Cond Res* 1:11-13, 1987.

25. Hoeger, WW, Hopkins, DR, Barette, SL, and Hale, DF. Relationship between repetitions and selected percentages of one repetition maximum: A comparison between untrained and trained males and females. *J Strength Cond Res* 4:47-54, 1990.

26. Issurin, VB. Training transfer: Scientific background and insights for practical application. *Sports Med* 43:675-694, 2013.

27. Kawamori, N, and Haff, GG. The optimal training load for the development of muscular power. *J Strength Cond Res* 18:675-684, 2004.

28. Kraemer, WJ, Deschenes, MR, and Fleck, SJ. Physiological adaptations to resistance exercise: Implications for athletic conditioning. *Sports Med* 6:246-256, 1988.

29. Kraemer, WJ, Fleck, SJ, and Evans, WJ. Strength and power training: Physiological mechanisms of adaptation. *Exerc Sport Sci Rev* 24:363-397, 1996.

30. Kraemer, WJ, Hatfield, DL, and Fleck, SJ. Types of muscle training. In *Strength Training,* 2nd ed. Brown, LE, ed. Champaign, IL: Human Kinetics, 49-73, 2017.

31. Kravitz, L, Akalan, C, Nowicki, K, and Kinzey, SJ. Prediction of 1 repetition maximum in high-school power lifters. *J Strength Cond Res* 17:167-172, 2003.

32. LeSuer, DA, McCormick, JH, Mayhew, JL, Wasserstein, RL, and Arnold, MD. The accuracy of prediction equations for estimating 1-RM performance in the bench press, squat, and deadlift. *J Strength Cond Res* 11:211-213, 1997.

33. Mayhew, J, Ware, J, Cannon, K, and Corbett, S. Validation of the NFL-225 test for predicting 1-RM bench press performance in college football players. *J Sport Med Phys Fit* 42:304, 2002.

34. Mayhew, JL, Ball, TE, Arnold, MD, and Bowen, JC. Relative muscular endurance performance as a predictor of bench press strength in college men and women. *J Appl Sport Sci Res* 6:200-206, 1992.

35. Mayhew, JL, Johnson, BD, LaMonte, MJ, Lauber, D, and Kemmler, W. Accuracy of prediction equations for determining one repetition maximum bench press in women before and after resistance training. *J Strength Cond Res* 22:1570-1577, 2008.

36. Mayhew, JL, Prinster, J, Ware, J, Zimmer, D, Arabas, J, and Bemben, M. Muscular endurance repetitions to predict bench press strength in men of different training levels. *J Sport Med Phys Fit* 35:108-113, 1995.

37. Mayhew, JL, Ware, JR, and Prinster, JL. Test & measurement: Using lift repetitions to predict muscular strength in adolescent males. *Strength Cond J* 15:35-38, 1993.

38. Medicine, American College of Sports. American College of Sports Medicine position stand: Progression models in resistance training for healthy adults. *Med Sci Sports Exerc* 41(3):687-708, 2009.

39. Morán-Navarro, R, Pérez, CE, Mora-Rodríguez, R, de la Cruz-Sánchez, E, González-Badillo, JJ, Sanchez-Medina, L, and Pallarés, JG. Time course of recovery following resistance training leading or not to failure. *Eur J Appl Physiol* 117:2387-2399, 2017.

40. O'Connor, R, O'Connor, B, Simmons, J, and O'Shea, P. *Weight Training Today.* St. Paul, MN: Thomson Learning, 1989.

41. Pearson, DR, and Gehlsen, GM. Athletic performance enhancement: A study with college football players. *Strength Cond J* 20:70-73, 1998.

42. Plisk, SS, and Stone, MH. Periodization strategies. *Strength Cond J* 25:19-37, 2003.

43. Poliquin, C. Football: Five steps to increasing the effectiveness of your strength training program. *Strength Cond J* 10:34-39, 1988.

44. Pollock, ML, Gaesser, GA, Butcher, J, Després, JP, Dishman, RK, Franklin, BA, and Garber, CE. ACSM position stand: The recommended quantity and quality of exercise for developing and maintaining cardio-respiratory and muscular fitness, and flexibility in healthy adults. *Med Sci Sports Exerc* 30:975-991, 1998.

45. Reynolds, JM, Gordon, TJ, and Roberg, RA. Prediction of one repetition maximum strength from multiple repetition maximum testing and anthropometry. *J Strength Cond Res* 20:584-592, 2006.

46. Rhea, MR, and Alderman, BL. A meta-analysis of periodized versus nonperiodized strength and power training programs. *Res Q Exerc Sport* 75:413-422, 2004.

47. Richens, B, and Cleather, DJ. The relationship between the number of repetitions performed at given intensities is different in endurance and strength trained athletes. *Biol Sport* 31:157, 2014.

48. Rydwik, E, Karlsson, C, Frändin, K, and Akner, G. Muscle strength testing with one repetition maximum in the arm/shoulder for people aged 75+-test-retest reliability. *Clin Rehabil* 21:258-265, 2007.

49. Santos, WDND, Vieira, CA, Bottaro, M, Nunes, VA, Ramirez-Campillo, R, Steele, J, Fisher, JP, and Gentil, P. Resistance training performed to failure or not to failure results in similar total volume, but with different fatigue and discomfort levels. *J Strength Cond Res* 35(5):1372-1379, 2021.

50. Schoenfeld, BJ, Grgic, J, Ogborn, D, and Krieger, JW. Strength and hypertrophy adaptations between low-vs. high-load resistance training: A systematic review and meta-analysis. *J Strength Cond Res* 31:3508-3523, 2017.

51. Schoenfeld, BJ, Peterson, MD, Ogborn, D, Contreras, B, and Sonmez, GT. Effects of low-vs. high-load resistance training on muscle strength and hypertrophy in well-trained men. *J Strength Cond Res* 29:2954-2963, 2015.

52. Shaw, CE, McCully, KK, and Posner, JD. Injuries during the one repetition maximum assessment in the elderly. *J Cardiopulm Rehabil Prev* 15:283-287, 1995.

53. Sheppard, JM, and Triplett, TT. Program design for resistance training. In *Essentials of Strength Training and Conditioning,* 4th ed. Haff, GG, and Triplett, TT, eds. Champaign, IL: Human Kinetics, 439-469, 2016.

54. Shimano, T, Kraemer, WJ, Spiering, BA, Volek, JS, Hatfield, DL, Silvestre, R, Vingren, JL, Fragala, MS, Maresh, CM, and Fleck, SJ. Relationship between the number of repetitions and selected percentages of one repetition maximum in free weight exercises in trained and untrained men. *J Strength Cond Res* 20:819-823, 2006.

55. Siff, MC. *Supertraining.* Denver, CO: Supertraining Institute, 2003.

56. Simão, R, Farinatti PdTV, Polito, MD, Maior, AS, and Fleck, SJ. Influence of exercise order on the number of repetitions performed and perceived exertion during resistance exercises. *J Strength Cond Res* 19:152-156, 2005.

57. Stone, MH, O'Bryant, H, and Garhammer, J. A hypothetical model for strength training. *J Sport Med Phys Fit* 21:342-351, 1981.

58. Stone, MH, and O'Bryant, HS. *Weight Training: A Scientific Approach.* Minneapolis: Burgess, 1987.

59. Stone, MH, Stone, M, and Sands, WA. *Principles and Practice of Resistance Training.* Champaign, IL: Human Kinetics, 2007.

60. Tan, B. Manipulating resistance training program variables to optimize maximum strength in men: A review. *J Strength Cond Res* 13:289-304, 1999.

61. Ware, JS, Clemens, CT, Mayhew, JL, and Johnston, TJ. Muscular endurance repetitions to predict bench press and squat strength in college football players. *J Strength Cond Res* 9:99-103, 1995.

62. Whisenant, MJ, Panton, LB, East, WB, and Broeder, CE. Validation of submaximal prediction equations for the 1 repetition maximum bench press test on a group of collegiate football players. *J Strength Cond Res* 17:221-227, 2003.

63. Williams, TD, Tolusso, DV, Fedewa, MV, and Esco, MR. Comparison of periodized and non-periodized resistance training on maximal strength: A meta-analysis. *Sports Med* 47:2083-2100, 2017.

64. Young, WB. Transfer of strength and power training to sports performance. *Int J Sports Physiol Perfor* 1:74-83, 2006.

65. Zatsiorsky, VM, Kraemer, WJ, and Fry, AC. *Science and Practice of Strength Training,* 3rd ed. Champaign, IL: Human Kinetics, 2020.

66. Zourdos, MC, Jo, E, Khamoui, AV, Lee, S-R, Park, B-S, Ormsbee, MJ, Panton, LB, Contreras, RJ, and Kim, J-S. Modified daily undulating periodization model produces greater performance than a traditional configuration in powerlifters. *J Strength Cond Res* 30:784-791, 2016.

Chapter 24

1. Armitage-Johnson, S. Providing a safe training environment for participants, part I. *Strength Cond* 16:64-65, 1994.

2. Bates, M. Choosing the right equipment. In *Health Fitness Management,* 2nd ed. Bates, M, ed. Champaign, IL: Human Kinetics, 2008.

3. Children's Healthcare of Atlanta. Emergency action plans. https://images.template.net/wp-content/uploads/2015/09/11195620/Emergency-Action-Plan-for-Sports-Sample-Template-jpg. Accessed September 17, 2020.

4. Coker, E. Weightroom flooring. *Strength Cond J* 11:26-27, 1989.

5. Department of Homeland Security. Active shooter preparedness. www.cisa.gov/active-shooter-preparedness. Accessed September 17, 2020.

6. Greenwood, M. Facility maintenance and risk management. In *Essentials of Strength Training and Conditioning,* 2nd ed. Baechle, T, and Earle, R, eds. Champaign, IL: Human Kinetics, 2000.

7. Greenwood, M. Facility and equipment layout and maintenance. In *NSCA's Essentials of Personal Training,* Earle, R, and Baechle, T, eds. Champaign, IL: Human Kinetics, 2004.

8. Greenwood, M. Facility organization and risk management. In *Essentials of Strength Training and Conditioning,* 3rd ed. Baechle, T, and Earle, R, eds. Champaign, IL: Human Kinetics, 2008.

9. Holcomb, W, Kleiner, D, and Chu, D. Plyometrics: Considerations for safe and effective training. *Strength Cond* 20:36-41, 1998.

10. Hudy, A. Designing the strength and conditioning facility. In *Essentials of Strength Training and Conditioning,* 4th ed. Haff, GG, and Triplett, NT, eds. Champaign, IL: Human Kinetics, 2016.

11. Kroll, W. Facility design: Developing the strength training facility. *Strength Cond J* 11:53-55, 1989.

12. Kroll, W. Facility design: Evaluating strength training equipment. *Strength Cond J* 12:56-65, 1990.

13. Kroll, W. Facility design: Selecting strength training equipment. *Strength Cond J* 12:65-70, 1990.

14. Kroll, W. Facility design: Structural and functional considerations in designing the facility: Part I. *Strength Cond J* 12:51-58, 1990.

15. Kroll, W. Facility design: Structural and functional considerations in designing the facility: Part II. *Strength Cond J* 13:51-57, 1991.

16. Kroll, W. Facility design: Aesthetics of the strength training facility. *Strength Cond J* 13:55-58, 1991.

17. National Institute for Occupational Safety and Health. *Criteria for a Recommended Standard: Occupational Noise Exposure.* NIOSH Pub. No. 98-126. Cincinnati: Author, 1998.

17b. National Strength and Conditioning Association. *Essentials of Strength Training and Conditioning,* 3rd ed. Baechle, TR, and Earle, RW, eds. Champaign, IL: Human Kinetics, 2008.

18. Occupational Safety and Health Administration. Emergency action plan. www.osha.gov/SLTC/etools/evacuation/eap.html. Accessed September 17, 2020.

19. Patton, R, Grantham, W, Gerson, R, and Gettman, L. *Developing and Managing Health/Fitness Facilities.* Champaign, IL: Human Kinetics, 1989.

20. Polson, G. Weight room safety strategic planning - part IV. *Strength Cond* 17:35-37, 1995.

21. Sawyer, T, and Stowe, D. Strength and cardiovascular training facility. In *Facility Design and Management for Health, Fitness, Physical Activity, Recreation, and Sports Facility Development,* 11th ed. Sawyer, T, ed. Champaign, IL: Sagamore, 2005.

22. Tharrett, S, McInnis, K, and Peterson, J. *ACSM's Health/Fitness Facility Standards and Guidelines,* 3rd ed. Champaign, IL: Human Kinetics, 2007.

23. Tharrett, S, and Peterson, J. *ACSM's Health/Fitness Facility Standards and Guidelines,* 4th ed. Champaign, IL: Human Kinetics, 2012.

Chapter 25

1. Abbott, AA. Aquatic emergencies. *ACSMS Health Fit J* 21(4):35-39, 2017.

1a. Abbott, AA. CPR/AED—Just certified or truly qualified. *ACSMS Health Fit J* 23(1):37-41, 2019.

2. Abbott, AA. Fitness professionals: Certified, qualified and justified. *Exerc Stand Malprac* 23(2):20-22, 2009.

3. AED Challenge. 66% of responders can't pass CPR test 3 months after training. www.aedchallenge.com/articles/cprskilldecline.php. Accessed November 16, 2020.

4. American College of Sports Medicine and American Heart Association. Automated external defibrillators in health/fitness facilities. *Circulation* 105(9):1147-1152, 2002.

5. American College of Sports Medicine. *ACSM's Exercise Management for Persons with Chronic Diseases and Disabilities,* 4th ed. Moore, G, Durstine, L, and Painter, P, eds. Champaign, IL: Human Kinetics, 2016.

6. American College of Sports Medicine. *ACSM's Guidelines for Exercise Testing and Prescription,* 10th ed. Riebe, D, Ehrman, J, Liguori, G, and Magal, M, eds. Philadelphia: Lippincott Williams & Wilkins, 2018.

7. American College of Sports Medicine. *ACSM's Resources for the Exercise Physiologist,* 2nd ed. Philadelphia: Lippincott Williams & Wilkins, 2017.

8. American Heart Association. *Basic Life Support for Healthcare Providers.* Dallas: Author, 2015.

9. American Heart Association. *Basic Life Support Provider Manual.* Dallas: Author, 2016.

10. American Heart Association. *Heartsaver CPR AED Student Workbook.* Dallas: Author, 2015.

11. American Heart Association. *Heartsaver First Aid CPR AED Student Workbook.* Dallas, TX: American Heart Association, 2016.

12. Bates, M, Spezzano, M, and Danhoff, G. *Health Fitness Management,* 3rd ed. Champaign, IL: Human Kinetics, 2020.

13. Cotton, D, and Wolohan, J. *Law for Recreation and Sport Managers,* 7th ed. Dubuque, IA: Kendall Hunt Publishing, 2017.

14. Eickhoff-Shemek, J, Herbert, D, and Connaughton, D. *Risk Management for Health/Fitness Professionals.* Baltimore: Lippincott Williams & Wilkins, 2009.

15. Einspruch, EL, Lynch, B, Aufderheide, TP, Nichol, G, and Becker, L. Retention of CPR skills learned in a traditional AHA Heartsaver course. *Resuscitation* 74(3):476-486. 2007.

16. Hart, KE. Will your insurance cover an award of punitive damages? www.fwhtlaw.com/briefing-papers/will-your-insurance-cover-an-award-of-punitive-damages. Accessed November 16, 2020.

17. Herbert, D. *The Personal Trainer: A Tale of Pain, Gain, Greed & Lust.* Canton, OH: PRC, 2013.

18. Herbert, D, and Herbert, W. *Legal Aspects of Preventive, Rehabilitative, and Recreation Exercise Programs,* 4th ed. Canton, OH: PRC, 2002.

19. International Health, Racquet & Sportsclub Association. Terms of use. www.ihrsa.org/terms-of-use. Accessed November 16, 2020.

20. Malek, M, Nalbone, D, Berger, D, and Coburn, J. Importance of health science education for personal fitness trainers. *J Strength Cond Res* 16(1):19-24, 2002.

21. National Strength and Conditioning Association. Codes, policies, and procedures. www.nsca.com/codes-policies-procedures. Accessed November 16, 2020.

22. National Strength and Conditioning Association. *NSCA's Essentials of Training Special Populations.* Jacobs, P, ed. Champaign, IL: Human Kinetics, 2018.

23. Sharkey, B, and Gaskill, S. *Fitness and Health,* 6th ed. Champaign, IL: Human Kinetics, 2007.

24. Skinner, J, Bryant, C, and Merrill, S. *ACE's Medical Exercise Specialist Manual.* San Diego: American Council on Exercise, 2015.

25. Spano, M. Basic nutrition factors in health. In *Essentials of Strength Training and Conditioning,* 4th ed. Haff, GG, and Triplett, NT, eds. Champaign, IL: Human Kinetics, 175-200, 2016.

26. Statler, T, and Brown, V. Facility policies, procedures, and legal issues. In *Essentials of Strength Training and Conditioning,* 4th ed. Haff, GG, and Triplett, NT, eds. Champaign, IL: Human Kinetics, 641-656, 2016.

27. Tharrett, S, and Peterson, J. *ACSM's Health/Fitness Facility Standards and Guidelines,* 4th ed. Champaign, IL: Human Kinetics, 2012.

28. Triplett, NT, Brown, V, Caulfield, S, Doscher, M, McHenry, P, Statler, T, and Wainwright, R. NSCA Strength and Conditioning Professional Standards and Guidelines. *Strength Cond J* 39(6):1-24, 2017.

29. U.S. Department of Health and Human Services. *2015-2020 Dietary Guidelines for Americans,* 8th ed. www.health.gov/our-work/food-nutrition/2015-2020-dietary-guidelines/guidelines. Accessed November 16, 2020.

Appendix

1. Association of Fitness Studios. *AFS 2018 fitness studio operating and financial benchmarking report,* 15, 2018.

2. Bureau of Labor Statistics. *Occupational Outlook Handbook: Fitness Trainers and Instructors.* www.bls.gov/ooh/personal-care-and-service/fitness-trainers-and-instructors.htm. Accessed August 11, 2020.

3. International Health, Racquet & Sportsclub Association. *The IHRSA health club employee compensation and benefits report,* 47, 2015.

4. Moriarty, J. Personal trainer insurance: Cost, coverage & providers. Fit Small Business. https://fitsmallbusiness.com/personal-trainer-insurance. Accessed August 11, 2020.

5. Nutting, MA. *The Business of Personal Training.* Champaign, IL: Human Kinetics, 120-123, 2018.

6. Salary.com. Personal fitness trainer salary in the United States. www.salary.com/research/salary/alternate/personal-fitness-trainer-salary. Accessed August 11, 2020.

7. Schroeder, J. 2015 IDEA fitness industry compensation trends report. *IDEA Fitness Journal* 12(10):47, 2015.

Note: The italicized *f* and *t* following page numbers refer to figures and tables, respectively.

Brad J. Schoenfeld, PhD, CSCS,*D, CSPS,*D, NSCA-CPT,*D, is internationally regarded as one of the foremost authorities on muscle hypertrophy. He has worked with numerous elite-level athletes, including many top pros. Dr. Schoenfeld was the 2011 National Strength and Conditioning Association (NSCA) Personal Trainer of the Year. He was the recipient of the 2016 Dwight D. Eisenhower Fitness Award, which is presented by the United States Sports Academy for outstanding achievement in fitness and for contributions to the growth and development of sport fitness through outstanding leadership activity. He was also the 2018 cowinner of the NSCA Outstanding Young Investigator Award.

Dr. Schoenfeld earned his PhD in health promotion and wellness at Rocky Mountain University, where his research focused on elucidating the mechanisms of muscle hypertrophy and their application to resistance training. He has published more than 300 peer-reviewed scientific papers and serves on the editorial advisory boards for several journals, including the *Journal of Strength and Conditioning Research* and the *Journal of the International Society of Sports Nutrition*. He is the author of multiple fitness books, including *Science and Development of Muscle Hypertrophy*, *The M.A.X. Muscle Plan*, and *Strong & Sculpted*.

Dr. Schoenfeld is a full professor of exercise science at Lehman College in the Bronx, New York, and is director of the graduate program in human performance and fitness. He previously served as the sports nutrition consultant to the New Jersey Devils hockey organization.

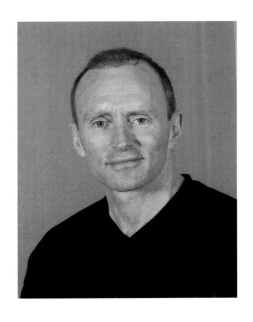

Ronald L. Snarr, PhD, CSCS,*D, NSCA-CPT,*D, TSAC-F,*D, is an assistant professor of exercise science at Missouri State University. He has over 15 years of personal training and strength and conditioning experience, having worked with athletes at the Olympic, professional, and collegiate levels; firefighters; police officers; adapted athletes; and others. Dr. Snarr earned his PhD in exercise physiology and human performance from the University of Alabama, his master's degree in exercise science from Auburn University at Montgomery, and his bachelor's degree from Pennsylvania State University. Dr. Snarr is also completing another master's degree in applied biostatistics with a focus on research design and methodology.

His current research focuses include high-intensity interval training, tactical athlete and adapted athlete performance, electromyography, and body composition. From these interests, he has published over 75 peer-reviewed manuscripts and presented at multiple national and regional conferences. He serves on the editorial board for *Personal Training Quarterly*. He is also currently authoring a textbook on scientific writing for the field of kinesiology. Dr. Snarr was named the recipient of the 2020 Junior Researcher of the Year Award by the Water's College of Health Professions at Georgia Southern University.

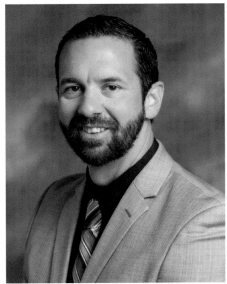

Courtesy of Georgia Southern University

CONTRIBUTORS

Anthony A. Abbott, EdD, CSCS,*D, CSPS,*D, NSCA-CPT,*D, TSAC-F,*D, FNSCA
Fitness Institute International, Inc.

Jamie L. Aslin, MS, ATC, CSCS, NSCA-CPT
Los Alamos National Laboratory

Chris A. Bailey, PhD, CSCS,*D, RSCC
University of North Texas

Alexis Batrakoulis, PhD, CSCS,*D, CSPS,*D, NSCA-CPT,*D, RCPT*E
University of Thessaly—Greece

Joseph J. Bonyai, MEd, CSCS
Lehman College

Megan A. Bryanton Jones, PhD, CSCS
Kinetic Advantage Consulting

Jason C. Casey, PhD, CSCS,*D
University of North Georgia

Kelli M. Clark, PT, DPT, MS
Florida International University

Jared W. Coburn, PhD, CSCS,*D, FNSCA
California State University, Fullerton

Gavin Colquitt, EdD, CAPE, CSCS
Georgia Southern University

Nicole C. Dabbs, PhD, FNSCA
California State University, San Bernardino

Jay Dawes, PhD, CSCS,*D, NSCA-CPT,*D, TSAC-F, FNSCA
Oklahoma State University

Michael R. Esco, PhD, CSCS,*D, CEP
The University of Alabama

Avery D. Faigenbaum, EdD, CSCS, CSPS, FNSCA
The College of New Jersey

Cassandra Forsythe, PhD, RD, CSCS
Central Connecticut State University

David H. Fukuda, PhD, CSCS,*D, CISSN, FNSCA
University of Central Florida

Brian T. Gearity, PhD, ATC, CSCS, FNSCA
University of Denver

Georgia H. Goslee, Esq.
Private practitioner

Carmine R. Grieco, PhD, CSCS,*D
Colorado Mesa University

David J. Heikkinen, PhD, CSCS,*D
Fitchburg State University

Eric R. Helms, PhD, CSCS
Auckland University of Technology

Margaret T. Jones, PhD, CSCS,*D, FNSCA
George Mason University

Kristina L. Kendall, PhD, CSCS,*D, CISSN
Edith Cowan University

Laura Kobar, MS, LAC, BHP
Arizona State University

Morey J. Kolber, PT, PhD, OCS, CSCS,*D
Nova Southeastern University

Cindy M. Kugler, MS, CSCS, CSPS
Bryan Health

Steven M. Laslovich, PhD, PT, DPT, CPed
University of St. Augustine for Health Sciences

Robert Linkul, MS, NSCA-CPT,*D, CSCS,*D, FNSCA
TrainingTheOlderAdult.com

Robert G. Lockie, PhD, TSAC-F
California State University Fullerton

Moh H. Malek, PhD, CSCS,*D, NSCA-CPT,*D, FNSCA
Wayne State University

Mike Martino, PhD, CSCS,*D
Georgia College

Kevin McCurdy, PhD, CSCS,*D, FNSCA
Texas State University

Don Melrose, PhD, CSCS,*D
Texas A&M University-Corpus Christi

Jonathan N. Mike, PhD, USAW, NKT-2
Grand Canyon University

Michael G. Miller, PhD, EdD, ATC, CSCS,*D, NSCA-CPT,*D, TSAC-F,*D, FNATA, FNSCA
Western Michigan University

E. Whitney G. Moore, PhD, CSCS,*D
Wayne State University

Mark A. Nutting, BS, CSCS,*D, NSCA-CPT,*D, RCPT*E
FitnessBusinessSpecialist.com

Douglas W. Powell, PhD, CSCS, TSAC-F, FAHA
University of Memphis

Benjamin H. Reuter, PhD, ATC, CSCS,*D
California University of Pennsylvania

Dean Robert Somerset, BSc. Kinesiology
Somerset Fitness, Ltd.

Michael D. Roberts, PhD
Auburn University

Brad J. Schoenfeld, PhD, CSCS,*D, CSPS,*D, NSCA-CPT,*D, FNSCA
CUNY Lehman College

Abbie E. Smith-Ryan, PhD, CSCS,*D, FISSN, FNSCA
University of North Carolina Chapel Hill

Ronald L. Snarr, PhD, CSCS,*D, NSCA-CPT,*D, TSAC-F,*D
Missouri State University

Paul Sorace, MS, CSCS
Independent personal trainer

Brian St. Pierre, MS, RD, CSCS, PN2
Precision Nutrition

N. Travis Triplett, PhD, CSCS,*D, FNSCA
Appalachian State University

Nick Tumminello, NSCA-CPT
Performance University

Wayne L. Westcott, PhD, CSCS
Quincy College

Chat Williams, MS, CSCS,*D, NSCA-CPT,*D, CSPS,*D, FNSCA
Youth Performance

Tyler D. Williams, PhD, CSCS,*D
Samford University

Anthony A. Abbott, EdD, CSCS,*D, CSPS,*D, NSCA-CPT,*D, TSAC-F,*D, FNSCA

Thomas R. Baechle, EdD, CSCS,*D, retired; NSCA-CPT*,D, retired

Travis W. Beck, PhD

David T. Beine, MS, ATC, LAT

Lee E. Brown, EdD, CSCS,*D, FNSCA

Jared W. Coburn, PhD, CSCS,*D, FNSCA

Matthew J. Comeau, PhD, ATC, LAT, CSCS

Joel T. Cramer, PhD, CSCS,*D, NSCA-CPT,*D, FISSN, FNSCA

J. Henry "Hank" Drought, MS, CSCS,*D, NSCA-CPT,*D

Roger W. Earle, MA, CSCS,*D, NSCA-CPT,*D, RSCC*D

Kyle T. Ebersole, PhD, LAT

JoAnn Eickhoff-Shemek, PhD, FAWHP

Todd Ellenbecker, PT, MS, SCS, OCS, CSCS

Tammy K. Evetovich, PhD, CSCS

Avery D. Faigenbaum, EdD, CSCS,*D, FNSCA

Ryan Fiddler, MS, CSCS

Sean P. Flanagan, PhD, ATC, CSCS,*D

John F. Graham, MS, CSCS,*D, FNSCA

Mike Greenwood, PhD, CSCS,*D, FNSCA

G. Gregory Haff, PhD, CSCS,*D, FNSCA

Erin E. Haff, MA

Patrick S. Hagerman, EdD, CSCS, NSCA-CPT, FNSCA

Everett Harman, PhD

Bradley D. Hatfield, PhD, FNAK

Allen Hedrick, MA, CSCS,*D, RSCC*E, FNSCA

Susan L. Heinrich, MS

David L. Herbert, JD

Kristi R. Hinnerichs (Fox), PhD, ATC, CSCS

Carlos E. Jiménez, MD

Phil Kaplan, MS

John A.C. Kordich, MEd, CSCS, NSCA-CPT, FNSCA

Len Kravitz, PhD, CSCS

Tom P. LaFontaine, PhD, CSCS, NSCA-CPT, FAACVPR

Moh H. Malek, PhD, CSCS,*D, NSCA-CPT,*D, FNSCA

Robert Mamula

John P. McCarthy, PhD, PT, CSCS,*D, CSPS,*D, FNSCA

Kevin Messey, MS, ATC, CSCS

David R. Pearson, PhD, FNSCA

Stacy Peterson, MA, CSCS

David H. Potach, PT, MS, CSCS

Sharon Rana (Perry), PhD, CSCS

Kristin J. Reimers, MS, RD

Peter Ronai, MS, CSCS, CSPS, NSCA-CPT

Jane L.P. Roy, PhD, CSCS

Eric D. Ryan, PhD, CSCS,*D, NSCA-CPT,*D, FNSCA

Douglas B. Smith, PhD

Torrey Smith, MA, CSCS,*D, CSPS,*D, NSCA-CPT,*D, TSAC-F,*D

Paul Sorace, MS, CSCS

Marie Spano, MS, RD, CSCS, CSSD, FISSN

Shinya Takahashi, PhD, CSCS

N. Travis Triplett, PhD, CSCS,*D, FNSCA

Vanessa van den Heuvel Yang, MS, ATC

Christine L. Vega, MPH, RD, CSCS, NSCA-CPT

Robert Watine, MD

Joseph P. Weir, PhD, FNSCA

Wayne L. Westcott, PhD, CSCS

Jason B. White, PhD

William C. Whiting, PhD, CSCS

Mark A. Williams, PhD, FAACVPR

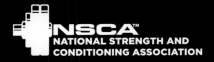
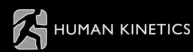